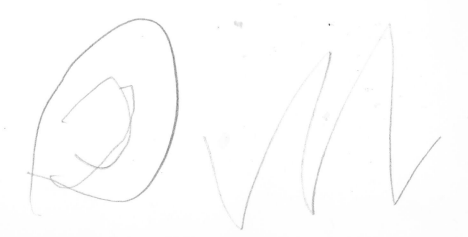

Bunnell's

SURGERY OF

THE HAND

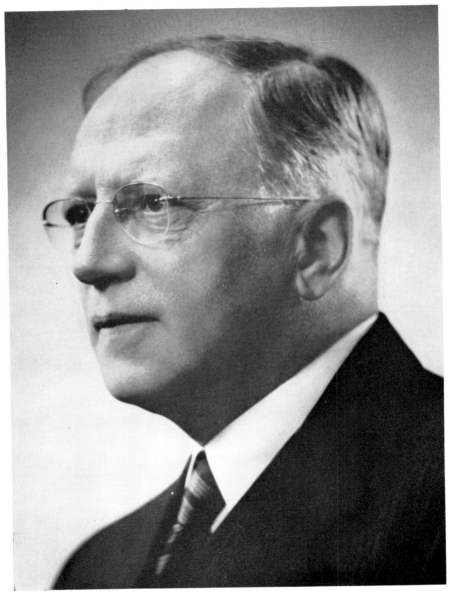

STERLING BUNNELL

1882 – 1957

Bunnell's
SURGERY OF
THE HAND

Revised by

JOSEPH H. BOYES, M.D.

Honorary member, American Orthopaedic Association, American Academy of Orthopaedic Surgeons, Western Orthopedic Association and Japanese Society for Surgery of the Hand; Member, Pacific Coast Surgical Association, American Society of Plastic and Reconstructive Surgery and American Society for Surgery of the Hand; Clinical Professor of Surgery, University of Southern California

FOURTH EDITION

J. B. LIPPINCOTT COMPANY
PHILADELPHIA AND MONTREAL

Preface to the Fourth Edition

Sterling Bunnell designed this book primarily to treat of reconstruction, with added sections for other necessary aspects such as infections, fractures and tumors and such personal interests as phylogeny and comparative anatomy of the hand. He assumed that the reader had adequate knowledge of the basic anatomy and the surgical principles and felt that hand surgery should be a composite of plastic, orthopedic and neurologic experience. The original edition was illustrated from his extensive experience. Subsequent editions included the reports of many others, particularly of the casualties of World War II.

This fourth edition is a complete revision, designed along the original lines, stressing principles over details and reconstructive rather than reparative surgery. Purposeful repetitions in previous editions have been deleted, and items of only sectional interest, such as local governmental regulations of disability allowances, have been discarded.

The terminology used in the previous editions describing the finger joints as proximal, middle and distal rather than the cumbersome anatomic terms of metacarpophalangeal and interphalangeal is still preferred. The names of the carpal bones and some of the forearm and hand muscles now conform to the accepted P.N.A. system.

The original plan of treating the reconstructive problems of the various tissue systems—skin, bones, joints, nerves and tendons—is followed again, but a new arrangement of chapters leads the reader through the comparative anatomy to embryology and congenital deformities before discussing the reconstruction of the systems.

New material has been added on splints, the surgery of the intrinsic muscles, the neurovascular pedicle transfer of tissues, tendon transfers, reconstruction of the thumb and trophic and vascular lesions. The principles of the surgical treatment of rheumatoid arthritis and gout are covered in the chapter on Joints.

A bibliography for each chapter lists articles considered worth while for further reading. An index has been provided which will help to locate the principal topics rather than catch words. Where a subject such as tendon repair is treated both from reconstructive and reparative standpoints, the text contains the necessary cross reference.

As in all endeavors, much help comes from others. Mrs. Bunnell has made many notes and records available. Dr. L. D. Howard has clarified questions on the use of some procedures described in the latest edition. The material in the chapter on tumors, which he originally provided, has been edited and condensed with his permission.

Thanks are extended to colleagues who provided illustrative material, especially to William H. Frackelton, M.D., Walter C. Graham, M.D., J. William Littler, M.D., Daniel C. Riordan, M.D., R. R. Schreiber, M.D., and L. Ramsey Straub, M.D. My associate, C. R. Ashworth, M.D., arranged the bibliography.

The typing of the manuscript by Miss Berle Draper has been done as a measure of the respect and the esteem which she and the revisor shared for Sterling Bunnell by reason of their previous experience in working for him.

JOSEPH H. BOYES, M.D.

Preface to the First Edition

We are now in a mechanized age, which means that millions of hands will be injured. It might be called the Age of Trauma. With the speed-up of industry and with mechanized warfare the manual worker will, from the very nature of his work, injure his hands. Hands lead the list of industrial accidents and are responsible for a large portion of compensation expense. From a social standpoint the functioning of this valued member is of vital importance to the manual worker for his very livelihood.

From an evolutionary aspect, our hands when we became bipeds were relieved from the duty of locomotion and were then free to develop into more useful instruments. By brains and hands man excelled over all other species; for other animals had as weapons only hoofs, claws, or teeth, while the hand of man could grasp any weapon. The brain developed the hand, but it is also true that in each one of us many of our mental processes have developed from the feeling and movement of our hands. In the case of the brilliant Helen Keller, both deaf and blind, her whole life was opened up through her hands. The special development of the human hand is largely responsible for the great handicraft of man.

The hand is so intimately rooted into our lives, thoughts, and expressions that it has become a part of our language, as evidenced by the following: handle, handy, secondhand, to give the hand in marriage, all hands on deck, rule with a strong hand, at hand, on hand. From the Latin *manus* are derived manage, management, mandate, manipulate, maintain, manner, manuscript, manufacture; from the Greek *cheiro* come the French word *chirurgie* and our English surgery.

Although the hand is composed mainly of tough material, it also includes exact machinery of much refinement and tissues of great delicacy and specialization. Such a mechanism is readily wrecked by trauma and infection, and it is little wonder that hands mangled by trauma, or those infiltrated and gutted by infection, later present difficult problems in reconstruction. After tendons and nerves have sloughed and the storm of infection is over all of the tissues contract, resulting in flexion contractures, and the movable parts become bound with cicatrix into a congealed hand. Much of this disability may be spared by correct early treatment of infections and injuries.

Malformation, injury, and infection swell the ever-coming stream of crippled hands needing repair. To recondition these members successfully is difficult. Surgical reconstruction of the hand requires special careful technic to minimize adhesion formation which is so prone to bind together the nicely adjusted moveable parts. It is a composite problem requiring the correlation of the various specialties—orthopedics, plastic and neurologic surgery—the knowledge of any one of which alone is inadequate for repairing the hand. Trauma involves all types of tissue, irrespective of the artificial divisions of our specialties. Usually in the same traumatized limb with flexion contracture, injury to tendons, bones, joints, and nerves, we must combine plastic, orthopedic, and neurologic surgery. As the problem is composite, the surgeon must also be. It is impractical for three specialists to work together or in series. There is no shortcut. The surgeon must face the situation and equip himself to handle any and all of the tissues in a limb.

In hand surgery the structures encountered are the same, though in miniature, as found elsewhere, so the same principles and problems met with here apply throughout the body. In reconstructing hands, though the cosmetics are important, the practical object is to restore enough function to the limb to allow the patient to return to wage earning and self-support.

Primarily this book was designed to treat reconstruction alone; but it has been expanded to include a little of other aspects that seemed necessary, and also along some lines where interest beckoned. An attempt has been made to keep it concise for the sake of the reader's time. Main principles have been stressed over details, as any able surgeon should improvise his own methods of operating. There are some purposeful repetitions for emphasis where the subject applies in different chapters, lest only that part be read at the time. An effort has been made not to overburden the text with historical references but merely to express the facts on a working basis. Knowledge develops from the thousands who precede, and to these we owe our gratitude. As many as practical are mentioned in the text and bibliography, but there are many more.

The terms metacarpophalangeal, proximal interphalangeal, and distal interphalangeal are too ponderous, and first, second, and third joints are ambiguous as counting may start from either end. Therefore, the terms proximal, middle, and distal joints or segments are used for fingers and proximal and distal for thumb. Also, to avoid ambiguity the digits are designated by name rather than by number. Angulating is used in the sense of describing an arc with the distal fragment.

Throughout the world in peacetime were myriads of hands in need of repair. The war is adding such an appalling number of crippled hands, depriving men of their earning power, that surgeons now have had thrust upon them this work of reconstruction. It is with a desire to aid in this work of restoration that this book is written.

I wish to express my appreciation to my colleagues, Major L. D. Howard, Jr., M.C., A.U.S., and Captain Donald R. Pratt, MC., A.U.S., for their cooperation and help in the surgery of hands and in the development of the use of removable stainless steel wire. To my associate, Doctor Howard, I am especially grateful for his contribution, the chapter on Tumors of the Hand.

Deep appreciation I feel for my wife, Elizabeth Bunnell, who with steadfast, wholehearted cooperation prepared the major portion of the manuscript. I wish also to acknowledge my gratitude to Mrs. Helen Loran for her valued help in this work, to Mrs. Douglas Young for her part in the photography, and to Miss Margot Beggs for her editorial work.

Grateful acknowledgment is due Mr. Ralph Sweet and Mrs. Rosebud Preddy for many of the illustrations.

I wish to acknowledge with thanks the permission received from the following journals to reproduce in part my articles published in them: The American Journal of Surgery, California and Western Medicine, Industrial Medicine, Journal of Bone and Joint Surgery, Surgery, Gynecology and Obstetrics, and Rocky Mountain Medical Journal.

Last but not least I feel a debt of gratitude to my publishers, J. B. Lippincott Company, who induced me to write this book and who have been splendidly cooperative throughout.

STERLING BUNNELL, M.D.

Contents

1. THE NORMAL HAND 1
   Skin and Creases 1
   Movements of the Arm 3
   Movements of the Wrist 3
   Movements of the Hand 6
   Mechanics of Muscle and Tendon Action 9
   Sensibility and Sensation 18
   Surgical Anatomy 20

2. PHYLOGENY AND COMPARATIVE ANATOMY AND EMBRYOLOGY 24
   Origin of Limbs 24
   Phylogenetics of Intrinsic Muscles of the Hand 24
   Pectoral Girdle 29
   Arm 32
   Forearm 34
   Hand 35
   Phylogeny and Differentiation of Muscles from Amphibia to Mammals . . . 40
   Strange Specialization for Adaptation of Manus 42
   Primate Hand 45
   Embryology and Development 48

3. CONGENITAL DEFORMITIES 55
   Incidence 55
   Classification 55
   Terminology 55
   Etiology 56
   Absence of All or Part of a Limb 64
   Shoulder, Arm and Forearm Deformities 65
   Clinarthrosis or Deviation in Alignment of Joints 72
   Congenital Dislocations 74
   Synostoses 74
   Deformities of the Hands 77
   Deformities of the Fingers 80
   Arteriovenous Abnormalities 93
   Knuckle Pads 93
   Principles of Treatment of Congenital Deformities 94

4. EXAMINATION OF THE HAND 98
   History 98
   Examination, Whole Arm 99
   Diagnosis 107
   Malingering 111
   Records and Reports 111
   Impairment of Function and Disability 116

x   Contents

5. PRINCIPLES OF RECONSTRUCTION 121
    General Considerations 121
    Principles 125
    Operative Technic 129
    Prognosis 147

6. SPLINTS AND FUNCTIONAL BRACING 150
    Splinting To Prevent Deformity 150
    Splinting To Immobilize 150
    Splinting To Protect Tendons 156
    Miscellaneous Plaster Splinting 157
    Splinting To Change or Convert Position of Joints 159
    Splinting To Substitute for Paralyzed Muscles 159
    Active Splinting by Spring or Elastic 160
    Types of Splints 162
    Splinting for Paralysis 173
    Internal Splinting 177
    Functional Bracing 180

7. SKIN AND CONTRACTURES 182
    Effect of Cicatrix 182
    Flexion Contractures 182
    Dupuytren's Contracture 231
    Volkmann's Ischemic Contracture 244
    Local Intrinsic Contracture in the Hand 256

8. BONES 265
    Correction of Deformities 265
    Bones of the Forearm 273
    Madelung's Deformity 280
    Reconstruction After Metacarpal Losses 282
    Carpal or Metacarpal Boss 292
    Traumatic Degeneration of Carpal Bones 293

9. JOINTS 298
    Why Finger Joints Stiffen 298
    Prevention of Joint Stiffness 299
    Mobilizing Stiffened Joints 300
    Surgical Repair of Joints 305
    Rheumatoid Arthritis 327
    Treatment of the Rheumatoid Hand 334
    Gout 348

10. NERVES 351
    Importance of Nerve Function in Upper Extremity 351
    Individual Nerves 359
    Treatment of Injured Nerves 379
    Cerebral Palsy 394

11. TENDONS 404
    Morphology 404
    Response of Tendons to Injury and Infection 405
    Healing of Tendons 407

11. TENDONS—(*Continued*)
Technic of Tendon Repair 412
Problem of Gliding 424
Free Tendon Grafts 432
Tendon Transfers 438
Postoperative Treatment 460
Evaluation of Results After Tendon Reconstruction 463
Special Situations Affecting Tendons 464

12. INTRINSIC MUSCLES OF THE HAND 482
Intrinsic Muscles of the Fingers 482
Intrinsic Muscles of the Thumb 508

13. RECONSTRUCTION OF THE THUMB 535
Loss of Thumb 535
Tubed Pedicles To Lengthen the Thumb 540
Pollicization Operation 543
Digital Transfer 553
Thumb Reconstruction 553
Résumé of Principles in Thumb Reconstruction 553

14. SHOULDER AND ELBOW 561
Shoulder 561
Elbow Region 580

15. WOUNDS, BURNS AND AMPUTATIONS 587
Wounds 587
Burns 608
Amputations 616

16. FRACTURES AND DISLOCATIONS 628
Special Aspects in the Hand 628
Injuries of the Wrist 630
Fractures of the Metacarpals and the Phalanges 650
Dislocations 657
Injuries of the Thumb 658

17. INFECTIONS 665
Pyogenic Infections 665
Special Infections 686

18. TROPHIC AND VASCULAR CONDITIONS 699
Trophic Conditions 699
Vascular Lesions 714

19. TUMORS 721
The Common Tumors of the Hand 721
Ganglia 721
Xanthoma 725
Epidermoid Cysts 727
Sebaceous Cysts 729
Vascular Tumors 730
Fibromas 733

19. TUMORS—(*Continued*)

The Common Tumors of the Hand—(*Continued*)

Neurofibromata 735

Epitheliomata 735

Lipomas 742

Enchondroma or Chondroma 743

Glomus Tumors 745

Bone Tumors 749

Muscle Tumors 762

Subungual Melanoma 763

Carcinoma of Nail 765

Tendon-sheath Tumors—Synovia 766

Peripheral Nerve Tumors 769

INDEX 775

Chapter 1

The Normal Hand

The hand is an organ of grasp as well as an organ of sensation and expression. By the use of our hands we learn shape, size and texture of objects and then combine this information with impressions from other senses to build in our brain the knowledge of our environment. We use our hands not only as tools for grasping, pinching and pushing, but with our brain directing the hands we manufacture tools for special purposes. Lower animals have specialized claws and hooves, whereas man can make and grasp any weapon. Our hands become extensions of the intellect, for by hand movements the dumb converse, with the specialized fingertips the blind read; and through the written word we learn from the past and transmit to the future. The normal hand is a pentadactylate mechanism of basic design; its finer motions and sensibility have been developed over the ages on the primitive amphibian pattern. It is not self-sufficient but needs the control of higher centers. It is the brain that sets man apart, but the brain acting through the mechanism of the hand has helped him to become the master of the universe.

To reconstruct a damaged hand, we must know the normal. Surgery of the hand is that of the upper limb, for though the hand's mechanical base may be at the elbow, its dynamic origin is in the brain. All movements of the shoulder, the elbow and the forearm are made to place the hand in a proper position for function. These parts may be normal, but without a mobile sentient hand they are of little use. Conversely, a normal hand without a stable elbow and shoulder is little more than a feeble helper.

The right hand is usually dominant; the arrangements of objects in the physical world, as in the turning of screws, doorknobs and bolts being such as to utilize supination, which is stronger than pronation. Left-handedness varies between 10 and 30 per cent of the population and is reportedly somewhat higher in young children and in some areas such as England. True ambidexterity or bilaterality is rare. Dominance is easily transferred in the young, after injury or paralytic disease.

SKIN AND CREASES

The skin on the volar surface of palm and fingers is tough and thick to stand wear. It covers a thick pad of fat with many fibrous septa. It is not very mobile and allows little plastic maneuvering. A system of creases, where the skin is adherent to the deeper layers, allows for closing of the hand without bunching up in folds.

On the dorsum, the skin is thin, soft and yielding, and its subcutaneous layer is loose and pliable. Covering a convex surface, it is flexible to allow for closure of the fist. Minute wrinkles at right angles to the line of pull take the place of creases as on the volar surface, and special redundancies over the finger joints allow the covering skin to stretch over these areas in maximum flexion. Over the thenar eminence a combination of longitudinal and transverse wrinkles allows the infinite combination of movements of this digit.

The palmar skin is without pigment and hair, but well supplied with sweat glands. On the dorsum, hair-bearing skin is present except over the distal and sometimes the middle segments.

Two flexor creases overlie the middle finger joint; but only one, and it slightly proximal, marks the level of the distal finger joint. A single crease in the proximal segment of the finger identifies the distal edge of the palm or web, which extends volarward to the middle third of the proximal phalanx. On the dorsum, the base of the cleft lies more proximal, and for cosmetic reasons this sloping appearance of the web should be reconstructed in syndactylism operations.

Two creases are normally seen in the palm: the proximal or thenar crease for use of the thumb; and the distal, running from the index middle finger cleft to the ulnar border, for use of the ulnar 3 fingers. A composite crease, the line extending from the radial end of thenar to the ulnar end of distal crease is often called the midpalmar crease. It represents the level of proximal finger joint action. Since the fingertips normally flex to touch this crease, a measurement of the distance which a finger pulp lacks of touching the crease can be used to record impaired finger flexion.

The thenar crease allows for the wide range of thumb motion. Thus longitudinal wrinkles for forward motion of opposition and reposition are present as well as transverse wrinkles at the base for flexion. The thumb index web is loose and pliable and has alternating oblique folds as the thumb is moved away from or toward the plane of the palm. Transverse folds appear as the thumb approaches the index finger.

On each finger the flexor creases divide the subcutaneous fat into 3 pads. Each crease extends only to the midlateral line. The skin is attached directly to the flexor tendon sheath at the level of the middle crease, and puncture wounds in this area enter directly into the sheath space.

The nails are specialized ectodermal organs for scratching, pinching and picking up small objects. They give added stability to the pulp. The pulps of the fingers contain a large number of sensory receptors. Skin grafts for replacement of pulp skin never have the fine quality of sensibility or stereognosis that is present in normal skin.

The fingernails require about 4 months to grow their length and may show transverse grooves partly down the nail from an illness within the last 4 months. At their sides and bases the nails curve more sharply, so this must be kept in mind in incising for paronychia. The lunula corresponds to what is practically a potential space, like an ungual bursa; the cellular attachment there is so slight that the space may readily fill with blood or pus. The nails overlie the distal phalanges intimately enough to give firm support to the finger pulp.

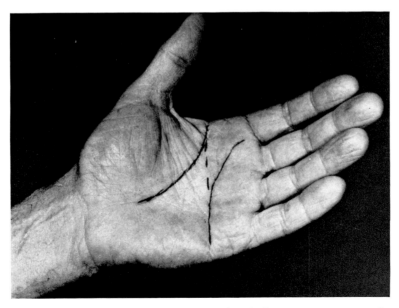

Fig. 1. Normal flexion creases of the palm. A thenar crease representing the level of motion of the thumb and an ulnar crease for motion of the middle, the ring and the little fingers. Motion of all fingers results in a combination or *distal palmar crease*. Lack of flexion of the pulp of a finger to this crease is a measurement used to record finger flexion.

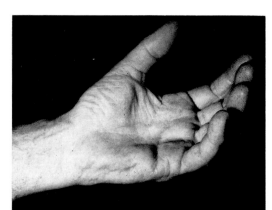

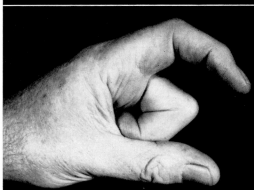

FIG. 2. Arches of the hand and flexor creases of the finger. (*Top*) The carpal and and the metacarpal transverse arches. As the fingers flex, their tips remain on same level because of the concave plane of the metacarpal heads. (*Bottom*) The flexor creases in a finger. Only the middle flexion crease lies directly over a joint, the proximal crease is at the level of the web, and the distal crease is well cephalad to the distal joint. When the finger is flexed, the creases are almost at right angles. Note the dorsal termination of the middle flexion crease, the optimum site for the midlateral skin incision.

MOVEMENTS OF THE ARM

A series of joints from shoulder to fingers give the hand a most unusual versatility. By a combination of the ball-and-socket shoulder, the elbow hinge and the rotary motion of the forearm, the palm can be placed to cover any part of the body except between the scapulae. The hand can push away or pull to the body from any of these positions.

The shoulder has a large range of motion angulating and rotating widely. Shoulder motions are complex, involving scapular movements on the chest wall as well as motion in the scapulohumeral joint. The clavicle acts as a strut for stability.

The elbow hinges in one plane until the last third of extension when the forearm angulates outward to form the carrying angle.

The 2 radio-ulnar joints furnish pronation and supination of the forearm through an arc of 120° to 150°. Rotation of the forearm is measured with the elbow at right-angle flexion, thus blocking rotary motions of the humerus. With the ulna fixed, the radius rotates around the axis of the distal ulna; but in pronation and supination a combination motion takes place, the ulna deviating opposite to the radius, so that the axis of motion, as in using a screwdriver, is more in line with the distal radius and the 2nd metacarpal.

Each radio-ulnar joint has the same amount of rotary motion. The proximal joint is a true swivel with an orbicular ligament, but at the distal joint the broad end of the radius rotates around the fixed ulna. On the head of the ulna opposite the styloid process is the articular facet comprising about two thirds of the surface. There are 3 ligaments at the distal ulna. One is a strong pivot ligament from styloid process to triquetrum; a second is a loose cufflike ligament around the radio-ulnar articulation, which clasps about the margins of the opposing facets. This ligament, as the radius rotates, tightens in its dorsal part on pronation and in its volar part on supination. Its volar portion is most important in preventing subluxation of the ulna. The third ligament is the articular disk, attached to the radius and pivoting on its attachment to the styloid process of the ulna.

MOVEMENTS OF THE WRIST

The wrist can angulate in any direction and by a combination can circumduct as a universal joint. Palmar flexion is normally greater than dorsiflexion, and ulnar flexion is usually double that of radial flexion. Lateral motions are greatest with the wrist straight or in slight palmar flexion. In normal use, the axis of motion in the wrist is not in a true dorsal volar direction but more from dorsoradial to ulnar volar. The strongest wrist

Dorsum

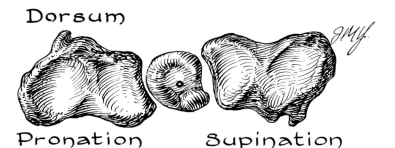

Pronation   Supination

Left

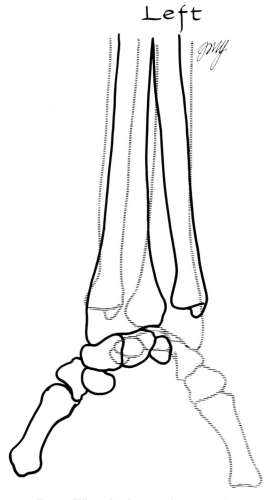

FIG. 3. The radius and the ulna seen from the wrist to show relations in pronation and supination. If the ulna is fixed, the radius performs an arc of slightly less than 180° about the center axis 0.

motors are the flexor carpi ulnaris and the opposing 2 radial wrist extensors.

The center for lateral motions appears to be more distal than that for anteroposterior motions. Detailed studies show wrist motions to be most intricate. Neither motion takes place through a single center, for both involve more than one joint.

ANTEROPOSTERIOR MOVEMENTS

Roentgenograms of a wrist in dorsal and volar flexion with center lines drawn through radius, capitate and lunate were measured to determine relative movements. Of 122° of movement between capitate and radius, 66° or 54 per cent took place between the lunate and the radius; thus the radiocarpal joint provides about one fifth more motion in this plane than the midcarpal joint.

LATERAL MOVEMENT

This movement is complex. The capitate moves with the hand and, as measured on the line of the radius, about 45° of motion takes place. Of this, about two thirds is ulnarward of the neutral position. However, the capitate in making this motion also moves in a dorsal volar direction, rocking on the concave surface of the lunate. In turn, the lunate rotates on the articular surface of the radius. In ulnar flexion the scaphoid is pushed radialward by the capitate and makes a dorsal revolution. In radial flexion the trapezium moving with the thumb ray pushes the scaphoid, causing it to make a volar revolution and a simultaneous shift ulnarward. Strict radio-ulnar motion is impossible at the radio-carpal joint because of the double curvature of the end of the radius; therefore, the functional midcarpal joint runs out the cleft between the thumb and the index.

FIG. 4. When the forearm is pronated and supinated, as in using a screwdriver, the motion involves not only a rotation of radius around ulna but also a lateral shifting of the ulna. The longitudinal axis for this total action is now near the ulnar border of the distal radius. (Adapted from Capener, N., J. Bone Joint Surg. 38B:128, 1956)

FIG. 5. In anteroposterior motion of the wrist, more motion occurs at the radiocarpal than the midcarpal joints. The axes of the capitate, the lunate and the radius are shown.

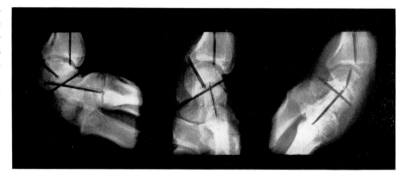

FIG. 6. In lateral movements of the hand at the wrist joint the capitate moves with the hand on the proximal carpal row, and the proximal row shifts on the radius. The thumb ray, the trapezium and the scaphoid form a separate unit, the rotary motion of the latter being volar in radial flexion and dorsal in ulnar flexion.

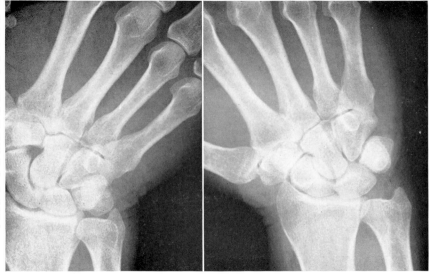

FIG. 7. Motions in the carpus on lateral movements. (Left) Ulnar deviation. (Right) Radial deviation. The lunate rotates volarward in the cup of the ulnar half of the radiocarpal concavity, while the scaphoid rotates volarward when the wrist is deviated radially.

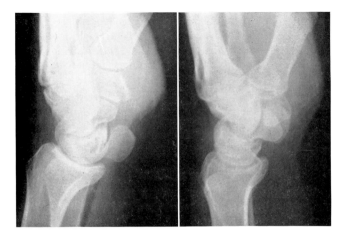

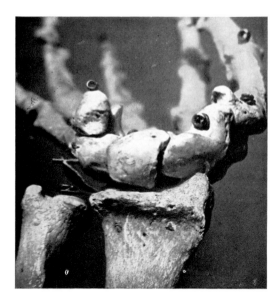

FIG. 8. Carpal arch and tunnel. On the radial side two bony ridges, the trapezium and the scaphoid, and on the ulnar side, the pisiform and the hook of the hamate, form the bony pillars. Spanning the roof of the canal, the volar carpal ligament completes the carpal tunnel through which pass all the digital flexor tendons and the median nerve.

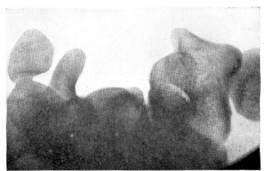

FIG. 9. Tunnel view of wrist, demonstrating borders of carpal canal. Such views can be obtained by directing the rays along the axis of the 3rd metacarpal, while the volar aspect of the wrist rests on the film holder, and the wrist is dorsiflexed about 60°. (Hart, V. L.: J. Bone Joint Surg. *23*:948)

The thumb ray moves with the proximal carpal row, and on radial flexion the tip of the thumb reaches ½ inch farther down the index than on ulnar flexion.

MOVEMENTS OF THE HAND

The hand can change from flat to slightly curved to a complete ball fist. The digits spread widely in opening, and their tips converge in closing. With the fingers we can pick up objects of any size from a tiny seed to an 8-inch ball.

The 2nd and the 3rd metacarpals constitute the fixed part or keystone of the arching hand. The index metacarpal is firmly fixed on the carpus, and the middle metacarpal is almost as solid. On the radial side the thumb moves freely through a wide arc, and on the ulnar side the ring and the little metacarpals have considerable mobility on the hamate.

ARCHES OF THE HAND

There are 2 transverse arches: one at the metacarpal heads, the other at the distal carpal row. The metacarpal arch is flexible, being in-

creased by action of the thenar and the hypothenar muscle groups pulling the outside rays forward. The arch gives strength to the hand in grasping round or irregular objects and causes the fingers to converge in flexion. As the fingers flex, the curve of the metacarpal arch increases, tipping the axes of the proximal finger joints. When opening the hand the flattening of the arch causes the fingers to spread. This spreading action of the long extensors may be mistaken for intrinsic muscle activity. Flattening the arch as by pressure or holding a rod prevents the tipping, and the fingers no longer converge. When the fingers are individually flexed, each tip points to the bony landmark of the trapezial ridge. A finger immobilized in flexion should be pointed to this area. Flexing all fingers together, they touch a line from the base of the thumb to hypothenar eminence.

The extended fingers are unequal in length; in semiflexion the tips form a straight line. If the open hand, lying on a flat surface, is gradually closed to make a fist, the tips of all the fingers will stay aligned on the same plane through most of the act, though at the end of the middle finger leads to touch the palm. In full extension the ring finger is usually next in length to the middle finger, but in many individuals the index finger is equal to or longer than the ring finger.

MECHANICS OF FINGER MOTIONS

The finger joints are sliding joints like the knee, so that in flexion the prominence of the joint is the distal condyle of the proximal bone of that joint. The proximal joints flex 70° to 90°; the middle joints 105° to 115°; and the distal joints 45° to 90°.

In extension all finger joints have some lateral motion which is lost in flexion. Lateral stability in the flexed position provides firmer grasp. This mechanism is most noticeable in the proximal joints and is due to the shape of the metacarpal heads and the disposition of the collateral ligaments. In the dorsal volar plane the metacarpal heads are narrow on the dorsum, the articulating surface when the proximal phalanx is in extension. Volarly, the metacarpal head is much wider and has a broad area to articulate with the phalanx. The obliquely placed collateral ligaments extend-

ing from dorsal aspect of metacarpal to volar aspect of phalanx allow considerable play laterally when the phalanx slides on the narrow metacarpal head; but when the joint is flexed, their direction is now that of a true collateral ligament, and the joint is laterally stable. More motion takes place ulnarward than radialward, especially in the index proximal joint. Ulnar deviation is accompanied by exo-rotation, and radial deviation by endorotation of the phalanx. The collateral ligaments vary in size and in points of intersection. On the index and the middle fingers the radial ligament is larger and more oblique than the ulnar collateral ligament, whereas in the ring and the little fingers they are more symmetric, more oblique and less well developed. In all

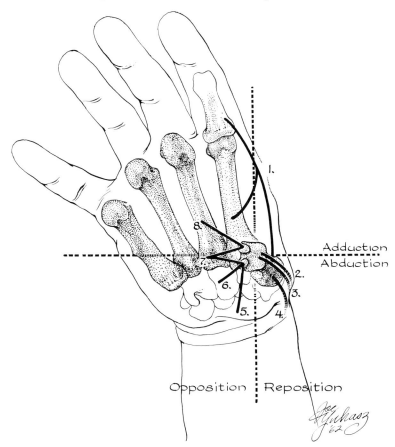

FIG. 10. Motions of the thumb. The thumb metacarpal as seen from above and foreshortened. (1) First interosseus muscle, (2) extensor pollicis longus, (3) extensor pollicis brevis, (4) abductor pollicis longus, (5) abductor pollicis brevis, (6) superficial head, flexor pollicis brevis, (7) flexor pollicis brevis, (8) adductor pollicis, transverse head. (Redrawn from Von Lanz and Wachsmuth, Praktische Anatomie, Fig. 240 B, Berlin, Springer, 1959)

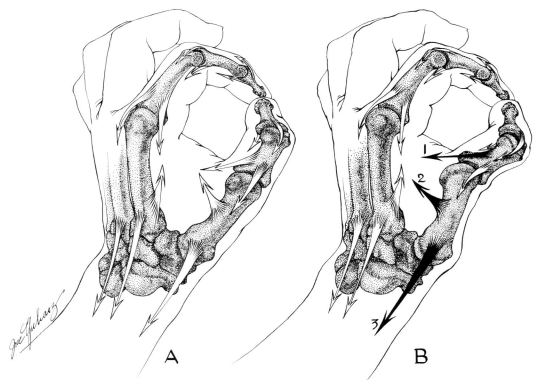

FIG. 11. Mechanics of pinch between thumb and index finger. (*Left*) Stabilization by muscle action creating balanced forces at each joint. (*Right*) Poor pinch with failure of longitudinal arch of the thumb from various causes (1) loss of adductor power from ulnar palsy, (2) dropping of 1st metacarpal from cicatricial contracture of 1st cleft or dislocation at metacarpocarpal joint, (3) loss of abductor pollicis as in radial palsy.

fingers the radial ligament attaches more distally on the metacarpal.

Lateral motion of the fingers results from action of the interosseus muscles, the 4 dorsal abducting the index and the ring fingers away from the middle one and moving the middle finger to either side. The 3 volar interossei draw the index, the ring and the little fingers toward the middle. The abductor minimi digiti acts as a dorsal interosseus to spread the little finger, and the abductor pollicis brevis has a similar function on the thumb. The oblique portion of the adductor pollicis muscle acts as a volar interosseus. Dorsal interosseus muscles have tendon insertions either to the base of the proximal phalanx or into the aponeurotic extensor hood mechanism or both. Though varying somewhat, a consistent pattern has been found. Volar interossei insert only into the hood. From a more volar position their tendons approach the digit at a greater angle

and thus provide more of a flexion component. The lumbrical on the radial side of each finger also has a strong flexion component, and it likewise inserts into the extensor machanism. Such muscle tendon units can flex the proximal joint and at the same time extend the 2 distal joints or impart lateral motion to the finger when the proximal joint is stabilized by the common extensor.

The profundus tendons, except the index, have a common muscle and interdigitate in the palm through the lumbrical origins. Therefore, if one of the fingers is held in extension, the other fingers cannot be fully flexed voluntarily. Such conditions occur if a flexor tendon is sutured to extensor over an amputated stump of a finger. Similarly, the extensor tendons interdigitate on the dorsum of the hand by the oblique interconnecting tendons. A finger held in flexion will then prevent the adjoining fingers from extending completely.

THUMB MOTIONS

The thumb can be spread away from the palm in the plane of the hand or at right angles to it. Extended, it can circumduct and describe an irregular circle. Starting with its tip at the base of the little finger in combined flexion and adduction, its tip can be scraped along the volar aspect of the fingers to the middle crease of the index, then in and slightly dorsal to the plane of the palm it extends and abducts and rolls over in a wide arc to oppose the fingertips. All the muscles of the thenar eminence enter into this complete series of actions; some stabilize, while others act as prime movers. It is an error to think that a muscle acts only to provide a motion similar to its name.

Most angular motion at the base of the thumb takes place in the carpometacarpal joint, though the trapezium also moves a little on the scaphoid. Rotation occurs at the metacarpophalangeal joint along with some angulation.

There is some variation in individuals in the range of motion in the 2 distal thumb joints. It is not uncommon to find only a few degrees of motion in the metacarpophalangeal joint, but these same individuals usually have a greater range in the interphalangeal joint. Thus the sum of angulatory movement in the 2 joints is approximately the same.

Extension of the distal joint of the thumb in some hands may be carried out even when extensor pollicis longus is not functioning. The flexor pollicis brevis and the adductor pollicis both send fibers of their insertions into the extensor aponeurosis over the base of the proximal phalanx. This action is similar to the lumbrical-interosseus action on the fingers. A contracture of these thenar and first cleft muscles can result in a flexed position of the metacarpophalangeal joint and a hyperextension of the distal joint, analogous to the deformity seen in the fingers.

MECHANICS OF MUSCLE AND TENDON ACTION

COORDINATION

A motion is rarely performed by a single muscle or tendon. A stable base for the moving part to work from must be controlled by muscle action. Such a kinetic chain for finger

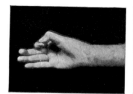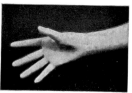

FIG. 12. Deformity of dropped metacarpophalangeal joint of the thumb in pinching against the index finger. A good O cannot be formed as the arch of the thumb breaks down. This phenomenon is seen after severance of the tendon of the abductor pollicis or of the ulnar nerve, but this case (as seen in the right-hand picture) is due to a third reason, there being a cicatricial flexion contracture between the first 2 metacarpals or a backward dislocation of the thumb metacarpal on the trapezium.

motions extends all the way to the trunk. This stabilizing action is through either a tonic contraction of opposing muscles pulling in the line of the limb or a voluntary contraction of a group to hold a joint in position so that more distal joints can be moved. When a fist is made, the wrist must be fixed in dorsiflexion so that the fingers can grip. If not, the wrist falls into palmar flexion and strength of grasp is lost. Clinically, the severance of radial wrist extensors results in loss of 50 per cent of the grasping power.

Pinching between the thumb and the fingers illustrates this necessary coordination of stabilizers and movers. For an adequate pinch the long abductor muscle of the thumb must stabilize the carpometacarpal joint in extension, and at the same time the adductor of the thumb must stabilize the metacarpophalangeal joint in flexion. If either of these factors of stabilization is missing, the longitudinal arch of the thumb is weakened, and the metacarpophalangeal joint will drop into hyperextension. The distal joint overflexes in an attempt to strengthen the pinch. Especially when the adductor pollicis is paralyzed, as from ulnar nerve lesions, this excessive flexion of the distal joint is noted. It serves to increase the effective power of the extensor pollicis longus which then acts as a supplementary adductor because of its oblique course over the dorsum of the wrist. In the finger a similar coordinated movement allows the interosseus to stabilize the proximal finger joint

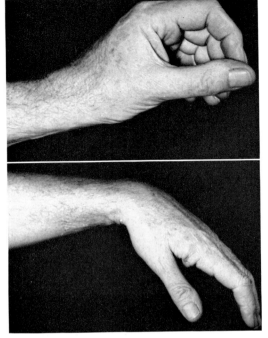

FIG. 13. Automatic motions. (*Top*) When the wrist is dorsiflexed, the fingers drop into semiflexion and the thumb in opposition. All muscles are in balance, and the hand is in the position of function. (*Bottom*) When the wrist palmar flexes, fingers extend and thumb goes into reposition. This is the position of rest; the muscles are still in balance but little practical function is possible.

so that the common extensor can extend the middle and the distal joints. The common extensor, by stabilizing the proximal joint in extension, allows the interosseus to impart lateral motion.

To use the hand many muscles from the trunk to the hand spring into action and hold or place the hand in a position to act. Thus coordination of many motor mechanisms is essential to carry out the simplest motion.

MUSCLE BALANCE

When all the muscles controlling the hand are in normal tone, the joints are approximately in their middle position. This is the position of function and the optimum position to perform a useful act. The forearm is in midrotation; the wrist is dorsiflexed so that the cleft between the opposed thumb and in-

dex finger is in line with the radius. The wrist is ulnar-deviated slightly so that the index metacarpal is a projection of the longitudinal axis of the radius. The thumb is opposed, with its metacarpal lying in a plane at right angles to the palm, and the fingers are bent; the degree of flexion increases from index to little finger. In this position the hand grasps a cylinder 1½ to 2 inches in diameter.

The wrist is the key joint in the position of function. If a hand is allowed to assume its own position of rest, almost always the wrist will be in slight palmar flexion. This upsets the balance of the rest of the hand. The proximal finger joints tend to remain in extension or even hyperextension with compensatory flexion of the middle and the distal joints. If the hand is allowed to rest unprotected as on a pillow, the thumb will be forced back into the plane of the palm and nearer the index finger. The wrist being the key joint, a simple volar wrist support will prevent the development of many disabling deformities of the hand.

Muscles are arranged about joints in pairs. Antagonistic motions may be carried out, but also by a combination of several muscles a circumduction can take place as in the proximal finger joints or at the wrist.

About the wrist only the extensor carpi radialis brevis acts in a true dorsal volar plane. Its antagonists are the flexor carpi radialis and the palmaris longus. The extensor carpi radialis longus, the abductor pollicis longus and the extensor pollicis brevis are all radial deviators of the wrist, with only the abductor being in the lateral plane. Combined with the extensor carpi radialis brevis, they bring the wrist into strong dorsal and radial flexion. This motion is opposed by the flexor carpi ulnaris, one of the strongest of the forearm muscles. This plane from radial and dorsal to ulnar and volar is the physiologic axis of wrist activity.

FORMS OF GRASP

Though the hand can grasp objects of varying size and shape, there are two basic forms of grasp. Napier has defined these as power grasp and precision grasp. Each form has certain characteristics. Power grasp is illustrated by gripping a wooden cylinder, such as a hammer handle. The wrist is dorsiflexed so that

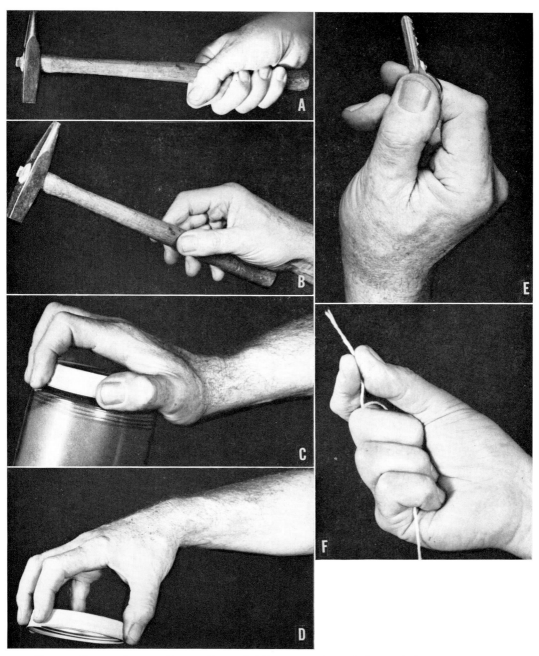

FIG. 14. Forms of grasp. Power (A) and (C) and precision (B) and (D) are the two basic forms of grasp. Note in power grasp the adducted thumb, in precision grasp the opposed thumb. The form of grasp is determined by the use desired not by the object itself. (C) To tighten or loosen a jar cap, the thumb is adducted, and the wrist is dorsiflexed for maximum power; when force is no longer needed the grip changes to the precision type (D). Key grip (E) or side pinch is a type of power grasp. Combination grasp (F), power with 3 ulnar fingers, precision with index and thumb. (Napier: J. Bone Joint Surg. *38-B*:902)

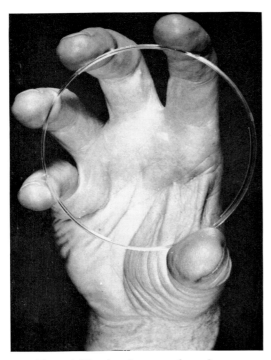

FIG. 15. The thumb moves through an arc from the side of the index to the tip of the little finger by a combination of muscles. In this photo the thumb is opposed to the middle finger.

the long digital flexors press the object firmly against the palm, and the thumb is clasped either over the clenched fingers or pressed tightly against the handle in adduction. In precision grasp, the wrist may be in either dorsal or volar flexion, the thumb is opposed to the semiflexed fingers, and the intrinsics provide most of the finger movement. The type of grasp depends not so much upon the object held as on the use planned for that object. The hand can change quickly from one type to another as the need varies. Combinations also are present, as when holding a rope with the ulnar 3 fingers, the thumb and the index are used to tie the ends.

The term "pinch," as denoting the close approximation of the pulps of thumb, index and middle fingers, is a weak form of precision grasp. Pinching with the thumb against the side of the index, called key pinch, is a form of power grasp. The strong adductor of the thumb and the 1st and the 2nd dorsal interossei provide the forces to close the 2 arms of the pincers in a firm and strong action.

MUSCLE POWER

The natural length of a muscle is that length of its fibers when lying free of all nerve supply and not stretched by the pull of any antagonist. It is approximately twice the maximally contracted length. The absolute power of a muscle is that force required to draw out the muscle from the maximally contracted state to its natural length. This force is proportional to the physiologic cross section, a section cutting each fiber at a right angle. Although easy to measure in parallel muscles, the physiologic cross section is difficult to determine in pennate muscles. The constant 3.65 kg. $\times$ cm^2 of the physiologic cross section has been accepted by Steindler for the power of muscle.

The number of fibers in cross section thus determines the absolute muscle power, whereas their length determines the amplitude of motion that they provide to the tendon. Force of muscle action times the distance or amplitude equals the work capacity of a muscle. A large mass of relatively long fibers, such as the profundus muscles, is thus capable of more work than a similar mass of short-fibered muscles, such as the wrist extensors.

The work capacity of the forearm muscles activating the wrist and the hand has been given as follows (von Lanz and Wachsmuth):

WORK CAPACITY OF MUSCLES IN MKG.

Flexor carpi radialis	0.8
Extensor carpi radialis longus	1.1
Extensor carpi radialis brevis	0.9
Extensor carpi ulnaris	1.1
Abductor pollicis longus	0.1
Flexor pollicis longus	1.2
Flexor digitorum profundus	4.5
Brachioradialis	1.9
Flexor carpi ulnaris	2.0
Pronator teres	1.2
Palmaris longus	0.1
Extensor pollicis longus	0.1
Extensor digitorum communis	1.7

AMPLITUDE

The distance through which a tendon moves when its muscle contracts can be measured directly. This excursion of the various tendons was measured in a cadaver. The amplitude of tendon motion for each individual joint and also for the complete motion of flexion and

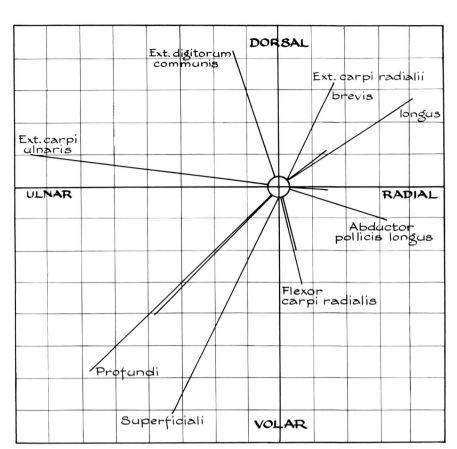

FIG. 16. The motions of the wrist and the relative power and direction of forces produced by the various muscles. The length of the line is proportionate to the work capacity of the designated muscle. Note that the plane of dorsiflexion is radialward, and that of volar flexion is ulnarward. The flexor carpi ulnaris is the most powerful muscle for wrist action and should be preserved in radial palsy operations to maintain effective action of the wrist in the proper plane. (Steindler A.: Post Graduate Lectures, Vol. 1, Springfield, Ill., Thomas, 1950)

FIG. 17 (Bottom). The power of a muscle is that force which will draw out the muscle from its maximally contracted state to its natural length. It is 3.6 kg. times the physiologic cross section. (Steindler, A.: Post Graduate Lectures, Vol. 1, Springfield, Ill., Thomas, 1950)

extension was noted. For each measurement the joint indicated was the only joint moved. Excursion of flexors was measured, starting with the wrist and the digits in full extension and for the extensors with the wrist and the fingers in full flexion as listed in the table on page 14.

Amplitude of wrist tendons was measured, starting with the wrist in the straight position (see table at bottom page 14).

An average total amplitude of excursion of tendons at various levels can be stated as in the table on page 15.

These figures agree quite closely with those

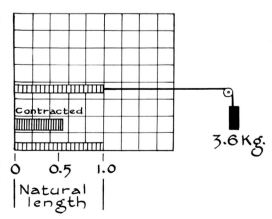

EXCURSIONS OF TENDONS

	Extensor Proprius and Extensor Communis (in mm.)	Flexor Profundus (in mm.)	Flexor Super- ficialis (in mm.)		Extensor Proprius and Extensor Communis (in mm.)	Flexor Profundus (in mm.)	Flexor Super- ficialis (in mm.)
Index Finger				*Little Finger*			
Distal joint ..	0	5	..	Distal joint ..	0	3.5	..
Middle joint .	2	20	16	Middle joint .	2	11	8
Proximal joint	15	15	16	Proximal joint	12	15	17
Wrist joint ..	38	16	16	Wrist joint ..	20	45	40
Full flexion of all joints ..	54	50	53	Full flexion of all joints ..	35	70	60
Middle Finger							
Distal joint ..	0	5	.				
Middle joint .	3	17	16		*Extensor Pollicis Longus*	*Extensor Pollicis Brevis*	*Abductor Pollicis*	*Long Flexor*
Proximal joint	16	23	26					
Wrist joint ..	41	38	46	*Thumb*	*(in mm.)*	*(in mm.)*	*(in mm.)*	*(in mm.)*
Full flexion of all joints ..	55	85	88	Distal joint	8	..	..	12
Ring Finger				Proximal joint ...	7	9		20
Distal joint ..	0	5	..	Carpomet- acarpal joint ...	6	7	5	8
Middle joint .	3	12	11	Wrist joint	33	14		23
Proximal joint	11	15	21	Totals	58	28	28	52
Wrist joint ..	39	45	40					
Full flexion of all joints ..	55	76	65					

given by Weber. As a working rule, one can remember that wrist motors average 33 mm., finger extensors 50 mm., flexor of thumb 50 mm., and finger flexors 70 mm.

After repair or transfer of a tendon some of the amplitude may be lost, due to scarring along the gliding surface or to contracture of the muscle itself. Thus the amplitude may no longer be sufficient to move all the joints through a full range but can move one or two of the joints to good degree. Knowledge of normal excursion values is most important in

selecting donor muscles for tendon transfers. A donor muscle should have at least as much amplitude as is necessary to carry out the desired motion. An even greater amount is desirable in most cases, for some loss of gliding ability will usually limit the newly transferred tendon.

Absolute amplitude as measured above should be differentiated from relative amplitude. This relative or effective amplitude may be sufficient to carry out a motion in the hand after transfer, because a new factor in muscle

Tendons	Palmar Flexion (in mm.)	Dorsi- Flexion (in mm.)	Total A.P. Motion (in mm.)	Radial Flexion (in mm.)	Ulnar Flexion (in mm.)	Total Lateral Motion (in mm.)
Extensor carpi radialis longus ..	16	21	37	8	16	24
Extensor carpi radialis brevis ...	16	21	37	4	12	16
Extensor carpi ulnaris	14	4	18	3	22	25
Flexor carpi radialis	20	20	40	2	4	6
Flexor carpi ulnaris	13	20	33	6	9	15

Average 33 mm.

	Above Wrist (in mm.)	Level of Metacarpals (in mm.)	In Proximal Segment Digit (in mm.)	In Middle Segment Fingers (in mm.)	In Proximal Segment Thumb (in mm.)
Wrist tendons	33	. .	. .	. .	. .
Flexion Fingers					
Flexor profundus	70	35.6	19.6	4.6	. .
Flexor superficialis	64	35.2	14.7	. .	. .
Extension Fingers					
Extensor digitorum communis and also proprius	50	16	3	. .	. .
Thumb flexor	52	32	. .	. .	12
Thumb Extensors					
Extensor pollicis longus	58	15	. .	. .	8
Extensor pollicis brevis	28	9	. .	. .	. .
Abductor pollicis longus	28	. .	. .	. .	. .

and tendon action is brought into play. Thus a muscle, normally acting on one joint and possessing a relatively short amplitude, may, when its tendon is transferred beyond that joint, then take on the characteristics of a biarticular or pluriarticular muscle. In this case, other muscles controlling the action of the intercalated segment or joint act as synergists to the action of the transferred unit and increase its effective amplitude.

An example of this added function when monoarticular muscles are changed to pluriarticular action is the use of an extensor carpi radialis for digital flexion. We know that this muscle has an amplitude of 37 mm., yet when its tendon is transferred to the flexors of the fingers it is capable of flexing the fingers to the palm and still allowing the hand to open

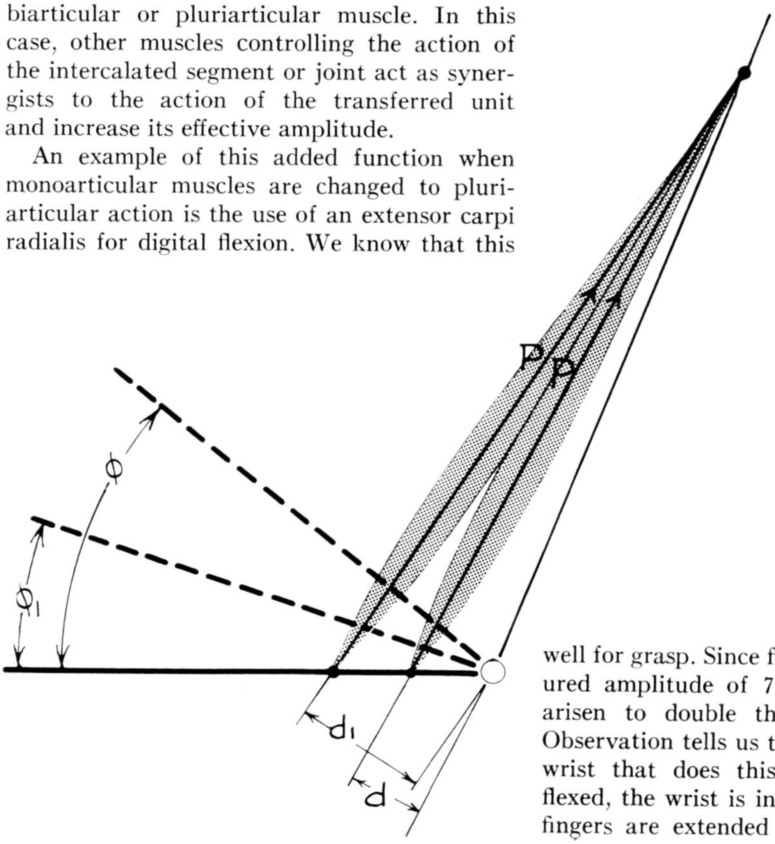

Fig. 18. The variability of lifting height. For the same muscle and the same contractile distance the power (PD; PD_1) increases with the distance ($d;d_1$). The lifting height ($\emptyset; \emptyset_1$) decreases with the distance ($d;d_1$). (Steindler, A.: The Traumatic Deformities and Disabilities of the Upper Extremity, Springfield, Ill., Thomas, 1946)

well for grasp. Since finger flexors have a measured amplitude of 70 mm., some factor has arisen to double the amplitude effectively. Observation tells us that it is the action of the wrist that does this. When the fingers are flexed, the wrist is in extension, but when the fingers are extended the wrist is dropped to

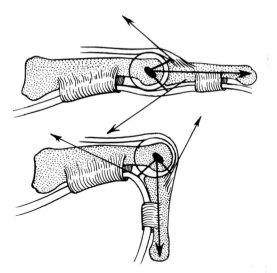

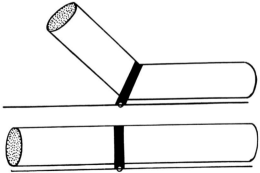

FIG. 20. The third form of tendon action diagrammatically shown as extensors would act under a retaining pulley such as the dorsal carpal ligament. (After Landsmeer: Acta. Morph. Neerl. Scand. III, Nos. 3 and 4)

FIG. 19. Mechanics of tendon action on a finger joint. The arrows represent the angles of approach in extension and in flexion. Movement of the extensor is directly proportional to the angular deviation of the joint. The flexor tendon spans the joint increasingly, so as flexion proceeds, the location of the pulleys determines the amount of this shift as well as the angle of approach.

neutral or palmar flexion. This interposed segment now working opposite to the action of the terminal moving parts has doubled the effective amplitude of motion. Arthrodesis of the wrist or lack of controlling muscles destroys this effect. The intervening joint must be under good control. Other examples are use of brachioradialis or pronator teres as digital extensors or flexors and flexor carpi radialis or ulnaris as digital extensors.

JOINT ACTION

Tendons passing across joints act to hold the bones together in a stabilizing effect or to move the joint. To move the joint there must be some length of lever arm between the insertion of the tendon and the center of motion of the joint. The greater the angle of approach of the tendon to the insertion the more angulatory effect there will be; the less the angle of approach, the more of a stabilizing effect. The angulating force is proportional to the sine; the stabilizing force, to the cosine of the angle of approach. As the joint flexion increases, the angle of approach increases. In some mus-

cle tendon units this is almost a right angle, such as the transverse adductor of the thumb, the biceps, the triceps and the pectoral muscles. Increasing this angle of approach, an expansion of the end of each bone of the extremity makes a prominence over which the tendons pass to go directly to an insertion on the next bone. In the flexors of the fingers, this terminal expansion of the proximal phalanx forces the flexor tendons over the prominence, and they are then held to the middle phalanx by the fibrous pulley of the tendon sheath.

In the finger the flexor tendons pursue this undulating course, moving volarward over the expansion of the bone and joint capsule and then dorsally to lie close along the phalanges held there by the 3 pulleys. The profundus tendon has a more advantageous angle of approach to the middle segment, because it is held in the loop of the superficial flexor. The dorsal and volar carpal retinacular ligaments likewise act as restraining bands, preventing bowstringing of the tendons as they pass across the wrist. Loss of any of these annular bands destroys the mechanical efficiency of tendon action.

Tendons pass across joints to act on the next distal segment in 1 of 3 patterns. The extensor tendon over the middle and the distal finger joints illustrates the simple type where the tendon passes over a convex gliding surface. Assuming that this is spherical, there is a direct relationship between the shortening of

FIG. 21. A flexor tendon held by restraining pulleys is a more effective force in flexion as this motion increases the angle of approach. The angle of approach can also be increased to a certain point by altering the sites of the retaining pulleys. In this diagram the distance AB increases as the joint flexes and represents an increased angle of pull. If the distances BC and BD were increased, a similar increase in effect would be seen. (After Landsmeer: Acta. Morph. Neerl. Scand. III, Nos. 3 and 4)

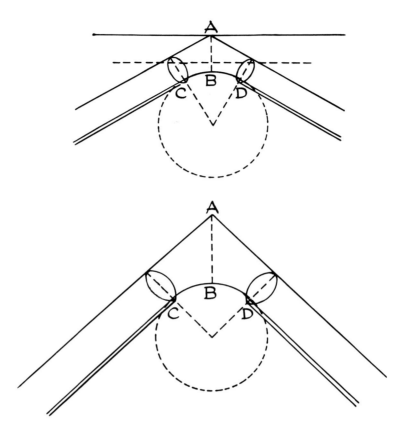

the tendons and the change of angle of the joint.

A second form, illustrated by a restraining loop or band, is seen in the action of the volar and dorsal carpal ligaments. A flexing tendon utilizing this mechanism likewise can be assumed to have its shortening take place in direct relationship to the change of angle of the joint.

A tendon running in a sheath with allowance for bowstringing at the joint level is seen in the flexors at the middle finger joint level. The rigid portion of the sheath is the surgical pulley mechanism. As flexion increases, the bowstringing increases; and the distance between the axis of the joint and the tendon tends to increase. Obviously, the distance of the free edge of the pulley from the joint level is also a determining influence on the amount of bowstringing. The pulley mechanisms in the finger are of utmost importance to the functioning of the flexor mechanism. Their preservation when possible and their reconstruction when necessary are important aspects of surgery of the hand.

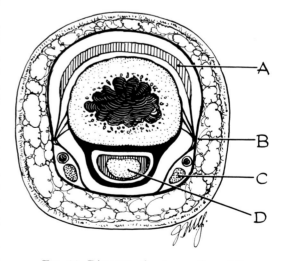

FIG. 22. Diagram of cross section of finger near middle joint: (A) extensor tendon; (B) conjoined fascias at midlateral line (? Cleland's ligament); (C) neurovascular bundle; (D) flexor tendons in the sheath. (After Skoog: Acta. Chiru. Scand., Supp. 139, 1948)

SECTION
FINGER TIP

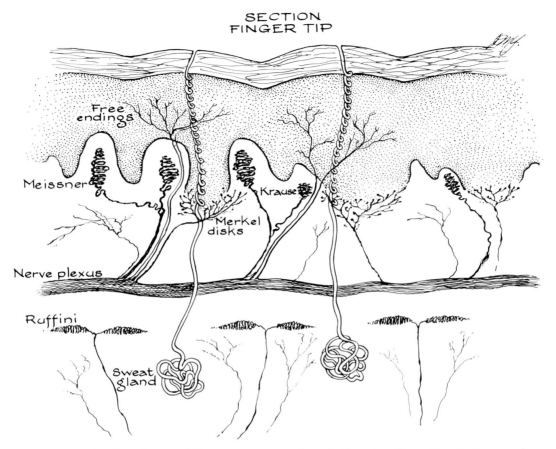

Fig. 23. The dermal plexus. Diagram of cross section of a fingertip, illustrating the types and the locations of the nerve endings of glabrous skin. (After Miller, Ralston *et al.*, Amer. J. Anat. *102*, 1958)

SENSIBILITY AND SENSATION

The hand is a sense organ capable of transmitting to our brain information as to size, weight, texture and temperature of the objects touched. The system of nerves subserving these functions also controls vasomotor, sudomotor and pilomotor activity.

To avoid confusion, a distinction should be made between sensation and sensibility. A normal hand possesses sensibility, but not sensation. Sensation has been defined as the cerebral mechanism activated by impulses in the afferent nervous system. It is defined by Winklemann as a product of spatial and temporal summation at the periphery and in the spinal cord and the interaction of central factors, such as emotion, experience and atten-

tion. Sensibility is the mechanism in the receptor area by which stimuli become coded into nerve impulses. Sensation would then be the correct interpretation of this complex pattern of impulses set up by these receptors (Noordenbos).

SUPERFICIAL SENSIBILITY

The 4 primary types of cutaneous sensibility are usually referred to as touch, pain, heat and cold. Elaborate methods have been devised for testing and recording function in the nervous system of the hand. For diagnostic purposes, such as determining nerve damage from a wound of the limb, the presence of paralysis of course indicates damage to a motor component of the nerve. Loss of sensibility to touch and pinprick are the simplest tests and usually are reliable. It is only in areas of skin where regeneration of the nerve is taking place that difficulty in interpretation arises.

The Dermal Network. The major part of nervous tissue in the skin is found in the dermal nerve network. The smaller branches of the nerves course through the subcutaneous tissues, and as they approach the surface in the subdermal layers they lose their myelin covering. Usually following the blood vessels, they then pass as fine fibers, some into the epithelial cells, some into the papillae, where they form twisted loops. Some fibers go directly to special regions or hair follicles without entering into the network. Certain hairless areas have high density networks, whereas in hairy skin the nerve network is decreased.

Hair follicles have a characteristic nerve supply, a double ring, one within another about the follicle neck. Each is supplied by more than one nerve fiber. As many as 9 fibers have been found going to one follicle. This random, multiple nerve supply is characteristic of the whole dermal network and of the so-called end-organs.

Meissner in 1852 described a corpuscle in papillae of distal glabrous skin. Like all endings, it is served by fibers from several nerves. Weddell believes that the network is really the receptor and that these corpuscles are not specific organs. According to Winklemann, they are found more on the fingertips than on the palm, and more on the radial than the ulnar side of the upper limb. Other forms of nerve endings such as Merkel-Ranvier, Krause and Dogiel have been described and given various functions. Not all observers agree even as to the presence of certain structures, though there is general agreement that separate receptors for the 4 basic modalities do not exist. Thus the concept that each type of stimulus was received only by a specific receptor and transmitted through a specific fiber has been abandoned. Head's divisions of sensibility into protopathic and epicritic types are still in use in describing certain findings in studies on regeneration of sensory nerves.

There is one form of sensory receptor in the body large enough to be seen with the naked eye and prominently in view in the tissues of the hand. The Vater-Pacini corpuscle occurs in the connective tissues below the skin of the fingers, the palm, the sole and the toes. It occurs in the genital areas but not in the lips or the conjunctivae. Extremely large bodies have been found in the mesentery. On the volar surface of the fingertip Winklemann counted as many as 120 per cu. mm. Corpuscles are found along nerve trunks, fascial planes and about joints, in the sacral and the epigastric plexuses, the pancreas and in paws and hooves of animals. Because the corpuscles lie deep in the tissues, they are probably not suitable for acute touch reception but are considered to be pressure receptors.

In the fingers, the characteristic dermal nerve network as found in the glabrous skin is most dense in the terminal parts. Zrubecky reports 23 Meissner type corpuscles per square mm. in fingertip, 9 per mm. on middle segment and 3 on the proximal segment.

On the side of the digit a transitional zone joins the volar to the dorsal part, where the Meissner corpuscle is less frequent and the nerve network more dense. On the dorsal hairy portions the characteristic follicle nerve supply is seen. No Pacinian corpuscles are found in the hairy regions.

The essential feature of the nerve supply that provides the hand with normal sensibility is the multiple innervation of the various receptors and the random supply of the skin areas. Nerve fibers from all directions interweave with other nerves so that each area may receive a supply from several sources. After nerve severance and regeneration, there is said to be a return of only one fiber to a specific receptor. Thus the summation of stimuli so necessary to provide normal sensation is no longer possible, and the stimulus is thus unidentifiable to the cortex, and paresthesia results.

DEEP SENSIBILITY

Nerve endings in muscle and tendons collect and transmit impulses which provide the ability to tell with eyes closed whether a joint is flexed or extended. In isolated lesions of the peripheral nerves in the hand, the loss is hardly noticeable because of overlap. A median nerve lesion may result in loss of joint sense only in the middle joint of the index and the middle fingers. In brachial plexus palsy, however, this loss of position sense may be severe.

TESTING SENSIBILITY IN THE HAND

For practical purposes testing for light touch with a wisp of cotton and for response to pinprick with a sharp point are sufficient for everyday clinical use. It is when there is a question of the amount and the quality of regeneration after nerve repair or when it is important to determine the impairment of function in the hand that more refined and more objective methods are required. All such tests using a stimulus such as pins, cotton wisp, cold or heat are to some degree subjective. They depend on cooperation and concentration of the patient and skill in the examiner. They provide no objective record. Distinguishing paresthesia from sensibility to touch is difficult. Hyperpathia, the pain response to non-noxious stimuli, is impossible to evaluate or measure.

The coin test of Seddon, Weber's 2-point discrimination test and inscribing numbers on the skin are useful for determination of the state of recovery of nerve function.

SURGICAL ANATOMY

LANDMARKS

Wrist. The styloid process of the radius is almost ½ inch more distal than that of the ulna and is easily felt. Its tip covers the upper one third of the scaphoid bone. The tip of the styloid of the ulna marks the level of the radiocarpal joint, and the curve of this joint rises proximal to the interstyloid line. The head of the ulna is prominent in pronation, but in supination the styloid process is what we feel in place of the ulnar head.

On the dorsum of the wrist the bases of the 1st, the 3rd and the 5th metacarpals can be easily felt. The most prominent central projection on the dorsum of the wrist is the styloid process of the 3rd metacarpal, which projects dorsoradially. This projection, which frequently receives the bruise in crushing injuries, is 1½ inches distal to and on a line with the prominent tubercle on the dorsum of the radius. Between these 2 points, as landmarks, is the carpus. The bases of the metacarpals can be located by a dorsal cross groove.

The tubercle of the radius, easily felt, lies between the tendons of the long extensor of the thumb ulnarward and the short extensor of the wrist. A line from this tubercle to the external epicondyle of the humerus naturally marks the septum between the extensor muscles of the fingers and those of the wrist. The long extensors of the wrist insert on the bases of the 2nd and the 3rd metacarpals, and the extensor ulnaris on that of the 5th. The snuffbox lies between the long and the short extensors of the thumb, and its floor is composed of the scaphoid and the trapezium. The radial artery crosses it beneath the tendons to dive through the 1st metacarpal cleft. Control of bleeding from this artery from here to the deep arterial arch in the palm is difficult.

The 2 sesamoid bones in the adductor and the short flexor tendons of the thumb are readily felt, and so is the joint between the 1st metacarpal and the trapezium bone. Occasionally, a sesamoid may be felt when present in the anterior capsule of the other metacarpophalangeal joints, especially in the index and even at the distal joint of the thumb. Of the 4 projecting hooks on the volar aspect of the carpus, the pisiform and the tubercle of the scaphoid are more easily felt, the hook of the hamate and the ridge of the trapezium bone being deeper in the heel of the palm. The tubercle of the scaphoid bone is at the base of the thenar eminence just beyond the distal flexion crease of the wrist and between the tendons of the long abductor of the thumb and the flexor carpi radialis. What usually passes for the tubercle of the scaphoid is the ridge of the trapezium. The scaphoid tubercle is slightly deeper and proximal. The pisiform bone is grooved at its base on its radial side, and there it overhangs and protects the ulnar nerve and artery after they have penetrated the transverse carpal ligament to a position volar to it. The 4 bony hooks or projections, mentioned above, together with the transverse carpal ligament bound and protect the channel of the wrist, through which run the flexor tendons and the median nerve. This channel is in the line of the forearm when the hand is ulnar flexed but is angulated 25° radialward when the hand is straight with the forearm. Therefore, the grip is stronger when the hand is in ulnar flexion.

The cleft of the extended thumb is on a cross-line with the superficial arch in the palm from the ulnar artery, and the deep arch from the radial artery is ½ inch proximal to it.

PLATE 1

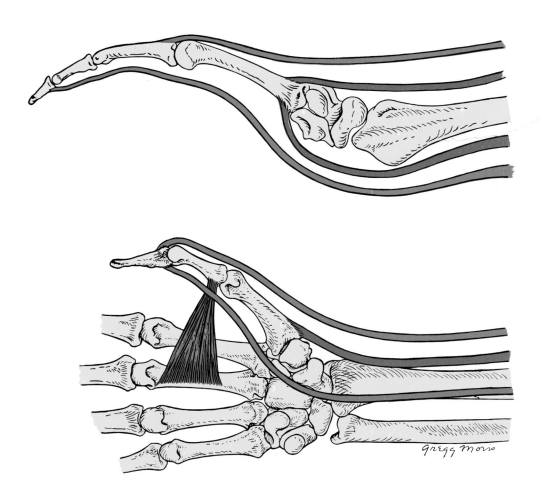

Principle of stabilization of the proximal joints so that the distal joints may be moved.
(*Top*) Wrist movers (*red*) stabilize the wrist so that the digit movers (*blue*) may act.
(*Bottom*) In pinching with the thumb, the abductor pollicis longus (*red*) stabilizes the carpometacarpal joint in extension. Also, the adductor pollicis (*green*) stabilizes the metacarpophalangeal joint in flexion. These two stabilizers hold the thumb in a firm arch so that the digit movers (*blue*) may act.

In transferring tendons for radial palsy, all three of the above stabilizers in red should be activated.

PLATE 2

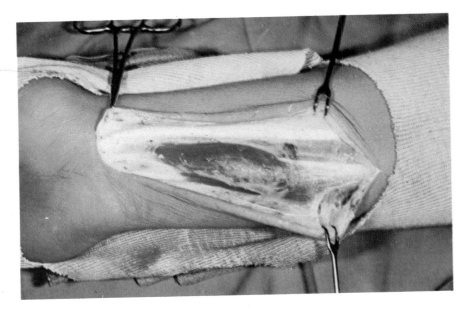

The palmaris longus muscle may be in an abnormal location; here its origin is at the wrist, and the tendon is proximal and short. The muscle and tendon are absent in 10 to 15 per cent of patients.

The webs of the fingers are ¾ inch distal to the proximal finger joints, and the digital arteries fork ½ inch proximal to the webs. The first dorsal interosseus muscle is prominent between the thumb and the index metacarpal. It is composed of 2 parts: the superficial belly, which can be felt to contract as the index finger abducts, and the deeper part when it flexes the proximal joint of the index. Both bellies contract when pinching between the thumb and the index finger either in the lateral or anteroposterior plane. Incisions in the dorsum through this cleft should be kept radial to this muscle.

The carpal bones together are concave in their volar aspect and convex in their dorsal. There is hardly any motion in the carpometacarpal joints with the exception of that of the thumb, and here the trapezium has in addition considerable motion as it moves with the metacarpal. Of the other carpometacarpal joints, that of the little finger has more motion than the rest by a slight degree. The metacarpals of the index and the middle fingers are fixed largely to the carpus, and those of the ring and the little fingers are movable and more or less oppose and arch the palm.

Volar Aspect of Forearm. The 2 superficial tendons—flexor carpi radialis and palmaris longus—can be made to stand out by flexing the wrist against resistance. Opposing the thumb also brings out the palmaris longus tendon. Beneath this tendon or slightly radial to it is the median nerve. This tendon is unique in running two thirds of the way up the forearm. It may be absent in 10 to 15 per cent of patients.

The deep fascia enclosing the long flexors in the forearm is tough and unyielding, so that pressure developing within its enclosure from trauma or obstructive venous engorgement squeezes out the blood supply, and Volkmann's ischemia results. Within this space the long flexor of the thumb and the flexor ulnaris muscle fill in the 2 lateral aspects. In between them, occupying mostly the ulnar half of the space due to the crowding by the flexor carpi radialis, are the 2 layers of flexor digitorum: superficialis and profundus. The superficialis tendons are muscled much farther distalward than are the profundus tendons, and each muscle slip runs down to a point, while those of the profundus end squarely across. The

profundus tendons are on the same plane and are parallel and larger, but the superficialis tendons of the middle and the index fingers cross each other. The floor of the space is formed by the pronator quadratus muscle and proximal to that the interosseous membrane, down which run the interosseous vessels and the nerve to the pronator quadratus. The flexor tendons travel straight through the wrist channel when the hand is ulnar flexed and then fan out to the digits. The tendon to the thumb runs through the radial bursa, and those to the fingers through the ulnar bursa.

Dorsal Aspect of Forearm. The long extensors of the fingers occupy the center of the dorsum of the forearm, and the long extensors of the wrist the radial part of the dorsum, the latter being especially prominent in the upper part of the forearm. Taking their origin from the interosseous membrane and adjoining parts of the bones deep in the forearm, the 3 extensor muscles of the thumb emerge from under the extensors of the fingers and roll over the extensors of the wrist to reach the thumb. Just within the V of the crossing of the long extensor of the thumb and the short extensor of the wrist is felt the radial tubercle. Arising in the same plane as the thumb extensors is the extensor indicis. The extensor proprius of the little finger is in the same deep plane with the extensor digitorum communis and the extensor carpi ulnaris. Higher in the forearm the supinator brevis is on the same plane with the thumb extensors.

At the wrist each extensor tendon has a separate synovial sheath, with the exception that the abductor pollicis longus and the extensor pollicis brevis share the same sheath and so do the extensor indicis and the 4 tendons of the extensor communis digitorum. Thus, there are 7 synovial sheaths on the dorsum, but only 2 on the volar aspect. The extensor digitorum communis and extensor of the little finger override the deep layer of oblique muscles and lie in a trough between the radial and the ulnar extensors of the wrist. The nerve supplying the muscles in the back of the forearm emerges from the supinator brevis and lies between the superficial and the oblique muscle layers.

Palm. The palm owes its toughness to the skin, the subcutaneous fat and the palmar fascia, and these durable tissues protect the more delicate structures beneath. The skin is so tough that it will not angulate for plastic maneuvers. The subcutaneous fat is in firm adherent lobules, each contained in a pocket of connective tissue. The palmar fascia sends septa and fibers to the skin and also deeply to the ligamentous tissues at the sides of the metacarpals. At the creases in the palm the skin is held tightly by these fibers to the palmar fascia. The same applies in the fingers. The attachments, reaching from the metacarpals to the skin, maintain the hollow of the palm. A description of the fascial septa in the palm may be found under Dupuytren's contracture in Chapter 7. In the distal part of the palm opposite each digital cleft is a soft prominence where the fat bulges through between the 4 slips of the palmar fascia as each of these continues down each finger. Because of the firmness we do not find in the palm hematoma or edema so often found in the dorsum of the hand.

Incisions to expose the contents of the palm are made through skin, fat and palmar fascia, thus exposing the blood vessels of the superficial arch and the volar digital nerves. The vessels of the superficial arch lie superficial to the nerves here, just as those of the deep palmar arch lie superficial to the deep branches of the ulnar nerve. Between these 2 sets of vessels and nerves are the superficialis and the profundus tendons and the lumbrical muscles.

A tiny nerve twig runs to the base of each lumbrical muscle, 2 of which are from the adjoining volar digital nerves from the median, but the other 2 from the motor branch of the ulnar nerve; they should not be harmed by the surgeon; nor should he injure the main motor branches from the median and the ulnar nerves. The former extends from the median nerve directly to beneath the deep fascia in the thenar eminence just beyond the volar carpal ligament, and it may be in 2 parts. The motor branch from the ulnar nerve leaves the main trunk just past the pisiform bone.

The transverse metacarpal ligament is a strong, flat band crossing between the heads of the metacarpal bones at their volar borders. It separates the interosseus muscles and spaces behind from the lumbrical muscles in front. The strong ligamentous annular sheaths of the flexor tendons arise from this transverse metacarpal ligament, commencing just proximal to the metacarpal heads. Opposite the joint is a short gap, and then the second annular sheath continues to halfway down the proximal phalanx.

The skin of the palm and the volar surface of the fingers contains more sweat glands than that of the dorsum of the hand and has an abundance of lymphatic vessels but is hairless and almost devoid of subcutaneous veins or pigment. Lymphatics and veins all run to the dorsum of the hand and on up the arm. In hand and forearm venous return is mostly external, as in the fetus, and in contrast with the upper arm.

Dorsum of Hand. On the dorsum of the hand there is more or less interdigitating of the tendons, so that even if one tendon is severed the finger may still extend. The tendon of the extensor indicis is smaller than the extensor communis tendon to that finger, while that of the extensor digiti minimi is larger. Both of these proprius tendons lie to the ulnar side of their respective communis tendon. The diagonal intercommunicating tendon slips, just proximal to the knuckles, aid in coordinating extension of the fingers, which should work together. Only the index and the little fingers extend freely alone.

Fingers. There is a set of 4 nerves and arteries down each finger, but the dorsal 2 of these are not of much importance. The volar pair is on a level with the anterior volar border of the flexor tendons, and the dorsal pair is on a level with the dorsal border of the extensor tendon. Unlike in the palm, the arteries lie dorsal to the volar digital nerves.

The flexor superficialis tendon becomes flat and partially surrounds the profundus tendon just before it splits into its 2 flat tendons of insertion. It forms a 3-legged sling over the proximal phalanx to help hold the profundus tendon in its bed. The annular ligaments in a finger, ensheathing the flexor tendons, are opposite the proximal halves of the proximal phalanges and the central thirds of the middle phalanges but are not present opposite the joints. They keep the tendons from bowing across the flexed fingers and add to the efficiency of their action. A description of the dorsal aponeurosis, which can be palpated readily on the back of the finger, may be found in Chapter 12, Intrinsic Muscles of the Hand.

BIBLIOGRAPHY

Bell, Sir Charles: The Hand, London, William Pickering, 1834.

Capener, N.: The hand in surgery, J. Bone & Joint Surg. *38B*:1, 1956.

Cirillo, N.: Anatomical clinical study of relation between articular skin folds and underlying bone structure in palm of hand, wrist, and elbow, Arch. Inst. biochim. ital. *10*:233, 1938.

Cirillo, N., and Baldesi, A.: Anatomical and clinical relation of blood vessel arcades and skin folds in human palm, Scritti biol. *13*:106, 1938.

Cirio, J. J.: Uniform criteria of movements of opposing flexion and extension of joints, Arch. Soc. argent. de anat. norm. y pat. *1*:144, 1939.

Cunningham, D. J.: Text-book of Anatomy, 5th ed., New York, William Wood & Co., 1928.

Ghigi, C.: Contribution of the study of the wrist, Chir. d. org. di movimento *24*:344, 1939.

Goff, C. W.: Comparative anthropology of man's hand, *in* De Palma: Clinical Orthopaedics, No. 13, Philadelphia, Lippincott, 1959.

Graziani, A.: Anatomical history of wrist—roentgen study, Radiol. med. *27*:382, 1940.

Imura-Kozi: Mechanics of elbow, forearm and wrist joints and arrangement of muscles involved, Tokyo Igakkwai Zassi *55*:401, 1941.

Jones, F. W.: Principles of Anatomy as Seen in the Hand, Baltimore, Williams & Wilkins, 1942.

Kirk, T. S.: Some points in mechanism of human hand, J. Anat. *58*:228, 1924.

Landsmeer, J. M. F.: Studies in the anatomy of articulation; II. Patterns of movement of bimuscular, bi-articular systems, Acta morph. Neerl.-Scand. *3*:304, 1960.

MacConaill, M. A.: Mechanical anatomy of the carpus and its bearing on some surgical problems, J. Anat. *75*:166, 1941.

Miller, M. R., Ralston, H. J., and Kasakara, M.: The pattern of cutaneous innervation of the human hand, Am. J. Anat. *102*:183, 1958.

Napier, J. R.: The prehensile movements of the human hand, J. Bone & Joint Surg. *38B*:902, 1956.

Noordenbos, W.: Pain, Amsterdam, Elsevier, 1959.

Ralston, N. J., Miller, M. R., and Kasakara, M.: Nerve endings in human fasciae, tendons, ligaments, periosteum, and joint synovial membrane, Anat. Rec. *136*:137, 1960.

Steindler, A.: The Traumatic Deformities and Disabilities of the Upper Extremity, Springfield, Ill., Thomas, 1946.

————: Postgraduate Lectures in Orthopedics, Diagnosis and Indications, Springfield, Ill., Thomas, 1950.

Stilwell, D. L., Jr.: The innervation of deep structures of the hand, Am. J. Anat. *101*:75, 1957.

Todd, T. W.: Atlas of Skeletal Maturation, St. Louis, Mosby, 1937.

Van Lamoen, E.: Een outleedkundig-functioned ondarzoek van let polsege-wricht, Thesis, Univ. of Leyden, 1961.

Von Lanz, T., and Wachsmuth: Praktische Anatomie, Berlin, Springer, 1959.

Winklemann, R. K.: Nerve Endings in Normal and Pathologic Skin, Springfield, Ill., Thomas, 1960.

Zrubecky, G.: Die Hand, das Tastorgan des Menschen, Stuttgart, Ferdinand Enke, 1960.

Chapter 2

Phylogeny and Comparative Anatomy

ORIGIN OF LIMBS

Inquiry into the origin of hands leads us down the animal phyla until we find the beginning of limbs in the primitive sharks. Here is the first sign—a lateral fold on each side, continuous from gill to anus, into which muscles grew in later development. The middle of each fold receded, but the two ends increased, so that it became the established order throughout all fishes to have 2 pectoral fins just behind the gills and 2 pelvic fins near the anus. Since then this tetrapod or 4-limbed architecture has persisted through all consecutive classes—amphibians, reptiles and mammals—up to man.

PHYLOGENETICS OF INTRINSIC MUSCLES OF HAND

From a search through the literature and by dissection of the hands of reptiles, mammals, monkeys and higher apes, including man, for the origin of the intrinsic muscles, the author concludes the following: Of all the muscles of the upper extremity, the intrinsic ones of the hand are primordial. They date back to the early fish where there was no arm but only a pectoral fin, the forerunner of the hand. Thus, the hand in phylogeny preceded the arm, which developed later from higher cervical segments. The fish has not yet a neck, the

bones of the pectoral fin articulating with the skull. Our intrinsic muscles are still supplied by the lower 2 nerves of the brachial plexus, and nerves remain true to their muscles. The arm developed later from the neck for terrestrial existence.

EARLIEST INTRINSIC MUSCLES MOVED FIN RAYS

The tetrapod or 4-limbed arrangement which became standard had its forerunner in the fish with pectoral and pelvic fins. The independent muscle action of the rays of the pectoral fin was made possible by the anlage of our intrinsic hand muscles. Watching pectoral fins in an aquarium, one sees versatility of movement as the fins are continually fanning the water. A wave of movement may run down or up a pectoral fin, causing the fish to rise or descend as if the fin were geared to the water. One of the earliest fishes that still persists and is closely allied to the early shark is the skate; it swims along by graceful undulations of its wings, which are merely glorified pectoral fins. The muscles that move these rays in fins are the anlagen of the intrinsic muscles of the hand.

ORIGIN OF PENTADACTYLISM

In the development from fish through amphibians to man, the multirayed fin of the

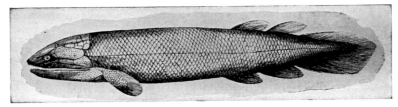

FIG. 24. Following the sharks, and just before the lung fishes, came the Crossopterygii, or fringe fins, with fleshy, jointed fins. It is conceded that this is the subclass which emerged from the water to become Amphibia, and developed lungs and limbs for terrestrial existence. (Jordan, D. S.: Fishes, New York, Appleton)

24

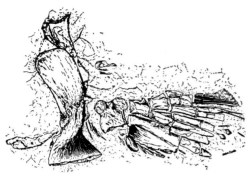

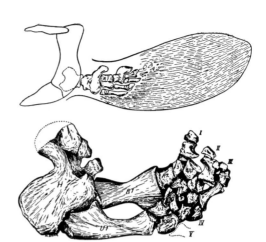

Original specimen of a pectoral fin of the fringe-fin fish, *Sauropterus taylori* Hall, from the upper Devonian of Pennsylvania—the conceded ancestor of the Amphibia and all the vertebrates that followed.

Comparison of the pectoral girdle and the limb of a crossopterygian fish with that of Eryops of the stegocephalian amphibians.

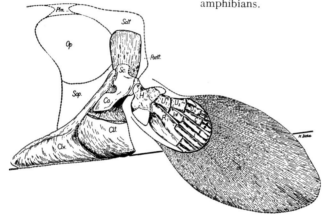

Median view of the right side of a reconstruction of the pectoral girdle and the paddle of *Sauropterus taylori*.

Fig. 25. How the pectoral fin of this early crossopterygian developed into the forelimb of the earliest known amphibian, Eryops, thus changing from the multirayed fin to the 5-digit type. (After W. K. Gregory) (The American Philosophical Society)

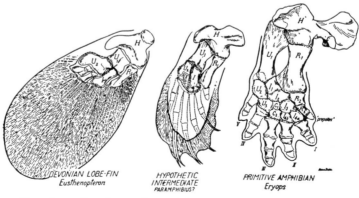

DEVONIAN LOBE-FIN
Eusthenopteron

HYPOTHETIC INTERMEDIATE
PARAMPHIBIUS?

PRIMITIVE AMPHIBIAN
Eryops

Transformation from the multirayed crossopterygian paddle to the pentadactylate hand of Eryops and all subsequent vertebrates.

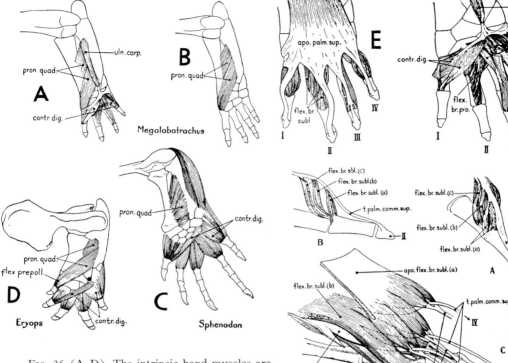

FIG. 26 (A–D). The intrinsic hand muscles are well developed in Amphibia, and, in fact, are the only muscles that control the digits. The arm muscles stop at the carpus or the metacarpus. The arm developed after the hand from higher cervical segments. The intrinsic muscles in man are supplied by the lower segments of the eighth cervical and the first thoracic nerves, and the arm by higher segments up to the fifth cervical. The surprising development of the intrinsic muscles in amphibians is shown in this dissection of the hand of the giant salamander of Japan, Megalobatrachus. Comparison of the deepest layer of forearm muscles and the contrahentes digitorum of Megalobatrachus with those of the reptile Sphenodon, and their inferred restoration in Eryops.

FIG. 26 (E–G).
(E) Dissection of the hand of Megalobatrachus, showing the superficial flexors and their attachment to the palmar fascia.
(F) The deep flexors and their relation to the ulnocarpalis.
(G) Dissection of the second digit of Megalobatrachus (A and B) and of the second, third and fourth digits in the reptile Sphenodon (C) to show the relation of the digital flexors to the palmar aponeurosis. (After R. W. Miner) (Bull. Am. Museum Nat. Hist.)

fish was reduced to the pentadactylate type. It is generally conceded that it was the crossopterygian fish called "fringed fins," relatives of the lung fishes, which emerged from the water, evolved to Amphibia and developed lungs and feet for terrestrial existence. Some lung fishes that persist today use their pectoral and pelvic fins in walking.

Fossils from upper Devonian in Pennsylvania prove that the fringed-fin fishes had jointed pectoral fins, each with an axis fringed with a series of soft rays. In the step from these fishes to the Amphibia, according to

W. K. Gregory, the most proximal segment of the stubby bones at the base became the humerus, and the next 2 segments became radius and ulna. The next several segments, still dividing, developed into the carpus. The main stem became the thumb, and the bones on the ulnar side became the other 4 digits. From the digit bones the many soft rays extended. The resulting pentadactylism persisted through the ages, with recession in some instances in various forms of amphibians, reptiles and mammals.

From the above it is apparent that the hand

Fig. 27. (*Top*) Ventral view of the right front foot of an alligator. In reptiles, as in amphibians, the hand is thick and meaty from the intrinsic muscles. All muscles controlling the digits are of the brevis type, except the long flexor profundus—the only forearm muscle which acts on the digits. Even it is still bipartite. In the gradation to mammals, the extensor brevis and the flexor sublimis became long muscles by fusing end to end over the carpus with the forearm muscles and then separating from the carpus. The predominance of the intrinsic muscles in reptiles is shown in these sketches from the hand of an alligator.

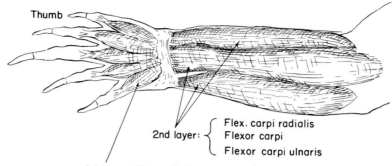

Thumb

2nd layer: { Flex. carpi radialis
Flexor carpi
Flexor carpi ulnaris

1st layer: Flexor digitorum brevis (sublimis).

(*Center*) Ventral view of the right front foot of an alligator.

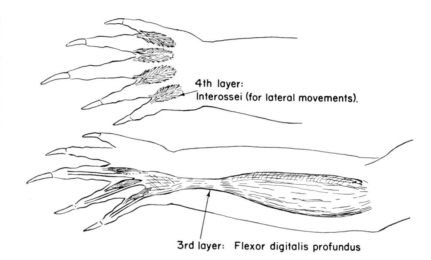

4th layer:
Interossei (for lateral movements).

3rd layer: Flexor digitalis profundus

(*Bottom*) Dorsal view of the right front foot of an alligator.

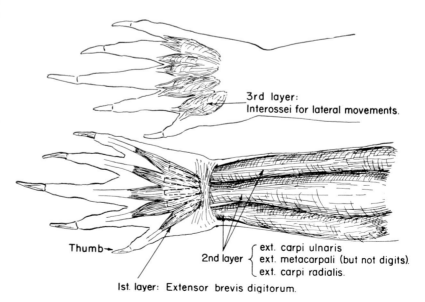

3rd layer:
Interossei for lateral movements.

Thumb

2nd layer { ext. carpi ulnaris
ext. metacarpali (but not digits).
ext. carpi radialis.

1st layer: Extensor brevis digitorum.

(J. Bone Joint Surg.)

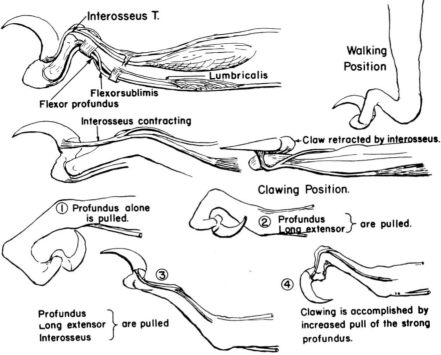

FIG. 28. The specialized retractile and clawing mechanism of the cat tribe is dependent on the interaction between the long extensors and flexors and the interosseus muscles. The latter retract the claw until the distal two phalanges overlap each other. These sketches are from the paw of a wildcat. (J. Bone Joint Surg.)

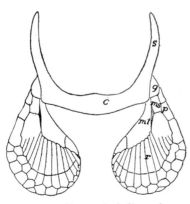

FIG. 29. Pectoral girdle and cartilaginous fin skeleton of the fish Scyllium. (c) coracoid region; (g) glenoid surface; (ms) mesopterygium; (mt) metapterygium; (r) radialis; (s) scapular region. (Kingsley, J. S.: Comparative Anatomy of Vertebrates, New York, Blakiston)

developed before the arm and from its very beginning contained intrinsic muscles. Muscles in fish are largely undifferentiated and are arranged in segmental myotomes. Those in the pectoral fin are developed from modification of the adjoining myotomes.

INTRINSIC HAND MUSCLES WELL-DEVELOPED IN AMPHIBIA

The intrinsic muscles of the hand are found to be already highly developed in the Amphibia, and in this class they have sole control of the digits. As yet no forearm muscles move the digits; all extensors and flexors of the digits are of the "brevis" type, their origin not reaching above the carpus. The same high development of intrinsic muscles runs through Reptilia, and even here the long flexor profundus is the only forearm muscle which has joined to the intrinsic muscles across the carpal ligament so as to move the digits.

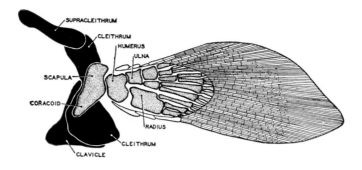

Fig. 30. Pectoral girdle and fin of Sauropterus, an upper Devonian crossopterygian fish. Interest in this type of fish fin lies in the similarity of relations of the proximal elements of the extremity to those found in the pectoral extremity of the tetrapods. Bones of dermal derivation are in black. (After Brown, Neal, and Rand: Comparative Anatomy, New York, Blakiston)

Long Forearm Muscles Assume Control of Digits

All other forearm muscles at this stage did not insert below the carpus or the metacarpals. It was an easy step, therefore, in the gradation to mammals for this tendinous attachment or connection across the carpus merely to loosen from the carpus, with the result that the long muscles in the forearm became continuous with the brevis muscles in the hand. This is apparently the development of the long extensors and the long flexor sublimis and profundus in man which now control our digits from the forearm. Recently, the author had 3 patients who had 1 and 2 slips of the atavistic extensor brevis. In the human foot there is still an extensor brevis, and the flexor sublimis is a brevis. Thus we see that the hand developed before the arm, and that the intrinsic muscles of the hand were primordial; some of them joined later with the forearm muscles to become long extensors and long flexors. All intrinsic muscles in the hand are supplied by the 8th and the 1st spinal segments. The arm, which has a higher segmental nerve supply as we ascend to biceps and deltoid muscles, developed later from the side of the neck at higher segmental levels.

Intrinsic Muscles of Hand From Amphibia Through Primates

The many layers of muscles and tendons in the hand of the Amphibia (6) have been consecutively traced by McMurrich and others in their gradual modification through reptiles (8) and mammals to man, who has only 5 layers in the palm. In mammals the intrinsic muscles persisted well in those which used their front extremities as hands. Some interosseous muscles became specialized, as in the cat tribe, to retract and erect the claws.

In monkeys and higher apes the intrinsic muscles of the hand are well developed, and their arrangement is so similar to that of man that the variations are small and rather exceptional. The 4 or 5 contrahentes of most mammals and monkeys, which are separated from the interossei by the deep branch of the ulnar nerve, have been reduced in man to only the adductors of the thumb. The contrahentes have origin in the carpus and the metacarpal bases. They insert on the metacarpal heads and the proximal phalanges and adduct toward the 3rd metacarpal. In monkeys, the 2nd to the 5th are often absent. The 2nd, the 4th and the 5th are poor in gibbons and absent in gorillas, orangoutang and man. The chimpanzee has only the 1st, the 4th and the 5th.

Palmar interossei in most mammals number 6 or 7; in primates 5 or 6; but in man there are only 3 because 4 have fused with the dorsal interossei, thus accounting for the latter's double insertion.

In primates the palmar interossei and the lumbricales insert in the lateral expansion of the extensor tendons, and the dorsal interossei insert only on the phalanges. The axis of the interossei in man and most primates is the 3rd digit, but in some prosimians it is the 4th.

The lumbricales in primates are variable in number and in the number of their heads, and they may have accessory fasciculi. In most, they are radial and 4 in number; the outer 2 are supplied by the median, and the inner 2 by the ulnar nerve.

PECTORAL GIRDLE

With the necessity for mobility in the primitive vertebrates came the 2 girdles—pectoral and pelvic—the first just behind the last gill and the second just in front of the anus. At first these were to furnish scaffolding for muscle attachments to move the fin and finally the limb. Later, in the Amphibia when the pectoral girdles separated from the skull and the spine, it became movable on the trunk by muscle attachments.

FISHES

In the early fishes the pectoral girdle, like the pelvic girdle, was simple and U-shaped. It formed outside the main body or myotomes. Later, nerves to the limbs grew past it and through it. Each side of the girdle was of 2 parts—the dorsal one, the scapula; the ventral one, the coracoid—and between them was the glenoid cavity, which articulated with the limb. The 2 coracoids were attached to each other by membrane or an intermediate bone. There developed an omovertebral bone and a suprascapula for attachment to vertebrae and the skull. The clavicle developed from the skin, and in different fishes many subplates developed, but in all there was the main ventral part, the coracoid, and the dorsal part, the scapula with the limb springing from between them.

AMPHIBIA

As amphibians emerged from the water, accommodating to the need for terrestrial locomotion, the girdle modified to become a trident; the ventral portion expanded broadly with a foramen through it or divided into precoracoid and coracoid, with the foramen formed between them and their union with the sternum. This change into bipartite coracoid also occurred in the pelvic girdle and here is still retained, the ilium being the dorsal part and the pubis and the ischium the ventral. The obturator foramen corresponds to the coracoid foramen.

In the amphibious stegocephalia, such as Eryops, there were a scapula, a coracoid, a clavicle, an interclavicle and also a cleithrum articulating between the suprascapula and the skull. However, this latter, with the need for

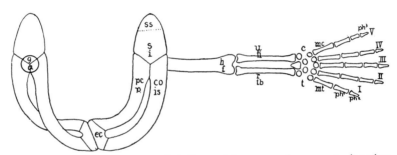

FIG. 31. Diagram of tetrapod girdles and free appendages, posterior view. Upper letters, pectoral; lower, pelvic appendages. (a) acetabula; (c) carpus; (co) coracoid; (ec) epicoracoid (no equivalent in pelvis); (f) femur; (fi) fibula; (g) glenoid fossa; (h) humerus; (i) ileum; (is) ischium; (mc) metacarpus; (mt) metatarsus; (p) pubis; (pc) precoracoid; (ph) phalanges, numbered; (r) radius; (s) scapula; (ss) suprascapula (no equivalent in pelvis); (t) tarsus; (tb) tibia; (U) ulna; (I-V) digits. (Kingsley, J. S.: Comparative Anatomy of Vertebrates, New York, Blakiston)

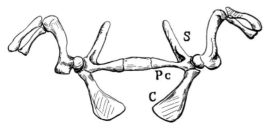

FIG. 32. Pectoral girdle of Southern snapping turtle: (S) scapula; (Pc) precoracoid; (C) coracoid.

a more mobile head and girdle, disappeared in all later amphibians, thus allowing the scapula to descend and liberating the head for free movement. This descent of the scapula is rehearsed in each human embryo. The median interclavicle was lost in some amphibians but retained in others and was passed on to the reptiles. In most amphibians the clavicle fused with the precoracoid.

The frog, which lands so hard on his front legs and chest, developed for this a very large

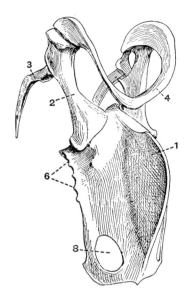

Fig. 33. Shoulder-girdle and sternum of a black vulture (*Vultur cinereus*) × ⅓ (Cambridge Museum): (*1*) carina of the sternum; (*2*) coracoid; (*3*) scapula; (*4*) clavicle; (*6*) surfaces for articulation with the sternal ribs; (*7*) xiphoid processes; (*8*) fontanel. (Reynolds, S. H.: The Vertebrate Skeleton, Cambridge Univ. Press, 1897)

broad girdle with flat, overlapping, platelike coracoids, epicoracoids, precoracoids and clavicles; the coracoid and the precoracoid were joined by a bar. A large proportion of the specialized parts of the various girdles were cartilaginous.

REPTILES

The reptiles retained the trident girdle. There usually was a foramen through the coracoid, though in some the foramen was formed by the presence of a precoracoid. The parts became more bony and differentiated for greater activity. The humerus, as in all vertebrates, sprang from the glenoid at the juncture between the scapula and coracoid. The platelike character of the interclavicle, the sternum and the broad coracoid and epicoracoid remained, as these animals largely slid along on the ground. In the turtle the scapula is only a little spike, extending backward; diverging forward from it as a Y is the coracoid and the clavicle fused with the large precoracoid. The crocodilia have only a broad coracoid, an interclavicle and a scapula. In snakes both girdles have been lost, though some remnants of the pelvic girdle are still to be found in pythons and boas, consisting of 2 rudimentary clawed bones.

BIRDS

Here there is special tremendous development of the keeled sternum for origin of pectoral muscles for flying. The scapula is firmly fixed to the sternum by a rodlike prop, the coracoid, and is also braced to it in front by the clavicle. The 2 clavicles are fused to each other at their sternal attachment, thus forming the wishbone. The scapula is only a small curved rod extending down the back for muscle attachment. The bird in flight lifts itself by its sternum through its pectoral muscles. Some of the moas, which are flightless, have even lost all vestiges of the upper limb and the pectoral girdle. The early prehistoric toothed bird, Archaeopteryx, had a pectoral girdle much like that of a reptile and, unlike

Fig. 34. Illustrating the fundamental similarity of the human (B) and the amphibian (A) pectoral girdle. In man, the coracoid element has degenerated into a process (coracoid) and a connective-tissue ligament, occasionally containing cartilage. (Redrawn after Huntington, Neal and Rand: Comparative Anatomy, New York, Blakiston)

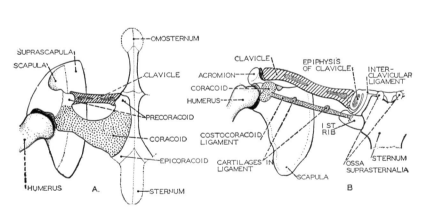

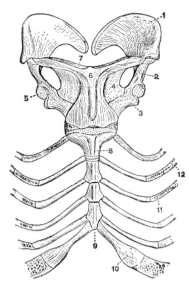

FIG. 35. Ventral view of the shoulder-girdle and the sternum of a duckbill (*Ornithorhynchus paradoxus*) × ¾ (After Parker): (*1* and *2*) scapula; (*3*) coracoid; (*4*) precoracoid; (*5*) glenoid cavity; (*6*) interclavicle; (*7*) clavicle; (*8*) presternum; (*9*) third segment of mesosternum; (*10*) sternal rib; (*11*) intermediate rib; (*12*) vertebral rib. (Shipley, A. E., and MacBride, E. W.: Zoology—An Elementary Text-book, Cambridge Univ. Press, England; New York, Macmillan)

other birds, had a foramen through the coracoid.

MAMMALS

In the amphibians and the reptiles, largely belly draggers, the breast plate was large with strong coracoid attachments. This applies also to birds, as their sternums are weight-bearing. However, mammals walk, supporting their weight on their limbs, not on their sternum, and their limbs are more movable. Therefore, they have lost all coracoid attachments to the sternum, and in many without clavicles the girdle is completely free from bony attachments. The coracoid process has become unattached, short and rudimentary. It still, though, retains ligamentous attachment to the sternum through the costocoracoid ligament, and occasionally pieces of cartilage are found in this. As the weight is transmitted through muscle attachments to the scapula, this bone is highly developed in mammals. The acromion is large and is prolonged as the spine of the scapula. The clavicle, when present—the only bony connection of the shoulder girdle to the sternum—is still attached to the coracoid process by the conoid and the trapezoid ligaments, which are all that remain of the primitive precoracoid fusion of the clavicle. The clavicle is attached mainly to the acromion. The clavicle commenced in fishes, was present in the Crossopterygii and in the earliest known amphibians. Ever since, it always has been attached to the scapula through an acromion.

The duckbill is such a primitive mammal,

dragging as it does on the ground, that, as expected, its pectoral girdle is more like that of a bird or a reptile. It has a broad sternal plate, with a coracoid bracing between it and the glenoid. There are an interclavicle, an epicoracoid, a precoracoid, an episternum and a supraclavicle. It is interesting that a mole, a much higher mammal but also a belly walker, has developed a similar broad, plate-like girdle. However, it is entirely composed of 3 flat, square bones—the clavicles and a sternum. These are also exceptional in that they articulate with the humerus instead of with the acromion.

CLAVICLE

This bone is well developed in mammals that climb, dig or fly but is absent in the runners and the swimmers. It is present in climbers, such as the marsupial opossum and the squirrel; in diggers, such as moles, armadillo and beaver; and also it is found in the bats which fly and in the primates. It is absent in most runners such as ungulates and carnivores, including dog and bear, but is rudimentary in the cat tribe. It is absent in swimmers such as whales, porpoises (Cetacea) and manatee (Sirenia). Only in man and the 3 higher apes does the clavicle furnish origin to the pectoral muscle.

ARM

In the primitive Amphibia both the front and the rear limbs were alike in bones, muscles and nerves; hence, the homologies between them that are still apparent in man.

CHANGE OF POSITION

In the change from the position of the fleshy fringe fin to that of the front foot of the amphibian, starting with the fin horizontal and directed backward, the radius forward and the ulna backward, the lower surface is destined to be the palm. When the fin is pronated, this surface faces the body; and when supinated, it faces outward. Starting in supination as the elbow forms, the limb there bends forward. The distal half then pronates, the radius crossing over the ulna, and as the forearm slopes toward the ground the wrist dorsiflexes so that the tip lies flat on the ground on the palm to be. This is the position assumed by the lung fish in walking on its fins.

The arm bones are cuboid in the fish, elongating in the amphibian. In the latter the limb is lateral to the body; the humerus points outward and somewhat caudalward and the forearm somewhat cephalad; the hand points forward with the palm down. In reptiles, the limbs incline more downward for greater body support.

Adaptation to Weight-bearing

In mammals the limbs retain the angles but project downward from the body for weight-bearing. This proves to be adapted to ease the jar in running or jumping. The scapula, the humerus and the forearm form a 2-angle zigzag which gives elasticity. The weight of the front of the body is slung on each side from scapula to ribs by a shock absorber, the serratus anticus. In the running animals which have the shoulder completely mobile on the trunk without even a clavicle, this arrangement is particularly fitting. While the pectoral girdle became detached from skull, vertebrae and sternum, the pelvic girdle in contrast became more and more firmly attached to the transverse processes of the vertebrae for propulsion.

Assuming Upright Posture

When the upright position is assumed, both the humerus and the scapula incline downward. The scapula in this vertical position, with elongation of its lower angle, is in better position for stabilization by muscles for arm raising. In the change through primates from the slightly stooped position of the anthro-

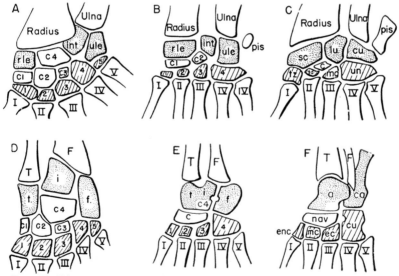

Fig. 36. Diagram of carpus (A to C) and tarsus (D to F) to show essential homologies between primitive tetrapod (A, D), primitive reptile (B, E) and mammal (C, F). The proximal row of elements is stippled; the central row (and pisiform) is unshaded; the distal row is hatched. Digits are indicated by Roman numerals, distal carpals and tarsals by Arabic numerals. (as) astragalus; (c, c1 to c4) centralia; (cal) calcaneus; (cu) cuneiform in carpus, cuboid in tarsus; (ec) external cuneiform (ectocuneiform); (enc) internal cuneiform (entocuneiform); (f, fbe) fibulare; (F, Fib) fibula; (i, int.) intermedium; (lu) lunar; (mc) middle cuneiform (mesocuneiform); (mg) magnum; (nav) navicular; (pis) pisiform; (rle) radiale; (sc) scaphoid; (t) tibiale; (T, Tib) tibia; (td) trapezoid; (tz) trapezium; (ule) ulnare; (un) unciform. (Romer, A. S.: The Vertebrate Body, p. 200, Philadelphia, Saunders)

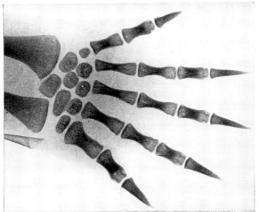

FIG. 37. Bones of the hands of reptiles. (*Top*) Florida turtle. Primitive type of hand, radiale, intermedium, ulnare, os centrale and carpals five. Phalangeal formula 2, 3, 3, 3, 2, differing from the primitive type of 2, 3, 4, 5, 3. (*Center, left*) Chuckwalla. Fairly primitive types of hand; phalangeal formula is typical of reptiles 2, 3, 4, 5, 3. (*Center, right*) Crested lizard. Fairly primitive type of hand; phalangeal formula is typical of reptiles 2, 3, 4, 5, 3. (*Bottom, left*) Collared lizard. Fairly primitive type of hand; phalangeal formula is typical of reptiles 2, 3, 4, 5, 3. (*Bottom, right*) Alligator. Carpals reduced by synostosis to three; phalangeal formula 2, 3, 4, 4, 2.

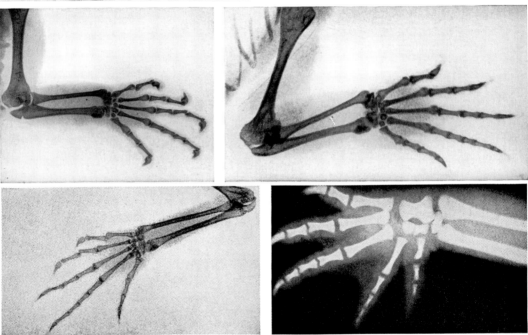

poid with shoulders forward, the posture of man is more erect, and both the shoulders and the hips have rolled outward. This explains the curve backward in the neck of the femur and the fact that the supraspinatus muscle in man pulls in the lateral plane, while that of apes works in the anteroposterior. Raising the arm laterally by this muscle is phylogenetically new, thus explaining why this tendon ruptures so frequently.

FOREARM

The radius and the ulna remain separate through most classes of animals. They are fused in the frog. In mammals that no longer have pronation and supination, as in many ungulates, the ulna has become rudimentary and fused with the radius which expands at its upper end for weight-bearing. The ulna shows only as a large olecranon which is always preserved for leverage and as a tiny rudiment of its upper shaft. Most other vertebrates have the movement of pronation and supination. In the elephants it is the ulna which enlarges for weight-bearing, the radius reducing to a minor bone.

HOMOLOGIES FROM CARPUS OF PRIMITIVE HAND

PRIMITIVE HAND	PRIMITIVE FOOT	HUMAN HAND	MAMMALIAN FOOT
Radiale	Fibulare	Scaphoid	
Intermedium	Intermedium	Lunate	Astragalus
Ulnare	Tibiale	Cuneiform	Calcaneus
Os centrale	Os centrale	Fused with scaphoid	Scaphoid
Carpals: I	Carpals: I	Trapezium	Inner cuneiform
II	II	Trapezoid	Mid cuneiform
III	III	Os magnum	External cuneiform
IV & V	IV & V	Fused as the unciform	Cuboid

From the primitive foot, the radiale gradually disappeared or formed the external tubercle of astragalus or became separate as the os trigonum. The tibia moved over to articulate on top of the astragalus. The tibiale became elongated for lever action as the calcaneus.

HAND

PRIMITIVE HAND

The primates retain more of the primitive pattern of hand first found in the earliest amphibians than do most animals except the turtle. In other mammals the hand has become highly specialized for running, flying, clawing, hanging, digging, swimming, etc. The primitive hand was pentadactylate and had 2 rows of carpal bones from 1 to 3 central ones. The 3 of the first carpal row—called radiale, intermedium and ulnare—are named from their relation to the forearm bones; starting with the thumb, the 5 in the distal row are called I, II, III, IV and V. From each of these extends a number of phalanges; the formula for the number of phalanges in each digit starting with the thumb is 2—3—4—5—3. The os centrale, probably originally of 3 bones, was soon reduced to 1.

The primitive hands and feet were similar. The homologies between the primitive hand and foot and the human hand and the mammalian foot are shown according to Keith in the table above.

CARPUS

The primitive pattern of hand was soon lost in amphibians, being present only in some stegocephalians. In modern amphibians some of the carpal bones are fused or absent, and the digits are reduced in number. In the frog the radius and the ulna are fused, and there are only 6 of the original 9 carpals.

In reptiles also some of the carpal bones are fused or lost, though all are retained in many turtles. In the crocodilia the original 3 carpals remain in the proximal row, but only 2 in the distal. The pisiform is present. In birds the carpals are reduced to 2: the radiale, which is fused with the intermedium as the scaphoid lunar, and the ulnare or cuneiform.

FIG. 38. Ichthyosaurus *communis*, Conyb. Lower Lias, England. Pectoral arch and right forelimb, ventral aspect; × ¼: (*cl*) clavicle; (*cor*) coracoid; (*h*) humerus; (*i*) intermedium; (*icl*) interclavicle (partly covered by clavicles); (*R*) radius; (*r*) radiale; (*sc*) scapula; (*U*) ulna; (*u*) ulnare. (After Zittel, K. A., Palaeontology, from Goodrich, E. S.: Studies on the Structure and Development of Vertebrates, New York, Macmillan)

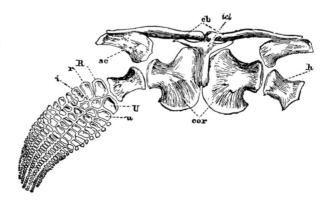

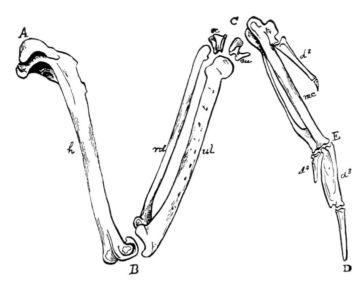

FIG. 39. Right wing bones of a duck: (h) humerus; (rd) radius; (ul) ulna; (C) carpus; (sc) outer carpal, scapho-lunare or radiale; (cu) inner carpal, cuneiform or ulnare, these two composing the wrist or carpus; (mc) the compound hand bone or metacarpus, composed of 3 metacarpal bones bearing as many digits—the outer digit seated on a protuberance at the head of the metacarpal, the other two situated at the end of the bone. (d^2) The outer or radial digit, thumb of 2 phalanges; (d^3) the middle digit of 2 phalanges; (d^4) the inner digit of 1 phalanx; (D to C) seat of flight feathers or primaries; (C to B) seat of secondaries. (Coues, Elliot: Key to North American Birds, Dana Estes and Co., 1903) (Legend abridged)

The carpus has been modified the most in mammals that bear weight on the digits. The Amphibia and the reptiles were plantigrade. In primates the carpus has changed but little from the primitive pattern. The os centrale, though present in the embryo of most mammals, fuses with the scaphoid before birth. In man it appears in the 6th week and fuses in the 8th. Carpals IV and V have fused in mammals, including man, to become the unciform. In primitive mammals there were 3 carpals and a pisiform in the first row and 4 in the second. Due to bearing weight longitudinally through the carpus, more of them fused or became lost. The scaphoid and the lunate support the radius, and the cuneiform supports

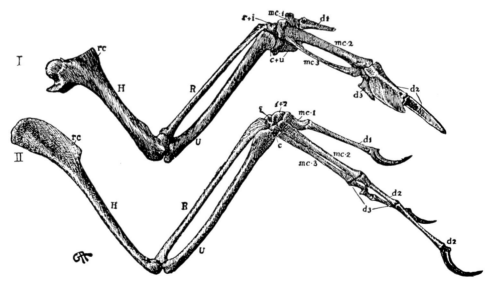

FIG. 40. Right forelimb of (I) pigeon and (II) *Archaeornis siemensi,* drawn by the author from the fossil in Berlin: (H) humerus; (R) radius; (U) ulna; (c) centrale; (d 1–3) first to third digits; (i) intermedium; (mc 1–3) first to third metacarpals; (r) radiale; (u) ulnare; (1 + 2) coalesced first and second distal carpals. (Heilmann, Gerhard: The Origin of Birds, New York, Appleton)

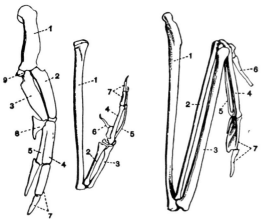

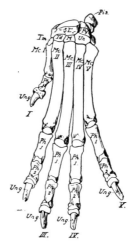

FIG. 41. Adaptations of the upper extremity in birds to environment. (*Left*) Penguin that flies under water; (*center*) ostrich, a flightless bird; (*right*) gannet, an able flyer. (*Right*) In the gannet, the distal phalanges of the pollex and the second digit have been omitted: (*1*) humerus; (*2*) radius; (*3*) ulna; (*4*) second metacarpal; (*5*) third metacarpal; (*6*) pollex; (*7*) second digit; (*8*) cuneiform; (*9*) sesamoid bone. (Reynolds, S. H.: The Vertebrate Skeleton, Cambridge Univ. Press, 1897)

FIG. 42. Left manus of the wolf: (*SL*) scapholunar (fused as in all carnivores); (*Py*) pyramidal; (*Pis*) pisiform; (*Tm*) trapezium; (*Td*) trapezoid; (*M*) magnum; (*Un*) unciform; (*Mc*) metacarpals; (*Ph*) phalanges; (*I*) pollex. (Scott, W. B.: A History of Land Mammals in the Western Hemisphere, New York, Macmillan)

the ulna. The scaphoid rests on the trapezium, the trapezoid and part of the os magnum; the lunate rests on the os magnum and usually also on the unciform; and the cuneiform on the unciform. In all carnivora, including seals and sea lions, the scaphoid and the lunate are fused; and in the hoofed animals the trapezium is lost. In the primitive pattern the trapezium, the trapezoid and the os magnum rest each on 1 metacarpal, and the unciform on the 4th and the 5th, but this modifies as the number of metacarpals is reduced.

The pisiform is not a true carpal, having developed as a sesamoid bone in a tendon at least as far back as in the reptiles. In crocodiles and in most mammals it articulates also with the ulna. In the carpus of most quadrupeds and also higher apes, the pisiform stands out as the most conspicuous bone. This and the tubercle of the scaphoid project for great muscle leverage in running, but the pisiform is rudimentary in man.

DIGITS AND PHALANGES

Amphibians and Reptiles. The primitive hand had 5 digits, but in all except the earliest

Amphibia these have reduced to 4 and in some to 3, although 5 in the foot. Throughout the reptiles, pentadactylism prevails, though in some of the dinosaurs, such as the ferocious Tyrannosaurus rex, there was a reduction to 3. The number of phalanges on each digit is distinctively quite constant in reptiles. The formula, commencing with the thumb, is 2—3—4—5—4 in the manus, and 2—3—4—5—3 in the pes. Crocodilia are an exception, with a formula of 2—3—4—4—3. There are also some that reverted into the sea, the marine reptiles, in which the number of phalanges was greatly increased. The arm and the carpal bones became short and flat, and the digits were joined in a paddle resembling a fin. It was quite unlike that of a fish and definitely a reversion of limb bones. One of these, the Ichthyosaur, had as many as 9 digital rays and totaled 100 phalanges, there being up to 26 in the 3rd digit. It is the only known species of animal (not a freak) to have had more than 5 digits.

Birds have an arm of humerus, radius and ulna. Extending from their 2 carpal bones are 3 fused metacarpals and 3 digits. The 1st metacarpal is a stub, supporting 2 or 3 phalanges as a thumb. The 2nd and the 3rd meta-

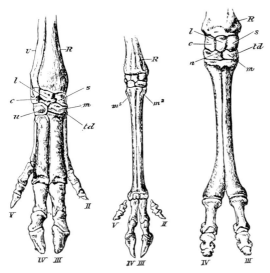

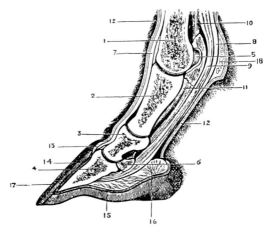

FIG. 43. Bones of the right forefoot of even-toed animals. (*Left*) Pig; (*center*) red deer; (*right*) camel. The metacarpi are fused. First the thumb is lost, then the two marginal rays, leaving the third and the fourth digits in the cloven hoof. (*U*) ulna; (*R*) radius; (*c*) cuneiform; (*l*) lunar; (*s*) scaphoid; (*u*) unciform; (*m*) magnum; (*td*) trapezoid. (Flower, W. H.: An Introduction to the Osteology of the Mammalia, New York, Macmillan)

FIG. 45. Manus of the horse: (*1*) metacarpal; (*2*) proximal phalanx; (*3*) middle phalanx; (*4*) ungual phalanx; (*5* and *6*) sesamoids; (*7*) extensor tendon; (*8*) flexor sublimis; (*9*) flexor profundus; (*17*) nail or hoof. (Flower, W. H., and Lydekker, Richard: An Introduction to the Study of Mammals Living and Extinct, London, Adam & Charles Black, 1891)

carpals are larger, fused at each end; they support an index finger of 3 phalanges. The 3rd digit springs from the side of the 3rd metacarpal and is very short, consisting of 1

or 2 phalanges. The primary wing feathers attach to the index phalanges and the 3rd metacarpal, and the secondaries to the ulna. The outstretched wing from the wrist distally can supinate, just as from the palm-down position with arms spread we can make our finger pulps face forward without turning the forearm. This aids in flying, like an aileron,

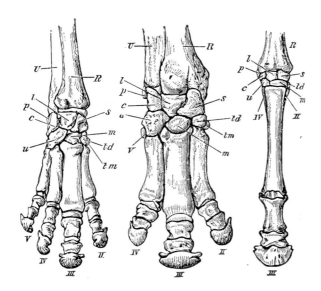

FIG. 44. Bones of the right forefoot of odd-toed animals. (*Left*) Tapir; (*center*) rhinoceros; (*right*) horse. The thumb is lost first, then the little finger, and then the two marginal rays, so that the horse walks on his long finger. (*c*) cuneiform; (*l*) lunar; (*s*) scaphoid; (*u*) unciform; (*m*) magnum; (*td*) trapezoid; (*tm*) trapezium. (Flower, W. H.: An Introduction to the Osteology of the Mammalia, New York, Macmillan)

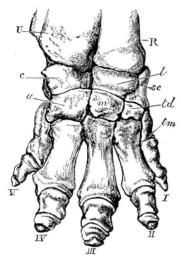

FIG. 46. Right manus of the elephant: (*c*) cuneiform; (*l*) lunar; (*sc*) scaphoid; (*u*) unciform; (*m*) magnum; (*td*) trapezoid; (*tm*) trapezium. The ulna (*U*) is the larger forearm bone. (Flower, W. H., and Lydekker, Richard: An Introduction to the Study of Mammals Living and Extinct, London, Adam & Charles Black, 1891)

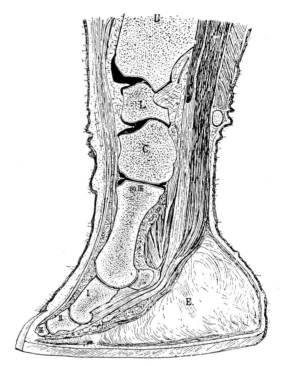

FIG. 47. *Elephas maximus.* Lengthwise frozen section of the front foot: (*U*) ulna; (*L*) lunate; (*C*) capitatum; (*m*III) third metacarpal; (*I, II, III*) phalanges of the third finger; (*E*) elastic pad. At the distal end of the third metacarpal is attached a sesamoid. Behind this lies the flexor muscle. (Note that the weight is borne on the digits and an elastic pad.) In front of the tendon is the extensor muscle. (Weber, Max: Die Säugetiere, Vol. 2, Jena, Fischer)

or a boatman holding back with one oar.

The turkey buzzard has a claw on the thumb, and the ostrich one on the thumb and the index. The cassowary has a formidable claw on its single digit. One of the earliest known toothed birds, the Archaeopteryx, had 3 long, separate, well-formed digits, each with a claw. The young of the modern hoatzin of South America are born with a large claw on the thumb and the index finger, with which they climb about on the limbs. These are lost in the adult. The Hesperornis, a prehistoric toothed water bird, had lost all of its wing except a rudimentary humerus, and some of the extinct large flightless Moas of New Zealand had not a trace left of wing or pectoral girdle.

Mammals show the greatest variation in number of digits; the lowest is in those that are the most specialized for running. Most carnivores walk on their metacarpal heads (the central pad) and their 4 terminal phalanges, the thumb having been lost or reduced to a dewclaw; the hoofed mammals walk on their terminal or ungual phalanges. The un-

gulates have been divided into odd and even-toed, the Perissodactyls and the Artiodactyls. In them, the marginal digits are those lost, the thumb being the first to go. In the odd-toed the 5th digit is then lost, leaving 3, of which the central or long digit is the largest, as in the tapir or the rhinoceros. On again losing the 2 marginal digits, only the middle one remains, as in the horse, in which the process can be traced from the 4-toed Eohippus of the lower Eocene. The even-toed or ruminants lost the index and the little digits, leaving the long digit and the ring digit which form a cloven hoof. The pig still has 4 toes, of which the 2 lateral ones are off the ground. Most rodents have lost the thumb. The pha-

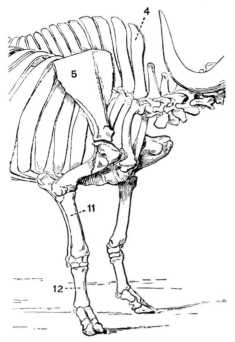

langes in land mammals are never more than 3 in each digit and 2 in the thumb, but in whales and porpoises they may be multiple.

PHYLOGENY AND DIFFERENTIATION OF MUSCLES FROM AMPHIBIA TO MAMMALS

Flexor muscles in the forearm in Amphibia were differentiated into a superficial and a deep layer. The superficial layer was divided into the radiali and the ulnari muscles from their respectvie bones, and an intermediary muscle, taking origin mainly from the inner humeral condyle. This primary differentiation has persisted, developing into the muscles of primates as follows:

Of the superficial layer the radiali split into pronator teres and flexor carpi radialis. The ulnari became the flexor ulnaris and the intermediate or condylar portion split into palmaris longus and flexor digitorum sublimis. The splitting was not quite so definite, as in some there were 2 or 3 palmaris longus muscles from the superficial parts of all 3 divisions; in some the sublimis came more from the ulnari, and in others more from the radiali.

The deeper layer, originally composed of one longitudinal and a number of deeper oblique muscles, finally reduced to the flexor digitorum profundus and the pronator quadratus.

In no amphibian, and in only a few reptiles, does any forearm muscle insert distal to the metacarpals. Several layers of brevis muscles move the digits, taking their origin from several layers of palmar aponeurosis. The flexor digitorum profundus which inserted into this aponeurosis was first to become continuous through it with the deeper brevis group to the digits. By the aponeurosis merely freeing itself from the carpus, the profundus moved the digits, and that brevis muscle became the lumbricales, as shown in the alligator.

The flexor digitorum sublimis appeared first in mammals. The arrangement of the tendons of the superficial brevis muscles, being per-

Fig. 48. Upper extremity of a Cape buffalo showing the vertical position of the scapula in quadrupeds. As in most ungulates, the weight is borne on the radius, the ulna, with the exception of the olecranon process, being rudimentary and fused. The carpus is reduced. The metacarpals are fused to one and the third and the fourth digits remain. (Shipley, A. F., and MacBride, E. W.: Zoology—An Elementary Textbook, Cambridge Univ. Press, England; New York, Macmillan)

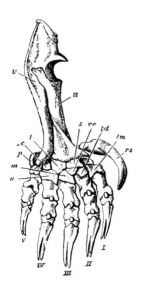

Fig. 49. Hand of the mole (*Talpa europaea*) specialized for digging, with extra breadth furnished by the radial sesamoid: (*c*) cuneiform; (*ce*) centrale; (*l*) lunar; (*m*) magnum; (*p*) pisiform; (*R*) radius; (*rs*) radial sesamoid; (*s*) scaphoid; (*td*) trapezoid; (*tm*) trapezium; (*U*) ulna; (*u*) unciform; (*I–V*) digits. (Flower, W. H.: An Introduction to the Osteology of the Mammalia, New York, Macmillan)

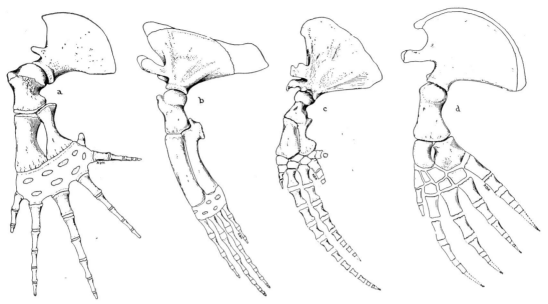

Fig. 50. Left pectoral limbs of mammals that reverted to sea life, cretacia. The arm bones are shortened. Joints are without spaces, phalanges are multiple, but of not over 5 rays.

(*a*) *Eubalaena balaena,* or right whale; (*b*) *Sibbaldus,* blue whale or rorqual; (*c*) *Globicephala,* pilot whale or black fish; (*d*) *Platanista,* fresh-water dolphin, River Ganges. (Howell's Aquatic Mammals, Springfield, Ill., Thomas)

forated for passage of the profundus tendons, was already present as the result of the divisions of the digital slips of the aponeurosis. The belly of the sublimis muscle, split from the profundus muscle as the condylar portion, was first inserted into the palmar aponeurosis from which the superficial brevis took origin, so all that was needed in order for the muscle to move the digits was a separation of the aponeurosis from the carpus and conversion of the brevis muscles into tendons. The superficial brevis muscles at the 2 borders of the hand developed into the thenar and the hypothenar eminences.

The extensor muscles on the dorsum of the forearm underwent similar changes. They were first divided into radial, ulnar and intermediate parts and did not reach beyond the metacarpals. They separated from a deeper layer, which eventually became the extensor proprius muscles to the digits, the extensor pollicis longus and the abductor pollicis longus being in series with these. The long forearm extensors joined with the brevis muscles on the dorsum of the hand that moved the digits.

Then, on the separation of the tendons from the carpus, the long muscles assumed the duty of extending the digits. The muscle bellies of the brevis became tendinous.

In certain mammals such as the ungulates with a reduced number of digits and absence of pronation, supination and lateral wrist movement, the muscles have been similarly reduced. In some, the tendon of the flexor digitorum profundus is prolonged proximally from the muscle to a bony attachment to act as a tenodesis and give a springlike recovery (horse and neurotrichus, a shrewlike mole). Most mammals have radiali, ulnari and intermediate flexors, both extensor communis digitorum and extensor proprius to all fingers and a long abductor and extensor of the thumb, if the latter is present. In marsupials, carnivora and moles, the palmaris longus—a muscle found only in mammals and the iguana—consists of 2, one reaching to the 1st digit and the other to the 5th. The latter tendon, as explained by its origin, may be perforated for the passage of the profundus tendon as in the sublimis.

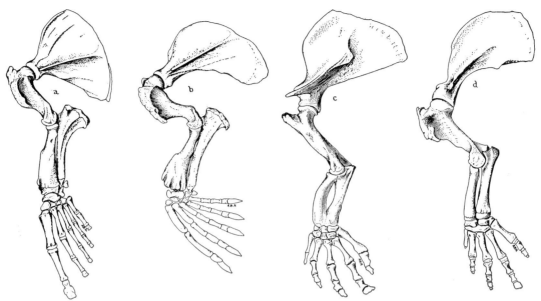

Fig. 51. Left pectoral limbs of mammals that reverted to sea life, pinnipeds and sirenians. The arm bones are well formed. The carpals are reduced by synosteosis. Digits are 5.

(a) *Zalophus*, sea lion; (b) *Phoca*, seal; (c) *Trichechus*, manatee; (d) *Halicore*, dugong. (Howell's Aquatic Mammals, Springfield, Ill., Thomas)

STRANGE SPECIALIZATION FOR ADAPTATION OF MANUS

It is remarkable what versatility of modification for special usage the hand shows in various animals, though in each it was built

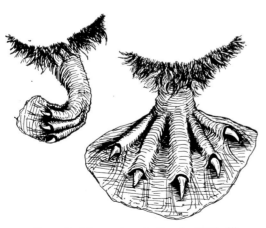

Fig. 52. The webs of the duckbill, like those of the seal, extend well beyond the nails, but fold back for use of the claws in digging.

on the same original fundamental structure heritage, the primitive hand. Animals of widely divergent classes may develop similar structures to live in similar ways. The following are some adaptations of the hand to the various environments.

For Running

From the elbow distalward the tendency is to reduction to a single bone in each segment, as in the horse, which has only the radius, a single metacarpal and the 3 phalanges of his long finger; or to a pair, as in the ruminants; and to provision with durable evergrowing hoofs to withstand the wear. The carnivora similarly are protected from wear with growing claws and 5 durable pads.

For Digging

The mole, the ant bear and the armadillo have long, strong claws and tremendous development of arms and shoulder girdle. The mole has an extra projection from the radial side of the radius to broaden his spade. It is a radial sesamoid of one of the 2 tendons of the palmaris longus going to the 1st digit, the other of

FIG. 53. Pterodactyl skeleton (*Nyctodactylus*). Wingspread 8 feet. Large deltoid attachment. What appears to be a recurved thumb is calcification of ligament. The main wing ray is the fourth, the fifth being absent. (Williston, S. W.: Am. J. Anat. *1*:299, 1902)

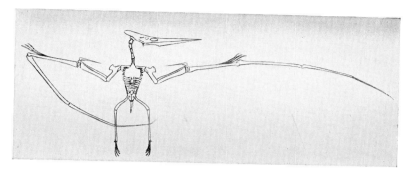

which goes to the 5th. The claws of the ant bear are so large and curved that it walks on the outer border of its hands with the digits and the claws in flexion.

For Fighting

The prehistoric reptile Iguanodon had the thumb developed into a formidable spike projecting at a right angle from the hand. Examples of modern weapons are the sharp erectile claws of the members of the cat tribe, the large claws of the bear, and the claw on the index finger of the cassowary.

For Hanging

The sloth moves slowly, hanging by its digits with the large claws, but it is helpless on the ground. With such existence its digits have been reduced to 3 in one species and 2 in another.

FIG. 54. Skeleton of a bat (*Vesperugo noctula*). The web spans from the tips of the digits to the foot. The thumb is free and the index and the long digits, including the metacarpals, are close together as the first of the 3 struts: (*u*) rudimentary ulna; (*m*) metacarpal; (*d 1–5*) digits; (*ph 1–3*) phalanges. (Flower, W. H., and Lydekker, Richard: An Introduction to the Study of Mammals Living and Extinct, London, Adam & Charles Black, 1891)

For Adhering

Suckerlike pads have developed in the fingers of tree toads, geckos and the Tarsus monkey for adhering to surfaces in climbing. In the last, the fingers are so long and slender that they can grip the limb from any direction.

For Acrobatics

The gibbon is the champion, swinging with its long arms from limb to limb, so that it seems fairly to fly through the trees. Its fingers are long for hooking over the branches. For this it does not use its small thumb.

For Biped Progression

The kangaroos and the jerboas, due to the great development of the hind legs, have forelimbs that are very small but are active for use as hands.

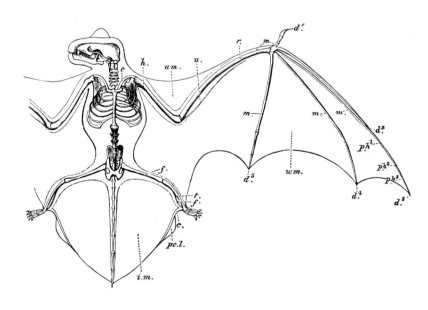

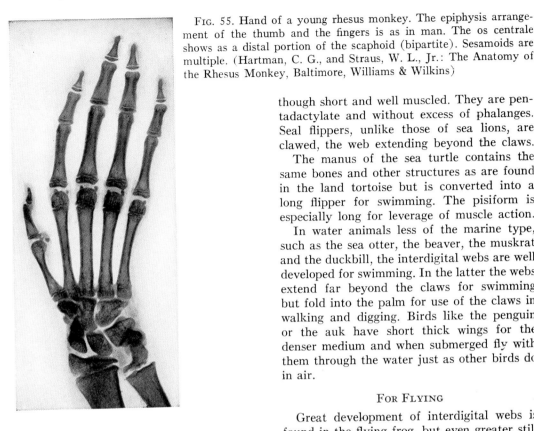

Fig. 55. Hand of a young rhesus monkey. The epiphysis arrangement of the thumb and the fingers is as in man. The os centrale shows as a distal portion of the scaphoid (bipartite). Sesamoids are multiple. (Hartman, C. G., and Straus, W. L., Jr.: The Anatomy of the Rhesus Monkey, Baltimore, Williams & Wilkins)

For Swimming

In swimming animals the front limbs are paddlelike, short, broad and fairly thick for use in a dense medium, in contrast with those with large, thin, light expansions of their front limbs for flying in the lighter medium, air. The marine reptiles mentioned above, like the mammalian Cetacea (whales and dolphins) and the Sirenia (mantee), had their front extremities developed to short, broad fins, the pelvic girdle being absent or reduced to 2 rudimentary bones. In Cetacea and Sirenia the arm bones are short and broad, and there are 5 digits, but there are only 4 in the finned whales. The carpals in Cetacea are mosaiclike and difficult to identify. The mantee have 2 rows with 3 in each. The phalanges in Cetacea, as in no other mammal, are multiple, ranging from 2 in the thumb to 11 in the 2nd digit. In whales the joints from the shoulder distally have lost their joint cavity and are fibrous. The arms and the flippers of seals have well-differentiated bones much as in land animals, though short and well muscled. They are pentadactylate and without excess of phalanges. Seal flippers, unlike those of sea lions, are clawed, the web extending beyond the claws.

The manus of the sea turtle contains the same bones and other structures as are found in the land tortoise but is converted into a long flipper for swimming. The pisiform is especially long for leverage of muscle action.

In water animals less of the marine type, such as the sea otter, the beaver, the muskrat and the duckbill, the interdigital webs are well developed for swimming. In the latter the webs extend far beyond the claws for swimming but fold into the palm for use of the claws in walking and digging. Birds like the penguin or the auk have short thick wings for the denser medium and when submerged fly with them through the water just as other birds do in air.

For Flying

Great development of interdigital webs is found in the flying frog, but even greater still in the bat and the extinct Pterodactyl. Bats have scapulae and clavicles like ours, but they have long, light arm bones. The metacarpals and the phalanges are greatly elongated as 3 struts for wings, which are merely the 2 layers of skin of the webs. The index and the long fingers are close together, forming the first strut, and the ring and the little fingers the other two, the phalangeal formula being 2—1—3—2—2. From the tip of the little finger the web spans to the ankle. The short thumb projects free and has a claw with which it pulls itself along on the ground. The vampire bat walks high on its feet and thumbs.

Pterodactyls, the prehistoric flying reptiles, ranging in size from that of a sparrow to some with a 25-foot wingspread, had 4 fingers. The first 3 were free, but the 4th was greatly prolonged as the single wing strut to hold the web which spanned from it to the foot. From the carpus there projected a thin bone toward the body; at first this bone was thought to be the thumb. If so, the wing would be held by the little finger. It was suggested that the small bone from the carpus was not the thumb but only an ossified ligament, and that the first of the 3 fingers was really the thumb. This was verified by finding that the phalangeal formula starting with this first finger, was 2—3—4—4—0, thus conforming closely to that of reptiles and indicating that it was the ring and not the little finger that made the wing of the Pterodactyl.

Other modifications for flight aside from those seen in birds are found in the broad web expansion between neck, hands and feet in the flying squirrel, the cabego and the flying phalanger. However, hands are not necessary for flying; the flying lizard and the flying snake of the Malays use spreading ribs for gliding.

For Versatility and Handicraft

Here man stands supreme.

PRIMATE HAND

The hands of the various primates, including man, are very similar and have changed the least compared with other mammals from the type of the primitive hand of early amphibians. Their minor variations are adaptations to their special activities.

Primates

Primates range from the lowest types, the Lemuridae, through the monkeys (arboreal in habit, especially in the Western Hemisphere, where many have prehensile tails) and up through the 4 types of anthropoid apes. Of these the gibbons and the orangoutang are lower in the scale, and the chimpanzee and the gorilla the closest to man.

The gibbon is a wonderful acrobat, with greatest development of arms for swinging through trees, and when it stands its arms reach to the ground. It is only 3 feet tall but has an armspread of 5½ feet.

The orangoutang is a large, heavy, arboreal dweller. Its arms reach down to its feet and attain a spread of 7½ feet.

The largest ape, the gorilla, is too heavy for much climbing. Its hands reach to the mid-tibia. It is gross in muscle and frame like Neanderthal man or a modern man with acromegaly; it is considered to be nearest to man.

The chimpanzee is high mentally and is of a lighter build and more agile both on the ground and in trees. Its hands reach to below the knees, while those of man, who has the longest legs, reach only to the mid-third of the thigh.

Thumb

Of all mammals only the primates have opposable thumbs. In other mammals the thumb is absent, rudimentary or like the other digits. In the feet of birds the hallux opposes the other toes, and in owls the 4th digit can be placed either with or opposite the other toes. Cuckoos, kingfishes, parrots and woodpeckers have 2 pairs of opposable toes. Hands of rodents are nimble; most are thumbless and grip with their fingers against a pad in the palm.

Strangely, the lowest primates, the slow-moving limb clingers, the Lemuridae, have the largest and most opposable thumbs, reaching the greatest development in the slow loris, in which the thumb can be spread to a right angle from the palm. Of the later monkeys and apes, the thumb is smallest and least opposable in arboreal forms, and even absent in some (as the spider monkey, whose need is supplied by the prehensile tail). Thumbs are much better developed in those that dwell on the ground. In the howling monkey the cleft in the hand is between the 2nd and the 3rd digits. In the potto the index is a mere stub, thus furnishing a wide cleft for the thumb.

In man, the thumb shows the greatest specialization and development in strength, opposition and size. Next in order come the great apes, the gorilla and the chimpanzee. Of the apes, the thumb of the orangoutang is shortest, the distal phalanx often being absent. Though the gibbon does not use its thumb in its acrobatics, it can oppose it for holding objects. As in the orangoutang, it is deeply cleft and narrow, showing weak muscle control.

The pollical index, or percentage of length of thumb to that of the middle finger, concerns length alone and not opposability or function. Ashley-Montagu determined in this the following figures:

Spider monkey (0), orangoutang (30.2), gibbon (35.2), chimpanzee (35.4), gorilla (37.4), old-world monkeys (av. 37.4), new-

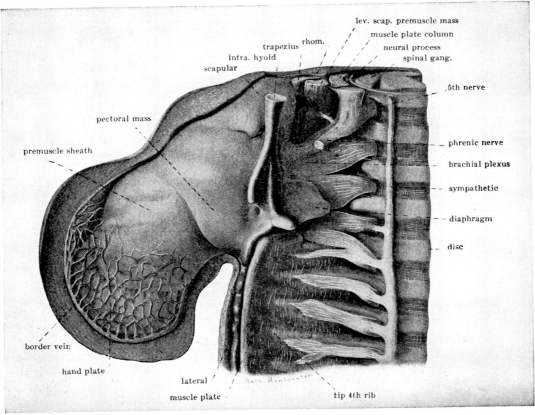

FIG. 56. Ventral view of the arm region of a human embryo. Length, 9 mm.; ovum size, 25 mm. dia.; age, 4½ weeks. (Lewis, W. H.: Am. J. Anat. *1*:157)

world monkeys (av. 47.4), baboons (48.8), Negro (56), Chinese-Japanese (57.2), Englishman (57.7).

The length of the hand compared with that of the arm is greater in other primates than in man, except in the gorilla, where it is the same. This ape and man are the only animals with an extensor pollicis brevis and a peroneus tertius muscle.

INTEGUMENT

In the Lemuridae there are pads over the finger ends, the metacarpal heads and the base of the palm. These pads diminish on ascending through the primates and are least in the apes. Apes walk on the ends of their proximal phalanges, thus developing knuckle pads, as seen occasionally in humans.

Crease patterns in the palms are conspicuous. There is often a longitudinal crease for curvature of the arches, and the transverse distal palmar crease runs completely across the palm, allowing only for flexion of the fingers as a whole. This is seen occasionally in the human hand. In man the distal of the 2 creases is for flexion against the thumb of the ulnar 3 fingers and the proximal for the radial 3, thus providing a differential action between the 2 sides of the hand.

Finger prints or papillary ridges on palm and the fingers began low in the primates and show increasingly with the use of the hand as a sense organ.

Fingernails took the place of claws in higher primates. Of the lower forms, in the aye-aye all digits have claws, and in marmosets all except the thumb, which has a nail. New-world monkeys have claws, and old-world ones nails. Apes have nails, though in the gibbon they are rounded. Some toenails in old people revert to claws.

FIG. 57. (*Top*) Embryo CIX; length, 11 mm.; age, 5 weeks; ovum, 30 mm. dia. Shows the beginning of the hand and the arm before interdigitation. The scapula is descending, having started opposite the fourth and the fifth myotomes. Its tip border is now at 6 C and its lower overlaps 2 ribs, the first 3 of which show. (Bardeen and Lewis: Am. J. Anat., *1*: Plate IV)

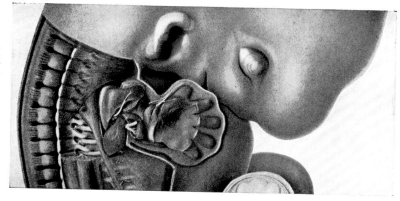

(*Bottom*) Diagram from the same embryo, showing the undescended scapula and the precartilage differentiated to form the arm and the hand bones. (Lewis, W. H.: Am. J. Anat. *1*:161)

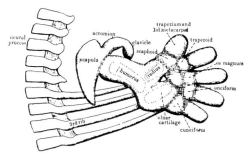

Syndactylism is found in many monkeys. The wrist of most primates has a much wider range of motion than in man. The gibbon can even flex its palm against its forearm. The bony carpal tunnel for restraining the tendons is much deeper and boxlike: There are only 8 carpal bones in man, the gorilla and the chimpanzee; but in the gibbon, the orangoutang and many monkeys there are 9, for the os centrale is still present.

MUSCLES OF THE PRIMATE HAND

Compared with lower mammals, there is in primates greater differentiation within the muscle masses, especially in the higher apes. There is much similarity in the various primates. The following variations in the individual muscles may help our conception of them in man:

Palmaris Longus. This may be absent in some (gorilla) and present in others (Rhesus monkey, chimpanzee). In the chimpanzee its palmar aponeurosis, just beyond the center of the hand, forms the flexor tunnels and sends no slips to the fingers.

Flexor Digitorum Superficialis. This is fused with the profundus in lemurs, and here a flexor digitorum brevis is still present. In baboons the superficial has only one muscle belly, but in the chimpanzee the bellies are separate for each finger. In the latter, the split of the superficial tendon is proximal to the metacarpal head, so all 3 tendons bear separately on the bone. The origin in primates is always largely from the humeral condyle.

Flexor Digitorum Profundus. In the gibbons the muscle is split longitudinally for the 3rd interdigital cleft, and in other apes for the 2nd. In Rhesus it is split on the 3rd ray, both sides pulling on this finger. In most primates the muscle has 5 tendons, the flexor muscle of the thumb as in other mammals not being differentiated.

Flexor Pollicis Longus. Man alone has enough differentiation to have a strong flexor of the thumb, separate from the common profundus muscle. In the gibbon, also, the muscle is separate but is weak. It is usually absent in the gorilla. In the chimpanzee and the orangoutang there is only a narrow tendon from the distal phalanx of the thumb to the transverse carpal ligament, though in some it reaches the flexor profundus belly to the index finger. It acts as a tenodesis, flexing the thumb automatically on tensing the abductor pollicis longus. In the Tarsus the muscle is almost separate, and in the baboon there is a common profundus.

Extensor Indicis and Extensor Minimi Digiti.

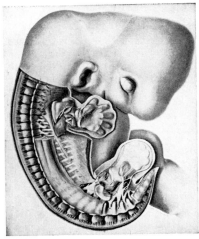
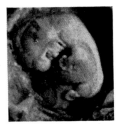
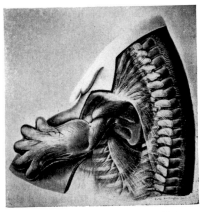

FIG. 58. (*Left*) Embryo CIX; length, 11 mm.; age, about 5 weeks. Hand forming within the paddle. (*Center*) Embryo CLXVII; length, 14.5 mm.; age, 5½ weeks; ovum, 33 x 30 x 20 mm. The hand is like a mitten. Scallops precede interdigitation. (*Right*) Embryo XLIII; length, 16 mm.; age, 6 weeks. Interdigitating. (Bardeen and Lewis: Am. J. Anat. *1*: Plate I)

In most mammals and lower primates and the gibbon there is a tendon to each digit from this deeper second layer of extensor muscles. In other apes there may be, in addition to the tendon to the index and the little fingers, an adjoining one to the middle or the ring finger.

Abductor Pollicis Longus. In most primates this muscle has 2 tendons: one to the metacarpal and the other to the trapezius (chimpanzee, gorilla, gibbon, but only one in the orangoutang), thus explaining this aberrant tendon in man.

Extensor Pollicis Brevis. This tendon on the ulnar side of the abductor pollicis is found only in man and some gorillas.

Extensor Digitorum Communis and **Extensor Pollicis Longus.** These muscles are as in man.

NERVES

The nerves are largely standard from amphibians to man, being exceptionally constant to the muscles supplied by them. In Amphibia the interosseous branch was the main median nerve, and the ulnar communicated with the median in the forearm. Later, the superficial branch became the main median nerve, and the ulnar increased in size to supply the hand. In many mammals and frequently in primates, there may be a large anastomotic branch between median and ulnar nerves at or below

the elbow. Otherwise, throughout primates, arm and hand nerves are practically the same.

EMBRYOLOGY AND DEVELOPMENT

Some knowledge of the embryologic development of the hand is necessary for an understanding of congenital deformities of the hand.

The embryonic period, by agreement, is said to comprise the first 7 postovulatory weeks, the change from embryo to fetus or the shift in emphasis from differentiation to growth taking place at the period when the cartilage of the humerus differentiates into bone marrow. From this time on, as far as the form of the hand is concerned, there is simple maturation and growth in size, all elements having been formed at the end of the embryonic period. Thus any deformity involving a change in number or arrangement of the basic elements was determined by this time.

A tabulation of the embryology of the hand, as found in the works of Bardeen and Lewis, Keibel and Mall, O'Rahilly and Gardner, shows the following developmental stages:

Postovulatory weeks

3 – 4   Limb bud and ectodermal ridge.

5   Condensation of mesenchyme for arm, forearm and some cartilage. Hand undifferentiated disk. Muscle groups visible.

6   Cavitation for elbow, carpal condensations and raylike condensations for fingers; dorsal grooves begin to develop in hand. Fingers still webbed. Metacarpal and carpal cartilage. Os centrale.

7   Now most of arm structures present. Shoulder migrating, fingers interdigitate, cavitation in wrist. Cartilaginous sesamoids present.

8   Thumb and fingers free. Some cavitation in fingers.

Since the number and the arrangement of the basic elements are all formed by the end of the embryonic life, some factor present before that time had to act to cause anomalies such as polydactylia or ulnar dimelia, in which the number of elements is increased. On the contrary, a decrease in number may result from failure of development after as well as during embryonic life.

Some typical deformities must have been determined early in the embryonic period, as they cannot have occurred after the involved structures had differentiated. Some examples are:

Abrachius	2½ weeks
Phocomelia ⎱	
Hemimelia ⎰	3 weeks
Polydactylism ⎱	
Lobster claw ⎰	3 weeks
Brachydactylia ⎫	
Syndactylism ⎬	6 weeks
Elevated scapula ⎭	
Brachyphalangia ⎱	
Symphalangism ⎰	7 weeks

OSSIFICATION

The tips of the distal phalanges are ossified in some embryos at 7 weeks. In the fetal period other bones of the hand ossify by bone collar formation followed by invasion of periosteal vessels. These appear in the metacarpals between 9 and 15 weeks, though the center for the mid-phalanx of the little finger may be delayed until full term (Gray, Gardner and O'Rahilly).

Ossification centers in carpus appear after birth, according to Marnbrand, 1945. Greulich and Pyle, 1950 as shown in the table on page 50.

The epiphysis of the thumb metacarpal is at the base, as in the phalanges, instead of at the distal end as in other metacarpals, al-

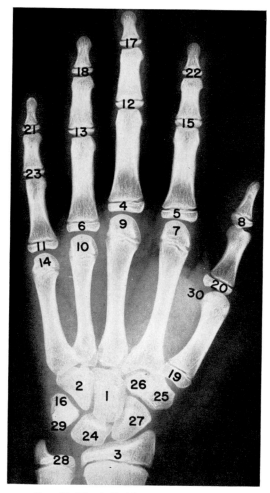

FIG. 59. The individual carpals and epiphyses numbered approximately in the order in which their ossification begins. (Greulich, W. W., and Pyle, S. I.: Radiograph Atlas of Skeletal Development of the Hand and Wrist, Stanford, Calif., Stanford Univ. Press)

though occasionally one is present at the base of the 2nd metacarpal or at each end of the thumb metacarpal. The styloid process of the 3rd metacarpal may develop from a separate center and may unite instead to the carpus.

MATURATION

A careful study has been made, notably by Todd, of the maturing of skeletal elements. He found that of the whole skeleton the hand showed the most constant changes chronologi-

	Appearance		Complete Fusion	
	Female	Male	Female	Male
Radius, distal end	1 yr.	1 yr.	16 yrs.	18 yrs.
Ulna	6–7	5–7	16	18
Capitate and hamate	By 1	By 1	. .	. .
Triquetrum	2	2–3	. .	. .
Lunate	2–3	3–4	. .	. .
Trapezium, trapezoid and scaphoid	4	4–6	. .	. .
Pisiform	8–9	10–11	. .	. .
Metacarpal epiphyses	1–2	1–2	14	17
Phalangeal epiphyses	1–3	1–3	14	17
Sesamoids	11	13	. .	. .

cally, and he made an atlas of standards for ages from 3 months to 19 years by which, from the appearance of the bones of the hand as shown roentgenographically, the age may be told. The criteria used were not the times of appearance of centers of ossification or the actual measurements of growth, as these depended on fluctuating conditions of health, which influenced ossification by affecting the mineral supply and the preparation of carti-

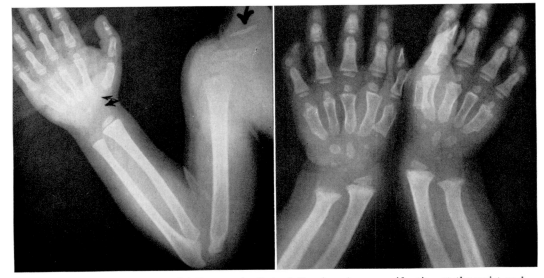

Fig. 60. (*Left*) Cleidocranial Dysostosis. Retardation in primary ossification at the wrist and accessory ossification center at the proximal end of the index metacarpal are two of the many generalized abnormalities which are sometimes found in association with this condition. Only the middle third of the clavicle has begun to ossify in this boy. (R. R. Schreiber, M.D., Los Angeles Orthopaedic Hospital)

Fig. 61. (*Right*). Hurler's type of osteochondrodystrophy. Gargoylism, dysostosis multiplex. The proximal ends of the metacarpals are moderately pointed. Phalanges may be thick. The ends of the radius and the ulna show mild variations in structure. Similar findings to those shown can also be found in Morquio's type of osteochondrodystrophy. (R. R. Schreiber, M.D., Los Angeles Orthopaedic Hospital)

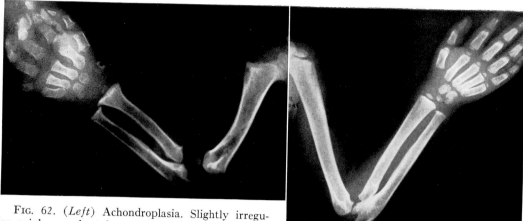

Fig. 62. (*Left*) Achondroplasia. Slightly irregular epiphyses, short bones, disproportionate elongation of the hands, progressive shortening in a proximal direction of the long bones (centripetal shortening). (R. R. Schreiber, M.D., Los Angeles Orthopaedic Hospital)

Fig. 63 (*Right*). Metaphysial dysplasia. Pyle's disease. Flaring of the ends of the long bones was more marked in the lower extremities in this case. Thickening of the calvarium and the facial bones was also present. Pease and Newton (Radiology *79*:233, 1962) found metaphysial dysplasia in 24 of 48 cases in a follow-up study of lead poisoning. (John L. Gwinn, M.D., Los Angeles Childrens Hospital)

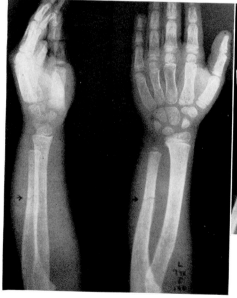

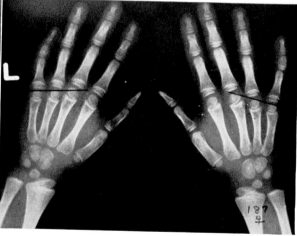

Fig. 64 (*Left*). Osteogenesis imperfecta of mild severity. Seven-year-old male of Mexican extraction with blue sclerae. Mother had a number of fractures as a child. Note relatively thin cortices, coarse trabecular pattern and fresh fracture of the ulna. Ulna is also short in this case. (R. R. Schreiber, M.D., Los Angeles Orthopaedic Hospital)

Fig. 65 (*Right*). Gonadal dysgenesis. Girl with Turner's syndrome. Metacarpal sign is positive bilaterally and is more pronounced on the left, which is often the case. The metacarpal sign is positive when a line drawn tangential to the ossified portions of the heads of the ring and the little finger metacarpals intersects the ossified portion of the head of the middle finger metacarpal. This sign is also evident clinically if a pencil is held across the ends of the ring and little fingers when the fist is clenched. Increased obliquity of end of radius and other changes in distal radius and ulna have been described but are not present here. (V. G. Mikity, M.D., Los Angeles County General Hospital)

lage for ossification; instead, they were based on the changes in shape and relative measurements of the phalanges, the metacarpals and —with lesser reliance—on the radius. These vary much with age in the growing shafts and in the penetration of bone into their epiphyses and cartilage. Before the epiphyses show, the shafts of the phalanges and especially the metacarpals are used.

At first the hand is short and broad; but, by growth of the shafts of the metacarpals and the phalanges, it lengthens considerably through the 1st year and continuously until matured. At birth the metacarpals and the phalanges have the roentgen appearance of short, wide, rectangular rods with similar lengths of digits and almost no differentiation in their contours. Through the years to maturity great differentiation occurs in each bone until they finally attain their shapely shafts and ends. Todd has tabulated these changes chronologically in his atlas in 40 standards for males and 35 for females. Their maturation is alike until the age of 10, when it progresses faster in the female, being complete at 16 compared with 19 in the male. The accuracy was tested for the ages most difficult to determine—between 8 and 14 years—by Newell, who found the margin of error for these ages to be 1 year. The accuracy is much greater in younger children.

Todd's work was carried on by Greulich and Pyle, who published a new Atlas in 1950. They found that bone development as shown in hands greatly speeded up with puberty, being stimulated by gonadal and related hormonth. In too early menstruation, it so speeds that the epiphyses close early and stunt the growth. An illness may make a transverse scar of dense bone near the epiphysis.

Unlike Todd, these authors found that in healthy children, the order of development of centers of ossification is in such constant sequence that anteroposterior films of the hand are used as "maturity indicators."

In the young and also on to adulthood, centers of ossification are a good guide. From puberty to late adolescence, the degree of fusion of the epiphyses is important. In the intermittent period, the shapes of the bones and other skeletal features are used as indicators.

BIBLIOGRAPHY

Ashley-Montagu, F. M.: On the primate hand, Am. J. Phys. Anthropol. *13*:291, 1931.

Bardeen, C. R., and Lewis, W. H.: Development of limbs, body wall, and back, Am. J. Anat. *1*:1, 1901.

Bardeen, C. R.: Studies of development of human skeleton, Am. J. Anat. *4*:265, 1905.

Bayer, L. M., and Newell, R. R.: Assessment of skeletal development of hand and knee between eight and fourteen years, Endocrinol. *26*:779, 1940.

Brooks, H. S.: On the short muscles of the pollex and hallux of the anthropoid apes, with special reference to the opponens hallucis, J. Anat. & Physiol. *22*:78, 1887.

Campbell, B.: Comparative anatomy of dorsal interosseous muscles, Anat. Rec. *73*:115, 1939.

"Challenger" Reports: Report on some points in the anatomy of the Thylacine, etc., Zoology *5*: part 14, 1881.

Chase, R. E., and DeGaris, C. F.: Brachial plexus in macacus rhesus compared to man, Am. J. Phys. Anthropol. *27*:233, 1940.

Christ, H. H.: A discussion of causes of error in the determination of chronological age in children by means of x-ray studies of carpal-bone development, S. Afr. Med. J. *35*:854, 1961.

Cummins, H., and Spragg, S. D. S.: Dermatoglyphics in chimpanzee; description and comparison with man, Human Biol. *10*:457, 1938.

Cunningham, D. J.: The intrinsic muscles of the mammalian foot, J. Anat. & Physiol. *13*:1, 1878.

———: The relation of nerve-supply to muscle-homology, J. Anat. & Physiol. *16*:1, 1881.

Francis, C. C.: Factors influencing centers of ossification during early childhood, Am. J. Dis. Child. *57*:817, 1939.

Frazer, J. E.: The derivation of the human hypothenar muscles, J. Anat. & Physiol. *42*:326, 1908.

Garn, S. M., and Rohmann, C. G.: Variability in the ossification of the bony centers of the hand and wrist, Am. J. Phys. Anthrop. *18*:219, 1960.

———: The number of hand-wrist centers, Am. J. Phys. Anthrop. *18*:293, 1960.

Garn, S. M., Rohmann, C. G., and Robinau, M.: Increments in hand-wrist ossification, Am. J. Phys. Anthrop. *19*:45, 1961.

Goodrich, E. S.: Studies on the Structure and Development of Vertebrates, London, Macmillan & Co., Ltd., 1930.

Gray, D. J., Gardner, E., and O'Rahilly, R.: The prenatal development of the skeleton and joints of the human hand, Am. J. Anat. *101*:169, 1957.

Gregory, W. K.: Present status of the problem of the origin of the Tetrapoda with special reference to the skull and paired limbs, Ann. N. Y. Acad. Sci. 26:317, 1915.

————: Further observations on the pectoral girdle and fin of Sauripterus taylori Hall, a Crossopterygian fish from the upper Devonian of Pennsylvania, with special reference to the origin of the pentadactylate extremities of Tetrapoda, Proc. Am. Philosoph. Soc. 75:673, 1935.

Greulich, W. W., and Pyle, S. I.: Radiographic Atlas of Skeletal Development of the Hand and Wrist, Stanford, Calif., Stanford Univ. Press; London, Oxford Univ. Press, 1950.

Greulich, W. W.: Value of x-ray films of hand and wrist in human identification, Science 131: 155, 1960.

Haines, R. W.: The law of muscle and tendon growth, J. Anat. 66:578, 1932.

Hartman, C. G., and Straus, W. L., Jr.: Anatomy of the Rhesus Monkey, Baltimore, Williams & Wilkins Co., 1933.

Hepburn, D.: The comparative anatomy of the muscles and nerves of the superior and inferior extremities of the anthropoid apes, J. Anat. & Physiol. 26:149, 1892.

————: The integumentary grooves of the palm of the hand and sole of the foot of man and the anthropoid apes, J. Anat. & Physiol. 27:112, 1892.

————: The adductor muscles of the thumb and great toe, J. Anat. & Physiol. 27:408, 1893.

Howell, A. B.: Anatomy of the Woodrat, Baltimore, Williams & Wilkins Co., 1926.

Howell, A. B., and Straus, W. L., Jr.: The brachial flexor muscles in primates, U. S. Nat. Mus. 80 (Art. 13):1, 1931.

Huxley, T. H.: Anatomy of the Vertebrates, New York, D. Appleton & Co., 1881.

Jones, F. W.: Attainment of upright posture of man, London, Nature, 146:26, 1940.

Keibel, F., and Mall, F. P.: Human Embryology, Philadelphia, J. B. Lippincott Co., 1912.

Keith, A.: Notes on a theory to account for various arrangements of the flexor profundus digitorum in the hand and foot of primates, J. Anat. & Physiol. 28:335, 1894.

————: Human Embryology and Morphology, London, Edward Arnold & Co., 1921.

————: The gorilla and man as contrasted forms, Lancet 210:490, 1926.

Kingsley, J. S.: Comparative Anatomy of the Vertebrates, Philadelphia, P. Blakiston's Son & Co., 1917.

Kollman, A.: Tactile apparatus in man and monkey, Arch. Anat. für Physiol. p. 56, 1885.

Lewis, W. H.: The development of the arm in man, Am. J. Anat. 145, 1902.

Lumer, H.: Relative growth of limb bones in anthropoid apes, Human Biol. 11:379, 1939.

Macalister, A.: On the arrangement of pronator muscles in limbs of vertebrate animals, J. Anat. & Physiol. 3:162, 1869; 3:308, 1870.

MacDowell, E. C.: Notes on the myology of the chimpanzee, Am. J. Anat. 10:431, 1910.

McGregor, A. L.: Contribution to morphology of the thumb, J. Anat. 60:259, 1925.

McMurrich, J. P.: Phylogeny of forearm flexors, Am. J. Anat. 2:177, 1903.

————: Phylogeny of the palmer musculature, Am. J. Anat. 2:463, 1903.

Midlo, C.: Form of hand and foot in primates, Am. J. Phys. Anthropol. 19:337, 1934.

Miner, R. W.: The pectoral limb of Eryops and other primitive Tetrapods, Bull. Am. Museum Nat. Hist. 51:145, 1924-1925.

Neal, H. V., and Rand, H. W.: Comparative Anatomy, Philadelphia, P. Blakiston's Son & Co., 1936.

Novack, C. R., Moss, M. L., and Leszczynska, E.: Digital epiphyseal fusion of the hand in adolescence: A longitudinal study, Am. J. Phys. Anthrop. 18:13, 1960.

O'Rahilly, R. O.: The developmental anatomy of the extensor assembly, Acta Anat. (Basel) 47: 363, 1961. Pfaff. P.: Experimental study of development of extremities of land animals, Morphol. Jahrb. 61:489, 1929.

O'Rahilly, R. O., Gardner, E., and Gray, D. J.: Ectodermal thickening and ridge in the limbs of staged human embryos, J. Embryol. & Exper. Morphol. 4:254, 1956.

————: The skeletal development of the hand, Clin. Orthrop. 13:42, 1959.

Rabl, C.: Extremitäten der Wirbeltiere, Leipzig, Verlag von Wilhelm Engelmann, 1910.

Raymond, P. E.: Prehistoric Life, Cambridge, Harvard Univ. Press, 1939.

Reynolds, S. H.: The Vertebrate Skeleton, Cambridge, At the University Press, 1913.

Schultz, A. H.: The skeleton of the trunk and limbs of the higher primates, Human Biol. 2: 303, 1930.

Snodgrasse, R. M., Dreizen, S., Parker, G. S., and Spies, T. D.: Serial sequential development of anomalous metacarpal and phalangeal ossification centers in human hand, Growth 19:307, 1955.

Sommer, A.: Muscles of the gorilla, Jenaische Zeitschr., N. F. 35:181, 1906-1907.

Sonntag, C. F.: On the anatomy, physiology, and pathology of the chimpanzee, Proc. Zool. Soc. London 1:323, 1923.

————: The anatomy, physiology, and pathology of the orangoutan, Proc. Zool. Soc., London *1*:349, 1924.

————: The Morphology and Evolution of the Apes and Man, London, John Bale, Sons, and Danielsson, Ltd., 1924.

Straus, W. L., Jr.: Phylogeny of human forearm extensors, Human Biol. *13*:23, *13*:203, 1941.

————: Homologies of the forearm flexors, urodeles, lizards, mammals, Am. J. Anat. *70*:281, 1942.

Todd, T. W.: Atlas of Skeletal Maturation, St. Louis, C. V. Mosby Co., 1937.

Troxell, E. L.: Thumb of man, Scient. Month. *43*:148, 1936.

Walsh, J. F.: Anatomy and function of muscles in the hand and with extensor muscles of thumb (Boylston Prize Essay, 1897).

Watson, D. M. S.: Evolution of Tetrapod shoulder girdle and fore limb, J. Anat. *52*:1, 1917.

Windle, C. A.: Flexors of digits of hand: Muscular masses in forearm, J. Anat. & Physiol. *24*: 72, 1889.

Young, A. H.: Intrinsic muscles of marsupial hand, J. Anat. & Physiol. *14*:149, 1879.

Zuckerman, S.: Functional Affinities of Man, Monkeys, and Apes, Harcourt-Routledge, 1933.

Chapter 3

Congenital Deformities

INCIDENCE

Congenital abnormalities occur in large numbers. In a 5-year period Ivy found an incidence of 8.5 per 1,000 live births; 60 per cent were males. The commonest deformities were clubfoot, cleft lip and palate, spina bifida and polydactylia. It has been reported that the incidence of hand deformity is 5.4 per 1,000 live births. Some of these must be minor anatomic variations, for Birch-Jensen, in a 1949 survey in Denmark, found only 1 hand deformity per 6,438 of the population. However, he did not count polydactylia or syndactylia, the two most common deformities. Many congenital abnormalities are incompatible with life; and if all fetal deaths are considered, congenital deformities account for most of the mortality in this period. Ivy's studies showed that 17.27 per cent of the live births with congenital abnormalites died within the first year of life.

Some abnormalities of the hand are repeatedly found together, e.g., syndactylia, polydactylia, brachydactylia and brachyphalangia. The defect is often bilateral, and the feet may be involved. Other deformities may be present, such as absence of the pectoral muscle, most commonly with brachyphalangia. There are many variations in degree and areas of involvement.

CLASSIFICATION

It is almost impossible to classify congenital abnormalities of the hand. The classification may be anatomic or based on hypoplastic or hyperplastic changes or on embryologic stages according to the periods when differentiation of the part takes place. A simple division may be that of anomalies resulting from inherited germ plasm defects compared with malfunctions due to extrinsic factors at certain stages of development. However, there is experimental evidence to show that teratogenic agents acting at the proper time and place not only may alter the development of the embryo but may also produce a change in the hereditary genes to produce a similar deformity in subsequent generations. Thus this apparently simple division may not be a clear separation of classes of deformity.

Skeletal Deficiencies

In the type of deformity in which a portion of the skeleton is missing, a reasonable descriptive classification has been made by O'Rahilly. The 2 major classes of terminal and intercalary deficiencies are further subdivided into transverse or paraxial. This system allows specific terms to be used to describe any form of congenital skeletal limb deficiency.

TERMINOLOGY

Many terms are used to describe the various deformities of the upper extremity. All are purely descriptive, and most are based on Greek roots:

Melos = limb	Clino = bent
Cheir = hand	Ectro = abortion
Daktylos = digit	Megalo = giant
Phoke = seal	Micro = small
Hemi = half	Pero = deformed
A = without	Poly = many
Acro = summit or peak	Syn (m) = together
Arachno = spider	

Some common deformities are thus described:

Ectromelia	with defective or absent limb
Brachymelia	short limb
Phocomelia	like a seal, hand(s) but no arm(s)
Perochirus	deformed hand
Syndactylia	webbed fingers
Symphalangia	fused phalanges
Brachydactylia	short fingers
Clinodactylia	bent or inclined finger(s)

Hyperphalangia is used to denote more than the normal number of phalanges in the longitudinal axis, while polyphalangia indicates more than the normal number in the transverse direction.

ETIOLOGY

Most deformities are explained on the basis of heredity, twinning, atavism or acquired defects from environmental changes.

HEREDITY

The hereditary transmission of congenital deformities is thoroughly established, but in many cases no deformity is known among the immediate relatives. The character may be recessive and appear sporadically when similar genes chance to meet. There is also the possibility of the isolated occurrence of the deformity in one individual only.

Almost all types may be inherited, except

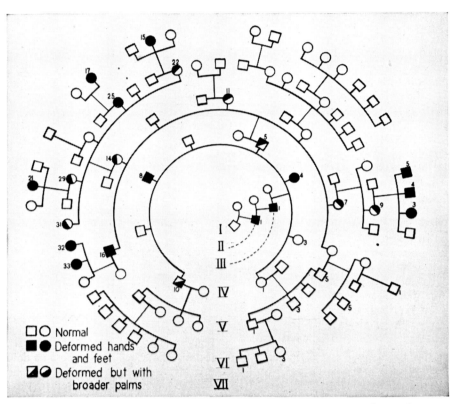

□○ Normal
■● Deformed hands and feet
◪◕ Deformed but with broader palms

FIG. 66. Six generations of malformed hands and feet. The pedigree chart shows the origin of the mutation from normal parents. Although in the 2nd and 3rd generations all offspring are affected, and in 2 families, IV-10 and V-11, all are normal, the chance errors are balanced if we total all offspring in affected families to date, which give 23 affected to 23 normal—exactly what one would expect for a simple, autosomal mendelian dominant. Hegdekatti concludes that: (1) This trait of malformation of hands and feet came into existence by mutation. (2) It is a single factor mutation which affects only hands and feet. It behaves as a single mendelian dominant in inheritance. (3) It seems that this trait is autosomal and not sex-linked. (4) There is some variation in the degree of malformation, the offspring exhibiting any degree regardless of that manifest by the parent. (After Hegdekatti: Malformed hands and feet, J. Hered. *30*:192-193, No. 5)

megalodactylia which is a hyperplasia instead of a defect, but reports indicate that the following deformities are almost exclusively hereditary: syndactylia, polydactylia, brachydactylia and brachyphalangia, ectrodactylia, split hand, clubhand, clinodactylia, symphalangia, lobster-claw hand and dyschondroplasias. Typical of the many reports on the hereditary aspects of these defects are the following:

R. M. Hegdekatti describes a closely intermarried family of a caste in India in which 23 members have normal and 23 others deformed hands, showing the ratio to be that of a mendelian dominant. In all marriages, an affected individual mated with a normal. With minor variations, the deformity was reduction of digits to one on each extremity.

Tubby reported 5 generations of cleft hand.

De Forest Willard reported 15 lobster claw hand children out of 22 in one family. In a family of 300, Hall found 100 with brachydactylia and brachyphalangia.

Of 78 of his cases, Kanavel found 37 to be hereditary.

Drinkwater traced short fingers through 7 generations; of these, all 25 who were living had short fingers.

Other deformities have been reported

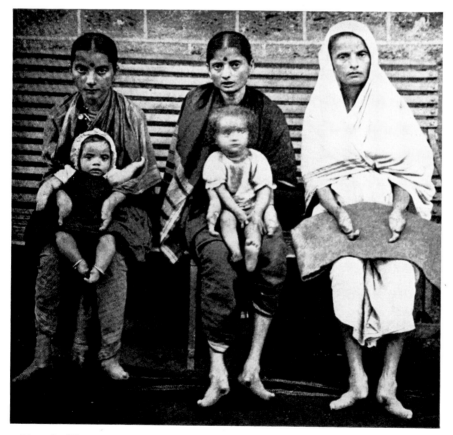

FIG. 67. Three generations of malformed hands and feet. The daughters and the mothers, and the grandmother on the right. The grandmother is V-14 in the pedigree chart, Fig. 66, and the deformed daughters are VI-22 and 25. The abnormal child is VII-17, and the normal child is VII-14. The marriage of an affected individual who is heterozygous for the dominant gene would be expected to yield one normal child to one abnormal. As deformed parents thus have some normal children, they believe that the deformed children are born to them because of a lack of religious zeal. (After Hegdekatti: Malformed hands and feet, J. Hered. *30*:192-193, No. 5)

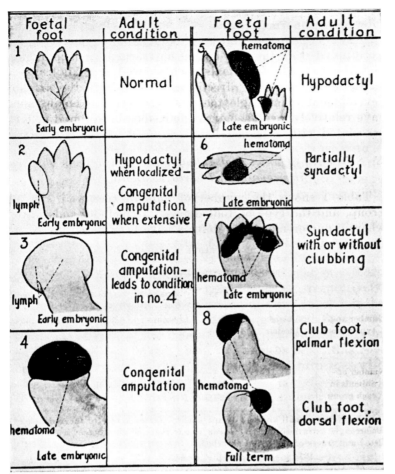

Foetal foot	Adult condition	Foetal foot	Adult condition
1 Early embryonic	Normal	5 hematoma Late embryonic	Hypodactyl
2 lymph Early embryonic	Hypodactyl when localized — Congenital amputation when extensive	6 hematoma Late embryonic	Partially syndactyl
3 lymph Early embryonic	Congenital amputation— leads to condition in no. 4	7 hematoma Late embryonic	Syndactyl with or without clubbing
4 hematoma Late embryonic	Congenital amputation	8 hematoma Full term	Club foot, palmar flexion / Club foot, dorsal flexion

FIG. 68. This chart illustrates early and late fetal abnormalities of the limbs and the abnormal structural conditions of the limbs at birth, and indicates the probable condition of these members in later life. The adult condition is indicated to the right of the illustrated abnormality. (Bagg, H. J.: Hereditary abnormalities of the limbs, their origin and transmission, Am. J. Anat. *43*:190)

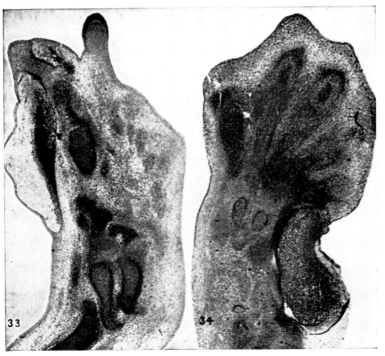

FIG. 69. (*Left*) Photomicrograph of a lateral section through the right hind foot of a 13.5 mm. fetus, showing the formation of a bleb on the surface of the foot. Note the escape of blood into this distended lymph space. (*Right*) Photomicrograph of a section of a fetal foot cut parallel with the dorsum of the foot, showing a small localized blood clot in the lower right of the illustration. The fetus is about the same age as the preceding. (Bagg, H. J.: Hereditary abnormalities of the limbs, their origin and transmission, Am. J. Anat. *43*:167-220)

FIG. 70. Double humerus with 3 hands and 16 fingers. (*Left*) anterior view with the forearms in supination. Note the common thumb for the distal and the middle hands; also the rudimentary finger in the web between the middle and the proximal hands. (*Right*) Posterior view, the proximal and the distal hands visible. (Stein, H. C., and Bettmann, E. H.: Am. J. Surg. *50*:337)

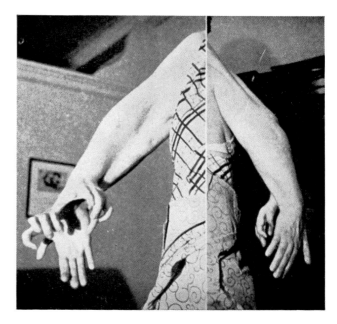

through 6 generations (Mohr and Wreidt) and 10 generations (Kellis).

A certain type of deformity may be transmitted with only slight variations through many generations, while in other families there may be much variation in the type of deformity. In the words of Bagg: "When considered as a general tendency to abnormal structure they approach mendelian expectation in behavior." The characters producing a deformity are apparently destructive and act as a hereditary influence to check development of a part at a critical stage, the nature of the resulting deformity depending on the degree of destruction and the embryonic stage in which it occurred. They may act on a certain anatomic site, such as the hand, the arm or certain rays; or selectively on a particular type of tissue, such as bone; or they may be linked with a syndrome of deformities, such as arachnodactylia.

There has been much discussion as to whether the transmission of congenital deformities is dominant or recessive in character. In some instances, as in the family reported by Hegdekatti, it appears to be clearly dominant; and in others, like Bagg's mice, recessive. There are so many instances in which the behavior is atypical that there are probably varying degrees of dominance or recessiveness—so-called qualified dominance or recessiveness—that the same effects are not always produced. Variations are produced by

mutation and when exaggerated are called deformities; thereafter these may be transmitted as mendelian dominants. A dominant gene can pass on a characteristic from one parent; but if a recessive gene is to be effective, it must meet a similar gene from the other parent.

Inherited Effects From Roentgen Rays. Bagg subjected mice to 5 light roentgen exposures on successive days and produced a strain prone to have deformities of the paws. He traced them through 19 generations and found the deformities to be mendelian recessive in nature. In 5,200 of these mice he obtained 432 with defects of the front or the hind paws, consisting of syndactylia alone in 9 cases; club and syndactylia, 29; club, 300; polydactylia, 93; amputation, 16; and hypodactylia, 27.

The rays apparently affected the hereditary characters of the germ plasm, resulting in arrest of development. On opening the pregnant females surgically, certain lesions could be seen through the transparent membranes of the uterus. He marked these fetuses so that the lesion could be checked with the deformity produced. The lesions varied from a bleb in part of the paw, or a bleb with some blood clot within it, to a hematoma on the side or the back of the paw. The greater the lesion the greater was the deformity, ranging through hypodactylia, polydactylia and clubhand. A mere bleb led to a mild deformity like syndactylia. A severe lesion, such as a hema-

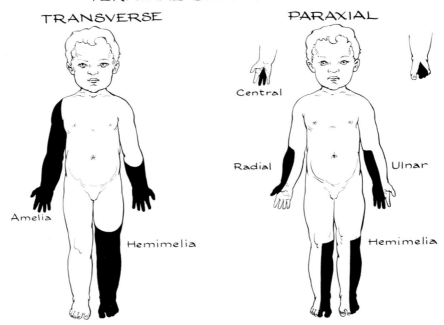

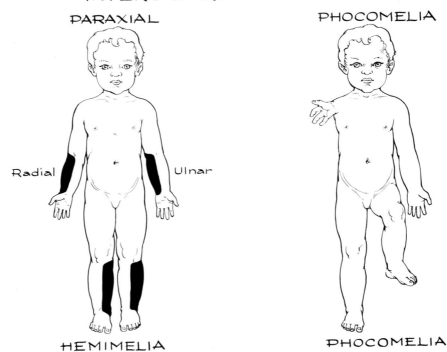

FIG. 71. Classification of skeletal limb deficiencies. Each of the two main classes may be divided: the terminal into transverse or paraxial, and the intercalary into paraxial or phocomelia. Paraxial deficiencies are designated radial or ulnar by reference to the missing component. (Hall, C. *et al.* from O'Rahilly: J.A.M.A. *181*:590)

toma which formed a spherical mass at the end of the limb, produced amputation. A dorsal hemorrhage would cause syndactylia with or without clubbing. Linked with these deformities were defects in eyes and kidneys. The deformities were noted in the 3rd and subsequent generations, and following these occurred as true mendelian recessives through 19 generations. Some inherited factor caused the lesion, or destruction at a certain period of embryonic development resulted in the deformity.

It is not the acquired characteristic which is inherited but the radiation so alters the gene mechanism as to produce the deformity.

In view of these findings it should be noted that up to 1961, there was no evidence that there have been more genetic abnormalities among the children of people exposed to atomic radiation at Hiroshima than there has been among the nonexposed.

Twinning and Reduplication

There is a tendency in low forms of life to grow a new appendage when one is broken off, and a double one when the limb is partially broken. Thus, a crustacean may develop 2 claws or a lizard 2 tails. This offers an explanation of polydactylia, marginal supernumerary digits, twin thumbs, or even twin or mirror hands. A small, partial congenital defect on one side in early fetal life is a plausible explanation. After finding such lesions in polydactylia and its association with clubhand and syndactylia, Bagg states:

Stochard and others have shown that a reduplication of embryonic parts may be brought about experimentally by a temporary arrest of embryonic development at a critical growth period. When a growing apical bud is arrested in development by pinching off or other methods, dichotomous growth occurs, and as a result the two adjacent axillary buds quiescent during the supremacy of the apical bud begin to develop twin branches. Similarly, Stochard has produced a reduplication of parts and marked degrees of twinning in trout embryo by arresting the development at a critical growth period.

Arndt and Schultz claim that minor stimuli cause irritation and result in overgrowth or division, while major stimuli cause inhibition and result in stunting, webbing or necrosis and loss. A case of twinning was reported by H. C. Stein and E. H. Bettmann; it is the most bizarre case on record. The right upper extremity of a 52-year-old woman was double in size and had 3 hands. There was a giant scapula, 9 × 9 inches, attached to the 4th cervical vertebra, where the spine was curved to the right; there were 2 radii and 3 ulnas.

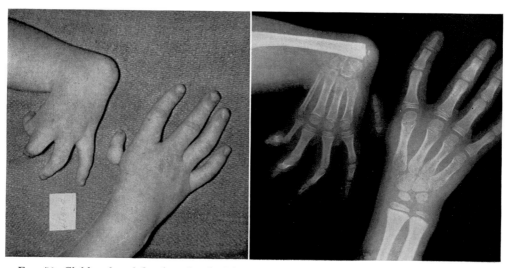

Fig. 72. Clubhand and floating thumb. The left can be classed as terminal paraxial radial hemimelia, and the right as an intercalary defect limited to the thumb.

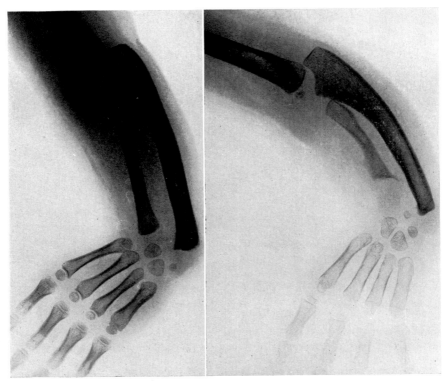

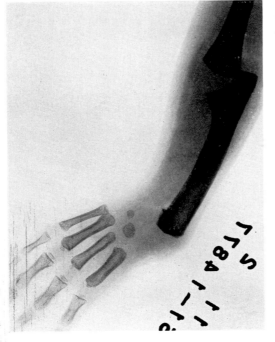

Fig. 73. Variations in extent of radial deficiencies. (*Top, left*) Proximal end and most of shaft present. (*Top, right*) Partial radial absence. (*Bottom*) Complete absence of radius. (D. C. Riordan, M.D.)

All 3 hands functioned and moved independently, and there were even 2 rudimentary fingers of a 4th hand located in a web between the hands. The hands were rotated 90° from each other.

Atavism is long-distance heredity—our phylogenetic development is re-enacted in the embryo. The explanation of certain deformities may be found in a search along the line from fish through a certain limited line of amphibians, reptiles, and mammals through primates.

In the fish there is only a hand but no arm, as in the deformity of phocomelia. The arm and the pectoral girdle developed later, as did also the neck. Thus the arm and the shoulder are supplied by higher segments (C-5, C-6 and C-7) than the hand (C-8, T-1). Phocomelia is an intercalary deficiency in which the arm is defective, the hand joining directly to the trunk. In the embryo we have first a hand but no arm, then a large hand with a short stub of an arm. As the arm and the hand bones form, they are short and broad as in the amphibia.

The shoulder in the embryo starts high, opposite its nerve segments, but descends, dragging its nerves caudalward— unless in the deformity of elevated scapula it remains in the primitive position. In the fish the shoulder girdle is high and attached to the head, the omovertebral bone joining the suprascapula to the occiput. In an individual with Sprengel's deformity, this bone joins the scapula to the 5th cervical vertebra. The elongation of the neck is related to the descent of the scapula; therefore, the cervical spine often is also deformed in this condition.

It is tempting to consider polydactylia a throwback to the multirayed fin, but this is doubtful in the usual case, as it is associated with other deformities.

Man still retains a hand much less specialized than the "hands" of most vertebrates and not far removed from the primitive amphibian type. The os centrale, present in most mammals, appears in the fetus and, if it does not fuse to the scaphoid, remains as the deformity of bipartite scaphoid. There is reason to regard the metacarpal of the thumb with its epiphysis at the proximal instead of the distal end, as in the others, as a fusion of the proximal phalanx and metacarpal. This may account for the frequent deformity of the 3-phalangized thumb.

Aside from true atavism, there are typical variations found repeatedly in other animals which are also seen in congenital deformities in man. Many reptiles have ribs as far as the skull. In man a cervical rib is a deformity. Though many mammals have more than 5 lumbar vertebrae, a 6th in man is a deformity. Similarly, in many animals the number of digital rays may be decreased, or phalanges in a digit may be increased or decreased—the tendency in our deformities. In man a defect or synostosis in the radius or the ulna is a deformity, but in many animals either the radius or the ulna is represented by a rudimentary remnant synostosed to the other bone. Synostosis between carpi and digital rays is common in reptiles, birds and mammals but is a deformity in man.

EFFECTS OF DISEASE OR CHANGES IN UTERO

There is no basis for the belief that insufficient amniotic fluid results in compression and bends the extremities or that constricting bands of amnion or umbilical cord strangle limbs, resulting in circular furrows or amputations. Bagg and others have shown the fallacy of these theories. Limbs are normally curved in utero and when there has been known lack of amniotic fluid, deformities have been absent. Clubfeet have been seen as early as in the 3rd month in utero and frequently in the 4th and the 5th months. Annular lesions and amputations, like clubfeet, often are accompanied by multiple deformities in the trunk and the extremities. These annular grooves, which are circular instead of segmented or longitudinal defects, may be of any depth and when complete appear as actual amputations with scars terminating the stumps.

The neurogenic theory of deformities is untenable with the possible exception of hypertrophied parts of limbs, such as megalodactylia, which are accompanied or caused by neurofibromata. Moore found that 91 per cent of 78 cases of various congenital anomalies had neurofibromata. Congenital deformities resemble paralytic deformities. Lesions in the spinal cord or the brain accompanying limb deformities are part of the general abnormal development and not the cause of the limb lesion.

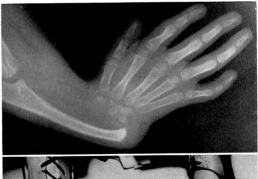

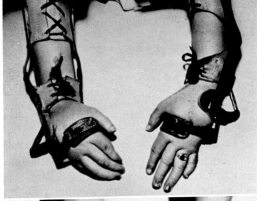

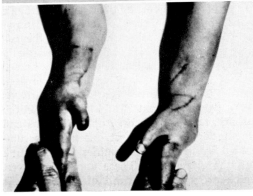

Fig. 74. Case S. P. (*Top*) Defect of the radius and clinarthrosis. (*Center*) Cumbersome splints. (*Bottom*) Clinarthrosis corrected by Z-plasty. (Plast. & Reconstr. Surg. *16*:169-173)

ACQUIRED DEFORMITIES

Dietary deficiencies can produce deformities in rats. Warkany and Nelson found 39.05 per cent of those born alive to have skeletal deficiencies when fed a specific test diet. Half of the deformities were in the forelegs with absence, shortening or fusion of digits or meta-carpals. Feeding 2 per cent pig's liver or ribo-flavin as late as the 13th day prevented the deformities. Feeding after the 15th day was ineffective because the structures had already been formed. Vitamin A deficiency results in blindness, and vitamin D deficiency causes bony curvatures and angulations.

Rubella in the first 2 months of pregnancy is alleged to cause deaf mutism, cataracts, heart defects, mongolism and microcephaly.

The "epidemic" of phocomelia in Germany in 1961 was apparently related to the use of a sedative drug of thalidomide type, ingested during the sensitive period before the 6th week of pregnancy.

Stochard produced many types of deformities in eggs of fish, amphibia and birds by lowering the temperature or the oxygen tension in early developmental stages. The deformity did not result from the specific damaging agent but depended on the developmental stage during which the injury took place.

Duraiswami produced many congenital deformities in chickens by injecting a little insulin under the shell of the egg at a very early stage. He found that he could prevent them by injecting nicotinamide and riboflavin in addition to the insulin. In the case of the clubfeet thus produced, the deformity was transmitted through 5 generations.

ABSENCE OF ALL OR PARTS OF LIMBS

ECTROMELIA AND ECTRODACTYLIA

Defects may be terminal or intercalary, transverse or paraxial or phocomelic in type. The defect may follow the ray or segment distribution. If it is a ray defect, there may be absence of one or several digits, usually either the marginal or the central portions of the hand, or absence of the radius or the ulna or their respective buds, including the digits. Often the thumb and its metacarpal are missing, or similarly the little finger. Absence of central rays is described under cleft hand.

When the defect is segmental, there may be absence of any or several segments in the limb. Even all 4 limbs have been missing up to the glenoid and the acetabular sockets, as reported by Price. The missing segment may be only one or several in a digit, or of a digit itself, or of several digits. The whole hand may be missing or represented by one or several fingers, rudimentary or not. If the whole arm is missing, usually the hand is also; but in some the forearm is missing, the hand being joined to a rudimentary humerus; or the whole arm may be missing, the hand joining directly to the trunk (called phocomelia from the seal, though really the seal has an arm). Absence of the arm, but not of the hand, corresponds to a defect from C-5 to C-7, but absence of radial and ulnar aspects of the arm to that of C-5 and C-6, and C-8 and T-1, respectively.

SHOULDER, ARM AND FOREARM DEFORMITIES

Congenital Elevation of the Scapula, Sprengel's Deformity

Failure of descent of the scapula is a type of atavism. At about the 4th week of embryonic life the scapula shows as a condensation of mesenchyme opposite the 4th and the 5th myotomes, later as cartilage opposite C-4 to C-7. It continues to migrate, reaching its permanent level at T-2 in the 3rd month. Any arrest before this time results in the deformity.

Symptoms. One shoulder appears to be higher, and the scapula is felt above its normal position. Sometimes the condition is bilateral, but, due to cervical scoliosis, the elevation on the concave side is masked. Occasionally, the defect is shown only in the muscles which elevate the scapula, but often there is an abnormal vertebral attachment, an omovertebral bone. This bone, normal in the fish, is triangular in shape, with its base at the upper third of the vertebral border of the scapula, and its apex is attached to the transverse processes of the lower 3 cervical vertebrae, either directly or through cartilage.

The scapula itself is shorter in the vertical plane and tilted so that its lower angle is near the spine, as in quadrupeds. The upper border and the coracoid process are curved forward. Cervical scoliosis, fused vertebrae and short neck, with cervical ribs, are often associated. Wryneck is present in 10 per cent of cases. The lower thirds of the trapezius and the serratus magnus muscles may be absent, and those that raise the scapula are usually overly prominent. The limb does not work very well in its distorted position and appears awkward.

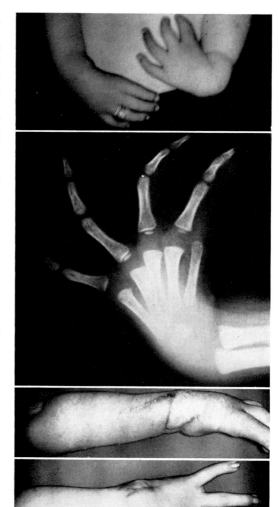

Fig. 75. Case B. A. (*Top*) Clinarthrosis bilateral. (*Second illustration*) Radius and ulna synostosis. (*Third illustration*) Clinarthrosis corrected by Z-plasty. (*Bottom*) Good alignment. (Plast. & Reconstr. Surg. *16*:169-173)

Treatment. Correction is difficult and unsatisfactory. For mild cases, early intermittent stretching may be of help. Myotomies are insufficient. Operative correction should be done early, at about the age of 3. For younger patients the magnitude of the procedure is excessive, and correction later is almost impossible. Paralysis may result if the brachial plexus is overstretched or if the scapula is attached with the plexus on tension. Arm action is dependent on stabilization of the scapula, and this depends on muscle balance, the clavicle being the only bony attachment of the extremity to the trunk.

The operation was described by Schrock. Through a curved dorsal incision greater than the length of the scapula and with its convexity toward the spine, the scapula is stripped sub-periosteally from its muscle attachments, displaced downward, attached by suture to the ribs, and allowed to re-acquire its muscle attachments at a different level. Enough muscles to free the scapula are stripped and may include trapezius, levator anguli scapulae, rhomboids, supraspinatus and infraspinatus, teres major and minor, serratus anticus and subscapularis. The subscapular nerve should be spared. It may be necessary to cut off the superior border of the spine, or even the acromion of the scapula. Some degree of improvement in appearance and function can be

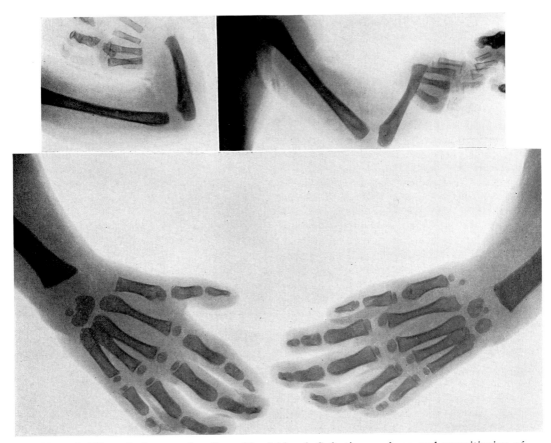

Fig. 76. Bilateral absence of radius with clubhand. Soft tissue release and repositioning of hand on carpus at age of 6 months. (*Bottom*) two years later, position was well maintained by simple splints. Arthrodesis will be done later if instability persists. (D. C. Riordan, M.D.)

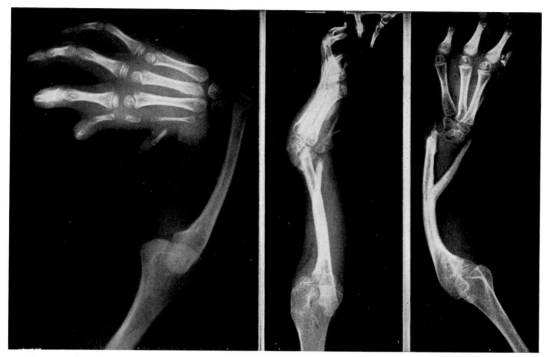

FIG. 77. (*Left*) Congenital absence of the radius. (*Center*) Same after Albee type of operation by S. L. Haas. (*Right*) Lateral view. (S. L. Haas)

expected. Woodward has reported some excellent results.

KLIPPEL-FEIL SYNDROME

In this strange syndrome, a part of which is congenital elevation of the scapulae, there is webbing of the skin between the head and the shoulders and beneath the arms. There may also be cervical ribs, large transverse vertebral processes and feeblemindedness.

DEFECTS OF THE RADIUS

Congenital absence of part or all of the radius is not uncommon and is considerably more frequent than absence of the ulna. As a skeletal deficiency it is classed as hemimelia and may be terminal or intercalary. It is often hereditary and associated with other deformities. Of 253 cases collected by Kato, most of total absence of the radius, 46 per cent were bilateral, and 38.8 per cent were unilateral. In

partial absence of the radius 0.8 per cent were bilateral, and 11.1 per cent unilateral. Any part of the radius may be absent, the shaft or either end, the retention of a rudimentary upper end being more frequent.

Defects in the Radial Bud. The defect is in the radial bud and, therefore, often includes the carpal and the digital rays of the radius and the radial part of the end of the humerus; or the arrangement may be segmental of C-5 and C-6, there being also a defect in the deltoid, the upper pectoral and the flexor muscles of the elbow. If the upper end of the radius is present, there may be ankylosis with the humerus or radio-ulnar synostosis. The radial bones of the carpus may be absent or fused. The thumb is usually absent, and sometimes the index finger. O'Rahilly noted absence of the scaphoid, the trapezium, the first metacarpal and the thumb in most cases in which the distal radius was absent. Thus these bones constitute the radial ray.

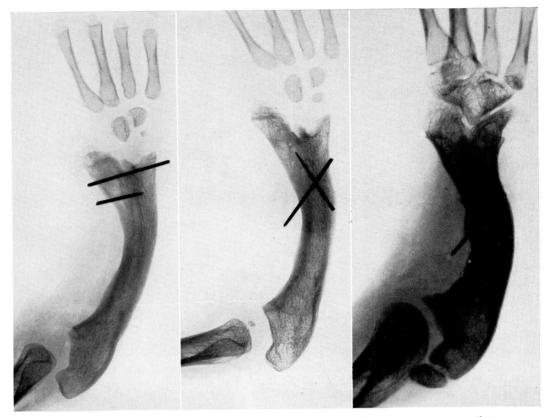

FIG. 78. Transplantation of fibular head and epiphysis. (*Left*) Operation at age of 4 years (1950). (*Center*) one year postepiphyseal transplant and correction of bowing. (*Right*) nine years after transplant; good stability and some wrist motion. (D. C. Riordan, M.D.)

In 77 cases of absence of the radius the scaphoid was absent in 82 per cent and the trapezium in 86 per cent. In 115 such cases, the 1st metacarpal was absent in 80 per cent, and the 2nd metacarpal was present in 85 per cent. The lunate, the trapezoid and the 2nd metacarpal were absent in only 15 per cent. This places the index finger in line with the cleavage plane between the ulnar and the radial buds.

The ulna is short and thick and curved radially. As the forearm grows without its radial support, the hand deviates radialward until it is at a right angle with the forearm. The distortion my be so great that the radial border of the hand is against the forearm. The fingers are flexed and, from muscle atrophy, disuse and loss of mechanics, are limited in voluntary and passive motion.

Clinarthrosis radialward, often to a right angle, occurs at the wrist in radial hemimelia, which means a defect of the radius or the radial bud. Similar clinarthrosis may occur in the presence of both radius and ulna. In radial clinarthrosis, even if the radius is present, the thumb is often defective or absent. In ulnar hemimelia, the clinarthrosis is ulnarward.

Treatment. One should endeavor to lessen the deformity and counteract that which accompanies growth. In mild cases, correction by manipulation without force may be maintained by an adjustable brace or repeated applications of plaster casts. Treatment begins as soon as possible after birth.

As a prelude to the bone treatment, a liberal Z-plasty may be necessary on the concave side to relieve the flexion contracture. Sometimes a small skin graft is necessary. Also, the deep fascia is severed across, and the tendons that flex the wrist radially are tenotomized or elongated, and a capsulectomy of the wrist joint is done. The tendons to the digits are protected. If the radius is absent, the wrist-moving tendons may be severed, as there will be an arthrodesis of the wrist later. If wrist motion is contemplated, they are elongated. The soft-tissue operation involves a radical release to place the carpus over the distal end of the ulna.

The wrist then will straighten and is held so temporarily by a Kirschner wire introduced through the palm, the carpus and the forearm bone. It is not difficult to maintain this straight position with a simple plastic gutter splint so that the arm will grow longer until the time for the bone operation of osteotomy on the curved ulna and either a bone graft of the radius or fusion of the ulna into the carpus. In this way the cumbersome and difficult-to-apply long elbow splinting is eliminated. Riordan was successful in correcting the alignment of the hand with the forearm by using repeated plaster encasements in the first year of life. He tried a series of casts but found that it was always necessary to release the tissues surgically in order to correct the deformity completely.

The next step is to correct the curvature of

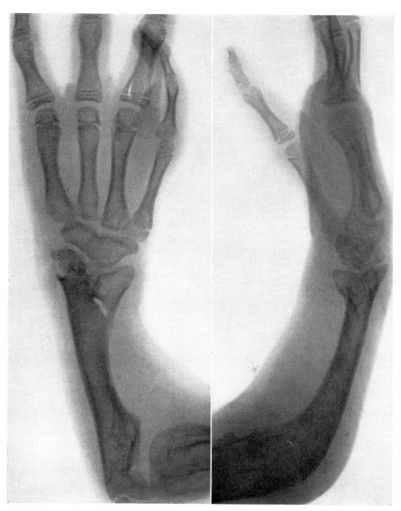

Fig. 79. Eight years after epiphyseal transplant with upper end of fibula.
(D. C. Riordan, M.D.)

the ulna. Sometimes an osteotomy at two levels is necessary. When the forearm alignment has been obtained, then some stabilizing procedure is necessary on the wrist.

If a movable wrist cannot be expected, the hand should be placed in the line of the forearm and there ankylosed with good contact, broadly and massively. It may be necessary to resect part of the carpus and to shorten the ulna to bring the hand straight with the forearm.

Various methods of obtaining this firm support, in joining the hand to the ulna, have been used; the most popular is that of Albee. A rod of bone is cut from the tibia. Both ends are wedged, one end being embedded in a notch in the ulna and the other into the scaphoid side of the carpus, to form with the ulna a Y-support for the hand.

Bardenheuer also made a Y-support of the carpus by splitting up the ulna a few inches and spreading it out. Steindler made a double osteotomy to the lower end of the ulna, removing the segment between. The lower osteotomy was made so oblique that on contacting it with the upper osteotomy the hand came straight.

Sayre shortened and sharpened the lower end of the ulna, removed the capitate and the hamate and thrust the ulna not only through the carpus but also between the metacarpals, since fastening it to the carpals alone is hardly sufficient.

Riordan grafted the upper end of the fibula

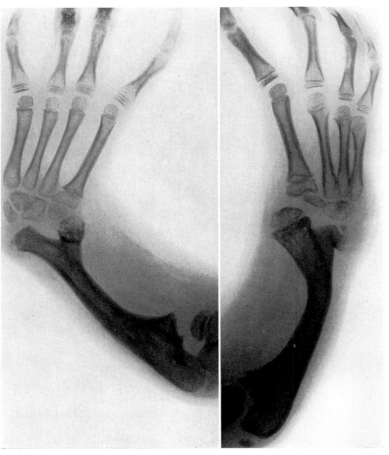

Fig. 80. Bilateral fibular graft done in 1955. Roentgenograms in 1960. (*Left*) Epiphysis closed. (*Right*) Epiphysis still open. (D. C. Riordan, M.D.)

FIG. 81. Case T. S. Mirror hand with clinarthrosis; flexion contracture on the radial side as in defect of the radius, although both the radius and the ulna are present. Clinarthrosis is primary whether or not there is defect of the radius. This was corrected by large Z-plasty, severing the wrist capsule and what wrist tendons were necessary, and by pinning the wrist straight by a Kirschner wire. (*Bottom picture*) Later, the head of the ulna was removed as it was causing further deviation, and a thumb was reconstructed from digit V. Digits VI and VII were filleted, deleted, and the skin was used to line the thumb cleft. Digit V, with all its blood, nerve and tendon supply, was circumscribed and osteotomized into position. (Plast. & Reconstr. Surg. *16*:169-173)

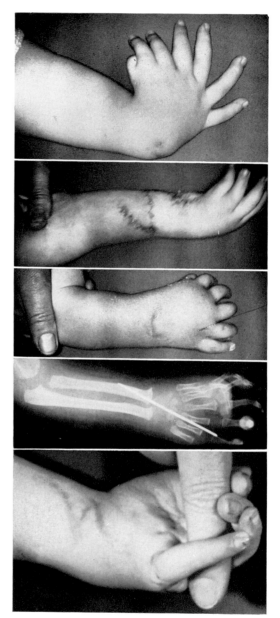

with the epiphysis into the shaft of the radius in such a way that the head of the fibula participated in the wrist joint, thus obtaining a movable wrist. The hope was that the epiphysis of the radius would grow. However, it is exceedingly doubtful that a grafted epiphysis will grow.

The operations are followed by long splinting, leaving the fingers and the thumb free so that function will stimulate growth.

DEFECTS OF THE ULNA

Defects of the ulnar bud of the arm occur much less frequently than defects of the radial bud. Accompanying defects, being along the ulnar side of the arm or the C-8 and T-1 segments, involve the ulnar digital rays. Like the radial defect, it is often hereditary, accompanied by other deformities and bilateral in almost half of the cases.

The ulnar side of the carpus may be absent or fused, and more digits may be absent than with a radial defect. The middle, the ring and the little fingers are frequently missing. In ulnar hemimelia, the thumb and the index rays usually are spared, but the pisiform, the hamate, the triquetrum, the capitate and the last 2 metacarpals usually are absent.

The defect is usually of the whole ulna but may be of the shaft or either end, though of these—as in the radius—it is usually the distal portion that is missing. At the elbow where the ulna should furnish joint stability, the unstable radial head in most cases dislocates up-

ward, the bone even crossing the humerus. In some, the radius is fused with the humerus. The trochlea is often missing, and if the upper end of the ulna is present, it may be fused with it, or there may be radio-ulnar synostosis. The arm is short, and the radius is curved ulnarward.

At the wrist it is the radius that gives stable support to the carpus, so that in defectiveness

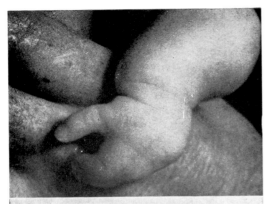

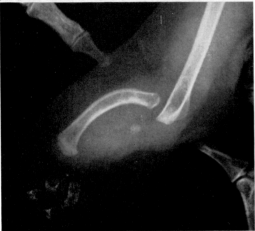

FIG. 82. Congenital absence of ulna with ulnar 2 rays missing, radius markedly bowed and elbow flail. Should have first incision of ulnar contracted structures, then osteotomy of radius and eventually arthrodesis of elbow.

of the ulna the deformity of the ulnar palmar deviation is much less marked than is the radial palmar deflection from defectiveness of the radius. It is only occasionally that the clubhand deflection from an ulnar defect reaches a right angle. Therefore, there is often good function of the hand. In fact, the greater disability may be in the elbow, due to pronation of the forearm.

Treatment. Early splinting and manipulation should keep the deformity in check for the first 3 years of growth. Surgery may not be necessary but if needed is similar to that used for radial defects, first correcting the soft-part factor of the deformity and then stabilizing the wrist by the methods men-

tioned. It is the radial epiphysis from which the growth of the forearm must come, so that this should be preserved, if possible, using only a bone graft extending from the shaft to support the carpus from the side. Ankylosis may be necessary at the elbow. If only the lower part of the ulna is missing, the radius may be made to unite with the upper fragments of the ulna as one bone.

Rarely, both the radius and the ulna may be missing, the carpus articulating with the humerus as a type of phocomelia, or the humerus itself may be missing, the forearm or the hand springing from the trunk. One or both clavicles may be absent or defective, allowing wider range of shoulder motion.

CLINARTHROSIS OR DEVIATION IN ALIGNMENT OF JOINTS

Bagg showed that an embryonic lesion on one side of a limb leads to contracture toward that side, due to a defect in development. Bones, muscles, nerves and vessels may be absent in the concave side. At the elbow, cubitus varus or valgus is sometimes seen, due to laxity of the ligaments. At the wrist, clubhand is frequent and is usually associated with a defect of the radius or the ulna, though it can occur when the bones are normal. The deviation, usually radial or ulnarward, may also be volar or dorsal or a combination and is frequently bilateral.

Clinarthrosis occurs often in the fingers, particularly the little finger. It is usual for the middle joint to be in flexion, while the proximal and the distal joints are in extension, though the whole finger may be in flexion. The little finger may overlap the ring finger. Lateral deviation of the fingers occurs when one phalanx, such as the middle, is rudimentary and wedge-shaped. Sometimes all fingers and toes show ulnar deviation in their proximal joints. Mild forms of arthrogryposis may manifest themselves in the hands.

TREATMENT

Conservative treatment is used first, starting early in life, manipulating and then gradually stretching the soft parts by splints or casts and holding them so until the limbs grow straighter. Surgery is deferred until age 6 or later and consists of freeing or severing the

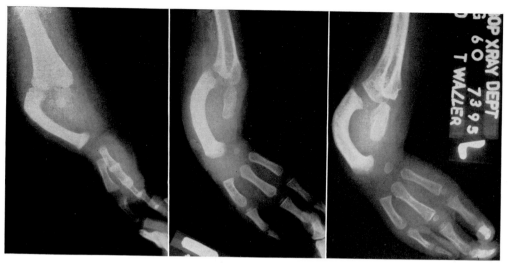

Fig. 83. Congenital absence of ulna. At first only a small ossification center is apparent (*left*). This increases in size, but note (*right*) the increased radial bowing, as if the short ulna were acting as a checkrein. Soft tissue release should be done early, excising all bands of contracting tissue extending from the ulnar remnant.

contracted parts and straightening curved bones by wedge osteotomy. In clubhand the bones are treated as for a defect of the radius and the ulna. The surgical treatment for congenital flexion of a finger is disappointing. All the tissues share in the contracture, tending to reproduce it. When lateral deviation in a finger is due to a rudimentary or a supernumerary wedge-shaped phalanx, the latter may be resected and the capsule of the new joint reconstructed. When all fingers deviate ulnarward at their proximal joints, soft tissue and ligamentous release followed by prolonged splinting is better than bony correction. Usu-

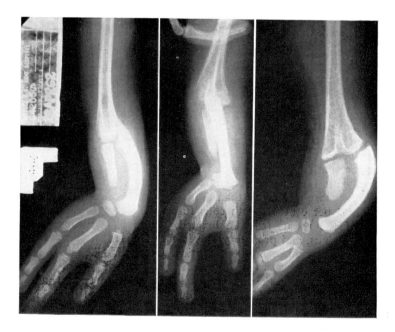

Fig. 84. (Same patient as Fig. 83.) At age 6 the deformity involves the humerus as well. Thumb, index and middle fingers function well. (Col. Anderson, Tripler General Hospital, Honolulu, H.)

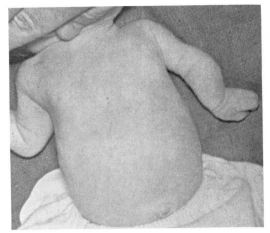

FIG. 85. Congenital absence of ulna and 2 ulnar digits. Note in this 2-month-old infant the bowing of the radius and the internal rotation of the arm.

ally, the common extensor tendons will have dislocated onto the ulnar groove and should be replaced.

CONGENITAL DISLOCATIONS

Any joint from shoulder to digit may be dislocated. Complete elbow dislocations are rare, though the radius is often dislocated upward, in front, at the side or behind the elbow, often bilaterally and in association with a defect of the ulna. A few cases are reported of bilateral dislocation of the wrist, though there are many such associated with a defect of the radius. Dislocations of thumb and finger joints are usually a part of other deformities.

SYNOSTOSES

Fusion of the humerus, with the radius or the ulna, or both, may occur either at a right angle or in extension. Radio-ulnar fusion is common, and in some is hereditary. In half the cases it is bilateral. The upper ends are fused far more frequently than the lower, and in only 2 per cent are both ends fused. The head of the radius may be luxated, giving cubitus valgus, and pronatory movements are frozen in the middle or fetal position. Occasionally, fusion occurs with a wide angle between the radius and the ulna.

Carpal fusions are fairly numerous, every possible combination having been described. The most common is between the lunate and

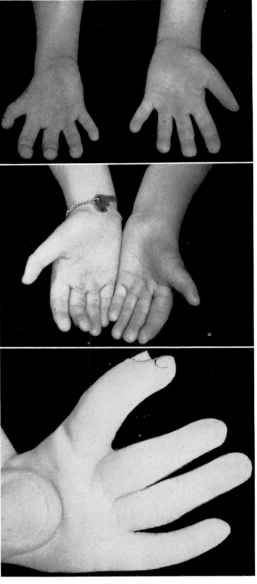

FIG. 86. Familial and hereditary deformities. (*Top*) Congenital deficiency of right carpus and thenar eminence in male. (*Center*) Sister showing bilateral deficiencies of thenar eminence. (*Bottom*) Daughter of the patient above, bilateral absence of thumb and duplication of index with clinarthrosis.

the triquetrum. This is almost racial in the Bantu tribe in South Africa (Minnarr). The lunate and the scaphoid are often fused, as in all carnivores. Fusions are numerous be-

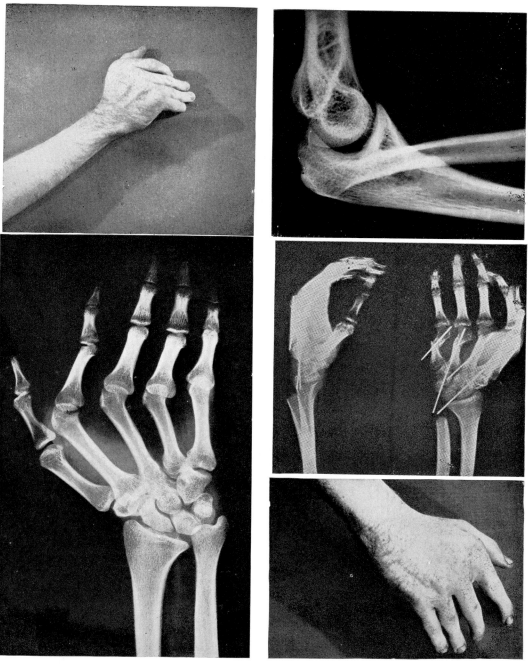

Fig. 87. Case C. S., aged 17. Congenital clinarthrosis of the proximal finger joints with synostosis of the upper radio-ulnar joint. The feet showed polydactylism and syndactylism. (*Left, top*) Right hand preoperatively. (*Left, bottom,* and *right, top*) Roentgenograms showing clinarthrosis and synarthrosis of the upper radio-ulnar joint. (*Right, center*) Roentgenogram 75 days postoperatively shows clinarthrosis corrected by wedge osteotomies secured by wires. The head of the ulna has been removed, together with the head of the radius, to allow pronation and supination. All flexor tendons were lengthened, and a plastic zigzag was done to let out the ulnar border of the skin. (*Right, bottom*) Postoperative appearance. Function much improved.

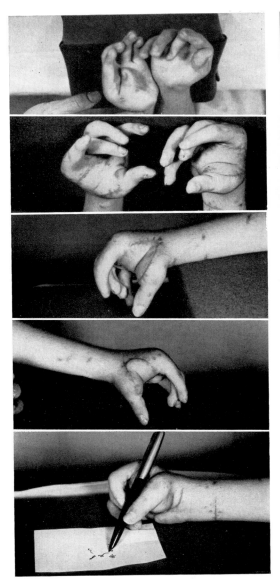

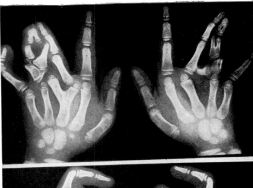

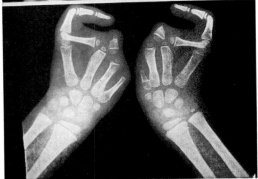

FIG. 89. Bizarre types of bilateral clinodactyly and ectrosyndactyly. (*Top*) Symphysodactylia is prominent. (*Bottom*) Ectrodactyly predominates. (S. L. Haas, Shriners Hospital)

FIG. 88. Case M. Y. (*Top*) Congenital clinarthrosis with flexion contractures of the hands, club feet and inability to raise the arms at the shoulders. The hands were operated on simultaneously, opening out the palms and the thumbs by releasing incisions and applying pedicle grafts. Osteotomies were done on the metacarpal necks to straighten the fingers, and also on the thumb metacarpals. Finger webs were corrected. There was much improvement in appearance and function, as shown in the 4 remaining illustrations.

tween hamate, capitate, multangular and carpus and metacarpus. Some carpal bones may be absent, such as the scaphoid, even without hemimelia. Many ossicles have been described in the carpus and the tarsus by O'Rahilly. The epitriquetrum, next to the triquetrum where it meets the lunate, the capitate and the hamate, is definitely established but rare.

Metacarpals may be fused completely or at one end only with a Y-separation at the other. Synostoses are frequent in syndactylia and polydactylia.

TREATMENT

Operative separation of the forearm bones at the elbow is often disappointing because of the marked tendency to re-fuse.

For synostosis of the elbow in extension a wedge osteotomy to flex the elbow to 70° will allow the arm to function and develop until successful arthroplasty can be done at adult

Fig. 90. Absence of thenar muscles and the 1st metacarpal. Thumb small, flail and attached only by skin. "Pouce flottant." When the opposite hand is normal, amputation of this nubbin should be considered.

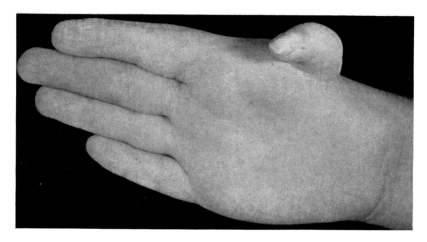

age. The osteotomy should be done above the epiphysial plate lest growth be prevented.

In synostoses of the upper end of the radius and the ulna there is often also a defect of the muscles of supination. A wide resection of the head of the radius and the interosseus ridges for the distance of the fusion, followed by interposition of soft parts, is necessary to give pronation and supination but often fails. One may free the radius of muscles and allow them to reattach in the position of supination or do a rotary osteotomy of the radius to the position of supination. Because of the poor late results it is probably better to sever the radius below the synostosis, interpose soft parts and put up the arm in supination.

DEFORMITIES OF THE HANDS

CLEFT, LOBSTER-CLAW AND MIRROR HANDS

Cleft hands and feet are often hereditary and bilateral. Tubby traced them through 5 generations, and Lewis and Embleton found that all but 13 of 130 cases were hereditary. Cloven front feet are among the natural variations in animals such as ungulates or the African chameleon. Functionally, the hand of man has 2 parts, as outlined by the 2 distal palmar creases—the proximal one for the radial 3 fingers grasping against the thumb, and the distal one for the ulnar 3 grasping against the palm. The division between median and ulnar nerve supply is a line down the

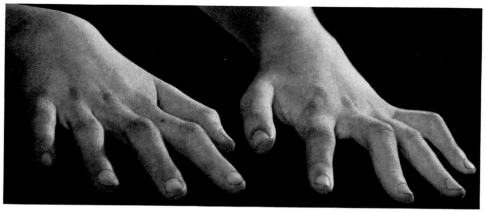

Fig. 91. Congenital flexion contracture of all the middle finger joints. For correction, spring splinting is better than surgery. (Jack Penn)

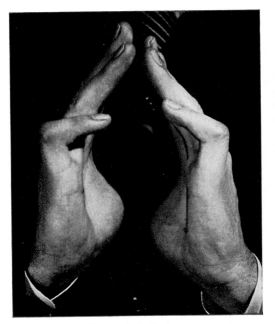

FIG. 92. Congenital flexion contracture, often a familial trait. In young children, directed splinting using the orthodontist's principles may provide much better extension and lessen the deformity.

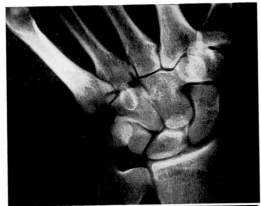

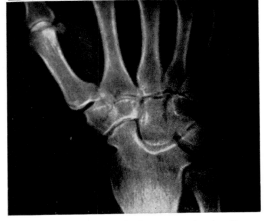

FIG. 94. Congenital synostosis in the carpus. (*Top*) The capitate and the lesser multangular are as one. (*Bottom*) Synostosis of the radius, the lunate and the navicular; also the capitate and the hamate.

center of the ring finger, while the divisions between the 2 fascial spaces and the functions of the intrinsic muscles divide it along the 3rd ray. With the radial bud are included the thumb and the index finger, and with the ulnar the index and the other fingers. The deformity of bifurcated hand may follow these natural divisions, there being a central defect of one or more rays from the 2nd to the 3rd.

Lobster-claw hand, having only a thumb and a little finger, results from a central defect of the intervening fingers. Their metacarpals and even part of the carpus may be missing, or these metacarpals may be rudimentary and at odd angles.

All these deformities belong to the class of central paraxial hemimelias.

Mirror hands are the result of twinning and are identical or nearly so, each being the mirror complement of the other. Even the carpus may be double. The thumbs are usually absent, the twinning being of the 4 or less digits supported by the ulna, though rarely the ulnar instead of the radial bud is the missing one. If the twinning is higher, there may be absence of

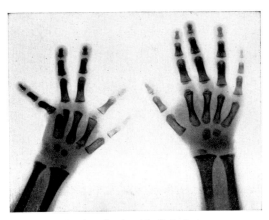

FIG. 93. Defect in the 5th digital ray; synostosis of the metacarpal and clinodactyly.

FIG. 95. Synostosis of carpal bones. Eleven-year-old girl with complete fusion of the lunate and the triquetrum on the left and partial synostosis on the right. These were an incidental finding on routine investigation because of mental retardation. (R. R. Schreiber, M.D., Los Angeles Orthopaedic Hospital)

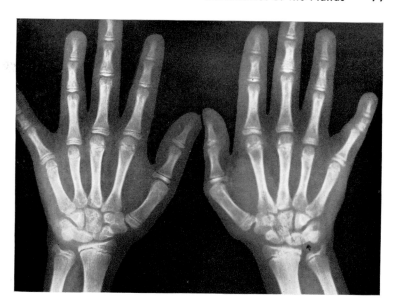

the radius but doubling of the ulna. Extra, aberrant fingers may be present, or the total number of digits may be 10 or less. In Saviard's case there were 10 digits on each of the 4 extremities. Bradford and Lovett saw a case with 15 fingers and 13 toes.

Treatment. In cleft or lobster-claw hand, the appearance may be improved by narrowing the cleft. This may also aid in function. The central metacarpals of the missing digits are excised, especially if they are more or less transverse, and the 2 parts of the hand are made to approach each other. If the digits cannot be opposed, they can be positioned by osteotomy and, if muscles are not present to make them work against each other, tendon transfers are done (Chap. 11).

FIG. 96. Chondro-ectodermal dysplasia. Ellis-Van Creveld syndrome. The tubular bones become progressively shorter distally in a centrifugal manner. There are 6 radiants. There is synostosis of 2 of the metacarpals. The large central carpal bone probably represents fusion of the hamate and the capitate bones and is a constant feature in this syndrome. This girl also had congenital heart disease and a short stature. The combination of polydactyly, syndactyly, massive central carpal bone and centrifugal shortening of the tubular bones is practically diagnostic. (John Gwinn, M.D., Children's Hospital, Los Angeles)

For mirror hands, amputation is done to leave 1 digit as a thumb and 4 remaining fingers. Selective amputation with filleting of the digit provides skin for cleft use as well as a pseudothenar eminence.

The carpus is made to rest centrally on the ends of the forearm bones.

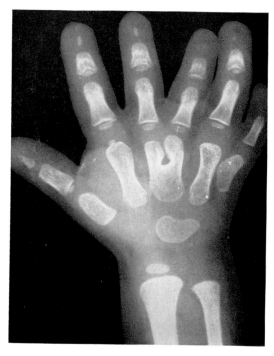

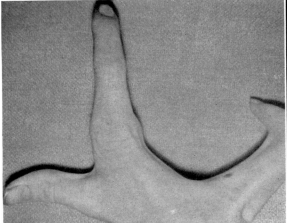 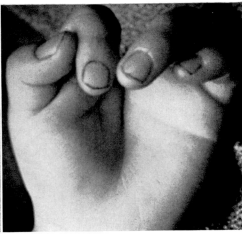

Fig. 97. Cleft hands or forms of terminal paraxial central deformities. Similar deformity in the feet (*bottom*).

Wrist arthrodesis is often necessary, as absence of wrist extensors occurs with the absence of the radial half of the forearm.

Clump or drumstick hand is an exaggeration of syndactylia. If allowed to remain, the abbreviated and bound digits will not develop. Therefore, early in life they should be separated and enough skin furnished to cover their denuded surfaces. This should be done in stages for the different clefts. The digits, when separated and working against each other, then will have a chance to develop.

DEFORMITIES OF FINGERS

POLYDACTYLIA

This deformity, probably the most common of all hand anomalies, is frequently hereditary and accompanied by other deformities, such as syndactylia, brachydactylia, brachyphalangia, hyperphalangia, symphalangia and other aberrations. Deformities of the digits, the terminal parts of a limb, are much more common than defects of the limb itself and are more varied. Polydactylia tends to be marginal, either of the ulnar or the radial borders, or to be centrally arranged in the hand, and it consists usually of doubling of 1 or more digits, making 6 or more. It is most common of the little finger at the ulnar margin of the hand, next of the thumb, and least of the central digits. An extra digit usually but not always has a separate metacarpal, and this may be fused to the adjoining one. The extra little finger may be full size or sometimes merely a tab of skin. It may stand out at any angle.

The thumb, when involved, often has 3 phalanges instead of the customary 2, and so may be confused with a finger. The epiphysis of the normal thumb metacarpal, being basal like a phalanx, suggests that either the metacarpal is absent or has fused with the proximal phalanx, taking on the proximal epiphysis of the latter. A bifid thumb is common, the forking being at any level of phalanx, joint or metacarpal, though usually at the distal joint. The fork may be as a Y of phalanx or metacarpal and at varying angles. The extra thumb may be symmetrical and equal in length with the other thumb, or may come off as a rudimentary thumb at the radial side. Occasionally, the thumb is triple; then the central member is the largest.

Treatment. After ascertaining the condition of the bones by means of roentgenograms, treatment must consider both cosmetic and functional factors. In the latter, those digits that oppose each other will be the most useful. One should ascertain that the digits preserved have tendons and muscle attachments, or preserve tendons and muscles of any digit to be amputated and transfer them to a remaining digit. In amputating median supernumerary fingers it may be necessary to remove the metacarpal to narrow the hand and bring the adjoining fingers together. In a bifid thumb a central wedge of soft tissue can be removed, so that the 2 ends can be later fused as one; or the radial member may be amputated and the other aligned by osteotomy.

Syndactylia

This deformity is the next most common in the hand. In the fetus the fingers do not grow out from their webs until the 7th week. Often hereditary and almost twice as frequent in males, syndactylia may involve any 2 digits or all, though rarely the thumb, and most commonly the middle and the ring fingers. It may be symmetrically bilateral, as in almost half the cases, and may occur in the toes at the same time. It is frequently associated with

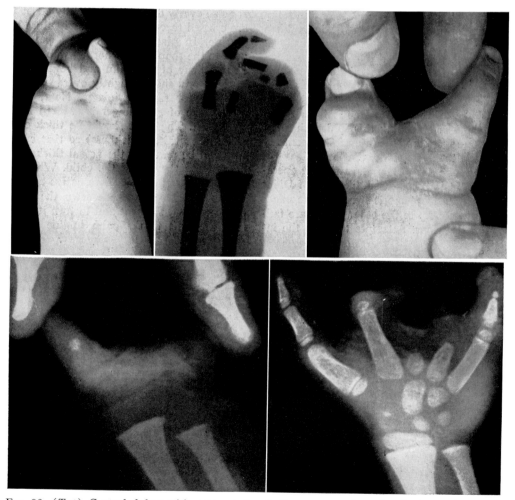

Fig. 98. (*Top*) Central defect with contracted soft tissues, opened out by Z-plasty. (*Bottom*) Other examples of central paraxial deficiencies.

other deformities of the same hand and with defects elsewhere in the body and is often combined with many other types of finger aberrations. The joining of the fingers may be of any degree of length or thickness of web. There may be a thin web or a broad attachment of the fingers and the nails, showing as a deep or shallow depression between them, or the attachment may be so intimate that the bones are fused. The fusion may also involve the tendons and the digital nerves and sometimes may extend proximally to include the metacarpals and the carpal bones. The double nail is broad, with a groove between its 2 parts. It is rare that only the ends of the fingers are fused together (acrosyndactylia). The joints of the adjoining fingers, if opposite each other, allow good motion; but if not, the joints fail to coincide, thus preventing flexion. When only 2 fingers are webbed, they are usually of equal length, but they change to the normal length ratio after they are separated surgically. Even short webs interfere with free finger movements. In an adult, the length from prominence of knuckle to web is from 2.0 to 2.5 cm. Webs exceeding this in length show when the fingers are spread as a skin contracture across the distal end of the palm.

Treatment. The plastic flap-swinging operations as commonly pictured, like that of Didot in which the dorsal flap is swung to one finger and the volar flap to the other finger, are failures for 2 reasons. Attempts to draw the insufficient skin too tight cause necrosis or even gangrene, and the scar running down one side and up the other contracts, as all scars do. This draws down the skin of the hand, reproducing the web. Since the scar is under tension, especially as the finger grows, it distorts the finger with a lateral curvature and a rotary twist and draws the nail and the matrix on one side back into a point. The way to avoid this deformity is first to establish the depth of the cleft and second to furnish additional skin by partial-thickness grafts. Where possible, suture lines should be curved for slack, instead of straight down the finger. The depth of the cleft is fixed by first outlining a dorsal and a volar pointed skin flap. Then the web is slit through, and by blunt pressure the cleft is made overly deep. The 2 slightly offset flaps are crossed through the cleft and sutured side to side. In planning these flaps one should imitate the shape of the normal web, its being in the plane of the palm and beveled to the dorsum, and should slightly overdo the depth to allow for some shrinkage. Next, the denuded side of each finger is covered by free skin graft. The graft should be thick enough (about two thirds thickness) so that contracture will be minimal, the actual thickness depending on the age of the child. When there is only one web, a good alternative method is to raise one broad pedicle from the back of each proximal segment and to turn it forward into the cleft to the palm to line the cleft

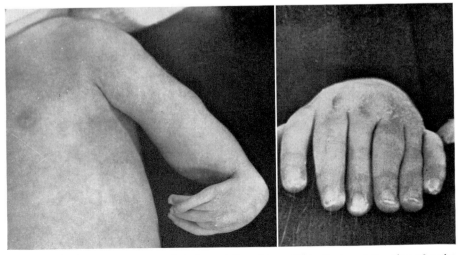

Fig. 99. Mirror hand. Central digit is an index finger. Note flexion deformity of wrist from the lack of radial wrist extensors. See Fig. 100.

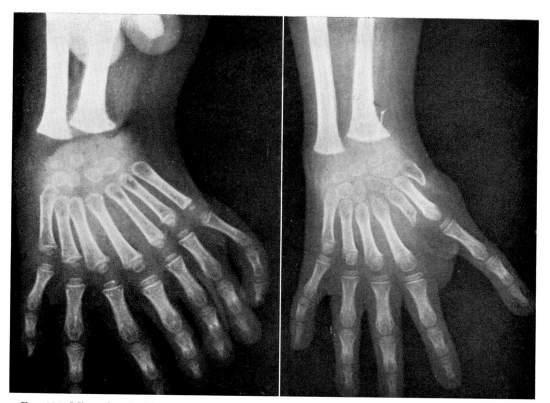

FIG. 100. Mirror hand with double ulna and duplication of middle, ring and little fingers of one hand. (*Right*) The 1st and the 3rd rays have been filleted and skin from the first digit used for a pseudothenar eminence and that from the 3rd for a cleft. Tenodesis to keep wrist in functioning position.

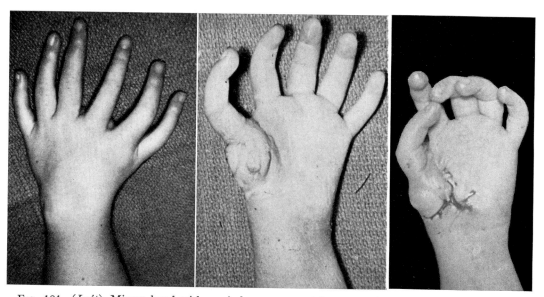

FIG. 101. (*Left*) Mirror hand with no index component but normal forearm. (*Right*) The most radial digit was filleted to provide skin for a pseudothenar eminence, and the next digit was osteotomized, shortened and rotated into position on the base of the most radial metacarpal. (*Center*) First stage. (**Right**) Position and lengh of new thumb at completion of osteotomy and shift of metacarpal.

smoothly. Similarly, a transverse flap from the redundant skin on the dorsum of the hand can be laid across an interdigital cleft.

In repairing cicatricial webs, as often after burns, free grafts are needed because flaps of scar tissue will not live; but for congenital webs the above double flap method is best. Quite short, broad webs can be corrected by the Pieri Z plastic.

A denuded cleft is often pictured as closed

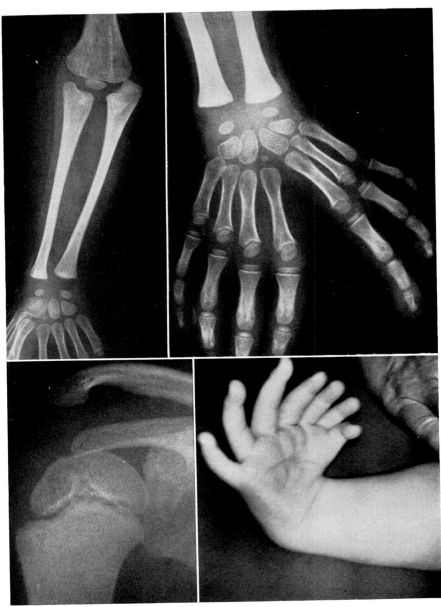

Fig. 102. Case B. B., aged 5. Double ulna, mirror hand, cleft humeral head. The radial buds are missing, and the cleft involves even the humeral head. Note the cleft carpus. The index finger marks the division between the radial and the ulnar buds. (*Additional picture on facing page*)

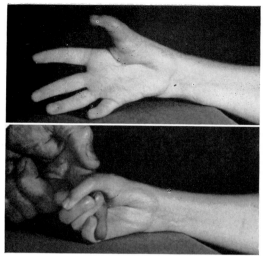

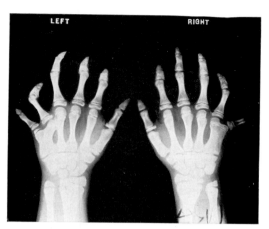

FIG. 104. Polydactyly with synostosis of the metacarpals and brachyphalangia of the supernumerary digit. (Robert Newell, Stanford Univ. School of Medicine)

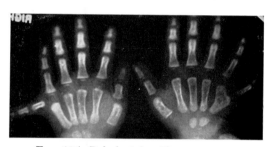

FIG. 105. Polydactyly. The supernumerary digit is on the outer side of the hand and with clinodactyly.

FIG. 102 (*Continued*). Digits 1 and 2 were filleted and deleted. Digit 3 was osteotomized to place it as a thumb, and the filleted skin from digits 1 and 2 was used to cover in the new thumb cleft.

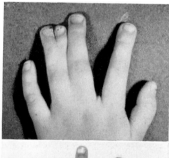

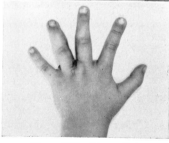

FIG. 103. Case Baby J. H. (*Top*) The supernumerary digit was excised, and the depth of the cleft was established by a double skin flap. (*Bottom*) The fingers were separated by wavy incisions, and skin grafts covered the denudations.

in by one piece of skin inlay graft, using a wax stent molded to the proper shape of the web and the fingers. The fallacy of this method is that each border of the cleft will contract to a short U, thus drawing down 2 webs, one on the dorsal and the other on the volar aspect of the cleft. This can be partially avoided by cutting a liberal, rounded redundant piece projecting from each side of the graft, so that there will be plenty of depth to the cleft and much slack skin on the volar and the dorsal aspects. However, the pointed double flap method is better.

Before the skin grafts are applied, the hand should be immobilized on a well-padded skeleton hand splint which gives free access to the clefts. The fingertips are held to the splint by adhesive or a stainless steel wire suture. The grafts are sutured in place with 4/0 or 5/0

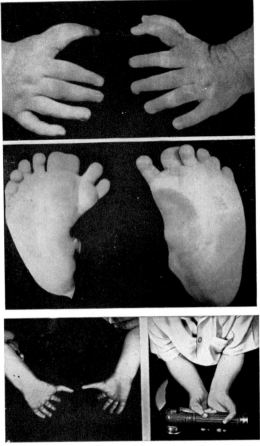

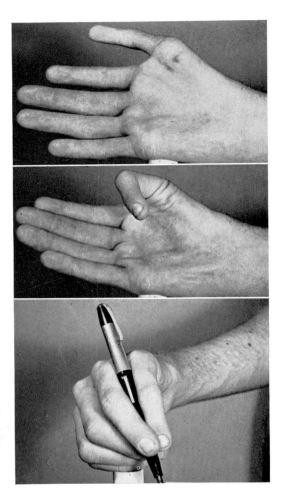

FIG. 106. Case D. O. (*Top*) Polydactylism of all 4 extremities. Instead of a thumb, there are, as often happens, 2 fingers, each with 3 phalanges. (*Center*) The feet of the same patient. (*Bottom, left*) The supernumerary digits have been removed. (*Bottom, right*) Showing grasping ability of the thumbs.

FIG. 107. Five-fingered hand. Independent action of the radially placed finger and good function.

plain catgut, and the digit is wound spirally with a coarse mesh gauze to provide even firm pressure. This material is sutured in place. A separate layer of nonadherent gauze is placed over the area, and dressings are applied. Even pressure is maintained with steel wool pads. One should never hold the fingers apart by wax, sponge rubber or other pads for fear of pressure necrosis. The fingers are held apart by the splint; the dressings are merely applied. Following thick skin grafts, splinting should be prolonged one to several months to avoid contracture from irritation of early movement. Children's joints do not stiffen readily. On wrapping the hand and the splint, both should be enclosed in a plaster-of-Paris casing that extends up the arm to the axilla with the elbow at a right angle. The fingertips must be available for inspection of the state of circulation.

When a double nail is split, a strip of the cut border should be removed, including a similar width of the matrix, and the skin reshaped around the nail edge by swinging a pointed flap from the side of the pulp around

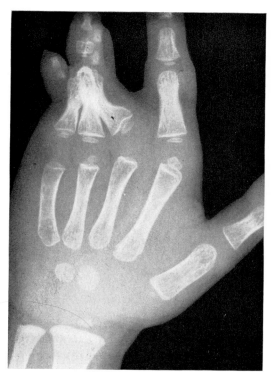

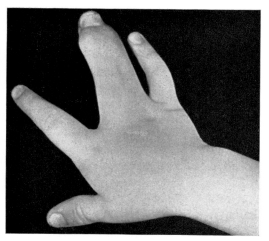

FIG. 110. Syndactylism with fusion of terminal phalanges and a common nail.

FIG. 108. Synostosis of proximal phalanges of 3 fingers.

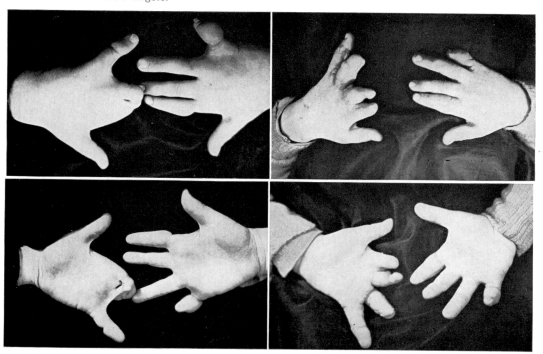

FIG. 109. Case H. L. (*Left*) Acrosyndactylism. (*Right*) Postoperative view. Right hand: annular grooves were corrected by zigzag plastics and redundant tissue was excised. Left hand: the groove around the little finger was corrected. The fingers were separated, determining the depth of each cleft by suturing points of skin across it. The sides of the fingers were skin-grafted.

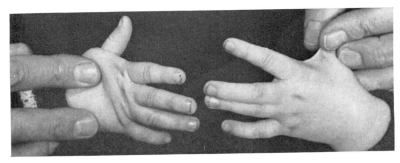

FIG. 111. Syndactylism of middle and ring fingers with shallow first cleft.

the angle of the nail. The same is done for secondary repair of scars on the side of a nail.

When 2 fingers are joined together broadly, there may be a common tendon, nerve and vessel. Joint capsules will be deficient on the open side, and the circulation may be jeopardized if both sides of such a digit are operated on at once. Thus, in badly fused fingers, it may be necessary to operate on only one at a time. If there is only one tendon, it should go to the better finger, and a tendon graft placed in

the other later. The single nerve should go to the radial side if in the index, the middle or the ring finger and to the ulnar side if in the little finger. If the joints will be left without a capsule on one side, it is better not to operate on the fingers but to leave them double— especially if there is good function.

The age at which to operate is important. Infant fingers are short, and the rate of growth is greatest in the first and early years. A scar made along the side may contract as the finger

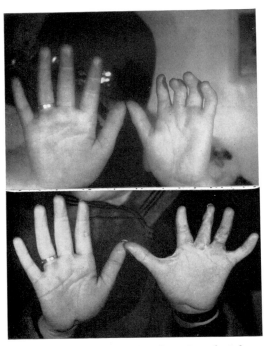

FIG. 112. Brachyphalangia and syndactylism, with contractures from incomplete operation. (*Bottom*) Corrected surgically.

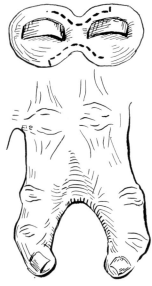

FIG. 113. **Incorrect** operation for webbed fingers. There is not sufficient skin, and the linear scar down one finger and up the next is later drawn by contraction from a long V to a short U, reproducing the web and distorting the fingers in rotary and flexion contracture, as shown in the lower illustration. (J. Bone Joint Surg. *14*:44)

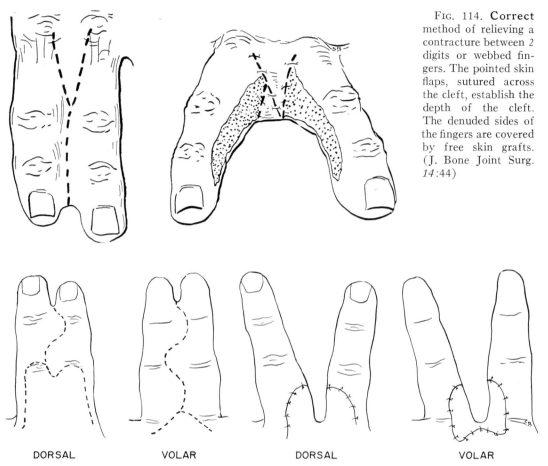

FIG. 114. **Correct** method of relieving a contracture between 2 digits or webbed fingers. The pointed skin flaps, sutured across the cleft, establish the depth of the cleft. The denuded sides of the fingers are covered by free skin grafts. (J. Bone Joint Surg. *14*:44)

DORSAL   VOLAR   DORSAL   VOLAR

FIG. 115. Pantaloon method of correcting syndactylism, establishing depth of the cleft when only 2 fingers are webbed. A broad pants-shaped flap is raised from the dorsum and laid across the cleft to establish its depth. A pointed volar flap is raised to fit into the notch so as not to have a suture line paralleling the web. The remainder of the web is severed by a wavy line, the volar incision corresponding to the dorsal one to avoid a linear scar. Such skin flaps as possible are sutured and the remaining denudations are covered by whole thickness or thick split grafts.

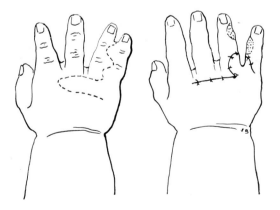

FIG. 116. Method of repairing syndactylism when only one cleft is involved. A transverse flap is raised from the redundant dorsum of the hand and laid across the cleft. The fingers are separated by a wavy incision, front and back. As much skin is sutured directly around each finger as possible, and the remainder of the denudation is skin-grafted (*dotted areas*).

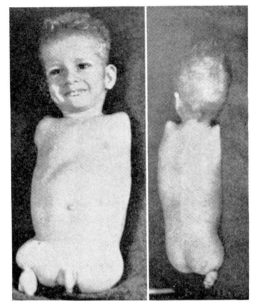

FIG. 117. Phocomelia and amelia. The type of deformity reported in the thalidomide cases. (Killingworth, W. P., and Engledon, R.: Amer. J. Dis. Child. 63:916)

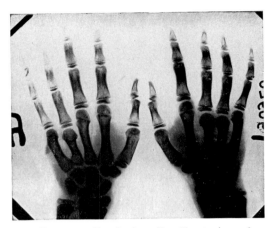

FIG. 119. Brachydactylia. Shortening of several metacarpals, of which the epiphyseal lines appear closed.

grows, just as after a Didot operation, and require one or more plastic operations later. If the fingers are clumped together or limited by inequality of the joint levels, they cannot function and will not develop unless they are

freed. Even the whole arm will be short if the hand cannot function. In this type of defect, operation should be done early, but scars should be so curved that contractures from growth will be lessened. Since scars do not grow as fast as the hand, contractures will develop. If there is good function, the fingers will develop normally, and operation may be delayed until the kindergarten age of 5 or more. The shorter the web and the freer the motion, the better it is to wait until the fingers and the arm attain sufficient size.

BRACHYDACTYLIA

From arrest in development in the embryonic hand, one or all digits may be short. Usually some phalanges or metacarpals are

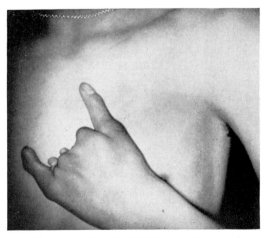

FIG. 118. Case T. M. Frequently, aplasia of the fingers or brachydactylia is associated with absence of the pectoral muscle, as in this case.

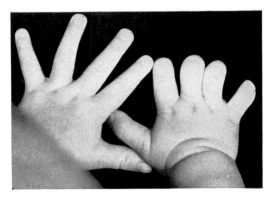

FIG. 120. Brachyphalangia.

short or absent. The distribution of short hand bones may be grouped on either side or in the middle of the hand or across any row of phalanges or of the metacarpals, though most commonly the middle phalanges are involved. Accompanying brachydactylia there is often absence of a part or all of the pectoral muscle.

HYPERPHALANGIA

In contrast with polydactylia or extra fingers is hyperphalangia or an excessive number of phalanges in a digit. The digit may be of normal length. The thumb is commonly affected, having 3 instead of 2 phalanges. Variation in the number of phalanges is common in vertebrates and can be expected as a frequent anomaly.

SYMPHALANGIA

Here the defect is in the development of the finger joints, there being bony or fibrous fusion between the phalanges. This is end-to-end fusion of phalanges contrasted with synostosis which is side-to-side fusion. Drinkwater traced this condition through 14 generations.

ARACHNODACTYLIA

The hand is long and slender with long slender fingers suggesting the legs of a spider; the phalanges and the metacarpals are excessively long, and the fingers are held in flexion as if the bones exceeded the tendons in length. Other long bones in the body are also elongated and thin, and these long bones may be affected alone without elongation of hands or feet. The condition is suggestive of endocrine disturbance, such as achondroplasia or fragilitas ossium (marble bone with blue sclera); several times the latter condition has been found in association.

The spider hand is only a part of a syndrome; these people, from laxity of ligaments, are double-jointed and clumsy. The lens of the eye dislocates. They are tall, slender and weak, have underdeveloped musculature and

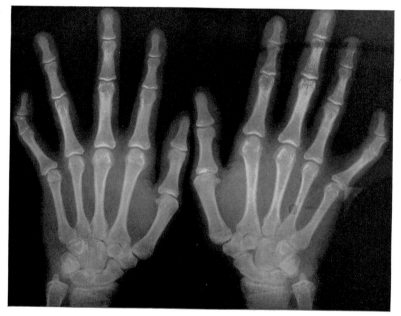

FIG. 121. Brachydactylia of little finger. Hypoplasia of the middle phalanx of the little finger is most commonly associated with mongolian idiocy. It is seen occasionally in cretins, achondroplastic dwarfs, normals and in progressive myositis ossificans. This 13-year-old girl also exhibits the long, slender radiants of arachnodactyly. She did have kyphoscoliosis, but further facts are lacking. (R. R. Schreiber, M.D., Los Angeles Orthopaedic Hospital)

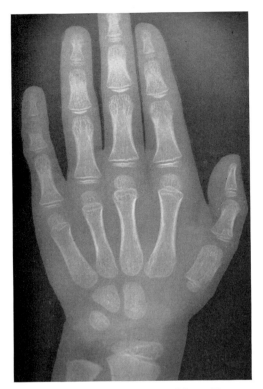

FIG. 122. Progressive myositis ossificans. Hypoplasia of the thumb metacarpal and congenital deformities of the great toes are unaccountably found in a majority of cases. This 6-year-old boy developed massive extraskeletal ossification of the trunk. Shown here are hypoplasia of the thumb metacarpal and a conical or "push-up" epiphysis of the proximal phalanx of the thumb, the latter of no known significance. (R. R. Schreiber, M.D., Los Angeles Orthopaedic Hospital)

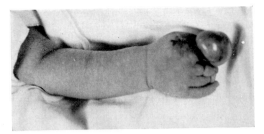

FIG. 123. Case Baby A, aged 6 months. Several annular defects in the fingers and the toes. In the right index finger, the lymphatic return is so obstructed that an amputation of this plumlike, red, edematous end was necessary. Z-plasties were done on the ring finger, one side at a time.

may have infantilism, congenital heart disease, scoliosis, kyphosis or pigeon breast.

ANNULAR GROOVES AND CONGENITAL AMPUTATIONS

These are ring-shaped defects and do not arise from intra-uterine adhesions or amniotic bands. They may be shallow in the skin and the subcutaneous tissues only or may involve the deep fascia or be to any depth. They are single or multiple and often occur in the central or the lower part of the forearm and high in the upper arm. They may occur in a finger, or there may be a rudiment of a finger separated from the hand by a groove. If a ring is shallow, it causes edema of the part distal to it, but if deep it may so constrict the limb during embryonic growth that actual amputation results, and granulation tissue or a scar terminates the stump. The causative factor must have been present before the 8th week of development.

Treatment is for cosmetic reasons and to relieve the distal edema. Merely excising the tissues of the groove and suturing the skin borders together fails, because the circular scar contracts, reproducing the constriction. Instead, after excising the tissues of the groove one should create as broad and as long an approximation of subcutaneous tissue and skin as possible by making diagonal cuts alternately in each skin margin to the deep fascia and undermining the skin and the subcutaneous tissue for a distance in the plane between the deep and the superficial fascia. The skin and the whole thickness of subcutaneous tissue are brought together broadly and crowned, so that a zigzag juncture is made. This succeeds by avoiding a circular constricting scar and furnishes maximal area of contact for re-establishing lymphatics. It is safer to work in 2 or 3 stages when the entire circumference of the digit or the arm is involved.

DYSCHONDROPLASIA

The metacarpals and the phalanges may show effects of symmetrical aberrant growth, such as being short, curved, with thick, irregular ends with multiple, knobby exostoses and deformities of joint surfaces, causing distor-

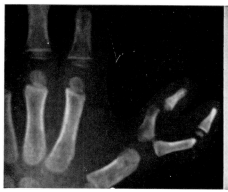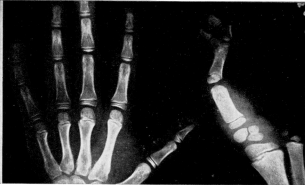

FIG. 124. Bifid thumbs. (*Left*) Equal twinning of the proximal joint. (*Right*) Asymmetrical twinning of the proximal phalanx and absence of all other digits.

tion. This condition does not show itself at first, but, being a defect in the parts about the epiphysial plate, it becomes evident as the child grows. It is not confined to the hand but affects the bones throughout the body. It is hereditary and associated with other congenital deformities, of which it is just another type.

MEGALODACTYLIA

This uncommon deformity consists of hyperplastic, giant overgrowth of one or several of the digits. It usually involves the index or the middle finger or the thumb, but usually not the metacarpals. It is not commonly associated with other deformities, is seldom bilateral and usually is not hereditary. In some cases it is due to bony overgrowth with normal-appearing soft parts; in others it results more from abnormal excess of fat, lymphatic and fibrous tissue, like a tumor. Large neurofibromata have been found in these digits frequently enough to suggest a causal nerve trophic effect on the overgrowth. Megalodactylia may be associated with lymphangioma or hemangioma due to the excessive blood and lymph supply.

When the deformity is too unsightly, amputation is indicated. A giant finger may be amputated, including its metacarpal; if a central ray is involved, the hand is narrowed by jogging the marginal ray into its place. The abnormal fat and fibrous tissue may be reduced in size by multiple excisions, and an attempt to limit bone growth can be made by destroying the epiphyses.

ARTERIOVENOUS ABNORMALITIES

Arteriovenous angioma may be congenital in the hand and may be progressive, leading to amputation. The vessels and multiple communications between the arterial and the venous systems may be demonstrated by arteriograms. Amputation of the affected part may be necessary if it is a terminal part, such as a finger.

Other vascular anomalies such as hemangiomata are discussed in Chapter 19, Tumors.

In the hand usually one can dissect these out completely. If involved skin or other affected tissue is preserved, there may be difficulty in healing. Skin grafts may be necessary.

KNUCKLE PADS

Knobs on the dorsum of the fingers opposite the middle joints are not rare. They may

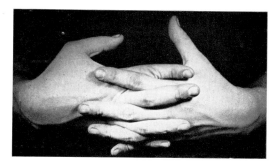

FIG. 125. Congenital absence of the extensor pollicis longus.

be the size of a bean and may appear on a few or all of these joints. On palpation they appear to be on the bone but on dissection are seen to be composed of thickening of all the tissues, the ligamentous capsule of the joint and skin. For this reason it is difficult to remove them. The ligament and the undersurface of the skin may be pared thin, but removal is unsatisfactory.

Considering that the anthropoid apes walk on these knuckles and have these pads, atavistic occurrence in the human is not at all surprising. Some have considered that they are caused by trauma. They are often associated with Dupuytren's contracture.

PRINCIPLES OF TREATMENT OF CONGENITAL DEFORMITIES

Many deformities such as segmental defects, brachydactylia and arachnodactylia cannot be benefited by treatment.

Deformities of the hand are often only a part of the problem. Other congenital lesions may be present but not yet apparent. Ivy reported that of all live births with congenital defects, 17 per cent died during the first year. When a defect is present from birth the compensatory adaptability is tremendous, and a physical defect may so direct or stimulate mental activities that the individual may succeed in life even better than if his pursuits had been along physical lines.

If the appearance of a conspicuously deformed hand can be improved, it is well to do it before 5 or 6—before schooling starts—for the parents' sake and to ward off complexes in the child, because of cruel ridicule from other children. Thus, angulations can be corrected by splinting, supernumerary digits removed, ugly, wide clefts narrowed, and simple webbing removed.

Special treatment has been mentioned for each of the individual deformities so that what follows concerns principles in general.

As a rule, function takes precedence over appearance. To obtain maximal function, the limb should be aligned so that it can be used, and one or more digits should be made to be opposable pincers for grasping. In deformities with digits bound together, as clump-hands, or when in syndactylia the joints do not coincide for bending or the clefts are too narrow

or too wide for grasping, or the digits do not oppose enough to hold objects, the hand will fail to develop properly. Early development in the growing age is so important that surgical corrections to give function should be done early in such cases. If, however, the deformity is such as to allow adequate function, it is best to defer operation until the age of 6 or more.

The rate of growth of digits and hands is so great from infant to adolescent life that longitudinal scars made in infancy will not grow as rapidly as the rest of the digit or the hand. If incisions must be made in infancy, they should be transverse or widely zigzagged to allow for growth, instead of being longitudinal with the finger or the limb.

Whenever possible, conservative treatment is best in infancy, surgery being delayed until bone centers have developed and the hands are larger. By prolonged mild splinting or frequent applications of plaster of Paris, many deformed limbs can be gradually straightened and held so until they grow straight. Deformities, a defect of a forearm bone or dyschondroplasia can be held in check.

Roentgen studies should always be made. Ossification centers may be delayed in appearing. Films of the other hand or a normal hand of the same age should be compared. See Chapter 2 for normal ossification times.

A defect is a defect. It is impossible to replace parts that are missing, and there is no natural tendency to grow them. We may build a post for a thumb for the fingers to work against, but usually one can merely modify for better cosmesis and function those parts that are already there.

First, the deformity must be overcome; if this cannot be done by splinting, surgery on the soft parts is needed. As the soft parts—muscles, tendons and nerves—may share in the defect with the bones, these must be freed, divided or transferred as required. Skin grafts may be necessary. Tendon lengthening, rather than tenotomy, preserves the tendons for function. In realigning bones to straighten limbs or make digits opposable, cuneiform or rotary osteotomy is used, and bone grafts may be needed. In the absence of a thumb, a digit, usually the index finger, can be pollicized, transferring it on its neurovascular pedicle and with tendons intact. A finger used for a thumb will be too long. Therefore, the epiphyses on each side of the metacarpophalangeal joint should be eradicated. It is not enough to remove a small piece on each side of the plate; the whole plate should be curetted out through an incision on each side. The cavity may be filled with cancellous bone or chipped-up pieces from the adjoining bone.

For mirror hand one should retain 4 fingers and use one of the others for a thumb, selecting the fingers carefully. Osteotomy of a finger so as to parallel the others, and of the digit selected to be the thumb to oppose them, may be done. By filleting the fingers to be removed, enough skin for a thumb cleft and a pseudothenar eminence can be obtained.

In the absence of fingers, the metacarpals may be phalangized, using skin grafts for covering. A cleft may need widening by a plastic zigzag or a skin graft, or widely divergent digits may be brought nearer by excising the intervening obstructions, such as a cross-lying supernumerary metacarpal. If a supernumerary marginal or central digit is removed, its tendons should be spared for transfer to wherever they may be needed, as to another digit for tendon loop or tendon-T transfer to furnish adduction, or for a pulley transfer for opposition. A finger should not be removed if the adjoining one will be damaged and its function impaired.

To protect growth, in operations on bones in the young one should keep away from the epiphyses and delay arthroplasties to adult age, as excessive growth makes them unsatisfactory in children. Pedicled skin grafts are not suitable for infants. However, a free skin graft of the split-thickness type is satisfactory. Infant skin is thin; therefore, the dermatome graft of 0.010 to 0.012 at this age may remove the full thickness. Full-thickness grafts are seldom required but can be obtained from the antecubital fossa more readily and more satisfactorily than from the abdomen. Small split grafts are taken from the inner side of the forearm. Grafts from these two areas are of better color and consistency than those from the inguinal region.

Surgical correction of most congenital deformities of the hand requires multiple stage operations, often the last one being performed during adolescence. An understanding of this at the onset of treatment prevents many misunderstandings and creates better relations with the parents and the patient.

BIBLIOGRAPHY

Albaugh, C. H.: Congenital anomalies following maternal rubella in early weeks of pregnancy, J.A.M.A. *129*:719, 1945.

Albee, F. H.: Formation of radius congenitally absent; condition seven years after implantation of bone graft, Ann. Surg. *87*:105, 1928.

Alonso, S.: Supernumerary forearm and hand; complete aplasia of corresponding clavicle—surgical therapy, Rev. méd. Rosario *29*:786, 1939.

Bagg, H. J.: Etiology of certain congenital structural defects, Am. J. Obst. Gynec. *8*:131, 1924.

————: Hereditary abnormalities of the limbs; their origin and transmission, Am. J. Anat. *43*:167, 1929.

Bardeen, C. R., and Lewis, W. H.: Development of the limbs, body wall and back of man, Am. J. Anat. *1*:1, 1901.

Bardenheuer, B.: Verh. Deutsch. Ges. Chir. *23*:85, 1894.

Barsky, A. J.: Congenital anomalies of the hand, J. Bone Joint Surg. *33-A*:35, 1951.

————: Congenital Anomalies of the Hand and Their Surgical Treatment, Springfield, Ill., Thomas, 1958.

Bellelli, F.: Bilateral tri-phalangeal thumb, Riforma med. *55*:1001, 1939.

Birch-Jensen, A.: Congenital deformities of the upper extremities, Copenhagen, Munksgard, 1949.

Boppe, M., and Faugeron, P.: Treatment of syndactylias by total free skin graft, Paris med. *1*:522, 1939.

Brucer, M.: The great fallout controversy (editorial), J.A.M.A. *179*:66, 1962.

Caral, W. L. L., Prakken, J. R., and von Zwijudogt, H. A.: Knuckle pads—two cases, Acta dermat.-venereol. *21*:87, 1940.

Cohn, B. N. E.: True oxycephaly with syndactylism, Am. J. Surg. *68*:93, 1945.

Cohn, I.: Skeletal disturbances and anomalies, Radiology *18*:592, 1932.

Davidson, A. J., and Horwitz, M. T.: Congenital clubhand deformity associated with absence of radius; its surgical correction; case report, J. Bone Joint Surg. *21*:462, 1939.

Davison, E. P.: Congenital hypoplasia of the carpal scaphoid bone, J. Bone Joint Surg. *44-B*:816, 1962.

Drinkwater, H.: Phalangeal anarthrosis (synostosis ankylosis) transmitted through fourteen generations, Proc. Roy. Soc. Med. *10*:60, 1916-1917.

Duraiswami, P. K.: Experimental causation of congenital skeletal defects and its significance in orthopedic surgery, J. Bone Joint Surg. *34-B*: 646, 1952.

————: Comparison of congenital defects induced in developing chickens by certain teratogenic agents with those caused by insulin, J. Bone Joint Surg. *37-A*:277, 1955.

Entin, M. A.: Reconstruction of congenital abnormalities of the upper extremities, J. Bone Joint Surg. *41-A*:681, 1959.

Fischer, F. J., and VanDemark, R. E.: Bilateral symmetrical brachymetacarpalia and brachymetatarsalia, report of a case, J. Bone Joint Surg. *27*:145, 1945.

Flatt, A. E.: Treatment of syndactylism, Plast. Reconstr. Surg. *29*:336, 1962.

Fox, M. J., and Bortin, M. M.: Rubella in pregnancy causing malformation in newborn, J.A.M.A. *130*:568, 1946.

Frantz, C. H., and O'Rahilly, R.: Congenital skeletal limb deficiencies, J. Bone Joint Surg. *43-A*: 1202, 1961.

Greenthal, R. M.: Congenital malformation in infant caused by rubella early in pregnancy, Arch. Pediat. *62*:53, 1945.

Haas, S. L.: Three-phalangeal thumbs, Am. J. Roentgenol. *42*:677, 1939.

————: Bilateral complete syndactylism of all fingers, Am. J. Surg. *50*:363, 1940.

Hall, C. B., Brooks, M. B., and Dennis, J. F.: Congenital skeletal deficiencies of the extremities, J.A.M.A. *181*:590, 1962.

Hanley, T.: Congenital deformity of the carpus associated with maldevelopment of certain thenar muscles, J. Bone Joint Surg. *39-B*:458, 1957.

Harrison, R. G., Pearson, M. A., and Roaf, R.: Ulnar dimelia, J. Bone Joint Surg. *42-B*:549, 1960.

Hefner, R. A.: Crooked little fingers, minor streblomicrodactyly, J. Hered. *32*:37, 1941.

Hegdekatti, R. M.: Congenital malformation of hands and feet in man, J. Hered. *30*:191, 1939.

Heikel, H. V. A., Aplasia and Hypoplasia of the Radius, Supp. 39, Acta Orthopedica Scandinavica, 1959.

Henry, M. G.: Anomalous fusion of the scaphoid and the greater multangular bone, Arch. Surg. *50*:240, 1945.

Hill, L. L., Jr.: Congenital abnormalities—phocomelus and congenital absence of radius, Surg., Gynec. Obstet. *65*:475, 1937.

Hodgson, A. R.: Congenital retardation in development of carpal navicular, first metacarpal and styloid process of radius, Brit. J. Surg. *31*:95, 1943.

Huber, J.: Multilating gangrene of fingers of

infant three weeks old, Bull. Soc. pédiat. Paris *37*:54, 1939.

Hucherson, D. C.: The Darrach operation for lower radio-ulnar derangement, Am. J. Surg. *53*:237, 1941.

Humphries, S. V.: Congenital proximal radio-ulnar synostosis, S. Afr. M. J. *15*:486, 1941.

Ivy, R. H.: Congenital anomalies, Plast. Reconstr. Surg. *20*:400, 1957.

Johnson, H. M.: Congenital cicatrizing bands; report of a case with etiologic observations, Am. J. Surg. *52*:498, 1941.

Kanavel, A. B.: Congenital malformation of the hands, Arch. Surg. *25*:1; 1932; *25*:282, 1932.

Kato, K.: Congenital absence of radius, J. Bone Joint Surg. *6*:589, 1924.

Katzeff, M.: Arhrogrypsis multiplex congenita, Arch. Surg. *46*:673, 1943.

Kelly, J. W.: Mirror hand, Plast Reconstr. Surg. *30*:374, 1962.

Killingsworth, W. P., and Engledon, R.: Congenital absence of the four extremities, Am. J. Dis. Child. *63*:914, 1942.

Kite, J. H.: Congenital deformities, Arch. Surg. *49*:126, 1944.

————: Congenital deformities, Arch. Surg. *51*: 177, 1945.

Lapidus, P. W., Guidotti, F. P., and Coletti, C. J.: Triphalangel thumb; report of six cases, Surg., Gynec. Obstet. *77*:178, 1943.

Lapidus, P. W., and Guidotti, F. P.: Triphalangeal bifid thumb; report of six cases, Arch. Surg. *49*:228, 1944.

Levin, B.: Gonadal dysgenesis, Am. J. Roentgenol. *87*:1116, 1962.

Lewin, P.: Congenital defects of long bones of extremities, Am. J. Roentgenol. *4*:431, 1917.

MacCollum, D. W.: Webbed fingers, Surg., Gynec. Obstet. *71*:782, 1940.

Mead, N. G., Lithgow, W. C., and Sweeney, H. J.: Arthrogryposis multiplex congenita, J. Bone Joint Surg. *40-A*:1285, 1958.

Meyerding, H. W.: Correction of congenital deformities of the hand, Am. J. Surg. *44*:218, 1939.

Moore, B. H.: Macrodactyly and associated peripheral nerve changes, J. Bone Joint Surg. *24*:617, 1942.

————: Peripheral-nerve changes associated with congenital deformities, J. Bone Joint Surg. *24*:282, 1944.

Morrison, J. E.: Aetiology of congenital abnormalities, Ulster M. J. *14*:1, 1945.

Nylen, B.: Repair of congenital finger syndactyly, Acta chir. scand. *113*:310, 1957.

Olcott, C. T.: Arachnodactyly (Marfan's syndrome), with severe anemia, Am. J. Dis. Child. *60*:660, 1940.

O'Rahilly, R.: Radial hemimelia and the functional anatomy of the carpus, J. Anat. *80*:181, 1946.

————: An analysis of cases of radial hemimelia, Arch. Path. *44*:28, 1947.

————: Morphological patterns in limb deficiencies and duplications, Am. J. Anat. *88*:135, 1951.

————: A survey of carpal and tarsal anomalies, J. Bone Joint Surg. *35-A*:626, 1953.

O'Rahilly, R., Gardner, E. J., and Gray, D. J.: The skeletal development of the hand, Clin. Orthop. *13*:42, 1959.

Osbeck, F.: Therapy of "knuckle pads" with carbon dioxide snow, Dermat. Wschr. *110*:457, 1940.

Patterson, T. J. S.: Congenital ring constrictions, Brit. J. Plast. Surg. *14*:1, 1961.

Pino, R. H., Cooper, E. L., and Van Wien, S.: Arachnodactyly and status dysraphicus, a review, Ann. Int. Med. *10*:1130, 1937.

Riordan, D. C.: Congenital absence of the radius, J. Bone Joint Surg. *37-A*:1129, 1955.

Rocher, H. L.: Absence of hand, Jour. méd. Bordeaux *116* (pt. 2):115, 1939.

Rushforth, A. F.: A congenital abnormality of the trapezium and first metacarpal bone, J. Bone Joint Surg. *31-B*:543, 1949.

Sachs, M.D.: Familial brachyphalangy, Radiology *35*:622, 1940.

Shafar, J.: Hereditary short digits (with report of two cases of chondroosteodystrophy), Brit. J. Radiol. *14*:396, 1941.

Smith, S., and Boulgakoff, B.: Case of polydactylia showing certain atavistic characters, J. Anat. *58*:359, 1924.

Snedicor, S. T.: Surgical problems in hereditary polydactylism and syndactylism, J.A.M.A. *114*:2542, 1940.

————: Surgical problems in hereditary polydactylism and syndactylism, J. Med. Soc. New Jersey *27*:443, 1940.

Starr, D. E.: Congenital absence of the radius; a method of surgical correction, J. Bone Joint Surg. *27*:572, 1945.

Stein, H. C., and Bettmann, E. H.: Rare malformation of arm, Am. J. Surg. *50*:336, 1940.

Stenstrom, J. D.: Congenital malformations of extremities, Canad. M. A. J. *51*:325, 1944.

Stiles, K. A., and Dougan, P.: Pedigree of malformed upper extremities showing variable dominance, J. Hered. *31*:65, 1940.

Stochard, C. R.: Developmental rate and structural expression, an experimental study of twins, double monsters and single deformities and the interaction among embryonic organs during their origin and development, Am. J. Anat. *28*:114, 1920-1921.

Taussig, H. B.: A study of the German outbreak of phocomelia, J.A.M.A. *180*:1106, 1962.

Thomas, H. B.: Agnogenic congenital clubbing of fingers, Am. J. M. Sci. *2-3*:241, 1942.

Timoney, F. X.: Macrodactyly; case, Ann. Surg. *119*:144, 1944.

Touraine, A.: Origin of congenital defects—syphilis, heredity or induction, Progrès Méd. *74*:30, 1946.

Vaidya, D. R.: Amelia, Indian Med. Gaz. *74*:286, 1939.

Warkany, J.: Congenital malformations induced by maternal nutritional deficiency, J. Pediat. *25*:476, 1944.

————: Factors in etiology of congenital malformations, Am. J. Ment. Defic. *50*:231, 1945.

Warkany, J., and Nelson, R. C.: Skeletal abnormalities in the offspring of rats reared on deficient diets, Anat. Rec. *79*:83, 1941.

Warkany, J., and Schraffenberger, E.: Congenital malformations induced in rats by maternal nutritional deficiency; preventive factor—(riboflavin), J. Nutrition *27*:477, 1944.

Whitman, A.: Congenital elevation of scapula and paralysis of serratus magnus muscle, J.A.M.A. *99*:1332, 1932.

Woodward, J. W.: Congenital elevation of the scapula, J. Bone Joint Surg. *43-A*:219, 1961.

Zadek, I.: Congenital absence of extensor pollicis longus of both thumbs; operation and cure, J. Bone Joint Surg. *16*:432, 1934.

Zumoff, B.: Congenital symmetrical finger contractures, J.A.M.A. *155*:437, 1954.

Chapter 4

Examination of the Hand

The examination of a hand may be part of a diagnostic investigation, a study of current compared with past condition, or an evaluation of functional impairment prior to disability evaluation. Whatever the reason for the examination, accuracy in observation and recording is essential. Descriptions of the hand should be detailed and specific. Ambiguous or vague terms should be avoided, and clear, definite statements used. Motions are measured, not estimated; and a uniform method of mensuration is used, so that valid comparisons are possible. Use of terms such as good, poor, moderate, severe and slight are avoided when some objective measurable quantity can be used. Impaired flexion of a finger should be described in terms of how much the pulp lacks of flexing to touch a specific area of the palm or as the actual range of motion of the joints measured with a goniometer.

HISTORY

For diagnosis, examination begins with the history. The date of accident or onset is noted, followed by questions as to what happened, what was the injuring force or object and how was it applied, what was the position of the hand when struck and what other parts were injured. The immediate effect of the injury is recorded. Was there swelling, ecchymosis, bleeding or deformity? What loss of function was noted? Was there pain? If so, where was it specifically? What was done by the patient? What type of first aid was given? The time of hospitalization and the time away from work give indications of the severity of the injury and the motivation of the patient. Detailed records of any operation are necessary, including what was done and by whom. Roentgenograms, laboratory reports and photographs of the parts from the time of injury to examination aid in filling out the details. If infection followed the original wound, reports of bacteriologic studies should be available. The time of final healing indicates the amount of scar.

An account of the past history, including illness, previous accidents or previous operations, should not be omitted. Any systemic disease that might influence the possibility of reconstruction should be noted. Inquiry as to the condition of the hand before the accident is important. Lastly, we should know whether the patient is right- or left-handed and what are his hobbies as well as his specific occupational requirements for function.

A disability of the hand with gradual onset and without any specific traumatic incident often presents a difficult diagnostic problem. The history in these patients is extremely important. Underlying systemic diseases such as diabetes, gout and arthritis are often manifested in the hand. Careful questioning may elicit some unusual use of the hand which acted as the inciting agent or the history of some degenerative process which has finally reached a point where ordinary use becomes an abnormal strain. Tendons worn by passing over roughened bony prominences or weakened by synovial disease may rupture with ordinary motions. Careful evaluation of an alleged injury must be made, as it is a human failure to relate the presence of swellings of any kind to trauma. Every man with the palmar fascial thickening of Dupuytren tries to related his disease to the use of a hand tool or the handle of a golf club.

Although trauma may not be the cause of the patient's whole disability, aggravation of some underlying disease by trauma is possible. Treatment may be possible only for the aggravation, in which case the basic disease process with its disabling factors persists. In these cases the surgeon must be able to distinguish the two causes of the impairment of function so that administrative personnel can apportion the cost of disability properly.

Fig. 126. Motions of the elbow are measured with the long-armed goniometer placed in the midline of the upper arm and the forearm. Full extension is 180°; a 30° loss of extension would be noted as 150°/180°. Flexion is measured as the included angle between the upper arm and the forearm.

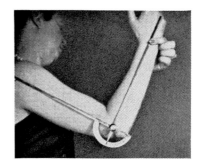

EXAMINATION

WHOLE ARM

Every examination of the hand should start with the shoulder. Long disuse or protection of the hand in a sling may result in inability to raise the arm to the vertical and in limiting external rotation at the shoulder. The ability to raise the arm should be tested in the antero-posterior and the lateral planes, and notes should be made of both internal and external rotation at the shoulder. At the elbow, limitation of extension and flexion and the degree of pronation and of supination should be included. Muscles, tendons, bones, joints, skin and nerves should be checked throughout the arm and especially in the forearm. The size of these muscles is an index of the use of the hand, and local and general atrophy or fibrosis is indicative of special conditions.

OBSERVATION

It is good routine when examining the hand to gain what one can by observation first. Sketches of the hand from various aspects to show scars, deformities and abnormal positions are helpful, and notations on the sketch point out details brought out by palpation or other tests.

This conveys much of the general condition of the hand—posture, deformities and amputations. Observations should include the general trophic condition or state of nutrition of the hand, color, cyanosis, coldness, presence and size of pulse. One should decide whether it is due to strangulation by scar tissue, impoverishment from obstruction of blood or lymph vessels, to some trophic condition from injury of the nerves, or to vaso-motor causes. Wear is an indication of work and should be compared with that in the other hand, as should swelling and edema. Fortunately, there usually is a basis for comparison, as the two hands should be similar.

Among deformities to be noticed is the position of the hand in its various joints. Are the joints in the position of function, and if not, what is the cause? Is flat hand present, with loss of the carpal and metacarpal arches? Does the thumb oppose well, or is it at the side of the hand, and are the proximal finger joints in hyperextension, or are the finger or any other joints in abnormal position?

MOVEMENTS

In testing the movements a conception of what the patient can and cannot do may be gained quickly by first having him, unclothed, perform at command all the normal movements in their full range from the shoulder down. It is best not to touch the patient in

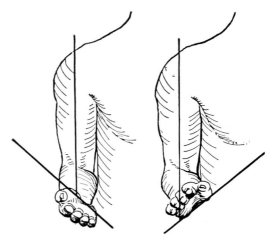

Fig. 127. Pronation and supination are measured with the elbow firmly at the side and at a right angle. The angle between the midline of the upper arm and the plane of the *heel* of the palm is compared with the normal and converted to percentage. Do not be confused by position of the thumb and the fingers.

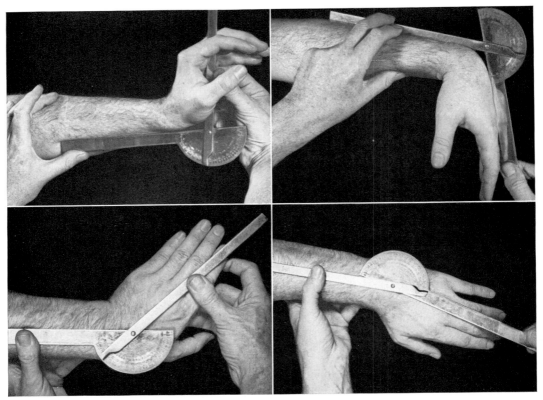

FIG. 128. The 4 motions of the wrist. (*Top, left*) Dorsiflexion of the wrist measured by placing the arms of the goniometer on volar surfaces, with fingers relaxed. (*Top, right*) Palmar or volar flexion is measured, using the dorsum of the forearm and the hand. (*Bottom, left*) Ulnar deviation is determined by the angle between the midline of the forearm and the line from the center of the wrist to the head of the 3rd metacarpal. (*Bottom, right*) In measuring radial deviation the hand must be kept in the true plane of the forearm. Abnormal values are recorded when dorsiflexion is allowed.

this test; with his own limb the physician can show the patient what to do.

The patient is told to do the following: raise the arms vertically, face the palms outwardly and then face the palms inwardly; with arms forward turn palms up and around and return to palms up; circumduct the arm through the normal range; with elbows forming right angles, rotate the shoulders internally and externally, or similarly, for rotation, touch the dorsal spine and the back of the neck, respectively, with the hand; shrug the shoulders; move the scapulae around and lean with the hands against the wall. He is told to flex and extend the elbow; and with his elbow resting on his knee or on a table to turn to the palm-up and then the palm-down positions.

To test the hand, he is instructed to flex the wrist dorsally, volarly, radially and ulnarly; to dorsiflex the wrist and extend the fingers; and to volar flex the wrist with the fist closed. He is told to extend his fingers and to flex them completely. With the fingers he should touch the distal and also the volar parts of the palm and demonstrate lateral motion. He should flex their proximal joints and at the same time extend their distal two. The thumb is put through the complete range of circumduction, from back of the hand to opposition and on to touch the base of the little finger. It is fully extended, fully flexed and made to scrape in the straight position across the palm and to make a strong 0 with the index finger. Knowing the normal ranges, by these tests one can determine quickly just what the patient is unable to do and wherein lies his disability.

The manner of moving is indicative. If he will not try, one suspects malingering. If he cannot make the hand move, a dissociation between hand and mind is suggested. He may be protecting the hand from the pain of causalgia or Sudeck's atrophy, or the dissociation may be from long disuse. Moving of the hand with great tremor and sweating indicates neurosis or vasomotor instability. Accompanying these conditions there is much actual stiffening of the joints.

In recording movements one should give in degrees the angle of flexion and that of extension but should specify in each instance whether it is voluntary or passive. Without this the figures are ambiguous and hence useless. Whenever necessary, the similar measurement in the normal or other hand should be given for comparison, expressing this as numerator and denominator.

Fingers. Movement of the fingers as a whole should be recorded. One can state that each finger lacks so many inches of full extension when measured at the tip. This measurement is taken from a plane surface laid on the dorsum of the hand. Similarly, for flexion we state that each finger lacks so many inches of flexing voluntarily to the distal crease in the palm and so many inches passively. This measurement is taken from the composite distal palmar crease to the nearest part of the pulp of the finger. Roughly, one can express the degree of motion of a finger in the proportion of the arc that the fingertips describe in passing from full extension to full flexion; thus, the fingers may flex through the first two thirds of their normal range of flexion, or in another case may lack their last third of extension.

One should also give in table form, and expressed in degrees, the measurements of each of the individual finger joints. This should be done for both extension and flexion and for voluntary and passive movements, remembering that unless voluntary or passive are specified, measurements are useless. To measure the degree of flexion of a finger joint, the goniometer is laid along the dorsum of the finger each way from the joint. The phalanx proximal to the joint measured is held from moving by the examiner, but care

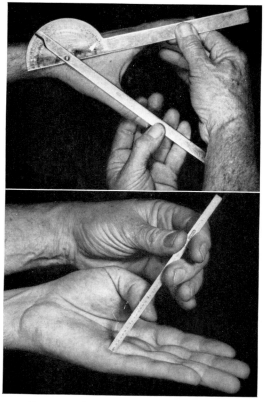

FIG. 129. (*Top*) Abduction of the thumb is designated as the angle between the 1st and the 2nd metacarpals with the thumb spread at right angles to the palm. (*Bottom*) Lack of flexion-adduction is the distance that the thumb lacks of reaching the palm over the head of the 5th metacarpal.

must be taken not to hold this on a strain of extension while the measurement of flexion is being taken, or vice versa, for fear of erroneously recording automatic movements. Flexion of individual joints may be greater, testing each joint separately, than if the joints are measured with the finger as a whole flexed.

Tables are convenient forms on which to record motions of the various joints.

It may be noticed that the fingers flex completely to their bases but do not flex in their proximal joints; or if their proximal joints flex well, the fingers may touch the palm proximally or a certain distance proximal to the distal crease in the palm but may lack so much of touching the distal crease. One can state how far proximal or distal to the distal crease in the palm the fingers touch. To express the practical degree of flexion of fingers one may state something such as the following: "The hand cannot hold 1 or 2 of the examiner's fingers but can grasp 3 of them weakly and 4 of them strongly" or "can grasp 1 or more of the examiner's fingers strongly."

Bones. Note should be made of any deviation from the normal in contour, length and alignment, especially as regards position of function and muscle balance. The bones must be right for correct mechanics. Roentgenograms of hands should be taken in 3 views: anteroposterior, lateral and oblique. Several views of the carpus with the hand in various positions may aid in diagnosis.

Thumb. In describing the thumb, its position with reference to the hand is noted—whether it is at the side or in back of the hand, or in a position forward from it. Measurements are made of limitation of extension, of flexion and adduction and of opposition. Of these, the former is measured by placing the 2 hands palm to palm, with the fingers reaching equally; then the normal thumb is fully extended and bent backward voluntarily. From this the examiner marks a point in space where the injured thumb would be in a similar symmetrical position and measures with a ruler how many inches the thumb lacks of reaching this point both voluntarily and passively. In testing for flexion and adduction, the normal thumb is made to reach as far as it can down the ulnar border of the hand. Measurements then are taken in the injured hand of how far the thumb fails to reach this point.

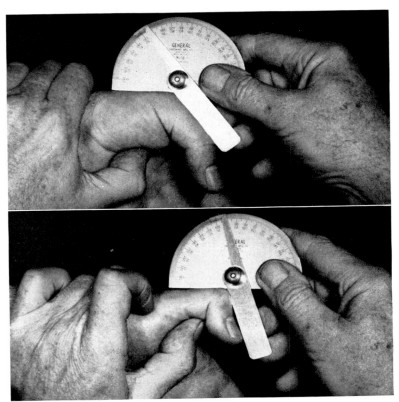

Fig. 130. Flexion of thumb joints. Each joint is stabilized by holding the segment proximal to it in a neutral position and the flexing angle measured on the dorsum of the digit.

Fig. 131. Flexion of the 3 finger joints. (*Top*) For proximal joint flexion the wrist is stabilized by the examiner's hand, and the patient flexes only the proximal joint. If the middle and the distal joints are flexed simultaneously as in making a fist, the proximal joint measurement will be diminished. (*Center*) The proximal phalanx is held firmly, and the patient exerts maximum power on the middle joint. If voluntary flexion is greater when the proximal joint is in flexion than when it is in extension, the intrinsic muscles are contracted. (*Bottom*) Flexion of the distal joint is measured while the 2 proximal joints are held in 180° extension.

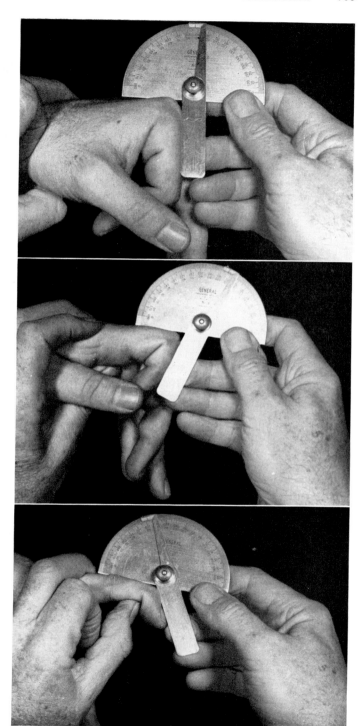

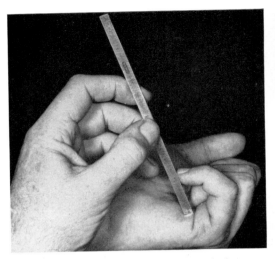

FIG. 132. This left little finger lacks 1 inch of flexing to the distal crease of the palm. Note that it is the point of the pulp where the measurement is taken, not the edge of the nail.

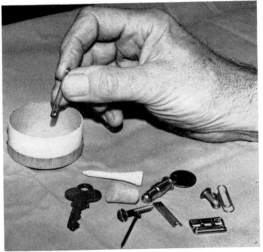

FIG. 134. Moberg's picking-up test. Articles of various shape, size and texture are picked up between the thumb and the fingers, with eyes open and then eyes closed. The loss of tactilegnosis is made readily apparent.

The above are expressed in this way: "The thumb lacks of extension so much and of flexion and adduction so much."

Opposition is expressed in two measurements: one is the farthest distance forward from the hand that the pulp of the thumb will reach when it is opposite the base of the middle finger; or, if it cannot abduct that far, the measurement can be made opposite the base of the index finger. The other is the angle that the nail makes with the palm when so doing. The normal angle is zero in full opposition, as then the nail is parallel with the palm; when the thumb is at the side of the hand, the nail normally is at a right angle to the palm.

The spread of the thumb can be expressed by the angle between the first 2 metacarpals, by the angle that the thumb makes with the radial border of the palm, or by how far the tip of the thumb spreads from the radial border of the palm or the index finger. Measurements are also taken of limitation of both voluntary and passive extension and flexion of both the proximal and the distal joints of the thumb.

In recording limitations of motions of joints, it should be stated whether the joint shows signs of inflammation, such as general tenderness or swelling throughout its circumference, or whether limitation is due to some special adhesion or shortness of capsule which may show by local pain or tenderness. If there is any suspicion of joint or bone trouble, roentgenograms should be taken.

CONTRACTURES

Cicatrices of skin are recorded by measurements of size and by sketches with accurate proportions. The digits and the wrist are bent in the opposite direction to ascertain if the scar whitens on tension and to bring out the lines of tension in the scar where keloids will form. Firmness and degree of fixation of the skin to the firm underparts is tested by attempting to slide the skin, or by having a tendon move beneath the skin while the skin is held. Scars contract, so that one must be alert to the results of this, such as deformity

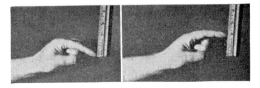

FIG. 133. A graphic way of describing the effective range of motion is to measure the amplitude of motion at the tip of a finger.

Fig. 135. An outside measuring caliper to which 2 steel points have been welded registers the distance between the 2 points when used in the Weber 2-point discrimination test.

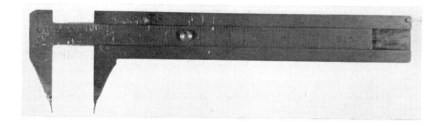

of joints and bones and circumferential strangling of vascular and nerve supply, resulting in defective nutrition and hampering movable parts in general. In a flexion contracture one should ascertain which of the various tissues is causing the contracture. In contractures one should record an estimation of the size of the defect of the skin or the nerve by imagining the amount of extra material necessary to allow the limb to extend fully.

Tendons

Tendons generally can be felt to move beneath the surface, especially if the movement is against resistance. Tests should be made to ascertain whether a tendon is severed or adherent, or perhaps trying to work against an adherent antagonist or to move a stiffened joint. One should test to ascertain if one tendon is adherent to a parallel tendon, such as superficialis to profundus, or whether the tendon bows across the joint from loss of an annular band.

Pain and Tenderness

When pain and tenderness are present, their location and cause can be sought for by straining the parts of the hand in different directions until it is ascertained what particular tissue causes the pain. This may be a tendon, a muscle, a joint, a ligament or a

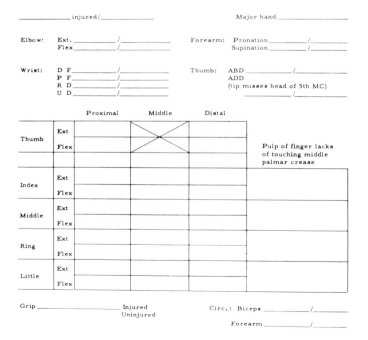

Fig. 136. A chart for recording the measurements of the elbow, the wrist and the hand. Printed forms facilitate recording and easy comparison with former examinations. Using the letter size sheets, the blocks are planned to fit standard typewriter spacing.

bone, or it may prove to be a neuroma or a tender nerve. Activation of a certain muscle may produce the pain either by contracting voluntarily against resistance or by overstretching the muscle passively, indicating the cause of the pain to be at the insertion or origin of the muscle. Or the pain may be located by squeezing bones together, moving them against each other, or by shoving up in turn through the carpus and the bones of each separate ray.

A tender area should be outlined accurately with ink. To do this, the end of the finger or the eraser on a lead pencil approaches the area from all sides, pressing intermittently as it goes, each spot where the tenderness commences being marked with ink.

In testing the grip, one should obtain an average from three trials with each hand without the patient's seeing the instrument. Note should be made whether he is right- or left-handed. Further tests can be made for skill and endurance.

In examining the hand one should cover all tissues, skin, bones, joints, tendons, blood vessels and nerves and not overlook the factors of nutrition, vasomotor changes or functional conditions.

Practical Use

The practical aspects of function for use of the hand in work should always be kept uppermost: the width of the spread for grasp, the opposition of the thumb and the size of the object that can be held. Notes should be made of how much of each finger the thumb can touch and if the joint positions will permit use. Important functions are grasping (1) with the hand as a whole, (2) between the thumb and the fingers and (3) between the palm and the fingers, large and small objects with strength, firmness and agility.

Nerves

Examination should cover the 3 nerves of the hand and their branches for motor, sensory and trophic functions. Areas of anesthesia to light and coarse touch and of analgesia to pinprick should be plotted accurately on sketches as should those of paresthesia, hyposensitiveness and hypersensitiveness and the exact spots of sensitive neuromata.

These simple tests are easy to perform and,

when simply studying the injured hand, are adequate for determining proximal lesions of nerves. If the examination is being done for evaluation of impairment of function, such as is required as a part of disability evaluation, then the functional capacity of the hand must be determined by more detailed and elaborate methods. Sensory disorders, particularly in the median innervated area may seriously impair the prehensile function of the hand. Motions may be almost normal, and protective sensibility as determined by cotton wisp and pinprick may be present, and yet the hand may not be able to function well as a precision gripping mechanism.

Moberg, who has made a special study of this problem, uses the term tactile gnosis for that combination of sensibilities required for useful function. He attempts to evaluate this by testing the gripping function, both for gross and precision sensory grip, and by determining the presence or the absence of protective sensibility. A careful history is elicited of any difficulty at work, and the surface of the hand is observed for signs of wear or areas of lack of use. The ability to button clothes, tie shoe laces, dress and wind a watch are demonstrated. A picking-up test is used, in which the subject picks up between his thumb and fingers and transfers to a container an assortment of small objects, first with one hand, then the other and then with eyes closed. The speed of doing this is measured, and the various surfaces of the digits used are noted. Gross grip is tested on objects of varying size such as a doorknob, a bottle and the handles of tools, such as hammer and axe. Three tests which have been used are the digit writing test, in which numbers are inscribed on the skin surface with a blunt pencil; the coin test (Seddon) in which the subject is asked to distinguish a smoothedged from a milled-edged coin; and the 2-point discrimination test (Weber). Only the last gives results that are more nearly accurate than the picking-up test, but care and skill on the part of the examiner as well as cooperative subject are required. All tests are affected to some degree by subjective factors. A purely objective test, using ninhydrinimpregnated paper to register an impression as a permanent record has been described by Moberg. As a test of recovery after nerve suture, its usefulness is limited, and special care and skill are required in its use.

Motor function is shown in the action of the intrinsic muscles of the hand. Areas of trophic change, due to lack of nerve function, can be outlined by sight and touch. Signs of vasomotor disturbance, such as sweating, pallor, flush, cyanosis, blotchiness and pathologic skin texture, should be included.

Signs of nerve lesions are so typical that often a glance will lead to the diagnosis. Postural deformity, atrophy of muscles and skin, and anesthetic areas are characteristic of lesions of each single nerve, of a combination of nerves, or of the brachial plexus. Ulnar palsy shows the typical clawing of the last 2 fingers, intrinsic atrophy, especially of the 1st interosseus and the hypothenar muscles. Median palsy shows the thumb at the side, atrophy of muscles of opposition, the feel of skin atrophy and anesthetic areas in the median instead of the ulnar distribution. Combined median and ulnar palsy shows atrophy of all of the intrinsic muscles, the thumb at the side, loss of the metacarpal arch, clawing of all fingers, the feel of skin atrophy and an anesthetic area over the whole volar surface. In contrast, radial palsy shows wrist, finger and thumb drop. Muscle atrophy and paralysis up the arm are typical for each nerve, hand paralysis for lower brachial palsy and shoulder paralysis for upper brachial palsy. These gross signs quickly orient the examiner before he makes a studied survey.

DIAGNOSIS

The examination and the diagnosis of a hand take time and thought. A mental impression develops as data is gathered during the survey; at its conclusion one lists as the diagnosis all of the features which are pathologic.

The Lesion May Be Higher

One should not assume that the disability in the hand is always due to changes there; Instead, it may be the result of a general ailment which has an effect on the hand. Various diseases of the spinal cord—such as syringomyelia, poliomyelitis, and the various atrophies of the cord or dystrophies of the muscles—may show themselves in the hand.

It is not unusual for the examiner to direct all his attention to pain or circulatory or nerve changes in the hand, only to find that the difficulty is due to scalenus anticus syndrome, cervical disk, or perhaps an overpulled brachial plexus. The effect of trauma or pressure from a tumor located in the nerves of the arm may produce symptoms in the hand.

Not only should one be alert to the possibility of symptoms in the hand originating elsewhere but, in order to avoid the sin of omission, in the case of injury to a part, one should always seek some other injury incurred at the same time. The diagnosis of conditions in the hand is often obscure, but if any one questionable point is found, it pays to study all its ramifications thoroughly.

Limitation of Movement

Many different factors can limit the normal range of motion of a digit. First, one should determine whether it is voluntary or passive motion that is limited. In the former case, the nerve, the muscle or the tendon that should execute the motion fails to do so. In the case of passive limitation, the trouble may be in the joint itself or in a flexion contracture that hinders the motion; or it may be that the antagonistic tendon or muscle is holding back the motion because it is adherent or too short. In other words, one should determine which is to blame—the activating apparatus or the hold-back apparatus.

If passive motion is greater than voluntary motion, the tendon is not pulling. If passive motion is equal to voluntary motion, the trouble is in the joints or is due to fixation of the opposing tendons or tissues. If voluntary motion is limited and passive motion is complete, the joints and the opposing tendons or tissues are exonerated. However, if voluntary motion is limited and passive motion is also limited but not so much, then both of the above factors are to blame, but the primary trouble is that the tendon does not pull and the joints or the opposing tendons or tissues have become involved secondarily and are contributing to the limitation of motion.

If a digit does not extend voluntarily but can be extended passively, the extensor tendon or tendons are severed or are adherent proximally, or their muscle is injured, or the radial nerve or its posterior interosseous branch is injured. If the tendon is adherent on the dorsum of the hand, the position of the wrist will not affect the lack of extension of the finger; but if it is adherent above the wrist, flexion of the wrist will make the finger extend. If flexion of the proximal finger joint causes extension of the middle finger joint, the extensor tendon is adherent on the dorsum of the hand. This can be tested by holding the proximal joint passively fully flexed. Then the finger extends stiffly in its distal two joints, resisting any attempt to force it into flexion.

If there is neither voluntary nor passive extension of the digits but still the digit can be extended voluntarily if the wrist is flexed, either the flexor tendons or the muscles are too short or are adherent above the wrist. Again, if the digit will not extend voluntarily or passively unless the proximal finger joints are flexed, it can be assumed that adhesions hold the flexor tendons in the palm. If, however, the digit will not extend voluntarily or passively, irrespective of the position of the wrist or the proximal joints, either the finger joints are to blame or there is a flexion contracture within the finger, such as would be caused by adhesions to its flexor tendons or by contracture of the other volar tissues.

If the finger extends well in the proximal joint but poorly voluntarily in the distal 2 joints, although they extend passively, the intrinsic muscles or tendons are to blame—either through severance, adhesions or loss of nerve supply. When fingers will not flex completely on a voluntary basis but do so passively, the flexor tendons are not pulling. However, the intrinsic muscles in the hand still should be able to flex the proximal finger joints unless they, too, are injured. If there is no voluntary flexion at all of the middle or the distal finger joints, the flexor tendons are either severed or adherent, or the trouble lies in the muscle or the nerve supply.

If the adhesions are in the palm or the forearm, flexion of the proximal joints will allow the fingers to be extended. If this has no effect on the extension of the distal 2 joints, the adhesions to the tendon are within the finger, or there is flexion contracture within the finger itself. If the adhesions are in the forearm, the fingers will extend if either the proximal finger joints or the wrist is flexed.

LOCATING POINT OF ADHESION

To locate the point at which a tendon is adherent anywhere from the forearm to the digit, commence proximally. In the case of an extensor, first tense the tendon by holding the wrist passively on a strain in flexion. If the adhesion is above the wrist, the tendon will tense firmly, and the digit cannot be flexed passively. However, it can be flexed readily if the tendon is relaxed by dorsiflexing the wrist. If it is not affected by wrist motion, tense and relax the tendon by flexing and extending the proximal finger joint. If tension limits flexion of the distal 2 joints, and relaxation does not, the adhesion is in the dorsum of the hand. If not, try the middle finger joint to determine if an adhesion over the proximal finger segment limits flexion of the distal 2 joints. An adhesion to a flexor tendon is located in the same way, using the reverse movements of wrist, proximal and middle finger joints in turn, first tensing and then relaxing the tendon proximally. Where an adhesion is present, the tension produced will be so firm that there will be no slack for motion distally.

JOINT STIFFNESS

If, when in full flexion, the fingertips touch the bases of the fingers or the distal end of the palm only but cannot touch the remainder of the palm, the proximal finger joints may be to blame, or the extensor tendons are adherent, or the intrinsic muscles of the hand which should flex these proximal joints are not functioning. The usual cause for limitation of passive flexion of these proximal joints is contracture of their collateral ligaments from prolonged immobilization of these joints in the straight position, especially in the presence of inflammation, edema or reaction from trauma. If, when the fingers flex, their tips touch the proximal portion of the palm but cannot flex to the distal crease in the palm, then the middle or the distal joints, or both—or limitation of excursion of the flexor or the extensor tendons—are to blame.

THUMB LIMITATION

Limitation of spread of the thumb from the hand is usually due to the accumulation and the contraction of scar tissue between the first 2 metacarpals as the effect of trauma, infection in the thenar space or ischemic contracture of intrinsic muscles. If there is loss of voluntary opposition of the thumb, but this is present passively, the median nerve is injured, affecting its motor thenar branch, or the opponens pollicis and the flexor brevis pollicis muscles have been injured. If the thumb does not oppose either voluntarily or passively, the cause may be cicatricial adhesions between the first 2 metacarpals, a dorsal scar or fixation by adhesions of the tendon of the extensor pollicis longus muscle. It also may be due to ankylosis of the carpometacarpal joint, or it may be postural as part of a flat hand from flat splinting. If the base of the thenar eminence rides forward and there is not proper muscular control of the thumb, the tendon of the abductor pollicis longus has been severed, or the hand has been displaced backward by a midcarpal dislocation.

If a thumb extends forward in the palm and cannot be brought to a position to the side of and behind the hand, the cause may be holding back by cicatrix of the thenar eminence, cicatrix between the first 2 metacarpals, a midcarpal or a carpometacarpal dislocation or a lack of pull from lack of action of either the extensor pollicis longus or the abductor pollicis longus.

If one finger has been injured, so that its flexion is much limited, and the other fingers —especially the adjoining ones—do not flex completely, the cause is usually that the flexor tendon of the injured finger cannot be drawn proximally through its full excursion by the common flexor profundus muscle. Therefore, being held, this common muscle cannot flex the adjoining fingers fully. This also occurs when the one finger has a short amputation stump and the flexor profundus tendon is adherent within it, since the amplitude of motion of the tendon in moving the short stump is much limited, thus robbing the adjoining fingers of the ability to flex completely. This condition in which one tendon holds back the others can be tested easily by grasping the same finger in the other hand, holding it in extension, and instructing the patient to make a fist. The same degree of limitation of flexion in the other fingers will be seen in the good hand as in the injured one if the diagnosis is correct. Similarly, when one extensor tendon is adherent in the dorsum of the hand, or the proximal finger joint of one finger is held in flexion contracture, the extensor digitorum communis muscle may not be able to extend the adjoining fingers. When extensor tendons are adherent on the dorsum of the hand, the fingers flex in their distal 2 joints, but the proximal joint remains straight.

When the proximal finger joint is pressed in flexion and it is found that the distal 2 finger joints cannot be flexed, the extensor tendon is adherent on the dorsum of the back of the hand. However, when the proximal finger joint is pressed in extension and the distal 2 finger joints cannot be flexed passively, the cause is contracture or adhesions of the intrinsic muscles of the hand.

INTRINSIC MUSCLES

If the intrinsic muscles (interossei and lumbricales) are working, the distal 2 finger joints extend well when the proximal joint is straight. Also, the lateral bands can be felt to move voluntarily when the finger is straightened against resistance, and each finger shows lateral motion.

If intrinsic muscles have contracted, as in intrinsic contracture local in the hand, the proximal finger joints will be held flexed, the distal 2 straight and the thumb clumped into the palm. A test for short interossei is to hold the proximal finger joint fully extended, in which case the distal 2 joints cannot be forced into flexion; when the proximal joint is allowed to flex, the distal 2 joints flex freely.

Loss of lateral motion in a finger is due to loss of function of the interossei or the lumbricales muscles, or to the cicatrix of a flexion contracture at one side of the base of the finger.

When fingers cross each other on flexion, this is due to a tipping of the axis of the proximal finger joint. This may be from malunion in rotation of a fracture of the metacarpal, or it may be due to amputation of either the middle or the ring fingers, including the head of the metacarpal. This robs the adjoining metacarpals of the side support of the missing head, so that the axes of the proximal finger joints of these adjoining fingers tip toward each other. A cause which may act alone or modify the above is surface or deep scar contracture, on either the dorsal or the volar aspect, which may roll the metacarpal heads toward each other.

If a finger which flexes well passively can flex voluntarily in its proximal and middle joints but not in its distal joint, either the profundus tendon is not working, or else the profundus and the superficialis tendons are adherent to each other, so that the motion affects the middle joint only. In this case, if the finger is held in partial extension in its middle joint, some flexor action may be seen in its distal joint.

To test for the presence of the flexor superficialis tendon, have the patient hold the finger with the proximal and the middle joints fully flexed. The distal joint then can be passively moved freely. If the profundus holds the finger in this position, the distal joint is held firmly. Another test is to hold all fingers passively in full extension except the tested one so as to tighten the profundus tendons. If the patient can flex the middle joint, the superficialis is working.

If, in a hand at rest, the finger bends back passively without resistance, its flexor tendon is either severed or too long. Similarly, if the proximal joint of the finger flexes passively without resistance, the long extensor is either severed or too long. If, in such cases, the wrist is flexed passively and the finger in question does not extend, or if the wrist is dorsiflexed passively and the finger does not flex, the opposing tendon is either severed or too long.

If, on instructing a patient to flex his fingers, it is found that he merely stiffens his fingers into a spasm and that they will not flex passively, the patient is tightening both flexors and extensors simultaneously instead of carrying through the motion with the flexors and inhibiting the tension of the extensors. This may be recognized readily by finding solid resistance on tapping the back of the fingers; they should be free to flex passively. The patient may or may not be malingering, according to whether or not he responds to an explanation and instruction.

Some hands are atrophied, cold, bluish, stiff and indurated. It may be from the enormity of the injury of the arm, from Volkmann's ischemic contracture, or from interruption of much of the nerve supply or of the main blood vessels. It may be due also to a girdling scar of the arm in general or at one site. Excessively long immobilization in treatment for a fracture or other injury of the arm may be the cause.

If a hand is in the position of nonfunction (flexed wrist, cocked-back fingers, and thumb at the side), the cause may be postural from holding the wrist flexed, from injury, infection or paralysis, or it may be from malunion of the lower part of the forearm bones or dislocation of the carpus, thus tightening the extensors of the digits.

FLEXION CONTRACTURE

Limitation of extension of the digits by flexion contracture may be due to many causes, affecting any or all of the various tissues from the skin to the capsule of the joint. Usually, one tissue is primarily and the others secondarily involved, until finally all are involved. If the skin itself is contracted, it will whiten on attempts at extension, but it will not do so if the contracture is due to deeper tissue. Commonly, flexor tendons become adherent within a finger, or, due to past infection in the finger, there is contracting cicatrization in all of the tissues in its volar aspect. A median longitudinal volar scar is frequently to blame. If the history indicates that the finger was forcefully overextended and contracture is found within the finger, the cause is usually contracting cicatrization resulting from a rupture of the anterior capsule of the joint, usually the middle one. If the fingers and the wrist were both overextended, the contracture is usually due to shortening of the forearm flexor muscles following overstretching or multiple rupture within these muscles.

If the flexion contracture is due to the condition described by Dupuytren, it will be seen to be in the palmar fascia, involving the skin in the characteristic cross-wrinkles and hard plaques, with loss of subcutaneous tissue. The bands may run down the fingers. If the contracture is of the type described by Volkmann, there are signs of shortening of the flexor muscles of the forearm, so that the fingers cannot be extended unless the wrist is flexed. These muscles will show atrophy and hardness, and the hand will show nerve changes and the typical position of flexed wrist, clawed fingers and thumb at the side.

There will be a history of venous obstruction at the elbow.

In making a diagnosis, errors will be frequent if one jumps to a conclusion too quickly. All possible causes for limitation of motion, flexion contracture, nerve lesions, etc., should be sought and weighed carefully before any commitment is made.

MALINGERING

Under some conditions it may be more remunerative to a patient to remain disabled. One must distinguish the common tendency to exaggerate pain and loss of function following an injury from true hysterical states or malingering.

The anesthesia may be glovelike or sleevelike instead of conforming to the anatomic nerve supply, or a patient can be caught off guard when instructed to keep his eyes closed and to answer "yes" when he feels a pin prick and "no" when he does not. Anesthesia should be accompanied by objective trophic changes such as smooth satiny skin and lack of perspiration. Paralysis without atrophy is not natural. Even disuse results in lessened circumference of the forearm muscles. Signs of wear such as calluses belie a history of complete lack of use.

When asked to move his hand in a certain way he may show not the slightest effort to move it—a finger laid on the muscle will verify this—or he may tighten both flexors and extensors at the same time so that his digits do not move. If the examiner can induce him to relax, one can move the finger rhythmically and feel voluntary resistance from the patient's efforts to show that it cannot move. By diverting his attention, the finger can be moved passively through the complete range. The patient may hold that position on command, showing that he has power of complete flexion. Some who are not malingerers develop the habit of tightening both flexor and extensor tendons when they attempt to flex. However, as a rule they can be taught to correct this. The usual position of the hand held by a malingerer is that used in thrusting the hand through a sleeve. Tests using electric current make it difficult for the patient. He sees his allegedly paralyzed muscles snap into action with no sign of reaction of degeneration when the galvanic or faradic current is applied. If the current is fairly strong and is applied over the nerves at the eblow, the digits will show full flexion in spite of his efforts to prevent them from moving. However, only rarely does a malingerer admit that he is faking, even in the face of a clear demonstration.

RECORDS AND REPORTS

Accurate records provide the baseline for comparison with previous examinations and permit an evaluation of methods of treatment. Quick sketches and a few specific notes describing color, warmth and such practical functional attainments as being able to button clothes, tie shoes, hold a toothbrush and a comb portray the condition more graphically than do mere figures. Actual measurements of ranges of motion are necessary but present only part of the picture.

A Picture in Words

When presenting the findings of the examination, the diagnosis and the recommendations for reconstruction, a well-written report is necessary.

One should endeavor to include in the report all necessary data and a true picture of the condition of the patient, taking care to make the report clearly understandable to medically educated laymen as well as physicians.

One should begin by stating the nature of the case and should simplify the report of the actual examination by indicating first of all the area affected by the pathology e.g., "In the right upper extremity, the thumb, the wrist and all proximal are normal"; or "The injuries are limited to the right hand and forearm and the left hip." The report should be well organized, each group of factors being covered separately under specific headings such as appearance, deformity, scars, motions of the wrist joint, motions of the fingers, motions of the thumb, the bones and the joints, and the condition of the nerves and the general nutrition of the hand. The lesions of hands are so variable that the grouping is individual for each case. Simple, straightforward, descriptive language is preferable to ultrascientific terms, since the object is to convey the information as directly as possible. A common fault is to crowd a report with measurements that do not paint the picture, even to those familiar with them. A few summarizing descriptive sentences clarify the picture for the reader.

As a preliminary to giving the measurements of flexion and extension of fingers, generalizations are useful, e.g., "Voluntary flexion of the fingers is considerably limited, as shown in the following table, although passive flexion is of good degree."

The measurements should follow these word pictures to provide accurate details.

Ambiguity and Clarity. Ambiguities should be avoided. For example: If the examiner describes the finger joints as 1st, 2nd and 3rd joints, he may be misunderstood, as not all people start to count at the same end of the finger. Similarly, if one speaks of the 1st, the 2nd and the 3rd fingers, some people will count from the thumb. It is preferable to use the terms proximal, middle and distal finger joints, and the terms index, middle, ring and little fingers and thumb. When the measurements of limitation of motion are given, one should give the reason why the motion is limited and carry the complete thought through. This spares the reader from carrying the figures in his head and thinking out the diagnosis. For instance, in speaking of the left middle finger, after stating the exact degree of limitation of flexion in distance from fingertip to palm and the degree of flexion of each individual joint, one adds "because both flexor tendons to that finger were severed in the palm and are now pulling in a limited excursion through intervening scar tissue." Also, measurements of the degree of limitation of extension of that finger are followed by such a statement as "because the distal portions of the flexor tendons have become adherent in the distal part of the palm, thus preventing extension of the finger." In this way one can associate for the reader the technical data with the conclusions to be deduced from them.

Practical Use. One should keep always in mind the practical use of the hand, including position of function, spreading of the thumb from the fingers to reach around an object, and flexion of the thumb and the fingers for

grasping it firmly, the size of objects that can be grasped, the strength of the grip and the actual use of the hand. It is equally important to give the area of sensory loss, because a hand without sensation in the area supplied by the median nerve is unfit for work.

Conclusion. At the conclusion of the report, the diagnosis is given by listing the various features of the hand that are pathologic, the cause, whether due to injury or disease, and whether an injury aggravated some underlying disease or deformity. The prognosis is stated, especially from the standpoint of use of the hand for work and whether improvement can be expected with additional time and use. If further treatment or reconstructive surgery can improve the condition, an estimate of what can be done, how long it will take, how much it will cost and what the eventual result will be all help to determine the future course of treatment.

IMPAIRMENT OF FUNCTION AND RATING OF DISABILITY

There is much confusion in the use of the terms "impairment" and "disability." They are not synonymous, and though impairment of function may be a contributing factor to disability, it is not necessarily an indication of the amount of disability.

To clarify the use of these terms and provide a uniform basis for evaluation and rating of permanent disability, a committee of the American Medical Association has suggested that the terms be used with specific meanings.

Permanent impairment means any anatomic or functional abnormality or loss which a person is found to have after maximal medical rehabilitation has been achieved. It is one factor in the estimation of permanent disability.

Permanent disability is an appraisal of a person's ability to engage in gainful activity, as affected by age, sex, education, economic and social environment, motivation and the physical impairment resulting from the anatomic or functional abnormality or loss as determined medically. Lacking measurable factors, except the medical, it is apparent that in many instances the impairment of function will be the disability. However, it should be

AMPUTATIONS

	Digit	Hand	Impairment of Upper Extremity	Whole Man
Forequarter amputation	....	....	....	70%
Disarticulation at shoulder joint	....	....	100%	60%
Amputation of arm above deltoid insertion	....	....	100%	60%
Amputation of arm between deltoid insertion and elbow joint	....	....	95%	57%
Disarticulation at elbow joint	....	....	95%	57%
Amputation of forearm below elbow joint proximal to insertion of biceps tendon	....	....	95%	57%
Amputation of forearm below elbow joint distal to insertion of biceps tendon	....	100%	90%	....
Disarticulation at wrist joint	....	100%	90%	....
Midcarpal or mid-metacarpal amputation of hand	....	100%	90%	....
Amputation of all fingers except thumb at metacarpophalangeal joints	....	60%	54%	....
Amputation of *Thumb*				
At metacarpophalangeal joint or with resection of carpometacarpal bone	100%	40%	....	....
At interphalangeal joint	75%	30%	....	....
Amputation of *Index Finger*				
At metacarpophalangeal joint or with resection of metacarpal bone	100%	25%	....	....
At proximal interphalangeal joint	80%	20%	....	....
At distal interphalangeal joint	45%	11%	....	....
Amputation of *Middle Finger*				
At metacarpophalangeal joint or with resection of metacarpal bone	100%	20%	....	....
At proximal interphalangeal joint	80%	16%	....	....
At distal interphalangeal joint	45%	9%	....	....
Amputation of *Ring Finger*				
At metacarpophalangeal joint or with resection of metacarpal bone	100%	10%	....	....
At proximal interphalangeal joint	80%	8%	....	....
At distal interphalangeal joint	45%	5%	....	....
Amputation of *Little Finger*				
At metacarpophalangeal joint or with resection of metacarpal bone	100%	5%	....	....
At proximal interphalangeal joint	80%	4%	....	....
At distal interphalangeal joint	45%	2%	....	....

FIG. 137. The values of impairments of function for amputation of the upper extremity. These are *not disability* factors. See text. (J.A.M.A.)

stressed that they are separate and distinct evaluations or ratings. Rating of permanent impairment is a medical function, while evaluation of permanent disability is an administrative decision.

EVALUATION OF IMPAIRMENT

It is the surgeon's role to evaluate impairment only as it affects the patient's personal efficiency in ordinary daily living. It is not meant to include any evaluation of social or economic relationships but is based on the loss of those functions common to all men. Therefore, the impairment from severance of the flexor tendons of the left index finger must be the same whether the man is a Russian concert violinist or a primitive tribesman from New Guinea. The value of these impairments is based on an appraisal of the effect of the injury or the disease on the daily activities of self-care, normal postures, ambulation, elevation, traveling and nonspecialized hand activities.

Appraisal of Impaired Function. Appraisal of a hand should be based on loss of useful function. Sensibility and motion are about equal in value. A hand without sensibility to touch, pain and movements of muscles and

All Joints	Amputated	IMPAIRMENT OF HAND Ankylosed in		
		Full Extension	Position of Function	Full Flexion
Thumb	40%	30%	23%	40%
Thumb Index	65%	53%	43%	65%
Thumb Index Middle	85%	71%	59%	85%
Thumb Index Ring	75%	62%	51%	75%
Thumb Index Little	70%	58%	47%	70%
Thumb Index Middle Ring	95%	80%	67%	95%
Thumb Index Middle Little	90%	76%	63%	90%
Thumb Index Ring Little	80%	67%	55%	80%
Thumb Index Middle Ring Little	100%	85%	71%	100%
Thumb Middle	60%	48%	39%	60%
Thumb Middle Ring	70%	57%	47%	70%
Thumb Middle Little	65%	53%	43%	65%
Thumb Middle Ring Little	75%	62%	51%	75%
Thumb Ring	50%	39%	31%	50%
Thumb Ring Little	55%	44%	35%	55%
Thumb Little	45%	35%	27%	45%
Index	25%	23%	20%	25%
Index Middle	45%	41%	36%	45%
Index Middle Ring	55%	50%	44%	55%
Index Middle Little	50%	46%	40%	50%
Index Middle Ring Little	60%	55%	48%	60%
Index Ring	35%	32%	28%	35%
Index Ring Little	40%	37%	32%	40%
Index Little	30%	28%	24%	30%
Middle	20%	18%	16%	20%
Middle Ring	30%	27%	24%	30%
Middle Ring Little	35%	32%	28%	35%
Middle Little	25%	23%	20%	25%
Ring	10%	9%	8%	10%
Ring Little	15%	14%	12%	15%
Little	5%	5%	4%	5%

FIG. 138. When more than one digit has been amputated the values are combined as in this table; and if ankylosis of the digits occurs, the impairment will depend upon the position in which the joint is fixed. For impairment values from ankylosis of individual joints of a finger see following tables. (J.A.M.A.)

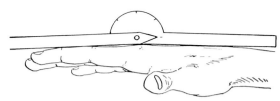

FIG. 139. Estimating impairment from limited motion or ankylosis of a single joint. (J.A.M.A.)

METACARPAL JOINT OF ANY FINGER
TECHNIC OF MEASUREMENT: FLEXION, EXTENSION
Restricted Motion

1. Place patients hand in neutral position as shown in Fig. 1.

2. Center goniometer over dorsum of metacarpophalangeal joint as shown in Fig. 1. Record goniometer reading.

3. With patient attempting to make a fist as shown in Fig. 2, follow range of motion with goniometer arm. Record end of arc of motion.

4. Consult Restricted Motion Table for corresponding impairment of finger.

Example: 30 degrees active flexion from neutral position (0°) OR from maximum extension = 37% impairment of finger.

Ankylosis

1. Place goniometer base as if measuring neutral position shown above. Measure deviation from neutral position with goniometer arm. Record goniometer reading.

2. Consult Ankylosis Table for corresponding impairment of finger.

Example: Metacarpophalangeal joint ankylosed at 30 degrees flexion = 45% impairment of finger.

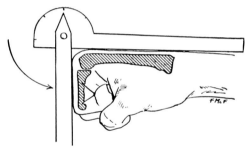

FIG. 140. Table of values to go with Figure 139 in estimating impairment of a finger from restricted motion or ankylosis. (J.A.M.A.)

METACARPOPHALANGEAL JOINT OF ANY FINGER

IMPAIRMENT
OF FINGER

AMPUTATION—At Joint 100%
RESTRICTED MOTION TABLE
Average range of FLEXION-EXTENSION = 90°
Value to total range of joint motion = 100%

Degrees of Joint Motion
LOST   RETAINED

Flexion from neutral
position (°) to:..

	LOST		RETAINED	
0°	90	0	55%
10°	80	10	49
20°	70	20	43
30°	60	30	37
40°	50	40	31
50°	40	50	24
60°	30	60	18
70°	20	70	12
80°	10	80	6
90°	0	90	0

Ankylosis Table
Joint ankylosed at:

0° (neutral position)	55%
10°	52
20°	48
*30°	45
40°	54
50°	63
60°	72
70°	82
80°	91
90° (full flexion)	100

* Position of function.

THUMB
When BOTH JOINTS are Involved

1. CALCULATE *separately* and record impairment of thumb contributed by EACH joint.
2. COMBINE impairment values, using combined values table, to ascertain impairment of thumb contributed by BOTH joints.

IMPAIRMENT
OF THUMB

Example—Ankylosis
Interphalangeal joint: ankylosed at 40 degrees flexion .... =   35%
Metacarpophalangeal joint: ankylosed at 50 degrees flexion .... =   35
(35 *combined* with 35 = 58)   58%

Example—Ankylosis and Restricted Motion
Interphalangeal joint: ankylosed at 40 degrees flexion .... =   35%
Metacarpophalangeal joint: 50 degrees active flexion from neutral position (0°) OR from
  maximum extension .... =   9
(35 *combined* with 9 = 41)   41%

Example—Restricted Motion
Interphalangeal joint: 40 degrees active flexion from neutral position (0°) OR from
  maximum extension .... =   23%
Metacarpophalangeal joint: 50 degrees active flexion from neutral position (0°) OR from
  maximum extension .... =   9
(23 *combined* with 9 = 30)   30%

Example—Amputation and Restricted Motion
Interphalangeal joint: amputated .... =   75%
Metacarpophalangeal joint: 50 degrees active flexion from neutral position (0°) OR from
  maximum extension .... =   9
(75 *combined* with 9 = 77)   77%

3. CONSULT following table to ascertain impairment of HAND contributed by THUMB.

FIG. 141. If both joints are involved, the impairments cannot be added but must be combined. This table illustrates use of the combined values table, a portion of which appears as Figure 146. (J.A.M.A.)

THUMB

Impairment of Thumb	Hand		Impairment of Thumb	Hand
0% —	1% = 0%		52% —	53% = 21%
2% —	3% = 1%		54% —	56% = 22%
4% —	6% = 2%		57% —	58% = 23%
7% —	8% = 3%		59% —	61% = 24%
9% —	11% = 4%		62% —	63% = 25%
12% —	13% = 5%		64% —	66% = 26%
14% —	16% = 6%		67% —	68% = 27%
17% —	18% = 7%		69% —	71% = 28%
19% —	21% = 8%		72% —	73% = 29%
22% —	23% = 9%		74% —	76% = 30%
24% —	26% = 10%		77% —	78% = 31%
27% —	28% = 11%		79% —	81% = 32%
29% —	31% = 12%		82% —	83% = 33%
32% —	33% = 13%		84% —	86% = 34%
34% —	36% = 14%		87% —	88% = 35%
37% —	38% = 15%		89% —	91% = 36%
39% —	41% = 16%		92% —	93% = 37%
42% —	43% = 17%		94% —	96% = 38%
44% —	46% = 18%		97% —	98% = 39%
47% —	48% = 19%		99% —	100% = 40%
49% —	51% = 20%			

NOTE: Impairment of HAND contributed by THUMB may be rounded to the nearest 5 per cent ONLY when it is the *sole* impairment involved.

FIG. 142. Relating impairment of a thumb to the whole hand. (J.A.M.A.)

FINGERS

Impairment of Hand Index Finger		Impairment of Hand Middle Finger	
0% —	1% = 0%	0% —	2% = 0%
2% —	5% = 1%	3% —	7% = 1%
6% —	9% = 2%	8% —	12% = 2%
10% —	13% = 3%	13% —	17% = 3%
14% —	17% = 4%	18% —	22% = 4%
18% —	21% = 5%	23% —	27% = 5%
22% —	25% = 6%	28% —	32% = 6%
26% —	29% = 7%	33% —	37% = 7%
30% —	33% = 8%	38% —	42% = 8%
34% —	37% = 9%	43% —	47% = 9%
38% —	41% = 10%	48% —	52% = 10%
42% —	45% = 11%	53% —	57% = 11%
46% —	49% = 12%	58% —	62% = 12%
50% —	53% = 13%	63% —	67% = 13%
54% —	57% = 14%	68% —	72% = 14%
58% —	61% = 15%	73% —	77% = 15%
62% —	65% = 16%	78% —	82% = 16%
66% —	69% = 17%	83% —	87% = 17%
70% —	73% = 18%	88% —	92% = 18%
74% —	77% = 19%	93% —	97% = 19%
78% —	81% = 20%	98% —	100% = 20%
82% —	85% = 21%		
86% —	89% = 22%		
90% —	93% = 23%		
94% —	97% = 24%		
98% —	100% = 25%		

Ring Finger

0% —	4% = 0%
5% —	14% = 1%
15% —	24% = 2%
25% —	34% = 3%
35% —	44% = 4%
45% —	54% = 5%
55% —	64% = 6%
65% —	74% = 7%
75% —	84% = 8%
85% —	94% = 9%
95% —	100% = 10%

Little Finger

0% —	9% = 0%
10% —	29% = 1%
30% —	49% = 2%
50% —	69% = 3%
70% —	89% = 4%
90% —	100% = 5%

NOTE: Impairment of HAND contributed by FINGER may be rounded to the nearest 5 per cent ONLY when it is the *sole* impairment involved.

FIG. 143. Relative impairment of hand contributed by finger amputations, restricted motion or ankylosis. (J.A.M.A.)

joints is devoid of stereognosis, protection against injury and trophic control and is unfit for work.

The basic motions are opening for grasp by extending the thumb and the fingers apart, and closing to hold objects firmly and for prehension. This is by opposition, the fingers working against the palm or against the thenar eminence and the thumb, the latter encircling, or by the fingertips pinching against the tip of the thumb. Another function is that of hook action with the fingers, and still another the lateral or rotary control of tools by wide surface of grasp—the width of the palm. Firmness of grip depends on the number of fingers and the way they grasp, and on stabilization of the wrist in dorsiflexion.

For any function, the arm must be able to place and hold the hand where it can work, the hand and the arm being interdependent. The hand can be considered to be a tool that holds other tools.

Limitation of motion expressed in percentage of degrees lost from the normal complete range of motion does not describe impairment fairly. Digits fixed in extension may have one fifth of their range of motion, but this is useless because they cannot oppose each other for practical grasp. For fingers, the last half of the range of flexion, that is from semiflexion to full flexion, is more useful than the first half. For the thumb the midrange of its extension and flexion and of opposition is more useful. Fingers in full extension or strong flexion contracture or a thumb fixed at the side of the hand lose their value and are in the way. The loss of an index or a little finger results in little impairment. However, the index finger

HAND

Impairment: Hand	Impairment of Upper Extremity	Impairment: Hand	Impairment of Upper Extremity	Impairment: Hand	Impairment of Upper Extremity
0%	= 0%	34%	= 31%	68%	= 61%
1%	= 1%	35%	= 32%	69%	= 62%
2%	= 2%	36%	= 32%	70%	= 63%
3%	= 3%	37%	= 33%	71%	= 64%
4%	= 4%	38%	= 34%	72%	= 65%
5%	= 5%	39%	= 35%	73%	= 66%
6%	= 5%	40%	= 36%	74%	= 67%
7%	= 6%	41%	= 37%	75%	= 68%
8%	= 7%	42%	= 38%	76%	= 68%
9%	= 8%	43%	= 39%	77%	= 69%
10%	= 9%	44%	= 40%	78%	= 70%
11%	= 10%	45%	= 41%	79%	= 71%
12%	= 11%	46%	= 41%	80%	= 72%
13%	= 12%	47%	= 42%	81%	= 73%
14%	= 13%	48%	= 43%	82%	= 74%
15%	= 14%	49%	= 44%	83%	= 75%
16%	= 14%	50%	= 45%	84%	= 76%
17%	= 15%	51%	= 46%	85%	= 77%
18%	= 16%	52%	= 47%	86%	= 77%
19%	= 17%	53%	= 48%	87%	= 78%
20%	= 18%	54%	= 49%	88%	= 79%
21%	= 19%	55%	= 50%	89%	= 80%
22%	= 20%	56%	= 50%	90%	= 81%
23%	= 21%	57%	= 51%	91%	= 82%
24%	= 22%	58%	= 52%	92%	= 83%
25%	= 23%	59%	= 53%	93%	= 84%
26%	= 23%	60%	= 54%	94%	= 85%
27%	= 24%	61%	= 55%	95%	= 86%
28%	= 25%	62%	= 56%	96%	= 86%
29%	= 26%	63%	= 57%	97%	= 87%
30%	= 27%	64%	= 58%	98%	= 88%
31%	= 28%	65%	= 59%	99%	= 89%
32%	= 29%	66%	= 59%	100%	= 90%
33%	= 30%	67%	= 60%		

NOTE: Impairment of UPPER EXTREMITY contributed by HAND may be rounded to the nearest 5 per cent ONLY when it is the *sole* impairment involved.

FIG. 144. An impairment of the hand contributes to the impairment of the upper extremity, according to this table. (J.A.M.A.)

UPPER EXTREMITY

Impairment of Upper Extremity	Impairment of Whole Man	Impairment of Upper Extremity	Impairment of Whole Man	Impairment of Upper Extremity	Impairment of Whole Man
0%	= 0%	34%	= 20%	68%	= 41%
1%	= 1%	35%	= 21%	69%	= 41%
2%	= 1%	36%	= 22%	70%	= 42%
3%	= 2%	37%	= 22%	71%	= 43%
4%	= 2%	38%	= 23%	72%	= 43%
5%	= 3%	39%	= 23%	73%	= 44%
6%	= 4%	40%	= 24%	74%	= 44%
7%	= 4%	41%	= 25%	75%	= 45%
8%	= 5%	42%	= 25%	76%	= 46%
9%	= 5%	43%	= 26%	77%	= 46%
10%	= 6%	44%	= 26%	78%	= 47%
11%	= 7%	45%	= 27%	79%	= 47%
12%	= 7%	46%	=28%	80%	= 48%
13%	= 8%	47%	= 28%	81%	= 49%
14%	= 8%	48%	= 29%	82%	= 49%
15%	= 9%	49%	= 29%	83%	= 50%
16%	= 10%	50%	= 30%	84%	= 50%
17%	= 10%	51%	= 31%	85%	= 51%
18%	= 11%	52%	= 31%	86%	= 52%
19%	= 11%	53%	= 32%	87%	= 52%
20%	= 12%	54%	= 32%	88%	= 53%
21%	= 13%	55%	= 33%	89%	= 53%
22%	= 13%	56%	= 34%	90%	= 54%
23%	= 14%	57%	= 34%	91%	= 55%
24%	= 14%	58%	= 35%	92%	= 55%
25%	= 15%	59%	= 35%	93%	= 56%
26%	= 16%	60%	= 36%	94%	= 56%
27%	= 16%	61%	= 37%	95%	= 57%
28%	= 17%	62%	= 37%	96%	= 58%
29%	= 17%	63%	= 38%	97%	= 58%
30%	= 18%	64%	= 38%	98%	= 59%
31%	= 19%	65%	= 39%	99%	= 59%
32%	= 19%	66%	= 40%	100%	= 60%
33%	= 20%	67%	= 40%		

NOTE: Impairment of WHOLE MAN contributed by UPPER EXTREMITY may be rounded to the nearest 5 per cent ONLY when it is the *sole* impairment involved.

FIG. 145. Whole man impairments result from upper extremity impairments, according to this scale. (J.A.M.A.)

is more independently mobile, and both index and little fingers give width of grip for leverage. The middle finger does the work of the index finger and soon can be educated for this. The ring finger and especially the middle finger are more valuable; the latter is the stronger, but the loss of either leaves a gap. A stiff finger in any position is in the way. Normally, the motion of the 3 finger joints should amount to 3 times 90 or 270°, the middle joints flexing more and the distal less than 90°. Full flexion allows a slender rod to be grasped, but partial flexion permits only larger objects to be grasped. If the proximal

	1	2	3	4	5	6	7	8	9	10	11	12	13	14	15	16	17	18	19	20	21	22	23	24	25	26	27	28	29	30	31	32	33	34	35	36	37	38	39	40	41	42	43	44	45	46	47	48	49	50
1	2																																																	
2	3	4																																																
3	4	5	6																																															
4	5	6	7	8																																														
5	6	7	8	9	10																																													
6	7	8	9	10	11	12																																												
7	8	9	10	11	12	13	14																																											
8	9	10	11	12	13	14	14	15																																										
9	10	11	12	13	14	14	15	16	17																																									
10	11	12	13	14	15	15	16	17	18	19																																								
11	12	13	14	15	15	16	17	18	19	20	21																																							
12	13	14	15	16	16	17	18	19	20	21	22	23																																						
13	14	15	16	16	17	18	19	20	21	22	23	23	24																																					
14	15	16	17	17	18	19	20	21	22	23	23	24	25	26																																				
15	16	17	18	18	19	20	21	22	23	24	24	25	26	27	28																																			
16	17	18	19	19	20	21	22	23	24	24	25	26	27	28	29	29																																		
17	18	19	19	20	21	22	23	24	24	25	26	27	28	29	29	30	31																																	
18	19	20	20	21	22	23	24	25	25	26	27	28	29	29	30	31	32	33																																
19	20	21	21	22	23	24	25	25	26	27	28	29	30	30	31	32	33	34	34																															
20	21	22	22	23	24	25	26	26	27	28	29	30	30	31	32	33	34	34	35	36																														
21	22	23	23	24	25	26	27	27	28	29	30	30	31	32	33	34	34	35	36	37	38																													
22	23	24	24	25	26	27	27	28	29	30	31	31	32	33	34	34	35	36	37	38	38	39																												
23	24	25	25	26	27	28	28	29	30	31	31	32	33	34	35	35	36	37	38	38	39	40	41																											
24	25	26	26	27	28	29	29	30	31	32	32	33	34	35	35	36	37	38	38	39	40	41	41	42																										
25	26	27	27	28	29	30	30	31	32	33	33	34	35	36	36	37	38	39	39	40	41	42	42	43	44																									
26	27	27	28	29	30	30	31	32	33	33	34	35	36	36	37	38	39	39	40	41	42	42	43	44	45	45																								
27	28	28	29	30	31	31	32	33	34	34	35	36	36	37	38	39	39	40	41	42	42	43	44	45	45	46	47																						
28	29	29	30	31	32	32	33	34	34	35	36	37	37	38	39	40	40	41	42	42	43	44	45	45	46	47	47	48																					
29	30	30	31	32	33	33	34	35	35	36	37	38	38	39	40	40	41	42	42	43	44	45	45	46	47	47	48	49	50																				
30	31	31	32	33	34	34	35	36	36	37	38	38	39	40	41	41	42	43	43	44	45	45	46	47	48	48	49	50	50	51																			
31	32	32	33	34	34	35	36	37	37	38	39	39	40	41	41	42	43	43	44	45	45	46	47	48	48	49	50	50	51	52	52																		
32	33	33	34	35	35	36	37	37	38	39	39	40	41	42	42	43	44	44	45	46	46	47	48	48	49	50	50	51	52	52	53	54																	
33	34	34	35	36	36	37	38	38	39	40	40	41	42	42	43	44	44	45	46	46	47	48	48	49	50	50	51	52	52	53	54	54	55																
34	35	35	36	37	37	38	39	39	40	41	41	42	43	43	44	45	45	46	47	47	48	49	49	50	51	51	52	52	53	54	54	55	56	56															
35	36	36	37	38	38	39	40	40	41	42	42	43	43	44	45	45	46	47	47	48	49	49	50	51	51	52	53	53	54	55	55	56	56	57	58														
36	37	37	38	39	39	40	40	41	42	42	43	44	44	45	46	46	47	48	48	49	49	50	51	51	52	53	53	54	55	55	56	56	57	58	58	59													
37	38	38	39	40	40	41	41	42	43	43	44	45	45	46	46	47	48	48	49	50	50	51	51	52	53	53	54	55	55	56	57	57	58	58	59	60	60												
38	39	39	40	40	41	42	42	43	44	44	45	45	46	47	47	48	49	49	50	50	51	52	52	53	54	54	55	55	56	57	57	58	58	59	60	60	61	62											
39	40	40	41	41	42	43	43	44	44	45	46	46	47	48	48	49	49	50	51	51	52	52	53	54	54	55	55	56	57	57	58	59	59	60	60	61	62	62	63										
40	41	41	42	42	43	44	44	45	45	46	47	47	48	48	49	50	50	51	51	52	53	53	54	54	55	56	56	57	57	58	59	59	60	60	61	62	62	63	63	64									
41	42	42	43	43	44	45	45	46	46	47	47	48	49	49	50	50	51	52	52	53	53	54	55	55	56	56	57	58	58	59	59	60	60	61	62	62	63	63	64	65	65								
42	43	43	44	44	45	45	46	47	47	48	48	49	50	50	51	51	52	52	53	54	54	55	55	56	57	57	58	58	59	59	60	61	61	62	62	63	63	64	65	65	66	66							
43	44	44	45	45	46	46	47	48	48	49	49	50	50	51	52	52	53	53	54	54	55	56	56	57	57	58	58	59	60	60	61	61	62	62	63	64	64	65	65	66	66	67	68						
44	45	45	46	46	47	47	48	48	49	50	50	51	51	52	52	53	54	54	55	55	56	56	57	57	58	59	59	60	60	61	61	62	62	63	64	64	65	65	66	66	67	68	68	69					
45	46	46	47	47	48	48	49	49	50	51	51	52	52	53	53	54	54	55	55	56	57	57	58	58	59	59	60	60	61	62	62	63	63	64	64	65	65	66	66	67	68	68	69	69	70				
46	47	47	48	48	49	49	50	50	51	51	52	52	53	54	54	55	55	56	56	57	57	58	58	59	60	60	61	61	62	62	63	63	64	64	65	65	66	67	67	68	68	69	69	70	70	71			
47	48	48	49	49	50	50	51	51	52	52	53	53	54	54	55	55	56	57	57	58	58	59	59	60	60	61	61	62	62	63	63	64	64	65	66	66	67	67	68	68	69	69	70	70	71	71	72		
48	49	49	50	50	51	51	52	52	53	53	54	54	55	55	56	56	57	57	58	58	59	59	60	60	61	62	62	63	63	64	64	65	65	66	66	67	67	68	68	69	69	70	70	71	71	72	72	73	
49	50	50	51	51	52	52	53	53	54	54	55	55	56	56	57	57	58	58	59	59	60	60	61	61	62	62	63	63	64	64	65	65	66	66	67	67	68	68	69	69	70	70	71	71	72	72	73	73	74
50	51	51	52	52	53	53	54	54	55	55	56	56	57	57	58	58	59	59	60	60	61	61	62	62	63	63	64	64	65	65	66	66	67	67	68	68	69	69	70	70	71	71	72	72	73	73	74	74	75

COMBINED VALUES TABLE

These combined values are based on the formula: A% + B% (100% — A%) = combined value of A% and B%. The guides to the table are percents ranging from 1 to 100 printed down the side of the page, and across the bottom. To combine any two values locate the larger of the two on the side of the page and read along that row until you come to the column indicated by the second value at the bottom of the page. At the intersection of this row and column is printed the combined value. For example, to combine 35% and 20% read down the side of the page until you come to the larger value, 35%. Then read across the row you have located until you come to the column indicated by 20% at the bottom of the page. At the intersection of this row and column is the number 48. We say that 35% and 20% combine to 48%. Due to the construction of this table, the larger value must be read at the side of the page.

If three or more values are to be combined, select any two and find their combined value as above. Take this combined value and the third value and find their combined value. This process can be repeated indefinitely with the value obtained in each case being the combination of all the previous values.

FIG. 146. A sample of the combined values table used in arriving at percentages of impairments when two or more values are to be combined. (J.A.M.A.)

joints are limited, half flexion of them is the better position.

The wrist is most useful in the first 40° of dorsiflexion. With the wrist dorsiflexed the digits flex best, which is useful, but with the wrist flexed they extend better. Ranges of motion in the hand near the position of function have the greatest value. Measurements of joint limitation are compared with the ranges of motion in the other hand as is strength of grip, with 3 or more trials on the dynamometer with each hand without the patient's seeing the dial.

If there is solid fixation of pronation and supination, slight pronation is the optimal position (writing, typewriting, bench work, etc.), but if there is motion, the power to supinate is more valuable than the power to

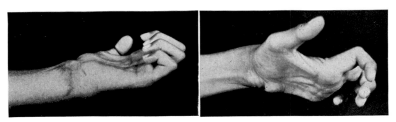

FIG. 147. The deformity of imbalance from median and ulnar palsy is accentuated when adhesions bind the flexors proximal to the wrist.

pronate. It means more range of this motion, since supination is the first to be lost. Pronation can be done by means of gravity. Pronation, supination, and certain limitations of wrist motion can be overcome or compensated for by movements of the arm and the shoulder.

Evaluation of impairment should be based on the practical functions enumerated above; these are necessary for all the various activities of the hand. Other factors to be considered are strength, speed, endurance and coordination, all of which depend on composite functions. It is possible to make actual tests of these, but at the present time the simpler methods are used. Pain is such an intangible, subjective factor that it is better to base ratings on objective symptoms; even gripping is under control of the applicant. Pain can be evaluated best by the doctor who has followed the case, as this factor is too easily exaggerated by someone coming only for a rating. It should be commented on by the doctor for better evaluation. The nutritional factor is real, but too much attention paid to vasomotor disturbances, with repeated medical examinations and court hearings, only fixes and encourages the aberration.

The tables of values are based on an estimate that loss of the upper limb is 70 per cent impairment of the whole man. Similarly, disarticulation of the wrist equals 100 per cent of the hand and 90 per cent impairment of the upper limb. Further, a 90 per cent impairment of the upper limb is considered to be a 54 per cent impairment of the whole man. Values for restricted motion of each joint and for ankylosis in various positions have been determined.

When multiple digits are involved, a system of combining values before estimating loss of the next higher unit is used.

Relative values for impairment of other functions such as sight, hearing and cardiac lesions have been determined, and studies relating to impairment from lesions of the peripheral nerves are being made.

RATING OF DISABILITY

In theory, an award for permanent disability is based on decreased earning power and is intended to tide the man over in support of himself and his dependents until he has adapted himself to his new situation. It is not compensation for loss of a part, though it may be based on loss of parts.

The doctor alone has the right to describe and appraise the impairment, but the courts determine the award. The rating should be based on loss of function, but the award is modified by certain social factors.

Awards are usually expressed in weeks of compensation figured from the percentage rating of disability, each per cent corresponding to the number of weeks, such as 2 or 5. They also vary in that other factors are considered, such as major or minor hand, age and occupation. For the first factor, 10 to 5 per cent may be allowed for a major over a minor hand down to 1 per cent for a finger. Rate schedules are graded for age on the basis that from 15 to 25 years of age a boy is still learning and is adaptable both physically and mentally, i.e., he can learn a new trade. Below 40 the disability rate decreases with the age in years, but after that age it increases because learning a new trade or adapting oneself physically becomes more and more difficult; thus, the same impairment may be rated at 5 per cent at the age of 15 and 20 per cent at 70. The loss of a hand makes some occupations impossible but has little effect in others, so that schedules are made listing the various occupations with each type of disability. From 12,000 to 18,000 specific occupations are listed; in some schedules these are grouped in 9 classes and arranged in tables for each type of disability.

There have been schedules in Europe for a long time. In this country, the United States Veterans' Administration has one coordinating main disabilities with each of 9 grades of occupation, the rates being higher for the skilled worker. Earl D. McBride gives a complete and excellent system in *Disability Evaluation*, as also does Henry H. Kessler in his book *Accidental Injuries*. These cover the subject in a masterly way.

BIBLIOGRAPHY

Bertelsen, A., and Capener, N.: Fingers, compensation and King Canute, J. Bone Joint Surg. *42-B*:390, 1960.

Bradburn, H. B. Chase, R. A., and Fessel, J. M.: The hand in systemic disease, J. Bone Joint Surg. *44-A*:1395, 1962.

Bulletin of U. S. Bureau of Labor Statistics No. 333, pp. 72-150; Bulletin No. 359, Standard Permanent Disability Schedules, pp. 17-30.

Commission on Medical Rating of Physical Impairments; a guide to the evaluation of permanent impairment of the extremities and back, J.A.M.A. Special Edition, 1958.

Kessler, H. H.: Accidental Injuries: The Medico-Legal Aspects of Workmen's Compensation and Public Liability, ed. 2, Philadelphia, Lea & Febiger, 1941.

McBride, E. D.: Disability Evaluation, ed. 6, Philadelphia, Lippincott, 1963.

Moberg, E.: Objective methods for determining the functional value of sensibility in the hand, J. Bone Joint Surg. 40-B:466, 1958.

————:Evaluation of sensibility in the hand, Surg. Clin. N. Amer. 40:2, 1960.

————: Peripheral nerves and hand function; editorial, J. Bone Joint Surg. 43-B:423, 1961.

————: Criticism and study of methods for examining sensibility in the hand, Neurology 12:8, 1962.

Rice, C. O.: The Calculation of Industrial Disabilities of the Extremities, Springfield, Ill., Thomas, 1952.

Chapter 5

Principles of Reconstruction

GENERAL CONSIDERATIONS

The main function of the upper extremity is to place and control the hand. It is the hand that does the work and is the important part of the arm. A prosthesis is a poor substitute for a hand, and even with the best prosthesis an arm without a hand is of very limited use. This point of view is of direct and major importance when the nerves of the arm share in the injury. Rowley Bristow said, "The surgery of the upper extremity is the surgery of the hand."

When we consider what a wonderful mechanism the hand is, it is not surprising that its successful reconstruction by surgery is unusual. Let us think of the hand as a marvelously functioning piece of live machinery and regard it with due respect. Though its tissues are tough and compact, its tendons, tendon sheaths, pulleys, joint surfaces and flexible joint capsules all glide on each other so easily and smoothly that there is little that the hand cannot do, so refined are the motions of which it is capable. If infection or trauma insults these perfected parts, a tissue reaction occurs, binding the gliding surfaces together, thickening and stiffening the joint capsules, contracting the tissues of the finger and strangulating the nerves and the vessels. Loss of function must result.

Hands in need of repair range from those with only a simple severance of a nerve or a tendon to those with extensive crippling in which all the structures have been damaged—the tissues tightly contracted by cicatricial tissue, joints stiffened in nonfunctioning positions, flexion contractures, and great lengths of tendon and nerves that have sloughed and been reduced to scar tissue. Thus, repairs are not limited to nerves and tendons but must include all tissues.

To diagnose and reconstruct a crippled hand an intimate knowledge of the anatomy, the mechanics and the physiology of the normal hand is necessary. When the normal is known, whatever pathologic state exists in the injured hand will be clearly evident.

In the skin, the creases and the areas of redundancy conform with the movement. Each of the joints from shoulder to fingertips has its range of motion, which allows the hand or the limb as a whole to move into almost any desired position. There is a nicely adjusted muscle balance between the long extensors, the long flexors and the intrinsic muscles in the hand, which determines the posture of the hand at rest, and on which the use of the hand depends. Any imbalance is readily noticeable.

The mechanics of the joints and the tendons, the carpal and the metacarpal arches, the angles of approach of tendons at each joint, the restraining pulleys, the tendon sheaths are all remarkably adjusted, so that the hand and its digits, working in relation to each other, can fulfill innumerable functions. Every tissue in the hand is perfectly specialized for its purpose—skin, nerves, joints, bones, muscles and tendons—in such complexity and perfection that an adequtae conception of and regard for the normal will influence the outcome of surgery—whether it wrecks or reconstructs. Success in the repair of a hand crippled by injury requires the correlation of plastic surgery, neurosurgery and orthopedic surgery, because injuries affect every tissue in the limb without

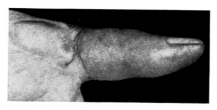

Fig. 148. The encircling scar. Such a digit can seldom be reconstructed when it is nourished so poorly.

regard for medical specialties. The hand surgeon must be versatile in all three.

For a viewpoint of attack, let us consider the skin as the covering, the bones as the scaffolding, the joints as the hinges, the muscles as the motors, the tendons as the ropes, and the nerves as the wiring. Our problem is composite, as it includes all of these; it deals with deformities, disturbed mechanics, disturbed nutrition, paralysis, anesthesia, trophic and vasomotor conditions, contractures, cicatrices and defects of all tissues. The same tissues are found in both extremities. The problem in the lower extremity is largely to give stability; that in the upper is to give useful motion.

The surgeon should weigh well the amount of improvement he expects to accomplish and should avoid undertaking a surgical reconstruction just because it is possible technically.

Operation is contraindicated unless the whole ordeal of repair is amply justified by the improvement to be gained. Consideration should be given to the value of amputation of some parts, remembering that it is the function of the hand as a whole unit with which we are concerned.

The aim should be to give the patient sensation, position and the function of opening and closing the hand for grasp. He should be given placement of the hand by the arm and as much strength and refinement of motion as possible. A stable shoulder and elbow provide the firm base on which we can develop and reconstruct a terminal moving mechanism.

Individual reactions to reconstructive sur-

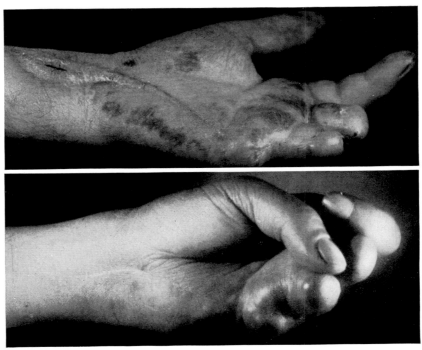

Fig. 149. Case A. T. Showing the great improvement in the nutrition of the hand from dissecting out all of the deep cicatricial tissue within the hand. This octopuslike internal scar bound blood, lymph vessels and nerves, causing the poor nutrition shown in the top picture.

The hand had been almost severed by a saw, following which infection developed. The tendons and the nerves sloughed out, robbing the hand of all motion and sensation, except that supplied by the radial nerve. Restoration of good function was accomplished by repair of the nerves and the tendons, but the point exemplified here is the improvement in nutrition as shown in the bottom picture, due mainly to excision of the deep cicatrix. (J. Bone Joint Surg.)

gery of the hand vary greatly. Some hands overheal with keloid formation and deep cicatrization, resulting in binding adhesions, contractures and stiff joints, while others remain limber. The joints of some persons who have a high cicatricial index, often the thin and the arthritic, sometimes the fat, and those over the age of 50 or those who age more quickly will stiffen on slight surgical provocation. Ample material should be available to fill in the defects of each tissue. The state of nutrition of a limb is all-important in the final result.

IMPORTANCE OF POSITION OF FUNCTION

Throughout reconstruction one should keep in mind that the hand should be brought into the position of function and should never lose this position and that the hand always should

be kept moving or it will stiffen. If the hand is left too long in a cast or in a rigid splint, or in a splint with joints on a strain, the joints will stiffen. Hands are peculiar in that they need function if they are to thrive and not stiffen. The natural state of a hand, and the only one in which it will thrive, is that of motion.

In hand reconstruction much can be done if one will give the time, exercise proper care and have patience. This is no work for the novice. Ordinary surgical procedure is too rough, so that it is necessary in this work to use as nearly as possible an atraumatic technic. In hand reconstruction certain main principles must be kept in mind. The rest depends on a host of tiny but important details. Hand surgery is not a tissue specialty but an anatomic or regional one like that of the eye and

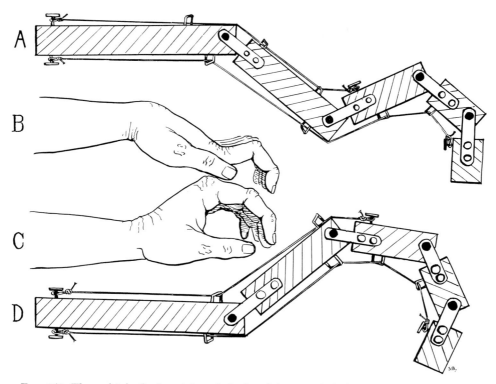

FIG. 150. The wrist is the key joint of the hand for muscle balance. If the wrist is flexed, the hand assumes the position of nonfunction (B) and, if dorsiflexed, the position of function (C). In either case, the muscles are in balance. (A and D) This manikin of hinged blocks for bones and of strings for tendons shows how the hand automatically assumes the position of nonfunction when the wrist is flexed and the position of function when the wrist is dorsiflexed.

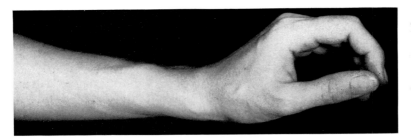

Fig. 151. The position of function. This should be the position for immobilization of a hand and the goal of all corrective splinting and operative procedures.

the ear. The hand surgeon should choose between free and pedicle skin grafts according to the tissue beneath and should place the borders of his pedicles with the conception of a moving hand, that is, without contracting keloid scars coinciding with lines of push and pull, and he should make his pedicles aseptic to avoid stiffness. At dissection, valuable observations of the understructures can be recorded for the whole repair problem. Some other structures, like nerves and deep flexion contractures, can be repaired at the time of the pedicle. If he operates to repair a nerve, he can repair many other deep structures at the same time, instead of having to make 2 extensive dissections. Often on uncovering a forearm and a hand, the findings cause one to change the plan of procedure from nerve repair to tendon transfer or arthrodesis or a bone operation with plastic swinging of flaps included. It is all one composite problem, and the full responsibility to the patient should be held by one surgeon. The mechanical unit of the hand, that is, of bone, joint and muscle action, is from the elbow down. The dynamic control of the hand starts at the opposite cerebral cortex. The main function of the whole arm is to place the hand where it can work.

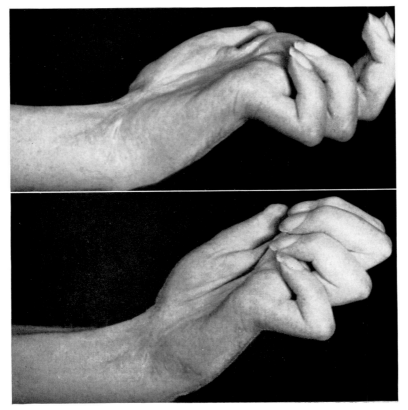

Fig. 152. The flexed wrist, here held by scar contracture, has thrown the fingers out of balance and intensified the deformity resulting from the median and ulnar nerve palsy. The thumb is at the side of the hand, and the fingers are clawed,

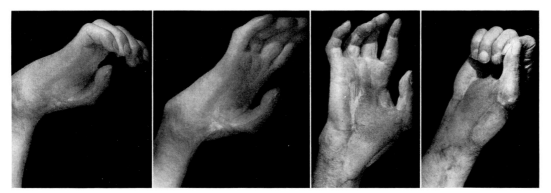

FIG. 153. Restoring the position of function and replacing cicatrix. The 2 left illustrations show the result of severe crushing a year previously; healing required 6 months. The wrist is volar-flexed, the thumb position is lost, and the fingers with proximal joints are straight and stiff. Dense scar binds the wrist and the thumb and limits motion.

Gradual traction brought the proximal joints into flexion; the cicatrix was replaced by pedicle graft; and the deep scar was excised to allow the flexor tendons to function. The wrist was brought into dorsiflexion.

The 2 right illustrations show the improvement in appearance and position and range of digital motion following reconstruction. (Surg., Gynec. & Obs. *39:254*, No. 9)

PRINCIPLES

PLAN

A definite plan of procedure should be thought out, giving the chronologic sequence and the serial order of each of the operative procedures and courses of treatment. Consideration is given to the time schedule that the patient can arrange and the expense that he can bear.

Primary needs are the restoration of position of function, motion, sensation, nutrition and a good covering. The digits should have noncicatricial, workable ends. The thumb or some digit should oppose the fingers, and the hand should open and close for grasping. The arm should work well to place the hand where it is needed, including raising at the shoulder and supinating in the forearm.

RESTORING POSITION OF FUNCTION

First, the wrist and the fingers must be brought into positions of function. That is, the wrist should be cocked up in dorsiflexion and the fingers partially flexed, especially in their proximal joints. The thumb should be in the position to oppose the fingers. A hand with a straight wrist and extended proximal joints and the thumb at its side is practically useless. In the absence of a thumb, some digit should oppose the others for prehension. While the limb is undergoing healing from infection or injury, the position of function should be maintained.

PREVENTION OF STIFFENING

Whenever possible, a hand should be given as much exercise as possible. This predisposes to limber joints and mobile tissues. Hands are peculiar in that they are prone to stiffen, evidently because the joints are fitted together so accurately, and there are more close-fitting gliding parts than elsewhere in the body. Joint ligaments are just long enough, and if, from any cause, a hand remains swollen and immobile, the serum-soaked ligaments become short and thick, binding the joint. From the fluid of edema, fibrin settles between the movable tissues and within them—muscles, tendons and joints alike. Fibroblasts invade, and the whole becomes organized and shrinks, and a congealed hand results. The proximal finger joints stiffen in the straight position because of their collateral ligaments. These are tight in flexion, but shorten so much when they are relaxed with the joint in the straight position that they prevent flexion.

Splints stiffen hands if they are kept on too long, if they hold a joint on a rigid strain, or if they hold a hand in a position of nonfunction. Errors of position in splinting are holding the wrist flexed, fingers straight, palm flat and thumb at the side or clumped close into the hand. Rigid splinting, nonuse, edema and dependent position stiffen hands. Elastic or spring splints allow the necessary movement that makes a hand thrive. Stiffening is more easily prevented than cured. Hand patients must be urged continually to keep the hand active by exercise, occupational therapy or work.

Wrist Is Key Joint. When the hand is held flexed in the protective position, the extensors of the digits are tightened, hyperextending the proximal finger joints, drawing the thumb back and to the side of the hand and flattening the metacarpal arch; in this position the intrinsic muscles are too far off center to act. Shortening of muscles from disuse exaggerates the effect. The muscles are in balance in this position of nonfunction, but if the wrist is dorsiflexed, they will be in balance in the position of function. The position that the hand assumes is determined by the muscle balance which changes with the position of the wrist.

Open wounds on hands cause stiffness. The longer raw tissue is exposed, the stiffer the hand will be. Early closure of wounds and avoidance of any raw tissue, sinus or raw stem of a pedicle keeps hands limber.

LIBERATION OF SCAR

Hands that are bound, compressed or strangled by extensive scars have poor nutrition, as both the deep and the surface cicatrices interfere with the function of nerves, lymph vessels and blood vessels. The contracted cicatrix should be excised en bloc, allowing the structures to relax and the skin margins to recede. Excision of the deep cicatrix liberates the strangulated nerves, vessels and moving structures. The area should be covered with good skin by the pedicle method. This liberation from both deep and superficial cicatrices changes the whole appearance and consistency of the hand, restoring its nutrition and again allowing it to thrive. After a pedicle has been applied and the tissues have become soft and pliable, reconstruction of the deep structures is carried out. An essential part of this phase is the wide excision of deep cicatrix binding the movable structures. Just as the external scar binds and strangles the hand, so the deep

cicatrix impairs the function of reconstructed tendons and ligaments.

Before operating on the deeper parts (tendons, bones and joints) the surface plastic work should be completed, and good skin should replace cicatrix, for if one operates through scar, the wounds will not heal, infection will be more likely, and the repaired deep structures will slough out. Skin before deep structures should be the unbreakable rule.

Joints must be mobilized before tendons are repaired. One cannot expect a newly repaired tendon to move a stiff joint; nor should the surgeon repair a bone and a tendon or a joint at the same time. The bone demands postoperative immobilization; tendons and joints require mobilization.

TIMING OF OPERATIONS

After trauma, infection or an operation, some induration of the tissues is present, and the time required for this to recede varies with the cause and with the individual patient. A secondary operation on such indurated tissues results in a summation of scar tissue. It is best to wait until all inflammatory signs have disappeared, the tissues are soft and supple, the joints limber and the danger of latent infection is past. Steindler has described the ideal state as morphologic quiet and an equilibrium of the soft tissues.

Time in itself is an essential factor in reaching this state. While waiting, attention is paid to proper positioning, encouragement of active voluntary motion and the use of corrective or substitutional splints. Passive manipulation and the usual physiotherapy procedures are of no value in speeding the return of normal tissue equilibrium. Heat, as usually used, is excessive, and the hand remains red, swollen and edematous.

ORDER OF PROCEDURES

Operative procedures should be directed first toward restoring the position of function; then a good skin and soft-tissue covering should be provided. If pedicle grafts are applied, adequate time should be allowed for the newly transplanted skin and fat to soften. Nerves should be repaired before tendons and bones, and joint reconstruction should precede tendon work. Motor nerves severed in the arm or the forearm should have priority of repair.

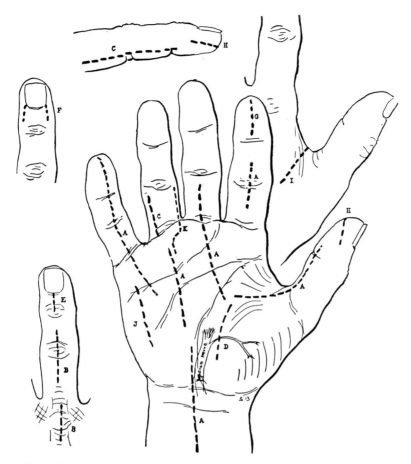

FIG. 154. A chart of pernicious or *incorrect incisions in the hand*, any of which will do harm. (A) Median longitudinal incisions which cross flexion creases at right angles and result in flexion contractures. These are prevalent but pernicious. (B) Median incision on dorsum of finger which later leaves a scar that contracts and hinders flexion of the finger. When present, it is impossible to fashion a proper skin flap under which to repair the extensor tendon. (C) Anterolateral incision in finger which is directly over and endangers vessels and nerves. It is the usual one pictured for draining tendon sheaths, but instead should be mid-lateral. (D) Incision which thoughtlessly severs the motor thenar nerve and so robs thumb of power of opposition. (E) Median longitudinal incision through matrix which will produce a rigid nail. (F) Incisions for paronychia often pictured, but erroneous, as they do not drain the bottoms of the clefts formed by the borders of the base of the nail, which curve strongly forward. (G) Median longitudinal incision in pulp for drainage of a felon. It will not drain, because due to cleavage planes the pus progresses in spite of it and points dorsilaterally. Also, the scar resulting is in the tactile surface. (H) Alligator-mouth incision wrongly placed too far anteriorly, which leaves a scar in the tactile surface. (I) Incision across a web injures the web which itself has a function of complicated foldings to allow for movements of thumb. (J) Incision often made for drainage of pus in sheath of tendon to little finger. However, the tendons converge sharply in the palm to pass between the ridge of the trapezium and the unciform process of the unciform bone. (K) Incision continuous from finger to palm severs the nerve, thus rendering half of the finger permanently anesthetic. (J. Bone Joint Surg. *14*, Jan., 1932)

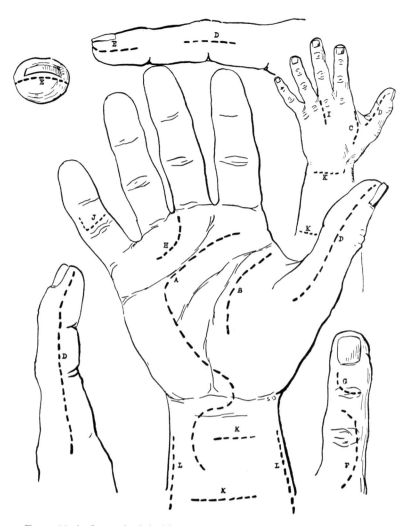

Fig. 155. A chart of advisable or *correct incisions in the hand,* which will afford access and will not cause disability. (A) Incision opening the palm or draining the middle palmar space, parallels flexion creases, exposes by triangular flap, enters between median and ulnar nerve supplies and may be extended through the ulnar side of the carpal ligament up the forearm. Curve crossing creases in wrist avoids contracture. (B) Drainage for thenar space, parallels thenar crease. Must not sever the thenar motor nerve. Pedicles between it and the palmar incision must be wide enough to nourish intermediate skin. (C) Usual drainage for thenar space. Should be radial to the interosseus muscle and not sever the radial artery in cleft. (D) Midlateral incisions in digits spare nerves and vessels and do not cause flexion contractures. (E) Drainage for pulp abscess, posterior to tactile surface. Should sever the vertical fat columns and not cause tenosynovitis by nicking sheath of flexor tendon. (F) Flap exposure to avoid overlying the extensor tendons. (G) Exposure of insertion of the extensor tendon. (H, I) Drainage of collar-button abscess. Avoid the volar nerve. (J) Flap drainage of subcutaneous abscess. One arm is median to nerve and the other blocks upward extension of infection. (K) Transverse incisions parallel wrinkles, thus avoiding conspicuous keloid formation. (L) Drainage for quadrilateral space in the forearm. Made anterior to bone and the radial nerve and posterior to the dorsal branch of the ulnar nerve. (J. Bone Joint Surg. *14,* Jan., 1932)

FIG. 156. Anterolateral scar with contracture. Incisions must not cross flexion creases. The mid-lateral incision in the finger will not cause this deformity.

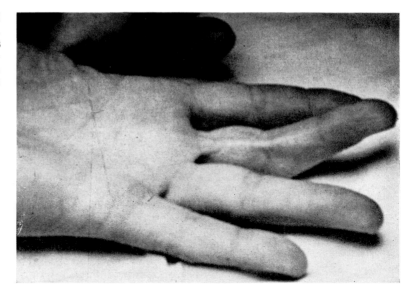

The building up of scar tissue is avoided by allowing sufficient time between operations. Careful follow-up observations are made over many months, and a year or more should elapse after the last procedure before the permanent impairment of function is estimated.

OPERATIVE TECHNIC

THE PRELIMINARIES

Skin Preparation. A thorough preparation of the skin of the hand and the arm should be carried out before any operative procedure.

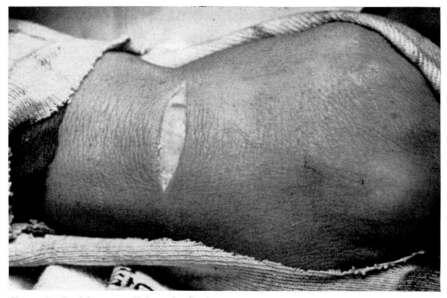

FIG. 157. Incisions parallel to the flexion creases. Here a transverse incision is used to expose the dorsal carpal ganglion.

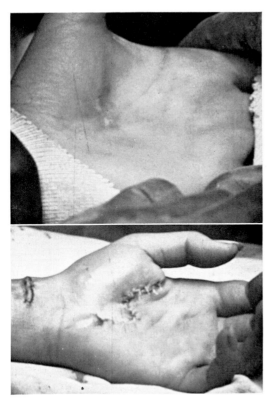

FIG. 158. (*Top*) A scar in the palm which crosses the thenar flexion crease. (*Bottom*) After excision, the wound is enlarged by extensions *paralleling* the crease in bayonet fashion.

The extremity should be cleansed with soap and water, a brush used on thick horny skin and the nails trimmed. Hands that have not been used or that have been painful and tender will be covered with scales of piled-up epidermis. This must be removed by repeated washing and scrubbing before the final preparation in the operating room.

As an added protective measure, after the uninflated tourniquet is placed on the upper arm, the hand and the arm up to the cuff are painted with an iodine solution; the standard $2\frac{1}{2}$ per cent tincture is commonly used. The solution is flowed on from a swab as from a paint brush, thoroughly covering all areas; it must be allowed to soak into the thick horny palmar skin and the crevices of the nails. Care is taken to prevent the iodine from running beneath the cuff of the tourniquet. The solu-

tion as applied remains on the skin, and no attempt is made to remove it with alcoholic solutions. The danger of burns from iodine on the skin is remote when care is used and the solution is not allowed to soak into a drape or beneath the tourniquet cuff.

Draping the Arm. The hand and the arm, covered with the iodine solution, are covered with a sterile sleeve of stockinette, long enough to be unrolled over the tourniquet cuff. The arm board is covered with a sheet of sterile aluminum foil, and over this a double-thickness surgical drape with a turned-back cuff is placed beneath the upper arm. This folded portion is brought around the upper arm and fastened with a clamp over the uninflated cuff; the closure should be loose to allow for the distention of the rubber bag tourniquet. Additional drapes are placed over the arm and over the body of the patient. Drapery material should be of some color other than white to cut down reflecting light and reduce eye fatigue.

The Arm Board. Surgery of the hand involves working on relatively small parts in a confined area. For this type of work in the manual arts, the part is usually held firmly in some form of clamp or vise on a sturdy work bench. From a study of the optimal area of use for 2-handed work at a bench, an arm board was designed to facilitate surgery on the hand. It is heavy so that it is not easily moved by inadvertent bumping; it can be firmly attached to the operating table and yet is adjustable to compensate for arms of various sizes. A fixed leg braces it on the floor. Since it has a firm base, the assistant is able to position the hand for the surgeon by pressing it firmly onto the immovable work bench, which becomes the vise of the artisan. The sides of the arm board are cut out to form a rest for the surgeon's and the assistant's elbows and forearms, and an extension tray is provided so that the instruments can be placed within easy reach.

Keeping Off the Skin. It is not practical to use skin clips in the stockinette or towels around the wound edges, since many different incisions are required, and frequent changes of position are necessary. It is better for the surgeon and the assistant to develop the habit of always holding the parts with a piece of gauze or toweling rather than the gloved hand.

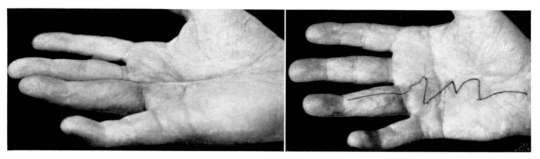

Fig. 159. (*Left*) A median longitudinal scar resulting from operation for Dupuytren's contracture. (*Right*) Correction by multiple Z-plasty.

Skin preparation is never perfect, and the skin surface should not be touched if possible.

Holding by Assistant. The assistant should hold the hand immobile with the part being operated on in a plane at a right angle to the line of vision of the surgeon. The assistant's forearm should be braced on the table, and he should so hold the limb that the skeletal segment which is being operated on does not move. If he holds it 1 or 2 joints beyond, movement will result. In presenting a finger, the assistant should hold the fingertip with gauze so as to present a clear lateral surface for incision and should brace the dorsum of the patient's finger with his finger. A sling of toweling holds the other fingers flexed and out of the way. To present a palm, one hand presses the forearm at the scaphoid down on the board to keep it supinated, and other flattens the fingers. An assistant should change quick, and on time, from one position to another and then freeze motionless. He should not brace on the trunk of the patient as this will transmit respiratory movement, and he should guard against making any athetoid or other movements. Some assistants are so in sympathy with what the surgeon is doing that each time the surgeon aims his stroke the assistant will move in harmony. Whenever he sees the surgeon about to make a stroke, he should become immobile so that the stroke will hit its mark. For some simple cases, the hand may be fastened immobile to a spreading hand splint. Sometimes holding the limb is quite difficult, as when the surgeon is approximating nerve ends for suture and the elbow and the wrist must be flexed. In this situation it is hard for the assistant to brace solidly on his

elbows, and the surgeon often must work in cramped positions, taking even an upside down look at things. Such parts of an operation are long and difficult. When in a tight and awkward place, after hours of tedious work, it is well to realize that there is no such thing as giving up. The surgeon must always succeed.

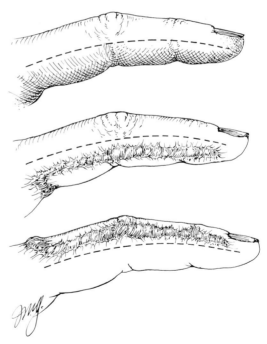

Fig. 160. The midlateral line of the finger (*top*) is not subject to push and pull, and contracture will not occur. When scars are excised from either the volar (*middle*) surface or the dorsal (*bottom*) surface, the excision should be extended to bring the junction of the replacing graft and normal skin in this line.

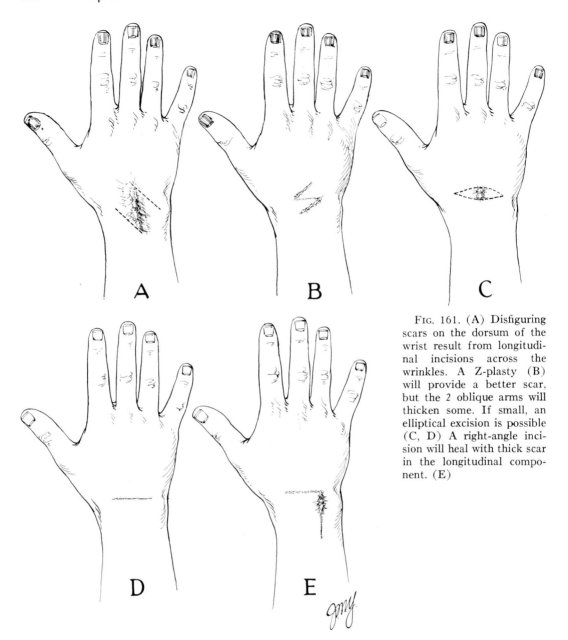

FIG. 161. (A) Disfiguring scars on the dorsum of the wrist result from longitudinal incisions across the wrinkles. A Z-plasty (B) will provide a better scar, but the 2 oblique arms will thicken some. If small, an elliptical excision is possible (C, D) A right-angle incision will heal with thick scar in the longitudinal component. (E)

Tourniquet. It is impossible to dissect a hand properly without the aid of ischemia from a tourniquet. It is also dangerous. Without a tourniquet the field is covered with blood, which is opaque; therefore, instead of progressing with the dissection the surgeon will be fumbling, traumatizing the tissues by sponging constantly, and the tissues will be crushed by too many hemostats. Could a jeweler repair a watch immersed in ink? Dissection of a limb in which the blood is held back by a tourniquet makes it possible to see every little nerve and vessel or other structures and to dissect with accuracy and minimal trauma. At the end of the operation the tourniquet is removed, the wound is held under steady gauze pressure and elevated for a few minutes; this allows the small vessels to be stopped by clot,

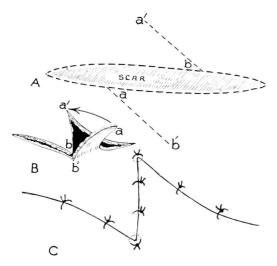

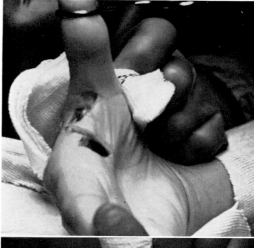

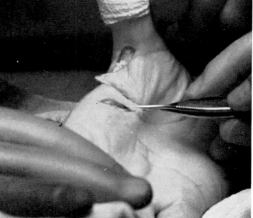

Fig. 162. The ever-useful zigzag plastic. By it, the transverse slack is utilized to relieve the line of tension. *a* is transposed to *a'* and *b* to *b'*. Intermittent tension causes keloid, but, after the zigzag plastic, the tension is spent, merely opening out the angles of the scar.

and only a few hemostats will be needed for the larger vessels.

Paralysis has often resulted from the use of an Esmarch bandage as a tourniquet. Each turn adds to the pressure, and when the turns overlie each other narrowly, actual nerve crushing may result. Spiegel and Lewin found 18 cases in the literature and reported 3 cases in which some type of tourniquet had been used. Most paralyses were temporary, ending in 3 to 6 weeks, but 5 were permanent. This paralysis from direct pressure usually does not include loss of sensation to temperature and pain and sympathetic action. None of the cases resulted from the use of a pneumatic tourniquet. The pneumatic band of a blood-pressure apparatus, applied smoothly and inflated to 300 mm. Hg, may be used safely for periods up to 2 hours.

All of the dissection and much of the repair work should be done before the tourniquet is released, though in extensive cases it is sometimes necessary to do the actual tendon and nerve suturing afterward. After the limb is given a breathing spell of 10 minutes, the tourniquet can be reapplied for another period.

Fig. 163. Z-plasty to relieve a web between thumb and index. The increase in length increases the depth of the cleft.

It is important that tissues devoid of blood supply be kept cool. One should avoid hot solutions and guard against overheating from inefficient lights.

APPLICATION. First place the cuff of a blood-pressure band or a pneumatic tourniquet around the limb near the shoulder, not tight, with the tubes proximal. The cuff may be reinforced with a bandage, because the bag may bulge irregularly under inflation. Not until the limb is completely sterilized and draped is it rendered ischemic by winding it with a bandage. The blood is expressed by winding from fingertips upward with a sterile rubber Esmarch, Ace or other elastic bandage. If one

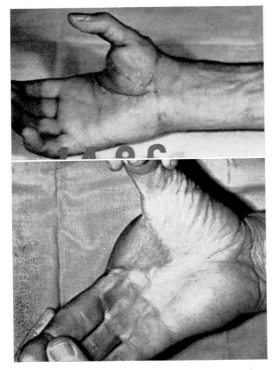

FIG. 164. For adduction contractures of the thumb, pedicle grafts are often necessary. The pedicle extends from the base of the cleft on the palmar side to the base on the dorsum. (See next figure.)

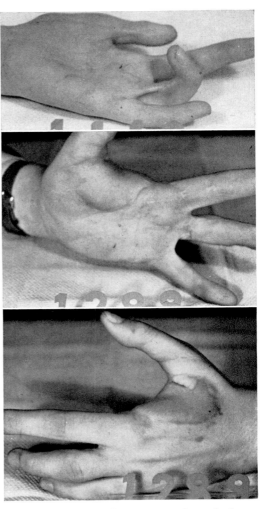

FIG. 165. (*Top*) A homemade explosive blew off the index ray, the cicatrix bound the thumb to the side of the middle finger, and a volar scar on the ring finger resulted in a flexion contracture of that finger. (*Center*) A tubed pedicle from abdomen replaced the thumb cleft scar, and its end was "waltzed" onto the ring finger. (*Bottom*) The pedicle extends to the depth of the cleft both on palm and on dorsum.

of these is not available, even gauze will do. Tourniquet time is precious, so the limb is not wound until the last minute before the operation. The elastic bandage should be kept sterile, since it may be needed again.

The pressure in the bag is raised to 300 mm. of mercury (in a child, to 250, and in an infant, 150 mm.); the tubes are clamped with rubber-protected clamps, or an adequate valve is used, and the Esmarch bandage is removed. It is necessary to leave a space of at least 1 inch between the Esmarch bandage and the blood-pressure cuff, for if the bandage is wound right up to the cuff, the fat is squeezed up beneath the cuff, and the pressure within the latter will be so lowered on removal of the Esmarch bandage that troublesome bleeding will occur during the operation. A pressure of 300 mm. of mercury corresponds to 5½ pounds, one of 258.5 mm. to 5 pounds, and one of 310 mm. to 6 pounds. One pound pressure is equivalent to 51.7 mm. of mercury.

Better than the standard blood-pressure machines are the commercial tourniquets available. Those with reservoir facilities, such as the Robbins and Zimmer, have the added advantage of maintaining an even pressure in spite of minor changes in cuff position. The gauges should be checked periodically.

TOURNIQUET IN INFECTIONS. The Esmarch bandage should not be used to express the blood from infected hands before applying a tourniquet, for this will express bacteria and their products into the general circulation. Therefore, in infections, the blood is emptied from the arm by holding it for several minutes in a vertical position before inflating the pneumatic tourniquet. The inflation should be done very rapidly so that the heart will not get in

several beats, forcing more blood into the arm before the systolic pressure level is reached.

Anesthesia. Selection of the type of anesthesia depends on many factors. Block and local anesthetics are often used for short, relatively simple, clean procedures. General anesthesia is essential for extensive work and usually when infection is present; use of block anesthesia in the presence of infection carries a risk of spreading the infection higher up the extremity. Local anesthesia, if instilled only in the line of incision, can be used to drain

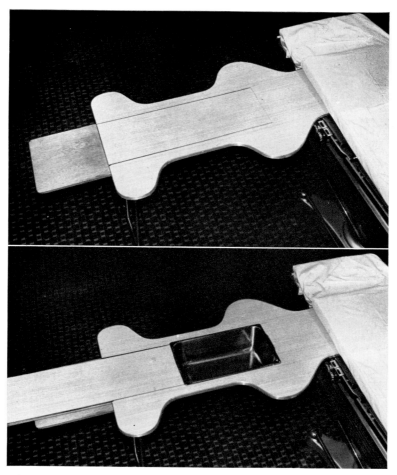

FIG. 166. An arm board for surgery on the hand. (*Top*) The long tongue slides beneath the mattress, allowing variation for different length of patients' arms. On the left is a sliding tray upon which the instrument tray is placed. (*Bottom*) When the slide is withdrawn, a pan can be inserted for collection of irrigating or wash solutions.

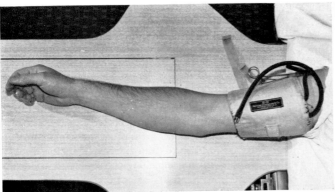

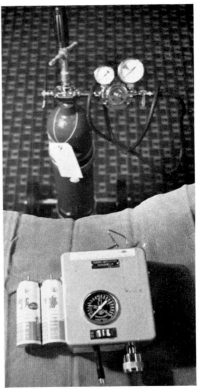

FIG. 167. A tourniquet is essential. Here a rubber bag around the upper arm, with tubes away from the surgical field, is held in place with a cloth cover and 2 straps. On the right are 2 available methods of supplying adequate volume and pressure to the tourniquet. On the table, the Robbins, which utilizes Freon gas in disposable cans; above, the Zimmer valve set, which connects to tank supply of oxygen. In all tourniquet apparatus, the accuracy of the valves should be checked periodically.

some infections. Ethyl chloride spray suffices for simple incision and drainage and removal of Kirschner wires.

A general anesthetic, even for extensive reconstructions lasting many hours, is best, for it allows the surgeon to work unhampered by the distractions of a conscious patient. Pentothal Sodium induction and light gas-oxygen anesthesia are adequate and safe when administered properly. Postanesthetic complications should be infrequent, for most patients can be ambulatory within 1 or 2 days, even after a prolonged operative procedure.

BRACHIAL PLEXUS ANESTHESIA. When done properly, this type of anesthesia is satisfactory, and there is no complaint of pain from the tourniquet such as accompanies the peripheral blocking of median and ulnar nerves. Two per cent procaine or lidocaine (Xylocaine) with epinephrine gives a prolonged anesthesia and allows extensive surgical procedures to be done. Certain risks, such as puncturing the pleura and the apex of the lung, are inherent in the method. Unrecognized pneumothorax can be fatal. Some risk of hemorrhage is also present.

AXILLARY BLOCK ANESTHESIA. Another method providing excellent anesthesia and carrying less risk than brachial plexus block

has become popular, particularly in emergency work, where proper preparation of the patient is not possible. Palpating the neurovascular bundle on the inner aspect of the arm at the level of the pectoral fold, the needle is inserted on both sides of the artery, and the anesthetic agent is injected directly into and around the major nerves.

BLOCK ANESTHESIA. This anesthetic is especially useful for routine work on fairly simple cases where the operation does not last longer than 2 hours. It should be used only on quiet, cooperative patients who have self-control and will not bother the surgeon—toward the end of the first hour the pneumatic tourniquet causes some pain, though this is entirely bearable by the normal individual. The worst of the pain lasts only about 15 minutes, and for this an additional injection of narcotic drug and a few words of encouragement generally suffice.

A tourniquet on the upper arm is used in conjunction with the block anesthesia, and, in addition, 3 drops of epinephrine per ounce are added in all block anesthesias except that of a digit. Epinephrine (Adrenalin) should never be injected into a digit—this often results in gangrene because the ischemia which must be removed serially lasts too long. A good routine is to block the ulnar nerve at the elbow and the median and the radial nerve above the wrist. Anesthesia results in 1 to 5 minutes, and after working on the hand for a while,

one can also operate painlessly on the forearm, the tourniquet furnishing the higher anesthesia. To inject the ulnar nerve, the arm is held in supination by an assistant with the elbow not quite in full extension and resting on a folded towel. By palpation the ulnar nerve is trapped between the finger and the internal epicondyle. Here it is penetrated with a quick jab by a fine hypodermic needle aimed

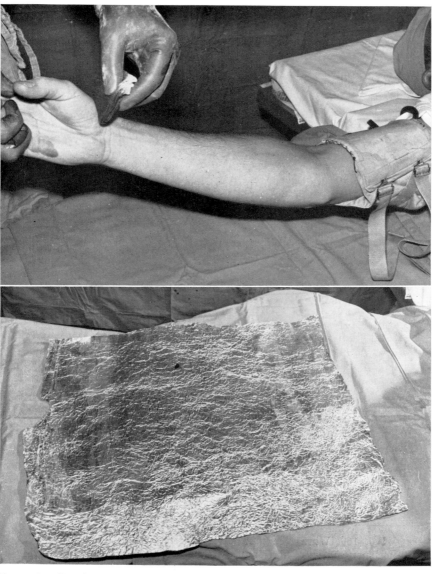

Fig. 168. (Top) Final skin preparation is with iodine. (Bottom) A sheet of aluminum foil separates the 2 layers of sterile drapery.

just distal to the palpating finger. When the patient announces that pain runs to the little finger, 2 ml. of the anesthetic is injected in the nerve and about 5 ml. around it.

To inject the median nerve, the arm is steadied by an assistant, with the dorsum of the lower part of the forearm resting on the folded towel. Two inches above the wrist the fine needle is made to penetrate the skin just radial to the palmaris longus tendon; then with a few quick ½-inch jabs the median nerve is located, as announced by the patient when he feels a pain in the thumb or the first 3 fingers. It is injected as was the ulnar nerve. Usually, the median nerve may be found just to the radial side of the palmaris longus, but sometimes under the palmaris longus or as far radial as under the tendon of the flexor carpi radialis.

To inject the radial nerve, the sharp edge of the curve of the lower end of the radius is used as the guide. The anesthetic is placed subcutaneously in the deep layer of fat, start-

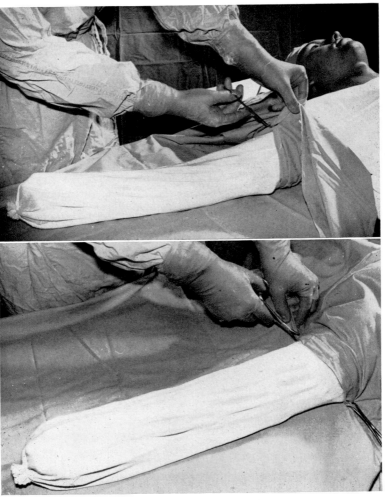

Fig. 169. When skin preparation is complete, a sterile sleeve of stockinette is unrolled from fingertips to above the tourniquet, and the cuff of a folded sheet is brought around the arm. A second sheet (*bottom*) covers the patient and the upper arm.

FIG. 170. Block anesthesia. The ulnar nerve (*top*) is trapped with a finger behind the internal condyle, and the anesthetic solution is injected directly in as well as around the nerve. The median nerve can be blocked at the wrist (*bottom*) if the wrist is slightly dorsiflexed over a folded towel and the mass of volar tendons fixed by the operator's fingers. A quick jab into the nerve to produce a shocklike sensation in thumb or fingers indicates correct site of placement of anesthetic solution.

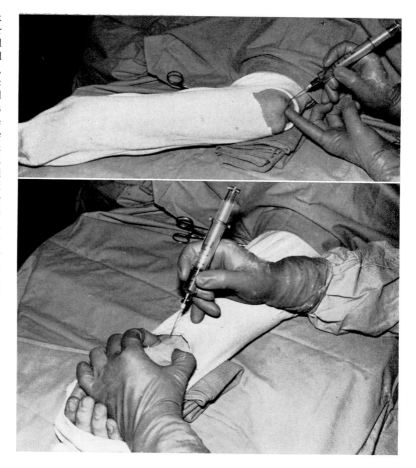

ing at the edge of the radius 2 inches above the wrist where the nerve emerges. No attempt is made to hit the radial nerve itself.

If done awkwardly, injection of the ulnar nerve occasionally has resulted in postoperative tingling for a few weeks or in breaking the needle.

When the arm is draped for the operation, the border of the sterile sheet which encircles it should be at least 2 inches above the epicondyle of the humerus to allow injection of the ulnar nerve.

Occasionally, it is desirable to block the median nerve in the channel under the transverse carpal ligament, or to block the ulnar nerve as it grooves the inner side of the pisiform bone. However, at the latter site one may puncture the blood vessels that accompany the nerve.

When anesthesia of a digit is required, the volar digital nerves can be blocked before their bifurcation at the distal part of the palm. In addition, an infiltration block should be done on the dorsum of the hand. Distal to this, epinephrine should not be used. The finger can be blocked at its base by 1 ml. of anesthetic solution near each volar digital nerve, entering dorsally where the skin is thin, and another 1 ml. subcutaneously across the dorsum. When the tourniquet is removed, this anesthesia will disappear quickly because of the absence of epinephrine. Finger blocks are dangerous. On all operations, the tourniquet is used around the upper arm. Tourniquets on the forearm are inefficient, and the use of rubber bands and such at the base of a digit is dangerous. Gangrene of a finger has occurred from a rubber-band tourniquet and local digi-

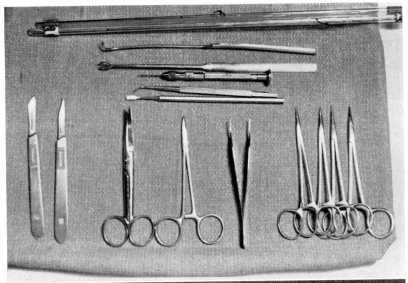

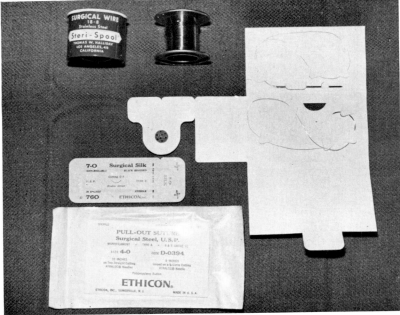

Fig. 171. Basic instruments include small dental chisel, dissecting probe, a machinist's pin vise and drill and wire sutures precut in 12-inch lengths and autoclaved in glass tubes to prevent kinking. In lower photo is wire as obtained on spools, a fine silk suitable for nerve suture and a prepackaged "pull-out-wire" kit, also shown opened on the right.

tal block, even though epinephrine was not used.

Block anesthesia should not be used for infected hands, but it is very useful in treating fresh injuries in an office or first aid station and allows thorough excision and closure of wounds.

LOCAL ANESTHESIA. In reconstructive surgery the tissue is in need of maximal vitality. As local anesthesia reduces this, it is better to use block anesthesia, although the latter is dangerous in the presence of infection except in the line of incision. If used in a digit it should not contain epinephrine. Local anesthesia, using 1 per cent lidocaine, is often useful in operating on small areas of the hand and the forearm or in removing skin grafts. Hands are so sensitive that it is considerate to the patient to use for at least the first injection a needle as fine as No. 30. A thrust through thick volar or palmar skin is painful, so that the needle, even when injecting the volar parts, should be introduced through the thin skin of the sides of the finger or the dorsum of the hand.

Ethyl Chloride Freezing. When used in conjunction with a tourniquet about the arm, freezing will last long enough and cause sufficient anesthesia to drain a small area of infection or to operate on a paronychia, removing the nail. Freezing without the aid of a tourniquet is very satisfactory for removing skin for Thiersch grafts and does not harm the grafts.

The Operative Procedure

Only the basic technical points will be mentioned here. For details of specific problems reference should be to the respective chapters on these subjects.

Incisions and Dissections. Incisions should be planned so that they do not overlie or parallel tendons and are remote from deep structures to be repaired. Whenever possible, they should parallel the flexor creases of the skin. An incision in the skin has little if any relationship to the direction of the deep structures. In every instance, the direction of the skin incision is chosen with reference to skin lines; once the skin is divided, an essential step is the undermining of the skin edge so that the opening is now as much in the direction at right angles to the skin incision as it is in the direction of the original cut. This development of the incision allows dissection and exposure of the deeper structures to be carried out in an entirely different plane. This is most important in areas such as the dorsum of the wrist where the skin is loose and pliable and where the important deeper structures are at right angles to the skin creases. Skin incisions that cross flexion creases at right angles violate this first axiom of plastic surgery and will thicken and become keloidlike.

Incisions. Before incising a hand, due consideration should be given to the choice of incision. Incisions made thoughtlessly may cause damage or lead to contractures if wrongly placed, because the hand is unusually mobile and because it is packed with structures that should not be severed.

The creases and the folds of the skin should be safeguarded. Unfortunately, there is still an urgent need to warn against making the all-too-prevalent pernicious median longitudinal incisions in the hand and incisions that cross natural creases at a right angle or nearly so. These lead to keloids and contractures, due to the irritation of intermittent traction and compression at each movement. Such incisions do harm whether they are in the hand or the wrist. If made along the volar aspect of a finger, the resulting scar draws the finger into flexion. The cut pulleys allow the tendons to bow across the finger on flexion, the special gliding surfaces of the pulleys have been cut through, and a long length of adhesions binds the tendon. In the finger pulp, median incisions will not drain infections, and scar is left on the tactile surface. Incisions through the matrix result in a split and ridged nail. On the dorsum of a finger if the scar is median it overlies the tendon, resulting in adhesions. The scar limits flexion and later makes it impossible to use a skin-flap incision for repair of the tendons. The hand in motion demonstrates that there are certain directions in which there is push and pull in the skin. Incisions coinciding with these may become irritated and form thick contracting scars.

Elastic and connective tissue fibers in the derma are arranged parallel with the flexion creases. Therefore, a scar across a flexion crease broadens due to traction by these fibers.

Lines of Langer generally conform to the flexion creases at the joints of the body. However, in the palm, the sole and a few other places they do not. Therefore, in planning incisions the only safe way is to be guided by the flexion creases as one sees them at the time rather than to depend on memorized lines of Langer. Incisions should parallel flexion creases.

A finger should be opened by midlateral incisions, not anterolateral as so often pictured, for these are exactly over the nerves and the vessels. Midlateral incisions, being just behind the 3 volar creases, are not subject to intermittent compression and tension and so may become almost invisible. The more volar or dorsal on the finger, the greater is the movement of the scar. In the palm there are 3 major folds which, if crossed, lead to contractures. The contents of a palm may be completely

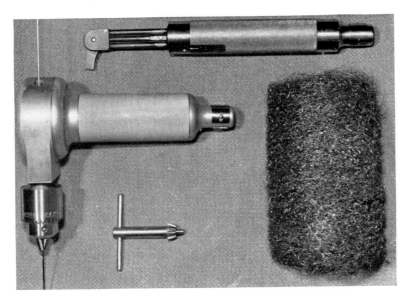

Fig. 172. A sagittal saw and drill head for use with Kirschner wire are useful accessories for the Stryker Electrosurgical unit. On the right is a pad of medium coarse steel wool used for compression dressings.

exposed by an L-shaped incision paralleling the distal crease and turning in an obtuse angle up the immobile heel of the palm to the carpus. Incisions on the back or the front of the wrist will become invisible if they conform to the creases but will make ugly keloids if they cross them. The cross incision may be prolonged longitudinally up the limb at one end and down it at the other, giving a wide double-flap exposure. This is a good way to uncover tissue beneath a transverse or diagonal scar or laceration, instead of making the usual longitudinal one crossing it at the center. An L incision heals better than an X, a Y or a T incision. It is rarely necessary to make a cross-extension over the volar aspect of a finger like an L. A midlateral incision combined with a cross incision at the distal crease of the finger has led to gangrene. On the dorsum of a finger, the incision may extend longitudinally down one side and then cross over abruptly and continue down the other side. In the pulp, a lateral or alligator-mouth incision is advisable, made posterior to the tactile surface. When incisions must cross creases, they should curve or zigzag to prevent contraction. In this way, the structures of the palm and the forearm can be laid open in one incision, being careful to enter between the two nerve distributions— the median and the ulnar along the 4th ray.

When choosing an incision regard should also be had for the deeper structures. No tiny nerves should be cut, such as the volar nerves of the digits and especially the motor thenar branch of the median nerve for opposition of the thumb, or the motor branch of the ulnar on which function of the intrinsic muscles depends. Even the nerve twigs to the lumbricals should be preserved. In making a transverse incision on the dorsum of the wrist, the skin on each side should be undermined freely, keeping rather superficial in the superficial fascia, because the branches of the radial nerve, as also the other cutaneous nerves in the forearm and the hand, lie deep in the superficial fascia. Utilizing wide undermining, a longitudinal incision through this fascia carries one into the deeper structures. An incision should not overlie a tendon, or the latter will be bound by a length of adhesions. If opened, all annular bands or pulleys should be slit through at one side, instead of through their central gliding surface. Incisions should be remote from tendon sutures or other repaired parts that might become adherent to the scar or exposed if the incision should separate. When possible, repaired parts should be separate from each other to reduce the local burden of healing and to prevent adhesions.

On entering a palm an L-shaped incision usually is made, following the distal crease and then turning proximally in the immobile heel of the palm to the center just beyond the wrist. This incision cuts through the palmar

FIG. 173. A hand drill with chuck and hollow shaft to use for insertion of Kirschner wire. (H. Weniger, San Francisco)

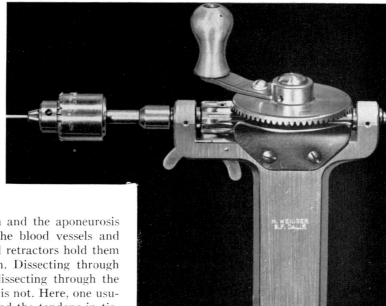

aponeurosis; as the skin and the aponeurosis are dissected off from the blood vessels and the nerves, small hooked retractors hold them out of the line of vision. Dissecting through normal tissue is easy; dissecting through the cicatrix left by infection is not. Here, one usually locates the nerves and the tendons in tissues farther proximal or distal where the cicatrix is less dense, and then follows them through the scar-bound mass. In dissecting with the scalpel down nerves, tendons or vessels, a trick is to use a sweeping, feathering stroke, with the edge of the scalpel always directed away from the structure that one does not wish to cut. Both the tissue being preserved and the tissue being cut from it should be held tense. This feather stroke of the knife is used throughout the dissection wherever the surgeon wishes to avoid cutting the structure he is uncovering.

Another useful instrument for dissecting out cleavage planes, nerves, vessels or tendons is the dissecting probe, by which one can lift connective tissue away from these structures. In following a small nerve, special scissors are useful. These are double-pointed, curved on the flat, and kept well sharpened. The point is repeatedly thrust along the nerve and then spread. It is better to dissect nerves from above downward, so as to preserve their branches. In excising deep cicatrix, a procedure which should accompany most reconstructive work, the surgeon should start at one side and go systematically across the whole area, excising the cicatrix en bloc, as for cancer, but preserving all of the essential structures, such as nerves, vessels, ligaments and tendons. If this cicatrix is left, it breeds

new cicatrix. It should be excised completely if possible, so that the wound is lined with well-nourished, normal-appearing tissue.

Hemostasis. Hematoma or postoperative bleeding resulting in a blood clot under the skin separates the structures and later leads to drainage and adhesions. The following procedures should be used to prevent this.

Hemostasis at the end of the operation should be as complete as possible. If oozing of blood is still present after this, multiple drains of tubing not over 3 mm. in diameter, with a small safety pin in each, should be placed between the sutures. These drains should not overlie repaired parts and should be removed on the following day or, if drainage is excessive, on the 2nd day. Also, one may rebandage the limb to force the blood out, pumping up the tourniquet until a voluminous waste or fluff dressing is applied, wound with elastic stockinette bandage snugly enough to check oozing but not so tight as to produce ischemia. A large fluff dressing is less likely to result in pressure necrosis than a thin one. Proper bandaging requires experience. A pad of steel wool or sponge rubber incorporated in the bandage furnishes useful pressure and splinting. After simple operations in which no large arteries have been severed, the tourniquet may be removed after the pressure dressing is in place.

Atraumatic Technic. This term was first used in 1921 to describe a system of operative technic designed to overcome the 2 great obstacles in reconstructive surgery of the hand. Infection and an excessive inflammatory reaction with resulting fibrosis are the major complications of reconstructive surgery. In the hand where this type of surgery consists of building up or restoring parts that move and glide on one another, infection and fibrosis are catastrophies. Finding that the technics which are satisfactory for excisional surgery were inadequate, Bunnell coined the term "atraumatic technic" to describe a whole method of approach based on careful handling of tissues, the lessening of trauma through improved manual skills and the expeditious use of tools, tissues and time.

Many free grafts of skin, bone, fascia and tendons are used in reconstructive hand surgery. Until these tissues develop a new blood supply, they provide ideal culture media for contaminating organisms. Asepsis in reconstructive procedures must be perfect. One cannot rely on local tissue resistance as one does in surgery of the face or the perineum. Extra care must be the standard, and errors in aseptic technic must be avoided at all costs.

Every wound heals with scar, and in long involved procedures many tissues are divided, fascial planes opened and dead spaces left to fill with fibrous tissue. Rough handling of tissue, tearing and stretching, the use of dull tools and an unsympathetic feel for the capacity of tissues may result in a mass of unyielding scar. This is of little importance in some regions, but in the hand scarring turns all the gliding parts into a functionally useless mass of cicatrix.

Additional scar tissue comes from suturing with too much tension, from foreign material, clusters of large catgut knots, an excess of suture ends, too many sutures, mass ligation, grasping excessive amounts of tissue in a ligature, tension on fatty tissue, too close proximity of suture line to buried grafts, hematomata, drying of tissues, use of hot solutions on sponges and prolonged exposure of tissues during operations.

EFFECT OF TRAUMA. In surgical procedures tissues are commonly torn, pinched, crushed, rubbed, scraped and picked to shreds. The wound surface is ragged and hemorrhagic with all semblance of normal surface obliterated. The tissues have lost their consistency and are flabby and shapeless. Treated with gentleness, the exposed tissues should be clean, moist and glistening, with each structure standing out clearly and retaining its natural color and consistency. Such tissues heal with minimal scarring.

HISTOLOGIC CONCEPTION OF TISSUES. If we think of the tissues as being a mass of succulent cells, joined by a fine meshwork of fibrous tissue with delicate nerve fibrils and blood vessels coursing among them, we will learn to handle them with gentleness and great respect. The eye specialist has learned to handle the tissues of the eye carefully with a delicate touch, using fine instruments and suture materials, and the brain surgeon has trained himself to produce minimal trauma as he works on the vital structures. General surgeons, especially when engaged in reconstructive procedures, must use these refined technics. The degree of force used in retraction must be gauged carefully. Dissection should be sharp, with clean incision of the tissues rather than blunt separation with clamp, scissors or gauze. Wiping the wound with sponges damages every surface cell. The use of a tourniquet obviates this constant trauma to the wound.

DELICACY, PLANNING AND TEAMWORK. An operation may be so prolonged by poor teamwork that the tissues dry out from exposure. Tremor on the part of an assistant prevents accuracy and leads to a moving field, loss of composure and repeated inaccurate strokes of an instrument. One motion should suffice. Repeated, aimless and ineffectual movements constitute an endless series of traumatisms. Dull needles require forcible pinching to make them penetrate tissues. Sharp-edged instruments should never be boiled and should be handled with care. Tissue forceps are used more as hooks, and hemostats are small and pointed to catch the minimal amount of tissue.

The duration of the operation should be reduced to a minimum. A well-thought-out plan, a good work table, capable assistants, sufficient lighting and a feeling of fixed purpose go a long way to maintain the surgical drive which is so necessary in complicated reconstructive work.

A very important factor in atraumatic technic is conservation of movement. Let each movement be studied, preplanned and purposeful, accomplishing its purpose in the single action. Thus there will be one traumatic impact instead of many. All movements should be direct and to the point. In order to reduce the operative time, the excursion of the surgeon's hand from one place to another should be rapid, but at the end of the motion when the tissue is acted on, the motion should be slower and under control. The motion should be refined, and the effort used should be the minimum that will accomplish the act. Gentleness must be the watchword throughout. Thought always should precede motion and, indeed, should anticipate the next motion.

False motions only complicate a procedure and upset composure. Watch a skilled mechanic at his work. He wastes no motions; each one accomplishes what it attempts. How far behind the mechanics we surgeons are in this aspect of our work!

In order to master conservation of movements in operating, the surgeon should practice it in everything he does in daily life, such as dressing and undressing, or working on his car. Why should he cultivate conservation of movement? It diminishes trauma and reduces operative time, and this lessens the duration of tissue abuse. It allows the surgeon to complete more difficult and extensive operations than would be possible otherwise. It develops skill. Once formed, this habit allows the mind to concentrate on the more important aspects of the operation. It fosters composure, and also it allows slower and more accurate movements.

If each movement accomplishes something, and if movements follow each other in rapid succession, the operation will be finished in a very short time.

THE STATIONARY FIELD. An important factor in atraumatic technic is a stable motionless field that the surgeon can work on. Fixing the arm and the hand on the firm unyielding armboard provides this. If the assistant fails to keep the limb in position, every movement of the surgeon becomes uncertain. This uncertain jogging or vibrating of the field makes it impossible to do accurate work. One never knows where the knife edge, the hemostat or the needle will meet the tissue. If the amplitude of the vibration is 3 mm., how impossible it is to be accurate within 1 mm. The miss of the instrument is equal to the amplitude of the jog. The surgeon is trying to do the impossible. Uncertainty is brought in. His composure is upset, and soon everyone in the room becomes irritated.

Usually the surgeon is not aware that it is the moving field that is causing the trouble. Tremor and a moving field account for many an inaccurate and repeated motion in surgery, thus adding materially to trauma. Tremor may be controlled by bracing, relaxation and poise.

BRACING AND LEVERAGE. The skilled manual worker uses bracing and leverage to gain control of finer movements. The best control is through wrist motions, provided that the shoulder, the elbow and the forearm are braced adequately. Watch the jeweler or the lapidary at work. His stool does not swivel, thus relieving the back muscles of strain; he sits with elbows and forearms braced, the piece on which he is working held firmly in a vise or a clamp; and he has sufficient light and, if necessary, additional magnification through lenses. All tremor is eliminated by an elaborate system of bracing. The surgeon can copy this system in his work, thus improving his accuracy, reducing fatigue and facilitating his efforts. Where the artist uses his mall stick, the surgeon using such instruments as scissors or a hemostat may brace them with an extended finger, with his forearm, his other hand, etc.

METHODS OF ACCURACY. The basic factor in the art of movements of skill is relaxation. The whole body is relaxed, and the only part that moves is that part doing the actual work. In addition, the whole body is balanced. Motion with the hands loses its refinement if the back is off balance; the consequent strain on the back muscles subconsciously diverts his attention and effort. When the body is relaxed and balanced, it can be ignored, and the surgeon can concentrate solely on the movement of his hand. If now he braces down on some of the fingers, his effort and attention can be concentrated on the specific part requiring surgery. In this way maximal refinement of motion is achieved, and tremor can be avoided.

IMPORTANCE OF ATRAUMATIC TECHNIC. If a Wolfe graft is not handled atraumatically, that part of it which has been abused turns black with necrosis toward the end of the first week. If the delicate membrane about a tendon (epitenon) becomes scratched, an adhesion between the tendon and its sheath forms at this point, preventing function. If nerve suture is not done atraumatically, fibrous tissue will form between the two ends and around the junction, encircling it tightly and preventing regeneration. If trauma accompanies the placing of grafts, serum forms about the grafts. This becomes infected, and the grafts slough out. If infection does not occur, the tissue reaction replaces much of the graft with scar tissue and binds it tightly. Many more disasters due to trauma could be cited, but suffice it to state once more than unless one uses atraumatic technic, the more difficult surgery of reconstruction cannot be accomplished. If mastered, it will greatly facilitate the simpler forms of surgery and result not only in an easier convalescence but also in very little local reaction. The reduction in the amount of local reaction is surprising.

Atraumatic technic has the advantage of ensuring an approximately reactionless healing and of reducing infection. We refer to the art of surgery, so why not make it an art and, like the artist, be engrossed in its technic?

PROCEDURES. In operating, the order followed is usually to make most of the skin incisions early and to the full distance needed. Then the nerves and the tendons are dissected out and deep cicatrix is excised. Some muscle belly is found available to move each tendon, and by tendon graft or transfer each tendon is connected to some muscle so as to restore all possible extension and flexion to the wrist and all the digits, opposition and adduction to the thumb, curvature to the arches, and proper muscle balance throughout. Where pulleys, ligamentous bands or tendon sheaths must be cut, they are cut through one side and repaired later if necessary. Skin margins, tendons, muscles, nerves or joints are truly freed, so that their complete movement is no longer hampered. The surgeon should actually accomplish this and not merely go through the motions of doing it. Tendons are repaired first, since they are tougher than the nerves which are repaired last because they must be protected from rebreaking and often must be sutured in awkward positions which must be maintained until the skin is closed and the limb immobilized.

If on closing it is found that the skin cannot be sutured without undue tension, as shown by a blanched appearance, some plastic maneuver is resorted to, so that by eliminating tension the skin will show good pink color throughout. Sometimes, to accomplish this it is necessary to make a parallel incision, undermine the skin and allow the edges to gap sufficiently for the closure. The denuded tissue thus exposed is covered by skin grafts.

At the beginning of the operation and throughout the time that the tourniquet is inflated the surgeon should work very rapidly. By conserving motions, making each one count, and keeping his mind on the main issues, the work can be done rapidly and accurately and still without detrimental haste. If one does not develop speed, it will be impossible to complete an extensive operation. There is usually time to complete all dissection and quite a little of the repair work before it becomes essential to loosen the tourniquet. When bleeding starts, the wounds are held firmly with gauze for a few minutes until clots form in the tiny vessels. Sponging should be by gentle pressure without any wiping motions which would express these clots, causing renewed bleeding. Elevating the limb at this stage is helpful. The larger bleeders, omitting the surrounding tissues, are accurately caught with mosquito hemostats and tied with very fine catgut. This is absorbed in a few days, leaving the tissue normal; silk or cotton leaves a permanent capsule of scar. Gross repair of tendons and nerves can be done without the tourniquet; but if this is found to be difficult, the limb can be rewound after 10 minutes and the tourniquet inflated again.

DRESSINGS. Postoperatively, the part of the limb that was operated on should be immobilized and the limb kept elevated because motion and the dependent position cause oozing.

The wrist should be immobilized in flexion following repair of the flexor tendons, but after repair of the extensor tendons the wrist and

FIG. 174. Sheet aluminum splints can be incorporated in dressings and are easily made either for right or left hand from the same pattern with a few blows of mallet.

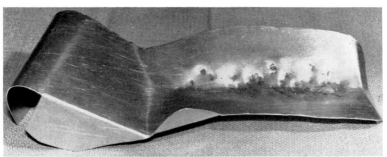

the fingers should be held in dorsiflexion. A slab of plaster of Paris laid on the dorsal or the flexor surface of the limb, respectively, will accomplish this. The joints should never be put up under full flexion because this will wreck them. Instead, as the plaster sets, the extreme of flexion is eased off a bit to relieve the strain. Only rarely should fingers be put up in flexion to prevent flexor tendons from breaking; the tendons will adhere too far proximally, and later it will be difficult to extend the digits. Flexion of the wrist is sufficient to rob the muscles of breaking force. After nerve repair, it may be necessary to flex various joints in order to prevent the nerve ends from being pulled apart. The elbow, the wrist and the finger joints can be maintained in flexion by a dorsal plaster-of-Paris half-circumference split. To flex the shoulder it may be necessary to hold the arm across the chest with adhesive plaster.

In most cases, the forearm should be in supination, care being taken so that this position is obtained when the first dressing is applied. Patients lying supine with arms outstretched on the armboard usually end up with the forearm in complete pronation. If plaster splinting is applied with the arm in pronation, it will be impossible when the patient becomes ambulatory for him to bring the forearm to the correct position without complete renewal of the fixation.

POSTOPERATIVE CARE. To lessen swelling postoperatively, the hand should be kept elevated on pillows considerably higher than the shoulder. Massive pressure dressings of waste, fluff and elastic bandage keep down edema and hematomas and act as a temporary splint until swelling has subsided and plaster can be applied. Twenty-four hours after operation the bandages should be loosened and any plaster cast opened along its full length and spread apart if by this time swelling has occurred. However, the dressings should be reapplied immediately to the proper degree of pressure. For this reason, at operation the casts should be bivalved or left open along the top and never made encircling. When after bone carpentry the bones are firmly repaired, it is well to dress the wound by binding a large mass of cotton waste about the hand. A nonpadded half-cast can be applied after 5 days. After arthrodesis, the skin at the side of the wrist may slough because of the swelling and the cast. Drains are removed if the discharge of blood is not excessive and there are no signs of hematoma. After simple operations the patients leave the hospital the following day, but it is better to keep patients for several days after extensive surgery. This gives them a chance to recover from the effects of the anesthetic and allows general bodily rest, which helps healing. Newly operated hands should not be allowed to hang down but should be kept elevated while the patient is in bed and in a sling when he is ambulatory. The patient who is undergoing prolonged treatment should be reminded occasionally to elevate his arm vertically lest, due to contracture of the great muscles that lower the arm, he lose the ability to do so.

The danger of ischemia always should be kept in mind; the necrosis or gangrene that follows leads to awkward complications. To remain alive, tissue must have an adequate blood supply at all times.

PROGNOSIS

LIMITATIONS OF SURGERY

It is hopeless to expect to make a perfect hand out of a cicatricial wreck. The state of nutrition of the hand and the amount of binding cicatrix throughout are the main factors in the prognosis. The greater the magnitude of the trauma, and the greater the intensity and the duration of the infection, the worse will be the material that the surgeon will have to build on. If there are too many unfavorable aspects to repair of a finger, such as annular scar, injured nerves, joints, tendons and skin, it is better to amputate.

THE RESULT

The result depends on several factors. Only by great care on the part of the surgeon and continued attention to the endless number of details involved in this tedious type of work will the reward of having grateful patients be obtained. Success depends to some extent on the patient as well. If fear of pain is paramount and will power is weak, he will not exercise the hand sufficiently or strongly enough to mobilize the tendons. One must take some punishment for the reward of a good result. There are other patients who are prone to form cicatrix and whose joints have an unusual tendency to stiffen. Results in these cases fall short of the average. Far better success can be obtained in children than in the aged, though procedures like arthroplasty give poor results in children.

The main factor influencing the return of movement and sensation and the restoration of tendon, joint and nerve function is the state of nutrition in the hand and the amount of cicatrix within it. In extreme cases, where the hand has been thoroughly gutted by infection and its contents replaced by cicatrix, its nerves and tendons destroyed, its joints stiffened, and its general nutrition greatly reduced, the surgeon should be able to restore position of function of the joints, a useful degree of sensation and the ability to grasp objects and to open the hand from 2 to 5 inches. If a finger is only slightly scarred and has flexible joints, one can replace a damaged tendon and probably give it flexion to within $1/2$ inch from the palm. If its joints are stiffened beyond repair, less is to be expected. However, when tissues are in excellent condition, the chances are good for restoring considerable useful function, often nearly approaching the normal and to the degree that there is no longer any interference with work.

To diagnose, measure, record and photograph a badly crippled hand properly requires an hour; to reconstruct it may consume a year. First it will be necessary to relieve flexion contractures and replace cicatrices by pedicled grafts. Over a period of weeks joints are placed in positions of function and mobilized. Many operations will be necessary, and time must elapse between each for nerves to regenerate and induration to subside. In an atrophic finger one must not repair the tendon or place a tendon graft until after the nerves have been repaired and have had time to regenerate; if they have not, the healing will be cicatricial, and the graft will degenerate or break. Operations themselves are several hours long and very fatiguing. As long as the tourniquet is on, the surgeon works under stress to accomplish as much as possible of the dissection before the tourniquet is released and the flow of blood obscures the operative site.

To the patient whose hand is a mere club with stiffened joints, no motion, no sensation and poor nutrition, it means much if the surgeon can restore to him even sensation and the ability to grasp. The loss of a leg is small compared with the loss of a hand.

BIBLIOGRAPHY

Allen, F. M.: Experiments concerning ligation and refrigeration in relation to local intoxication and infection, Surg., Gynec. Obstet. *68*:1047, 1939.

———: Surgical considerations of temperature in ligated limbs, Am. J. Surg. *45*:459, 1939.

———: Reduced temperatures in surgery; surgery of limbs, Am. J. Surg. *52*:225, 1941.

Ansbro, F. P.: Method of continuous brachial plexus block, Am. J. Surg. *71*:716, 1946.

Blalock, A.: Effects of continuous and of intermittent application of tourniquet to traumatized extremity, Arch. Surg. *48*:489, 1944.

Boyes, J. H.: Operative technic in surgery of the hand, Inst. Course Lect., Amer. Acad. Orth. Surg. *9*:181, 1952.

———: Operative technic of digital flexor tendon grafts, Inst. Course Lect., Amer. Acad. Orth. Surg. *10*:263, 1953.

Bruner, J. M.: Safety factors in the use of the pneumatic tourniquet for hemostasis in surgery of the hand, J. Bone Joint Surg. *33-A*:221, 1951.

———: Problems of postoperative position and motion in surgery of the hand, J. Bone Joint Surg. *35-A*:355, 1953.

Bunnell, S.: An essential in reconstructive surgery

PLATE 3

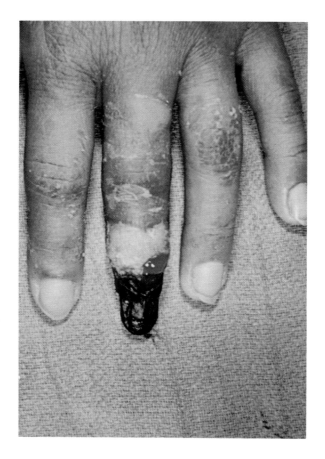

This finger tip became gangrenous after using a rubber band tourniquet and local anesthesia, without epinephrin, at the base of the finger to allow removal of a needle fragment. Protection of and preservation of optimum blood supply is a most important factor in all extremity surgery.

—atraumtic technique, Calif. State J. Med. *19*:204, 1921.

————: Reconstructive surgery of the hand, Surg., Gynec. Obstet. *39*:259, 1924.

————: Reconstruction of the injured hand, Rocky Mount M. J. *20*:269, 1938.

Cannon, B., and Peacock, E. E., Jr.: Plastic surgery: The hand, New Engl. J. Med. *263*:184, 238, 1960.

Clarkson, P. A., and Pelly, A.: The General and Plastic Surgery of the Hand, Oxford, Blackwell, 1962.

Cohn, J.: Crippled hand, Internat. Clin. *2*:225, 1934.

Cole, P. P.: Experiences in reparative surgery of upper limb, Brit. J. Surg. *28*:585, 1941.

Darrach, W.: Surgical approaches for surgery of the extremities, Am. J. Surg. *67*:237, 1945.

David, J. W.: Hand injuries, South. Med. Surg. J. *103*:258, 1941.

Griswold, R. A., and Woodson, W. H.: Brachial plexus block anesthesia of upper extremities, Am. J. Surg. *59*:439, 1943.

Hass, S. L.: Plastic restoration for loss of all fingers of both hands, Am. J. Surg. *36*:720, 1937.

Harmer, T. W.: Certain aspects of hand surgery, New Engl. J. Med. *214*:613, 1936.

Hawley, G. W.: Arm control for operations on upper extremity on Hawley table, J. Bone Joint Surg. *21*:794, 1939.

Hohmann, G.: Hand und Arm, pp. 1-251, München, Bergmann, 1949.

Iselin, M.: Chirurgie de la main, Paris, Masson, 1955.

Jansen, M.: Clawhand and clawfoot, Z. orthop. Chir. *58*:193, 1932.

Kaufman, P. A.: Gangrene following digital nerve block anesthesia, Arch. Surg. *42*:929, 1941.

Kendall, H. O., and Kendall, F. P.: Muscles, Testing and Function, pp. 1-131, Baltimore, Williams & Wilkins, 1949.

Kitlowski, E. A.: Preservation of tendon function by use of skin flaps, Am. J. Surg. *51*:653, 1941.

Klenerman, L.: The tourniquet in surgery, J. Bone Joint Surg. *44-B*:937, 1962.

Lance, M.: Importance of functionating positions; repair of extremities, Gaz. hôp. *113*:113, 1940.

Lange, Max: Orthopäedisch-Chirurgische Operationslehre, pp. 221-427, München, Bergmann, 1951.

Lipscomb, P. R.: Editorial, Surg., Gynec. Obstet. *113*:233, **1961.**

Littler, J. W.: Architectural principles of reconstructive hand surgery, Surg. Clin. N. Amer. *31*:463, 1951.

London, P. S.: Simplicity of approach to treatment of the injured hand, J. Bone Joint Surg. *43-A*:454, 1961.

Macintosh, R. R., and Mushin, W. W.: Local Anesthesia: Brachial Plexus, Oxford, Blackwood, 1945.

McLaughlin, C. W., Jr.: Gangrene of finger following digital nerve block anesthesia (with procaine hydrochloride), Am. J. Surg. *55*:558, 1942.

Mason, M. L.: Fifty years' progress in surgery of the hand, Surg., Gynec. Obstet. *101*:541, 1955.

Mayer, L.: The physiological method of tendon transplantation, Surg., Gynec. Obstet. *22*:298, 1916.

Murphey, D. R., Jr.: Brachial plexus block anesthesia; improved technic, Ann. Surg. *119*:935, 1944.

————: Stellate ganglion block; new anterior approach, Ann. Surg. *120*:759, 1944.

Murray, A. R.: Reconstructive surgery of the hand, Brit. J. Surg. *34*:131, 1946.

O'Neil, E. E., and Byrne, J. J.: Gangrene of the finger following digital nerve block, Am. J. Surg. *64*:80, 1944.

Paletta, F. X., Willman, V., and Ship, P. A. G.: Prolonged tourniquet ischemia of extremities: An experimental study of dogs, J. Bone Joint Surg. *42-A*:945, 1960.

Patrick, J.: Brachial plexus block anesthesia (procaine hydrochloride) in operations on upper extremity, Trans. Roy. Med.-Chir. Soc., Glasgow, p. 39 (1940-1941); in Glasgow Med. J., 1941.

Payr, E.: Treatment and restoration of totally crippled hands and extreme deformities of other members, Arch. klin. Chir. *200*:527, 1940.

Rank, B. K., and Wakefield, A. R.: Surgery of Repair as Applied to Hand Injuries, ed. 2, Baltimore, Williams & Wilkins, 1960.

Salsbury, C. R.: Some practical points in hand surgery, J. Okla. M. A. *26*:315, 1933.

Steindler, A.: Reconstructive Surgery of the Upper Extremity, New York, Appleton, 1923.

————: Mechanics of muscular contractures in wrist and fingers, J. Bone Joint Surg. *14*:1, 1932.

————: Mechanics of Normal and Pathological Locomotion in Man, Springfield, Ill., Thomas, 1935.

————: The Traumatic Deformities and Disabilities of the Upper Extremity, Springfield, Ill., Thomas, 1946.

Venable, C. S.: Osteosynthesis in presence of metals; studies on electrolysis, South. Med. J. *31*:501, 1938.

Chapter 6

Splints and Functional Bracing

The proper use of splints is an essential part of reconstructive surgery of the hand. After injury or infection or long periods of swelling and disuse, the hand is most likely to assume a nonfunctional position. When a proximal motor nerve is damaged, resulting in paralysis, the still-active muscles are no longer opposed by their normal antagonists, and the hand assumes an awkward and inefficient position. When a hand is not protected properly, the wrist falls into palmar flexion, the proximal finger joints hyperextend and stiffen and, if allowed to rest (as on a pillow or the chest), the thumb is forced back into the plane of the palm, the thenar muscles are stretched, and the first cleft muscles contract. It is rare to find the hand free of contractures in patients coming for reconstruction. Thus, the first step in reconstruction is the restoration of the position of function, the release of contractures and the mobilization of stiff joints. Splinting can accomplish much of this if the principles are understood and applied with patience and perseverance.

SPLINTING TO PREVENT DEFORMITY

The wrist is the key joint in the mechanics of the hand, and the proximal finger joint is of primary importance in the mechanical balance in a finger. After injury to the hand it is

a good rule to splint the wrist in the functional position of about 30° dorsiflexion. The application of a simple cockup splint, leaving the thumb and the fingers free, can prevent many deformities and hasten the recovery time. Therefore, unless there is some special reason why it cannot be done, one should make it a general rule to splint the wrist in the position of function during the immediate post-trauma period. This can be accomplished with a simple plaster slab applied on the volar surface over the dressing or by the use of a previously prepared metal or plastic splint. The proximal gutter should extend well up the forearm; the thumb should be free to fall forward, and the distal edge of the splint should stop at the distal palmar crease to allow full flexion of the proximal finger joints.

SPLINTING TO IMMOBILIZE

When required, complete immobilization of a part is carried out most satisfactorily with plaster of Paris. Splints made of plaster can be molded to the limb directly on the skin and provide complete fixation of the part. Padded plaster casings are inefficient; they allow some motion, the padding is displaced, and areas of localized pressure result, usually over the bony prominences. The plaster should not be applied circularly but should be laid

FIG. 175. (Left) Plaster slab applied after repair of flexor tendons to rob the muscles of strength

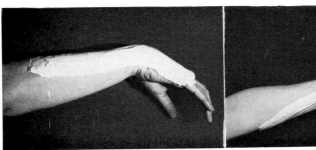

by keeping the wrist flexed and allowing the fingers to straighten and have some mobility. (Right) Plaster slab applied after repair of extensor tendons to hold the wrist and the proximal finger joints in extension until the tendons have joined.

on in flat slabs. With a little over half the circumference of the limb covered, an encircling wet gauze bandage is used to mold it into place. When the first layer of plaster is fairly hard, the gauze is cut its full length longitudinally to avoid constriction of the limb. Next, a layer of wax paper or cellophane is laid over the limb, and the back half of the cast is applied as a flat slab over it. Finally, another gauze bandage is wound around the entire cast. This bivalve is for safety; if the limb swells, the "lid" can be lifted and the cast spread apart, the lid being replaced afterward. In applying the nonpadded cast, the plaster is laid directly on the skin but is placed without any tension. It should be molded accurately to the curvature of the limb and around bony prominences, guarding the head of the ulna and the internal epicondyle from pressure. When encasing a hand, it is convenient, because of the many curves, to use multiple

small folded strips of plaster instead of a large slab. These fit the contours better and reinforce the cast wherever needed. One thicker strip is used to complete the cast. It is passed across the cleft of the thumb and the palm between the thenar and the distal palmar creases. This is made strong enough to withstand the wear of work but narrow enough to allow free motion of the thumb and the proximal finger joints. The joints should not move while the cast is being applied or pressure-producing ridges will form.

Position of Joints; Freedom for Movement

Joints never should be put up in a cast at their limit of flexion, because they will be damaged from pressure on the articular cartilages and tension on their ligaments. Instead, joints should be eased off a little from complete flexion. Unless there is reason to do

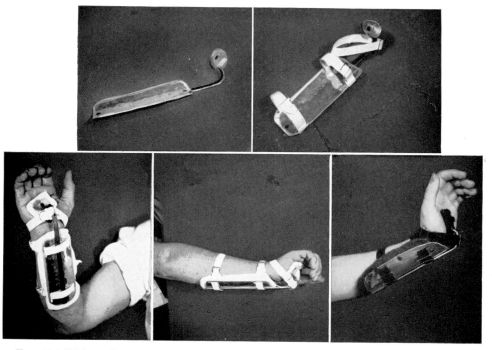

Fig. 176. Wrist splint, volar or cockup splint of aluminum sheet, steel rod and ovoid palm piece. One strap to the wrist must be oblique to keep the splint from displacing down the hand as it forces the wrist in dorsiflexion.

(*Top*) Splint easily made in an office. Straps are interchangeable through slits punched in the aluminum.

(*Bottom, left*) Volar view; (*center*) well padded with felt; (*right*) will give strong dorsiflexion if desired.

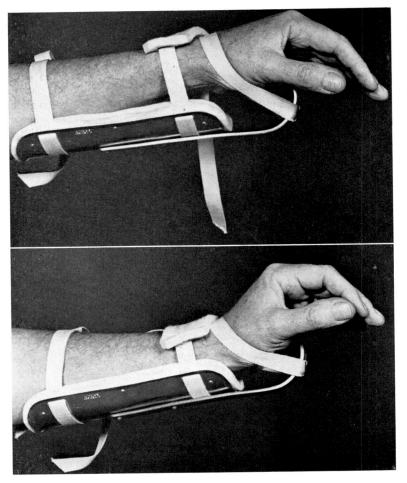

FIG. 177. Rigid cockup splint devised by Weniger. The oblique strap from the dorsum of the wrist to the apex of the curved volar piece is necessary.

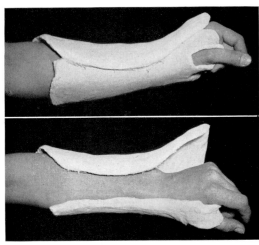

FIG. 178. Nonpadded plaster applied as volar and dorsal splints may be separated by waxed paper to allow swelling.

otherwise in making a cast, the joints should be placed in positions of function, and the thumb and the fingers should be free to move. The wrist should be moderately dorsiflexed and ulnarflexed, with the forearm slightly supinated, and the elbow should be at a right angle. In the palm the cast should end with a thick edge for wear—not a feather edge—and should stop at the distal palmar crease so that the proximal joints of the fingers are free to flex. The dorsum of the cast ends at the knuckles. The thumb should be in a forward position from the hand, and its proximal joint should be entirely free to move. If it is desired to stop the motion of pronation and supination, the cast should be continued to the axilla. This can be done by a sugar-tong U-ribbon of plaster taking in the upper arm and the elbow and held in place by a gauze bandage.

A cast on the hand either should run well

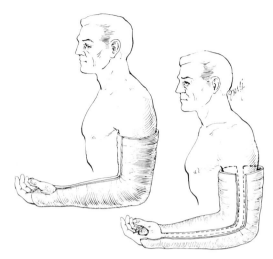

FIG. 179. (*Left*) Incorrect way to cut a tight cast. (*Right*) Only by making 2 complete cuts laterally can the front portion be lifted and pressure on the antecubital space relieved.

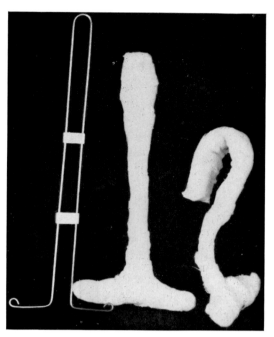

FIG. 180. The Böhler wire finger splint, bare, padded and bent to required position. Placed on the volar aspect directly on the skin and under a volar plaster slab from palm to forearm, it provides excellent fixation of a finger in any desired position.

up the forearm for good leverage in immobilizing the wrist or stop at the base of the hand so that the wrist will be free in all its motions.

Common mistakes in applying casts are to place the wrist straight instead of dorsiflexed, to prolong the cast beyond the distal palmar crease so that the fingers cannot be exercised, to disregard the transverse palmar arch and make it flat, to have the thumb at the side, and to leave the cast on too long.

DANGER OF TIGHT CASTS

Volkmann's ischemia is caused by pressure on the veins in the antecubital space, so that all elbow casts should provide adequate space for the elbow. It is advisable first to lay a small fluff of sheet wadding along the crease of the elbow and to apply the plaster in such a way that this region will be free from pressure. Movement of the elbow while the plaster is setting works a plaster ridge into this crease. In relieving pressure which develops in a right-angle elbow cast, it is wrong to slit the cast along its anterior and posterior longitudinal lines because this will not relieve the pressure on the front of the elbow. Instead, two midlateral cuts should be made the full length of the cast, one along the inner and the

other along the outer side, the front half being lifted from the rear half through its full length. It is impossible to relieve the pressure in an elbow cast by making one full-length longitudinal lateral cut and then attempting to spread the cast, for a right-angle cast will not spread in both arms of the angle at the same time. If the cast is applied following an

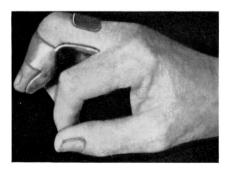

FIG. 181. Splint for rupture of extensor insertion. Shown here made of aluminum, it may be of plastic or plaster of Paris. (See Chap. 11, Rupture of Tendons.)

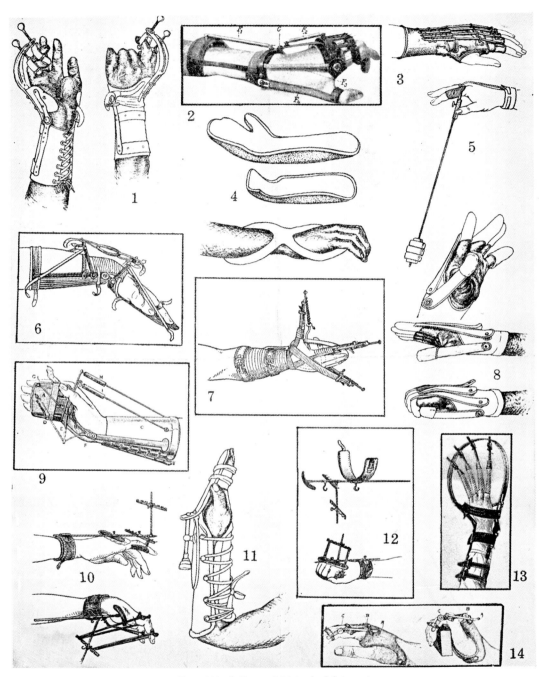

FIG. 182. Splints of historical interest.

(1) To extend the fingers (after Rey, J., 1927)
(2) Radial palsy (Gocht, 1917)
(3) Radial palsy (Radike, *et al.*, 1919)
(4) Radial palsy (after Lange, M., 1943)
(5) To exercise the metacarpophalangeal joint (Krukenberg, H., 1892)
(6) Volkmann's contracture (Schanz, 1908)

(7) Fractures (Bardenheuer, 1889)
(8) To extend the fingers (redrawn from Herzog, M. B., 1944)
(9) Volkmann's contracture (Bigg, H. A., 1869)
(10) To extend and flex the fingers (Schanz, 1908)

(Continued on facing page)

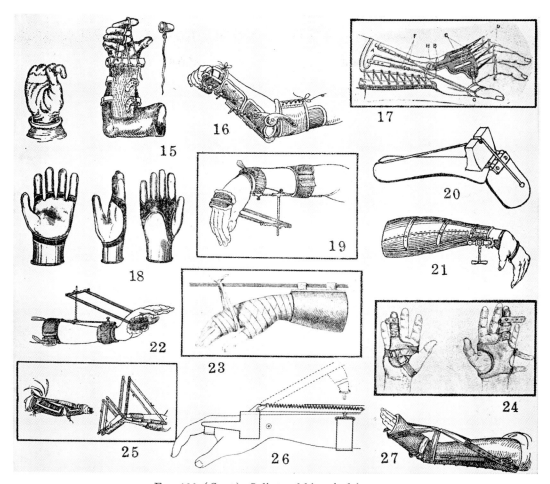

Fig. 182 (*Cont.*). Splints of historical interest.

(11) Volkmann's contracture (redrawn from Corret, P., Presse méd., 1938)

(12) To flex the finger (Schanz, 1908)

(13) To extend the fingers (Howitt, F., 1934)

(14) To flex the fingers (Dumoulin & Roederer, 1922)

(15) To flex the fingers (after Fabricii, Opera Chir., 1647)

(16) To immobilize the hand and the forearm (Gerson, K., 1905)

(17) Radial palsy (Bigg, 1869)

(18) To extend the fingers (after Wilson, W. J., 1949)

(19) To flex the wrist (Reibmayer, A., 1886)

(20) To flex the wrist (redrawn from Puzey, C., 1880)

(21) To flex the wrist (Schanz, 1908)

(22) To dorsiflex the wrist (Reibmayer, A., 1886)

(23) To dorsiflex the wrist (Hoffa, 1891)

(24) Dupuytren's contracture (Tubby, A. H., 1896)

(25) Volkmann's contracture (Schanz, 1908)

(26) To dorsiflex the wrist (after Von Recklinghausen, 1920)

(27) To dorsiflex the wrist (Schanz, 1908)

(American Academy of Orthopaedic Surgeons, Inc.—Orthopaedic Appliances Atlas, vol. 1, pp. 325, 326, Ann Arbor, Mich., Edwards)

injury or operation, the arm should be elevated for the first 1 or 2 days. Frequent inspections are imperative, as there is always danger of pressure points, ischemia or gangrene. The digits should be exposed to view when a cast is applied so that one can ascertain the condition of the circulation. Painful, cold, cyanotic, anesthetic swollen tips of an extremity are the danger signs. A hand which has been operated on must never be enclosed

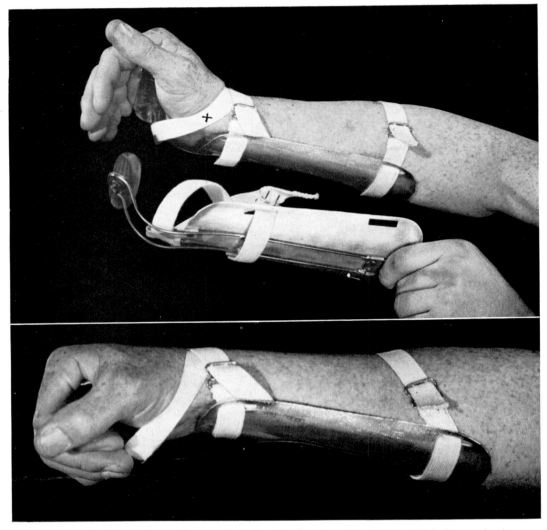

FIG. 183. Spring cockup splints made of flat blued spring, size 0.045 × ⅝ inch, or of a loop of piano wire, size 0.015 inch. This splint gradually causes the wrist to assume a position of dorsiflexion. An oblique strap (X) through the chamber in the neck piece and looped over the back of the wrist is essential to hold the splint in place. Spring splints allow exercise. (*Top*) Dorsiflexion; (*bottom*) flexion.

in a complete encircling nonpadded cast, as it is sure to swell and need relief. The cast should be bivalved, as described above, or made with an intervening sheet of wax paper or cellophane separating the volar and the dorsal slabs to allow easy spreading when swelling occurs.

SPLINTING TO PROTECT TENDONS

After repair of flexor tendons, a flat slab of 8 layers is laid on the dorsum of the hand and the forearm to hold the wrist in flexion. Following repair of extensor tendons, a similar slab is laid on the volar aspect to hold the fingers and the wrist in dorsiflexion. After a plastic operation on a youngster for syndactylia, burn contractures, etc., in which full-thickness grafts or vulnerable skin flaps are used, the hand and the fingers first should be fastened on a skeleton splint made of metal. Outside this there should be a casing of plaster of Paris enveloping two thirds of the circumference of the hand and the circumference of the arm. This is completed by adding a removable lid as a bivalve over the hand. For ease of inspection of the fingertips, a glass microscope slide can be placed in the cast as a window. In children, to prevent slipping, the plaster cast should extend to the axilla with the elbow at a right angle.

MISCELLANEOUS PLASTER SPLINTING

When traction is applied to the digits by extension splints or by the Böhler wire method, there is nothing better than nonpadded plaster of Paris about the hand and the forearm as a foundation to give attachment and stability to the extension. This may be on either the volar or the dorsal aspect. Embedded in it is the wire outrigger from which the fingers are pulled into flexion or extension. To draw the distal 2 finger joints into extension, a layer of felt is placed under the plaster across the backs of the row of proximal finger segments to act as a fulcrum. Similarly, after a recent wound is excised and the tissues repaired, an encircling cage of Cramer wire embedded in the front and the back of the plaster affords air dressing and, when enclosed by gauze, gives adequate protection from outside injury.

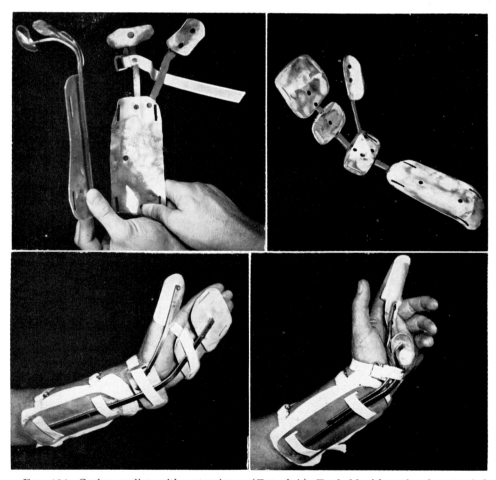

Fig. 184. Cockup splint with extensions. (*Top, left*) To hold either thumb extended. (*Top, right,* and *bottom, left*) To hold the wrist in dorsiflexion and all digits in extension after repair of extensor tendons. (*Bottom, right*) To hold the wrist in dorsiflexion and the index finger in extension after repair of the extensor tendons.

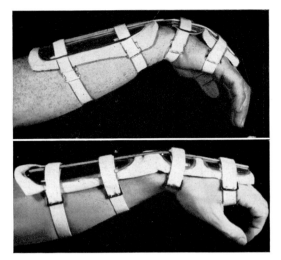

FIG. 185. (*Top*) Wrist splint, dorsal or flat splint. Holds wrist in flexion after repair of flexor tendons or when gradually straightening wrist after median or ulnar nerve suture. (*Bottom*) Can be bent to any angle. Easily made in the office. Straps are washable and replaced through slits. An extension to hold the fingers in flexion can be added.

For holding a finger for rupture of the insertion of the extensor tendon, with the distal joint in extension and the middle joint in flexion, plaster is better than any other material. Three layers of extra-fast-setting plaster, 4 inches wide and the length of the finger involved, are notched on both sides at the level of the middle and the distal joints. This plaster is dipped in warm water and laid on the flexor surface of the finger, with the digit in the correct position. Narrow 1-inch strips of plaster are used to reinforce the bends and the angles of the dressing, leaving the dorsum of the middle joint and the nail exposed. If the plaster is applied to the straight finger and then the joints are bent, there is danger of forming a ridge in the plaster where it folds on the flexor side of the middle joint and the dorsal aspect of the distal joint. Pressure here may result in ischemic necrosis of the skin. The finger should be placed in the correct position first, and then the plaster may be applied.

Splints that are used to immobilize inflamed or healing parts after infections, fractures or reconstructive procedures—particularly such procedures on the skeleton—must be stationary. However, if a hand is kept absolutely still, it atrophies and stiffens. Thus this type of splinting must be discontinued as soon as possible. It is also important not to immobilize more of the hand than is necessary. Every part that is not directly involved in the injury

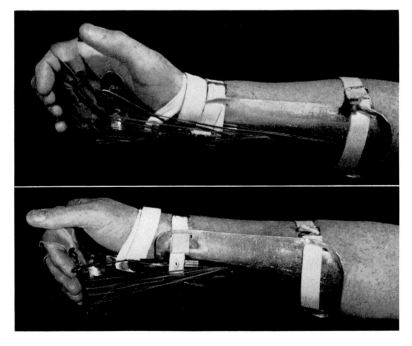

FIG. 186. Spring cock-up splint with attached outrigger to draw proximal finger joints into flexion. As the joints flex more, the rubber bands are connected directly to the hook in the belly of the splint. (*Top*) Dorsiflexion of the wrist and extension of the proximal finger joints. (*Bottom*) Flexion of the wrist and flexion of the proximal finger joints.

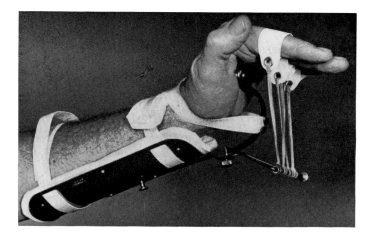

Fig. 187. Spring cockup splint with outrigger which can be attached at any point along the volar bar to control the direction of pull of the traction loops. Note the oblique strap to the gooseneck. (H. Weniger, San Francisco)

must be free to move and should be exercised regularly. A wrist fracture can be immobilized completely and yet leave the digits free to move through their full range of motion. To allow finger motion, splints must stop at the distal crease of the palm and not extend down to the webs, or the proximal joints will be restricted.

SPLINTING TO CHANGE OR CORRECT THE POSITION OF A JOINT

Purposeful, directive splinting can be used to change the angle of a joint or to overcome a contracture. The familiar method of casting for correction of clubfeet can be used to force joints into new positions and correct deformities. Plaster can be wedged or applied at frequent intervals, holding the parts in the corrected position until the plaster hardens. The same slow steady pressure used by the orthodontist can be used to change a joint position. Splints with a hingelike action centered at the joint can be activated by springs, coils or nonelastic straps arranged so as to exert a constant pressure on the restraining tissues. A slow steady pressure causes tissues to grow longer rather than stretch. Intermittent pressure such as that from passive manipulations or inexpertly applied elastic mechanisms causes fibrous tissue to hypertrophy. Just as the scar tissue across the flexion crease responds to the push-and-pull effect of the underlying joint motion by forming a keloidlike mass, the deep cicatrix which is preventing a joint action will thicken when it is intermittently stretched and relaxed. However, if the force put on it is constant, such fibrous

tissue atrophies, stretches and, in effect, grows longer. A tenodesis under constant strain, as in a weight-bearing joint, usually will give way, whereas fascial strips across the paralyzed abdominal wall, when placed at proper tension, hypertrophy and form a massive tendonlike cord (Lowman).

Splints can be made to provide the proper points of fixation and leverage to allow this steady force to be applied. A wrist in a straight or slightly palmar-flexed position can be brought into the correct position of function by using a cockup splint with a goosenecklike bar. A strap from the apex of this curve to the dorsum of the wrist, if kept constantly tight, draws the heel of the palm volarward and distally while the 2 points of counter pressure, the palm and the forearm, remain fixed. Thus the wrist is dorsiflexed. This steady force of the tight strap can be given additional force by making the gooseneck bar of spring steel. Such a splint requires delicate adjustment and an intelligent, cooperative patient.

Splints to draw a joint into flexion or extension should have 3 padded areas for broad pressure: one at the level of the joint to act as a fulcrum, and the other two on the opposite side of the limb as far from the fulcrum as possible to give maximal leverage.

SPLINTS TO SUBSTITUTE FOR PARALYZED MUSCLES

Early recognition of paralysis of some of the muscles that move the hand permits the substitution of some kind of apparatus to provide the motion until recovery occurs or reconstruction is carried out. Applied early, such

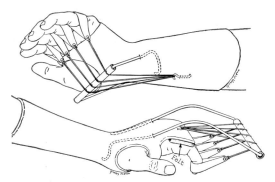

Fig. 188. Plaster-of-Paris splints with wire outriggers with rollers. (*Top*) To flex the proximal finger joints. The outrigger may be bent proximalward as the fingers become more flexed. (*Bottom*) To extend the distal two finger joints. Note felt for fulcrum. The rubbers exercise the fingers.

splinting prevents contractures of the still-activated muscles, which are no longer opposed by their antagonists, and prevents the secondary joint ligament and soft-tissue contractures which usually follow.

Splints of this type must be light in weight and easy to apply and wear. They are usually activated by rubber bands or springs. In radial palsy, a dorsal splint covers the forearm, and a bar beneath the fingers is connected to the splint by a spring steel extension. This spring is strong enough to extend the fingers in their proximal joints but weak enough so that the normal flexors can easily overcome its pull and flex the fingers completely. A similar extension provides a loop around the thumb to hold it in abduction and extension. For median palsy, to hold the thumb in opposition, an elastic loop can be drawn toward the pisiform and here fastened to a wrist strap. Abduction and opposition of the thumb can be maintained by a small semicircular band on which the thumb rests, held in proper position by a projecting wire from a wrist support. To allow motion, this bar can be swiveled at its base attachment. To prevent clawing in ulnar palsy, it is necessary to block hyperextension of the proximal joints either by pressure on the dorsum of the proximal segments of the ring and the little fingers or by a volar sling. In all paralyses, the principle of the splint is to substitute for the lost motion with just enough force so that

when the opposing normal muscles are relaxed, the parts will fall into the corrected position, and yet allow the normal muscles, when activated, to carry out the full range of motion.

ACTIVE SPLINTING BY SPRING OR ELASTIC

A system of using elastic or spring-powered splints to coax joints into proper position and maintain them there was outlined in earlier editions of this book. The principles underlying this system must be understood if the expected results are to be obtained. It is necessary to diagnose the cause of the limited motion. No active splint can overcome a bony mechanical block to a joint movement or overcome a deformity where the basic skeletal features are misaligned. When metacarpals are allowed to heal with marked dorsal bowing, the distal ends are depressed into the palm, the proximal joints are hyperextended, and the collateral ligaments become taut and fibrosed. It is folly to expect any splint activated by rubber bands or springs to restore flexion to these joints. The basic deformity in the longitudinal arch must be corrected surgically. Similarly, to expect a lightweight splint of this type to overcome deep scarring where a flap of skin and soft tissue is needed to replace the lost parts is to waste time, effort and money. Active splinting is best for those myogenic contractures of the normal muscles which follow paralyses and for the secondary ligamentous and soft-tissue fibroses which result from long immobilization with persistent edema. Even in these, the application, the splints and the forces used must be studied carefully. The basic factor used in overcoming a contracture of soft tissue is slow, persistent, steady force just under that which would cause a rupture of the tissues. The use of an active or dynamic splint allows some motion so that the hand can be used; also, the pumping effect helps to relieve edema, and ischemia from prolonged tension does not occur. It is the unusual patient who can understand and apply and persevere in the wearing of a properly used splint in these conditions. In many cases it is necessary to compromise by using a nonelastic force, such as a web strap, adjusted by the patient and worn for long periods. A simple example is the finger limited in flexion in its middle joint following injury to the flexor

FIG. 189. Clamping this unit to the standard elbow splint, the hand and the forearm are put into as much supination as possible and the set screw on the axle tightened. The twisted flat spring forces the part into more supination on the torsion-bar principle.

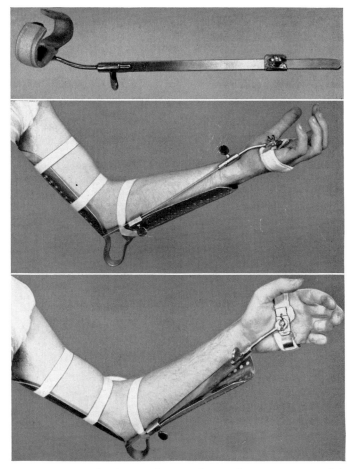

tendons. Before tendon reconstruction is carried out, a full range of passive flexion must be present. Intermittent passive flexion by manipulation will not help, but a web strap worn around the hand and kept snug by adjustment at the buckle can be worn day and night, being removed 3 or 4 times a day in order to bathe the hand in lukewarm soapy water and maintain extension. The strap is adjusted by the patient, who is warned to keep the tension just under that which produces pain and swelling. The strap is worn all night, principally to maintain the motion gained during the day. Once the full range of motion has been obtained, the force is changed to elastic or spring tension of such strength that the normal opposing muscles can just overcome it. Thus a short period of semirigid splinting draws out the contracture, and the active dynamic splinting maintains the correction. This same method of following steady force by

elastic traction can be used to overcome wrist, thumb and proximal joint contractures.

In active splinting the splint should be light and should not interfere with occupational therapy or work. If the hand is kept in the position of function, the digits can be used for grasping. If there is little movement, the hand is useless, but in the position of function it will be used more and more and will improve continuously.

The splints are designed to be lightweight, simple and economical. Attachments are available to allow several corrective forces to be utilized at the same time. They are manufactured by H. Weniger, 70 12th Street, San Francisco, Calif.

FITTING OF SPLINTS

The forearm piece should fit the forearm whether on the volar or the dorsal aspect. If on the dorsum, a hollow should protect the

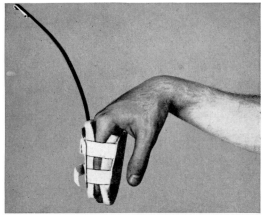

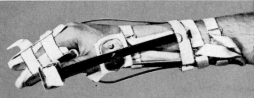

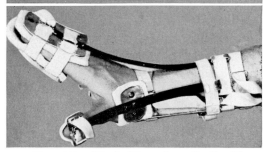

Fig. 190. (*Top*) "Pancake splint" with spring bar to promote dorsiflexion of the fingers and the wrist as for contracture of the long flexors of the forearm. A thumb piece (*center*) can be added. The springs allow exercise (*center* and *bottom*).

Figure 191 shows a similar splint with a rigid bar to provide steady force in overcoming a contracture.

head of the ulna from pressure. The elbow should be allowed full flexion without impingement of the splint in the flexion crease.

The palm piece should fit the metacarpal arch and allow the proximal finger joints to flex to a right angle.

A dorsal hand splint should be curved transversely to fit the back of the hand and should not impinge on the wrist on dorsiflexion.

A finger splint should follow the natural curve of the finger, usually when semiflexed.

A thumb splint should follow the natural curve of the thumb when semiflexed and hold the thumb in moderate opposition.

If splints are movable, the pivots should coincide exactly with the centers of movement of the joints, and the surface of the 2 end segments of the splint should ride the finger or the hand segments perfectly throughout the complete movement.

There should be no blanched areas where circulation is decreased. There should be no tight encircling of the hand because of the danger of local ischemic contractures in the hand.

There should be no pressure across the antecubital space of the elbow; this could lead to Volkmann's ischemic contracture.

Excess tension of circular straps causes edema and should be avoided.

When possible, a splint should fit a hand in the position of function and not force the hand into some position of nonfunction.

TYPES OF SPLINTS

VOLAR WRIST OR COCKUP

The cockup wrist splint is made in many forms and of many materials. It is a basic splint in that it can be used as the foundation for attachments such as extensions or outriggers for additional control of the digits. It is composed of a forearm piece connected by a neck to a palm support and is held to the hand and the forearm by encircling straps or laces. The forearm piece varies from one longitudinal strip of metal with 2 curved cross bars to a complete encirclement of the forearm. Usually it consists of a curved metal sheet over the lower two thirds of the volar aspect of the forearm. Straps and buckles encircling the forearm at each end hold it in place. The palm piece is oblique and may be a spindle-shaped rod or a rod curved to fit the arch of the palm, curved up at the sides or not, or it may be ovoid in shape. There may or may not be a strap from it encircling the hand. The palm piece should be riveted to the neck in such a way that its obliquity can be changed to fit either hand. The neck may be either an integral part of the splint as a whole or, preferably, a flat rod that can be bent to the desired curve. When a wrist is being forced into dorsiflexion by a cockup splint, it will be

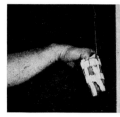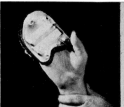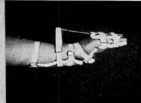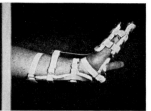

Fig. 191. Splint to extend the wrist and the fingers when the flexor muscles are too short, as in Volkmann's ischemic contracture. The 2 left-hand pictures show how, with wrist flexed, the fingers are straightened between 2 padded metal sheets strapped together; the dorsal sheet has an extension arm. (*Center, right*) While a cockup splint draws the wrist into dorsiflexion, the proximal finger joints gradually are straightened by drawing the extension arm to the forearm with a web belt and buckle. (*Far right*) The extension arm is bent as necessary finally to extend both wrist and fingers.

found that the splint slips distalward and ceases to maintain dorsiflexion. This can be prevented by having a web belt and buckle fastened to the prominence of the curve of the neck of the splint, encircling the wrist in a direction diagonally dorsal and proximal-ward. If a wrist is to be held firmly for a long time, a form-fitting leather casing laced along the dorsum is excellent. If it leaves the proximal joints of the digits free for full motion, it does not interfere too much with work. It is also possible to pound out of sheet aluminum a form-fitting encasement that reaches two thirds around the hand and the forearm and is either incorporated in the leather wristlet or held in place with one strap at the wrist.

Spring Cockup Splint

A spring cockup splint differs only in the neck piece, which may be either 2 piano spring wires (0.105 inch) or ribbon spring steel (0.047 x ⅝ inch). For greater spring they are fastened rather proximally on the forearm piece. The spring wire is looped on itself and bent into the proper curve. To the sharp U loop is brazed a flat piece to which the hand piece is riveted. The compartment for the oblique strap about the wrist is made from a prolongation from the forearm piece. The wires are riveted to the forearm piece by 2 strips of metal curved about each wire. Flat spring steel is preferable. After having been given the proper gooseneck bend, it is fastened by riveting. This spring splint is excellent for bending the wrist into dorsiflexion.

Extensions to Cockup Splint. These may be riveted to the neck or the forearm piece. They are to hold the thumb or the fingers in extension after the repair of extensor tendons and consist of a metal rod with a metal gutter at the end or a flat piece for several fingers. Also, the palm piece can be prolonged distally to support the proximal finger joints.

To Flex the Proximal Joints. A flat rod is riveted or fastened by a screw clamp to the belly of the cockup splint. On the end of the rod is mounted a triangle of stiff wire that extends beyond the fingers as the outrigger. Over this is threaded a piece of metal tubing that acts as a roller. Over the proximal segment of each finger is a soft leather loop to which is attached a rubber band or, for stronger traction, a piece of nonelastic cord. The bands pass over the roller to a hook in the belly of the splint. As the proximal finger joints bend, the wire outrigger is bent backward to pull proximalward, always at a right angle to the finger segment.

Dorsal Wrist Splint

Three separate pieces of aluminum or other sheet metal are molded to the dorsum of the hand, the wrist and the forearm, respectively, and riveted to a malleable metal strip. Slits punched through the edges of the sheet metal hold the removable web belts with buckles in place. The metal strip can be bent so that this flat splint will hold the wrist in any desired position from palmar flexion to dorsiflexion. In the latter case, the flat splint may be prolonged to the fingertips by an additional metal cross-sheet and strap to keep the fingers in extension.

Flat wrist splints are especially useful after

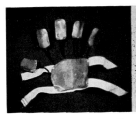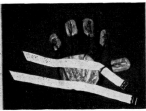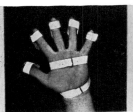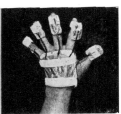

FIG. 192. Spreading hand splint. This is useful after operations for syndactylia or skin grafting for scarring from burns. When sterilized, it can be applied during the operation, compression bandages being applied to all surfaces.

repair of the flexor and the extensor tendons to keep them relaxed during the month of healing. They are useful after nerve suture to allow the flexed wrist to extend gradually.

For the purpose of gradually forcing a wrist into dorsiflexion, the spring cockup splint with the oblique wrist band is used; the padded dorsal wrist splint will suffice to force the wrist gradually into palmar flexion.

FOR PRONATION AND SUPINATION

Pronation and supination of the hand and the forearm can be brought about by the torque of a flat ribbon of spring steel. This unit is clamped to a standard elbow splint in the upper part of the forearm and clasps the hand distally as a flat padded bracelet. The degree of spring tension is set at a swivel with a set screw.

HAND SPLINTS

A large rubber sponge or pad of steel wool bound to the palm of the hand with a bandage is useful postoperatively. It furnishes pressure over the dressings and immobilizes the hand and the fingers.

Hand-Spreading Splint. This is useful after plastic operations, and especially after operations between the fingers as in syndactylia. It consists of a sheet of metal molded to the dorsum of the hand and held there by 2 encircling straps, one of them around the wrist. Soldered to this sheet are 5 diverging malleable metal rods, each extending down the back of a finger or the thumb and supporting the digit by a shallow gutter piece at its end. At the end of the operation, after padding, each finger is fastened to its respective gutter by a piece of sterile adhesive tape. In this way, the fingers and the thumb are held spread and extended.

It makes them easily accessible for dressings in the interdigital clefts.

Palm Splints. Incisions in the distal crease of the palm are slow to heal because of motion. This is especially true after operations for Dupuytren's contracture. The distal crease in the palm can be immobilized with either a volar or a dorsal splint after such operations.

The volar splint is a sheet of metal, somewhat triangular in shape, that has been hammered to fit the contour of the palm, to which it is fastened by 2 encircling straps. The center of this splint is laid open by making 2 crosscuts and bending the 4 points forward and away from the palm to allow ventilation and accommodate dressings.

The dorsal splint for Dupuytren's contracture, which is more efficient, consists of a sheet of metal molded to fit the dorsum of the hand, to which it is strapped. Five parallel metal rods soldered to this and joined at their ends by a crossrod extend as far as the middle joints of the fingers. A web strap woven in turn over the volar aspect of each finger and over the back of each rod will hold the proximal finger joints in extension. Thus, the palm is immobile and exposed for dressings, and the middle and the distal finger joints are free to move.

If one desires to splint only 1 or 2 fingers to keep the distal palmar crease from moving, a flat metal or plastic dorsal splint can be cut out to fit the back of the hand with 1 or more prolongations down the proximal finger segments. The hand and the fingers to be splinted are fastened to this with adhesive plaster. The palm is free for dressings.

FINGER SPLINTS

General Types. With sheet aluminum, a

ball-peen hammer and a lead block, one can fashion various types to gutter splints—curved or straight, volar or dorsal. Most finger splints are of the gutter type. Some have a flat extension overlying the palm or the dorsum of the hand to include the proximal finger joint for additional stability, and in some the extension reaches the wrist, where it has a cross-piece of sheet metal, curved partially about the wrist and completed with a strap. Other finger splints consist of a half gutter along the volar surface; these are curved on themselves around the end of the finger to cover the dorsum as well. This type of splint may cover only the finger or may have an extension of one of the arms running up either the palm or the dorsum of the hand. In this type of splint the dorsal arm may be a spring to bend the finger backward, and the volar arm may be just long enough to include the distal segment of the finger.

The above splints may have cross ribbons of metal partially encircling the wrist, the hand or the fingers, and some dorsal splints may have an encircling loop of metal under the pulp of the finger to hold the distal joint in extension.

Fig. 193. (*Right*) The palmar splint allows finger motion but keeps the palmar creases immobile. (*Bottom left* and *right*) The dorsal splint immobilizes the proximal joints and therefore the palmar tissues. It is useful as a postoperative splint after resection of fascia for Dupuytren's contracture.

A simple finger guard can be made by 2 straight, narrow, crowned strips of metal, riveted or fastened together at their centers at a right angle to each other and then curved over the end of the finger to form 4 strips the length of the finger. This splint may be curved on the edge to fit the curve of a finger. It is useful as a protective basket.

Adhesive plaster or web straps and buckles hold the various above-mentioned splints in place.

To Straighten a Finger. A simple method is to use a strip of blued spring steel. One end is bent over the end of the finger to engage the pulp. The other is drilled for a cord about the wrist. It is laid over a strip of felt along the dorsum of the hand and the finger. Adhesive plaster prevents it from slipping off the finger, or a transverse piece may be riveted

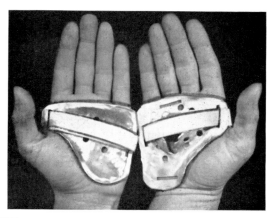

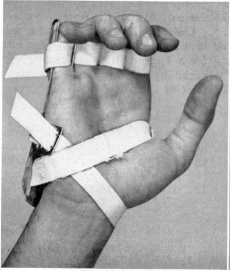

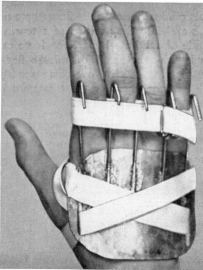

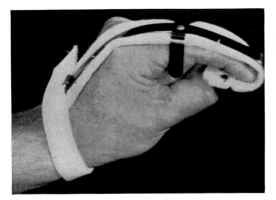

FIG. 194. Clock-spring splint to promote extension or substitute for loss of voluntary extension of a finger. The wrist strap can be adjusted to vary the tension. (H. Weniger, San Francisco)

to it to clasp the proximal segment of the finger. This is particularly useful in drawing out a myostatic contracture.

Safety-Pin Splint. This is useful for a moderately crooked finger. It consists of 2 parallel spring or solid steel wires, a little farther apart that the width of the finger and fastened together at each end by a crosspiece of galvanized sheet iron soldered to them. One crosspiece curves over the volar surface of the distal segment of the finger, and the other rests on the palm just distal to the distal crease. Both are well padded. A web strap with a buckle crosses over the dorsum of the finger at the middle joint, loops around each rod and passes backward over the finger, being buckled to itself. This gradually draws the finger between the 2 rods and into the position of extension. When made of solid steel rods, the force can be applied with exactness, and middle finger joint contractures can be overcome readily. This splint is preferred for the treatment of ruptures of the middle slip of the extensor

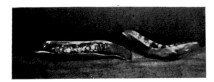

FIG. 195. Aluminum sheet can be molded on a lead block with a ball-peen hammer into the desired shape for either the volar or the dorsal surface of a finger.

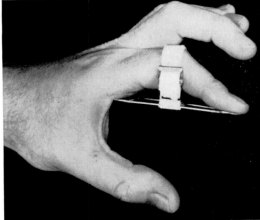

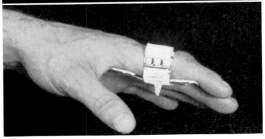

FIG. 196. The safety-pin splint to overcome contracture of a finger. Parallel rigid wires are connected at each end by soldering them to galvanized plates. The strap loops over the finger and back to the buckle. See Figure 197 for method of application.

apparatus, in which case the distal transverse crosspiece must not extend beyond the distal flexion crease of the finger.

Gutter Splint. A volar gutter splint which is straighter than the finger can also be used for a finger that is moderately crooked. An encircling adhesive strap opposite the middle joint of the finger gradually draws the digit straight.

A piano wire is bent on itself, leaving a space a little greater than the finger. A cross strap of tin is soldered to each end with another cross strap opposite the middle finger segment. This was devised by Oppenheimer. It lies on the dorsum with the pulp end of the finger over the distal tin and the proximal end held by a wrist strap. One pad is placed over the middle phalanx, and one over the dorsum of the hand.

To Flex a Finger. To draw a finger into

FIG. 197. Safety-pin splint
with side bars of spring wire.
This splint allows motion of
available flexors, the spring returning the finger to the extended position.

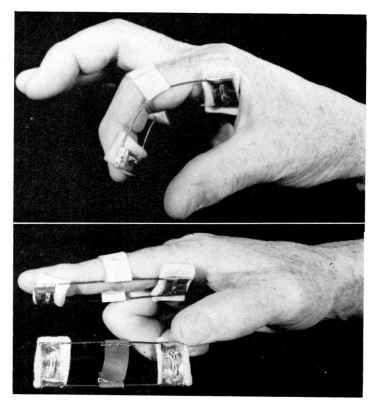

greater flexion, one can use either a volar or
a dorsal gutter splint with more of a curve
than the finger has. It is fastened firmly at
each end with encircling adhesive straps.

To Flex the Metacarpophalangeal Joints.
In most crippled hands these joints have stiffened in the straight position. Elastic traction
should be used to flex them. Many splints have
been devised. The simplest is a plaster-of-
Paris volar slab with an outrigger of a loop of
wire forming a transverse bar in front of the
proximal finger segments. Leather cuffs over
the backs of the proximal finger segments are
pulled by rubber bands that pass over this
outrigger rod and are fastened proximally to
a hook in the belly of the splint. As the proximal finger joints are flexed, the wire outrigger
is bent so that the pull will always be at a
right angle to the proximal finger segments.
At first the pull is at a right angle to the palm,
but finally it is proximalward.

Nachlas made a splint for this purpose with
an outrigger that slides along the forearm
piece to give the correct direction of pull.

Luckey made one with an outrigger that is
adjustable for 3 set positions.

A simple method uses the standard cockup
splint with the addition of an adjustable outrigger of wire that can be bent as desired as
the proximal joints flex. To avoid friction as

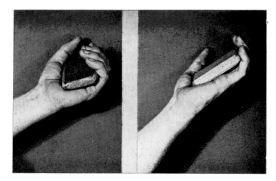

FIG. 198. To exercise newly repaired tendons and stiff joints, a rounded rectangular
block of wood furnishes the right fulcrum
on which the middle finger joints (*left*) and
the distal joints (*right*) can act. A rubber
ball exercises primarily the proximal joints.

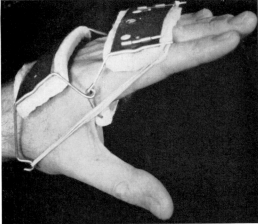

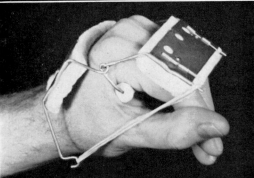

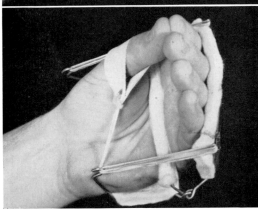

Fig. 199. The basic knuckle-bender splint. Used with rubber bands as shown, cockback of the proximal joints, as seen in ulnar or combined ulnar and median palsy, is prevented, and the long extensors extend the 2 distal joints. The palmar surface is open, and the hand can be used. (*Bottom*) An additional loop can help to maintain the thumb in opposition. The palmar bar is curved to fit the transverse metacarpal arch.

the rubber bands pull over the outrigger rod, metal tubing is slipped over the rod to act as a roller. Of course, the hand piece of the splint must not extend beyond the distal crease in the palm.

Glove-Traction Method. For this a web strap and buckle is riveted to the wrist of the glove so that the buckle lies on the volar aspect of the carpus over the scaphoid tubercle. A cord is fastened to the tip of each glove finger. Two of these cords are looped through the buckle, and then each is tied with a bowknot to one of the other two cords. By tightening these cords, the patient can gradually increase the flexion of the fingers. Rubber bands may be used.

Knuckle-Bender Splint. This was devised to apply the principle of elastic traction to the metacarpophalangeal splint, to flex the proximal finger joints and carry the motion through to completion. The 3 points of pressure are over the backs of the distal ends of the proximal finger segments, the back of the bases of the metacarpals and across the palm, along and curved into the distal palmar crease. For these points of pressure 2 padded ribbons of sheet metal cross the dorsum, and a padded transverse curved piece is placed against the hollow of the palm. The palmar piece is of wire rod (0.082 inch in thickness) and is turned up at each end dorsally until it is opposite the center of motion or imaginary axis of the proximal finger joints. Here it is looped on itself for a pivot and prolonged to the dorsum of the hand to be integrated there with the transverse metal ribbon. The distal metal ribbon over the proximal finger segments is soldered at each end to 2 such short wires, each of which ends in a loop linked to a loop of the crosspiece wire.

The hinge of the splint is in the axis of the proximal finger joints. The wire rods, to reach from here to the dorsal plane of the hand where they fasten to the cross ribbons, must angulate there to conform to the dorsal contour. Motor power is furnished by a rubber band over the end of the wires at each side. The wires along the dorsum of the hand are prolonged proximally and bent volarward to end in hooks at the plane of the palm to keep the rubber bands from pressing the skin and to give better leverage.

FIG. 200. Elastic knuckle-bender splint to restore muscle balance and position of function in combined median and ulnar palsy. This flexes the proximal finger joints, draws the thumb into opposition, and, by a detachable wire outrigger with a roller of metal tubing, corrects the position of clawfinger. (*Top*) Position of intrinsic muscle, minus; (*bottom*) position of intrinsic muscle, plus.

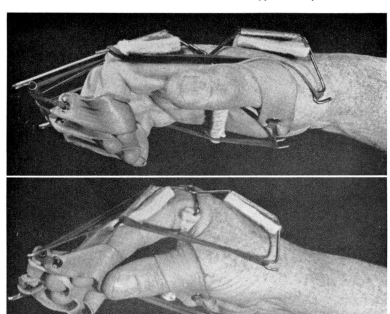

The splint will pull through from the straight position of the metacarpophalangeal joints to the completely flexed one. This splint is simple, cheap and easy to make of wire, sheet metal, felt and rubber bands. It is light and comfortable and goes through the coat sleeve; it is on the hand only and does not interfere with the use of the hand.

The knuckle bender as a basic splint may be combined with an Oppenheimer or a spring cockup splint so as to dorsiflex the wrist and flex the proximal finger joints at the same time. These are the 2 key joints of the hand to obtain the position of function.

Other attachments for the knuckle-bender splint are an extra segment to flex the middle finger joints or an outrigger to draw the fingers into extension. A reverse knuckle bender is made to draw the proximal finger joints into extension, as needed in local ischemic contracture in the hand.

A combination knuckle-bender and Oppenheimer splint is used to draw the wrist into dorsiflexion, the proximal finger joints into flexion, the thumb into opposition and the distal 2 finger joints into extension.

Knuckle-Bender Splint for Clawhand. The knuckle-bender splint is excellent for correcting the clawhand in median and ulnar palsy. It flexes the proximal finger joints, and to hold the thumb in opposition, it is necessary only to lift the rubber band on the thumb side over the thumb so that it will press on the dorsum, holding the thumb forward. To oppose the thumb more positively against resistance, a leather loop about the base of the thumb is pulled by a rubber band toward the rear wire hook on the opposite side. It is looped about this and drawn forward to hook over the distal projecting wire end. If the joints are not rigid, thin druggist rubber bands on the splint will suffice to substitute for muscle balance.

To extend the middle finger joints of clawhand, an outrigger of wire bent into a U is made to slip over the sheet metal ribbon on the backs of the fingers. Over the crossbar of this U is a tube roller. Leather cuffs over the finger ends are pulled by rubber bands over the roller. The bands are fastened to drill

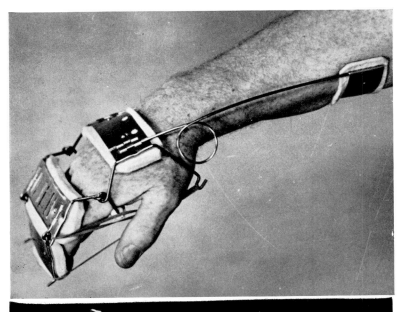

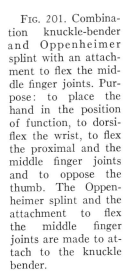

Fig. 201. Combination knuckle-bender and Oppenheimer splint with an attachment to flex the middle finger joints. Purpose: to place the hand in the position of function, to dorsiflex the wrist, to flex the proximal and the middle finger joints and to oppose the thumb. The Oppenheimer splint and the attachment to flex the middle finger joints are made to attach to the knuckle bender.

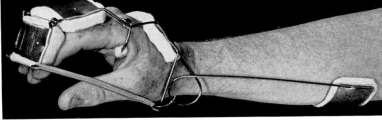

holes in the sheet metal over the fingers. This splint will flex the proximal finger joints and extend the distal two joints. It will draw the thumb into opposition. The metacarpal arch is curved by the pressure of the curved palmar piece. It places the hand in the position in which the intrinsic muscles should place it.

Web Strap Method. Later, even more flexion can be gained by strapping the fingers in flexion with a long, narrow web belt and buckle that encircles the fingers in various directions. It is held in place on the hand by a figure-of-eight turn around the wrist.

To Hold Thumb Extended. The thumb can be held in extension by a supporting outrigger rod and gutter riveted to the forearm piece of the cockup splint. A flexed thumb can be drawn gradually into extension by applying a padded flat spring looped over the end of the thumb and fastened with adhesive straps. The spring may end at the wrist or be fastened

well up the forearm for good leverage. A spring is usually bent so that the metacarpophalangeal joint is used as the fulcrum. This may be used in conjunction with a cockup splint.

To Hold Thumb in Opposition. The thumb may be held in the position of opposition by looping a ½-inch wide piece of adhesive tape around the padded dorsum of the distal end of the metacarpal and drawing the thumb toward the pisiform bone. The 2 arms of adhesive tape are continued, one around the back of the hand and the other around the back of the forearm. The resultant force is in line with the pisiform. This strapping aids in correcting flat hand. Another method is to use the elastic band and the leather cuff for opposition with the knuckle-bender splint, looping the rubber around the proximal hook and over the distal projecting wire.

To Hold Thumb in Adduction. To hold the

FIG. 202. Combination of knuckle-bender splint to flex the proximal finger joints, an outrigger to extend the distal 2 finger joints and an Oppenheimer splint to dorsiflex the wrist. The object is to place the hand in the position of function. The extra segment is shown above.

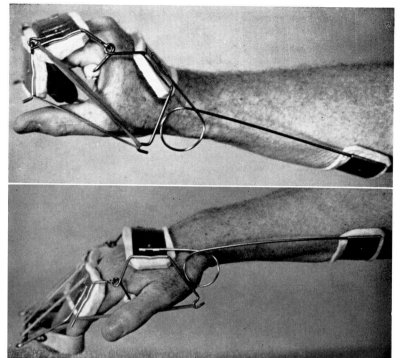

thumb near the hand, as after strain of the adductor muscles, a narrow web belt and buckle encircles the head of the first metacarpal, crosses itself in the depth of the first interdigital cleft and loops around the ulnar border of the hand.

To Draw Fingers and Wrist into Extension. The simplest method is to lay a plaster slab over the dorsum of the forearm, the hand and the proximal finger joints. A thick layer of felt should be placed under the plaster over the finger joints, since this part will act as the

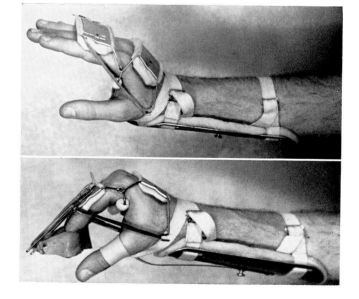

FIG. 203. Combination of knuckle-bender splint to flex the proximal finger joints and oppose the thumb, an outrigger splint to extend the distal 2 finger joints and a spring cockup splint to dorsiflex the wrist. The object is to bring the hand into the position of function.

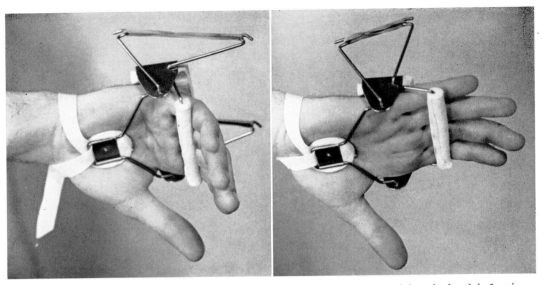

FIG. 204. Reverse knuckle-bender splint to extend the proximal finger joints in local ischemic contracture in the hand.

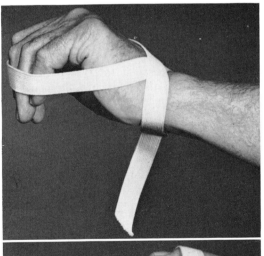

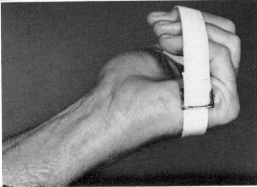

fulcrum. Embedded in the plaster are the 2 ends of a wire U. The crosspiece of the U is straight, and over it is slipped a piece of metal tubing that acts as a roller. This outrigger is placed so that it will pull the finger ends by leather cuffs and rubber bands in such a direction that the fingers will extend. The rubber bands run over the roller and continue proximally to attach to a hook previously embedded in the plaster. The plaster slab is fastened to the forearm by adhesive plaster or web belts and buckles.

In Volkmann's ischemic contracture, the flexor muscles to the fingers are too short. However, the fingers can be straightened by flexing the wrist. They are fixed so by strapping on them, front and back, 2 well-padded, flat, sheet-metal plates. Extending 7 inches proximalward from the dorsal plate and riveted to it is a flat rod, preferably of spring steel. This rises well above the dorsum of the

FIG. 205. (*Top*) A web strap applied as a figure-of-eight which can draw the proximal and the middle finger joints into flexion. (*Bottom*) When the proximal joints flex well and more flexion of the middle joints is desired, the strap is applied as a loop.

forearm. A cockup splint is applied to draw the wrist gradually into dorsiflexion; a web belt and buckle encircling the forearm and the rod from the dorsal finger plate draw the rod to the forearm, thus straightening the fingers at the proximal joints. The effect is to lengthen the forearm muscles that flex the fingers.

SPLINTING FOR PARALYSIS

When there are no fixed contractures, all that is necessary is to substitute just enough spring or elastic power for the paralyzed muscles to balance the loss of the muscle tone. In this way muscle balance will be restored, and the hand will assume the position of function. Active movements of the hand keep the muscles in good condition. The spring substitutes are sufficient to keep the paralyzed muscles from being continuously overstretched. If no splinting is used, the healthy antagonists will overstretch the paralyzed muscles. Then, when the nerve regenerates, it will have to re-innervate the muscle and, an even greater task, to shorten it against the pull of a strong antagonist.

For Radial Palsy

Only the wrist, the proximal finger joints and the base of the thumb should be supported

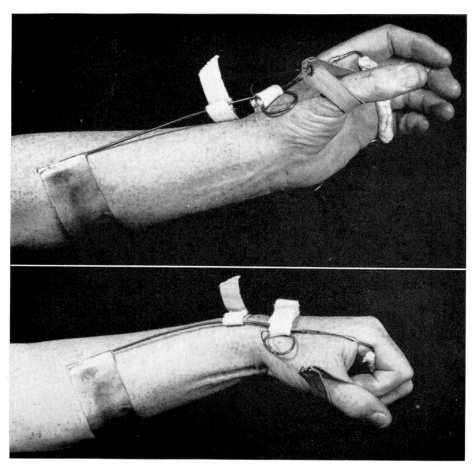

Fig. 206. Spring splint for radial palsy modified from an Oppenheimer splint in that the thumb is held in a leather cuff by a light, 0.033-inch, spring steel wire; the main wires are as light as 0.069 inch. This restores muscle balance in the position of function and allows the hand to be free to work.

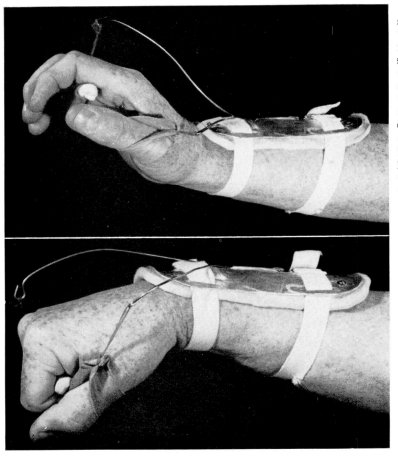

FIG. 207. Spring wire suspension splint of Thomas for radial palsy, modified by using lighter spring wire for the thumb, 0.045 inch, and a flat spring steel with one twist for lateral movement for the wrist. The crossbar should be arched and at the plica of the palm. This splint gives perfect freedom of action and perfect muscle balance.

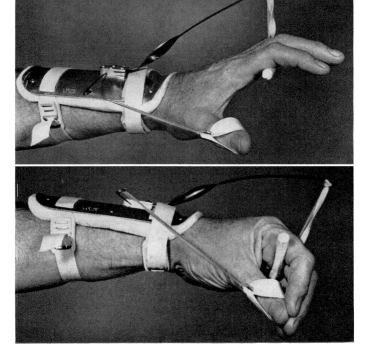

FIG. 208. Thomas suspension splint for radial palsy; extension power is provided by a twisted flat spring and a rubber band.

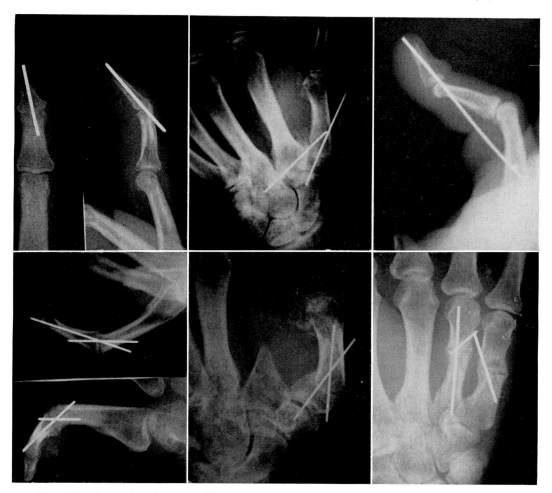

FIG. 209. Internal splinting by Kirschner wires placed in various directions. The wires are cut off beneath the skin so as to avoid infection. After union has occurred, they are removed under procaine.

(*Top, left*) To arthrodese the distal finger joint. (*Top, center*) To arthrodese the metacarpocarpal joint of the thumb. (*Top, right*) To splint for rupture of insertion of the extensor tendon in a finger (Pratt's method). This holds the distal joint in hyperextension and the middle joint in flexion. (*Bottom, left*) To arthrodese the middle finger joint. (*Bottom, center*) Angulatory rotary arthrodesis of the base of the metacarpal of the thumb. (*Bottom, right*) To fix fractures of the metacarpals.

(*Continued on page 176*)

in extension. Two splints are useful, the Oppenheimer splint and the suspension splint described by Thomas.

Oppenheimer Splint, Modified. This is made of light spring wire, bent into a rectangle but open proximally, the distal crosspiece being curved to fit under the distal fold in the palm where it will support the proximal finger joints. At the proximal end a volar

cross ribbon of metal forms a bridge between the wires and curves under the forearm. Just above the wrist a web belt and buckle loops about each wire and crosses over the dorsum. At the wrist each wire is made into an open loop for extra spring, and here the splint is bent backward to hold the wrist in dorsiflexion. It is necessary to place another web belt and buckle through these 2 loops and around

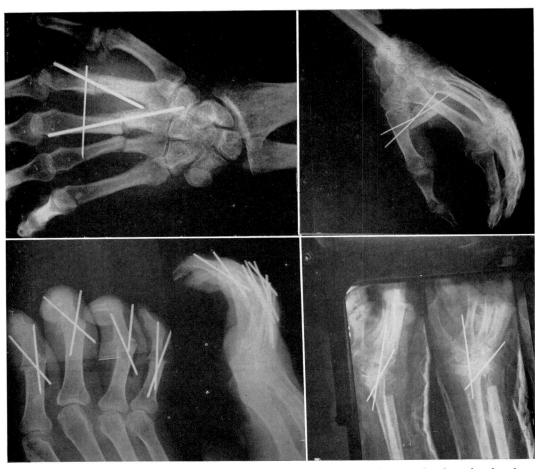

Fig. 209 (*Cont.*). (*Top, left*) To fix the metacarpals. (*Top, right*) To arthrodese the thumb with the bone block in the position of opposition. (*Bottom, left*) To arthrodese the middle finger joints, as after a burn. (*Bottom, right*) To arthrodese the wrist.

the dorsum of the wrist or the splint will not remain in place. Brazed to one wire is a short, very light (0.033 inch) spring wire that acts as an outrigger for the thumb. A leather cuff loops about the thumb and pulls from the outrigger by a rubber band. The old model with the wire ring held the thumb too rigidly, and the splint wires were too stiff.

The Suspension Splint for Radial Palsy (Modified from F. Bryan Thomas Splint). The forearm piece may be a plaster slab or a padded hammered piece of Duralumin (hollowed on each side to allow for the prominence of the head of the ulna). It ends at the wrist and is strapped to the forearm. From the

forearm piece extend 2 light spring wires, 0.063 inch in diameter for the hand and 0.056 inch in diameter for the thumb. Each terminates in a loop from which a rubber band extends, for the hand, to a curved padded crosspiece (rubber over a metal rod) and, for the base of the thumb, to a leather cuff. One wire arches over the hand, supporting the bases of the fingers and also the wrist in extension. The rubber band passes across the apex of the second interdigital cleft, and the cross rod provides support along the plica of the palm. The other wire arches in a plane at right angles to the first to give slight extension to the base of the thumb. The wires should not arch so far from the hand that they prevent passing it through a coat sleeve. This splint does all that is necessary and gives remarkable freedom of motion. If the wires emerge from the center and there is a bilateral hollow for the ulnar head, the splint is interchangeable for either hand.

SPLINT FOR COMBINED MEDIAN AND ULNAR PALSY

The knuckle bender changes the clawhand position, which is intrinsic minus, to that of intrinsic plus as seen in intrinsic contracture. It also opposes the thumb and, with the finger extension device, unclaws the fingers. It does everything that the intrinsic muscles can do except give lateral finger motion. It furnishes just the needed correction for the combination of median and ulnar palsy, especially when the long flexor muscles in the forearm are active.

SPLINT FOR ULNAR PALSY

For this all that is necessary is to furnish elastic flexion to the proximal joints of the ring and the little fingers by means of leather loops and light rubber bands running to a wristband.

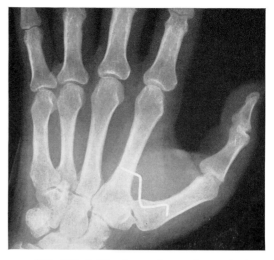

FIG. 210. A Kirschner wire used as a strut to maintain abduction of the 1st metacarpal after relieving adduction contracture. After the replaced skin pedicle is well healed, the strut can be removed by making a small incision on the dorsum, dividing the wire in the middle and extracting the 2 halves.

INTERNAL SPLINTING

Internal splinting means pinning the bones together with Kirschner wires. For arthrodeses of metacarpals and phalanges, the wires should

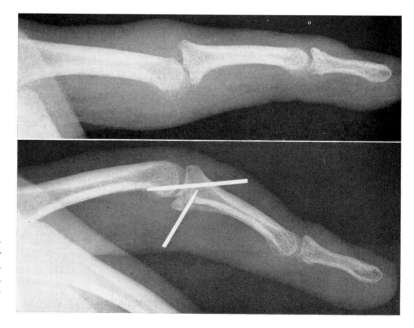

FIG. 211. Use of internal splint of Kirschner wire to maintain reduction of fracture dislocation of middle finger joint.

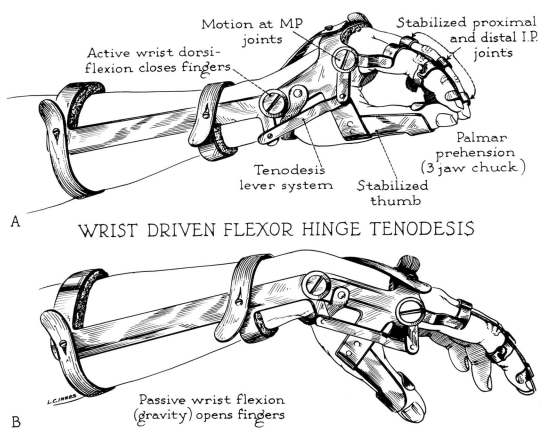

Active wrist dorsi-
flexion closes fingers

Motion at MP
joints

Stabilized proximal
and distal I.P.
joints

Palmar
prehension
(3 jaw chuck)

Tenodesis
lever system

Stabilized
thumb

A

WRIST DRIVEN FLEXOR HINGE TENODESIS

B

Passive wrist flexion
(gravity) opens fingers

FIG. 212. Ony an active wrist dorsiflexor is needed to activate the mechanism that brings the thumb and the index and the middle finger pulps into contact. Passive volar flexion opens the fingers for grasp. (Nickel, V.: J. Bone Joint Surg. *45-A*:933)

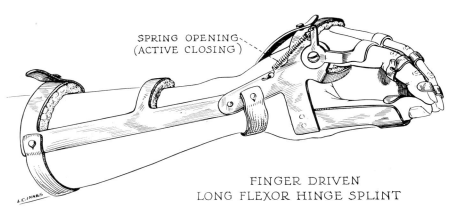

SPRING OPENING
(ACTIVE CLOSING)

FINGER DRIVEN
LONG FLEXOR HINGE SPLINT

FIG. 213. A retained finger flexor can be used, utilizing spring power for extending the fingers away from the fixed thumb. (Nickel, V.: J. Bone Joint Surg. *45-A*:933)

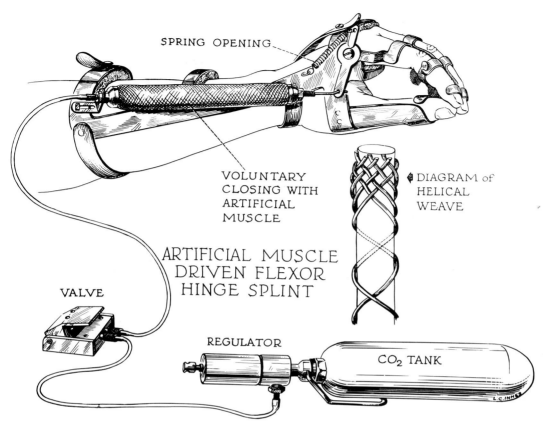

SPRING OPENING

VOLUNTARY
CLOSING WITH
ARTIFICIAL
MUSCLE

DIAGRAM of
HELICAL
WEAVE

ARTIFICIAL MUSCLE
DRIVEN FLEXOR
HINGE SPLINT

VALVE

REGULATOR

CO_2 TANK

FIG. 214. In this apparatus, the flexor power for the finger unit is the force supplied by the "artificial muscle" which increases in diameter but shortens in length when inflated. (Nickel, V.: J. Bone Joint Surg. *45-A*:933)

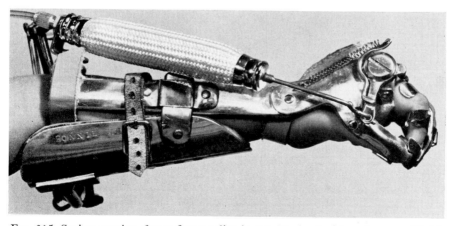

FIG. 215. Spring-opening, finger-flexor splint in use. It also is driven by an artificial muscle. (Nickel, V.: J. Bone Joint Surg. *45-A*:933)

cross and penetrate each fragment while the bones are held tightly together; otherwise, the crossed wires will cause distraction. An arthrodesis of the wrist is held in the same way.

After fracture, osteotomies, jogging or reconstruction by bone grafts, metacarpals may be pinned longitudinally, transversely and obliquely through each other and into the carpus or the wrist, if necessary. If the wrist is used, exact immobilization by a plaster cast is necessary until the wire is removed. The best treatment for Bennett's fracture is pinning with 1 or 2 Kirschner wires. An exact degree of pronation and supination, as in applying a pedicle graft to the hand, can be maintained by a strong Kirschner wire drilled through both the radius and the ulna.

All pinning operations should fix the bones firmly and immovably together. Infection may occur about wires that are left protruding through the skin; hence, they should be nipped off beneath the skin and later removed through a small nick in the skin. If wires are left protruding from fingers, they should be kept sterile and dry with dressings.

FUNCTIONAL BRACING

This term is used to describe the use of splints and braces in the severely paralyzed hand. By a combination of parts to hold certain areas immovable and yet allow other joints to move either by some remaining muscle power or by the use of springs, a hand with only a trace of motion can be restored to some usefulness.

Faced with the problem of the severely paralyzed postpolio patient, Vernon Nickel and his co-workers at the Rancho Los Amigos center in Los Angeles ulitized a fundamental principle of reconstructive surgery in restoring some function to these hands. In these almost flail hands the problem is to restore some basic motion that can be made with the minimal number of joints and the least number of muscles. They chose precision pinch, that is, the approximation of thumb pulp to index and middle finger pulp, as the basic function that is most useful and, by means of splints, placed the hand in this position. At first many contractures had to be overcome, but when the importance of early preventive splinting

was recognized, it was found to be possible to apply the splints early and prevent deformity.

The voluntary act of pinching in this position can be restored even if there is only one muscle functioning in either the fingers or the wrist. This muscle effect is transferred either through a mechanical linkage in the splint or surgically to provide opening or closing of the combined index and middle finger unit at the metacarpophalangeal joint level. These 2 digits are fixed at their middle and distal joints either by the splint or by surgical arthrodesis, and their only remaining motion is in the proximal joints. By placing the thumb in the fully opposed position and fixing it with an intermetacarpal bone block and arthrodesing its 2 joints, a post is provided against which the fingers can pinch. Either extension or flexion of the fingers can be procured through a linkage so that voluntary dorsiflexion of the wrist or some motion in the other fingers can control the action. The opposing force is supplied by springs. Once the splint has been worn and the patient learns to use this basic function, fusion of the interphalangeal joints and tendon transfers or tenodeses are done to eliminate portions of the apparatus. In this way many people are provided with a motion that is useful.

This external and internal splinting is not a substitute for tendon transfers when sufficient stabilizers and movers are available; it is a salvage procedure for the severely crippled.

In some patients the force available from remaining muscle power was so poor that some mechanical means was necessary to provide the motion. Cables activated by opposite shoulder movements as with a prosthesis can be used. An "artificial muscle" utilizing a helical woven cover over a cylinder inflated with CO_2 has been devised. Control of this can be by motion of a lower extremity or almost any other part of the body. In these ways, by a most ingenious combination of splints, surgery, prosthetic and orthotic appliances, a crude but basic function of the hand has been restored.

BIBLIOGRAPHY

Adams, B. D.: Device for fixation of hands and arms from certain operative cases, New Engl. J. Med. *210*:423, 1934.

Anderson, M. H.: Functional Bracing of the Upper Extremities, Springfield, Ill., Thomas, 1958.

Bennett, R. L.: Orthotic devices for weakness of the upper extremity, South. M. J. *50*:791, 1957.

Bunnell, S.: The knuckle bender splint, U. S. Army Med. Bull., p. 230, Feb. 1946.

————: Active splinting of the hand, J. Bone Surg. *28*:732, 1946.

————: Spring splint to supinate or pronate the hand, J. Bone Joint Surg. *31-A*:664, 1949.

————: Splinting the hand, Am. Acad. Orth. Surg. Instruct. Course Lect. *9*:233, 1952.

————: Splints for the hand *in* Orthopaedic Appliances Atlas, vol. 1, p. 211, Ann Arbor, Mich., Edwards, 1952.

Bunnell, S., and Howard, L. D.: Additional elastic hand splints, J. Bone Joint Surg. *32-A*:226, 1950.

Funston, R. V.: Suggestions from the brace shop, J. Orth. Surg. *2*:345, 1920.

Hart, V. L.: Simple and efficient finger splint, J. Bone Joint Surg. *19*:245, 1937.

Jelsma, F.: Finger splint that will not impair hand function, Am. J. Surg. *50*:571, 1940.

Koch, S. L.: Four splints of value in treatment of disabilities of hand, Surg., Gynec. Obstet. *48*:416, 1929.

Lewin, P.: A simple splint for baseball finger, J.A.M.A. *85*:1059, 1925.

Littler, J. W., and Tobin, W. J.: Thumb abduction splint, J. Bone Joint Surg. *30-A*:240, 1948.

Louis, W.: Hand splinting; effect on the afferent system, Thesis, Am. J. Occup. Ther., vol. 16, 1962.

Lowman, C. L.: Use of fascia lata in repair of disability at wrist, J. Bone Joint Surg. *12*:400, 1930.

Lyford, J., III: Two small wire splints for treatment by traction of fractures and deformities of fingers and metacarpal bones, J. Bone Joint Surg. *24*:202, 1942.

Marble, H. C.: Purposeful splinting following injuries to hand, J.A.M.A. *116*:1373, 1941.

Nachlas, I. W.: A splint for the correction of extension contractures of the metacarpophalangeal joints, J. Bone Joint Surg. *27*:507, 1945.

Neviaser, J. S.: Splint for correction of clawhand, J. Bone Joint Surg. *12*:440, 1930.

Nickel, V., and Perry, J.: The flexor hinge hand, Proc. West. Orth. Assn., J. Bone Joint Surg. *40-A*:571, 1958.

Nickel, V., Perry, J., and Garrett, A.: Development of useful function in the severely paralyzed hand, J. Bone Joint Surg. *45-A*:933, 1963.

Oppenheimer, E. D.: Splint for correction of finger contracture, J. Bone Joint Surg. *19*:247, 1937.

Polya, E.: Simple apparatus for relief of some palsies of upper extremities, Surgery *8*:464, 1940. Correction: *8*:1023, 1940.

Pratt, D. R.: Suggestions on immobilization of hand, Bull. U. S. Army Med. Dept. No. 86, 105, 1945.

Rozov, V. I.: Splint for therapy of lesions of extensor tendons of fingers, Ortop. i travmatol. *11*:98, 1937.

Saxl, A.: Splint for treatment of torn extensor sheath of a terminal tendon, Zbl. Chir. *63*:304, 1936.

Schottstaedt, E., and Robinson, G. B.: Functional bracing of the arm, J. Bone Joint Surg. *38-A*:477, 1956; *38-A*:841, 1956.

Schnayerson, N.: Finger splint for extension or flexion, J.A.M.A. *110*:2070, 1938.

Smythe, N., and Wynn Parry, C. B.: The use of lively splints in upper limb paralysis, J. Bone Joint Surg. *37-B*:591, 1955.

Snelson, R., and Conry, J.: Recent advances in functional arm bracing, correlated with orthopedic surgery for the severely paralyzed upper extremity, Orth. Prosth. Appliance J. *12*:41, 1958.

Stark, H. H., Boyes, J. H., and Wilson, J. N.: Mallet finger, J. Bone Joint Surg. *44-A*:1061, 1962.

Thomas, F. B.: A splint for radial (musculospiral) nerve palsy, J. Bone Joint Surg. *26*:602, 1944.

Wheeler, W. E. de C.: Splints for fingers and thumb, Lancet *2*:546, 1940.

Chapter 7

Skin and Contractures

EFFECT OF CICATRIX

Scarring of the skin and the deeper structures follows most open injuries of the hand and always follows delayed healing of wounds and infection. This cicatrix draws to itself the surrounding normal tissues and hampers nutrition of more distal parts by strangling the deeper structures, the nerves and the lymph and the blood vessels. Because of the dense bed on which it lies, the surface scar is avascular, hard and easily injured. It may interfere with local blood supply so severely that its center breaks down. Localized to the forearm or the wrist, the girdling effect may be most evident; but even when limited to only one side of the limb, it can, by drawing the surrounding tissues to it, effectively interfere with the flow of blood through incoming arteries and returning veins.

FLEXION CONTRACTURES

Contractures from burns involve primarily the skin and, to a lesser extent, the deeper tissues, whereas those from infections are from within outward, starting primarily in the deeper tissues and involving the skin secondarily. Skin cicatrix may follow sloughing from injury or infection or poorly chosen lines of incisions.

EFFECT OF INFECTIONS

Stage of Destruction. The longer infection lasts or healing is delayed, the greater is the growth of granulation tissue and, consequently, the greater the eventual contracture. Therefore, we should terminate infections quickly by prompt diagnosis, by choosing incisions which will drain each fascial space or tendon sheath adequately and still never cross flexion creases at a right angle, as this leads to flexion contracture. During healing, the position of function should be maintained by splints, and intermittent exercises should be started early.

The greatest damage from infections occurs in enclosed tunnels, such as in the wrist or the fingers. When tissue in such enclosures swells, blood is excluded, and ischemia occurs, resulting in necrosis and sloughing, followed by contracture. Such spaces should be opened laterally for decompression and drainage.

When the palmar space is infected, the intrinsic muscles of the hand are bathed in pus and become paralyzed; muscle balance is upset; and the clawhand position results. As the infection travels along the ulnar nerve in the forearm, additional damage occurs, and deformity increases. Subsequently, the cicatrix encases these structures, and the flexion contracture is fixed.

Stage of Healing and Contraction. Inflamed and granulating tissue throughout the hand and the forearm gradually contracts, binding all of the tissues together in a dense scar. Just as the area of skin involved may shrink to two thirds or one half its size, so the deeper tissues—including the deep fascia and the deep connective tissue which surrounds all structures—solidify, contract and shorten in all directions. Infected muscles shorten and fibrose, and so do the parts of joint capsules that were involved in the infection. Tendons are reduced to contracting scars firmly attached to the surrounding tissue. Tendon sheaths proliferate greatly, attach themselves to their surroundings and contract; thus, all of the tissue may share in drawing the joints into flexion. In the hand this applies particularly to the wrist, the cleft between the first 2 metacarpals and the distal 2 joints of the digits.

Granulation tissue is "baby" cicatrix; contracting cicatrix is in the "adult" stage. Therefore, if a burn is allowed to granulate for long, or if any wound is allowed to remain open, granulation tissue piles up, and when eventually it is epithelialized, contracture is inevitable. All wounds should be closed early by skin grafts, sliding flaps or pedicle flaps. In skin grafting after burns, the granulation tissue should be scraped off first.

Secondary Effects of Contractures. Infection follows blood and lymph vessels and nerves, especially the ulnar nerve. Granulation tissue forms around these structures and in the final contraction strangles them, impairing their function. The lessened nerve supply results in atrophy of all the tissues, stiffening of the joints and adherence of tendons. The lessened blood and lymph supply results in impoverishment of tissues, in edema and cyanosis. The whole hand becomes firm, atrophic, cyanotic and poorly nourished. In this so-called congealed hand the joints become stiffened and the tendons adherent, and there is pain, paresthesia, diminished sensation and distress when cold.

In skin, the irritation of the scar from intermittent tension results in keloid formation. Thus, where a scar crosses a flexion crease, every effort of extension increases the keloid formation and, in turn, the contracture. The same is true of the deep cicatrix of connective tissue, in some persons more than in others.

Secondary to contractures, muscle balance is upset; while one group of muscles is overstretched and weakened, the opposing group is allowed to contract and become fixed.

In flexion contractures many tissues are involved. Some are primarily affected; and others, including all from the skin to the capsules of the joints, follow secondarily due to the flexed position. If the skin whitens when stretched, the skin is the primary cause of the contracture, the deep structures being contracted secondarily. If the skin does not whiten, the deep tissue is the primary cause, the skin being affected secondarily.

Role of Tendons in Contractures. A sloughing tendon is replaced eventually by a contracting cicatrix, which attaches to the surrounding tissue and draws the joints into flexion. The tendon sheath proliferates greatly and similarly attaches itself and contracts. Such a firm cord cannot be drawn out by continuous traction. Physiotherapy is useless. The damage found at operation is always worse than is expected. When a tendon is severed by sloughing, its end always becomes fixed. It is only when a tendon is severed in a sheath, and without infection, that it becomes rounded over without any attachments. When severed in paratenon formation or in the presence of infection, the epitenon and the endotenon layers of the tendon end always proliferate and attach to the surrounding tissue, contracting and often resulting in a flexion contracture. The distal end of a flexor tendon left in a finger often will attach, contract and draw the finger into contracture. That part of a flexor tendon distal to an adherent portion always becomes attached throughout the length of the finger and limits extension of the finger. Similarly, any free tendon end left in the tissues predisposes to contracture from its tendency to reach out, attach itself to the surrounding tissue and then contract.

GENERAL PRINCIPLES OF TREATMENT

For contractures and cicatrices, conservative methods of treatment alone (such as long-continued, constant, mild traction) will draw stiff joints into the position of function and will elongate soft cicatrices and contracting muscles but will not draw out adherent cicatricial tendons—nor will physiotherapy, even if used for years. The traction method is advisable for mild cases and for preliminary use in the more severe ones. It will place stiff joints in the position of function so that the patient may use the hand and thus will improve it by exercise.

In contemplating repair of a contracted hand one should picture the normal hand first, with, of course, a clear concept of its anatomy and physiology. Only then can one perceive and calculate the defects in skin and deeper structures, nerve, lymph and blood supply, muscle balance and nutrition. The surgeon's conception of the hand should include the range of motion of each joint and of the hand and the digits as a whole, including function from a practical standpoint. The creases and the folds in the skin are for the definite purpose of accommodating movements that may be executed throughout their full range without resistance of binding or friction. Some of the details of the normal hand have been given in Chapter 1. With these in mind it is easier to assess the defects and the problems involved in the hand to be repaired.

The first procedure is to furnish new skin and to correct the contracture. The structures inside the hand are liberated, and good pliable skin provided by means of a pedicled skin graft is substituted for the tight, binding cicatrix.

First, the scar, both deep and superficial, must be excised completely down to normal tissue. The borders of the surrounding skin should be undermined in the plane between the deep and the superficial fascia, allowing the taut skin to retract freely. Superficial fascia and skin will stretch, but the deep fascia will not. New good material is needed to fill in the defect. This may be furnished by the sliding skin flap or by the pedicle skin graft which provides both skin and subcutaneous tissue. Free grafts of skin will not suffice when deeper structures are involved and the bed is cicatricial or of tendon, ligament or bone. The limb should be decompressed and freed from any binding scar so that all will be warm, soft and pliable, and muscles will roll freely under yielding skin. Superabundant blood supply is essential for reconstruction of all tissues, tendons, nerves and joints and for obtaining union in bone. This is absent in cicatrix, but by liberating tissue and covering by good pedicle skin, the blood supply is restored.

For contractures from burns, where the deeper structures are less involved, thick free grafts are generally used. This results in marked improvement in the general nutrition of the hand. At this procedure, enough of the deep cicatricial structures are excised or severed to overcome the contracture of the joints. The hand is placed on a previously prepared metal splint in the position opposite to the contracture, and a skin graft is applied. Tendon grafting or repair is omitted at this skin-grafting stage.

Frequently, the contracted joints cannot be extended at once because the nerves have shortened. However, with gradual continuous extension over a period of a few weeks, they will elongate readily.

The second operation is done a few months later when the new skin has sufficient vitality. At this stage an essential step in reconstruction is the bloc excision of all deep cicatrix. The tendons, the nerves and the vessels are not only dissected out from the scar tissue, but also the extensive deep connective tissue cicatrix which reaches out like an octopus with all its tentacles and binds and strangles is excised until only good tissue is left. By freeing the nerves from encircling scar and liberating all the deeper tissues, great improvement in the nutrition results. The state of nutrition of a limb is the most important factor influencing the return of function as regards tendons, joints and nerves. Simply replacing the covering skin and the subcutaneous fat with a pedicle graft may result in improvement in nutrition of the hand, but the deliberate excision of this deep scar is essential to restore the function of the deeper structures and provide a good bed for nerves and tendons. If this step in the staged repair of a badly crippled hand is omitted, the tendon and nerve repairs or grafts will not function at their best.

If in contractures the joint capsule is still holding, it should be severed or excised in its shortened part. If merely severed, the edges usually will rejoin. They may also do this if excised, unless prevented by splinting. If the joints of the digits are injured or destroyed, they may require capsulotomy, arthrodesis or arthroplasty to put them in the position of function or to give them more motion. Similarly, the wrist may be placed in moderate dorsiflexion and, if painful or showing too little movement, either ankylosed or given motion by arthroplasty. The treatment of joints and ligamentous contractures may be found in Chapter 9, Joints.

Tendons in contractures, if reduced to scar tissue, should be excised and replaced by free tendon grafts. Tendons that have been severed for several months must be dealt with in the same way, because the proximal ends will have retracted and the distal portion will have degenerated from disuse and will be adherent. Consideration of tendons in contractures may be found in Chapter 11, Tendons.

The skin is only a part of the problem. If, when the pedicle skin is placed, careful notes on the condition of the deeper structures are not made, the later deep repair will be handicapped. All dissections of the hand should be done under the ischemia produced by a pneumatic tourniquet. This should spare the deep structures—nerves, tendons, blood vessels, pulleys and joint capsules—from injury. Severance of the motor thenar nerve destroys opposition and of a volar digital nerve, sensation. Incisions that parallel tendons cause adhesions along the full length of the tendons.

Skin replacement should be planned so that, when the deep structures are repaired later, a flap may be turned back rather than placing the scar directly over the repair. The hand should be treated as a unit. Trauma has no respect for the specialties. Surgery of the hand is a regional and not a tissue specialty, and the same surgeon should carry out all the stages of reconstruction.

The Hand Is a Tactile Organ. In the hand, sensation is equal in value to motion. The hand is a specialized sense organ. This is especially true of the area supplied by the median nerve. The pulps of the thumb and the index and the middle fingers are the eyes of the hand. Their tips are covered with specialized skin in which the sensory receptors are more numerous, and two-point discrimination is most refined. When one constructs a new thumb or finger using pedicle skin from the abdomen, or places a patch of this on the tactile surface of a digit, the ability to distinguish touch or pain will return, but not to the same degree found in normal finger skin. Therefore, whenever possible, it is well in these strategic areas to transpose normal skin from the vicinity on its neurovascular pedicle to furnish this quality of sensation. The nerve attachments should accompany the skin flap. When a finger is to be discarded, its volar skin may be utilized, transferring it as a pedicle with blood vessels and nerves intact to the digit which is in need of tactile covering. In reconstructing a thumb it is of great advantage to do it by transferring another digit with its blood vessels and nerves so that it will have normal sensibility.

Nerve supply eventually comes into grafted skin so that light touch and pin prick can be felt, though usually not with normal acuity. In pedicled skin, return of sensation extends gradually from its proximal to its distal part; but return of sensation in free grafts usually comes in all areas at about the same time, and the thinner the graft, the quicker the return of sensation, though in a digit this is more likely to be serially.

The Hand Is a Mobile Organ. Normally, the hand can assume any position without placing any strain on the skin covering it; but, in surgery, this fact is too often ignored, being applied to the hand merely as a surface patch replacing a cicatrix. The borders of the patch, if they coincide with the directions of push and pull, are subject to irritation and will form thick, contracting, keloidlike scars. Before any incision in the hand is made, this problem should be considered. Incisions should parallel the wrinkles or the flexion creases wherever possible and should never be made across them at anything approaching a right angle. A median longitudinal incision anywhere in the hand has a pernicious effect. This is particularly evident in the hands, which are mobile, but applies to skin throughout the body. It applies especially to the borders of a skin graft whether the graft is free or pedicled.

On the dorsum of the hand is fine cross-wrinkling that provides the extra length of skin from the forearm to the fingernails necessary when one makes a fist with the wrist in flexion. Gross wrinkles cap the knuckles to allow free movement. This must be kept in mind in plastic surgery of the skin. An example of error is the placing of a pedicle graft as a circular patch on the dorsum of the hand so that the distal border parallels the thumb web and the proximal border forms a line across the back of the hand. The border along each web, because of the motion of push and pull, thickens to a keloid contracture, and the proximal border contracts so that the thumb cannot oppose and the metacarpal arch cannot curve. There is a transverse as well as longitudinal stretching of the dorsal skin. In fact, the whole area of dorsal skin of hand and fingers is one third greater on making a fist.

The volar aspect is cleft by deep folds. These take up the slack of skin on making a fist. The total volar skin area of a fist and flexed wrist is very small compared with the skin area of the hand when spread apart with the wrist dorsiflexed. These folds are transverse in the fingers, the thumb, the palm and the wrist and in the palm are also oblique to accommodate closing and spreading between the thumb and the last 3 fingers. If a surgeon bears in mind the importance of these structures, he cannot place an incision or a border of a pedicle or a free skin graft directly across either the deep volar folds or the fine dorsal wrinkling. He must picture the hand as mobile and arrange his scars to accommodate motion in any direction.

When new skin is supplied to the hand, the amount should be ample to cover the hand and

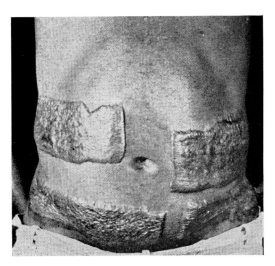

FIG. 216. Keloid formation in donor areas occurs in some individuals when the cut is deep into the derma.

the wrist in complete flexion and also in complete extension and dorsiflexion, including any additional slack needed to allow full pronation and supination at the same time. Transversely, the palm should have sufficient skin to accommodate for the full spread, as should the dorsum for opposition of the thumb and a fully curved metacarpal arch.

Whenever a scar or the borders of either a pedicle or a free graft may cross a flexion crease at a right angle, that is, coincide with the direction of push and pull, a zigzag or curved line should be made. A cross slit may be cut and a tongue of skin drawn into it, or the patch may be patterned with indentations and blunt points. Instead of allowing a scar to parallel the web, a long tongue of the graft should be laid across the web. To fill a thumb cleft, the pedicle graft across it should be long and diamond-shaped, the points or the angles reaching to the juncture, or hinge, of the first 2 metacarpals both in front and in back. Longitudinal scars or graft borders about the

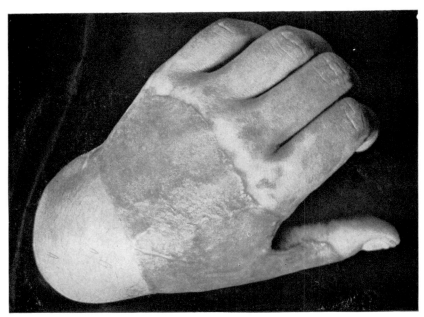

FIG. 217. Free graft of skin on the dorsum of the hand in which the error was made of allowing its border to coincide with the web of the thumb. Due to the irritation from push and pull, flexion contracture developed. The graft should have been prolonged as a long point well around the web, on the volar surface.

wrist are bad in any part of its circumference, as the wrist is a universal joint. In fingers the flexion creases extend back only to the midlateral line. Along this line a scar may become invisible; but if the scar is placed more volar or more dorsal to it, it will thicken and contract, because it will be subject to the irritation of push and pull. In applying free grafts to replace scar from burns along the dorsum of a finger, one should either zigzag the borders or furnish enough skin to allow the borders to follow the midlateral line of the finger on each side.

Plastic Repair of Skin in Flexion Contractures. In flexion contracture the amount of skin over the contracture is too small. The size of this defect in the amount of skin present can be estimated only by picturing the hand in the extreme contrary position with the contracture entirely excised and the surrounding skin liberated so that it is free to retract to its normal tension. Then the skin defect is seen to be greatly in excess of what one would guess at first glance. For instance, the minimal defect in a strongly flexed wrist is 3 inches in diameter. Contractures are greatest along directions of push and pull, as they are caused by this irritation. The length and the breadth of the defect are ascertained by comparing

measurements with the other hand, with all of the joints placed in the position opposite to that caused by the contracture. Comparative distances between a series of similar points are taken longitudinally down the wrist, the palm or the fingers and transversely in various lines across the palm with the 5 digits fully spread or across the dorsum with all fully flexed. In estimating the size of the pedicle, one third more is added to allow for the tightness of the skin about the contracture. Before a hand can be placed in the contrary deformity, the deep portion of the flexion contracture must be relieved, whether it is fascia, tendon or joint capsule. Only in mild contractures or small scars of the hand can sufficient good skin to cover the defect be obtained from the vicinity by sliding or swinging skin flaps. Usually, it is necessary to resort to the free or pedicled graft method.

KELOIDS. These scars are composed of thick cicatricial tissue covered by a thin layer of epidermis and contain some sweat and sebaceous glands. They are the result of overhealing; instead of healing to the surface and stopping, the tissues continue to pile up well above the surface level. The richness of blood vessels and luxuriant growth give the red color. After $1\frac{1}{2}$ years the cicatrix usually

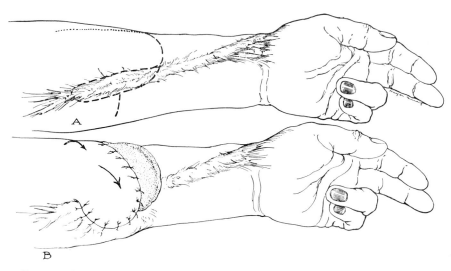

FIG. 218. Breaking a line of tension. The scar is partially excised and cut across to relieve tension. A flap of skin is swung across the line of pull, a split-skin graft covering the denuded area.

softens, sinks to the normal level and whitens. Keloids usually occur in dark-skinned races, though they are often seen even when there is white skin and red hair. Burns are prone to form keloids, evidently from the irritative effect of tissue that has been partially burned.

In the hand, scars from incorrectly placed incisions may result in keloids. Whether the resultant scar will be practically invisible or will be a conspicuous keloid contracture depends on whether the incision follows the folds or natural wrinkles in the skin or crosses them at a right angle or even obliquely.

Keloids and hypertrophic scar contracture

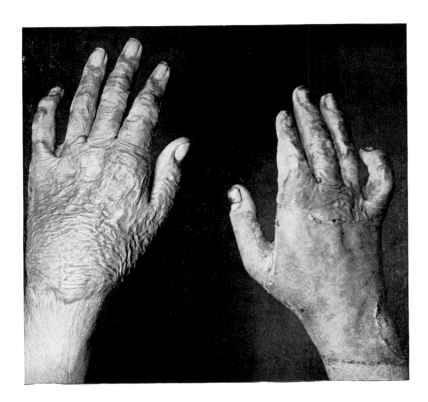

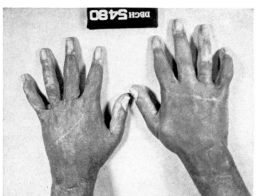
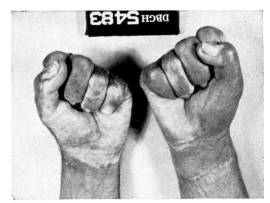

FIG. 219. Thick keloid-type scars from burn. Scars were excised and replaced with thick split-skin grafts. (*Top*) Left hand, preoperative; right hand after one stage had been completed. (*Bottom*) Postoperative, extension and flexion. (From W. B. Macomber, M.D.)

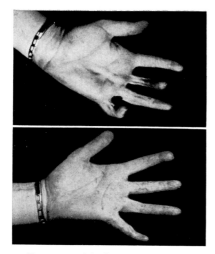

FIG. 220. Flexion contractures in the ring and the little fingers from falling in the fireplace at 10 months of age. At the age of 29, the keloids were excised, grafting whole skin in their place, while the hand was kept immobile on a spreading metal splint. (*Top*) Preoperative and (*bottom*) postoperative conditions.

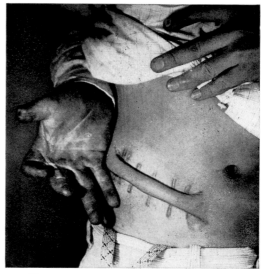

FIG. 221. To relieve this traumatic flexion contracture, new pedicled skin is needed to fill the defect after the scar has been excised.

form in response to postoperative irritation, either from something rubbing on them or from the irritation of intermittent tension and compression incurred when folds or creases of the skin continually open and close in the normal motion of the hand. This is often demonstrated in an L-shaped scar; the line of the L following the creases will be practically invisible, while the other line will be conspicuous, even to the degree of a contracting, thick keloid. This principle, which applies throughout the body, is usually overlooked, as evidenced for instance by the usual oblique direction of the McBurney and inguinal hernia scars, which could have been practically invisible if made transversely.

Deep cicatricial tissue reacts just as does skin in its response to intermittent tension. When a deep cicatrix spans a joint so that it is pulled each time the joint straightens, it forms in the line of tension a firm, thick, contracting cord of scar tissue which limits the motion of joints and draws them into extreme positions.

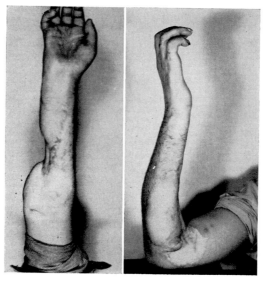

FIG. 222. (*Left*) Hand and arm had been caught in the rollers of a printing press. The gears ground out the inner side of the forearm, making an irreparable gap between the ends of the median and the ulnar nerves and a gap in the flexor muscles. (*Right*) Applied pedicle and amputated through the forearm.

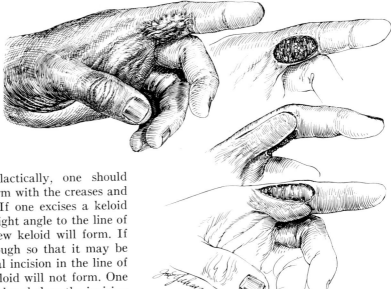

FIG. 223. Excision of scar and closure of defect by local flap, based proximally. The donor area then was covered with split-skin graft. This is especially useful when the primary defect exposes tendons, ligaments or joints.

Treatment. Prophylactically, one should plan incisions to conform with the creases and the folds in the skin. If one excises a keloid scar, that is, one at a right angle to the line of the skin wrinkles, a new keloid will form. If the keloid is short enough so that it may be removed by an elliptical incision in the line of the wrinkles, a new keloid will not form. One can excise a short keloid and close the incision by a zigzag plastic with some improvement. The cross-line of the zigzag will not form a new keloid, but the 2 short oblique ones will. Immobilization for 3 weeks postoperatively helps to lessen development of new keloid.

Radiation can be used prophylactically following excision of keloid; it, too, will help to reduce the new growth.

EXCISION OF SCAR. Small scars may be excised. The surrounding skin should be widely undermined, so as to detach it and make it possible to draw the skin margins together by suture. The undermining should be in a plane between the superficial and the deep fascia,

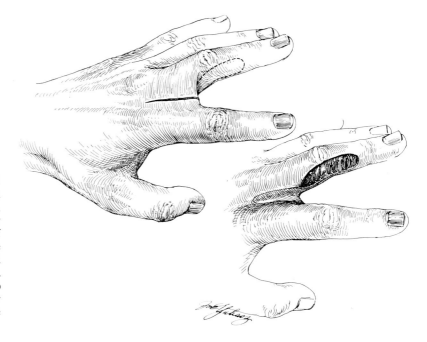

FIG. 224. A dorsal web, such as often results from burns, can be corrected by swinging a tongue of good skin from the anterolateral aspect of one of the fingers. A split-skin graft to the remaining raw area completes the closure.

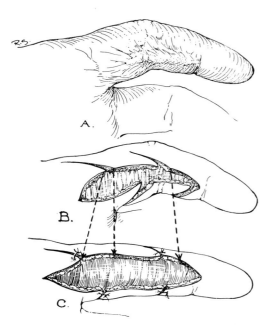

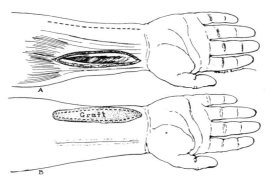

FIG. 226. Method of obtaining skin to close a wound. After an operation on the forearm, adding grafts or removing scars, it may be impossible to close the wound. By making a parallel incision, the broad ribbon of skin is sideslid enough to cover. The denuded area is skin grafted.

FIG. 225. A volar scar on a finger can be excised, and the skin margins relieved (A and B), but unless the resulting juncture of graft and skin is in the midlateral line, contracture will recur. (C) The excision is inadequate, and the scars will be anterolateral.

because the superficial fascia and the skin will stretch, but the deep fascia will not. If the scar parallels the creases in the skin, simple excision is all that is necessary, but, if it crosses them, some maneuver should be done whereby the resulting scar will parallel the creases if at all possible. This may be done by excising with a wide ellipse in the right direction, by a sliding skin graft or by a Z-plasty. When a scar shows a narrow line of contracture from tension, one may swing a flap of good skin across the line of tension, resort to a V to Y plasty, or employ the most useful method of Z-plasty. The problem is to elongate the skin in the line of tension at the sacrifice of the slack skin in a line at a right angle to this. By transposing the 2 pointed flaps in the Z-plasty, the straight line of pull is converted to a zigzag line so that the tension expends itself in merely broadening the angles of the

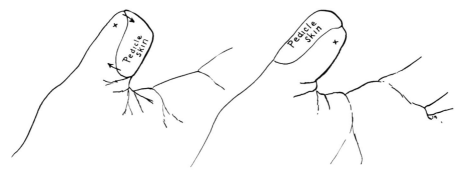

FIG. 227. (Left) Pedicle skin here covers the important surface of a thumb stump. Such skin never has the sensibility of normally innervated skin. (Right) A transposition places good skin on the tactile surface. A better way is an island transfer (Chap. 10).

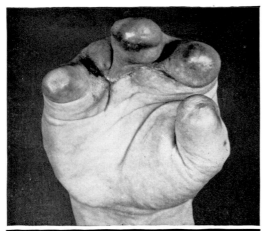

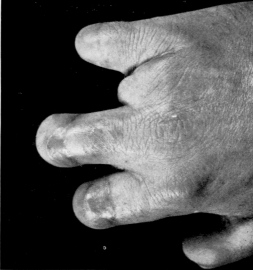

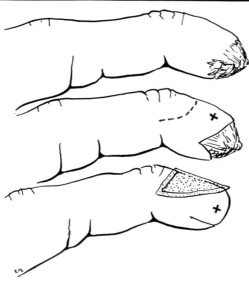

FIG. 228. When stumps of digits are cicatricial, a band of skin taken from across the dorsum can be drawn over to replace the poor end much like drawing a cap down over one's face. The part left denuded is covered by skin graft, which in outline resembles a nail. (*Top*) Preoperative and (*center*) postoperative views. (*Bottom*) Diagram of operation. (From W. B. Macomber, M.D.)

scar. By drawing the skin together crosswise to the line of tension, like fitting 2 crowns together, the skin is made greater in length in the line of tension.

Z-plasties are good for web contractures anywhere, but especially about the elbow and the axilla. If there is insufficient skin, these may be combined with a free skin graft in a part that does not move. For a long contracture, multiple oblique cuts alternating on each side convert the web into a long zigzag line free from tension. By the Z-plasty, which means transposing one flap for another, poor skin at a place of motion may be replaced by good skin, the poor skin being displaced to an area from which it can be removed by multiple excision.

In opening out a finger that has flexion contracture after the scar is excised from the volar surface, it will be found that the skin is too tight along the sides to allow the finger to straighten. One or 2 diagonal cuts into this border of skin allow the finger to straighten, as the points of skin so produced slide proximalward and can be sutured there. The resulting defect is closed by graft. Adequate excision to allow the resulting suture line to lie midlateral is necessary.

A small area from which skin has been excised can be closed by swinging a skin flap from the neighborhood over the defect. The bed from which the skin flap came can be closed by an immediate split graft. In this way one can cover with good skin areas that must stand the wear, clefts, or structures that would be vulnerable to infection or that have just been repaired. This procedure applies to the volar and the dorsal surfaces of the fingers and the dorsal surface of the hand and the arm. A contracture of one finger may be replaced by a skin flap from the side of the adjoining finger, skin grafting the donor site.

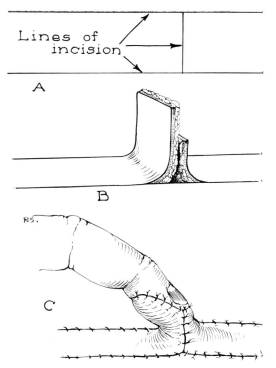

Lines of incision

A

B

C

R.S.

FIG. 229. A simple closed stem flap for covering finger pulp losses.

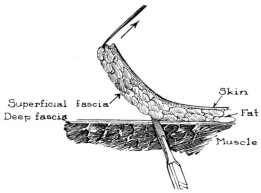

Superficial fascia
Deep fascia

Skin

Fat

Muscle

FIG. 230. To mobilize skin for pedicles, flaps or other shifting, the undermining is done in a fairly bloodless plane between the deep and the superficial fasciae. Only the latter of the two will stretch.

The palm, being thicker and stiffer, does not lend itself well to the swinging of skin flaps, because the torsion of the inelastic base of the flaps cuts off the blood supply. In the fingers, the flap usually is swung from the side, but its pedicle must be proximal.

If the flexion contracture of the finger is narrow, the Z-plasty may relieve it. By the above procedures as much as possible of the surface is covered, and the remainder is skin grafted.

Where skin tension is too great to close a wound after the deep structures have been repaired, as in the forearm, one can make an extra incision paralleling the wound and an inch or more from it. The intervening skin is undermined and can be slid across so that the wound can be closed without tension. The edges of the supplementary incision now gape widely, but the area can be covered by an immediate split-skin graft placed over good subcutaneous tissue away from the area where the deeper structures were repaired.

In raising skin flaps, the undermining should

be made just superficial to the deep fascia and liberally enough beyond the base of the flap so that the flap can be turned without tension. There should be sufficient subcutaneous tissue to carry blood supply. In an extremity, the base of the flap should be proximal whenever possible. A rounded flap is more viable than a pointed one, and the base should be broad enough for the length of the flap to ensure vitality. The ability to judge this can be gained only by experience. The inclusion in the flap of a large artery and vein ensures a better blood supply. In applying dressings care should be taken not to place undue pressure over the base of the flap.

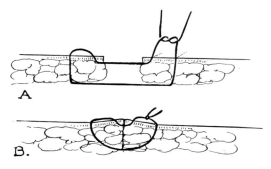

A

B.

FIG. 231. Far and near retention suture placed in the palm to prevent the tough skin edge from rolling in.

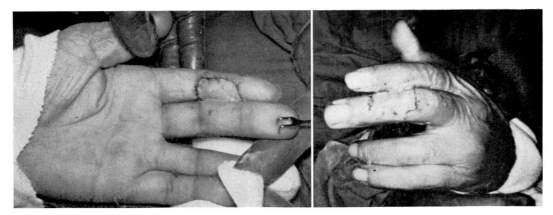

FIG. 232. (*Left*) A cross-finger flap for a defect on the volar surface of the index finger. A flap of skin from the dorsum of the middle segment of the adjoining finger is turned on a hinge at the midlateral line to cover the defect. All raw areas are covered with split-skin graft from the forearm. (*Right*) Cross-finger flap to restore pulp of middle finger. The flap from the dorsum of the ring finger is hinged on the radial side at the midlateral line. The connected fingers are in a semiflexed position, in balance and not under strain. The stem of the pedicle and the donor area are covered with a split-skin graft.

In plastic work, certain principles are essential. Hematoma should be avoided by hemostasis, brief tube drainage or suction, and gentle, prolonged pressure by voluminous, well-fitted waste or fluff wrapped with an elastic bandage. Steel wool, medium coarse grade, provides excellent compression, stays flexible longer than gauze or cotton waste and allows air to circulate, preventing maceration. For accurate healing, immobilization is necessary, as is avoidance of any raw area. Overstretching of skin results in necrosis. Skin flaps should be ample in size and provided with good circulation. Skin should be undermined widely enough to prevent tension. In plastic work one should be liberal and radical, as tension is fatal.

DEFORMITIES OF FINGER ENDS. Tender cicatricial finger ends are unfit for work. A small abdominal skin flap in one stage will place good skin there, but, because it is abdominal skin, sensibility will be poor. The volar skin of a toe as a free or a pedicle graft or even a small thick piece of toe pulp may be grafted as one grafts a portion of an ear to fill a defect in the nose. In loss of the distal part of the pulp, the nail and the distal phalanx may be shortened and the volar skin sutured to the nail.

Where possible, a cicatrix in a place which should be a tactile area may be replaced by normal innervated skin by transposing as a pedicled flap the skin from the side of a finger, the side then being skin grafted. A terminal scar on a finger stump may be replaced by dorsal skin from the stump by making a transverse incision across the dorsum. A ribbon of this skin attached at each end, a form of double pedicled flap, is slipped over the end of the stump to replace the scar, a skin graft being placed on the dorsum, which in outline resembles a nail.

CROSS FINGER FLAPS. For closing a finger amputation or replacing a cicatrix and flexion contracture of a finger, cross finger flaps are useful and furnish good tactile skin. The flap usually is taken from the dorsum or the side of the finger, raising the flap to cover the dorsum of the donee finger and turning the flap downward and over to cover the volar surface. One Kirschner wire through the phalanges holds the position. The skin graft on the donor area should be held on with a stent, thus avoiding clots beneath it.

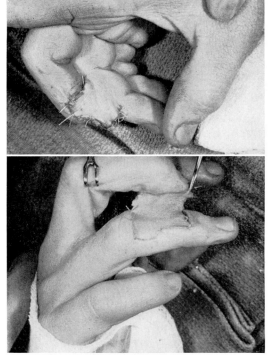

FIG. 233. Cross-finger flap to restore contour of pulp. (*Top*) Flap from dorsum of ring finger. (*Bottom*) The split-skin graft sutured in place. The pedicle is divided in 2½ to 3 weeks.

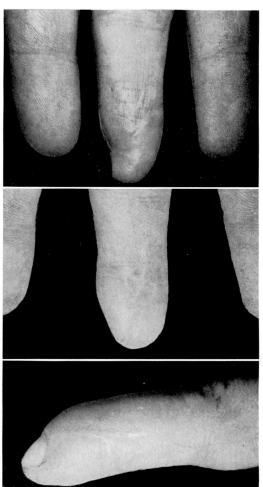

FIG. 234. Same patient as Figure 233. (*Top*) Preoperative. Loss of pulp on radial side of middle finger. (*Center* and *bottom*) Postoperative views of volar and radial aspects.

A fingertip may be covered by a skin flap from the thenar eminence, suturing it with the finger in flexion. Although this is useful in children, stiffness of the finger in flexion occurs commonly in adults.

FILLING DEFECTS. Hollows, as in the forearm, may be filled in several ways. Subcutaneous fat may be partially cut loose and rolled out under the skin to fill the defect, or the hollow may be filled with a pedicle skin flap. Another method is to bury a dermal graft with ½ inch of fat taken from the inguinal region, preserving Scarpa's fascia to keep the undersurface of the fat intact. First, a skin graft is taken to get the dermis and the fat beneath, and then it is laid back in place. A free graft of fat may be absorbed, but the fat of a pedicle graft will not be. Dermal grafts shrink about one fourth.

UTILIZING FINGER SKIN. To replace a scar on another finger, the dorsum or the palm of the hand, or both, the skin of a useless finger may be used. The finger is slit along the dorsal or the volar aspect, filleted, preserving its nerve and blood supply, and laid over to fill the denudation. To cover both surfaces, the finger may be split. This argues for not discarding viable fingers at the time of an accident.

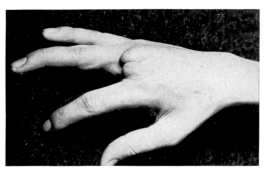

FIG. 235. Fillet of long finger to cover the dorsum of the hand. Dog ears left for circulation were excised later. Note how the tip of the finger is laid out as a W to handle the pad. (L. D. Howard, M.D.)

If it is desired to place the skin of a finger remote from the base of the finger, as across a thumb cleft, the skin may be detached entirely or circumscribed with the exception of the 2 volar digital nerves and vessels, which are used as the pedicle from the palm. In one instance this succeeded when only one of the volar digital arteries was present; in fact, a whole digit may transferred on a neurovascular pedicle. (See Island Flap, Chap. 10.)

CONTRACTURE OF THUMB CLEFT. This contracture ranges from mild to extreme and often involves all the muscles and the tissues between the first 2 metacarpals, including the carpometacarpal joint capsule. Ischemic contracture is the worst.

The zigzag plastic procedure will suffice for mild contractures from a scar or a burn of the web. Often a flap of skin from the dorsum of the hand may be swung well across the depth of the cleft, and the denuded part of the dorsal skin grafted. The cleft may be opened widely and a large diamond-shaped free skin graft used to close it. Whenever relieving webs by this method, whether in thumb clefts or between fingers, the points of the diamond should be prolonged far proximal on each side to avoid shrinking to form another web. A free graft in a thumb cleft wears so poorly that a pedicle graft is preferable.

A pedicle graft here should also be a long diamond reaching to the angle between the

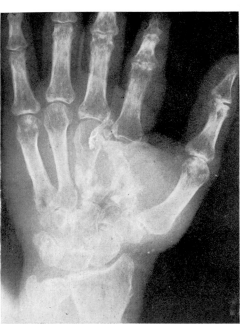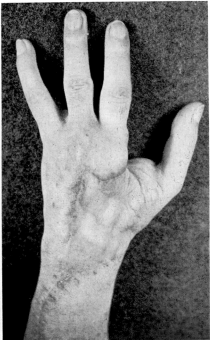

FIG. 236. The index finger which, from a gunshot wound, was beyond repair, was discarded, and the cicatrix of the cleft and the dorsum were replaced by volar skin by filleting the finger. Later use of the long finger was restored by bone and tendon graft. (L. D. Howard, M.D.)

first 2 metacarpals both in front and in back so as to be free from push and pull on its borders. This can be done by an expansion on a tube, but also by a direct abdominal flap, splinting the cleft wide open. The skin of the other arm has been used, but the scar here is objectionable.

The contracture from deep scar will recur at once unless the first 2 metacarpals are held apart. This may be done temporarily by inserting 2 crossed Kirschner wires through the first 2 metacarpals or by inserting a temporary strut in the cleft. The position may be made permanent by a bone-graft spreader fitted into slots in the 2 metacarpals or between them as a triangular bone block wedge in the position of moderate opposition.

SUTURING SKIN. Any of the various suture materials can be used, but stainless steel wire produces so little reaction that it has been adopted almost to the exclusion of other materials.

Needles should be slender and with cutting edges. Curved ones are used in the palm and in awkward places, but straight ones are used wherever possible, as they are time-saving. The Bunnell needle is spear-pointed, 0.020 inch in width and 2½ inches in length and is flexible enough to bend somewhat when the

occasion demands. The same needle is used in sewing tendons.

In the palm the skin is rigid, and the edges have a tendency to curl in; therefore, interrupted end-on mattress sutures are placed first, penetrating straight through each skin border at a right angle ¼ inch from the wound and returning to catch the edge of the wound itself. This is followed by a continuous simple over-and-over stitch for exact coaptation. This mattress method is useful elsewhere in the hand and the forearm wherever retention sutures are used. Often one can catch the deeper structures also, so as to obliterate dead space and prevent slithering of the layers of the wound. Stainless steel wire No. 34 is used for retention sutures, and No. 36 for the finishing apposition stitch. The latter should enter the skin 2 or 3 mm. from its border, depending on the skin thickness, and continue on through the skin, diverging from the incision so as to encircle a sufficient mass of subcutaneous tissue to cause the skin edges to rise up slightly. Of course, the stitch up through the opposite skin edge should embrace the same amount of subcutaneous tissue and emerge at exactly the same distance from the skin edge as on the other side. Sufficient subcutaneous tissue in the grasp of the stitch makes a thicker

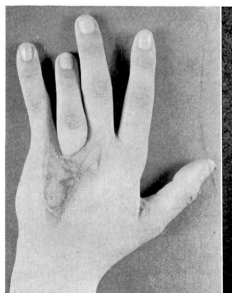
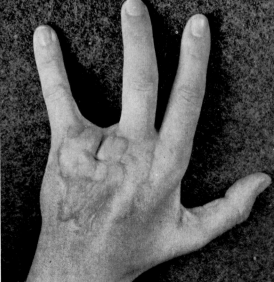

FIG. 237. Use of fillet of finger skin for dorsal defect. (L. D. Howard, M.D.)

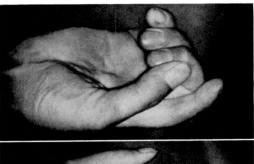

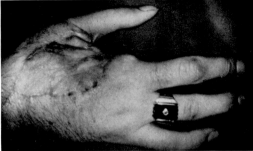

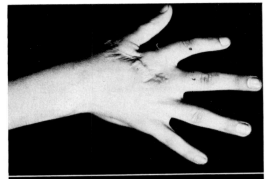

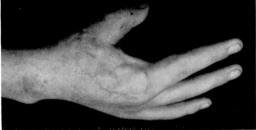

FIG. 238. Case L. P. (*Top*) Three years previously, a tractor had rolled on his hand, fracturing the second metacarpal and so extensively lacerating the thumb cleft that the cicatrix bound the thumb to the hand, greatly interfering with function. The index finger was useless. (*Bottom*) The scar was excised, including the metacarpal and the phalanges of the index. The index was filleted and laid down over the thumb cleft. The thumb was positioned on the carpus and temporarily pinned there.

FIG. 240. (*Top*) The hand had been caught in the chain and cogs of a gasoline lawn mower, with resultant fracture of the first 2 metacarpals and injury to the radial sides of the thumb and the index finger. The cleft was contracted and the index finger useless. Excised the cicatrix, opening up the thumb cleft. Removed the metacarpal and the phalanges of the index finger, filleted it, and laid it over the thumb cleft. Transferred the first interosseus muscle to the proximal phalanx of the middle finger. Transferred the profundus of the index to the thumb for a flexor and fused the metacarpocarpal joint of the thumb. (*Bottom*) The patient obtained full function and cosmetic appearance.

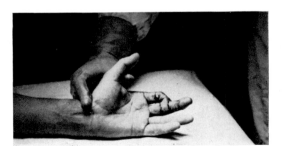

FIG. 239. Index with irreparable bone and tendon damage was filleted and its skin used to replace scar on volar surface of middle finger. Three weeks later the pedicle was divided, and amputation of the index ray completed.

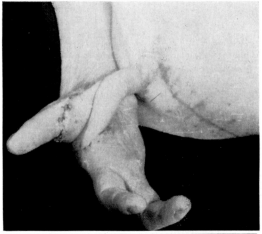

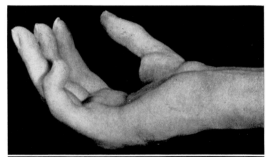

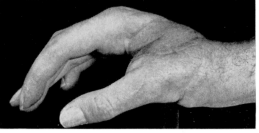

FIG. 242. Opening thumb cleft with pedicle graft. Note extent of graft on both volar and dorsal surfaces.

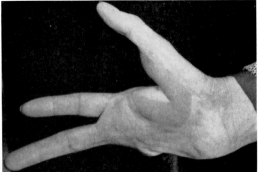

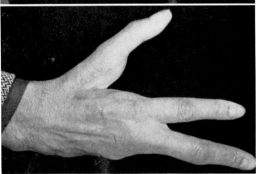

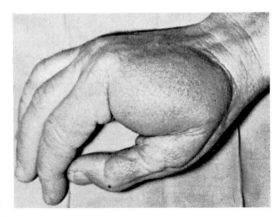

FIG. 241. Reconstruction of thumb cleft by tubed pedicle requires skin to extend from "hinge to hinge." This hand now requires adductor and opponens transfers to complete the restoration of all possible function.

FIG. 243. Ten years previously, a large direct abdominal flap was applied to the dorsum, along the ulnar side of the thumb and an extended point onto the palm. Patient is now obese, and the fat in the flap increases as did the abdominal fat. Two stages are required to remove excess fat.

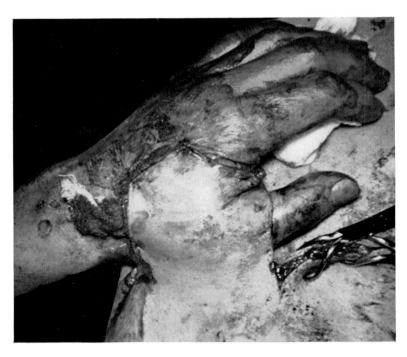

Fig. 244. Direct abdominal patterned flap to restore first cleft. Primary closure of the belly wall is facilitated by turning back a temporary flap from the dorsum of the 1st metacarpal area to cover the pedicle raw surface.

wall between the inside repaired structures and the outside and, by this broad attachment, prevents scars from spreading. Stitches placed too far from the skin edge allow the edge to infold. The tissues of the hand have so much movement that sutures should not be removed before the 9th day or incisions will break open. To protect the suture line from parting or stretching, the skin tension may be relieved by a butterfly of adhesive plaster crossing the wound or by strips of gauze painted to the skin with collodion. Whenever plastic maneuvers have been done, it is advisable to splint the hand until the skin has healed firmly, lest movement cause necrosis of such parts of low vitality as the points of skin or the ends of skin flaps.

Skin Grafts. Wherever the area of cicatrix is extensive one should excise all scar tissue and replace it with good skin by means of some method of skin grafting. When the cicatrix is unusually extensive, running well up the arm, it may not be practical to excise all of it. In such a case, the surgeon should determine the locations of the main lines of tension. These lines should be broken by excision and cross-cuts. The skin should be allowed to gape

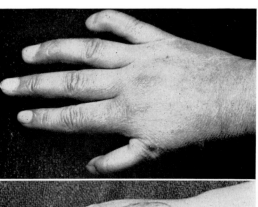

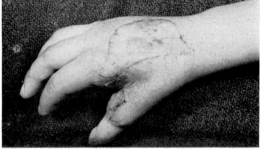

Fig. 245. Widening of first cleft by sliding flap from dorsum of hand and covering donor area with full-thickness skin graft. Congenital hypoplasia of the right thumb and adduction contracture. (*Bottom*) four weeks after operation. (From T. Tajima, M.D., Niigata University, Niigata City, Japan)

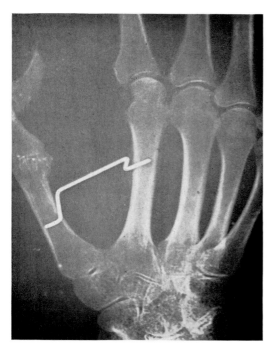

FIG. 246. When adduction contracture of thumb is released and first metacarpal spread, position can be maintained easily by inserting a Kirschner wire strut.

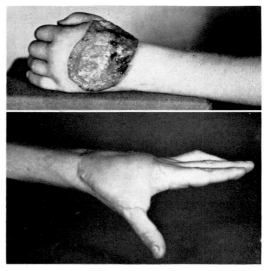

FIG. 247. (*Top*) Hand had been drawn into the rollers of a washing machine that kept rolling on the dorsum. (*Bottom*) Excised and skin grafted. Later, a pedicle was applied. A 2-inch gap in the extensor tendons was filled by grafts from the palmaris longus of both arms. The hand opened and closed well.

widely by freeing its margins, and the denuded areas should be grafted. Occasionally, in broad cicatricial areas, the tension can be relieved by cross-cuts across the whole area, dividing it into segments. Then split grafts are laid over the defects so produced. Occasionally, the tunnel method may be used, placing the split-skin graft over a wide flat stent of wax or metal placed through the tunnel, or even embedded under the skin without a through-and-through tunnel and later slit widely open.

The choice of the type of graft to be used depends on the bed to receive the graft, on the use to which the part must be put and on the time, the operations and the expense incurred. Skin furnished by the pedicle method is by far the best and is necessary in contractures resulting from infection, because in these the deeper tissues are involved, and the bed to receive the skin graft is cicatricial or may be of bone, tendon or joint capsule. Cicatrices from most burns have a good vascular bed, as the damage was inflicted from without. Free full-thickness grafts or thick split grafts are usually satisfactory.

A pedicle graft with its subcutaneous tissue will bring vascularity to the deeper cicatricial tissues, so that the pedicled graft is better than the free graft in withered limbs with poor nutrition. In areas subjected to much movement where there are flexion creases, pedicle grafts are especially indicated, in contrast with split of Thiersch grafts, though full-thickness grafts here are often quite satisfactory. Where there is much wear and hard usage, as over the volar aspect of the digits and the palm, pedicle grafts wear better than do free grafts. The pedicle graft method requires a series of operations and hospitalization of many weeks; consequently, there is more time and expense involved than with the free graft, which is done in one operation.

The pinch graft is mentioned only to be condemned, for it yields unsightly, irregular poor skin, and the donor areas are not only extensive and hideous but are spoiled for yielding subsequent crops of skin. It is easier and better to cut the regular split-skin graft and separate it into postage-stamp-sized pieces, which are scattered over the granulating surface.

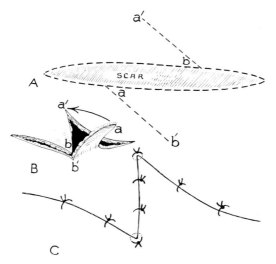

FIG. 248. Excision of scar and release of tension by Z-plasty. The included angle (a) and (b) is usually about 60°.

PEDICLE SKIN GRAFTS furnish good skin and subcutaneous tissue and relax all tissues within the limb, thus improving nutrition and bringing blood supply to the part. They may be applied to avulsed or denuded areas as a primary procedure and may be applied to cover any wound from days to weeks after the injury, provided that the wound is clean. They stand the wear and tear of rough usage as soon

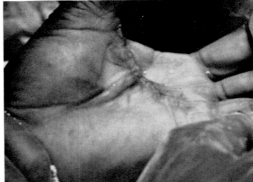

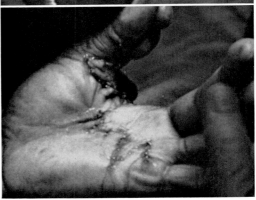

FIG. 250. (*Top*) From a laceration crossing the flexor creases a keloid scar limits the thumb and extends to the base of the ring finger. (*Bottom*) Multiple Z-plasties designed so that transverse components of the resulting scar will parallel the flexion creases relieves the contracture.

as nerve supply returns to them and furnish a bed under which tendons, whether old or newly repaired, will glide. They do not shrink, and they grow with the individual, as often seen in grafts which were placed when the patient was a child. They carry hair and all the structures of the skin and do not pigment excessively, as free grafts occasionally do. Skin which has been well transplanted by the pedicle method lies flat without excessive subcutaneous tissue, and its borders are quite inconspicuous if they do not cross flexion creases abruptly. One frequently sees poorly made pedicle grafts that show a domelike swelling from excess of subcutaneous tissue and often cover only a part instead of the whole of the cicatricial area. Thus they are often surrounded by a ring of scar tissue, and

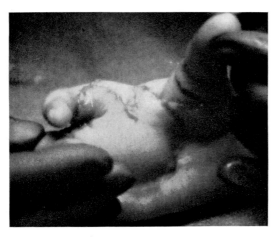

FIG. 249. A previously applied pedicle resulted in a line of contracture from thumb to index. A double Z-plasty allows opening of the cleft.

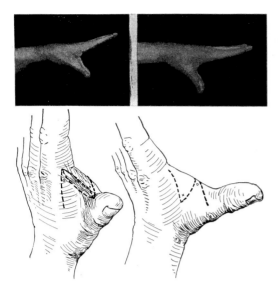

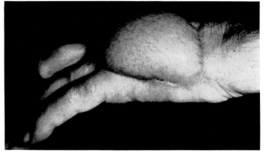

FIG. 252. "Biscuit" flap. Too thick, too small and showing lack of concept of moving areas of hand. Will require 2 or more operations to revise flap before attacking the impaired deeper structures.

FIG. 251. Keloid web contractures from an electric flash burn, corrected by a Z-plasty (*top, right*). The procedure is illustrated in the diagram below.

should be used in planning so that the borders of the graft will never limit normal, complete, free movement of the hand. Pedicle skin should lie flat on the hand. Too much fat is parasitic, being an additional burden on the

the border may be conspicuous and even thickened to keloid or flexion contracture where it crosses a flexion crease. The surgeon should err on the side of thoroughness—complete removal of all scar, freeing edges by undermining and furnishing ample coverage.

The blood supply of a pedicle flap is primarily in 2 locations. Large vessels are just above the deep fascia, but there is an abundant blood supply close to the skin. For a pedicle the size of a hand one may dispense with the deep layer of vessels except at the base of the pedicle, relying on those close to the skin for the flap which is on the hand. Redundant fat should be trimmed off so that the graft will be flat. A graft that is too puffy with fat can be leveled by raising half of it at a time and removing the fat. Pedicle grafts are often made excessively thick so that they stand out in a grotesque dome, the idea being to furnish ample skin. However, except in a few special cases such as clumped fingers, this idea is fallacious, because skin itself will grow to cover any area at normal tension. It is the borders that are unyielding and contract instead of elongating. It is they and not the skin itself that hamper motions. Great care

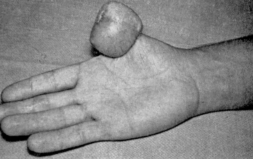

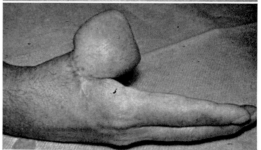

FIG. 253. Another example of error in pedicle application. The thumb had been amputated at the proximal joint. Had the wound simply been closed, the patient doing unskilled labor could have returned to work in a few weeks. Instead, this was the result after 10 months and 6 operations.

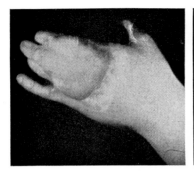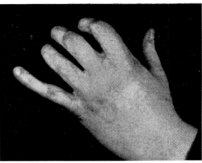

Fig. 254. (*Left*) Poor pedicle graft. Redundant, scanty and with webs. (Right) Same graft improved by raising up, removing excess of fat and replacing. The webs were restored by laying points of skin through the clefts.

blood supply. It should be trimmed fairly thin, leaving only enough to place a layer between the tendons if needed. Abundant blood supply, as seen on cross section, is between the fat and the skin, so that it is safe to trim away the redundancy. To correct excessive fat in a previously applied pedicle requires 2 operations.

For gunshot wounds or any wound with large skin destruction, reconstruction of the hand usually necessitates the preliminary placement of a pedicle skin graft just as is required for deep repair anywhere in the body.

Prevalent faults of pedicles are that they are domelike or, on the other hand, too scanty to replace the cicatrix entirely, that they are made merely as patches with borders paralleling lines of push and pull without regard to the mobility of the hand, and they may not be aseptic.

Hands are prone to stiffen. Besides prolonged splinting and edema, a major cause of stiffening is an open wound. The products of this inflammation, even in the course of a few weeks, result in considerable stiffening. Therefore, wounds in hands should be closed early by primary or secondary closure or by skin grafting. This is especially important in applying pedicles to the hand. The open pedicle method, that is, the septic pedicle in which the stem is raw with exposed granulations,

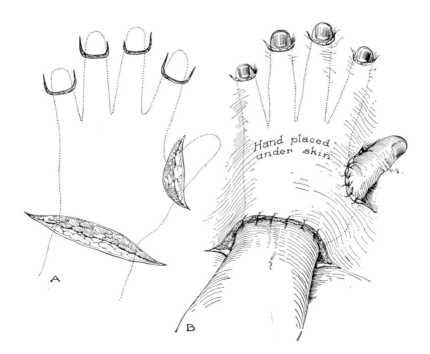

Hand placed under skin

A

B

Fig. 255. The obsolete pocket-graft method of covering the dorsum of the hand. Direct pedicled grafts or free grafts are more appropriate, cleaner and give better results.

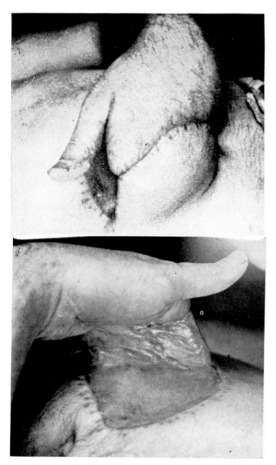

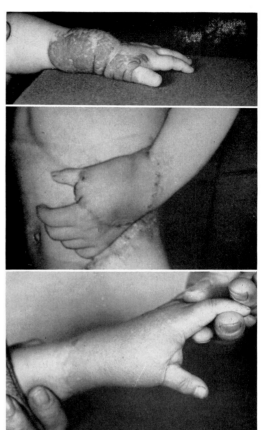

FIG. 256. Stump of hand covered by a direct flap. All raw surfaces are covered by skin graft. Here it is advisable to have much subcutaneous fat to have enough skin to cover the several digits, some of which may be phalangized. (W. B. Macomber, M.D.)

FIG. 257. Infant, age 10 months. (*Top*) Hemangioma. (*Center* and *bottom*) Excision and thick skin graft. A year later, the graft made contracture. Therefore, it was excised and a pedicle was applied.

should never be used. The open stem of a pedicle is equivalent to an open wound in the hand. The lymphatic vessels carry the products of inflammation directly into the hand, resulting in undesirable stiffening—the arch enemy. All pedicles to hands should be rendered aseptic by closure. This can be done either by tubing or by skin grafting over all raw surfaces. This fosters clean wounds and finer scars. Neat, careful suturing of pedicles yields clean healing instead of dirty borders.

It is important also, in order to prevent stiffening, to avoid collections of serum or blood. Careful hemostasis, placing drains for 24 hours and avoiding dead spaces, will allow prompt healing.

When one is confident in the use of pedicles, some operations on the deeper tissues may be done at the same time as the pedicle graft. This includes nerve suture, capsulectomy, excision of deep cicatrix, bone carpentry and even placing a bone graft such as a thumb post. Time is saved in this way, but elaborate reconstructions should not be attempted.

Pedicle grafts are of various types: pocket graft, flap graft and tubular pedicle. In the

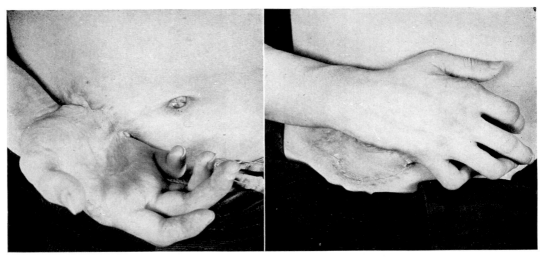

FIG. 258. Direct closed stemless abdominal flap showing incision for pattern before delayed detachment. (L. D. Howard, M.D.)

pocket type, the flap of skin is raised from the abdomen or the inner part of the thigh for the dorsum or from the hip for the palm. The hand is placed under this so that the denuded area on the hand is covered by the flap of skin. This flap should have 2 or more pedicles to maintain its blood supply. It can be cut to a pattern to cover all the digits and the back of the hand as a whole, being cut and replaced 2 weeks ahead of time for better vascularity. The objection to this method is that a dirty wound is unavoidable. The skin of much of the hand is in contact with the raw undersurface from which the flap is raised.

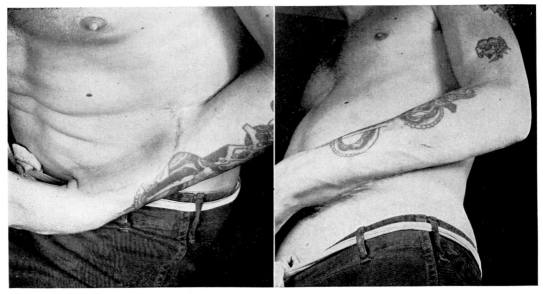

FIG. 259. Direct stemless abdominal pedicle. Incision for pattern is shown preparatory to detachment in 2 stages. (L. D. Howard, M.D.)

Compresses and constant care are necessary to keep it clean.

It is not practical to use a Thiersch skin graft on the area under a pocket graft unless this is done a week in advance and the pedicle is replaced at once; such grafts usually slough away because of the excess of inflammation. An experienced surgeon finds little advantage in pocket grafts.

Flap grafts are the type used most frequently for the forearm and the hand, although a tube pedicle is better adapted for elongated flaps covering digits and complicated surfaces. If a flap graft is made with a broad flaring base and, according to its blood supply, not more than 2 or 2½ times its width, previous preparation is unnecessary. If made in a direction not paralleling the blood supply, or if made in a bizarre shape, wider at the end than at the base, elongated or interdigitated, the blood supply should be developed slowly by repeated steps, i.e., delayed. In these delayed pedicle flaps, portions of the borders are successively cut, undermined and replaced at intervals of from 5 to 10 days, until the vessels in the base hypertrophy sufficiently to support the whole flap. If the graft is applied in the first procedure (pedicle in one), which, including detachment, takes about 5 weeks and is the usual method, much time is saved. There is an advantage, too, in applying the hand close against the abdominal wall so that the abdominal skin moves with the hand; the fixation of the hand to the abdomen can be made simply by elastoplast or adhesive plaster wrapped about the arm, the hand and the body.

Pedicle flaps should be located in the lower or the upper part of one side of the abdomen or the lower chest, or may be made to extend all the way across. As the blood supply is vertical, the flaps should be vertical. There is a rich thoracico-epigastric vascular system arising above from the lateral vein and the superficial superior epigastric vessels from the mammary. Arteries and veins course downward to meet those coursing upward from the superficial circumflex iliac and the superficial inferior epigastric from the femoral. Sometimes these vessels may be outlined through the skin, though this is not necessary. Pedicles are lost due to lack of venous drainage more than to lack of arterial blood. There is cyano-

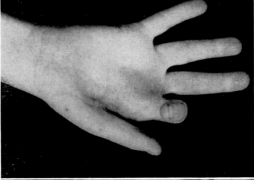
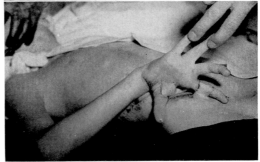

Fig. 260. A smoke bomb had exploded in the hand, leaving a cicatrix in the thumb cleft and a flexion contracture in the index finger. A double pedicle was applied, relieving each of these contractures simultaneously.

sis, blistering, thrombosis and finally gangrene. Heparin may be of aid in impending thrombosis. Flaps may be turned either up or down to fit the denuded area. If a flap is turned down, it should be placed in the inferior epigastric region; if turned up, it should be placed in the superior epigastric region. A turned-down flap should not be placed in the superior epigastric region, and a turned-up flap should not be placed in the inferior region, as sometimes the blood supply between these 2 regions fans out in a capillary bed, the long lateral vein being incomplete. If pronation and supination are limited, it may be necessary to use the longer tube pedicle in order to reach. The hairy pubic region should be avoided. Flaps from the other arm or forearm or the acromio-pectoral region are possible but seldom used.

In addition to its stem, a pedicle flap should be one fourth larger than the area to be

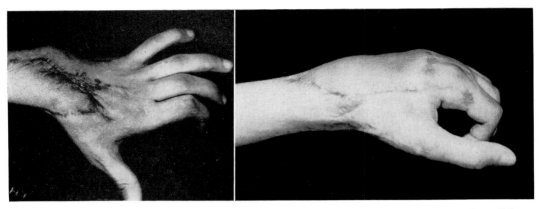

FIG. 261. (*Left*) A shotgun had been discharged with the wrist over the muzzle. A pedicle was applied. The extensor tendons were freed and capsulectomies were done. The volar cicatrix was excised. Three tendon grafts from the foot were used to join the severed flexors and the median nerve was sutured. (*Right*) The hand was in a good position for grasp and had enough movement for useful function.

covered, because skin retracts. Excessive fat should be trimmed off until the graft is flat. The stem of the pedicle should be short. If made long, it should be detached in stages. The donor area may be closed or partially closed by sliding, undermining freely. If when

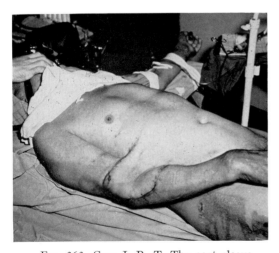

FIG. 262. Case J. R. T. The coat sleeve had drawn the antero-external part of the elbow into gears, fracturing the radius and the humerus and severing the radial nerve. A pedicle was applied and later tendon transfers to give extension of wrist, fingers and thumb. A useful hand resulted.

pulled taut the skin beyond the margin is still loose, the undermining should extend further. All remaining open areas of donor site and pedicle are closed with split-skin grafts. Sutures of the margins are left long to tie over pads to keep firm pressure on the grafts, thus avoiding edema and seepage. More external pressure is built up by waste or steel wool, snugged on by adhesive plaster so placed that it may be turned down for inspection. Petrolatum gauze or nylon is placed next to the skin graft, and a firm stent is sewed in place.

The hand is held in perfect position on the abdomen, and its limits—radial, ulnar and fingertip—are marked on the abdomen as a check against shifting. After the skin is painted with compound tincture of benzoin, broad adhesive is placed around the upper arm and the chest, another down the back of the upper arm, around the elbow and along the forearm to around the chest, and 2 more strips diagonally about the forearm, the upper arm and the chest. The pedicle site is kept free for inspection. Padding should not be placed between the adhesive and the arm, since it will pack and allow movement to pull the pedicle off to some extent, nor should all be closed in with adhesive plaster, as the wounds will become foul from lack of aeration. When the hand is attached to the far side of the abdomen, only a thin pad is placed in the axilla,

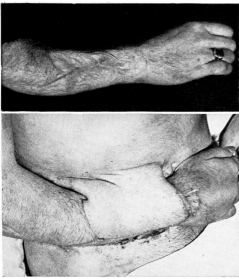
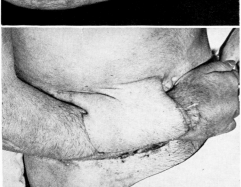

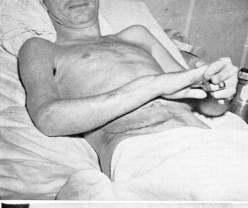

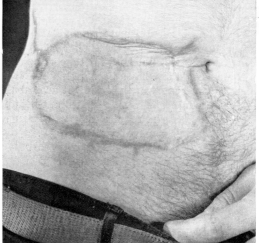

FIG. 263. Direct flap pedicle to the forearm to replace cicatrix preliminary to tendon transfer. All raw surfaces have been skin grafted. The 5 illustrations show the successive steps. (W. B. Macomber, M.D.)

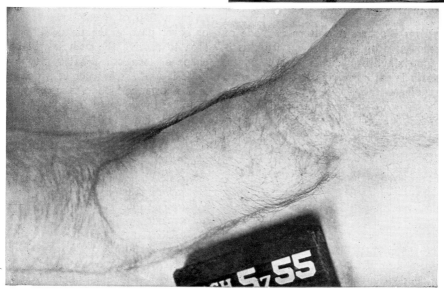

but when it is attached to the near side, the triangle formed by the arm and the chest should be firmly packed with padding and strapped to the chest for immovable anchorage. It is important to pack every angle and interstice with wadding held by outside wrappings of elastoplast or adhesive plaster so that the hand, the arm and the abdomen are one firm body, moving as a unit. Skin grafts over donor areas and undersurfaces of pedicles should have stents tied over them wherever possible. Walking is permitted in some cases after a week. In 3 weeks the pedicle is detached from the abdomen. The stem can be cut off long and replaced on the abdomen. If the stem is cut long on the hand, its blood supply will be jeopardized, since an area on the hand will hardly support a similar area of stem. It is safer to sever such a stem in 2 stages. This does not hold for tube or delayed pedicles, as they have been prepared. It is best to cover most of the recipient area at the first procedure and make flaps blunt-pointed and broad. Pedicles require early and frequent inspection and constant vigilance against displacement. Periodic cleansing with soap and water should be done whenever indicated.

To replace cicatrix on both sides of a limb simultaneously, both by flap graft, 2 flap grafts are prepared on the abdomen, pointing in opposite directions. The 2 flaps may be made by 1 broad S-shaped incision.

A simpler aseptic method that does not necessitate skin grafting is the stemless method developed by Blocker. A pattern is made of the denuded area on the hand left from excision of cicatrix and from freeing of skin edges. This pattern is outlined lightly with a scalpel on the abdomen. Either the lower or the upper half of this area is raised and turned back along a midline crossing the pattern, thus exposing raw surface the shape and size of the pattern. The similar denudation on the hand is applied to this, suturing around the complete circumference of the wound. After 3 weeks the other half of the flap is detached from the abdomen, cutting along the line originally outlined by the scalpel. This should be done in 2 stages a week apart, cutting first the sides of the flap and then the end. Next the hand is also detached from the abdomen to which it had been temporarily sutured in half the circumference of the wound. The skin flap, half of which has grown to the hand by

now, is laid down flat to cover the remaining half of the denuded area on the hand.

Dressings are packed closely all around to prevent edema and to hold the tissues together firmly. Two small tube drains may be placed with strings extending out for removal on the following day. Suction through the drainage tubes collapses dead spaces and prevents hematoma formation. The flap pedicle is the method of choice in most cases, since it is simpler and quicker than the tubed pedicle. It eliminates the 3 weeks or more of preparation of the tube.

The tubular pedicle has some definite advantages over the pocket and the open-flap pedicle grafts. The first is that it is aseptic because there are no raw areas exposed. Therefore, this method gives narrower and more inconspicuous borders and less stiffening in the hands than do the septic methods. Another advantage is that the tubular pedicle is longer and allows much more freedom of attachment during the 2 or 3 weeks the limb is fastened to the trunk. Also, it fits into awkward places and shapes where a flap would not. The fourth advantage is that the tubular pedicle can be waltzed from one place to another about the body. For this, the wrist is a convenient vehicle. The more often the pedicle graft is waltzed, the better becomes its vitality. Considerably more technical detail is required to use the tubular type of pedicle graft successfully. To make a pedicle fit a hand, one may swing a flap of normal skin to line a cleft or cover part of the denudation so that the area to receive the pedicle will be better in shape or location. Whatever type of pedicle graft is used, it is safer to proceed in stages. This allows the blood vessels in the part which is to be the base to hypertrophy. Each step requires from 1 to 3 weeks, depending on how radical the change in blood supply is.

It is common to find at the donor site a wide, unsightly cicatricial area which could have been avoided and is entirely out of proportion in importance to the site which was repaired. In order to remedy one scar, one should not produce a worse one in another area. Disregard for the cosmetic side of surgery is unfortunately prevalent.

TECHNIC OF TUBULAR PEDICLE GRAFT. The pedicle should be cut in such a way as to leave the smallest possible scar in the donor area. Those pedicles which are made longitudinal to the neck or the abdomen leave scars that are atrocious. If the pedicle on the side of the abdomen is made exactly parallel with the creases (that is, transversely), it will leave the smallest scar, but the pedicle will be somewhat taut. Here, therefore, a compromise is made, and the line of the pedicle is usually a little oblique, which gives a much slacker ped-

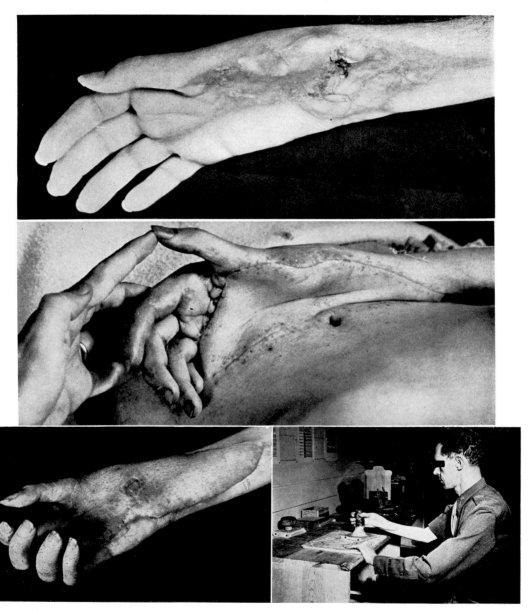

FIG. 264. (*Top*) Defect from a gunshot wound of all tendons on the radial side, the median nerve and part of the radius and the carpus. (*Center*) Direct abdominal flap applied, skin grafting raw surfaces. Detachment from the abdomen was done in 2 stages. Partial incision across the flap is shown. (*Bottom, left*) Result. (*Bottom, right*) Flexor tendon grafts from the long extensors of the toes were placed in all 5 fingers motivated by the brachialis anticus muscle. Opposition of the thumb was by the flexor ulnaris and adduction of the thumb by a tendon loop transfer from the extensor communis of the index finger. (William H. Frackelton, M.D.)

icle. A useful site for a pedicle is the acro-miopectoral region, where it can be made par-alleling the skin creases. All who have made tubular pedicles have experienced necrosis and separation of skin edges at the angles. If the pedicle is made in the simplest way, that is, with 2 parallel incisions, each angle will have entering into it 4 arms of incision, and the suture line of the pedicle will directly overlie that on the abdomen. The result will be that the angles break down and that the suture lines which overlie each other will reflect back and forth like 2 burning logs in the fire and so prevent good healing.

The following technic, which produces only 3 arms meeting at an angle and rotates the suture line of the pedicle away from that in the abdomen, will give much better healing. The cuts for this are simple; at each end of the lower incision a short diagonal incision is made, running downward and toward each other for about 1½ inches, making a point of skin at each end. Next, the skin all around is undermined, keeping exactly in the cleavage plane between the deep and the superficial fascia and extending for 12 inches or more above and below the pedicle and also some-what beyond each end of the pedicle. This thorough freeing will allow the skin edges to come together beneath the pedicle and to be sutured without tension.

First, each of the 2 pointed flaps should be

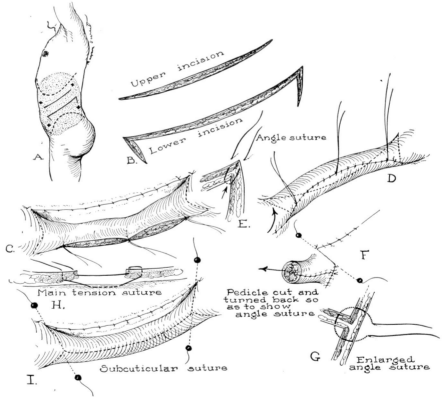

Fig. 265. Preparation of a tubular pedicle.

(A) Shows incisions, wide area of undermining (dotted), 4 points for rubber tube drains.

(B) Incisions to have a flap of skin in each angle and to place the 2 main suture lines so that they will not appose each other.

(C) Three guide sutures are placed on the pedicle. The main abdominal incision is closed as in (H) and the tips of the flaps are fastened as in (E).

(D) Suture lines do not appose.

(F) A subcuticular suture is used in the angle to avoid channelways through the skin that would carry infection. By the flap method, the vulnerable X juncture is replaced by a T juncture as shown in (G) and (I).

PLATE 4

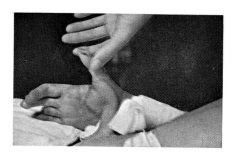 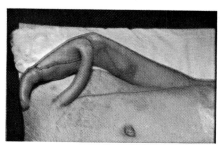

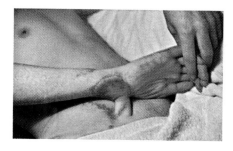 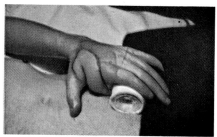

(*Top, left*) Double pedicle abdominal tube applied following excision of severe cicatrix of the palm with extensive loss of thenar muscles, flexor tendons and nerves. The tube was applied to the wrist when divided.

(*Top, right*) Application of a double pedicle tube to a severe injury of the hand and the forearm.

(*Bottom, left*) One-stage single pedicle abdominal tube applied to the wrist. At the time of application, the ends of the divided median and ulnar nerves were overlapped by suture. At the time of division, the nerves were sutured.

(*Bottom, right*) One-stage single pedicle abdominal tube applied to the web space to relieve contracture between the thumb and the index finger. At the time of division, the tube easily may be draped into the palm if required.

(Shaw, D. T., and Payne, R. L.: Repair of surface defects of the upper extremity, Ann. Surg. *123:722*)

PLATE 5

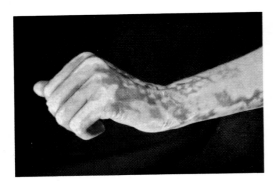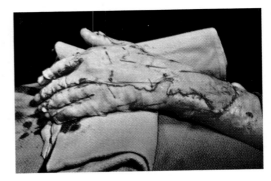

Cicatrix from burns replaced by thick free skin grafts. Case 1: (*Left*) Limit of flexion showing blanching. (*Right*) Extensive skin grafts supplied.

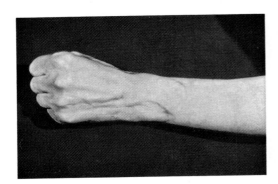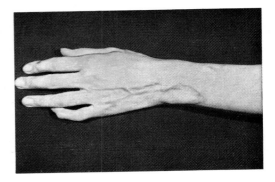

(*Left*) Postoperative. Complete flexion without blanching. (*Right*) Excellent appearance. Veins show through skin. (Geo. V. Webster, M.D.)

sutured by its point to the end of the upper incision of the pedicle, and the abdominal wound the length of the pedicle closed under the pedicle. The edges of the pedicle are sutured to each other to form a tube, after first placing a guide suture at each end of the tube (1¼ inches from each end) and a third at the middle. Commencing at the point of each of the flaps, the upper border of the pedicle is sutured down the adjoining border of each pointed flap for the width of the pedicle and to the first guide suture. Then the remaining short arm of incision at each end is also closed by suture.

It will be seen that the suture line of the pedicle is rolled outward so that it does not face the abdomen, and a point of skin lies across each of the angles between the pedicle and the abdomen. Only 1 border of this triangular flap is in a dark, covered place. A pad of gauze separating the pedicle from the abdomen aids in keeping the skin surfaces apart and in protecting this vulnerable line of suture. Even so, it has often been found that this suture line has sloughed out en masse; evidently, the sweat and the infection from the dark angle followed in along the stitches, causing necrosis of the suture line. To obviate this, we use stainless steel wire as suture material and sew this arm of the incision subcutaneously without any stitch in the angle penetrating through the skin which could carry in infection. The No. 34 wire is fastened with a shot over a button at each end. The remainder of the suturing is done with No. 36 stainless steel wire. In closing the abdominal wound it is first necessary to place wide encircling retention sutures of heavier wire to relieve the strain on the suture line. These stitches each catch the deep fascia in their encirclement so as to obliterate dead space and stop slithering.

It is essential to place a tube drain through a stab wound at each corner of the wide area of undermining of the skin. This stab wound should be made only superficially with a pointed scalpel and carried in through the fat by a spreading hemostat, because in some cases a deep stab of a knife has cut a deep vessel, resulting in a large hematoma.

Of course, it is essential to obtain good hemostasis on closing this extensive abdominal wound. Before the pedicle is made into a tube, sufficient fat should be trimmed away from it with sharp scissors so that its edges can be approximated without any tension. A pedicle which is tight at the middle or at its ends is sure to slough. However, if one trims away too much fat from the pedicle, it will be too baggy and will fill up with hematoma.

Instead of making the 2 angle flaps on the same side of the pedicle, the rear flap, if made above the pedicle, will bring the pedicle into a more vertical position and hence make it looser (Howard). Another method is to omit these flaps but to stagger the angles to make a continuous suture line. The lower cut may be longer so as to roll the pedicle out as described in making the tube pedicle in 1 stage. Also, the incisions for the pedicle may be curved to give more slack and staggered at the end to avoid X junctures.

The after-care of the pedicle is important. The suture lines are kept rolled apart and as many layers of gauze are kept between the pedicle and the abdomen as is possible without causing too much pressure under the pedicle. The aim is to obtain primary healing.

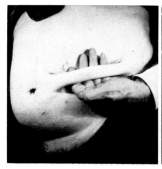 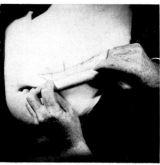 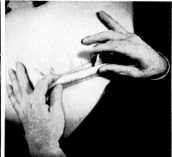

FIG. 266. Tubular pedicle on abdomen. (*Left*) Pedicle is loose by being slightly oblique. (*Center*) Flaps of skin lie across the angles. (*Right*) The 2 suture lines do not appose each other. This ensures against dampness and infection being reflected between them.

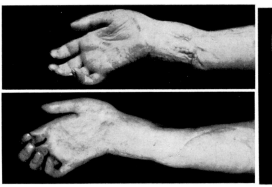
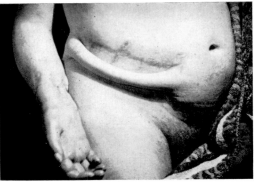

FIG. 267. Case T. L. Cicatrix from a shotgun wound followed by infection. The cicatrix was excised as a preliminary operation and replaced with good skin by the tubular pedicle method. (*Top, left*) Cicatrix. (*Right*) Pedicle ready. (*Bottom, Left*) Cicatrix replaced by pedicled skin.

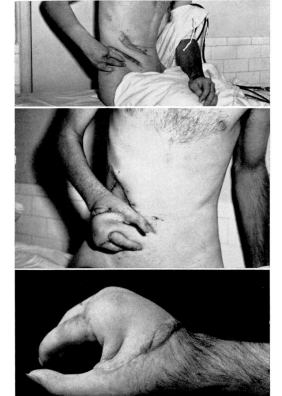

FIG. 268. Case J. W. G. A log had fallen on the hand, crushing off the index and the long fingers. A tubular pedicle was prepared and applied, replacing the extensive cicatrix.

This conserves time, often allowing the pedicle to be transferred at the end of 2 weeks. However, 3 weeks are preferable, as better blood supply is assured. The blood supply can be tested by temporarily clamping one end of the tube. A soft springy rubber-shod intestinal clamp is useful for this purpose. The patient should remain in bed throughout the first 2 weeks because the motion incurred in walking might separate the skin at the angles of the pedicle; if this happens, he should remain in bed until these angles have healed. To transfer a pedicle before all raw areas have been covered is to court failure.

A tube pedicle should never be made crossing the midline of the body, because only a few blood vessels traverse this line. If on separating one end of the pedicle on the abdomen a flap of skin for extra good measure is carried along with the pedicle, this flap often necroses at its end. An excellent method for avoiding this and increasing the area of skin transferred is, at the end of 2 weeks, to cut such a flap of skin as a pancake extension of the pedicle and raise it from the abdomen and replace it. At this stage one should not detach the base of the pedicle itself, as through this runs the nourishment for the newly constructed flap. Two weeks later this flap and the base of the pedicle can be detached from the abdomen and transferred. It will be found to be quite viable to its very tip. If a tube pedicle is short and thick, a pancake may be raised with one end of it directly, without any step cuts, and another pancake may be taken with it when it is detached from the abdomen. As a rule, if a pedicle is 8 inches long it should not be less than 2 inches wide, this being the proportion whatever the size. If greater length is needed, a central part of one of the borders is left uncut for central blood supply (method of Jerome Webster) but severed after 2 weeks. By using several intermediate pedicles a very long thoracico-abdominal tube can be built. Later, these secondary pedicles are severed until there is 1 long tube. A healed pedicle may be gradually elongated by a pad beneath.

In transferring a pedicle to the hand, whichever end will make the easier and more natural connection with the hand is severed from the abdomen. Any twist or strain of the pedicle will result in necrosis. After closing the wound in the abdomen by undermining freely, using retention and approximation sutures and usually 1 small drain, the length of the pedicle to be attached to the hand is opened out, excising both the linear suture line and the cicatricial core of the pedicle. Enough fat is trimmed away from the pedicle, using curved flat scissors so that the skin will lie flat, but not enough is taken to jeopardize a good blood supply to the pedicle throughout. A few light longitudinal incisions in the fat allow the pedicle to unfold.

It is advisable to place a few tiny rubber drains beneath the pedicle on the hand, lest a hematoma should form and spoil the result. There should not be the least tension, especially across the pedicle. The tip of the pedicle should not be too pointed, and it should be slightly redundant to ensure enough material's being present in case of necrosis of the edge. Usually, only part of the area to be covered in the hand is covered by the pedicle at this stage; but it is planned so that after 3 weeks, when the other end of the pedicle is freed from the abdomen, it can be laid down over the remainder of the part of the hand to be covered. For the first contact at least 3 linear inches of the pedicle should be placed.

If it is seen that the skin beneath the pedicle is tense, a relaxing strap should be used for a week or so. This runs around the neck and the shoulders and under the knees, buckling the patient forward.

The arm and the hand should be fastened firmly in place so that their position will not shift in the patient's sleep, kinking or straining the pedicle enough to cause necrosis. This can be done by adhesive tapes or, better, by plaster. Instead of encircling the body with this, as with a body cast, the plaster may be fastened to the abdomen and the arm by broad adhesive strips laid first on the skin. Each of these strips has attached to it, passing through holes, many short lengths of cloth tape. As

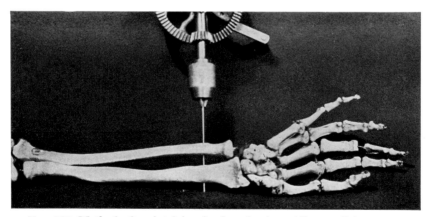

Fig. 269. Method of maintaining fixed supination while a pedicle skin graft is attached to the hand. Useful also in arthrodesis of the wrist and other conditions of the forearm bones, to hold the position of pronation or supination without the aid of a cast to the axilla with the elbow at a right angle. In the case of arthrodesis, the ends of the wire should be embedded in the plaster cast.

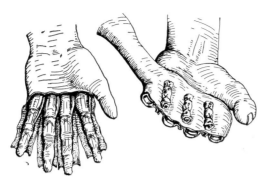

FIG. 270. Covering the volar or the dorsal surface of all fingers with pedicled skin by what may be called the mitten method. The cicatricial skin of each digit is split down the midline and folded back until that from each pair of adjoining fingers can be everted and sutured. The pedicle opened out is then applied over all, using bolsters tied very loosely to make it dip into the interspaces. The sutures that evert (see text, p. 218) should also catch a bit of the opposite fat of the pedicle. The pedicle should be ample in size because much more skin is needed than appears to be necessary.

the plaster-of-Paris slabs are laid on the abdomen these short lengths of tape are folded into them. Thus, a cast, half encircling the body, is made; it will not slip on the skin, and it includes the arm but leaves the pedicle open and free for dressings. Another way is to lay a scultetus bandage beneath the patient; as the plaster strips are laid on the abdomen and the arm, the several tails of the bandage are drawn up and embedded in the plaster. The cast about the arm is placed directly on the skin, free from padding except about the elbow, but an open slit is left along the forearm and the hand lest the cast need to be spread to relieve pressure. Two web belts encircle the plaster and the body. Occasionally, with this arrangement, the patient is allowed to be ambulatory. For some tube pedicles fixation by adhesive plaster may be sufficient. Where the hand must be held exactly right, plaster of Paris is preferable.

The arm and the abdominal members may be constructed separately so the hand can be perfectly adjusted to the pedicle, and then the

2 casts may be joined together. Sometimes, for a youngster, one thigh is included. If the forearm must be held strongly supinated, a heavy Kirschner wire drilled across through the radius and the ulna is used.

In transferring skin by the pedicle method we are frequently straining the last degree of vitality of the tissue. Too much padding mats and allows a pull on the pedicle. Tissue that is overstrained is white or too pale at the time of operation. Extra time spent then in relieving circulation is well repaid; if this care is not given, the white tissue may be black—"from ivory to ebony"—on the following day. One may see a black border of necrosis backed up by a wide zone of red, swollen tissue which may show blistering. This red, dusky, boggy area is from local thrombosis from too much lowering of the circulation. If the skin is merely red and blistered, it may live, though its quality may suffer. Necrotic skin does not blister. Warm compresses will help, but extreme caution should be taken whenever using heat, by lights or compresses on pedicles, because without nerve supply and with lowered circulation, they are exceedingly vulnerable.

When actual necrosis occurs in a skin flap, the surrounding wound becomes infected and does not do well. The necrotic mass acts at a nutrient focus disseminating infection, and much time is wasted in waiting for it to slough away. Therefore, when real necrosis is discovered, it is best just as in treating a pressure sore from a cast to excise it and do an immediate split skin graft. If the end of a pedicle necroses and must be detached, it may be reattached to the hand immediately as a shorter pedicle before infection occurs.

When sutured over, a free, blind end of a pedicle often necroses a little at its end. Rather than suture it over, it is better to embed it in some nearby skin, in which case it will obtain additional circulation and will live.

In transferring a pedicle for purposes of waltzing, a semicircular cut is made in the skin to receive it, and this flap is folded back, providing a raw, circular area to which the end of the pedicle is attached. Exact coaptation without intervening hematoma is obtained by means of several running stainless steel wires, No. 34, that catch each opposing surface alternately and are fastened on each side by shot on the surface of the skin. Greater blood supply may be obtained by raising a long tongue or broad flap instead of a semicircle of skin and inserting it down the seam of the tube. On again detaching the pedicle, this flap is replaced. A broad attachment is needed to carry a large tube, and, if the tube in turn carries a flap, the attachment should be similarly broad.

With a tube pedicle one may cover several digits, swing the pedicle from one digit to

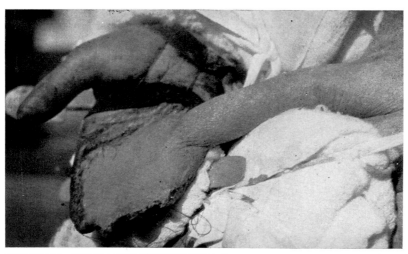

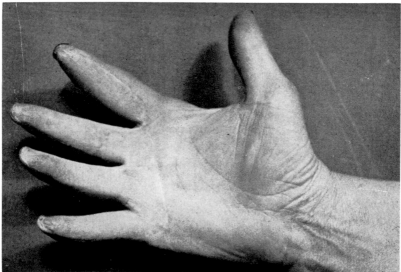

Fig. 271. Case V. B. The hand had been caught between hot rollers in a laundry mangle, denuding the skin from the whole volar aspect of all of the fingers. In the healing, each finger was drawn into sharp flexion contracture by the cicatrix which completely covered the volar surface of each.

First, the fingers were united by suture to each other by everting the volar cicatrix, and a tubular pedicle skin graft was applied to all the fingers and the distal part of the palm as a whole, as shown in the top picture. Later, this mitten was interdigitated and the skin laid smoothly on the full length of each finger, as shown in the bottom illustration. (J. Bone Joint Surg., p. 45, Jan., 1932)

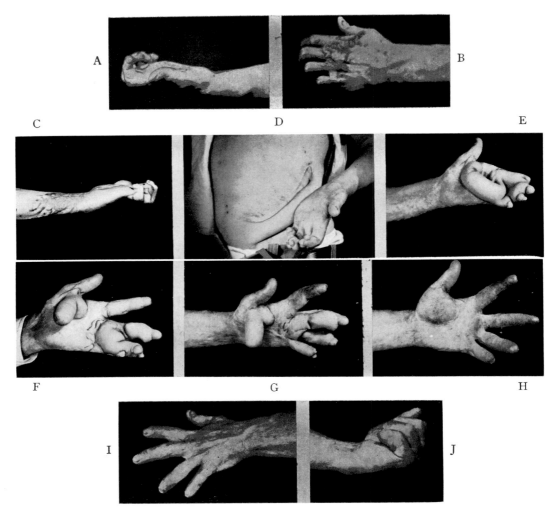

FIG. 272. Case M. J. R. (A, B, C) From a gasoline burn, the hand was reduced to a useless club, with flexion contracture of the fingers, webs, the thumb bound to the hand and much cicatrix. (D) Pedicle has been prepared, and, after excising the volar aspects of the fingers and extending them, they were covered with Thiersch grafts. The webs were relieved by tunnel grafts. (E) The volar skin was split along each digit, laid back and sutured together like a mitten, and the whole volar surface of the fingers was covered by the pedicle. On serving the pedicle from the abdomen, the end was placed in the cleft of the thumb. (F, G) Interdigitating the digits. (H, I, J) A year and a half from the accident, he had a useful hand, with good nutrition, sensation and motion restored.

another, or split the pedicle to cover 2 at a time.

Covering All Fingers at Once. If all volar surfaces of the fingers are to be covered at once, the cicatricial skin of each finger may be cut along the midvolar line and folded to the side, where it is sutured with eversion to the similar flap from the adjoining finger. This converts the hand into a mitten, over which a broad, redundant flap of pedicle can be placed longitudinally or transversely. To cover the dorsum of each finger, the incisions are made along the dorsal surfaces. The interdigitations are made later. Usually, it is found that the skin has shrunk to such an extent that the base of the pedicle must be swung around to cover the last finger.

A more satisfactory method is as follows: Raise and replace in stages a pancake flap, as part of either a flap pedicle or a tube pedicle, interdigitate it and suture it back in place. The hand is not converted to a mitten, merely denuded, and the interdigitations are sutured over the respective fingers. If needed, the base of the pedicle may be used to cover the palm or the dorsum with or without a separate attachment.

Still another method, occasionally useful, is to fix the denuded fingers widely spread on a splint and then cover all of their volar or dorsal aspect with a flap pedicle. The hand is turned over, and the raw areas of the pedicle between each 2 fingers is covered over by skin graft. In the next stage the pedicle flap is interdigitated, and the ribbons of skin are sutured into the sides of the fingers.

Tube Pedicle Without Undermining. A simpler preparation of tube pedicle in which undermining is not necessary and a fairly cosmetic scar is left is to raise the strip or the tube through 2 parallel incisions and to use split-skin grafts underneath it. The skin graft should reflect around each angle to cover also the small triangular raw area under each end of the tube, thus eliminating poor healing in the angles. For narrow tubes, the abdominal skin should be closed beneath by undermining, but for tubes of large diameter the skin-graft method is much preferable. To prepare a tube pedicle either by undermining or by skin graft requires about an hour.

Dressing such a pedicle is important. The smallest hematoma spoils a skin graft. First, petrolatum gauze covers the graft and angles under the pedicle, then flat folded gauze. A gauze roll parallels the pedicle on each side. Gauze, cotton waste or steel wool fills in all angles, and the whole is held firmly in place over pedicle and all by adhesive plaster. By skin grafting rather than closing by undermining, a much larger tube pedicle can be made, such as 15 × 9 inches, and the scar is not too deforming.

Tube Pedicle in 1 Stage. Taking advantage of the rich vertical blood supply in the lower abdomen, Darrel Shaw succeeded in making and applying many tube pedicles in 1 operation. A blunt flap with a length-width ratio of 2½ : 1 was raised with the superficial inferior epigastric vessels in its base. It was tubed and applied to the hand, and the denuded area was closed by undermining and drawing the skin together to leave a vertical scar. The tube could be rotated 90° either way, without twisting, to fit the hand if one arm of the incision was elongated and the margins were sufficiently staggered when the skin was closed. The open part of the pedicle faced to the side of the longer incision according to the amount of staggering. The pedicle was severed after 3 weeks only if it covered most of the defect; otherwise, this was done after 5 weeks or in stages to allow sufficient time for the circulation to compensate. Of course, a tube pedi-

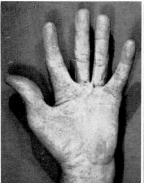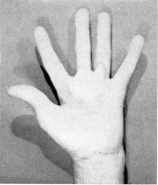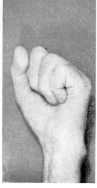

Fig. 273. Case T. J. B., aged 56. The hand had been burned by x-rays under the fluoroscope. (*Left*) Condition 2 years later, with complaint of great pain. (*Center* and *right*) The burned area was excised widely and deeply and replaced with good skin by the tubular pedicle method. Complete relief of pain and good function resulted.

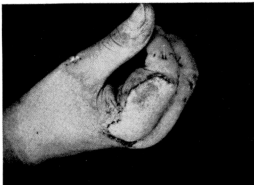

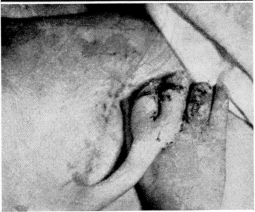

FIG. 274. Case J. L. The back of the fingers and the hand had been gouged out by a shaper, fracturing a phalanx. Tight scar over the backs of the fingers. The proximal joints functioned somewhat, but the middle joints did not. A tubular pedicle was prepared and in 2 extra steps interdigitated and applied to the fingers. The middle joints remained stiff, but there was good function in the hand. Preparatory interdigitation prevents shrinkage of the skin graft.

cle prepared in 1 stage is not the equivalent of the usual double-based tube pedicle and so is not as viable, because the principle of the tube pedicle is that there is a pre-prepared longitudinal blood supply. The tube pedicle in 1 stage is essentially a tubed flap.

Operating Beneath a Flap. In operating after a pedicle graft has been placed, it is heresy to incise directly through the graft. Instead, half of the border scar should be ex-

cised and the graft rolled back. If tendons are adherent beneath, a slice of fat may be folded down from under the undersurface of the graft and laid across under the tendons. In placing new tendons under a graft for gliding, they may be passed directly through the fat by tunneling. In operating through an area covered by a free skin graft, it is necessary to incise directly through it, for one cannot turn this back as a flap unless it has thick, vascular subcutaneous tissue beneath it.

FREE SKIN GRAFTS are either full thickness or partial thickness. The great advantage is that they can be applied at one operation, thus saving weeks of hospitalization and the inconvenience of step operations and the attachment of the pedicle graft. They are easier to use on children than the pedicle grafts. Unless the full thickness is taken, the donor area need not be closed. Thin split grafts will take even on a granulation surface. Full-thickness grafts furnish good quality skin if they are placed on a good bed of subcutaneous tissue. The cicatrix left from infection is not suitable. They are devoid of subcutaneous tissue and are not so durable as normal skin in parts which receive wear. Tendons will not glide under them. They shrink, especially if thin, and they often pigment. Free grafts are adaptable for shallow superficial cicatrices, such as those from burns, but are less adaptable over the cicatrices resulting from infections.

In placing free grafts, as with pedicle grafts, due regard to the movements of the hand will enable the surgeon to avoid placing the graft borders in lines of push and pull. Patches are put together with transverse, not longitudinal, junctures. In the fingers, the borders should be midlateral or they will thicken and contract; they should be zigzagged and wavy when in lines of irritation.

Homografts take temporarily but melt away in 2 to 6 weeks.

Full-Thickness Grafts (Wolfe Graft). Full-thickness grafts will not take over tendons, bones or joint ligaments; nor will they grow if gross infection is present, such as is always found in granulating tissue. They will sometimes take on the bed of a freshly excised area. A vascular aseptic bed is desirable. The usual source of full-thickness grafts is the abdominal skin, but the inner side of the thigh and the arm and that just above and below the clavicle furnish a thin, fine quality of skin that is useful in certain places, such as over the dorsum of a finger. An excellent donor site for full-thickness skin is an ellipse taken from along the fold of the elbow. The skin margins, with slight undermining, are sutured, and a right-angle elbow splint is applied. Many full-thickness grafts are prone to pigment. Some become black, some brown and some yellow, but the majority remain the natural color of the skin. In persons with the tendency to tan darkly in the region usually covered by clothing, one can expect pigmentation of these grafts when they are placed on the hands or the face, which are always exposed. A full or three-quarter thickness skin graft from good, pliable skin

will make better skin and contract less than a piece of split skin of the same thickness taken from thick skin such as that over the back. From tough skin, tough skin is generated. Care should be taken in placing a full-thickness or even a split graft not to have its border cross a flexion crease in such a way that it will become a keloid.

Full-thickness grafts require 3 weeks or more to heal. Frequently, during healing they retain their pink color and are clearly well vascularized. Often, however, during the healing the surface turns brown or black; but if one keeps the limb immobilized long enough, this surface necrosis will crust away, showing good, pink, vascular skin beneath. Sometimes a part may merely turn red and blister. Dead

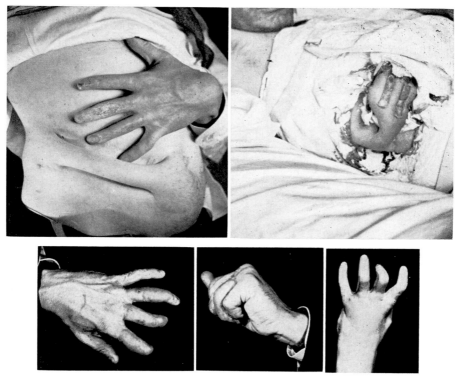

FIG. 275. A surgeon removed a foreign body from a child's hand under the fluoroscope. The hand of each was burned severely. Damaged skin must be excised and replaced by good skin. (*Top, left*) X-ray burns on the dorsum of the fingers and pedicle ready to apply. (*Top, right*) Pedicle on the dorsum of the fingers. Bolsters hold it between the fingers. (*Bottom, left* and *center*) New pedicled skin in place. Returned to practice. (*Bottom, right*) Hand of child after receiving new pedicled skin.

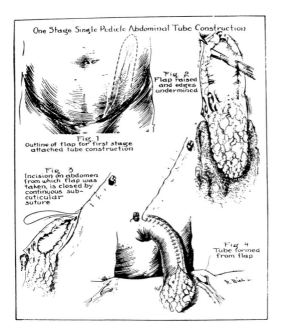
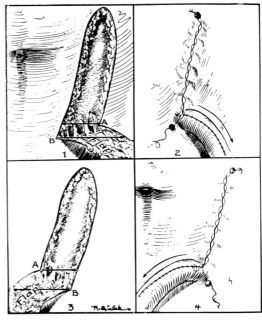

FIG. 276. Tubular pedicle made and applied in one operation (Shaw). (*Left*) (1) Flap is made in line of vessels. (2) Undermining to close. (3, 4) Stainless-steel wire is used. (*Right*) Methods of rotating pedicle either way. (1, 2) To left. (3, 4) To right, by making one incision lower and staggering. Shaw, D. T., and Payne, R. N.: J. Surg., Gynec. & Obstet.)

skin does not blister, so that if these areas are given a chance, eventually they will show good vitality. The skin of the blister should not be removed but merely pricked and used as a dressing. If removed, the skin beneath will necrose.

Full-thickness grafts are cut to exact size. A pattern of the place to be covered is cut from thin lead or tin foil and laid on the donor site. The pattern is not that of the cicatrix but of the area of denudation after the skin edges have been undermined and allowed to retract. The graft should be the same size as the area to be covered, because the lymph vessels remain open and the cells thrive best with tissues at normal tension. The skin is removed with a generous layer of subcutaneous tissue; the surrounding skin is undermined on the deep fascia, slid together and sutured, catching the deeper layers with the retention suture to prevent hematoma. Holding the graft tensely over the pulp of the finger, all of the subcutaneous fat is clipped away with sharp scissors.

Another method of taking a full-thickness graft and covering the defect is to use the dermatome, set for full thickness. When enough skin is cut for the graft, the dermatome is reset for a thin graft, and the cut is continued for a similar area. The thin graft is laid over the area from which the full-thickness graft was taken. Keloids may develop in those susceptible when the cut is deep in the derma. The graft is sutured in place, usually with fine catgut. It is essential to immobilize the hand on a splint or in plaster, because any motion will interfere with healing. This must be continued for 3 and sometimes 4 weeks. Another essential is to apply mild, even pressure to the graft. Steel wool provides excellent compression. The whole hand and the splint, with the exception of the area of the graft, should be enclosed in plaster of Paris. A sheet of wax paper is laid over the opening in the plaster, and a slab of plaster laid on it for a lid. Children especially need protection by plaster. The graft is not inspected until after the 10th day and after that at intervals of several days to a week.

Partial-thickness Grafts (Split Grafts). In questionable beds, grafts of partial thickness are more likely to take than are those of full thickness. The more questionable the vascular-

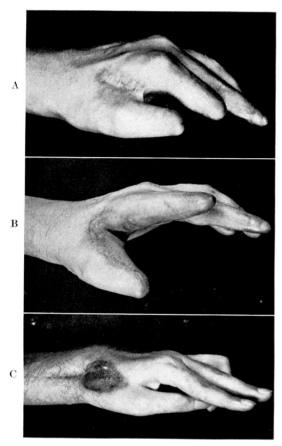

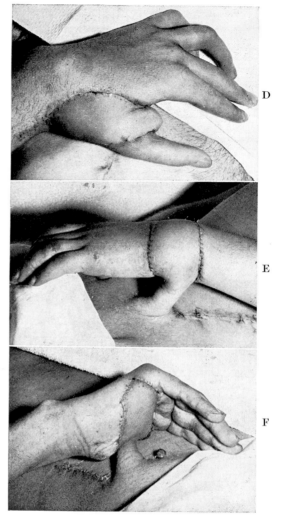

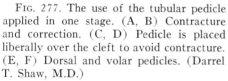

FIG. 277. The use of the tubular pedicle applied in one stage. (A, B) Contracture and correction. (C, D) Pedicle is placed liberally over the cleft to avoid contracture. (E, F) Dorsal and volar pedicles. (Darrel T. Shaw, M.D.)

ity and the asepsis of the bed, the thinner should be the graft. Thicker split grafts give a much better quality of skin than do thin ones, because they contain more skin structures. The thickness of a skin graft is relative. A three-quarter thickness graft from thin skin yields better coverage than the same thickness from thick skin such as that in the back. For the palm, a thick graft is best, but for the dorsum a thinner one will do. Thiersch grafts do not furnish all the necessary structures to grow into good skin, as they include very few hair follicles, sweat and sebaceous glands and fat. To obtain the best quality of skin the surgeon should select the greatest thickness of skin that will survive in that area. Thin skin or Thiersch grafts will grow even on granulating surface, where thicker grafts usually fail. Thiersch grafts heal in 10 days, but the thicker grafts require 3 weeks or more. The thinner the graft, the greater will be the contracture. Full-thickness grafts contract very little, and the contraction takes place in the layer between the graft and the host. Some hairs are carried with them. Thin or Thiersch grafts are useful for quick closing of raw granulating areas, fresh wounds or places from which skin flaps have been swung. By closing in raw areas with grafts, infection is terminated, and the too luxuriant growth of granu-

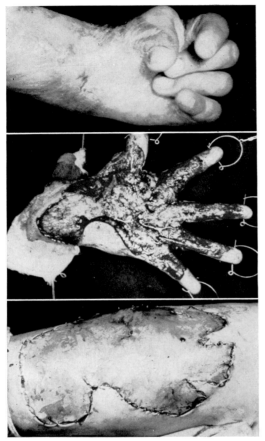

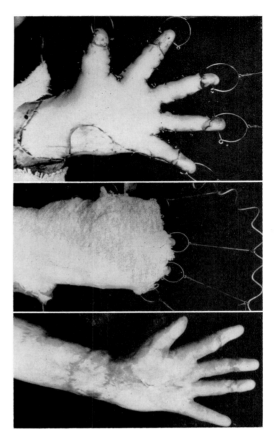

FIG. 278. (*Top*) A 5-year-old girl with severe flexion contracture from burns. (*Center*) After excision of scar. (*Bottom*) The extent of full-thickness skin removed from inner thigh and the area covered with split-skin graft. (From T. Tajima, M.D., Niigata University, Niigata City, Japan)

FIG. 279. (Same patient as Fig. 278.) (*Top*) Full-thickness graft in place. (*Center*) Compression dressing with digits maintained on "banjo." (*Bottom*) One month after operation. (From T. Tajima, M.D., Niigata University, Niigata City, Japan)

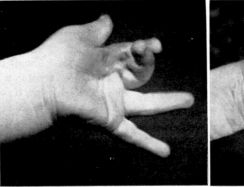

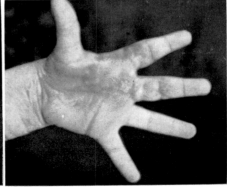

FIG. 280. Case R. B., age 3. (*Left*) Flexion contracture from a brush burn by an electric wringer. (*Right*) Correction by excision of cicatrix and replacement by full-thickness skin from the abdomen.

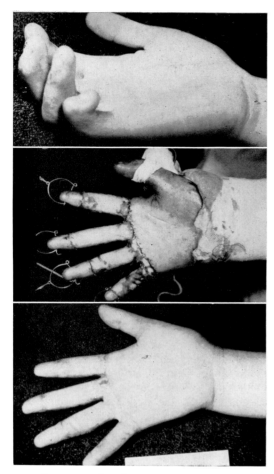

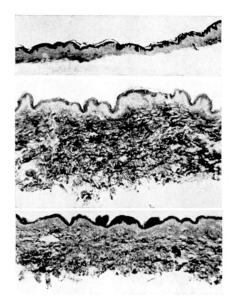

FIG. 282. Skin grafts of varied thickness. (*Top*) .010 inch—.25 mm. From an adult. (*Center*) .018 inch—.46 mm. From the abdomen of an adult male. (*Bottom*) .030 inch—.76 mm. From the thigh of a 65-year-old male. (Padgett, E.: Skin Grafting, Springfield, Ill., Thomas)

FIG. 281. (*Top*) Burn scar and flexion contracture of fingers in a 17-year-old girl. (*Center*) Excision of scar, relieving contracture, and covering with full-thickness skin graft. Eighth day after operation. (*Bottom*) Six months later. (From T. Tajima, M.D., Niigata University, Niigata City, Japan)

lations, which later leads to contracture, is avoided. At a later date, this poor Thiersch graft can be excised and good skin laid in its place. It will be found that by that time the Thiersch will have shrunk to a very small area, having drawn the good surrounding skin toward itself. To graft when luxuriant granulations are present, ischemia is provided by a tourniquet, and the granulations are scraped off with the handle of a scalpel. The graft and the pressure dressing are completed before the tourniquet is removed. When all granulation tissue has been removed, the grafted area will

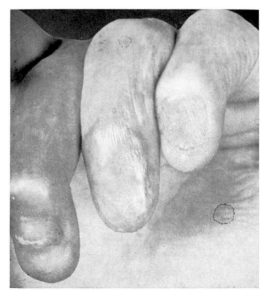

FIG. 283. When nails and matrices are too deformed, as from burns, they may be excised and replaced by skin grafts with fairly good cosmetic effect. (L. D. Howard, M.D.)

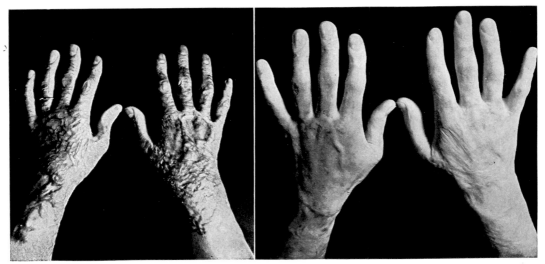

FIG. 284. (*Left*) Keloids from burns sustained in an airplane crash. (*Right*) Condition 6 months after excision and replacement with thick, free skin grafts, using the dermatome. (William H. Frackelton, M.D.)

be found to be soft, pliable and free from cicatrix. It is the granulating area that turns to cicatrix.

Split grafts scale excessively at first and appear very rough, but later they become softer and more like normal skin, and their area is much reduced by shrinkage. Even after a year, thick or full-thickness grafts seem to acquire some subcutaneous tissue.

In repairing contractures of the hand by split or full-thickness grafts, all surface scar and underlying cicatrix should be excised to good skin borders all around. Then the skin should be undermined; it will be found to be adherent at the periphery of the defect and, as it is undermined widely, it will retract. Enough deep cicatrix should be excised so that the hand or the wrist can be placed into

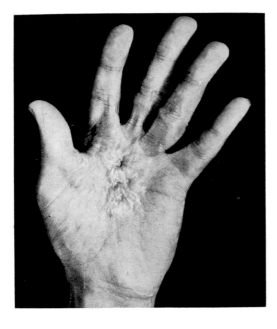

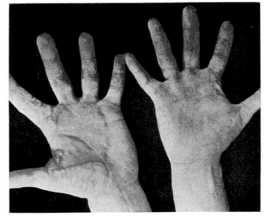

FIG. 285. (*Left*) Contracture in the palm from burn. (*Right*) Replaced by thick, free skin graft. The points of the graft pass over the clefts to prevent webbing. (W. B. Macomber, M.D.)

the position opposite to that of the deformity and should be fixed there by splinting. Care should be taken not to overstretch nerves. Tendons should be freed enough each way to allow the joints to bend sufficiently. Tendons, bones and joints should be covered by drawing over them thin layers of vascular tissue. Finally, the split graft is applied and sutured in place.

A calibrated dermatome, of which there are many models, is the best instrument for cutting a graft.

The following figures from Padgett will help to obtain grafts of proper relative thickness.

0.010 0.012	Not over this in an infant
0.014 0.016	This may be too deep for a child of 6
0.016 0.018	Not over this in a child of 12 to 14
0.018 0.020	May be too deep in a woman with her abdomen stretched by pregnancy or on the inner side of the thigh or the arm.

With a dermatome it is possible to remove the full thickness of skin, including all skin elements. Therefore, the above figures should be kept in mind. If full thickness is desired, the donor site may be covered over at once by a thin split graft. Grafts applied to dirty granulations should be dressed with the inserted catheter technic. (See Burns, Chap. 15.)

Placing Free Grafts. Split grafts contract, so that they should be sutured in place. Careful approximation of the edges to the skin makes thinner, less visible scars and often makes a later excision unnecessary.

For many wounds of the fingers only a small graft is needed. This can be cut readily with a G. V. Webster knife, using disposable razor blades. As a donor, the inner aspect of the forearm area provides skin of good quality and texture and color similar to the fingers. A keloidal reaction in the donor area is unusual.

Dressings for Skin Grafts. A good dressing for donor areas is fine mesh gauze impregnated with 5 per cent scarlet red ointment. All clots should be washed away and pressure applied to the dressings. Whenever such a thick graft is taken that fat globules show in the donor site, a thin graft should be applied to the donor site to replace the thick one. Otherwise, healing will be greatly prolonged. If the area

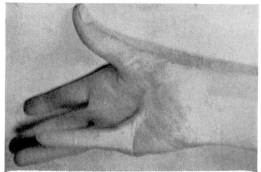

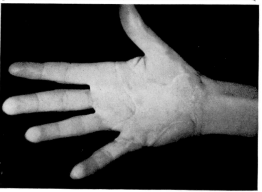

Fig. 286. Case M. E., when young, had placed her hand on a hot stove. Cicatrix was excised, skin borders were undermined and a new cover was supplied by thick, split graft. Care was used to place the margins where they would not form contractures.

becomes infected, it can be cleared in a few days by boric acid compresses, followed by a bland ointment or air dressing. Even late it may be advisable to cover a donor site with a thin graft. The skin graft itself is fastened in place by sutures and then held against its bed by wrapping a strip of wide-meshed material spirally about the finger or the limb. The wrapping may be fastened to the skin at each end by sterile adhesive plaster or a stitch. A layer of nonadherent gauze is placed over this, usually with Xeroform ointment. Even pressure is applied outside the gauze. The wide-mesh material allows changes of dressings and prevents the graft from slithering. Even pressure prevents the formation of a hematoma which might separate the graft from the bed and ensures freedom from edema and close approximation between these structures so that they will grow together quickly. If bleeding

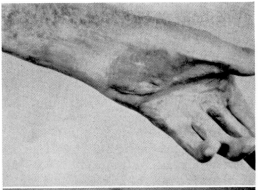

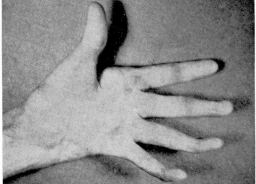

Fig. 287. Case F. A. G. (*Top*) The palm and the fingers had been burned on a stove 15 years previously. (*Bottom*) Contracted scar replaced by a split graft.

contracture with thick keloids of the palm and the fingers. Burns and inflammable liquid frequently involve the dorsum of the hand and the fingers and also much of the circumference of the wrist. The thick, broad, contracting keloids that form limit flexion of the fingers and motion of the wrist. The nail matrices are distorted. After mild burns the fingers may flex with some strain, but in doing so the tight skin over the knuckles blanches. There is a complaint of aching, a stiff feeling, limitation of motion and weakness of grip. A pattern of keloid encountered frequently is along the radial aspect of the thumb and the thenar eminence, around the heel of the palm and down the volar surface of the little finger, evidently because this region of the hand is more prominent. The thumb and the little finger are drawn into flexion and toward the wrist. Burns over the back of the fingers, the hand and the forearm draw the hand into a claw with hyperextension of the wrist and the bases of the fingers and flexed, webbed, attenuated fingers. The contraction of the dorsum of the hand reverses the metacarpal arch, draws the thumb back so that it cannot oppose and hyperextends the proximal finger joints. Dorsal webs extend an inch or more down the fingers, preventing spreading. Fingers may be drawn into flexion by volar keloids.

The middle finger joints become strongly flexed when the middle tendinous slip is burned, allowing the flexors to pull unopposed. These joints are nearest the flame. When the backs of the joints are roasted, ankylosis occurs. Even the phalanges or the metacarpals may be exposed. When the proximal finger joints are hyperextended, the hand claws as the distal 2 finger joints draw into flexion from pull of the long flexors. When the middle finger joints are held in tight flexion, the distal finger joints hyperextend because of upset muscle balance and tight skin. The whole hand may be so encased in cicatrix that the nutrition is very low. If joints are exposed, they should be covered by a pedicle skin flap from the abdomen. A hand encased in cicatrix must be covered by new skin, one side being covered at a time—the position of flexion and opposition is needed for the dorsum and that of extension for the volar aspects.

Burned fingers present many problems. If there is voluntary extension of the middle

cannot be stopped, the limb should be rendered ischemic and kept so until the graft is placed and a pressure dressing applied. The smallest blood clot will spoil the overlying graft. All clots should be washed out by squirting salt solution with a syringe beneath the skin graft just as the pressure is being applied.

A method that ensures excellent takes is one combining immobility, pressure and wetness. The last is furnished by instilling solution through rubber tubes embedded in the dressings.

Absolute immobilization by splint is necessary for free grafts, especially for the thick ones.

Contractures From Burns. Scars from burns may overheal and contract, leaving excessive contracture deformities. Burns of the hand and the arm occur in certain typical ways. The child puts his hand on the hot stove or catches it in a hot mangle, resulting in flexion

FIG. 288. After the contracting scar has been excised and full extension obtained, immobilization can be maintained by a fine Kirschner wire through the phalanges and into a metacarpal.

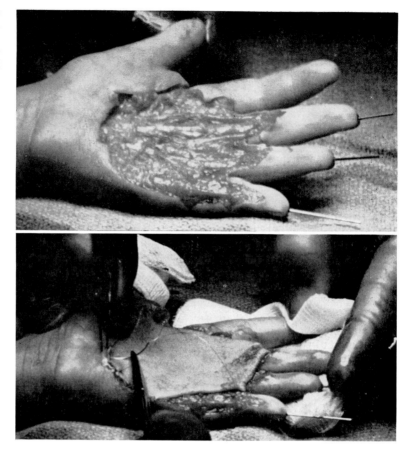

joint, a split-skin graft will suffice. An excellent finger covering is made from a full-thickness graft from above the clavicle or the inner side of the arm, but intermediate thickness split skin will be quite satisfactory.

If the middle joint has a fairly good covering but cannot extend because of loss of the middle tendon slip, the 2 lateral bands can be sutured together on the dorsum to provide extension. However, the distal joint will not flex. A new extensor tendon cannot be supplied for the middle joint until the finger is covered by pedicle skin, as the tendon will not slide under split skin. A good joint must be present. With loss of extensor tendon and partial or complete ankylosis of the middle finger joint in strong flexion, the joint should be placed into mild flexion by force or osteotomy under anesthesia, and there it should be ankylosed, being fixed by 2 crossed stainless steel pins.

When the distal finger joint is hyperex-

tended, it should also be placed in mild flexion and ankylosed. Fingernails deformed from burns are difficult to repair. Crosscutting the skin dorsally, freeing the skin and grafting the space so left has not helped. The whole nail and the matrix should be removed and a skin graft substituted.

Capsulectomy may be necessary to allow the proximal joints to flex. This can be done through a skin graft. It can also be accomplished by removing the collateral ligaments from beneath the aponeurotic hood and applying a skin graft at once.

Contracting keloids form especially in places where there is much motion, producing intermittent tension and compression of the scar; they are greatest on the dorsal or the palmar surfaces of the hand and worst over the joints. Often the dorsal aspect, and at times the volar aspect, of the lower and the upper arms shows marked keloid formation from burns. This is especially so where the keloid spans the axilla, the elbow or the wrist and is subject to intermittent motion. Often a scar runs across the inner aspect of the elbow and down to the radial border of the thumb and becomes tight on extension of the elbow and on supination and extension of the wrist and the thumb.

TREATMENT. Tissue that has been partially burned but recovers, as in the deeper portions of a burn, is so changed that it develops contracting keloids. It is this layer that contracts. As early as a burn can be cleaned it should be covered by thin temporary grafts; otherwise, time will be lost and granulations will pile up, eventually causing contractures in this thick layer of cicatrix. If such an area is excised down to good tissue and the region is covered over by a free graft of skin, there will no longer be the tendency to re-form keloid. Therefore, the treatment of contractures from burns is excision of the damaged skin and the thick subcutaneous cicatrix and substitution of good skin in its place. In burns the greatest damage is superficial, having been received from without; is lessens progressively with the depth; therefore, unlike contractures from infection and injury which stem from within, on excising contractures from burns one usually finds a good vascular bed underneath, well fitted to receive the free graft. However, for deep burns that extend down to the firmer tissues, tendons, ligaments and bones, pedicle grafts are necessary. Where possible, the whole keloid is cut away and replaced by as thick a free skin graft as will take, the deep intermediary or full-thickness yielding the best skin, three-quarter thickness for the dorsum but full thickness for the palm.

On the dorsum of the fingers the bed may be so poor that the pedicle graft may be necessary. For milder contractures here, the skin may be cross-cut in several places, allowed to gape and then covered in by free grafts of intermediary thickness. Of course, the fingers should be put up in flexion. If keloids are present, it will be found that under the thin skin of the keloid there are thick plaques and bands of cicatricial tissues. These bands cover the dorsum and run down the backs of the fingers and often between them as webs. Often over the extensor tendons there is a good areolar layer which will support a free skin graft.

The method of choice when the deep structures are uninvolved is to excise all the burned area of the dorsum of the hand and the fingers and cover the denuded area with one large piece of three-quarter thickness skin. It is important to excise all plaques of cicatricial tissue and the deepest white cicatricial layer, as this is the cause of the contracture. When it is removed, the fingers will flex. If the burn is not deep, all veins and subcutaneous fat should be preserved as the skin is dissected off. The new skin will be very pliable, and the veins will show through it. The forearm and the hand are placed on a splint which is rounded domelike for the palm so that the fingers will be spread and semiflexed, and the dressing is applied with firm compression. The proximal finger joint, long held in extension by cicatrix, may need capsulectomy and at the same time be grafted over by a thick split-skin graft.

If the skin is cut in 2 pieces, the juncture should be zigzagged across the back of the hand instead of longitudinal with it so that it will not thicken to keloid. On the fingers the graft margin should be either zigzagged or midlateral even at the expense of some good skin, as in this line there is no push and pull. It should be noticed that flexion creases in the fingers extend to the midlateral line only. Any border of a skin graft that is either anterior or posterior to this midlateral line, unless zigzagged, is prone to thicken.

Burned skin is removed under the ischemia of a tourniquet, as bleeding is excessive. The tourniquet may be released temporarily for ligation of large vessels, but should be inflated again so that the field will remain absolutely dry for the skin graft and until after the pressure dressings and also a slab of plaster to immobilize it are fastened in place. Not until then is the tourniquet removed.

Special care is taken in arranging the grafts at the webs. Wherever possible a strip of skin from the dorsal or the volar surface of the web or the side of the finger is laid across the depth of the cleft. If a graft border loops around a web on the dorsum, it should be deeply zigzagged. It is best to place long tongues of skin graft across a web, prolonging them on both surfaces of the hand to allow for shrinkage. When correcting webs after a hand has been skin grafted, it is best to do only the 2nd and the 4th clefts first, using long, pointed skin grafts held in place by stents, and to do the 3rd cleft at a later time. Dissecting deeply on both sides of a finger may jeopardize the circulation.

When deep structures are involved, the skin over the dorsum of all the fingers and the hand must be replaced by skin and subcutaneous tissue by means of a pedicle graft.

If possible, when a flexion contracture is excised and replaced by new skin, the limb should be put up in splints or plaster in the position opposite that of the original flexion contracture and maintained so for 3 weeks.

Where burns are too extensive to be replaced completely by good skin, the lines of tension in them where whitening occurs on extension should be excised or cut across. The gap so produced should be covered by good skin, usually by a free graft but often by swinging a flap of good skin across the line or by a pedicle graft. The amount of new skin necessary can be reduced to a minimum by placing it in these strategic places which break the lines of tension. An arm may be hidebound from extensive contracture from burn. By making several longitudinal incisions the length of the burn of the limb, thus breaking in about 3 places the circumferences which are too short, these wounds gape, relieving tension. They are covered at once by split grafts.

Deeply burned hands do not flex well because of the contracture of the collateral ligaments and the dorsal aponeurosis of the proximal finger joints, and contracture of the transverse metacarpal ligaments as well. Normally, when making a fist the breadth of the hand increases $\frac{1}{4}$ inch at the knuckles. If it cannot do this, flexion is limited. Therefore, in deep burns of this region, the transverse metacarpal ligaments should be divided.

Another complication is contracture of the interosseus muscles, either from involvement in the depth of the burn or due to ischemic contracture. (See Local Ischemic Contracture in the Hand.)

DUPUYTREN'S CONTRACTURE

In 1610 the condition now known as Dupuytren's contracture was first described by Plater. In 1808 it was referred to in the lectures of Henry Clive, and in 1818 Sir Astley Cooper wrote that it was due to hypertrophy of the palmar fascia. In 1831, Baron Guillaume Dupuytren, after dissecting a hand with this affliction, described the thickening of the palmar fascia.

INCIDENCE

Statistics compiled by various authors— Keane, Anderson, Black, Byford, Kanavel, J. S. Davis, A. A. Davis, Meyerding, Bruce Gill, Skoog, Conway, Boyes and Posch—establish the incidence of this condition.

Dupuytren's contracture occurs predominantly in Caucasian males of North European stock. In 60 per cent of one series the onset was between 40 and 60 years of age. The youngest patient reported was 11 years of age. Males predominate (89.3% in Skoog's series). All the digits can be affected, the ring and the little fingers most often, but even the thumb in many cases. It appears bilaterally in 40 per cent of patients, and handedness is not a factor in its appearance.

With few exceptions, authorities agree that the condition is more prevalent in people who do not use their hands for manual work than it is in manual workers, the percentages being 55 and 45, respectively.

ETIOLOGY

The etiology of Dupuytren's contracture is still unknown, although many theories have been advanced. However, there are certain aspects that stand out conspicuously. It is prevalent in males and in the aged. It is definitely hereditary, there being numerous instances of many in a family being afflicted with the condition and of its having cropped out in families in as many as 4 and 7 consecutive generations. The numerous instances of family history are far too common to be coincidental. An instance of 2 brothers with identical bilateral Dupuytren's contracture has been recorded. Couch reported identical Dupuytren's contracture in identical twins. Certain diseases, such as gout, arthritis deformans, rheumatic tendency and diabetes, have been associated more repeatedly with Dupuytren's contracture than others. Skoog found that in epileptics 42 per cent had Dupuytren's contractures.

People with this condition show a marked tendency toward limitation of motion in their joints on slight provocation. Apparently, the condition is associated with a diathesis which leads to overgrowth and thickening and con-

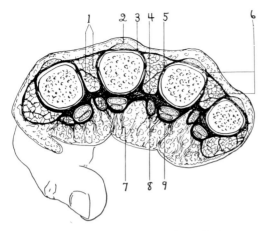

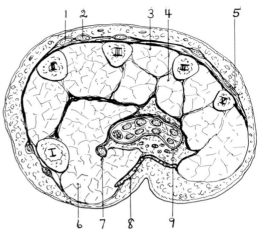

FIG. 289. Cross section of fresh frozen palm in a plane just proximal to the distal palmar creases. To show (black) the extensive system of ligamentous septa and fluted arches in the distal half of the palm, which bind firmly the tendons, the palmar fascia and the skin to the bones. Palmar fascia has here fused to the 4 large arches or pulleys of the flexor tendons, and also to the radial side of each, to the fascia forming the 4 lesser arches of the lumbrical canals.

(1) Anterior and posterior interosseus muscles. (2) Extensor tendon. (3) Dorsal aponeurosis. (4) Pre-interosseus fascia. (5) Attachment to metacarpal of dorsal aponeurosis and septa from pre-interosseus fascia. (6) Cleavage spaces between metacarpals and surrounding fascia. (7) Fibrous connections between palmar fascia and skin. (8) Lumbrical canal or lesser arch. (9) Tendon pulley or greater arch.

FIG. 290. Cross section of fresh frozen hand in a plane through the center of the metacarpals. Here the hand is largely of muscles, the passageway for the flexor tendons and the median nerve being small.

(1) Extensor communis digitorum. (2) Extensor indicis proprius. (3) Posterior interosseus muscle. (4) Anterior interosseus muscle. (5) Extensor minimi digiti proprius. (6) Thenar muscles. (7) Radial bursa and flexor pollicis longus. (8) Palmar fascia. (9) Ulnar bursa. Between palmar fascia and ulnar bursa are volar digital nerves and vessels.

tracture of ligamentous tissue, as in the collagen diseases.

The condition is usually bilateral and may be associated with contracture of ligamentous bands elsewhere. There may be thickening and contracture of the connective-tissue septum between the 2 corpi cavernosum, known as strabismus of the penis or induratio penis plastica (Peyronie's disease) in about 3 per cent of cases. There is the association in 5 per cent of cases of a similar condition in the plantar fascia of the foot with the maximal contracture in each instance greater on the medial side of the sole than on the outer side. It is more pronounced over the internal than the external plantar nerve. The latter corre-

sponds to the ulnar nerve in the hand. In the foot the nodules are flatter, the toes usually are not contracted, but there may be a tendency toward cavus. In one case of Dupuytren's contracture there was a subcutaneous tight, fibrous band running down the front of the left shoulder and arm. Often with Dupuytren's contracture there are "knuckle pads" over the middle joints of the fingers.

There is often the desire to claim that a Dupuytren's contracture is due to trauma from labor, and some early writers held this view. Although it is the usual and natural assumption of a patient to ascribe the condition to trauma, as it may be temporarily more conspicuous after trauma, it is clear that the cause of the condition is unrelated to trauma. Arguments against trauma as a cause are that the condition is idiopathic in origin and associated with other similar conditions and with a general tendency for the ligamentous tissues to undergo contracture. It is usually bilateral, though the right hand is more subject to

FIG. 291. Palmar fascia and fascial septa in the distal part of the palm. Eight arches and tunnels are seen with septa between, the 4 smaller fascial tubes each containing a lumbricalis muscle, vessels and nerves. In Dupuytren's contracture, the palmar fascia and the septa undergo fibrous hypertrophy.

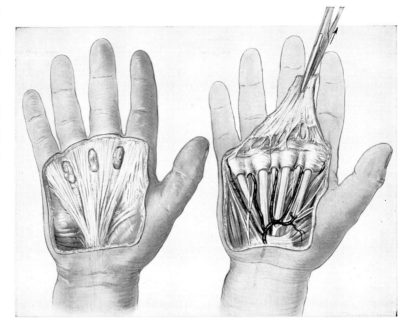

trauma. The fact that it occurs more frequently in those who do not perform manual labor than in those who do is quite conclusive. There are many injuries of the palm, but the incidence of Dupuytren's contracture following such injuries is so small that it must be considered to be coincidental. If trauma is a factor, the racial distribution cannot be explained.

SYMPTOMS

Symptoms from Dupuytren's contracture are not great, and often the contracture may be well established without producing any pain or discomfort. Sometimes the subjective sensations precede the occurrence of lump or contracture; in other cases a constant pain in the palm directs the patient's attention to a small lump forming in the skin. The usual symptoms complained of are a dull ache in the palm, a numb feeling, or tingling. The patient may complain of cramping; only a few complain of pain. If they do, it is best to look for some other cause, such as a carpal tunnel syndrome or gout. The hand may feel stiff in the morning, but, when the round cell stage is over, the condition is usually painless. At first there may be only a small nodule in the region of the distal crease in the palm opposite the ring finger. Here the skin may be felt to

be thickened, and soon a subcutaneous contracting band may be felt in the line of the palmar fascia. The skin at the distal crease rises in a transverse fold and on one or both sides of it there may be a crescentic dimpling, as the contracting fibrosis draws a funnel-like fold of skin inward. At first there may be no actual contracture of the fingers, though if each finger of each hand is bent backward and the degree of extension compared, some comparative limitation of extension will be noticed in the affected hand.

The progression of the contracture may be rapid or slow. In some instances considerable contracture occurs within a year, while in others the course may spread over 20 years. Occasionally, there are exacerbations, and there may be recessions, some of which seem to be brought about by incidents in the patient's general health, such as sicknesses or operation. Usually, first the ring finger commences to flex in its proximal joint. This may soon be followed by flexion contracture of the proximal joints of either one or both of the adjoining fingers, in which case subcutaneous bands of thickened palmar fascia can be felt running to one side or the other of the respective fingers. The middle joint of one or more fingers often shares in the contracture and sometimes eventually flexes to an extreme de-

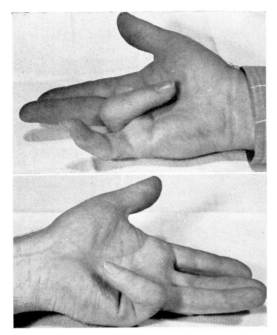

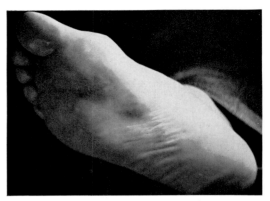

Fig. 293. Nodules in the plantar fascia seldom require excision. They may appear before the hands are involved and have been mistakenly excised as "tumors."

Fig. 292. Dupuytren's contracture is not always symmetrical and may affect the middle joint extension of a single finger.

gree. Rarely does the distal joint contract, but, because the flexion of the middle joint upsets the muscle balance, it often hyperextends.

As the contracture develops in the palm, the skin over the thickening fascial bands becomes firm with induration. Instead of having the normal resilience or softness from the subcutaneous fat, it feels hard, thick and tight to the thickened palmar fascia. Broad plaques of such induration spread out along the course of the thickened fascial bands in the region of the distal crease in the palm. They also appear in the volar skin of the proximal and the middle segments of the fingers, and frequently there may be a plaque of skin running between the thenar eminence and the radial end of the distal crease of the palm. Here there is often a separate fascial band contracting parallel with the web between the thumb and the index finger. Another band may form over the thenar eminence parallel with the long axis of the thumb and extending down its radial border. There may even be an isolated plaque near the pisiform bone.

With one or several fingers firmly hooked in flexion contracture, there is the danger that the patient will be unable to let go when his hand catches hooklike on the grab rail of a streetcar or on some other moving object. Many are unable to work because of the contracture. The patient may complain that in washing his face his finger pokes into his eye, or that in shaking hands with people the finger in their palm leads to embarrassing misinterpretation. When fingers remain strongly flexed, the deep folds of the skin macerate, and the deep crescentic, funnel-like puckerings of the skin of the palm may become infected.

The ring finger is the one most frequently affected and the little finger the next. Following this in frequency is the middle finger; the index finger is affected only occasionally. Contracture of the thumb is even more unusual. Tabulations from the 2,612 hands involved give the following relative frequency of involvement of the various digits:

Thumb	97
Index	143
Middle	622
Ring	1,616
Little	1,372

The ring and the little fingers are often contracted at the same time, and less so the ring and the middle fingers. The contracture usually starts in the distal crease in the palm, though occasionally in the proximal segment of a finger.

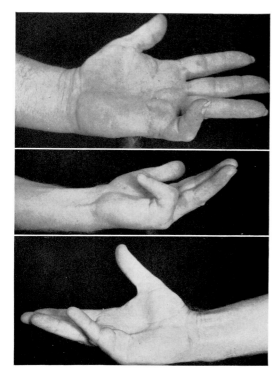

Fig. 294. Various manifestations of Dupuytren's contracture in the little finger. (*Top*) Middle joint contracture. (*Center*) Proximal and middle joints in flexion. The distal joint most often stays in extension or hyperextension. (*Bottom*) Proximal joint only restricted in extension.

Dupuytren's contracture is present bilaterally in the majority of cases. Case compilations by A. Kanavel, J. S. Davis and H. W. Meyerding place this majority at 48.3 per cent, 53 per cent and 64 per cent, respectively. Studies relating specifically to onset rather than to condition at examination show that 44 per cent gave a history of bilateral onset of the disease. In 22 per cent of the remainder, less than 1 year elapsed between the appearance in the first and in the second hand. Careful histories show that 40.7 per cent occur in the left hand of right-handed individuals; thus the simultaneous onset and the almost equal occurrence in the hands does not bear out the previous belief that it occurs more frequently in the major hand.

DIAGNOSIS

Dupuytren's contracture is so typical that

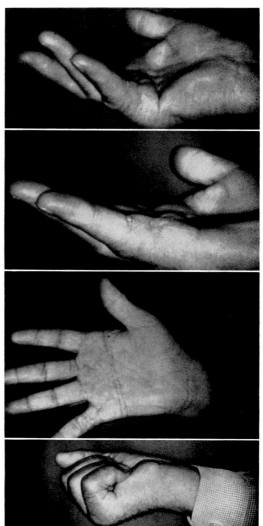

Fig. 295. Case G. C. (*Top*) Dupuytren's contracture of 1 year's duration. Fasciotomy was done in the office with the result shown in the second picture, allowing the skin and the nerves to lengthen out. Then formal resection of the palmar fascia was done through a transverse incision along the distal crease. The result is shown in the bottom 2 illustrations.

there should be no difficulty in its diagnosis, unless it is present in combination with other conditions in the same hand. The characteristic features are loss of fat between the contracting bands and the epidermis, hard nodules

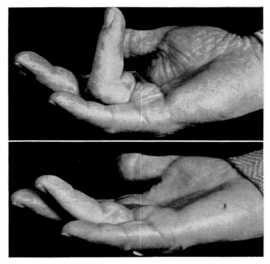

FIG. 296. Subcutaneous fasciotomy in palm with release of contracting band to ring finger.

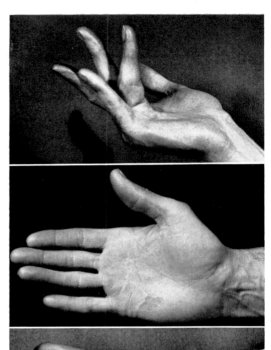

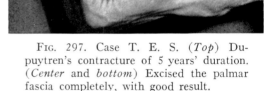

FIG. 297. Case T. E. S. (*Top*) Dupuytren's contracture of 5 years' duration. (*Center* and *bottom*) Excised the palmar fascia completely, with good result.

and induration in the skin, transverse skin folds and crescentic puckerings, and the arrangement of the contracting cords corresponding to the natural bands of the palmar fascia. There is absence of tendon involvement, and the digits can flex completely.

Shortened tendons result in flexion of the distal joints which are, if anything, extended in Dupuytren's contracture. In tendon shortening, motions of the digits will be found to be affected by the position of the wrist joint.

In spastic conditions, unlike Dupuytren's contracture, the proximal joints are usually in extension, and the distal 2 joints in flexion. Also, Dupuytren's contracture is usually bilateral. The presence of plantar thickening and especially of "knuckle pads" should aid in diagnosis.

PATHOLOGIC CHANGES

Palmar Fascia. The contracting bands in Dupuytren's contracture are merely an exaggeration of the normal palmar fascia and its attachments. Normally, these structures hold the volar and the palmar skin firmly in relation to the skeletal framework, the fibrous bands from the sides of the metacarpals and the phalanges to the volar and the palmar skin arching over and encircling alternately first the tendons and then the vessels, the nerves and the lumbricales. The palmar aponeurosis divides into 4 slips, 1 for each finger. The deep fascia that envelops the whole hand is attached to all bony prominences and is thickened in the palmar aponeurosis which is part of it. Thus the latter is continuous with the thin fascia over the thenar and the hypothenar muscles. It is also fairly thick where it spans the area between the thenar eminence and the main palmar fascia and the base of the index finger. In the distal third of the palm the longitudinal septa which pass vertically from the floor of the palm to the overlying palmar fascia divide the palm into a series of longitudinal tunnels by arching over the structures that pass to the fingers. There are 8 such arches; the 4 opposite the metacarpals enclose the flexor tendons, and those smaller ones be-

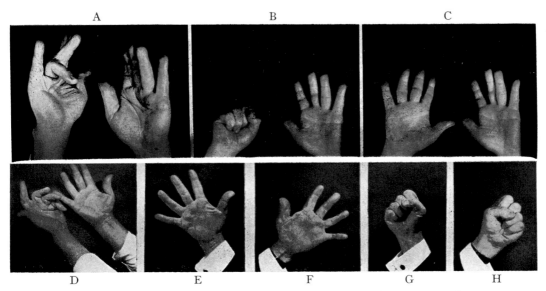

FIG. 298. Case A. M., age 58. (A) Dupuytren's contracture, May 2, 1927. Also present: similar contracture as strabismus of the penis. (B, C) Same case December 8, 1927. Right hand has been operated on. (D) Same case. Left hand has progressed. (E, F, G, H) Same case February 18, 1936, both hands postoperatively.

tween and opposite the interspaces each enclose the vessels, the nerves and a lumbrical muscle. These 4 smaller channels are known as the lumbrical canals. One of these septa which is so membranous that it is not important, extending between the metacarpal of the middle finger and the fascia beneath its tendons, is longer than the others, reaching proximally to the distal end of the transverse carpal ligament or slightly farther and dividing the midpalmar and the thenar spaces. The above vertical septa fuse with the firm fascia covering the floor of the palm over the interosseus muscles at the sides of the metacarpals and also the adductor muscles of the thumb. They also attach to the deep transverse metacarpal ligament, the capsules of the proximal finger joints and the annular ligaments over the tendons. Superficially, the fibers run vertically to all parts of the skin covering the palmar fascia, and especially to the folds in the palm. Between these fibers are many globules of fat. In each finger the palmar fascia divides roughly into 3 bands, 1 running broadly down the center and attached to the skin for the length of the finger and the other 2 running down each side of the finger to be attached to the ligamentous tissue and the periosteum at the sides of the phalanges, the annular sheaths

and the joint capsules as far distal as but not including the distal joint. Just proximal to the webs of the fingers there is a thin transverse ribbon of the deeper layer of the palmar fascia called the natatory ligament, with the fibers spanning the bases of all of the digits superficial to the nerves and the vessels. The palmar fascia proximally converges into the tendon of the palmaris longus. Strangely enough, in about one sixth of the cases of Dupuytren's contracture, this tendon may be absent.

Changes in the Fascia. In Dupuytren's contracture a part or all of this palmar fascia and its vertical attachments undergoes continuous thickening and contracture by proliferation of cicatricial tissue, drawing the proximal and the middle joints of the fingers into flexion contracture, puckering in the skin of the palm—especially at the creases—to crescentic, funnel-like depressions and binding down the whole structure tightly to the sides of the metacarpals and the adjoining ligamentous tissue. The greatest proliferation is usually at the level of the distal crease in the palm and is attached to the proximal margin and sides of the vaginal ligaments encircling the flexor tendons. The short fibers from the palmar fascia to the skin so proliferate and contract that they squeeze out all subcutaneous fat and

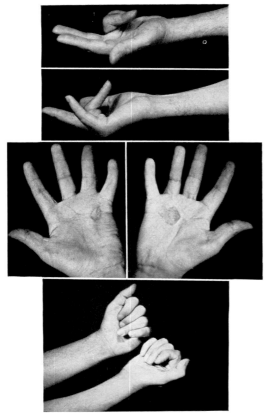

FIG. 299. Case H. W. S. Bilateral Dupuytren's contracture. Complete palmar fascia was dissected out through a transverse incision and from the ring and the little fingers through lateral incisions. Some skin grafts were placed in the palms. The 3 bottom pictures show the good results.

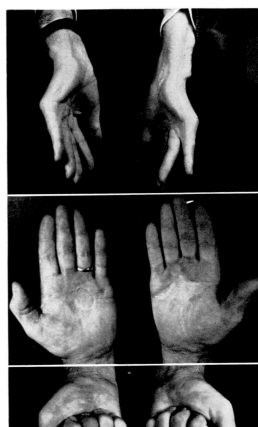

FIG. 300. Case F. B. Bilateral Dupuytren's contracture, 10½ years' duration. Excised all palmar fascia through one transverse palmar incision. Excised cicatricial skin and made full-thickness grafts from the creases in the elbow. Cicatricial tissue was also removed from the fingers.

even the sweat and the sebaceous glands and the blood and the lymph vessels, so that a thick plaque of tissue forms between the epidermis and the palmar fascia. Microscopic cross section of the skin in Dupuytren's contracture shows great thickening of the cornified layer, thinning and flattening of the stratum mucosum and obliteration of the papillae of the corium, which normally extend up deep into the epidermis. The papillae have been pulled downward and obliquely by the contracting fibers. Descending deeper, in the early stage, some round cell infiltration of the connective tissue suggesting inflammation is seen; later, nothing but dense cicatricial tissue which has squeezed out all the fat and the deeper structures of the skin is present. This tissue is somewhat more cellular and vascular in the early cases, when it has even been mistaken for fibrosarcoma, but eventually becomes thick, dense cicatrix. All is fibroblastic and closely resembles a fibroma. In some areas, the cells are numerous, and in others there is largely intercellular matrix in longitudinal arrangement. From the irritation of repeated attempts to extend the fingers, these contracting bands, which are like deep keloids even microscopically, thicken and contract the more. In places, such as the distal crease in the palm, an area just proximal to the web of the thumb or the volar skin of the proximal segments of the fingers, the cicatrix under the skin may thicken to a solid, broad plaque that strangles out all fat and normal structures and is covered by a mere thin layer of epidermis. When a digit remains in flexion contracture, all of the tissues in its volar aspect—skin, nerves and joint capsules—become secondarily contracted so that even after the palmar fascia and bands are excised, the finger cannot be straightened completely.

TREATMENT

Dupuytren treated the contracture named after him by multiple transverse incisions through skin and fascial bands. Later, as in tenotomy operations, Adams severed these bands subcutaneously; but, though there was temporary relief, the contractures reappeared. Many other methods were tried unsuccessfully. Irradiation resulted in temporary softening of the bands, but recurrence followed.

Radical resection of the fascia became popular when asepsis and surgical technics improved. The object of radical operation was to remove en bloc all of the cicatricial contracting tissue, including the palmar fascia, its connecting fibers to the skin, the septa to the sides of the metacarpals and the transverse metacarpal ligament and the lateral and the median bands running down the fingers.

Great difficulty is encountered in achieving healing per primam. The skin left after excision of the fascial bands is merely thin epidermis without good blood supply, and it is in the part of the hand where there is the greatest motion. Unless careful precautions are taken, this skin will slough, leaving necrotic and eventually raw areas, which greatly delay convalescence and leave contracting scars where these are most undesirable. Splinting is necessary to allow these areas to heal, and the longer the hand is splinted and the wounds in it allowed to remain open, the greater will be the stiffening of the joints and other tissues. In such a case it may take a year before the fingers will flex completely, for patients with

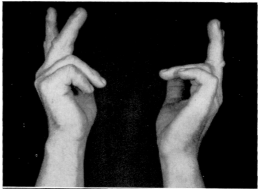
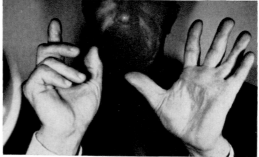

FIG. 301. Case A. D. Bilateral Dupuytren's contracture. The left hand was operated on, excising the palmar fascia from the palm and the fingers and skin grafting a spot in the palm.

Dupuytren's contracture are prone to stiffening of the joints and contraction of the ligamentous tissues.

This "radical" operation should be done when the disease is at an early stage before the skin over the contracture has lost its vitality and before the skin, the nerves and the joint capsules have secondarily become too short to allow the fingers to be extended after the contracted fascia has been removed. The best results are achieved in the younger age groups.

However, operation is not indicated until the skin of the palm is becoming fibrous or until digital contracture has begun. Operation is indicated when the hands can no longer imitate the position of prayer.

Radical operation in the full-blown disease, especially in the older age group, carries a considerable risk.

Since 1946 most surgeons have taken a more conservative approach, and partial and limited

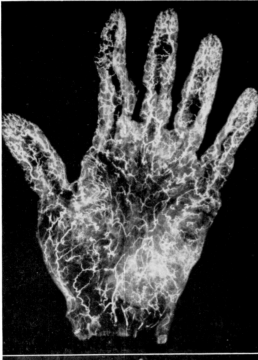

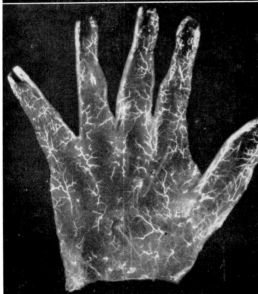

FIG. 302. Angiogram of the blood supply of (*top*) the volar and (*bottom*) the dorsal aspects of the skin of the hand. That of the palm shows that for Dupuytren's contracture a straight incision across the palm paralleling the distal crease in the palm interferes the least with the central sparse blood supply. (Stark and Conway: Plast. Reconstruct. Surg. *12*:358)

bands are the result of reactive hypertrophy, similar to that seen in the response of fascial tissues elsewhere, and that once the active site of the disease is removed in the nodule, release of the tension on the band by fasciotomy allows it to soften and atrophy.

Consideration of factors other than the lesion itself will help to select a method of treatment that promises some relief from the contracture without too much risk. One should realize that this disease is not a tumor or an infection. Radiation has given no lasting benefits, and, as yet, local injections of steroids have not been of value. No other local therapy, physiotherapy or splinting is of any use. Sur-

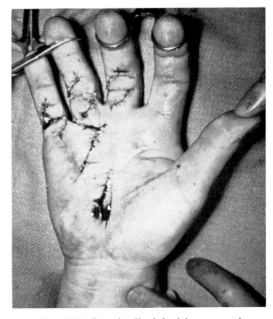

FIG. 303. Longitudinal incisions over involved fascial bands are closed with multiple Z-plasties to elongate the contracted skin.

excisions are done more often than the complete fasciectomy. Luck popularized the subcutaneous fasciotomy described by Adams but later added excision of the "nodules," which he feels are the active lesion of the disease. His theory is that the thickened collagenous

gical release is the only method available. This is a disease that in many patients results in more inconvenience than disability. Therefore, to submit them to a radical operation followed by months of impaired motion and discomfort is hardly justified. Most surgeons will evaluate carefully the particular patient, with age, general physical condition, occupation and hobbies being considered. The tendency to stiffen postoperatively is well known and probably is more likely to occur in the heavy-set patient with thick skin folds. A study of postoperative edema in Dupuytren's showed that half the patients have a measurable degree of edema after 3 months; the occurrence of edema is unrelated to the length of time of tourniquet application or the type of dressing.

Treatment is symptomatic in the sense that the cause of the disease is unknown, and its progress often slow. The aim is to provide sufficient relief of the symptom, the flexion contracture, to allow the hand to open well for grasp and not to jeopardize its more important function of closing around objects.

All types of conservative operations from the simplest fasciotomy to limited and partial resections have been described.

Operative Technic. All procedures are done under the ischemia of a blood pressure cuff tourniquet, and a compression type of dressing and immobilization are used in the immediate postoperative period.

SUBCUTANEOUS FASCIOTOMY. This operation is most appropriate for linear bands in the palm which hold proximal joints flexed. A cataract or myringotomy knife can be used, but a tenotome modeled after that of Adams with a straight backed blade is more satisfactory. Entering the palm over the hypothenar eminence, the blade is passed just beneath the skin, and the vertical fascial bands which pucker the skin are severed with the blade sweeping parallel with and just below the skin. This same freeing of the skin attachments is carried out over the aponeurotic band so that the skin is relaxed and free to allow extension of the digit when the band is cut. The knife is placed over the band and, with the involved finger forcibly extended, pressure is made directly down or toward the dorsum of the hand. A sawing motion is risky, and one should never pass the blade beneath the band and pull upward. Once the taut band is severed, the finger will extend, and there is little danger of severing the neurovascular bundles, which always remain soft and resilient. Usually, the band is severed at 2 levels: at the middle palm and at the distal palmar crease. Blind fasciotomy distal to this crease or in the fingers should not be done because of the danger of injury to the digital nerves.

FASCIOTOMY COMBINED WITH PARTIAL LOCAL EXCISION. After severing all palmar bands, small incisions in the proximal segments of the fingers will allow division or excision of this portion of the involved fascia under direct vision. Both these methods are very useful in hands with linear bands extending to the middle joints and in elderly patients. Many of these individuals are retired from active work, and some are cardiac cripples. Therefore, moderate improvement in extension of the fingers is very satisfactory.

LIMITED EXCISION means the removal of the thickened fascias without attempting to excise all the palmar aponeurosis or the uninvolved fascia.

When the palm and the proximal segments of 1 or 2 of the digits are involved, this may be done through a transverse palmar incision and a longitudinal incision, converted to a Z-plasty on closure, in each finger.

The principle of using the Z-plasty to provide exposure and to lengthen the shortened skin is also used in the case of a linear band from the palm to the finger. A longitudinal incision the full length of the fascial involvement is closed with multiple Z-plasties, making the transverse components of the resulting scars in such a way that they lie at the same level as the normal palmar and digital creases.

RADICAL FASCIECTOMY. Preliminary subcutaneous fasciotomy of the main fascial bands in the palm under local anesthesia is advisable in cases showing marked contracture, where a discrete band holds the proximal finger joints in flexion. A splint, or a rubber sponge bandaged into the palm, is applied to lengthen skin, nerves and joint capsules gradually, and the radical operation is done after 10 to 14 days. The incisions are made at the site of the contemplated operative incision, and care is used not to interfere with areas to be utilized as skin flaps.

An L-shaped incision may be used, though a straight one across the palm along the distal crease seems to interfere the least with the blood supply. Arteriograms show many vessels around the periphery of the palm but few in the center. Most vessels to the palm come straight up from the depths, as do those that supply the skin over the mammary glands. Long flaps of skin in such places do not live.

Through this long transverse incision the skin is undermined distally between it and the contracting tissues to the bases of the fingers and, similarly, proximally to the very apex of the palmar fascia near the wrist. Laterally, the dissection is carried beyond the last nerve on the radial side and to the last nerve on the ulnar side. The dissection is a bit awkward, but it can be done and gives the best blood supply to the skin, namely, from the complete periphery. In the worst places, where there is no more fat, the skin is shaved very thin. A careful excision en bloc is made, taking all the thickened fascia. Commencing at one side of the hand and at the base of the palm, one dissects cleanly, removing every vestige of deep fascia. Dissection may be done with sharp, double-pointed scissors curved on the flat or with a knife, or at times with a probe. The palmar fascia is cut across where it converges to the tendon of the palmaris longus; the cut end is grasped with a hemostat, and, as the dissection proceeds in an orderly manner across to the other side of the palm and on distally to the bases of the fingers, this fascia is held taut and cut free until it is held only by the bands running on down the fingers. As each volar digital nerve and artery is reached, the fascial septum running between them and the flexor tendons is trimmed off very deep in the hand where it joins the ligamentous tissue at the side of the metacarpal and the transverse and the vaginal ligaments. Care is used not to open any tendon sheath or to sever the motor thenar nerve or any of the tiny nerves to the lumbrical muscles or, of course, the volar digital nerves. Always locate the nerves before cutting freely and preserve or carefully ligate the communicating vessel between the superficial and the deep arteries at the base of the finger. Eight septa in all, extending from the palmar fascia through ligamentous tissue to the skeletal framework, are excised. The septa arch first over the tendons and then over the nerves, the vessels and a lumbrical muscle to each cleft, and alternately so across the palm, thickening superficially into the palmar fascia. The proximal ends of the vaginal ligaments are trimmed cleanly and preserved. The thickened fascia over the lumbrical muscles and the hypothenar and the thenar eminences is also trimmed away. By blunt and sharp dissection the fascial bands are traced down from the palm into the bases of the fingers.

Next, each affected finger is opened through a midlateral incision or a volar midline incision which will be closed with a Z-plasty. First, the volar digital nerves and vessels are located and so protected; then all the thickened fascial bands are dissected out completely and excised. The digital nerve may be embedded in the mass or may spiral around it. The bands may attach to the side of the proximal or the middle phalanges, the vaginal sheaths or the ligamentous tissue at the side of the joint capsule. Often there is a deep volar-lateral band spanning the middle finger joint that, together with the anterior part of the joint capsule, must be excised before the joint will extend. The central band is often densely adherent to the skin along the volar aspect of the proximal and sometimes the middle finger segment. This skin may have to be shaved very thin. Unless all volar digital vessels are preserved in both the palm and the fingers, gangrene of a finger may result.

After every vestige of thickened fascia has been removed, the effect of secondarily contracted tissue will be seen. The finger should not be extended farther than the skin and the nerves will tolerate easily. In a sharply contracted middle finger joint it may be necessary to strip or excise the anterior and the anterolateral parts of the capsule of the joint before the latter will extend. Too much extension at this time may result in dislocation, which later may require amputation at the middle joint.

If a finger is too badly contracted to save, it may be amputated; but first it should be boned and all possible good skin used to cover in any area in the palm where the skin, because of too poor quality, is excised. If it is the little finger that must be amputated, its metacarpal should be removed obliquely at its base, the hypothenar muscles being reattached to the ring finger and slack gained by narrowing the hand. This is the best policy for the little finger if it is too badly contracted. The

FIG. 304. The mechanism causing Volkmann's ischemic contracture in unreduced supracondylar fractures of the humerus. The forearm displaces backward, the fold of deep fascia kinking the brachial artery and the veins around the lower end of the shaft of the humerus. Also, due to the backward displacement and the swelling about the flexed elbow, the skin is drawn tight across the antecubital space, compressing off the main venous return of the forearm, which is subcutaneous and anterior. The contents within the closed compartment of the deep fascia swell, making pressure so that blood cannot circulate in this closed compartment. The contents undergo any degree of necrosis, followed by contracture.

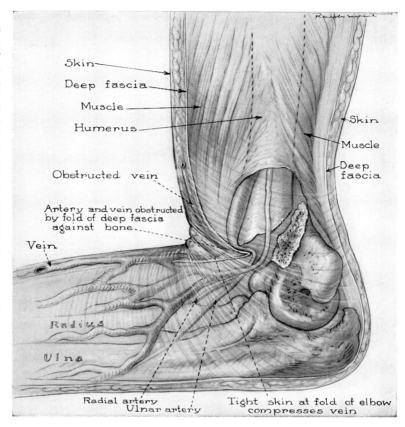

aim is to acquire primary healing, so as to avoid stiffening of joints and contracture from scar which follow prolonged convalescence. Therefore, skin which has been shaved too thin and is devoid of vascularity should be excised. This is especially true of the area in the region of the distal crease in the palm opposite the ring finger. The volar skin over the proximal segment of a finger, even if shaved very thin, often will live, because it is practically a full-thickness skin graft. In the palm and sometimes also in the fingers, it is better to cut away questionable skin and replace it with a thick split graft or by a full-thickness graft from the abdomen or the crease of the elbow. Where such grafts are used, absolute immobility by means of a dorsal splint and a compression dressing are necessary. Should the skin be too badly involved in an extreme case of Dupuytren's contracture, one may apply abdominal skin over the defect by the direct pedicle-flap method.

When the dissection of the hand is com-

pleted, the tourniquet is removed, while the wounds are pressed steadily with gauze for 5 minutes to allow clotting. The remaining bleeders are tied with fine catgut. At this stage the superficial palmar arch is seen to move with each heartbeat, and all the nerves and other structures of the hand free from fascial covering show as in an anatomic illustration. The incisions are closed with fine stainless steel wire, leaving small rubber tubes in place for drainage. Without this precaution and a compression dressing, hematoma generally follows such dissections and greatly detracts from the result. No attempt should be made to straighten the fingers completely at this time; if this is done, the skin will blanch and be given an additional strain in healing. Now that the contracted fascia is out, the fingers will readily straighten out gradually after the wounds have healed. A dorsal splint is applied which will immobilize the proximal finger joints but allow free movement in the middle and the distal finger joints so as to prevent stiffening and

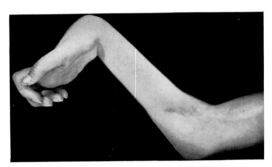

FIG. 305. The classic Volkmann's ischemic contracture following supracondylar fracture. Flexion contracture of elbow, pronation of forearm, flexion of wrist, hand flat, fingers hyperextended at proximal joints, clawing, and median and ulnar sensory loss.

keep the tendons gliding. Splinting for the first 2 weeks is necessary to immobilize the distal crease in the palm so that it will heal per primam. Instilling 2 ml. of hydrocortone into the palm decreases pain, swelling and stiffness.

Postoperative Treatment. On the following day the drains are removed. Steady, firm pressure by the steel wool mass is maintained throughout the first week and, if skin grafts have been used, for the first 2 weeks. Too early motion interferes with healing. The most mobile part of the palm, the distal crease, needs immobility to heal. Too prolonged splinting stiffens the fingers. The proper timing of immobilization and exercise ensures primary healing and limber joints. Motion in the middle and the distal finger joints should be allowed from the beginning and encouraged after the first week, to prevent adhesions of the tendons in the palm and the fingers.

In spite of the above precautions, some necrosis of the skin flap may occur at the distal crease in the palm, which will demand continuation of immobilization to allow healing. For the final healing a small flat metal or plastic splint can be shaped to the dorsum of the hand with a gutterlike extension extending over the proximal segment of the most involved finger. Adhesive plaster holds it in place so that the distal crease will not move and still the other fingers may be exercised.

It must be remembered that persons with Dupuytren's contracture have a tendency toward stiffening of the joints and contracture

of the ligaments so that the ability to flex the fingers may be slow in returning. If healing is primary and immobilization short, flexion may be complete in a month. If healing is delayed and immobilization correspondingly long, it may take a year before complete flexion of the fingers is attained.

Some patients will return later, showing more contracture in some of the parts where fascia had not been excised as not involved at the time, such as in some fingers or near the thenar eminence and sometimes also in a finger where the contracture was too extensive for complete removal. Apparently, Dupuytren's contracture spreads from the fascia in situ and, if this is completely removed, it will not recur at that site.

VOLKMANN'S ISCHEMIC CONTRACTURE

Richard von Volkmann of Halle described the condition in 1869, 1872 and 1881, referring to it as a rapid post-traumatic muscle contraction reaching its climax in a few weeks. In 1914, J. B. Murphy published such a comprehensive résumé of the subject that advances since have not been great. He advised slitting the deep fascia in front of the elbow within the first 36 hours after injury. The principal contributions since then have been made by Sir Robert Jones, Brooks, Jepson, Meyerding and E. B. Jones. Leriche and later Griffiths and Foisie stressed the vasomotor theory. Lipscomb has stressed the spasm of the traumatized brachial artery, and Seddon describes the lesion as an infarct.

DEFINITION

Following trauma, circulatory congestive interference occurs in either the whole lower arm or the volar fascial space in the forearm, and the limb swells. This squeezes out its blood supply, and ischemia results, affecting all of the enclosed tissues.

After an initial stage of partial necrosis, especially of the muscles, there follows progressive muscle fibrosis and contracture, strangling the vessels and the nerves and other tissues, resulting in flexion contracture, partial paralysis of the intrinsic hand muscles, glove anesthesia and impaired nutrition of the hand and the forearm. Varying in degree, the dam-

FIG. 306. Volkmann's contracture following fracture of both bones of the forearm at age 11. (*Bottom*) Limited rotation from synostosis and extent of finger flexion from automatic motions.

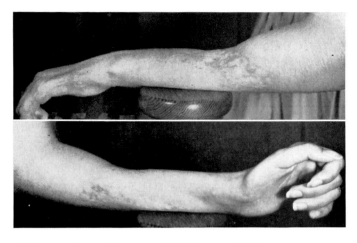

age occurs during the first 6 to 48 hours of ischemia, and the inevitable contracture continues progressively for weeks.

By far the majority had swelling in casts or other constricting dressings, but over 100 cases have been reported in which there was no outside constriction on the limb.

ETIOLOGY

Two thirds of the cases are under the age of 30, and most are between 2 and 16 years. The oldest patient on record was 50. In most cases the inciting injury is fracture, and by far the commonest of these is the incompletely reduced supracondylar fracture of the humerus. Less than one third are caused by fractures of the bones of the forearm, a small proportion by fractures higher in the upper arm and a few by dislocation of the elbow.

Supracondylar fracture is the most common extension fracture of children. C. F. Eichenberry showed how in this unreduced fracture the edge of the bicipital fascia kinked the vessels backward under the sharp, projecting fractured end of the humerus; every one of his 29 cases was caused by this supracondylar fracture.

The following causes, other than fracture, are in the minority but have been reported: damage to brachial or axillary artery, e.g., from gun shot wounds, embolus or rupture; subfascial hematoma from ruptured artery or hemophilia; trauma to forearm, such as contusion, crush or snake bite; exposure to cold; prolonged compression from an Esmarch bandage; or pressure incurred in a drunken stupor.

All of the above causes have in common

FIG. 307. Some of the cicatrix was excised and proximal skin was shifted to improve the contour of the forearm; the synostosis was excised, and a layer of extensor muscle interposed; the ulna was divided in its distal third and a ½-inch segment removed. There was much improvement in appearance and supination. Later the extensor carpi radialis longus was used for opposition of the thumb and the median nerve repaired, overcoming a 2½-inch gap.

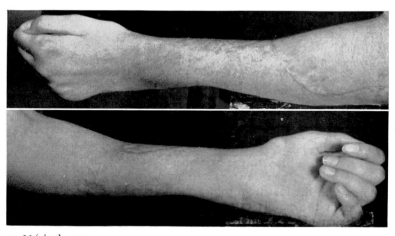

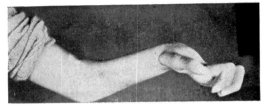

FIG. 308. A year ago, following a Colles'
fracture, a cast was applied. It was split in
4 days, and a new cast was applied. The
patient (then aged 41) had very little sleep
for a month, because of pain, after which
the cast was removed. The fingers were
drawn in then, but increasingly more for
a year. Sensation was lessened in the glove
area.

reactive swelling in the closed flexor fascial
compartment in the forearm, which becomes
so tight that blood is squeezed out. The tightness is usually from swelling in rigid casts or
constricting bandages but can be from the
fascia itself where no constricting dressing has
been applied. When due to a tight encircling
cast or vessel injury, the extensor group of
muscles may share in the contracture; but
when due to pressure in the volar fascial space,
the extensor group is spared.

There is an anatomic reason why this entity
is so typical in the flexor aspect of the forearm, though more casts are applied elsewhere
over the body. It is not found in the upper arm
or the upper leg and is quite rare in the lower
leg. In the forearm, the flexor fascial space is
closed in like a box, and its contents, under
swelling, have the blood pressed out just as in
the case of the swollen brain encased in unyielding dura mater or of the facial nerve that
reacts to exposure to cold by trying to swell
in the rigid facial canal and, from the ischemia
so produced, causing Bell's palsy.

The fascial space in the lower leg has a
vent on each side of the Achilles tendon and
so is involved only in cases of extreme swelling, as from obstruction of the femoral artery
and vein, a crush through the popliteal space
or even, in one case, cold from prolonged sitting on a cake of ice. In the case of popliteal
crushing, the toes became gangrenous. The
deformity in the foot from contracture of the
muscles in the calf is extreme equinus and
also flexion of the midtarsal joints and the
toes.

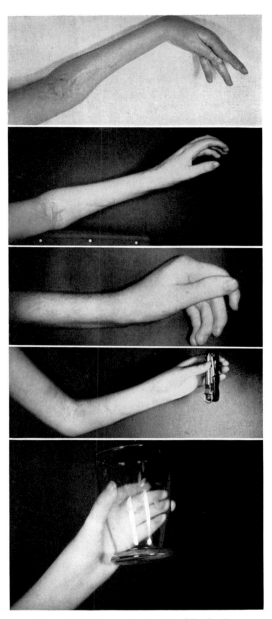

FIG. 309. Case A. V. V. (*Top*) From
supracondylar fracture at the age of 3,
there resulted a severe Volkmann's ischemic
contracture. The hand was useless. There
was no flexor action of any digit. The telltale scar is in the antecubital space. Arthrodesed the wrist, using iliac graft. Later,
transferred the extensor carpi ulnaris tendons to flex all digits and removed the head
of the ulna for pronation and supination.
A useful hand resulted, as shown in the 4
remaining pictures.

FIG. 310. (A) Intrinsic minus position from paralysis of the median and the ulnar nerves. (B) Intrinsic plus position from electrical stimulation of the median nerve. (C) Intrinsic plus position from electrical stimulation of the ulnar nerve at the elbow. (J. Bone Joint Surg. 35-A:88)

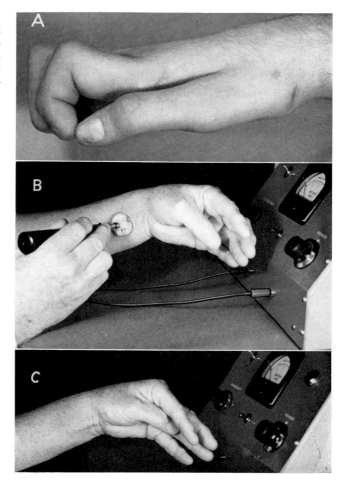

PATHOLOGIC FINDINGS

Before considering the mechanism one should review what has actually been found operatively in the acute stage. All authors report that the fascia in front of the elbow was very tight and that it spread widely on being split, allowing muscles under pressure, either pale or blue-black from extravasation, to protrude through the wound. In some cases a tight hematoma also was present.

Veins are always engorged. Tight skin across the front of the swollen elbow occludes the superficial veins and the folds of the bicipital fascia across the elbow, causes engorgement of the vessels either by direct pressure if there is only swelling or, in cases of supracondylar fracture, by pressing the vessels against the upper fragment. It is immaterial if the deep and the superficial veins communicate below

the elbow, for all veins are occluded as they converge and pass under the tight skin of the antecubital space. When an elbow is flexed, even when not swollen, the yield of the skin across its front is very slight.

The brachial artery in the antecubital space often is found to be ruptured, thrombosed or drawn out and reduced to a string. Some have claimed that the narrowing is due to a spasm effect from direct trauma, and in 1 case the vessel was seen to be normal again 6 months later. Smyth reports 4 cases of primary rupture of the brachial artery with supracondylar fracture, none of which had arterial deficiency. Often enough, the artery, the vein and the median nerve have been found to be actually torn in two by the projecting sharp edge of the upper humeral fragment but in other cases are merely squeezed between the tight fascia

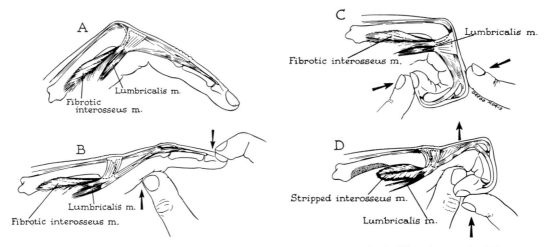

FIG. 311. (A) Intrinsic plus position with fibrotic intrinsic muscles holding the proximal finger joint in flexion and the distal 2 joints in extension. (B, C) Showing the test for intrinsic contracture. When the intrinsic muscles are tensed by holding the proximal joint in extension, the distal 2 joints cannot be flexed; but, when they are slackened by flexing the proximal joints, the distal 2 joints flex. (D) When the interosseus muscle is stripped and advanced, the distal 2 joints flex even when the proximal joint is held extended. (Am. J. Plast. Reconstr. Surg.)

and the swollen forearm or hooked backward by the fascial edge. Emboli have been found at the forks of the artery, resulting in Volkmann's contracture in 48 hours.

The whole contents of the anterior closed fascial space are found to be tensely swollen with edema and are ischemic, the main part of the blood present being in the form of either extravasation or hematoma.

The muscles, at first greatly swollen, show central necrosis of homogeneous appearance with few nuclei, but in their periphery there is inflammatory reaction with round-cell infiltration and, later, fibrosis. The surrounding connective tissue and intermuscular septa show similar reactive infiltration followed by fibrosis. Eventually, the necrotic muscle is absorbed and replaced by scar, and the whole mass undergoes contracture. Here and there, patches of active muscle tissue remain. Seddon describes the lesion as a massive arterial infarct and the involved area as an ellipsoid of necrosis. The flexor digitorum profundus and sublimis and the flexor pollicis longus are usually more badly damaged than are the pronator teres and the flexor carpi, perhaps because the former lie against the unyielding bones and interosseous membrane. In mild cases, nerves show destruction of axons and myelin sheaths; in more severe cases, they show fibrosis in the endoneurium. Pressure sores and sloughs are common accompaniments due to the swelling in casts, especially in the antecubital space and at the sides of the wrist. Fibrous tissue encircles, contracts and impoverishes lymphatics, blood vessels and nerves, resulting in poor nutrition throughout the anterior part of the forearm and the hand.

MECHANISM

There has been much experimentation and discussion as to the etiology of this unique entity. Arterial occlusion, complete or partial, venous obstruction, a combination of both of these and the additional factor of pressure from extrinsic or intrinsic causes, as well as vasomotor spasm, all have been studied in detail.

Arterial occlusion alone causes gangrene not simply of the contents of a fascial space but of the extremity, commencing in the digits. Arterial occlusion by emboli, gunshot wounds, etc., has resulted in muscle contractures in limbs as part of the picture. Brooks found that a tourniquet left on for 5 to 24 hours or a permanent stoppage of an artery caused

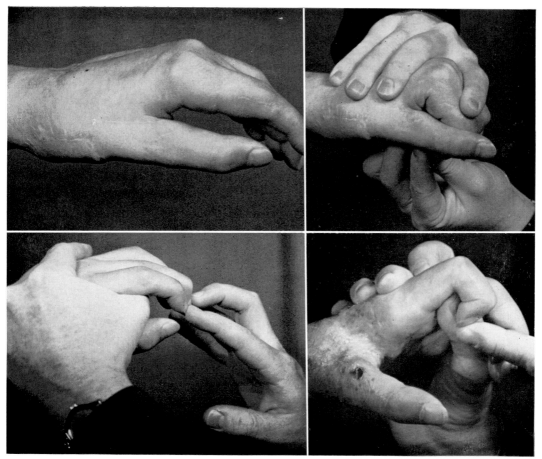

Fig. 312. Ischemic contracture of the intrinsic muscles in the hand due to impaired circulation following fractures from shell fragments of the shoulder, the forearm and the wrist.

(*Top, left*) Thumb in adduction contracture and fingers in the typical position produced by contracture of the interosseus muscles.

(*Bottom, left*) When the proximal finger joint is extended, the distal 2 joints cannot be flexed.

(*Top, right*) When the proximal finger joint is flexed, the distal 2 joints will flex.

(*Bottom, right*) Postoperatively, after the thumb cleft had been opened by a plastic maneuver and the interosseus muscles were stripped, the fingers then could flex while their proximal joints were held extended and the thumb cleft was wide.

temporary paralysis or gangrene but not a true Volkmann's contracture. Skin fared even worse than did muscle.

Ligation of all arteries to the rectus femoris produced atrophy only, but ligation of all veins resulted in contracture resembling that of Volkmann.

Occlusion of the artery entering the fascial space in the forearm does not rob the space contents of all its blood. From anastomoses about the elbow a backflow can enter the fas-

cial space through the posterior interosseous artery. Insufficient arterial supply causes the tissues to swell with edema; necrosis occurs first in the muscles. Total loss of arterial supply is not necessary.

Venous obstruction promptly brings about engorgement with blood. Capillary resistance is overcome at 60 mm. of mercury and, at 100 mm., petechiae appear, and extravasation of blood commences, accompanied by edema. In a closed space, even arterial inflow is re-

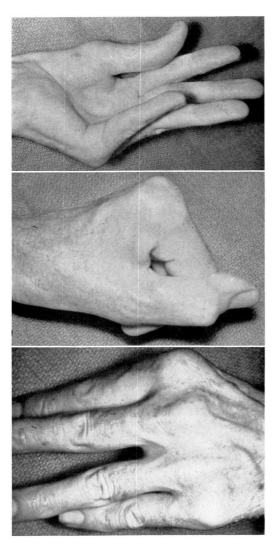

FIG. 313. Ischemic contracture confined to the hand. (*Top*) Limit of voluntary and passive extension. (*Center*) Flexion is almost complete. (*Bottom*) There is no ulnar drift, and the long extensors are in normal position over the metacarpal heads.

Jepson bandaged above the knee and ligated arteries and veins for varying lengths of time, obtaining contracture typical of Volkmann's contracture. Early drainage helped to prevent it. He concluded that increased venous pressure, impaired circulation and pressure were the causes. Ligation of the femoral artery and vein and the deep femoral vein caused the contracture.

A closed fascial space under pressure and, in addition, partial venous and arterial obstruction result in Volkmann's contracture. The circulation is slowed and congested but not stopped. Usually, the pulse is faint or temporarily impalpable at the wrist. There is still some, though insufficient, arterial inflow and venous outflow. This causes edematous swelling which provides the added factor of pressure in the closed space, impairing the arterial supply and causing the central necrosis of muscles, the inflammatory reaction and the partial damage of every tissue within the fascial space. Muscle is highly specialized tissue with little power of regeneration, and it is the tissue most affected. Early relief of pressure by fasciotomy often has checked the process.

The pressure within the closed fascial space is the result of swelling from edema, extravasation or hematoma, and these result from venous or partial arterial occlusion or both, as is so commonly produced by the unreduced supracondylar fracture. It may also come from any trauma to the contents of the anterior fascial space in the forearm. Whether from fracture of the forearm bones, contusion, crushing or thermal injury, the vicious circle is started. The greater the swelling, the more the circulation is reduced in the closed space. Casts become tight, especially in front of the flexed elbow. These and the tight antecubital skin, stretched from the swelling, occlude the superficial veins, and the tight fascia occludes the deep ones. All the veins, both superficial and deep, converge through the antecubital space. Partial arterial block and pressure complete the picture.

Of course, there is a wide range of degree of intensity of the circulatory interference, so that cases may be slight or severe. The process is a factor in producing the terrible crippling from severe infections of the hand and the forearm, because the intense swelling and the

duced, regulated only by the amount of outflow. Brooks found that venous occlusion caused hemorrhage, edema and degeneration of muscle fibers, resulting in acute inflammation progressing to fibrous contracture. He described more inflammation than degeneration but did not test it in a closed space. He concluded that venous obstruction is the primary cause of the condition.

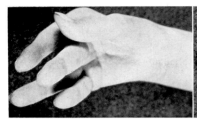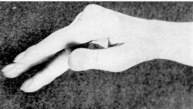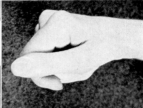

Fig. 314. (*Left* and *center*) Local ischemic contracture of the intrinsic muscles of the hand due to nerve and vascular injury in the upper arm. Fibrotic contraction of the interossei flexes the proximal finger joints and extends the distal 2, and of the thenar muscles clumps the thumb into the palm. It is necessary to excise or strip these muscles to restore balance. (*Right*) When the patient relaxes the interossei by flexing the proximal finger joints, he also can flex the distal 2 finger joints. (L. D. Howard, M.D.)

intrafascial pressure of the latter impairs the circulation within the closed fascial space. Contractures following muscle rupture or those affecting a few digits following contusion of the forearm muscles are quite different from Volkmann's.

Another conception of Volkmann's contracture, first stated by Leriche and concurred in by Griffiths and Foisie, is that the lowered circulation is due to local spasm of the brachial artery from 2 cm. above the elbow down to and including its bifurcation and, secondarily, to a spasm of its collateral vessels. The reflex is thought to be not through the ganglion but low in the nerves about the arteries themselves, started by the trauma at or near the elbow and lasting until relieved by stripping the sympathetics from the artery or, better, by segmental excision of the affected part of the artery, assuming that this is the trigger point that starts the reflex. Frequent reports of local narrowing of the artery and of cure by the above means support these claims.

Lipscomb in 1956 reported a large series of contractures, about half of which resulted from supracondylar fractures. He feels that the arterial injury is accompanied by a spasm of the collateral vessels and that this spasm is more important than the major vessel obstruction. Prompt decompression with resulting relief of the spasm prevents further damage.

Bunnell felt that the phenomenon was sufficiently explained by the closed-space concept without considering vessel spasm. Actual arterial damage is often found, and a local narrowing of the artery may occur from mechanical trauma or drawing out, or from the effects of pressure at the tight bend of the elbow. The fascia must be opened to expose the artery, and this in itself is known to cure the condition. Spasm scarcely explains why, of all parts of the body, the entity occurs in the closed fascial space in the forearm or why the digits or near tissues outside the space are not also involved. In many of the reported cases the cure did not follow the arterial operation at once but was delayed 18 to 24 hours, as after fasciotomy.

SYMPTOMS

Cases vary with the intensity of vessel occlusion; several factors determine the course. If occlusion is extreme, the course is acute; and in from a few hours to 2 days such severe damage is done that the whole life outlook of the child is changed, since he will be handicapped by a crippled hand. After 2 weeks of absorption of necrotic tissue and resolution, fibrous contracture continues through many weeks. If the cast is only moderately tight in the antecubital space or the cause, whatever it may be, is mild, the process may be insidious and, because the nerves are less affected, without much pain. The contracture follows even after weeks. It is most important to recognize the condition early and to act sufficiently promptly to avert the catastrophe.

The onset is usually sudden and severe, accompanied by much restlessness and the constant intense pain of tightness and of tissues dying from ischemia. The hand and the forearm are tense with edematous swelling and are

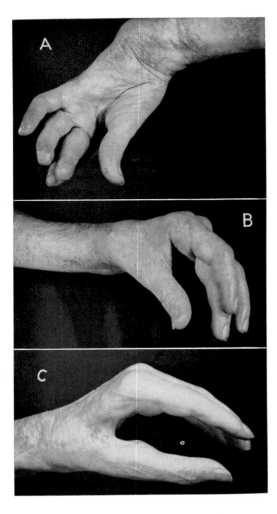

FIG. 315. This patient had sustained a belt-and-pulley injury with multiple fractures. A cast was applied for 3 months, with resulting severe ischemic contracture, of both the Volkmann type and the local type in the hand. All intrinsic muscles of the hand were involved, and the patient had no power to hold anything. The contents of the thumb cleft were excised. The cleft was held open by a bone-graft block, and a split-skin graft was applied to it. Tenotomies were done to all the lateral bands. (A, B) Showing the condition before operation; (C) showing the postoperative condition. The patient obtained a fairly useful hand. (J. Bone Joint Surg. *35-A*:98)

ture of the muscles as they shrink and reduce to fibrous tissue. At first they are greatly swollen, and much reactive hyperemia surrounds them in the process of repair. If the forearm is opened early, long, pale, gray-pink, friable, necrotic spindles of muscles can be drawn out. Finally, the necrotic muscle is absorbed and replaced by hard, contracted fibrous tissue, considerably shorter than the original muscle, and unyielding. Each muscle, tense and homogeneous inside from central necrosis, becomes encased in a sheath of fibrous tissue. This peripheral interstitial fibrosis binds and contracts all tissues in the fascial space.

The end-result of all this is a crippled hand and forearm. The extensor muscles are usually spared unless damaged from cast enclosure or high vessel damage, but the distal 2 finger joints are drawn into contracture, though the proximal finger joints are in extension. Because of the shortened flexor muscles, the digits cannot be extended passively until their flexor tendons are relaxed by increasing the flexion of the wrist.

Nerves are involved in the more severe cases, constituting about 60 per cent—the median the most and the radial the least—there being a numb feeling and paresthesia in glove distribution, and partial patchy complete anesthesia, reaching from the fingertips to anywhere from the bases of the fingers to the lower third of the forearm. As a result of lessened nerve action, the intrinsic muscles in the hand show atrophy and very little action, thus contributing to the typical claw posture. The clawing is exaggerated from firm contrac-

cold, cyanotic and numb. There is pale cyanosis in arterial occlusion, and darker cyanosis when the venous engorgement is primary. In late stages the hand may be cold and white, with hypesthesia and paresthesia. Because of muscle impairment, the patient has difficulty in moving the digits. There may be trophic skin changes at this stage. Muscles of the forearm are tender, and there is tense swelling over the whole mass of flexor muscles, especially in front of the elbow. The radial pulse is usually absent but may return in a few days.

On removing the cast, the forearm swells and becomes red; blebs and pressure sores may be present. Even on the 2nd day the fingers are semiflexed, and any attempt to extend them increases the pain. In 2 weeks there starts continuous and progressive contracture of the long, deep flexors of the fingers and the thumb.

The whole forearm and hand are shrunken. The forearm flexor muscles are hollowed and firm from fibrous atrophy. Usually, some of them function a little. The skin is smooth, cold and glossy. Fingers taper and may show trophic ulcers and deformed nails. Bones are porotic; in children, there may be retarded growth from damage to the epiphyses. All of the tissues show poor nutrition. Oscillometer readings are lowered and so are those of skin temperature. The pulse may have returned. Electrically, the muscles do not show polar inversion. Reaction to the faradic current is lessened or absent, and a greater galvanic current is necessary to produce contraction. The elbow may show flexion contracture.

TREATMENT

Supracondylar fractures should be set correctly very early, and partial reduction should be avoided. Kirschner wire traction or even open operation, at which time the vessels are freed, may be necessary. In a large series treated by overhead skeletal traction there were no cases of Volkmann's contracture (Dunlop). Fixation of supracondylar fractures by crossed Kirschner wires also avoids this complication. Acute flexion of the elbow is dangerous. Whenever applying a cast to an arm, the antecubital space should be kept free, even placing a soft fluff of cotton there to keep away the plaster. Pressure should be avoided along the course of the brachial vessels.

By recognizing early signs and anticipating the possibility early, when the damage is being done, circulation may be restored in time to avert the disaster. First, the limb should be freed of all encircling dressings, especially in the antecubital space. Right-angled arm casts should not be merely slit down their anterior or posterior surfaces and spread; they will not bend in 2 planes, and the pressure in the antecubital space will not be relieved. They should be split full length along both the lateral and the medial sides, and the 2 halves of plaster separated from each other, cutting all dressings down to the skin the full length. The arm should be elevated. Thorough fasciotomy is indicated. The flexor fascia should be split over the length of the muscle bellies and al-

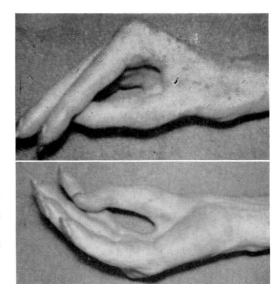

FIG. 316. Ischemic contracture in the hand. An excess of barbiturates caused a prolonged period of unconsciousness, and the hand was compressed for several hours. No forearm swelling or impairment. Flexion of index and middle fingers blocked by fixed thumb.

lowed to gape. There should be a jog in the incision at the crease of the elbow. The most important site for this is the antecubital space across the bicipital fascia. The arteries and the veins should be inspected carefully and freed from pressure or constriction. The fascia should be allowed to gape, but the skin should be reclosed at once by suture or skin graft, for, if left exposed, muscles are easy prey to bacteria. Repeated sympathetic block will increase the circulation. A supracondylar fracture should be reduced, though Fleming reports a cure by fasciotomy 48 hours after the onset, in which the fracture was not set until 1 week later. The pulse returned in 12 hours, and the fingers could be extended. Areas of pressure necrosis from casts should be excised and skin grafted, and the digits and the wrist should be splinted in extension and maintained in this position until the morbid process in the muscles has disappeared.

Conservative treatment should be given a good trial first. The contracted muscles and joints should be slowly, steadily and gently

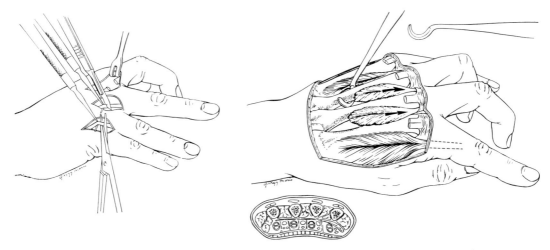

FIG. 317. (*Left*) Method for tenotomy of the lateral bands. This is done for severe interosseus contracture when very little function of the interosseus muscle remains. After operation, the hand is immobilized in the claw position. (*Right*) Method of stripping and advancing the interosseus muscles in order to slacken them, thus allowing the proximal finger joints to extend and the distal 2 to flex. The interosseus muscles of 2 of the clefts have been stripped. The insert shows a cross section through the middle of the hand. Stripping of the interossei is done only when these muscles still retain considerable function. The nerve supply should be spared. (J. Bone Joint Surg. *35-A*:90)

drawn out by splints until the contracted tissues grow longer. Forceful or intermittent traction is harmful. The splints should be removed several times a day for exercise of the fingers. When the contractures are drawn out, the muscle balance restored somewhat and exercise allowed, it is surprising to see the improvement in nutrition and use of the hand. First, the digits should be straightened by flexing the wrist, being splinted in this position between 2 flat, well-padded pieces of metal strapped on them front and back. Extending from the dorsal piece is a lever rod which, when drawn toward the back of the forearm, extends the fingers in their proximal joints. Then the cockup splint is added to dorsiflex the wrist gradually. Care must be used not to traumatize the insensitive fingers. Gentle pressure with a rubber sponge against their pulps can be used to draw them toward a dorsal extension splint. As long as there is improvement, even through several months, this method should be continued. As the posi-

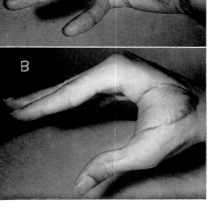

FIG. 318. (A) Showing ischemic contracture of the interossei and the thenar muscles, which was caused by suspending the arm by the wrist for 2 days in order to elevate it after an operation. (B) Showing improvement of the hand after some interossei had been stripped and others tenotomized, and the fibrous muscles in the thumb cleft had been excised and a pedicle graft applied. (J. Bone Joint Surg. *35-A*:98)

tion of function is obtained and the arm is used actively, more muscle bellies will become active. (For splints, see Chap. 6.) Sympathectomy relieves pain and increases blood supply.

After the limit of conservative treatment has been reached, operation is advisable. The problem is to place the hand into the position of function and, utilizing any active muscles available, to give flexion to the digits and opposition to the thumb. In mild cases, where some muscle power is still present but the limited motion is in the wrong range because of the contracture, a displacement of muscle origins distally lets the wrist and the fingers extend and allows active motion to be in a useful arc.

In more severe cases the damaged muscle should be removed, and motion supplied by tendon transfer.

When the forearm is opened, the fascia should be slit to liberate muscles, nerves and vessels. Muscles reduced to solid scar should be excised. For the deformity of pronation, the pronator teres and the pronator quadratus may be severed or, if fibrous, excised, and the forearm forced into supination. Flexion contracture of the elbow may be relieved by excising the scar tissue there, together with the anterior capsule of the joint.

Seddon recommends postponing reconstructive procedures until the tissue reaction is gone and then, after excising the damaged muscles, restoring flexor power by transfer of a wrist extensor to the profundi. He places great emphasis on the sensory loss and recommends nerve transfer, ulnar to median in the severe cases.

The median nerve is severely damaged in an ischemic contracture of the forearm. This loss of blood supply may be due directly to arterial block, as Seddon suggests, or due to compression and squeezing out of the blood supply by the surrounding damaged muscles. Some evidence indicates that early decompression of the nerve, done before the fibrous contracture takes place, may allow some recovery of the nerve.

Shortening of the forearm bones, as pre-

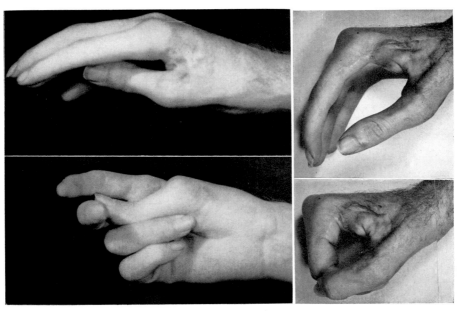

Fig. 319. The hand had been crushed and a cast applied. (*Left*) Showing the scars from pressure sores and the position in contracture of the intrinsic muscles of both the interossei and the thumb cleft. The contracted muscles of the thumb cleft were excised; the index finger was "filleted" and transferred on a neurovascular pedicle to cover the thumb cleft. (*Right*) Showing the postoperative result. (J. Bone Joint Surg. *35-A*:93)

viously recommended, is seldom indicated, since the muscle slide can give the same results. Tendon lengthening is not often done because it results in weakening of the power.

In some very severe contractures it may be necessary to fuse the wrist and thus make all the wrist movers available for transfer to the digits.

LOCAL INTRINSIC CONTRACTURE IN THE HAND

Fibrous contracture of the intrinsic muscles of the hand produces a condition quite similar to Volkmann's ischemic contracture of the forearm. Direct muscle injury, persistent spasm as in rheumatoid disease or prolonged parkinsonism, also may be causes. Bunnell called it intrinsic contracture, local in the hand.

The hand is in the normal position of function when there is proper balance between its long flexors, its long extensors and its intrinsic muscles. If the intrinsic muscles are paralyzed, the hand assumes the "intrinsic-minus" position, or that of the paralytic clawhand. The metacarpophalangeal joints are cocked back, the distal 2 finger joints are clawed, the metacarpal arch is lost, and the thumb is drawn to the side and back of the hand.

If, however, the intrinsic muscles overpull, as in spastic conditions, under electric stimulation or in fibrous contracture, the opposite or "intrinsic-plus" position is assumed. The proximal finger joints are flexed, the distal 2 finger joints are extended, the metacarpal arch is excessively curved, and the straight thumb is drawn by the short adductor muscles into the palm toward the third metacarpal.

This condition of intrinsic-plus position is recognized readily by simple tests.

The cause of the ischemic contracture is decreased blood supply in the hand, less from a complete arterial shut-off, which creates gangrene at the tips of the digits, than from a local congestion or lessening of the circulation, as in the Volkmann type. The most common cause is swelling of the hand in a plaster-of-Paris encasement or even in too tight an elastic bandage. The tightness may be over the whole limb, or it may be in the hand or in only a part of it. Just as in Volkmann's ischemic contracture, where there are often telltale signs of pressure such as scars from necrosis in the antecubital space and the sides of the wrist, so in this entity such scars commonly are found about the hypothenar eminence, the thenar eminence or the radial border of the hand.

The contracture also may follow gross damage to the great vessels and the nerves well up the arm, as is seen in the Volkmann type, and it may accompany Volkmann's ischemic contracture of the forearm, or it may occur entirely independent of it. In most cases, both the fingers and the thumb cleft are involved,

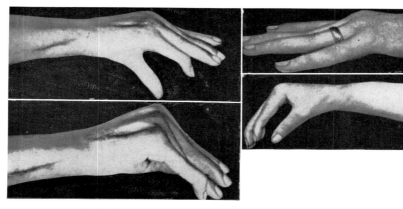

FIG. 320. (*Left*) Intrinsic contracture from crushing injury of arm and forearm and plaster immobilization for 2 months. (*Right, top*) Intrinsic contracture from fracture of humerus. Telltale scar of cast on ulnar border of hand. Similar scar on radial border. (*Right, bottom*) Extension of fingers following crushing injury of carpus.

but in some the involvement in either may be paramount. In a few, the contracture is more local from direct injury confined to part of the thenar eminence or in a lumbrical or an interosseus muscle.

SIGNS

This entity is recognizable by the characteristic posture of the hand with the proximal finger joints in flexion, the distal 2 joints in extension and the straight thumb in the palm. The thumb, from contracture of the adductor, blocks the complete flexion of index and middle fingers and, from shortening of the abductor brevis, may stand out from the palm. The diagnosis may be verified by the following test: For contracture of the interosseus or the lumbrical muscles, these are made taut by passively forcing the metacarpophalangeal joints into extension. Then tapping on the fingernail will meet with such resistance that the distal 2 finger joints cannot be flexed, while they flex readily if the metacarpophalangeal joints are held in flexion.

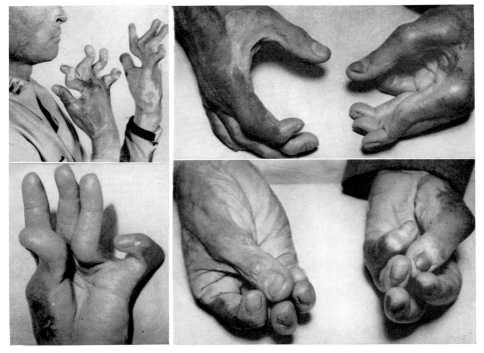

FIG. 321. Four years previously, the hands and the face of this patient had been burned severely in an airplane crash. Several skin-grafting procedures had been done on the hands. Following one of these, 1 year before the picture on the left was taken, the elastic bandages of the compression dressings had been left on for 12 days. When these were removed, the hands showed discoloration and necrosis in the thenar eminences. (*Left*) After 3 months, severe deformities from contracture of the intrinsic muscles developed. At that time, the patient was not able to hold even a piece of paper. (*Right*) Showing the postoperative results. Tenotomies were done on the lateral bands, and the fibrous musculature of the thumb clefts was excised. It was necessary also to sever the collateral ligaments and the volar capsule in some of the fingers and the capsule of the carpometacarpal joint of the thumbs, both in front and in back. Web contractures were attended to, and several of the middle and the distal finger joints were arthrodesed in the position of function. The result in appearance and function was very good, considering the extreme degree of previous crippling. (J. Bone Joint Surg. *35-A*:100)

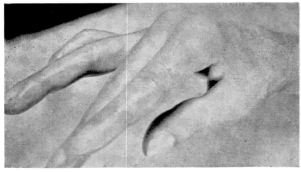

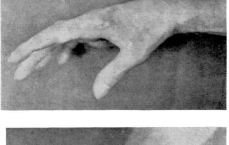

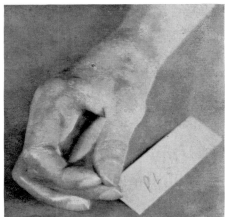

FIG. 322. (*Top, left*) Local ischemic contracture. History of tight cast holding the hand clumped because of fracture of the humerus. Contracture is worst in the thenar adductors and the interossei of the first 2 digits, but it affects all intrinsic muscles. (*Right, top* and *bottom*) Corrected muscle balance allows function and a position of function. The thenar adductors were disconnected, the interossei were stripped from the metacarpals and postoperative fixation was in the position of clawhand. (Donald R. Pratt, M.D.)

If there is contracture of the thenar muscles, the thenar eminence feels indurated, and an attempt to widen the angle between the 1st and the 3rd metacarpals meets with rigid resistance, since the adductors of the thumb and, secondarily, all other tissues have contracted.

SYMPTOMS

The main complaint is that the hand cannot be opened for grasping. The thumb is in the way and cannot be extended from its position in the hand, and the metacarpophalangeal joints cannot open from their flexed position. There may also be complaints of weakness, numbness, anesthesia, induration and signs of poor nutrition of tissues.

TREATMENT

Prophylactically, great care should be used to avoid swelling of the hand or the arm in tight encasements. When a hand is in a tight cast, the blood supply is squeezed out, and all intrinsic muscles are rendered ischemic and then contract. If the hand is clumped, the adductor muscles of the thumb suffer most. When the condition is discovered, relief should be undertaken immediately.

Later, in surgical correction, the aim is to

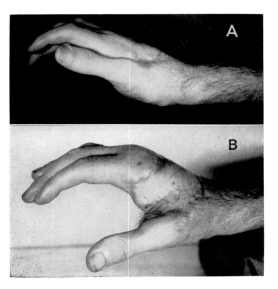

FIG. 323. (A) Following a direct crush to the hand and infection, contracture developed in the thumb cleft and in the interossei muscles. (B) The muscles were excised from the thumb cleft, and the position of the thumb was corrected by a wedge osteotomy. A pedicle graft was applied. The extensor proprius tendon was transferred to the lateral band of the index finger, with the result shown in this picture. (J. Bone Joint Surg. *35-A*:99)

release or divide the contracted interossei and to open out the thumb cleft. However, one cannot expect to restore voluntary action to fibrotic, contracted muscles.

Fingers. For the fingers, one should decide whether to advance the interosseus muscles, their function being retained as in the Steindler stripping operation in the foot or the muscle-slide operation for ischemic contracture of the forearm, or to discard them and tenotomize the insertion into the lateral bands. If the origins are stripped, the nerve supply which enters the volar aspect should be preserved.

In mild cases with good interosseus function, the elastic reverse knuckle-bender splint may extend the metacarpophalangeal joints, and there may be some tendency to recover.

The examiner can demonstrate function by feeling the lateral bands in action at the sides of the fingers, by noting ability to spread the fingers and pinch between them, as well as the ability to extend the distal 2 finger joints. If function is present, a stripping or advancement operation is indicated; but, if not, tenotomy must be done.

With a small curved periosteal elevator inserted through the dorsum, the interossei are separated from the metacarpals and allowed to advance distally until the proximal finger joints will extend and the distal 2 will flex. Stripping is from metacarpal head toward the base. Postoperative splinting in the intrinsic-minus position must be maintained.

If the intrinsic muscles are too fibrous to

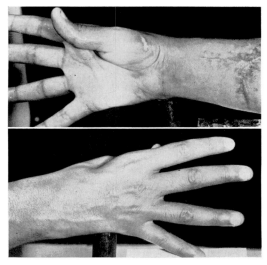

FIG. 324. Intrinsic contracture from severe lacerated wound of forearm. Proximal finger joints are not restricted but in full extension, flexion of middle and distal joints is impossible. Note telltale scars on thenar and hypothenar areas from pressure of bandages.

function or if a trial at stripping is not successful, tenotomies should be done through a short longitudinal incision in the dorsal aspect of each of the 3 finger webs until the fingers can be fully flexed when their metacarpophalangeal joints are extended. It may be necessary also to sever collateral or volar ligaments.

In severe cases, the primary deformity is the flexion of the proximal joints. This flexion

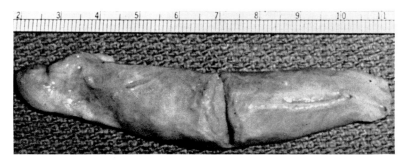

FIG. 325. Localized Volkmann's ischemia in forearm muscle. Three months after a compression injury of the forearm without fracture or open wound, a contracture of the profundi of the ring and the little fingers was present. This mass of "infarcted" muscle was excised, the palmaris longus tapped into the distal tendon, and full motion returned.

contracture cannot be overcome unless the muscle origins are displaced distally or the tendons are divided proximal to the joint level. Unless the proximal joints can be extended passively, there is no indication for the so-called release operation which divides the wing fibers of the extensor. Since it is the proximally inserted interossei attached to the phalanges that maintain the flexion, these must be divided. Only in mild cases, where the proximal joints can be extended passively and only the flexion of the middle joints is lacking, will tenotomy distal to the proximal joint level suffice.

Thumb. Skeletal traction for spreading of the thumb succeeds only in the mildest cases. Surgical repair is done by cutting across the thumb cleft from hinge to hinge, that is, from the juncture of the first 2 metacarpals in the front to that in back. Then the fascia of the cleft is excised, and the various contracted muscles are stripped from the bones and tenotomized or excised according to their degree of fibrosis. The first interosseus muscle may be stripped from both metacarpals, and the origin of the adductors of the thumb may be scraped from the 3rd metacarpal. All degrees of fibrous, degenerated, contracted muscle may be found. The pathologic changes are the same as those found in the muscles in Volkmann's ischemic contracture. Often the whole solid fibrous mass must be excised; even so, the first 2 metacarpals may not spread until the joint capsule is cut across. Here the deep branch of the radial artery should be identified and protected.

The spread of the thumb cleft must be maintained, either by the temporary insertion of 2 Kirschner wires crossing through the first 2 metacarpals or by a bone block pinned between them. New skin must be placed as a long diamond-shaped graft across the cleft from hinge to hinge, either by a free graft which is poor and unsightly or by an abdominal pedicle graft which furnishes fat to fill the space. This is usually done in 1 stage as a pedicle procedure. Tendon transfers for opposition and adduction of the thumb may be necessary later.

Spasm and later contracture of the intrinsic muscles in the hand frequently are observed in rheumatic hands, with grotesque deformity. Here it is not the result of ischemia but the end-result of the fibrosis from prolonged spasm and the inflammatory disease process. The intrinsic-plus sign is found early in rheumatoid hands. (See Chap. 9, Surgery of the Rheumatoid Hand, and Chap. 12, Intrinsic Muscles, for details.)

RESULTS OF TREATMENT

In severe contractures, results cannot be excellent, because there is too much induration, fibrous contracture, tissue damage and poor nutrition. However, a hand may be placed into a much better position for function and made so that it can open for grasping; thus the main disability of this condition may be overcome.

A summary of 25 cases with characteristic findings was reported by Bunnell in 1953.

BIBLIOGRAPHY

Barsky, A. J.: Surgical repair of unusual dermatological conditions, Surg. Clin. N. Amer. *19*: 459, 1939.

Blair, V. P., and Brown, J. B.: The use and uses of large split grafts of intermediate thickness, Surg., Gynec. Obstet. *49*:82, 1929.

Böhler, J., and Streli, R.: The use of flaps in the repair of the extremities, Minerva Chir. *16*: 1467, 1961.

Bojsen-Møller, J., Pers, M., and Schmidt, A.: Finger-tip injuries: Late results, Acta chir. scand. *122*:177, 1961.

Brenizer, D. G.: Skin and fascia grafting, Am. J. Surg. *47*:265, 1940.

Brown, D. O.: Repairs of limb wounds by the use of direct skin-flaps, Brit. J. Surg. *30*:307, 1943.

Brown, J. B.: Surface defects of hand, Am. J. Surg. *46*:690, 1939.

————: The closure of surface defects with free skin grafts and with pedicle flaps, Surg., Gynec. Obstet. *84*:862, 1947.

Brown, J. B., and McDowell, F.: Persistence of function of skin grafts through long periods of growth, Surg., Gynec. Obstet. *72*:848, 1941.

————: Skin Grafting of Burns: Primary Care, Treatment, Repair, Philadelphia, Lippincott, 1943.

Bunnell, S.: Contractures of the hand from infections and injuries, J. Bone Joint Surg. *14*: 27, 1932.

————: Plastic problems in the hand, Plast. Reconstr. Surg. *1*:265, 1946.

Byars, L. T.: Free full-thickness skin grafts; principles involved and technique of application, Surg., Gynec. Obstet. *75*:8, 1942,

Cannon, B., and Peacock, E. E., Jr.: Plastic surgery, the hand, New Engl. J. Med. *263*:184, 1960.

Clarkson, P., and Lawrie, R. S.: The management and surgical resurfacing of serious burns, Brit. J. Surg. *33*:311, 1946.

Converse, J. M.: Skin graft of dorsum of hand, Ann. Surg. *121*:172, 1945.

Conway, H.: Sweating function of transplanted skin, Surg., Gynec. Obstet. *69*:756, 1939.

Conway, H., and Stark, R. B.: Arterial vascularization of the soft tissues of the hand, J. Bone Joint Surg. *35*:1238, 1954.

Conway, J. H.: Technical details in skin grafting, Surg., Gynec. Obstet. *63*:369, 1936.

Cronin, T. D.: The cross finger flap—a new method of repair, Am. Surg. *17*:419, 1951.

Curtis, R. M.: Cross finger pedicle flap in hand surgery, Clin. Orthop. *9*:205, 1957.

Cuthbert, J. B.: The late treatment of dorsal injuries of the hand associated with loss of skin, Brit. J. Surg. *33*:66, 1945.

Davis, J. S.: Plastic Surgery, Philadelphia, Blakiston, 1919.

————: Use of small deep grafts in repair of surface defects, Am. J. Surg. *47*:280, 1940.

————: Address of the president; story of plastic surgery, Ann. Surg. *113*:641, 1941.

Davis, J. S., and Traut, H. F.: Origin and development of blood supply of grafts, Ann. Surg. *82*:871, 1925.

deHaan, C. R., and Stark, R. B.: Changes in efferent circulation of tubed pedicles and in the transplantability of large composite grafts produced by histamine iontophoresis, Plast. Reconstr. Surg. *28*:577, 1961.

DeJongh, E.: Simple plastic procedure of the fingers for conserving bony tissue and forming a soft tissue pad, Am. J. Surg. *57*:346, 1942.

Farmer, A. W., and Woolhouse, F. M.: Resurfacing of dorsum of the hand following burns, Ann. Surg. *122*:39, 1945.

Flatt, A. E.: The thenar flap, J. Bone Joint Surg. *39-B*:80, 1957.

Flynn, I. E.: Adduction contracture of thumb, New Engl. J. Med. *254*:677, 1956.

Gerrie, J. W.: Choice of skin grafts in plastic surgery, Canad. M. A. J. *44*:9, 1941.

Gillies, H.: Design of direct pedicle flaps, Brit. M. J. *2*:1008, 1932.

————: Experience with tubed pedicle flaps, Surg., Gynec. Obstet. *60*:291, 1935.

————: Practical uses of tubed pedicle flap, Am. J. Surg. *43*:201, 1939.

Gottlieb, O., and Mathiesen, F. R.: Thenar flaps and cross-finger flaps, Acta chir. scand. *122*:166, 1961.

Greeley, P. W.: Plastic repair of extensor contractures following deep second degree burns, J. Am. Soc. Plast. & Reconstr. Surg. *12*:79, 1943.

————: Plastic repair of burned hand, Am. Acad. Orthop. Surg. Lect., p. 169, 1944.

————: Plastic repair of extensor hand contractures following healed deep second degree burns, Surgery *15*:173, 1944.

————: Practical procedures for the correction of scar contractures of the hand, Am. J. Surg. *72*:622, 1947.

Hardy, S. B.: Principles in covering surface defects of the hand, Clin. Orthop, *13*:63, 1959.

Havens, F. Z.: Preoperative and postoperative care in skin grafting, Surg. Clin. N. Amer. *20*:1087, 1940.

Howard, L. D.: Contracture of the thumb web, J. Bone Joint Surg. *32-A*:267, 1950.

Kelikian, H., and Doumanian, A.: Skin grafts in hand surgery, Clin. Orthop. *9*:205, 1957.

Kiskadden, W. S.: Use of flaps and pedicles in repair of hand and arm defects, Am. Acad. Orthop. Surg. Lect., p. 180, 1944.

Kitlowski, E. A.: Preservation of tendon function by use of skin flaps, Am. J. Surg. *51*:653, 1941.

Koch, S. L.: Complicated contractures of hand; their treatment by freeing fibrosed tendons and replacing destroyed tendons with grafts, Ann. Surg. *98*:546, 1933.

Koch, S. L., and Kanavel, A. B.: Contractures due to burns; treatment with free full-thickness grafts and pedunculated flaps, Tr. Sect. Surg., Gen. & Abd., A. M. A., p. 208, 1928.

McCarroll, H. R.: Immediate application of free full-thickness skin graft for traumatic amputation of finger, J. Bone Joint Surg. *26*:489, 1944.

McCash, C. R.: Cross-arm bridge flaps in repair of flexion contractures of fingers, Brit. J. Plast. Surg. *9*:25, 1956.

Macomber, W. B.: Plastic considerations of burn scars and contractures of hand and forearm, Am. Acad. Orthop. Surg. Lect., p. 174, 1944.

Macomber, W. B., and Patton, H. S.: The split thickness graft—a useful adjunct in tube pedicle preparation, Surg., Gynec. Obstet. *84*:97, 1947.

————: Improved grafting technic for burns of the extremity, Am. J. Surg. *78*:684, 1947.

Macomber, W. B., and Rubin, L. R.: Late repair of massive tissue defects by the split skin-lined flap graft, Am. J. Surg. *73*:564, 1947.

Maltz, M.: New method of tube pedicle skin grafting, J. Internat. Coll. Surg. *3*:526, 1940.

Markee, J. E., Wray, J., Nork, J., and McFalls, F.: A quantitative study of the vascular beds of the hand, J. Bone Joint Surg. *43-A*:1187, 1961.

Mason, M. L.: Plastic surgery of hands, Surg. Clin. N. Amer. *19*:227, 1939.

———: Plastic surgery and repair with particular reference to cutaneous defects of hand, Indust. Med. *10*:47, 1941.

Moroney, P. B.: Conservation of the metacarpus by skin and bone grafting in three patients, Brit. J. Surg. *32*:464, 1945.

Moynihan, F. J.: Long term results of split-skin grafting in finger tip injuries, Brit. M. J. *2*:802, 1961.

Murless, B. C.: Fracture-dislocation of the base of the fifth metacarpal bone, Brit. J. Surg. *31*:402, 1944.

Padgett, E. C.: Full-thickness skin graft in correction of soft tissue deformities, J.A.M.A. *98*:18, 1932.

———: Skin grafting in severe burns, Am. J. Surg. *43*:626, 1939.

———: Calibrated intermediate skin grafts, Surg., Gynec. Obstet. *69*:779, 1939.

———: Skin grafting and "three-quarter"-thickness skin graft for prevention and correction of cicatricial formation, Ann. Surg. *113*:1034, 1941.

———: Skin Grafting from a Personal and Experimental Viewpoint, Springfield, Ill., Thomas, 1942.

Peer, L. A.: Fate of buried skin grafts in man, Arch. Surg. *39*:131, 1939.

Peer, L. A., and Paddock, R.: Histologic studies on fate of deeply implanted dermal grafts; observations on sections of implants buried from one week to one year, Arch. Surg. *34*:268, 1937.

Peer, L. A., and Walker, J. C., Jr.: The behavior of autogenous human tissue grafts, Plast. Reconstr. Surg. *7*:6, 1951.

Pickerill, H. P., and White, J. R.: Tube skin-flap in plastic surgery, Brit. J. Surg. *9*:321, 1922.

Preston, D. J.: Mechanical superiority of annealed stainless steel wire sutures and ligatures, Surgery *9*:896, 1941.

Rank, B. K.: Use of Thiersch skin graft, Brit. M. J. *1*:846, 1940.

Shaw, D. T., and Payne, R. L., Jr.: Repair of surface defects of the upper extremity, Ann. Surg. *123*:705, 1946.

———: One stage tubed abdominal flaps, Surg., Gynec. Obstet, *83*:205, 1946.

Sheehan, J. E.: Replacement of thumb nail, J.A.M.A. *92*:1253, 1929.

———: Use of free full-thickness skin grafts, J.A.M.A. *112*:27, 1939.

Soiland, H.: Lengthening a finger with the "on-the-top" method, Acta chir. scand. *122*:184, 1961.

Stracker, O.: Contracture of thumb in children, Wien. klin. Wchr. *44*:197, 1931.

Sutton, L. E.: Use of tubed pedicle flaps for study of wound healing in human skin, N. Y. J. Med. *40*:852, 1940.

Swanker, W. A.: Reconstructive surgery of the injured nail, Am. J. Surg. *74*:341, 1947.

Wright, C. S., and Guequierre, J. P.: Cutaneous diseases of the extremities and their relation to surgery, Am. J. Surg. *44*:322, 1939.

Zintel, H. A.: Resplitting split-thickness grafts with dermatome; method for increasing yield of limited donor sites, Ann. Surg. *121*:1, 1945.

DUPUYTREN'S

Adams, H. D.: Dupuytren's contracture, Lahey Clinic Bull. *2*:75, 1941.

———: Dupuytren's contracture, Surg. Clin. N. Amer. *22*:899, 1942.

Allen, R. A., et al.: Soft tissue tumors of the sole (Dupuytren's), J. Bone Joint Surg. *37-A*:14, 1955.

Arieff, A. J., and Bell, J. L.: Epilepsy and Dupuytren's contracture, Neurology *6*:115, 1956.

Barclay, T.: Edema following operation for Dupuytren's contracture, Plast. Reconstr. Surg. *23*:349, 1959.

Boyes, J. H.: Dupuytren's contracture, Am. J. Surg. *88*:147, 1954.

Callomon, F. F.: Induratio penis plastica; problem of its etiology and pathogenesis, Urol. Cutan. Rev. *49*:742, 1945.

Clarkson, P.: The aetiology of Dupuytren's disease, Guy's Hosp. Rep. *110*:52, 1961.

Clay, R. C.: Dupuytren's contracture: Fibroma of the palmar fascia, Ann. Surg. *120*:224, 1944.

Conway, H.: Dupuytren's contracture, Am. J. Surg. *87*:101, 1954.

Davis, A. A.: Treatment of Dupuytren's contracture, Brit. J. Surg. *19*:539, 1932.

Davis, J. S.: Dupuytren's contracture, Arch. Surg. *24*:933, 1932.

Deming, E. G.: Y-V advancement pedicles in surgery for Dupuytren's contracture, Plast. Reconstr. Surg. *29*:581, 1962.

Dudley, H. D.: Dupuytren's contracture, Northwest. Med. *38*:138, 1939.

Dupuytren, G.: Permanent retraction of the fingers produced by an affection of the palmar fascia, Lancet *2*:222, 1834.

———: Dupuytren's contracture; retraction of fingers following disease of palmar aponeurosis; description of disease; surgical therapy, Med. Classics *4*:127, 1939. (Reprint)

———: Permanent retraction of fingers produced by affection of palmar fascia, Med. Classics *4*:142, 1939. (Reprint)

Early, P. F.: Population studies in Dupuytren's

contracture, J. Bone Joint Surg. *44-B*:602, 1962.

Gill, A. B.: Dupuytren's contracture, Ann. Surg. *107*:122, 1938.

Granbard, D. J.: Dupuytren's contracture, J. Internat. Coll. Surg. *21*:15, 1954.

Greenberg, L.: Dupuytren's contracture of palmar and plantar fasciae, J. Bone Joint Surg. *21*:785, 1939.

Hamlin, E.: Limited excision of Dupuytren's contracture, Ann. Surg. *155*:454, 1962.

Hancock, J. D.: Dupuytren's contracture, Kentucky M. J. *38*:290, 1940.

Harper, W. F.: Distribution of palmar aponeurosis in relation to Dupuytren's contracture of the thumb, J. Anat. *69*:193, 1935.

Hayward: Surgery of Dupuytren's contracture, Med. Klin. *27*:1721, 1931.

Horwitz, T.: Dupuytren's contracture: A consideration of the anatomy of the fibrous structures of the hand in relation to this condition; with an interpretation of the history, Arch. Surg. *44*:687, 1942.

Howard, L. D., Jr.: Dupuytren's contracture, a guide to management, Clin. Orthop. *15*:118, 1957.

Hueston, J. T.: Incidence of Dupuytren's contracture, Med. J. Aust. *47 (2)*:999, 1960.

————: Limited fasciectomy for Dupuytren's contracture, Plast. Reconstr. Surg. *27*:569, 1961.

James, J., and Tubiana, R.: La maladie de Dupuytren, Revue chir. orthop. *38*:352, 1952.

Kanavel, A. B., Koch, S. L., and Mason, M. L.: Dupuytren's contracture, Surg., Gynec. Obstet. *48*:145, 1929.

Kaplan, E. B.: Palmar fascia in connection with Dupuytren's contracture, Surgery *4*:415, 1938.

————: Operation for Dupuytren's contracture based on anatomy of palmar fascia, Bull. Russian Med. Soc. N. Y., p. 78, 1939.

Koch, S. L.: Dupuytren's contracture, J.A.M.A. *100*:878, 1933.

Larsen, R. D., and Posch, J. L.: Dupuytren's contracture, J. Bone Joint Surg. *40-A*:773, 1958.

Luck, J. V.: Dupuytren's contracture, J. Bone Joint Surg. *41-A*:4, 1959.

McIndoe, A.: Surgical management of Dupuytren's contracture, Am. J. Surg. *95*:197, 1958.

Meyerding, H. W.: Treatment of Dupuytren's contracture, Am. J. Surg. *49*:94, 1940.

Meyerding, H. W., Black, J. R., and Broders, A. C.: Etiology and pathology of Dupuytren's contracture, Surg., Gynec. Obstet. *72*:582, 1941.

Moorhead, J. L.: Trauma and Dupuytren's contracture, Am. J. Surg. *85*:352, 1953.

Niederland, W.: The relation of Dupuytren's contracture to occupation, Arch. Gewerbepath. *3*:22, 1932.

Pederson, H. E.: Dupuytren's disease of the foot, J.A.M.A. *154*:33, 1954.

Riedl, L.: Dupuytren's contracture: Report of 30 cases—1932-1938, Zbl. Chir. *66*:1093, 1939.

Schroder, C. H.: Occupation and trauma in Dupuytren's contracture, Deutsche Z. Chir. *244*:140, 1934.

————: Heredity of Dupuytren's contracture, Zbl. Chir. *61*:1056, 1934.

Skinner, H. L.: Dupuytren's contracture; operative correction by use of tunnel skin graft, Surgery *10*:313, 1941.

Skoog, T.: Dupuytren's contraction with special reference to aetiology and improved surgical treatment: Its occurrence in epileptics; note on knuckle pads, Acta chir. scand., vol. 96, suppl. 139, 1948.

Smith, K. D., and Masters, W. E.: Dupuytren's contracture among upholsterers, J. Indust. Hyg. Toxicol. *21*:97, 1939.

Stern, E. L.: A new operative procedure for Dupuytren's contracture, Am. J. Surg. *54*:711, 1941.

Teleky, L.: Dupuytren's contracture as occupational disease, J. Indust. Hyg. Toxicol. *21*:233, 1939.

Tubiana, R.: Prognosis and treatment of Dupuytren's contracture, J. Bone Joint Surg. *37-A*:1155, 1955.

VOLKMANN'S

Brooks, B.: Experimental study of Volkmann's paralysis, Arch. Surg. *5*:188, 1922.

Brooks, B., Johnson, G. S., and Kirtley, J. A.: Simultaneous vein ligation, Surg., Gynec. Obstet. *59*:496, 1934.

Bruce, J.: Localized Volkmann contracture, J. Bone Joint Surg. *22*:738, 1940.

Bunnell, S.: Ischemic contracture, local, in the hand, J. Bone Joint Surg. *35-A*:101, 1953.

Bunnell, S., Doherty, E. W., and Curtis, R. M.: Ischemic contracture, local, in the hand, Plast. Reconstr. Surg. *3*:424, 1948.

Burman, M. S., and Sutro, C. J.: Brief communications; experimental ischemic contracture, Ann. Surg. *100*:559, 1934.

Cohen, H. H.: Adjustable volar-flexion splint for Volkmann's contracture, J. Bone Joint Surg. *24*:189, 1942.

D'Harcourt, J., and D'Harcourt, M.: A contribution to the study of Volkmann's ischemic contracture, Madrid Med. *6*:237, 1935.

De Nuce: Ischemic contracture, Rev. d'orthop. *20*:97, 1909.

Fleming, C. W.: Case of impending Volkmann's ischemic contracture treated by incision of deep fascia, Lancet *2*:293, 1931.

Foisie, P. S.: Volkmann's ischemic contracture, New Engl. J. Med. *226*:671, 1942.

Garber, J. N.: Volkmann's contracture as complication of fractures of forearm and elbow, J. Bone Joint Surg. *21*:154, 1939.

Glen, F. W.: Vascular injuries complicating supracondylar fractures of humerus in children, with case report, Bull. Jackson Mem. Hosp. *3*:29, 1941.

Griffiths, D. L.: Volkmann's ischemic contracture, Lancet *2*:1339, 1938.

————: Volkmann's ischemic contracture, Brit. J. Surg. *28*:239, 1940.

Guilleminet: Results of therapy on Volkmann's contracture, Lyon Chir. *36*:232, 1939.

Hill, R. L.: Volkmann's ischemic contracture in hemophilia, Tr. Hawaii Territor. Med. Assn., p. 26, 1929.

Hill, R. L., and Brooks, B.: Volkmann's ischemic contracture in hemophilia, Ann. Surg. *103*:444, 1936.

Holmes, W., Highet, W. B., and Seddon, H. J.: Nerve lesions occurring in Volkmann's contracture, Brit. J. Surg. *32*:259, 1944.

Horwitz, T.: Significance of venous circulation about elbow in patho-mechanics of Volkmann's contracture, Surg., Gynec. Obstet. *74*:871, 1942.

Jepson, P. N.: Ischemic contracture, Ann. Surg. *84*:785, 1926.

Jones, E. B.: Volkmann's ischemia; observations at open operation, Brit. M. J. *1*:1053, 1940.

Jones, Sir R.: Address on Volkmann's ischemic contracture with special reference to treatment, Brit. M. J. *2*:639, 1928.

Jones, S. G.: Volkmann's contracture, Am. J. Surg. *43*:325, 1939.

Laigle, L.: Evolution of ideas concerning Volkmann's syndrome, Médecine *19*:893, 1938.

Massart, R.: Volkmann's disease, ischemic contraction of the flexor muscles of the fingers: Pathogenesis and treatment, Presse Méd. *43*:1695, 1935.

Meyerding, H. W.: Volkmann's ischemic contracture, J.A.M.A. *94*:394, 1930.

————: Volkmann's ischemic contracture, Surg. Clin. N. Amer. *10*:49, 1930.

————: Fracture of elbow and Volkmann's ischemic contracture, Minn. Med. *22*:100, 1939.

Meyerding, H. W., and Krusen, F. H.: Treatment of Volkmann's ischemic contracture, Ann. Surg. *110*:417, 1939.

Middleton, D. S.: Discussion of Volkmann's ischemic contracture, Lancet, *2*:299, 1928.

Mitchell, W. J., and Adams, J. P.: Effective management for supracondylar fractures of the humerus in children, Clin. Orthop. *23*:197, 1962.

Paltrinieri, M.: Hematoma—ischemic contracture of Volkmann type in hemophilia; role of hematoma in contracture, Bull. sc. Med., Bologna *111*:203, 1939.

Parkes, A. R.: Traumatic ischaemia of peripheral nerves, with some observations on Volkmann's ischaemic contracture, Brit. J. Surg. *32*:403, 1945.

————: The treatment of established Volkmann's contracture by tendon transplantation, J. Bone Joint Surg. *33-B*:359, 1951.

Plewes, L. W.: Occlusion of brachial artery and Volkmann's ischemic contracture, Brit. M. J. *1*:1054, 1940.

Pollock, G. A.: Early operation for Volkmann's ischaemic contracture, Brit. M. J. *1*:783, 1944.

Pusitz, M. E.: Abortive treatment of Volkmann's ischemia, J. Kansas M. Soc. *35*:448, 1934.

Seddon, H. J.: Volkmann's Contracture: Treatment by excision of the infarct. J. Bone Joint Surg. *38-B*:152, 1956.

————: L'ischémie de Volkmann, Rev. chir. orthop. *46*:149, 1960.

Smyth, E. H. J.: Primary rupture of brachial artery and median nerve in supracondylar fracture of the humerus, J. Bone Joint Surg. *38-B*:3, 1956.

Stanford, S.: Traumatic ischemia in forearm and leg, Lancet *1*:462, 1944.

Steindler, A.: Ischemic contracture, Surg., Gynec. Obstet. *62*:358, 1936.

Chapter 8

Bones

In this chapter bones are considered from the standpoint of reconstruction, i.e., deformities, malunion, nonunion, acquired defects and avascular degeneration. See Chapter 16 for treatment of fractures and dislocations.

Operations on the bones should follow replacement of cicatrix by good skin and should precede the repair of tendons.

CORRECTION OF DEFORMITIES

MALUNION

When the bones of the forearm, the metacarpals or the phalanges are in abnormal alignment, the balance of the hand is disturbed, and there follows strain, pain and impaired function. In malunion, tendons pull at wrong angles and with the wrong leverage. If metacarpals unite with volar angulation, the flexor tendons will be relaxed and the extensor tendons tightened. The proximal finger joints then will go into hyperextension, and the distal 2 finger joints into flexion.

In a malunited Colles' fracture with the distal fragment cocked back and the proximal part of the radius protruding into the line of pull of the flexor tendons, there will be pain as the tendons pull around the bony prominence, and the muscle balance will be upset in that the flexor tendons will be too tight, and the extensor tendons too loose.

Angulation in a limb from malunion or dislocation upsets the balanced tension of the muscles spanning from forearm to digits, causing compensatory and opposite angulations of the joints serially down the limb. If the lower ends of the forearm bones are angulated volarward, or there is a dislocation backward of the carpus or of the metacarpals on the carpus, or malunion of the metacarpals with dorsal bowing, the consequent tightening of the long extensors in being stretched over these convexities hyperextends the proximal finger joints. This in turn tightens the long flexor

tendons, drawing the distal 2 finger joints into flexion. Correction of the alignment restores muscle balance, allowing the hand and the wrist to assume again the position of function. Where there are several deformities at different levels, the proximal lesion is corrected first.

If there is malunion of metacarpals and phalanges, the digits, when flexed or extended, may move entirely out of their normal course in either a spreading or a converging way, or the thumb and the digits may no longer move along their correct planes of motion and so may no longer oppose each other. Three roentgenographic views should be routine: anteroposterior, lateral and oblique. A true lateral of a finger can be obtained by taking each finger separately.

Deformities of malunion are rotary, angulatory or overlapping. In rotary deformity of the metacarpals or the proximal or the middle phalanges, the axes of the joints distal to the fracture will be tipped, so that on flexion the digits may cross each other. Normally, on flexion the fingers should converge toward the tubercle of the scaphoid bone.

Angular deformity is often quite conspicuous from a cosmetic point of view, whether it is in the anteroposterior or the lateral plane. In malunion of the metacarpals, the distal fragment is usually angulated volarward. The head of the metacarpal projects prominently in the palm, and when the dorsal aspect of the hand is viewed, it will be seen that that knuckle has dropped and is out of alignment with the other knuckles. There may be pain and tenderness in the palm due to pressure on the projecting metacarpal head.

The deformity in the proximal phalanx is usually dorsalward angulation of the distal fragment, in which case on full flexion the finger falls far short of reaching the distal crease in the palm. The angulation dorsalward is subtracted from the angle of flexion of the finger. If the deformity happens to be volar-ward, there is a similar loss of extension of the finger.

Overlapping deformity of a metacarpal or a phalanx results in shortening of the digit. Also, as the bone ends project against the flexor and the extensor tendons, there is a tendency, just as there is in angular deformity, for the tendons to be caught in the callus of the bony union. Much disability results from fracture of the phalanges because of adhesions of the flexor and the extensor tendons.

BONE CARPENTRY

Nonunion, malunion and defects in the metacarpals and the phalanges are corrected by physiologic bone carpentry. If necessary, any overlying cicatrix must be excised and a good covering furnished by sliding dorsal skin and skin grafting the donor site, by filleting a finger and laying its skin over the defect or by a preliminary pedicle graft from the abdomen. The malunited bones should be disconnected and rejoined in their normal alignment so that once more the fingers will extend and flex in their proper planes and the fingers and the thumb oppose each other in a functioning manner. The positions of the bones should be corrected so that the tendons will move in their proper straight courses, have their proper angle of approach to the joints, and that normal leverage and proper balance will be restored. Only when the mechanics of the hand are correct can good function be restored.

Delayed union is common after corrective osteotomies on metacarpals and phalanges. Firm fixation by pinning with Kirschner wires and the use of small key grafts will ensure union. A graft for this purpose may be a small, flat but thick chip of bone chiseled from one of the long bones such as the proximal half

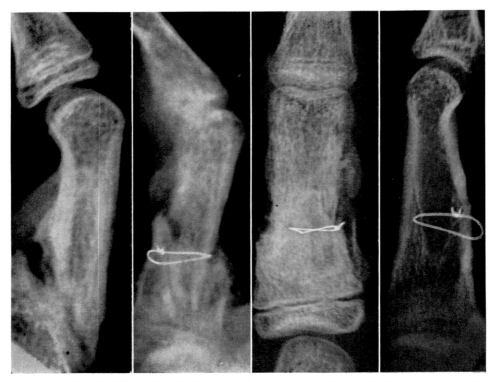

FIG. 326. Case R. M. D. (*Left*) Malunion of the proximal phalanx. Had been set 2 months previously on a roller bandage. Muscle imbalance caused the finger to be flexed. (*Center pictures*) Point of distal fragment was impaled into the proximal one, and bone chips from the ulna were packed about the juncture. One stainless-steel wire. (*Right*) Restoration of the shaft.

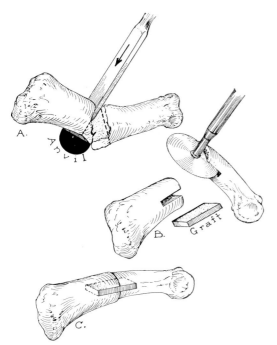

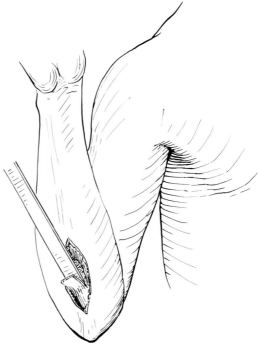

FIG. 327. Bone carpentry. A small key bone graft and a good fit ensure against nonunion. The point of an anvil is held under the phalanx to facilitate carving with an osteotome. A bone graft may be obtained easily by chiseling off a chip from the ulna of the same arm below the elbow.

FIG. 328. A convenient method of obtaining a small key bone graft from the ulna with which to unite a metacarpal or a phalanx.

of the ulna, which is uncovered through a short incision near the elbow. A saw cut is made in each bone end, and the bone graft is fitted in these two slits; the ends of the bone are shoved together over it. This spline or key graft is a traditional cabinet worker's method of joining materials; it stabilizes the junction and prevents deformity. Möberg has utilized this principle in the development of a key graft for forearm fractures.

In all bone surgery bony surfaces should be approximated so accurately and held in place so firmly that they will hold until a splint is applied. Such junctions will unite. If one attempts to join these bones by making the layers of bone too thin, even though dovetailing them, it will be found that the union will melt away because of insufficient blood supply. The surgeon's "cabinet work" should be accurate, but the parts of bone that are in contact should be massive. Frequently, bone

ends that are approximated inaccurately so that they are free to move do not unite; each time a vascular bridge forms, it will be sheared or broken until the repair effort ends and pseudarthrosis results. Certain mechanical aids facilitate the accurate shaping of bone ends; one is an anvil, with a pointed end, which fits behind the phalanx or the metacarpal and has a heavy base directly under the point. Both the base and the point are offset from the stem. The result is that when a sharp osteotome is driven across the phalanx, which is braced against the point of the anvil, the cutting will be as accurate as that used in carving an ornament out of ivory. It is important to hold the anvil exactly in the line of the chisel and the bone edge close against the anvil. The Stryker saggital saw is by far the best instrument for cutting these small bones. It is less dangerous, and its slender blade with an oscillating saw at the end fits well the width of a finger bone.

All the general principles regarding the re-

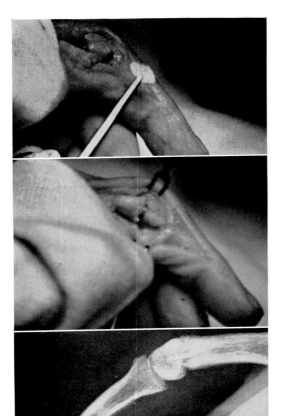

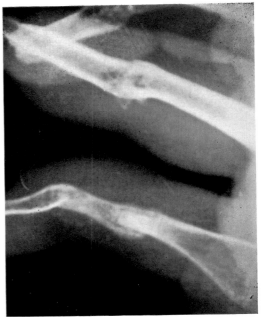

FIG. 330. Case E. S. Arthritic finger joint from an x-ray burn ankylosed by bone carpentry.

FIG. 329. (*Top*) Key bone graft (from ulna) for fracture of proximal phalanx. (*Center*) When fragments are shoved together over the spline, the fit is such as to maintain position without additional internal fixation. (*Bottom*) Healed in good position.

the point of a bone or a graft into a cancellous portion such as the carpus or the metacarpal head or the end of a phalanx so as to obtain firm fixation and ample contact to ensure union. As elsewhere, grafts should contact endosteum as well as periosteal and compact bone with maximal surface, thus obtaining blood supply and growth from each side. Fragments of these small bones may be fastened together by fine stainless steel wire through drill holes. This approximates the bones, but the fixation depends on splinting. It is preferable to pin them firmly to each other and to adjoining metacarpals.

In all metacarpal reconstruction the condi-

pair of bones apply equally to those in the hand. The periosteum should be preserved with its attachment to the soft parts intact with, if necessary, some additional osteoperiosteal or cancellous chips laid around the fracture line. Fortunately, ample bone is available for any size graft. A useful practice is to thrust

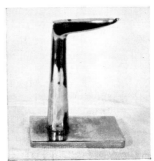

FIG. 331. A handy anvil for carving small bones with a sharp osteotome. When the point is placed under the bone, the heavy base is in the line of the stroke.

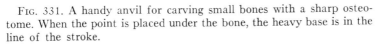

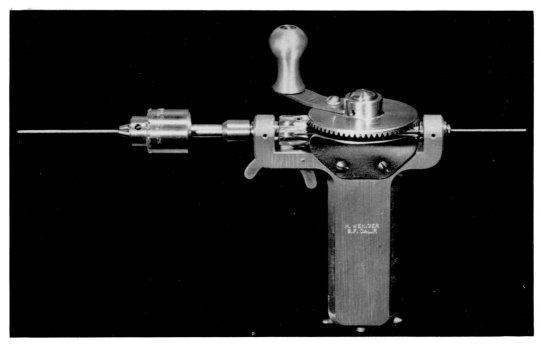

FIG. 332. Drill for pinning bones in the hand with Kirschner wires. (H. Weniger, San Francisco, Calif.)

tion of the surrounding soft parts must be considered. It the interossei are destroyed, the distal 2 joints of the fingers will not extend, i.e., the fingers will claw. In this case, one must either excise the ray or provide a substitute for the intrinsic muscles. If too many structures about the metacarpal are destroyed or are cicatricial, the ray should be excised.

GRAFTING FOR BONE DEFECTS

Defects left by curetting out cyst cavities where the main bone is still intact are filled readily by spongy bone obtained with a curette from the head of the tibia or the iliac crest. If the defect from a cyst or a tumor is across the shaft, a solid graft is necessary. Following gunshot wounds and many civil injuries there is often a defect in one or more metacarpals that necessitates bone grafting. Length, continuity and restoration of stability of the digits are accomplished readily by grafts.

Cortical bone from the crest of the ulna or the tibia provides good stability, can be shaped by saw or osteotome and is most useful in major defects of the metacarpals.

Cancellous bone from the ilium heals more rapidly and can be used to fill cyst cavities as well as used in block form. Taking some iliac cortex with it to provide stability makes this bone ideal for grafts.

Rib grafts have no advantage over iliac crest.

Grafts from cortical bone may be pointed at each end, shaped like a rolling pin for medullary insertion at each end, or stepped at each end for use as an onlay, the center of the graft in each case being of the thickness of the shaft. There are many ways of shaping and placing bone grafts in the hand, some by pinning and some by such close dovetailing that no other fixation is necessary.

Grafts of cancellous bone from the iliac crest, aside from their quick healing, have the advantage that holding pins may be thrust through them in any direction. When the bases and the shafts of several metacarpals need replacement, a flat outer slab of ilium is carved off, starting at the crest. One tapering edge is embedded in the carpus and the other in slits in the metacarpal necks.

Stabilization by Pinning. Approximation should be firm, both to ensure union and, at

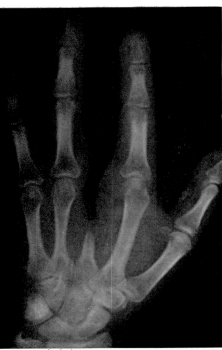

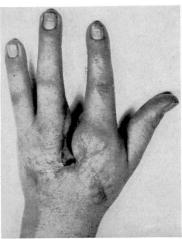

FIG. 333. (*Top*) A gunshot wound had destroyed most of the 3rd metacarpal and the surrounding structures, with loss of a finger. There was a painful neuroma and stiffening of all finger joints. (*Bottom*) The remains of the 3rd ray with cicatrix and neuroma were excised. The marginal or index finger was jogged over into its place, and the hand was narrowed, closing the cleft. Later, the extensor tendons were freed. A good, functioning hand results. (Walter Graham, M.D.)

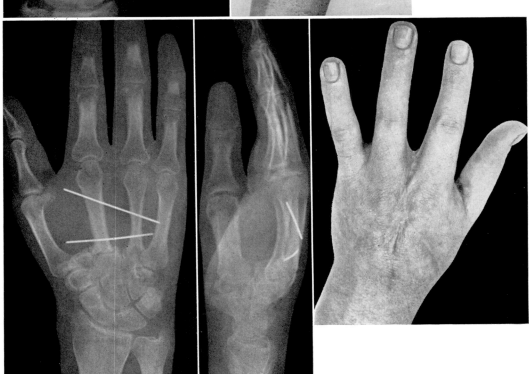

the same time, to allow the proximal finger joints to be placed in flexion without disaligning the bones. If bones are pinned firmly, very little external splinting is needed. Fine Kirschner stainless steel wires are drilled through the bones. They drill well if cut off obliquely with a wire cutter. Several are placed in different directions obliquely through the metacarpal and the carpus, obliquely through the 2 portions of bone or graft, transversely pinning several metacarpals together through heads, shafts or bases, or longitudinally down the center. When an oblique wire is placed, it may be pointed at each end. It is drilled into the open end of one bone and then reversed up through the open end of the other. In placing a longitudinal wire, the proximal finger joint is flexed, and the wire is drilled through the metacarpal head down the length of the metacarpal and the graft and on out the skin over the flexed wrist, which is then splinted. From here the wire is withdrawn until it just clears the articular cartilage of the head and is cut off at the wrist beneath the skin for withdrawal later. The wires usually are not left protruding through the skin, since movement leads to infection. They are clipped off just beneath the skin, to be removed as soon as union is apparent. Phalanges are usually pinned by 2 pins which are crossed to prevent distraction, routinely so for arthrodesis. As the pins are inserted, the bone ends should be clamped tightly together with 2 towel clips or with the special claw clamp that engages each bone by its points and screws the bones firmly together. Too often, nonunion results from distraction which is maintained by poorly placed cross wires. The first wire may be more or less longitudinal and the second placed obliquely after an extra hard squeeze by the clamp. Here a small key bone graft helps union.

The approach to the phalanges should be through midlateral incisions, that to the metacarpals through longitudinal dorsal incisions. Excellent exposure of the thumb metacarpal may be had by using a transverse incision along the creases around the base of the thenar eminence till over the metacarpal base and then extending distally along this bone. The muscles are stripped volarward from the metacarpal and then replaced.

On completing the bone operation, a nonpadded half plaster-of-Paris cast may be applied to the volar half or two thirds of the hand. Over the hand and also this part of the cast should be laid a piece of wax paper, and over this another slab of plaster, thus making a bivalve cast. The volar cast should fit around the hand and the fingers sufficiently—even to two thirds of their circumference—to hold the bones in place. Before 24 hours have elapsed, the dorsal part of the cast should be lifted a little to allow for swelling, spreading the cast if necessary. As the swelling gradually decreases, the dorsal part of the cast should be kept snugged up against the volar half. A circular nonpadded cast should never be placed about a digit which has just been operated on, since necrosis will be certain to occur.

If the bones have been fastened together securely so that they are firm, it is better as a first dressing to avoid plaster, filling all interstices with voluminous waste or fluffed gauze and wrap around with a bandage. After 10 days, when sutures are removed and the swelling is less, a half cast may be applied. When immobilized, proximal finger joints

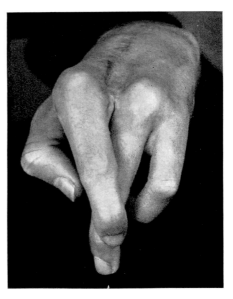

Fig. 334. Because of loss of support of the head of a central metacarpal, the joint axes tip so that the adjoining fingers cross on flexion. The index metacarpals should be jogged over onto the base of the metacarpal of the long finger.

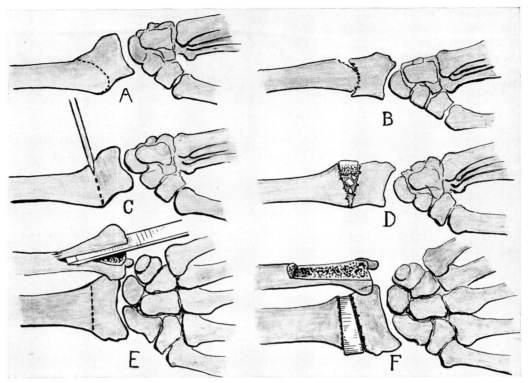

Fig. 335. Operations for malunion of Colles' fracture. (A, B) Osteotomy along the curve indicated gives angulation volarward and the desired lengthening of the radius. (C, D, E, F) Campbell's operation, utilizing part of the prominent ulnar head for a double-wedged bone graft to furnish angulation and elongation of the radius.

should be in flexion, if possible, lest they stiffen in extension.

A fresh fracture of a phalanx or a metacarpal will unite firmly in 3 weeks, but in a secondary repair using a bone graft it is best to immobilize for from 5 to 8 weeks, being guided by the roentgen appearance. Whenever plaster is applied to the hand, as much as possible of the undamaged digits should remain uncovered so that they will be free to move. This will not only prevent these digits from stiffening but will also keep the whole hand more mobile. Sometimes the bases of the 2 digits adjoining the finger operated on should be incorporated in the plaster, because movements of adjoining digits, since they are motivated by a common muscle, tend to angulate the bones. In order to leave a finger free to move, the cast should terminate at the distal crease in the palm or, for the thumb, at the thenar crease. For a fracture of a phalanx or a metacarpal, the cast should include the forearm, and the wrist should be in moderate dorsiflexion.

CROSSED FINGERS

Fingers cross on flexion for various reasons. Malunion of a metacarpal or a phalanx in rotation tips the joint axis so that the finger crosses or diverges, or loss of the support of the head of a central metacarpal allows the adjoining ones to rotate toward each other, tipping their axes so that the fingers cross. Excessive tipping causes the fingers to cross in moderate flexion but to diverge in full flexion.

When the intervening metacarpal head is missing, fingers may diverge on flexion due to contracting cicatrix on the dorsum, rolling the

2 metacarpal heads backward toward each other and tipping their joint axes. This may neutralize or nullify the effect of the missing head. Similarly, a volar contracting scar will exaggerate the crossing on flexion. Correct rotation is determined by ensuring that each finger points to the scaphoid tubercle in passive flexion. At the end of the operation a stainless steel wire may be placed through the finger pulps and the skin over the scaphoid tubercle as a definite guide. It will also keep the proximal finger joints in flexion. The plane of the fingernails is another good indicator, though that of the index finger is a little tipped.

BONES OF THE FOREARM

Deformities of angulation or rotation in the forearm may alter the mechanics of the muscles and thus affect the wrist and digital function. Therefore, the correction of this deformity becomes an essential part of the reconstructive plan.

DISLOCATION OF THE HEAD OF THE RADIUS

If the ulna is fractured in its upper third or the radius in its lower third and there is much angulation or overlapping, the head of the other bone must be dislocated. Forced supination to angulate the forearm backward, to break the ulna, dislocates the radial head forward from its orbicular ligament. On union of the ulna, the radial head blocks flexion and, being far from its pivot, pronation and supination also. Less commonly, the radial head dislocates backward.

Correction requires straightening the ulna by osteotomy and open reduction of the radial head. Cicatrix is cleared away for the reception of the radial head, and a new orbicular ligament of palmaris longus tendon is looped about the radial neck and fastened through a drill hole in the posterior border of the ulna. A Kirschner wire through the humerus holds the head temporarily while the tendon graft heals. In some cases the head of the radius cannot be made to pass the capitellum and must be resected. A tendon sling should be used in either case, and also some fixation of the fractured ulna by wire, bone graft or intramedullary pin.

EXCISION OF RADIAL HEAD

If the head of the radius is merely split or fractured without displacement, good pronation and supination may result. It should be treated by aspiration and the occasional injection of procaine and should be free to move. If one fragment is displaced, it should be removed; if the head is fractured off or there is comminution with displacement, the head should be removed. In children, however, excision should be deferred if possible until growth is attained—even though pronatory movement is checked temporarily.

In an old case pronation and supination may be gained by resecting the radial head, or, if it is fused to the ulna, by removing a short segment of the neck, taking great care to avoid the posterior interosseus nerve.

After resection of the radial head, there may be some complaint of pain and weakness, as reported by King, Lewis and Thibodeau, especially if too much of the radius was removed or if there is new bone formation. At the wrist the radius becomes relatively shorter than the ulna, and ulnar flexion may be limited. At the elbow the carrying angle is increased. Usually the hand does not deviate, though the ulnar head is more prominent. These complications can be prevented by removing only the head, keeping extraperiosteally and capping the neck over with fascia.

A dislocated radial head may be shoved back in place by Patterson's maneuver. The radiohumeral joint is strained open by ulnar flexion, extension and supination.

PRONATION AND SUPINATION

When the range of this motion is becoming limited, the forearm is usually in pronation. Supination or palm up is a very useful position and is more difficult to acquire than pronation because it is working against gravity. If the motion must be frozen, slight pronation is acceptable, but the ability to supinate is more desirable. Equal motion takes place at each radio-ulnar joint, so that restriction of either joint checks the motion. Therefore, removal of the head or a segment of the neck of whichever joint is to blame frees the motion. Motion is blocked when dislocation occurs at either radio-ulnar joint because the 2 parts of the pivot are apart; it is restored on reduction by placing them together again. In malunion of the radius and the ulna with much angulation, the motion is checked, since the pivots do not work in a parallel way. Synostosis anywhere between the radius and the ulna effectively prevents the motion.

In paralytic cases where there is a limited degree of rotary motion, a high rotary osteotomy on the ulna, as suggested by Milch,

will place the range of motion into the mid-position from which it can supinate sufficiently. Union and correct rotation can be ensured by a key bone graft. Blount successfully corrected the rotation by manual osteoclasis over an added wedge at the midforearm, casted in the corrected position for 2 months.

In applying an abdominal skin pedicle to

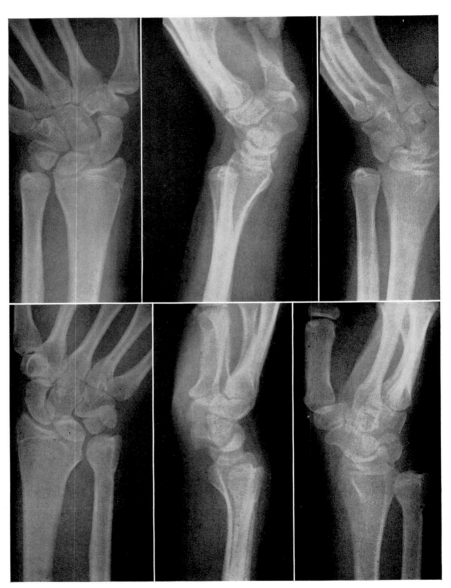

Fig. 336. Madelung's deformity. (*Top*) Left and (*bottom*) right in a young girl. Note the deformity of the radial epiphysis and the position of the lunate and the ulna.

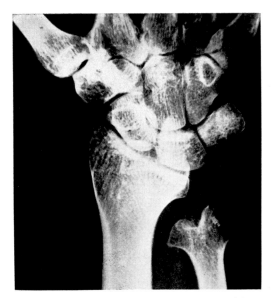

FIG. 337. Congenitally short ulna with bending of the end of the radius, probably from lack of support. Not Madelung's deformity.

the forearm or the hand, the forearm may be fixed in an exact degree of rotation by transfixing both bones with a Kirschner wire. Similarly, pronation and supination may be controlled, thus avoiding the necessity of applying the cast to the axilla.

To overcome a mild contracture, a torsion spring splint can be used. (See Chap. 6.)

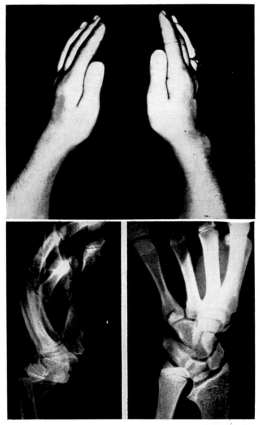

FIG. 338. Madelung's deformity. (*Top*) Comparison of the 2 wrists. (*Bottom*) X-ray appearance. (Robert Newell, M.D.)

SYNOSTOSIS BETWEEN RADIUS AND ULNA

Cross union may take place between the 2 bones at either radio-ulnar joint or anywhere along the shafts, usually opposite the site of a fracture. It occurs as bony growth along stripped-up periosteum, hematoma or interosseus membrane, especially after severe fractures in which the intervening soft parts were also injured, making a pathway for organized clot between the 2 bones. If in reconstruction both bones are exposed through the same incision, it is best to undermine the skin first so that each bone can be approached between different sets of muscles in order that direct communication between the 2 bones will not be established.

Treatment. For synostosis at the distal radio-ulnar joint, a segment of the neck or

the head of the ulna is removed, and, if necessary, a tendon graft sling is made to encircle the ulna and the flexor ulnaris tendon. At the proximal radio-ulnar joint, the head or a segment of the neck of the radius is removed, and a tendon graft is looped about the radius and fastened to a drill hole in the ulna in order to keep the bones from diverging.

If the synostosis is in the lower part of the forearm, a segment of the ulna just above it can be removed; if at the upper end, the same can be done to the radius.

Synostoses along the shafts should be excised very thoroughly because there is a strong tendency toward recurrence. Entering between the ulna and the extensor ulnaris muscle, the soft parts, together with their nerve supply, are reflected off the back of the bones and

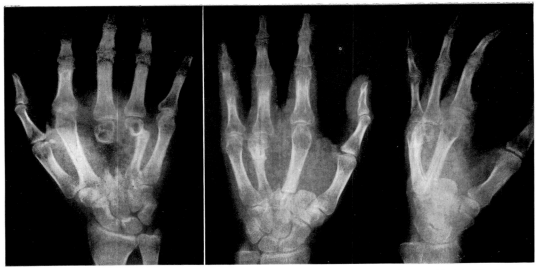

FIG. 339. Jogging a marginal ray over to take the place of a removed one. (*Left*) The long finger structures were injured so badly that they were excised. (*Right*) The index metacarpal was jogged over to narrow the hand, giving stability to the metacarpal arch. The ring metacarpal was repaired by a key bone graft. (Donald R. Pratt, M.D.)

the interosseous membrane, preserving the artery which perforates it. Part of each bone, as well as the synostosis and the interosseous ridges, is excised, and good muscle is sutured across the gap to separate the bones. Occasionally, a fascia lata covering of the bone may be needed if the surroundings are very cicatricial. There is so great a tendency for synostosis to recur that a little over half the circumference of each bone should be wrapped with a thin sheet of polythene. If one is radical and thorough, at least half range of motion can be expected.

MALUNION

In malunion of the radius and the ulna, the greater the angulation, the less pronation and supination will be possible, as their pivots and the bones which are the axles can turn only when in alignment. Ten weeks are usually required for healing of forearm fractures. If the cast is removed too early, the strong flexors and the force of gravity will cause the bones to angulate into pronation and flexion at the fracture site. Therefore, supination is checked the most. If only one bone is angulated, it is usually the radius.

Treatment is by open corrective straighten-

ing of the bones by osteotomy and bone graft or other fixation, shortening one bone if necessary to give the correct relative lengths of the bones for their participation in the wrist joint. The ulna at the wrist should be a little shorter than the radius. Rotary deformities are corrected, and the position is maintained with a key graft or a longitudinal spline as described by Möberg.

NONUNION

Nonunion of forearm bones is common, especially at the lower end of the ulna. Incomplete immobilization is usually the cause, but infection often plays a part. Fixation with small intramedullary Steinmann pins or a key graft and an onlay of cancellous bone and bone chips will ensure union. A case of nonunion in which the tissues over the fracture site are cicatricial first needs replacement of soft parts by a pedicle skin graft. After osteomyelitis, bone grafting should not be done until several months have elapsed. In an old case of nonunion lower than the middle of the forearm where the radius has united but a gap is still to be filled in the ulna, one can produce a synostosis between the lower fragment of the ulna and the radius. The upper end of the ulna will be long enough to give stability to the forearm, and there will be good pronation and supination.

OPERATIONS ON BONES OF FOREARM

The ulna, being subcutaneous throughout its length, is easy to approach. The neck of the radius can be reached between the anconeus and the extensor ulnaris, reflecting the supinator brevis and watching for the posterior interosseous nerve. It can also be reached rather deep in front between the brachioradialis and the pronator teres. The shaft is accessible between the extensors of the fingers and the wrist and the lower third of the radius between the extensors of the thumb and the brachioradialis, avoiding the nerve.

To place bone ends together without strain and with less chance of displacement, muscle

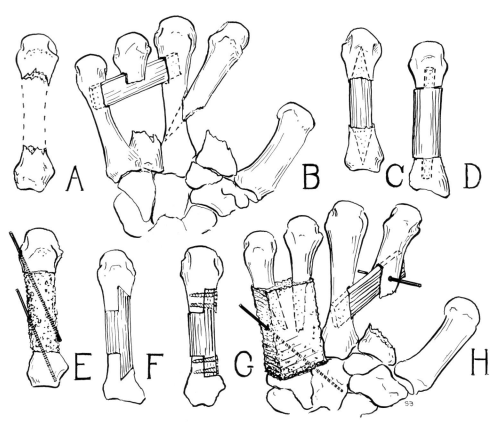

Fig. 340. (A) For absence of the metacarpal shaft, support for the metacarpal head may be supplied by various types of bone carpentry. (B) Transverse cortical graft from the ulna or the tibia. The index metacarpal may be spiked into the long finger. (C) Graft sawed from the ulna or the tibia may be spiked into the head and the base. (At one end a slot is cut so that the spike may be inserted without losing length.) (D) Cortical graft is nibbled with a rongeur like a rolling pin. Here, also, a slot is needed. If based on the carpus, pressure holds the graft into a slight indentation. (E) Iliac cancellous graft, based squarely, is pinned firmly in place. Cancellous bone has the great advantage of uniting in 5 weeks, whereas cortical grafts take 2 or 3 months. (F, G) Two types of inlay. (H) Iliac graft based on the carpus supports 2 metacarpal heads, and for stability is pinned by Kirschner wires. The index metacarpal is fixed to that of the long finger by a cortical bone graft.

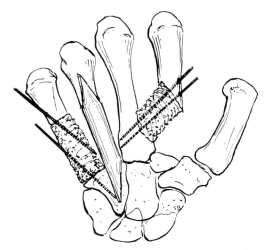

FIG. 341. For absence of the bases of the metacarpals, the bone graft, if cancellous from ilium, may rest pinned in place on the carpus; or if cortical, as in the 4th metacarpal, it may be spiked into place. For loss of the base of the index metacarpal, an iliac bone is pinned to the long metacarpal or to the carpus.

pull should be considered. The cross muscles are the brachioradialis, the pronator teres, the extensors of the thumb and the pronator quadratus. These have pronatory and supinatory effects and draw the bones together. In radial fractures above the pronator teres, the supinator brevis supinates the upper fragment, but below the pronator teres the pronator neutralizes this. Therefore, fractures above the latter should be put up in supination and those below it in the midposition. In all forearm fractures the flexors tend to flex and pronate the lower fragment. If low fractures are put up in pronation, the extensors of the thumb, which are supinators, will be tightened, displacing the upper end of the lower fragment forward. This is corrected by using the midposition. Full supination also displaces here, drawing the bones together by the pull of the pronator quadratus.

The use of an anvil and an osteotome facilitates separating and shaping the bone ends, and a Stryker saw is useful. Often there will be a strain in bringing the ends of one of the bones together because of inequality of

length. The interosseous membrane makes it impossible to displace the bone longitudinally, and, instead, the other bone must be shortened to suit, or the gap bridged by bone graft.

Often the head of the ulna projects too far in the wrist because of shortening of the radius from absorption, overlapping or angulation. This tips the hand radialward and interferes with anteroposterior, lateral and pronatory motions of the wrist. The head of the ulna should be excised, leaving the styloid in place. The ulna may be shortened. However, the ulna cannot be shortened above and drawn upward. The shortening must be done near its lower end by a long oblique or jogged osteotomy. Approximation and fixation should be firm, since nonunion here is frequent.

Secondary operations on forearm bones are so often followed by nonunion that grafting is generally resorted to, especially for nonunion. The bones are too small for sliding grafts, so that firm onlay grafts and stainless steel screws should be used. Good workmanship results in good union. In fresh fractures or old reconstructions of the radius and the ulna the bones may be held firmly in place by inserting a small intramedullary Steinmann pin. The point when drilled will follow the curve of the canal. The pin is introduced into the ulna through the olecranon and into the radius through the lower dorsal edge of the styloid process. Cancellous bone from the ilium may be laid over the juncture as an onlay, and additional bone chips may be packed around it.

A gap in one bone may be filled with a bone graft, preferably from the fibula, stepping it at each end and screwing it in place or threading it on an intramedullary Steinmann pin. A segment of ilium may be used, pinning it in place as is done with metacarpals. If the defect is small, the other bone may be shortened. Pronation and supination should be considered, remembering that the ulna does not turn but that the radius does. The ulna is the essential bone for stability at the elbow, and the radius is similarly essential at the wrist. A gap high in the radius or low in the ulna is not too crippling, and a low synostosis is a short cut when the gap is in the lower half of the ulna.

For absence of the lower end of the radius,

the upper shaft of the fibula together with its head was grafted. The head furnished a good socket for the carpus, and there was considerable motion after 2 years. Similarly, a fibular graft into the radius may be arthodesed into the carpus, removing the ulna head for freedom of pronation and supination. A simple method of fixation is to pass a Steinmann pin

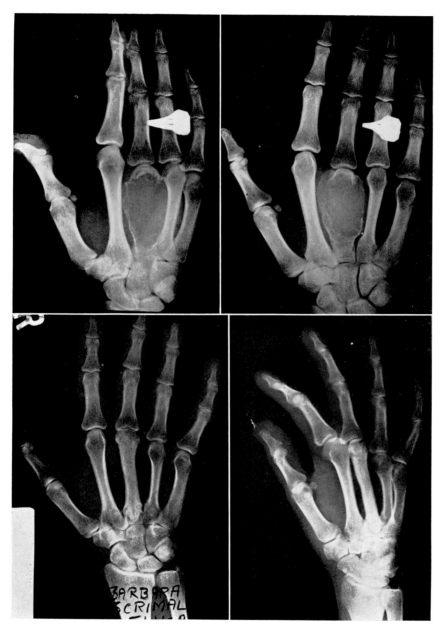

FIG. 342. (*Top*) Benign fibroma of metacarpal replaced by tibial graft. (*Bottom*) Roentgenogram 23 years after operation. Length and functional range of motion maintained. Original 3-year follow-up reported in Surg., Gynec. Obstet. *68*:936. (From D. H. Levinthal, M.D.)

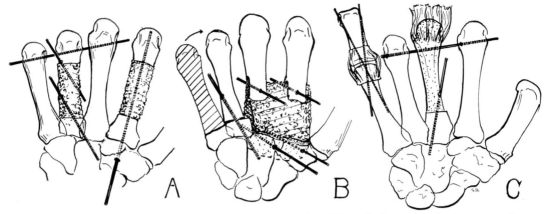

Fig. 343. (A) Methods of pinning iliac grafts in place. If made firm, capsulectomy may be done at the same time. As shown in the index metacarpal, the pin is inserted through the head and made to emerge through the skin back of the flexed wrist. It is withdrawn here just to clear the joint, and motion of the wrist is stopped with plaster.

(B) Using iliac grafts to support 2 metacarpals. The graft is slotted into the carpus, and each metacarpal is pinned in place. The metacarpal of the little finger has been jogged over to take the place of the ring finger and pinned there.

(C) Free graft of joint from toe or finger to act as the proximal joint of the little finger. Bones are pinned firmly into place. Free graft of the 5th metacarpal plus joint capsule to replace distal two thirds of a metacarpal and half of the proximal finger joint. Both operations have been successful.

through the carpus, the graft and the radius subcutaneously.

MALUNITED COLLES' FRACTURE

From malunion the muscle balance of the hand is upset. The tendons at the wrist pull around corners and at wrong angles of approach. The head of the ulna projects into the wrist, limiting motion, and the hand deviates radialward. Though arthritis may have resulted, much of the disability can be relieved by surgery.

Rixford's Operation. Through an incision on the radial side between the extensors of the thumb and the brachioradialis protecting the radial nerve, a curved osteotomy is done straight across the radius. This is made starting at the dorsal surface with a gentle curvature which is increased gradually until the volar surface is reached. When the distal fragment is drawn down around the curve and into place, the effect will be a correction of both angulation and length.

Campbell's Operation. Through the above exposure the radius is severed straight across at the fracture line. The lower end of the ulna is uncovered, and, with an osteotome, the outer posterior half is chiseled off from below upward as a long wedge the breadth of the radius. Its rounded surface is chiseled flat so as to wedge it in 2 planes. The radial fragments are pried apart, angulating the distal one, inserting the wedge so that there will be both angulatory correction and lengthening of the radius. The prominence of the ulna will also be eliminated. The styloid process and the triangular ligament are replaced by suture.

Postoperatively, the elbow should be immobilized at 90° to stop pronation and supination until union takes place. When a long projecting head of the ulna interferes with wrist motions and particularly when pain is present, the head of the ulna should be removed. If removed above the pronator quadratus, or if this muscle is weak, there will be instability unless a tendon sling is passed around the bone and the flexor ulnaris tendon.

MADELUNG'S DEFORMITY

DESCRIPTION

This entity, though first mentioned by Dupuytren in 1839, was described more extensively in 1878 by Madelung. The deformity is

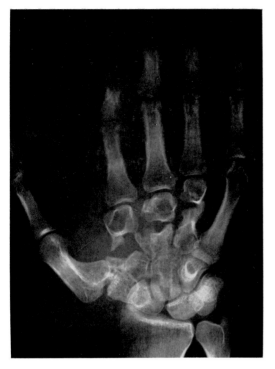

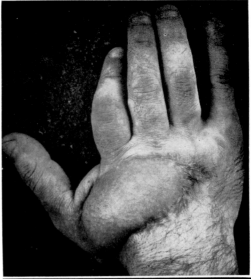

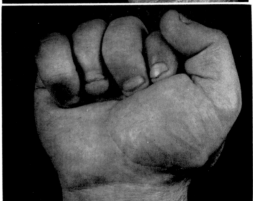

Fig. 344. Treatment overseas by direct flap; hand healed after arrival at home. In spite of x-ray appearance, no surgery was done because of good function and the absence of pain. (L. D. Howard, M.D.)

from an epiphysial growth defect in the lower end of the radius that does not make its presence known until the ages of 10 to 15, with 12 as the average. It is bilateral in two thirds of the cases and 4 times as frequent in girls. In at least 10 per cent it is hereditary.

Because of lessened and aberrant growth of the radial epiphysis, the lower end of the radius curves volarward and ulnarward and falls behind in growth compared with the ulna. Both radius and ulna are enlarged at their lower ends, and the relative increase of growth of the ulna makes this bone luxate from the radius and the triquetrum, project dorsally and distally and form a new facet on the side of the carpus. Epiphysial damage by injury, infection or rickets may imitate the condition, and in a few the curve has been dorsal.

Madelung's deformity has the appearance of a forward dislocation of the wrist, as there is a bayonet-like jog. The anteroposterior thickness at the wrist is increased. There is pain and muscle cramping until the deformity is established, and then a feeling of weakness or looseness. Due to the changed mechanics, dorsiflexion, abduction and supination at the wrist are limited, and flexion increased.

TREATMENT

Early treatment with a leather brace or the application of a series of plaster casts from the metacarpal heads to well up in the forearm will lessen pain and deformity. It is preferable to defer operation to obtain greater bone growth if fusion is contemplated. Otherwise, a wedge osteotomy of the radius is done. First,

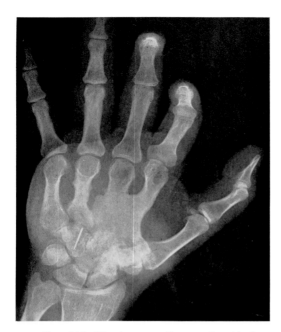

FIG. 345. Massive cancellous and cortical iliac graft to stabilize metacarpals destroyed by a gunshot wound through the palm.

the fibrous contractures are separated, and the ulna is shortened by removing its lower end. A tendinous sling placed about it and the flexor ulnaris tendon will check backward dislocation. The forearm is splinted in the position of a mild opposite deformity. The head of the ulna may be removed, including its periosteum but within the ligaments (Darrach), leaving them and the styloid process to re-form enough for radio-ulnar stability.

RECONSTRUCTION AFTER METACARPAL LOSSES

Severe crushing wounds, explosions and gunshot wounds perforating the hand result in much damage to the metacarpals and the surrounding tendons, nerves and intrinsic muscles. Restoration of hand function after these injuries is a serious problem. In this section will be discussed the principles involved in the decision between ablation of the part and reconstruction. From problems involving the 1st metacarpal and the thumb ray, see Chapter 13.

Injuries to the palm or the dorsum may involve wide destruction of skin with extensive cicatrix. Extensor and flexor tendons may be destroyed along with intrinsic muscles and the digital nerves. Metacarpals are often shortened or angulated with defects of the head or the base, or dislocated. Nutrition is poor, and the proximal points are usually stiff and in extension.

The degree of disability may be lessened by selective early treatment. Traction prevents malunion. Traction with the proximal finger joints in flexion prevents that joint from becoming stiff and straight. Early closure of wounds by skin graft avoids the general stiffening that results from long infection. Casts should not enclose too much of the hand; they should immobilize the injured parts but allow motion of the well parts. The hand should be maintained in the position of function, and the casts should not be kept on too long. Gunshot wounds through metacarpals present many problems in reconstruction.

EXCISION OF RAY

When a hand is badly crippled from injury which is primarily in one metacarpal, it is better to excise the whole digital ray, including the metacarpal, together with a block excision of the cicatrix around it. The finger itself should be conserved by filleting it, that is, boning it but preserving its nerves and vessels. The skin can be laid over the dorsum of the hand to replace the cicatrix. The hand can be narrowed with much improvement in nutrition, mobility and looseness. The skin will be ample and looser, and the movements of the adjoining fingers will not be held back by adherence of the tendons of the injured finger. When a metacarpal is excised, with the exception of the 4th, its base is preserved for attachment of the extensor tendons of the wrist. Otherwise, this insertion should be transferred to the next metacarpal.

If the metacarpal excised is of a central finger—the middle or the ring finger—the adjoining metacarpal heads can be snugged up against each other by suture and bandaged for mutual support to prevent the joint axes from tipping. A firmer metacarpal arch can be made by shifting the marginal metacarpal over, that is, the little for the ring and the index for the middle. The index metacarpal may be moved over, jogging it by osteotomy

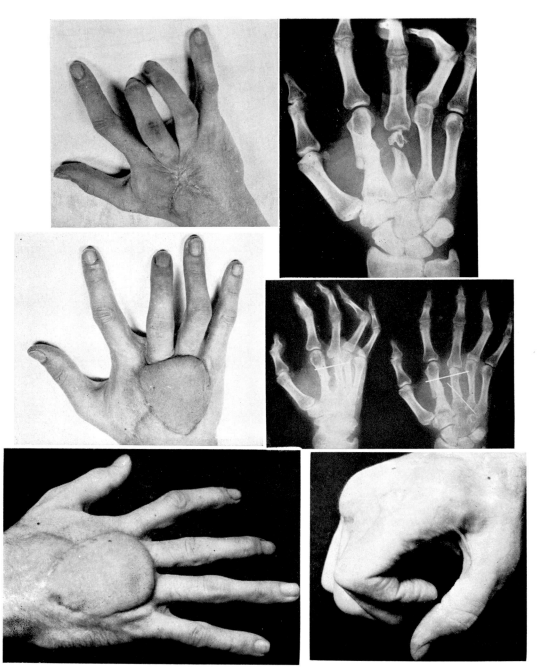

Fɪɢ. 346. Transplant of the 5th metatarsal with head and joint ligament to build out the 3rd metacarpal. (*Top*) Preoperative condition. The fingers could not flex, because their proximal joints were straight and stiff, and the extensor tendons were injured. (*Center, left*) A pedicle skin graft was applied. (*Center, right*) Later, a capsulectomy was done in the proximal joint of the ring finger, and the extensor tendon of the long finger was repaired by a graft. A new metacarpal was grafted from the 5th metatarsal. As the interossei to the long finger had been destroyed, the sublimis tendon was withdrawn into the palm, passed down through the lumbrical canals and sutured to the lateral bands of the long and the ring fingers to extend the distal 2 joints and to maintain flexion in the proximal joints. (*Bottom*) On discharge, the patient had 90° of voluntary motion in the new proximal finger joint (it flexed to 110° passively), and the grafted extensor tendon could extend the joint completely. The metatarsal functioned well as a metacarpal. (W. C. Graham, M.D.)

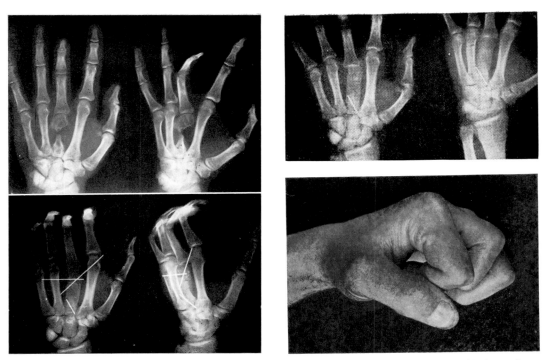

Fig. 347. Iliac bone pinned in place to fill a defect in the metacarpal shaft. (*Left, top*) Defect. (*Left, bottom*) Broad graft may be pinned in any direction. (*Right, top*) Union is firm in 5 weeks compared with 8 to 10 weeks with cortical bone. (*Right, bottom*) Flexion of the proximal finger joints is increasing. If bone is pinned firmly, capsulectomy may be done at the same time. (L. D. Howard, M.D.)

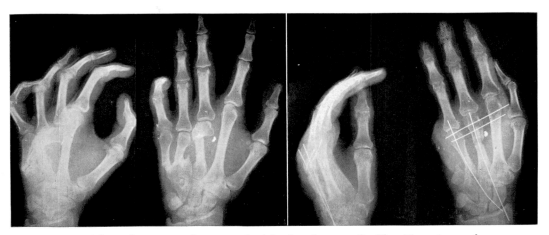

Fig. 348. The 3rd metacarpal was repaired by key bone graft. The 4th metacarpal was removed. The 5th metacarpal was jogged over to the place of the 4th, pinning all securely enough to do capsulectomies of the proximal finger joints. (Donald R. Pratt, M.D.)

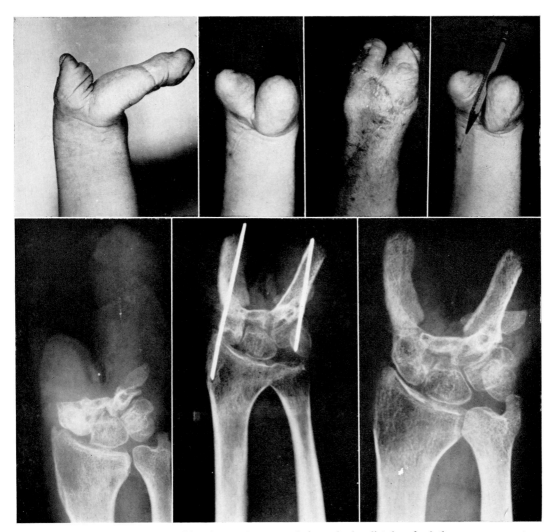

Fig. 349. Case D. W. Hand in planer. Amputated through the distal end of the carpus except for a nubbin of metacarpal, but left 2 boneless tassels of skin (*top, left*). Two posts of iliac bone were pinned on the carpus (see *bottom, center*). These were slipped into skin tubes and later supplied with tendons, crossing about the hand, and also a tendon T operation. The cleft formed was 1⅜ inches deep and had 1 inch of spread. The digits moved ½ inch to and from each other. He could hold objects ranging from a sheet of paper up to objects ½ inch in diameter and also could wear a prosthesis. (*Bottom*) X-ray views before, during and after operation. Two and a half years later, it was reported that he had very good function of these digits.

through its base. It is moved off itself and onto the stump of the middle metacarpal until parallel with the ring metacarpal. The 5th metacarpal may be readily dislocated over after severing its ligaments if the ring metacarpal is removed entirely, or it may be jogged

over on the stump of the ring metacarpal. Temporary fixation, with a buried Kirschner wire driven through the metacarpal and the carpus, maintains the position.

The decision to excise a metacarpal or a digital ray rests on the magnitude of destruc-

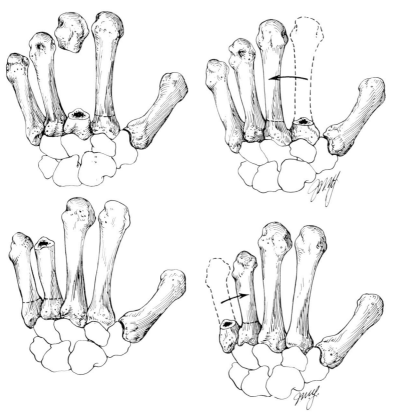

Fig. 350. (*Top*) Shift of marginal ray of the index finger to the middle finger, for loss of the 3rd metacarpal. (*Bottom*) Shift of the ulnar ray of the little finger to the base of the ring finger for loss of the 4th metacarpal. Alternately, the entire base of the 4th metacarpal can be removed, and the 5th jogged over on the common articulating surface of the hamate.

Fig. 351. Gunshot wound through the bases of the 2nd, the 3rd and the 4th metacarpals. (*Left*) Preoperative. Cicatrix was first replaced by pedicle skin. (*Right*) Two grafts from the tibia were united in 3 months. The 3rd metacarpal was straightened. Later, the extensor tendons were freed, and capsulectomy was done to the knuckles. J. William Littler, M.D.)

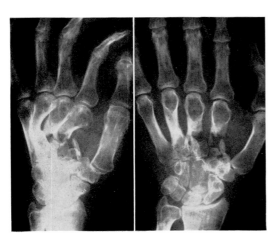

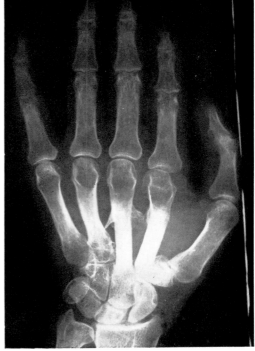

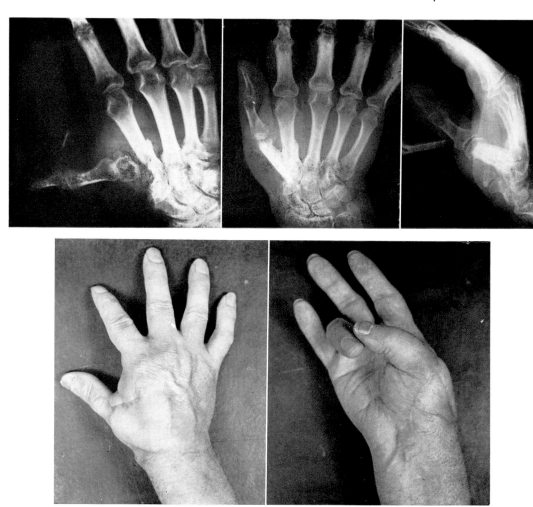

Fig. 352. Destruction by shell fragment of most of the 1st metacarpal, the base of the 2nd and the multangular bone. The free-floating thumb is useless. (*Top, left*) Preoperative. (*Top, center* and *right*) After the scar was excised and replaced by pedicle skin, the first 2 metacarpals were united to the carpus by a graft from the tibia in correct position. A new extensor pollicis longus tendon was grafted in, using the palmaris longus. (*Bottom*) Excellent functional result. (From J. William Littler, M.D.)

tion and scar tissue. If too many structures such as bones, joints, tendons and nerves are damaged, or if there is too much cicatrix, excision is advisable. Unless the interosseus muscles are active, flexion of the proximal finger joint, even when gained by capsulectomy, cannot be maintained unless specially compensated for. (See Chap. 12.) The presence of this function is manifested by the ability to move the finger laterally or to extend its distal joint or can be determined by feeling the interosseus tendons at the sides of the finger. If in doubt as to excision in the case of the ring finger, the fact that this is the finger that when stiff holds the others back the most should be the deciding factor. Severing the juncturae tendinae will help by freeing the adjoining tendons from this extensor tendon.

Loss of Metacarpal Head

When a head is gone from either marginal ray (index or little finger), the whole shaft

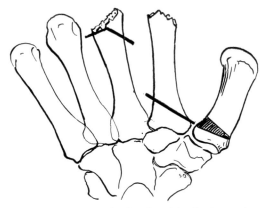

Fig. 353. If the heads of both the 2nd and the 3rd metacarpals are absent, the 2nd should be removed near its base. Whatever is left of the 3rd should be preserved to support a pad against which the thumb will work. A rotary angulatory osteotomy should be done on the base of the 1st metacarpal so that the thumb will work without strain against the ring and the little fingers.

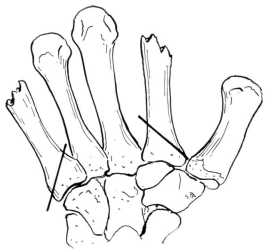

Fig. 354. If the head of either marginal metacarpal is gone, the remainder of that metacarpal should be removed obliquely at its base, leaving the insertion of the wrist extensor in place.

should be removed diagonally at its base, sacrificing the finger; or the proximal phalanx can be fused to the metacarpal shaft, retaining a short finger. The intrinsic muscles of the amputated ray should be reattached to the proximal phalanx of the next remaining ray.

If they do not reach, add a small strip of tendon graft. This will give valuable power to the new marginal finger to abduct from the midline. When removing the index finger, the first interosseus tendon is connected to the middle finger, and when removing the little

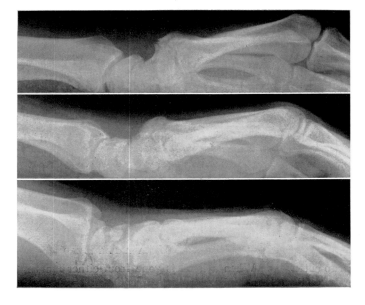

Fig. 355. Metacarpal or carpal boss. A slight change in the rotation of the hand to obtain several views illustrates the bony prominences, here at the 3rd metacarpocapitate joint.

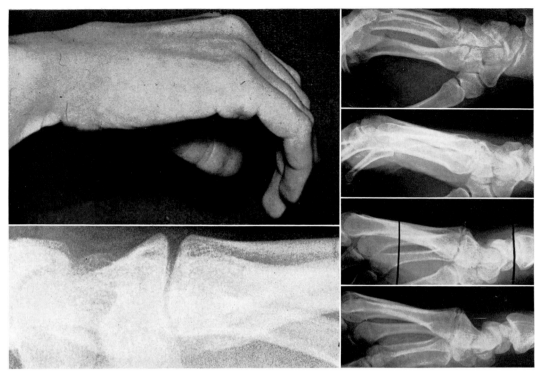

FIG. 356. (*Top, left*) Location of bony prominence of metacarpal boss. (*Right*) Four views in different degrees of rotation. (*Bottom, left*) The other wrist, which is normal.

finger, the hypothenar muscles are attached to the ring finger. If the head of a central metacarpal, middle or ring finger, is missing, the 2 adjoining fingers will cross on flexion, since they are no longer braced against the intervening metacarpal head and so will roll toward each other, tipping the joint axes. Therefore, after the shaft is removed, the adjoining marginal metacarpal is moved over for this bracing effect of the heads. The base of either may be left, or the entire ring metacarpal can be removed, since no wrist extensor inserts into it.

Replacement of a metacarpal head by a bone graft constitutes, also, an arthroplasty. There has been too much limitation of motion in such cases.

An arthroplasty in which one of the bones is a graft without a covering of articular cartilage results in poor motion and even shortening by absorption.

When surrounding tissues are in good condition, a new head and part of a shaft may be

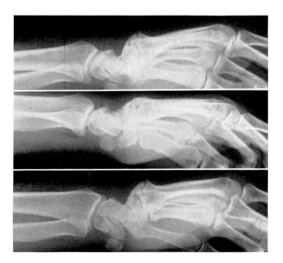

FIG. 357. Left hand of professional woman golfer. Severe pain on radio-dorsiflexion. The bony ridges of the index metacarpal and trapezoid show in the bottom photograph. Excision of impinging surfaces relieved most of the discomfort.

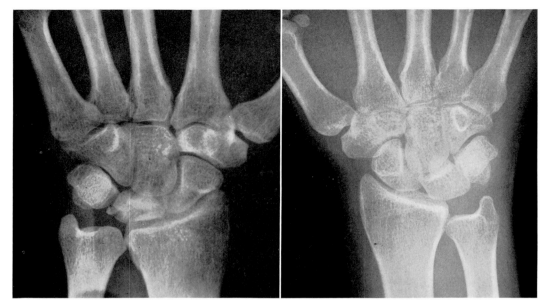

FIG. 358. (*Left*) Kienböck's disease or malacia of the lunate. This ulna is "normal," i.e., neither a plus nor a minus variant. (*Right*) "Minus variant" ulna. Note the position of the lunate. A wrist with this type of conformation is said to be more prone to develop lunate disease.

grafted in by taking the 5th metatarsal. It is removed obliquely at its base so as to leave the latter for weight-bearing. A phalanx can be used in the same way. Enough ligaments to form a new joint capsule should be carried with the head. The graft is pinned firmly in place. Such cases followed for 8 and 6 months (Graham and Bunnell) showed smooth joint motion of from 60° to 80°. A complete joint has been grafted. (See Chap. 9.)

If there is only partial loss of a metacarpal head, there may be left sufficient motion in this irregular joint for adequate function, but if motion is limited, an arthroplasty is indicated.

DEFECT OF SHAFT OF METACARPAL

If the damage is great, the remainder of the ray may be excised, filleting the finger and narrowing the hand, using the finger skin to replace the dorsal cicatrix. If surrounding structures are good, the metacarpal may be reconstructed by a linear bone graft. It is not necessary to gain length preoperatively by skeletal traction. It will be found that sufficient length is gained after complete excision of the surrounding cicatrix. If a graft that is

pointed at each end is inserted in the gap, some of this length will be lost. However, if one of the points is passed through a slot in one of the fragments, greater length will be conserved. It is advisable to have the metacarpal head on a level with the others, so that the soft parts will not form a sling, preventing flexion when that finger alone is flexed. When all are flexed together, such a sling does not interfere.

Loss of Base of Metacarpal. A linear bone graft is used to replace the defect. It is either rested on or driven into the carpus. Or, if long, the shaft may be united to the adjoining metacarpal to form a Y metacarpal on which 2 fingers are supported. This is successful in a marginal ray. Two heads may be mounted on one broad bone graft.

Defect of Distal Ends of Both the 2nd and the 3rd Metacarpals. The shaft of the index metacarpal should be removed diagonally at its base, but all possible length of the middle metacarpal should remain, since it is useful as a prominence opposing the thumb. If, then, the thumb does not work easily against the ring and the little fingers, a rotary angulatory

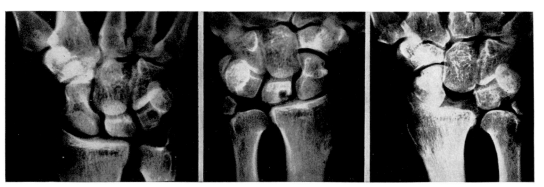

FIG. 359. Case W. M. (*Left*) Fracture of the lunate leading to Kienböck's disease. Nine months previously, the hand was forcefully supinated between a belt and a pulley. A line fracture shows in the lunate in a roentgenogram taken on February 3, 1941. After the accident, pain, swelling and limitation of motion were present. (*Center*) by December 3, 1941, the appearance was cystlike, having ruptured into the joint. Arthritis showed in the vicinity. The lunate was removed. The fracture still showed as a fine line. The radial half was much congested, there being solid granulations instead of a cyst. (*Right*) Appearance 9 months after removal of the lunate. The gap never closes. The patient worked 8 hours a day, though by the end of the day there was some lameness. His grip was $^{23}\!/_{40}$. Wrist movements were somewhat limited.

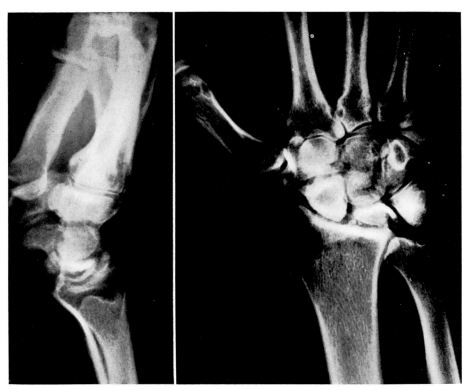

FIG. 360. Case D. A., age 25. Kienböck's disease. Three years previously, the patient forcefully struck his left hand, injuring the lunate. When seen, the wrist was too sore, painful and lame to work. X-ray views show the lunate to be degenerated, crushed and open to the joint, where there is much arthritis. The navicular is tipped, not fractured. The lunate should be removed to check arthritis.

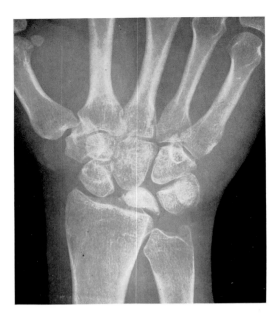

FIG. 361. The classic picture of Kienböck's disease. Note the short ulna, the collapse and the increased density of the lunate and the tail-like projection ulnarward of the bone. (From Drs. Kochsiek and Murasky)

osteotomy at the base of its metacarpal will relieve the strain.

LOSS OF BONY ALIGNMENT

To re-establish correct mechanics and muscle balance the bony framework must be restored to its normal alignment. Bowed or dislocated metacarpals must be straightened, and dislocations about the carpus must be corrected. The latter is done through the dorsum by a liberal excising of the cicatrix about the dislocation, excavating a space to receive the dislocated bone and pinning it in place with a subcutaneous, removable Kirschner wire. If the thumb metacarpal or the adjoining part of the carpus is dislocated backward, the thumb assumes a position close to the hand with the first 2 metacarpals parallel. Here the base of the metacarpal must be repositioned for proper mechanics.

The metacarpal problem usually comprises more than just the repair of the metacarpals. The long extensors of the fingers are densely adherent to the bone, and the proximal finger joints are stiff and straight. These 2 complications may be corrected at the same operation at which the metacarpal is repaired, provided that the fracture is not too close to the head of the metacarpal. Thus, the extensor tendons may be freed and gliding material placed between them and the bone, and capsulectomies may be done. Capsulectomy requires firm fixation of the metacarpal repair so that displacement will not occur; flexion of the proximal finger joints must be maintained postoperatively by splinting.

CARPAL OR METACARPAL BOSS

A firm, hard swelling on the dorsum of the wrist at the bases of the index and the middle finger metacarpals, tender to pressure and painful on dorsiflexion of the wrist, was designated *carpe bossu* by Fiolle in 1931.

The etiology is unknown, but bosselation may follow direct trauma to this area, the prominent point of the carpal arch where the 3rd metacarpal articulates with the capitate. In some the symptoms develop without direct trauma and are allegedly due to occupational strain.

Various authors have described the findings as being periostitis due to the pull of the extensor carpi radialis brevis which inserts near the prominent mass or to rupture of the dorsal ligament of the metacarpocapitate joint with later ossification beneath it. Foille described

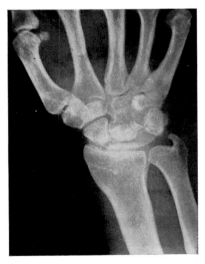

FIG. 362. Late Kienböck's disease of the lunate, with considerable arthritis and disability.

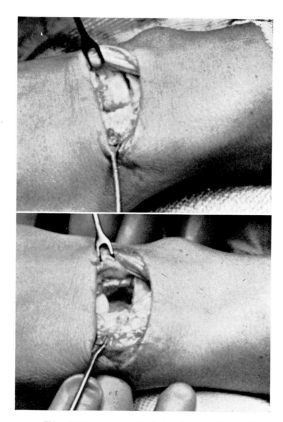

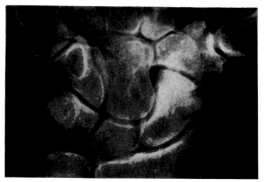

Fig. 364. Two cysts in the scaphoid following injury.

Fig. 363. Removal of the lunate through dorsal approach with transverse skin incision, digital extensors to ulnar side.

an exostosis at the bases of the index and the middle metacarpals. Lamphier reported 3 cases with prominent lips of bone on the adjoining surfaces of index and middle metacarpals and the capitate, all relieved by planing down the prominent bony masses. Curtiss apparently feels that the os styloideum—a supernumerary bone long known to anatomists—at the base of the 3rd metacarpal is present and may be confused with fractures or tumors. He considered reports of surgical excision to be discouraging and recommended conservative splinting.

Lateral roentgenograms reportedly show the bony exostoses or the os styloideum according to the authors' ideas of the pathologic process. This lateral view can be very confusing, and great care must be taken in localizing the involved area. It is best to take a series of views, rotating the hand a few degrees between each

view. Anteroposterior and oblique views are of little value.

In several personal experiences, the area involved has been either the joint between the 2nd metacarpal and the trapezoid or the 3rd metacarpocapitate joint. None had involvement of both as described by Lamphier, nor was the os styloideum present. Two patients with involvement of the index metacarpal base were golfers, and the condition was present only in the left hand. At operation, impingement of the base of the metacarpal against the capitate or the trapezoid could be demonstrated. Excision of this lip of the metacarpal relieves the symptoms.

TRAUMATIC DEGENERATION OF CARPAL BONES

In 1910, Preiser described a lesion in the scaphoid, and Kienböck reported a similar finding in the lunate. It has been called traumatic rarefying osteitis, traumatic malacia, traumatic nutritional disturbance, osteodystrophia cystica, localized osteitis fibrosa, necrosis, chronic osteitis, softening, traumatic atrophy and localized osteoporosis.

INCIDENCE

The condition occurs commonly in the lunate, one fifth as often in the scaphoid, and rarely in the capitate or the hamate. It is 3 or 4 times more frequent in males and is seen in the right hand about 5 times more often than in the left. It occurs mainly in manual workers between the ages of 20 and 50, particularly in those in their 30's.

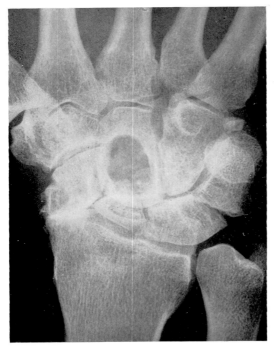

FIG. 365. Post-traumatic degeneration of the lunate and cyst in the capitate with subsequent arthritis of the wrist joint.

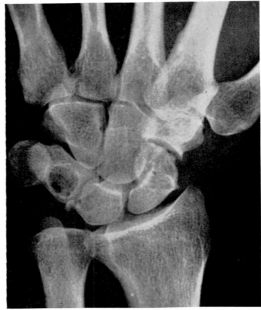

FIG. 366. Cyst in triquetrum and free fragment of adjoining lunate surface.

ETIOLOGY

The usual history is that of a fall on the dorsiflexed hand. Some patients tell of trivial or repeated injuries, and others do not recall having sustained an injury. In many cases the fracture line can be demonstrated through the lunate bone. Sometimes this line is very fine, and it is necessary to take roentgenograms in various directions to find it. It is usually in the radial margin and the proximal half of the bone. If the condition results from tearing off the blood supply from the lunate, one should expect to find it as a late result of all dislocations of this bone, but this is far from the case. However, the semilunar bone is very subject to strains of compression, and in a fall on the dorsiflexed hand it is directly between the head of the capitate bone and the radius. This direction of force is verified by the shape of the bone in late cases after crushing has occurred. When the ulna is shorter than the radius, the lunate is more vulnerable to compression. This so-called minus variant occurs in approximately 14 per cent of normal wrists; but Hultén reported it in 74 per cent, and Joeck in 64 per cent of cases with lunate necrosis. It seems quite probable that such a compression trauma, either with or without fracture, can precipitate this traumatic degeneration. The condition can hardly be classed with Osgood-Schlatter's, Legg-Calvé-Perthes' and Köhler's diseases or with Thiemann's disease of the phalanges, because these are all associated with the period of growth of the respective bones instead of with middle age.

Various untenable theories for the cause of the progressive degeneration have been advanced, such as embolism, infection and direct pressure. Loss of blood supply is more probable but does not explain the increased vascularity and the osteoporosis commonly seen in early cases. It is well known that there cannot be rarefaction of bone without hyperemia. Cutting off of circulation shows roentgenographically as relatively increased density.

Leriche maintained that all traumatism is accompanied by local alteration in the vasomotor equilibrium. This is a common occurrence, as seen in Sudeck's atrophy or even in the usual edema or hyperemia following trauma. Leriche maintained that there was first constriction and later dilation of the vessels, and that this was activated by "traumatic axon reflex." This hypothesis fits well the pathologic changes found and the clinical course. It is known that the cause of the necrosis is some circulatory disturbance, and that soon after trauma there are areas of hyperemic decalcification in the bones with other areas of relative increase of calcification from vessel obstruction.

Of all the carpal bones, the lunate and the scaphoid are unique in that they are covered mostly by articular surfaces. The area of their nonarticular surfaces, where vessels enter, is very small when compared with the other carpal bones, and these are the 2 bones which are most affected by post-traumatic degeneration. Instances of degeneration and necrosis in encapsulated regions are common, such as necrosis of the testis from swelling, the degeneration of muscles and nerves in the closed fascial space of the forearm in Volkmann's ischemia, Bell's palsy from inadequate circulation of the facial nerve when it swells in the unyielding facial canal, and of degeneration of the brain in increased intracranial pressure within the dural space. The lunate and the navicular bones can be considered to be encapsulated, since they are practically enclosed by articular surfaces and have only a few foramina for breathing purposes in the small nonarticular areas. Following trauma of explosive or compression type the vasomotor disturbances cause edema and swelling, thus raising the pressure within the bone so that circulation is excluded to the extent of causing central and patchy necrosis. This is followed by revascularization, sequestration, absorption and gradual substitution. The effect of synovial fluid on the healing mechanism of fractures is not fully understood.

Pathologic Changes

What appears roentgenographically to be a cyst usually is found to be a highly vascular granulating area. Occasionally, a fracture line may be seen to cross the bone through this area.

In the early cases there is little change in the roentgen appearance of the bone, but soon patches of osteoporosis and vacuolization become evident. These may coalesce later. The bone shows alternating areas of greater and lesser density, and, as a whole, the bone is apt to be slightly more dense than normal. There may be a central density with a peripheral zone of rarefaction or the appearance of a single vacuole, though it may prove to be a vascular area. The whole bone becomes slightly enlarged, as compared with the normal; but eventually it shortens and widens, and finally it may be crushed between the head of the capitate and the radius and spread out widely in the joint. If a fracture line is present, it is probably the result of the original compressive force, but in some cases it may be secondary.

Microscopic sections of the bone, removed after the condition has been established, show patchy aseptic necrosis accompanied by evidence of regeneration. The trabeculae are fragmented in disorderly manner, and there is fibrous replacement of bone. Connective tissue proliferates in the marrow, and at the same time there is osseous metaplasia. The vessels are hypertrophied, showing increased vascularity. The cartilage of the articular surfaces shows secondary erosion over the areas of greatest necrosis. Arthritic changes are regularly visible in roentgenograms, but arthritis becomes most severe in late cases in which the mechanics of the wrist joint have been upset by the lunate's being crushed out of shape. Arthritis in the early cases occurs in response to tissue reaction in the parts contiguous to the affected bone.

Symptoms

The initial symptoms are pain, tenderness, swelling and limitation of motion—especially on dorsiflexion of the wrist. The pain is through the wrist and radiates up the forearm; the tenderness is local over both the dorsal and the volar surfaces of either the lunate or the navicular bone. There is some general swelling of the wrist, but the edema is specially localized over the affected bone as can be recognized by pinching up a fold of skin. These symptoms may appear immediately following trauma or gradually thereafter. They may persist for a few days to several weeks and then usually subside for an interval that varies from weeks to years, after which the symptoms of the established condition increase and are progressive, causing considerable disability. In addition to the symptoms mentioned above, pain can be produced by pushing on the finger rays so that they press on the affected bone— in the case of the lunate, the middle finger especially, and for the scaphoid the index finger and the thumb. The roentgen appearance establishes the diagnosis. Some cases recover completely; others have recurrence in spells. However, many show prolonged disability, even up to 20 years. Of course, by that time there is marked hypertrophic arthritis. J. I. P. James even reports a case of rupture of the flexor profundus tendon of the index finger and the flexor pollicis longus in an advanced case of Kienböck's disease.

TREATMENT

Considering that in many instances a cure is brought about by conservative treatment in a cast for 6 to 8 months and that this usually brings at least temporary improvement, conservative treatment should be given a trial. A nonpadded cast is applied to the hand and the forearm, stopping at both the thenar and the distal creases in the palm to allow full motion of the digits. Successful treatment by drilling the bone has been reported. It is based on allowing the necrotic products to escape and bringing in a new blood supply. The usual treatment is to excise either the lunate or the navicular as soon as the condition has proved to be increasing or permanent. The sooner this is done, the less will be the resulting hypertrophic arthritis. Once the latter is established it is generally permanent. Following excision of the lunate bone there will be a certain amount of lameness and soreness of the wrist which will disappear eventually, though many patients will complain of some pain on prolonged use or overwork. Most cases show some diminution of grip. The same is true following the removal of the navicular bone. In some cases the disability will not be noticed, and in others a certain amount of lameness will follow. There will be less complaint from nonmanual workers.

Witt uses a Plexiglas prosthesis for the lunate, and Myrin reported 3 cases of Kienböck's as well as 2 scaphoid replacements in which Teflon prostheses were used.

Klutchareva reports some good results from merely scooping out the necrotic area and leaving the good bone. Filling the cavity by cancellous bone as Russe does for ununited fractures of the scaphoid may be better.

BIBLIOGRAPHY

Albee, F. H.: Bone-graft Surgery, Philadelphia, Saunders, 1915.

Bossaert, P.: A case of reversed Madelung's disease treated surgically, Acta chir. Belg. *59*:649, 1960.

Bravo y Diaz-Canedo, J.: Malacias of the navicular bone of the wrist, Arch. de med., cir. y especialid. *15*:921, 1934.

Bruner, J. M.: Bone graft replacement of multiple metacarpal loss, J. Bone Joint Surg. *39-A*: 43, 1957.

Buchman, J.: Traumatic osteoporosis of the carpal bones, Ann Surg. *87*:892, 1928.

Carter, R. M.: Carpal boss, J. Bone Joint Surg. *23*:935, 1941.

Colonna, P. C.: Bone grafting methods, Ann. Surg. *125*:96, 1947.

Curtiss, P. H., Jr.: The hunchback carpal bone, J. Bone Joint Surg. *43-A*:392, 1961.

Darrach, W.: Anterior dislocation of the head of the ulna, Ann. Surg. *56*:802, 1912.

————: Habitual forward dislocation of the head of the ulna, Ann. Surg. *57*:928, 1913.

Dornan, A.: The results of treatment in Kienböck's disease, J. Bone Joint Surg. *31-B*:518, 1949.

Dorosin, N., and Davis, J. G.: Carpal boss, Radiology *66*:235, 1956.

Eliason, E. L.: An operation for recurrent inferior radio-ulnar dislocation, Ann. Surg. *96*:27, 1932.

Evans, E. M.: Rotational deformity in the treatment of fractures of both bones of the forearm, J. Bone Joint Surg. *27*:373, 1945.

Frank, P.: The pathogenesis of necrosis of the semilunar bone and its relation to the effects of work on the wrist joint, Beitr. klin. Chir. *164*: 200, 1936.

Frassi, G. A.: On the surgical treatment of Madelung's deformity, Minerva Ortop. *12*:661, 1961.

Garcia, L. A.: Supernumerary muscle diagnosed as synovial cyst of carpus, Med. ibera *1*:882, 1936.

Gillespie, H. S.: Excision of lunate bone in Kienböck's disease, J. Bone Joint Surg. *43-B*:245, 1961.

Grettve, S.: Arterial anatomy of carpal bones, Acta anat. *25*:331, 1955.

Haüptli, O.: Die Aseptischen Chondro-Osteonekrosen, Berlin, Walter de Gruyter, 1954.

Henderson, M. S.: Chronic osteitis of semilunar bone (Kienböck's disease), J. Bone Joint Surg. *8*:504, 1926.

Horwitz, M. T.: Anatomic and roentgenologic

study of the wrist joint, Surgery 7:773, 1940.

Howard, L. D., Jr.: Problem of fractures of hand due to war wounds, Am. Acad. Orthop. Surg. Lect., p. 196, 1944.

Hucherson, D. C.: Darrach operation for lower radio-ulnar derangement, Am. J. Surg. 53:237, 1941.

Hultén: Enstehaug und Behandlung der Lunatummalacie, Acta chir. scand. (Schwd.) 76, 121, 1935.

Humphries, S. V.: Congenital proximal radio-ulnar synostosis, S. Afr. M. J. 15:486, 1941.

Hyman, G., and Martin, F. R. R.: Dislocation of inferior radio-ulnar joint as complication of fracture of radius, Brit. J. Surg. 27:481, 1940.

Ingebrigtsen, R.: Restoration of lost rotation of forearm and hand by intentional permanent defect in lower ulna, Acta orthop. scand. 25: 105, 1955.

Kienböck, R.: Über traumatische Malazie des Mondbeins und über Folgezustande, Fortschr. Geb. Röntgenstrahlen 14:77, 1910-1911.

Klutchareva, T. V.: The aseptic necrosis of the lunar and the scaphoid bones—Kienböck's and Preiser's disease, Ortop. i travmatol. 3:52, 1938.

Koetzle, D.: Zur Unfallbegutachtung der Mondbeinnekrose, Monatschr. Unfallh. 40:605, 1933.

Lamphier, T. A.: Carpal bossing, Arch. Surg. 81: 1013, 1960.

Leriche, R.: A propos du scaphoide carpien pommelo, Bull. mém. Soc. nat. Chir. 52:622, 1926.

Lewis, R. M.: Colles's fracture—causative mechanism, Surgery 27:27, 1950.

Lewis, R. W., and Thibodeau, A. A.: Deformities of the wrist following resection of the head of the radius, Surg., Gynec. Obstet. 64:1079, 1937.

Lievre, J. A., Camus, J. P., and Pouch, E.: Thiemann's disease (epiphysitis of the two digital phalanges); case report and general review, Rev. Rhum. 27:135, 1960.

Littler, J. W.: Metacarpal reconstruction, J. Bone Joint Surg. 29:723, 1947.

Logroscino, D., and De Marchi, E.: Vascularization and aseptic necrosis of the carpal bones, Chir. org. movimento 23:499, 1938.

McDougall, A., and White, J.: Subluxation of the inferior radio-ulnar joint complicating fracture of the radial head, J. Bone Joint Surg. 39-B: 278, 1957.

Macciocchi, B.: Genetic aspects of Madelung's dysmorphosis, Minerva ortop. 7:266, 1956.

Madelung, O. W.: Die spontane Luxation der Hand, Arch klin. Chir. 23:395, 1879.

Magos, L.: Preliminary communication: A physiological study of the effects of vibrations on the fingers, Brit. J. Industr. Med. 18:157, 1961.

Marek, F. M.: Avascular necrosis of the carpal lunate, Clin. Orthop. 10:96, 1957.

Milch, H.: So-called dislocation of lower end of ulna, Ann. Surg. 116:282, 1942.

————: Rotation osteotomy of ulna for pronation contracture of forearm, J. Bone Joint Surg. 25: 142, 1943.

Miyakawa, G.: Replacement of the shaft of the phalanx with iliac bone, J. Bone Joint Surg. 43-A:905, 1961.

Mollo, L.: Necrosis of the semilunar bone of the wrist, Chir. org. movimento 19:232, 1934.

Murray, G.: Small bone grafts of extremities, Canad. M. A. J. 48:137, 1943.

Oltramore, J. H.: Malacia of the scaphoid bone of the carpus; pathology and treatment, Schweiz. med. Wschr. 11:956, 1933; 63:956, 1933.

Persson, M.: Pathogenese und Behandlung der Kienböckschen Lunatummalazie, Acta chir. scand., vol. 92, Suppl. 98, 1945.

Preiser, G.: Zur Frage der typischen traumatischen Ernöhrungsstörungen der kurzen Hand und Fuss wurzel Knochen, Fortschr. Geb. Röntgenstrahlen 16:360, 1910-1911.

Rodholm, A. K., and Phemister, D. B.: Cyst-like lesions of carpal bones, associated with ununited fractures, aseptic necrosis, and traumatic arthritis, J. Bone Joint Surg. 30-A:151, 1948.

Santini, M.: Medicolegal evaluation in the so-called carpal boss; cauistic note, Minerva Med. 80:129, 1960.

Scharizer, E.: Therapy of Madelung's deformity, orthop. 87:209, 1956.

Siegling, J. A.: Progress in orthopedic surgery for 1944. A review prepared by an editorial board of the Am. Acad. Orthop. Surg., Arch. Surg. 51:174, 1945.

Sunderland, K.: Rotational movements and bony union in shaft fractures of the forearm, J. Bone Joint Surg. 44-B:340, 1962.

Vasko, J. R.: An operation for old unreduced Bennett's fracture, J. Bone Joint Surg. 29:753, 1947.

Wright, J. K.: Interphalangeal fusion following frostbite, Brit. M. J. 2:1432, 1955.

Chapter 9

Joints

Restoration of motion to the joints is one of the most common problems in reconstruction of the hand. Finger joints may stiffen after injury even though the insult was distant. Simple immobilization of a part of the hand in a position of muscle imbalance will result in stiffening and fibrosis of the joints. This tendency is greater in adults and the aged but varies with individuals. As some people form keloids in the skin, others have a tendency to form scar in the periarticular tissues. Much of this stiffening can be prevented by careful positioning and splinting of the damaged hand, prompt closure of wounds and early resumption of voluntary activity.

When the nerve supply of a part is impaired, the joints will stiffen easily. Degenerative changes follow quickly with erosion of cartilage, osteoporosis and fibrosis of capsules and ligaments. A nerve lesion with much accompanying pain, such as causalgia, is even more effective in producing stiffness of the joints.

Nutritional changes from impaired blood supply also help to stiffen joints, and when scar tissue from injury or infection is excessive and strangles the limb by its contracture, the effects of a lesion in the nerve and the vessel are compounded.

Overcoming stiff joints is essential if the hand is to function and is a prerequisite to any attempt to provide voluntary motion by tendon transfer or graft.

WHY FINGER JOINTS STIFFEN

The moving parts of the hand—especially the interphalangeal joints—are closely fitted structures with little tolerance. As the mechanism of a watch whose accuracy depends on an exact meshing of many moving parts fails when one small part is out of alignment, so the joints of the hand with their snugly fitted surfaces held together by elastic capsules and retaining ligaments become disabled from minor derangements. Anything altering the shape of the joint surfaces or the consistency of the soft parts limits motion.

The collateral ligaments of the metacarpophalangeal joint of a finger are especially vulnerable. With the finger in extension, the 2 collateral ligaments span the joint running from a dorsally placed proximal attachment on the metacarpal to a volar and distal insertion on the phalanx. In extension the ligaments allow lateral motion; but when flexed, the base of the proximal phalanx slides over the nonspherical curve of the metacarpal head and lies on the broad volar expansion of the metacarpal head. In this position no lateral motion is possible.

Because of the sites of attachments of the ligaments and the broader volar part of the head, the collateral ligaments are taut in flexion. Thus, whatever shortens the ligament, if such shortening takes place with the finger extended, will interfere with flexion. The restriction of flexion of the metacarpophalangeal finger joints is one of the most common complications of hand injuries.

When a hand remains swollen, from whatever cause, the movable parts are bathed in serofibrinous exudate. Fibrin is deposited between the various tissue layers and in the folds of the joint capsules, between the tendons and their sheaths, throughout the ligamentous tissue itself and between and within the muscles. While soaked in the exudate all these tissues swell with edema and become shorter and thicker. The fibrin seals them in this condition, and soon, as the fibroblastic growth transforms all to connective tissue, the ligaments become shorter and thicker. The folds of synovial membrane, the capsules of joints, the plicae of tendon sheaths and the tendons and their sheaths become plastered together with organized adhesions.

Swelling from edema may come from many causes; it may follow general traumatism to

Fig. 367. (*Top*) Preoperative position of nonfunction from shark bite in the upper arm, severing nerves and vessels. (*Bottom*) Correction to a position of function postoperatively by fusion of the wrist, capsulectomies, opening of the cleft of the thumb, a pulley tendon transfer for opposition, and transferring extensors of the wrist to flexors of the fingers.

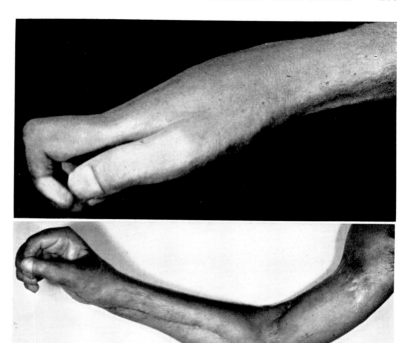

the hand or even an injury of the arm. It regularly accompanies fractures in the hand and the forearm, and even in the upper arm. Splinting a joint on a strain injures and stiffens it. Hematoma or general ecchymosis of the tissues causes edematous swelling, but the outstanding cause is infection. Functional disuse of the hand in itself may result in edema. The tissue fluids stagnate from the lack of pumping by muscle action.

Thus, edema is pernicious and may come from many causes. Edema alone may not cause a hand to stiffen, but when it is accompanied by immobilization so that the tissues are allowed to set in that condition, stiffening is inevitable.

PREVENTION OF JOINT STIFFNESS

To prevent stiffness one must prevent or reduce edema, avoid further injury from excessive manipulation or heat and strive for early motion of the part.

PREVENTION OF EDEMA

The hand should be elevated as long as necessary with the hand higher than the elbow, and the elbow higher than the shoulder. Lying in bed with the hand and the arm on a sloping bed of pillows or, if the patient is ambulatory, on an airplane splint will maintain the elevated position.

A fracture should be immobilized, including the joints above and below the fracture, but all uninjured parts should be free to move. Unless there are specific contraindications, the wrist should be in slight dorsiflexion.

Healing tissues require rest, so that massage and manipulations are avoided. Active motion when begun is limited to the tolerance of the parts. Application of heat in the form of hot epsom salt soaks or contrast baths promotes edema and swelling.

ACTIVE MOTION OF UNINJURED PARTS

All uninjured parts should be left free to move, and movement should be encouraged. If possible, the injured part is immobilized, the contiguous parts are left free, and the whole extremity is returned to use. A properly applied cast, as for Colles' fracture, should immobilize the wrist and the forearm but end at the distal crease of the palm to allow full extension and flexion of the fingers. The thumb should also be free. Movements of these parts should be started immediately, and the patient must be compelled to flex and extend all the digits voluntarily. If one finger is splinted in the balanced position of semiflexion, all the others can be moved through almost a normal range, in spite of the common muscles and the interdigitating tendons. If the required fixed position of the injured part should be that which prevents active motion of the remaining parts, then these parts should be moved passively. The motion must be maintained until the immobilization of the injured part is discontinued.

Some factors that cause stiffness are making plaster dressings too long, so that they cover uninjured digits, using too much padding which fails to immobilize completely and thus allows painful motion, and leaving splints on too long.

Constant vigilance is necessary. If left to himself, the patient will refrain from moving the uninjured parts because of discomfort or fear. Encouragement and a demonstration of what can be done will show him that his fears are ungrounded.

The prompt closure of open wounds is essential in preventing edema and stiffness. Temporary split grafts cover granulating wounds and allow healing and mobility to be regained. At a later stage, a more wearable full-thickness cover can be supplied.

The use of a sling should be avoided, as the shoulder will soon stiffen, and abduction and external rotation will be lost. When instructing a patient in the daily exercise of the uninjured parts, a plan of exercise for the shoulder and the elbow should be included.

MOBILIZING STIFFENED JOINTS

In long-standing flexion contractures all tissues, including the ligaments of the joints, share in the contracture, so that even when all

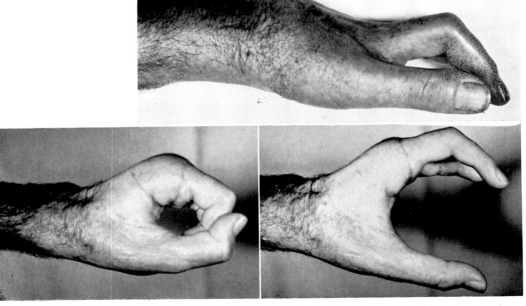

FIG. 368. (*Top*) Old dislocation of the metacarpals on the carpus, upsetting the muscle balance, thus resulting in a useless position of nonfunction. (*Bottom*) Dislocation reduced, restoring muscle balance in the position of function. A pedicle graft was applied to the dorsum of the hand and to the opened thumb cleft. Freeing of the extensor tendons and capsulectomies allowed the proximal finger joints to flex.

other restraining tissues are severed, the joint ligaments will still keep the joint from extending. Severance, excision or elongation of these ligaments by slow traction will be necessary.

THE POSITION OF FUNCTION

Following a severe injury or infection it is usual to find the wrist in flexion, the arches flat, the thumb at the side in the plane of the palm and the proximal finger joints extended. Usually, the 2 distal joints will be slightly flexed, and the forearm will be in pronation. A hand in such a position is useless, and what little motion is present is of no practical value.

The first procedure should be to bend these joints gradually until each is in the position of function; that is, with the wrist in dorsiflexion of about 30°, the carpal and the metacarpal arches well curved, the thumb in the position of opposition, and the proximal finger joints in flexion. If the fingers and the thumb show only ½-inch amplitude of motion in these positions, this motion will be useful, while in the position of nonfunction, the patient will not use his hand at all and, so to speak, will forget that he has one. Since the position of function allows him to pick up small objects, he will begin to use his hand. Under the stimulus of function, motion will increase, and he will use it more, so that a happy circle will be established which will lead to greater function.

Gaining and maintaining the position of function should be the goal in all hand surgery. At this position there is the greatest function. It is the starting point of all motions, and here the mechanics are most efficient. The position should be maintained throughout treatment for infections and the results of trauma.

Some authors describe the "position of rest" with the wrist slightly flexed and the proximal finger joints almost straight, as in sleep, but this has no place in reconstruction. One might as well describe the supine position of the body in contrast with upright posture. The position of function is dynamic with the muscles in normal tone.

Continuous Mild Traction. If flexion contracture is present from superficial or deep cicatrix, first it should be corrected by plastic procedures. The use of continuous mild traction to bend joints around to a better position or to gain more motion of flexion or extension differs greatly in results from the intermittent bending of joints, or the so-called pump-handle method. Intermittent force applied to the contracted ligaments merely stretches them, and like the rubber band these ligaments will shorten again immediately. In addition, there will be tiny tears and hemorrhages which will be followed by tissue reaction, resulting in further cicatricial contraction.

By the continuous mild traction method, however, a slight stretch is maintained on the restraining tissues until by cell multiplication they actually grow longer, so that the lengthening is permanent. The yielding of tissues to continuous mild force, together with adaptation by growth to the new position, is exemplified in the straightening of teeth by the orthodontist or in the extreme deformities seen after the loss of muscle balance or the elongation of tissues to make way for tremendous tumor growths. The orthodontist makes use of 2 mechanisms. The first is continuous spring tension, and the second intermittent bevel-action pressure in biting. The continuous mild traction to correct the deformity in the joint is applied to the limb by means of well-padded splints. This traction to bend joints should be maintained continuously, but it should be released every 1 or 2 hours by day, so that for short intervals the joints can be exercised to prevent stiffening. If traction is maintained constantly for too many weeks, joints will stiffen. Traction should be fairly gentle, yet firm enough to yield results. If it is too forceful, there will be pain, swelling and damage to the joint, including pressure atrophy of the articular cartilages. The skin that is pressed on should be watched for signs of ischemia, the first sign being a brownish color.

Continuous traction may be applied by means of plaster casts with intermittent wedging, by metal splints with web belts and buckles or by elastic or spring splinting. It is difficult for a patient to tamper with a cast and a patient who will not tolerate apparatus is less likely to try to remove them. They work well for clubfeet or clinarthrosis in growing limbs, but not so well in injuries from trauma in adults, since they cause stiffness. When using metal splints, the web belt and buckle is tightened or the splint is given a

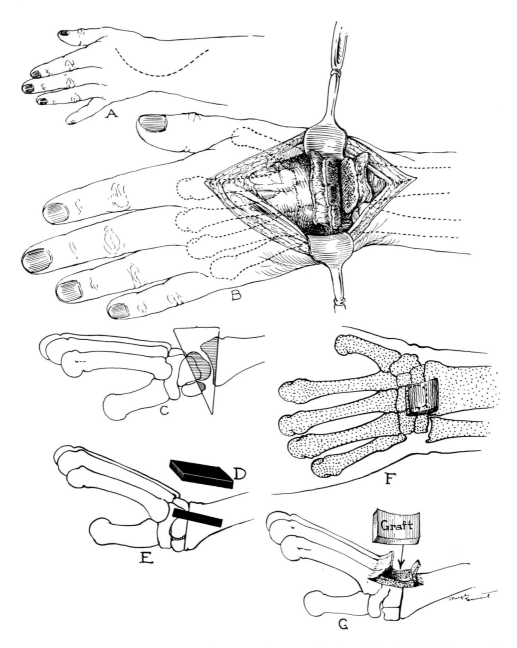

Fig. 369. Arthrodesis of wrist with preservation of radio-ulnar joint. (A) Incision curved to protect branches of superficial radial nerve. (B) The capsule is reflected both proximally and distally, along with a thin layer of bone. (C) Wedge resection to correct flexion deformity. (D and E) Bone graft of ilium used as a spline or key. Does not extend to metacarpals. (F and G) Epiphysial line can be preserved by a more superficially placed graft, extended distally into the bases of the metacarpals.

little more bend each day. This works well but, if persisted in too long, causes stiffening. The best results are obtained by elastic or spring traction, using rubber bands, spring wire or flat spring steel.

Elastic or Spring Splinting. This protects the joint from overstress. Elastic traction actually serves to exercise and mobilize a hand. The play of muscles and movable parts disseminates the stagnant fluids, allowing the tissues to return to normal. Elastic splinting is physiologic and effective. Elastic or spring splinting requires careful and frequent adjustment of the mechanism and fails in many instances because of 2 factors—wrong application and misunderstanding on the part of doctor and patient. In the case of very stubborn joints, all that can be accomplished is to bend them into a position of function so that their limited range of motion will be useful, or, if ankylosis is the eventual result, the joint will at least be in the right position.

When a joint is painful at its limit of flexion, this may often be cured by gradually drawing the joint into complete flexion. If maintained so for 2 weeks, until the restraining tissues elongate, the joint will flex without pain.

Various splints are described in Chapter 6.

Exercising Stiff Joints. While and after joints are being brought into positions of function, they should be exercised. Voluntary exercise and use of the hand by the patient throughout the whole day is far superior in result to the usual thermal and light treatments and forceful passive motion customarily applied only 1 hour a day. Daily forcing of finger joints causes reactive pain and swelling, and the joints become stiffer than ever. It is equivalent to spraining them daily. Such unphysiologic treatment seems to be based on early experiences with inanimate objects— forced movements will mobilize a rusty hinge or a stiff piece of leather. The patient will not hurt himself; his nerves are his protection against overstraining the joints. Before and while the hand is being exercised much can be gained by the use of mild heat, preferably by immersing the hand in lukewarm water. Adding soap to the water makes it easier to massage and work one hand with the other. Washing dishes is also helpful.

The hand may grip a cloth bag that is filled with dried rice and fastened to the wrist with an elastic. A flat block of wood, $\frac{1}{2}$ inch thick with rounded edges, or a rubber sponge which can be kept in the pocket is handy for exercising the joints. One can exercise to gain pronation and supination by rotating the forearm back and forth while holding a broomstick or a dumbbell in the hand. There is something about the natural use of a hand in light work that is the most conducive to the return of joint motion. However, there is an unavoidable time factor, for even with the best of treatment, a certain interval must elapse before the joints become mobile.

If gentle, passive physiotherapy may be beneficial for 2 or 3 weeks. However, in nerve lesions it must be used over long periods of time in order to maintain the position of the hand and the circulation of the joints and the tissues. The patient himself should be instructed to use his good hand to put his paralyzed hand through the proper motions.

When a joint is infected or injured it requires rest. One must judge carefully just when to change to gradual exercise, lest this cause a flare-up of the inflammation. Sometimes part of the swollen hand is so tender that a patient will not use any part of the hand. A cast which immobilizes just that part, such as the wrist, will allow the digits to be exercised without pain and so improve the whole hand.

Brisement Forcé. Forcing stiff fingers under anesthesia is dangerous and usually does harm. It not only produces more stiffness but traumatizes the joint so badly that it will never recover. Also, an osteoporotic bone is easily broken in this way. Only in very exceptional cases will the method be of advantage. If there is latent infection in the joint, as indicated by pain, swelling and tenderness, forcing the joint will cause an inflammatory flare-up. It is only when some particular adhesion is holding back the motion that the method succeeds. Of course, if on bending the joint with mild force, a single snap is heard, there is a chance of success; but if a general tear or yielding of the ligaments about the joint occurs, it is probable that increased stiffness will result.

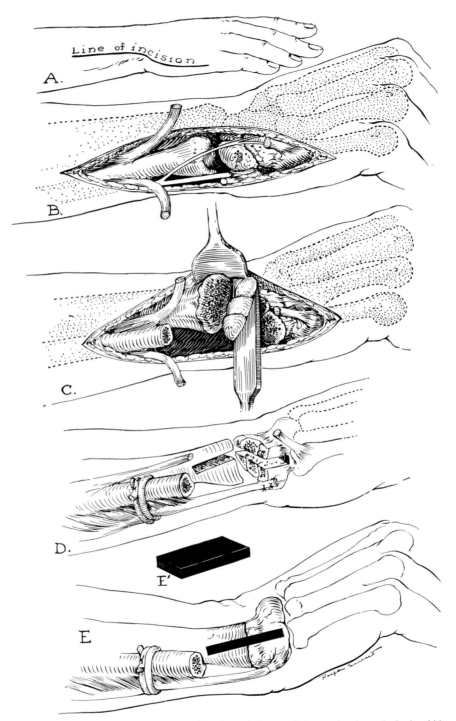

Fig. 370. Arthrodesis when the radio-ulnar joint participates in the ankylosis. (A) The joint is opened by the Smith-Petersen approach. (B) The tendons of the 2 carpi ulnari are severed, and the dorsal branch of the ulnar nerve is retracted. (C) The head of the ulna is excised, and the joint denuded so that it fits together at 30° of dorsiflexion. (D) The ulna, now free for pronation and supination, is lashed to the flexor ulnaris tendon to prevent displacement. (E) Bone graft from the tibia or the iliac crest is placed.

SURGICAL REPAIR OF JOINTS

Loose joints can be stabilized by grafting new ligaments to them, and their motion can be increased by capsulectomy or arthroplasty. Also, joints are rendered solid, painless and correctly positioned by arthrodesis.

Caution is essential; one must not operate on a joint in which the inflammatory process still lingers. Pain, tenderness, redness and edema are warnings that surgery may cause a flare-up.

Joints with intra-articular changes, including degeneration of articular cartilages, adhesions between the bones and destruction of synovia, usually require arthrodesis or arthroplasty. However, much improvement can be gained when the damage is extra-articular.

In all deformed hands coming for repair the surgeon must weigh the results to be gained from the many available procedures. The paramount goal should be the restoration of function, and for this the position of function is mandatory. This may be brought about by splinting, capsulectomy, arthroplasty and arthrodesis.

In planning tendon repairs and transfers, the surgeon must keep in mind the value of arthrodeses, as by these he may obtain the position of function when there are not enough tendons to give it. The fewer the tendons that are available, the greater the need for arthrodeses. By these, many a deformed hand may be placed in good position so that the few remaining tendons can furnish the ability to open and close for grasp. For loss of the deltoid, the arm is made useful by arthrodesing the shoulder. A flail elbow that is arthrodesed brings function to the hand. Arthrodesis of the wrist stabilizes the hand for use and makes the 5 wrist tendons available for the digits. The 3 large joints are rarely arthrodesed at the same time. Any one or 2 of the thumb joints may need arthrodesing, and any 1 or 2 of the 3 finger joints, leaving some joints for motion. When most joints are flail, a combination of functional bracing, transfers and arthrodeses, as in Chapter 6, may provide an essential function. In loss of nerves, muscles or tendons, enough joints in the limbs may be arthrodesed to give the position of function and allow the remaining available tendons to furnish prehension and what other motions they can.

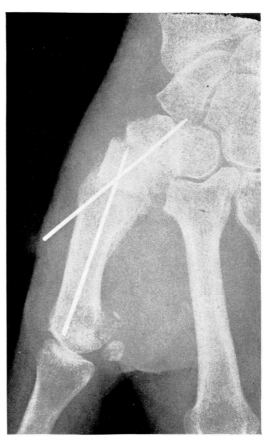

Fig. 371. The metacarpotrapezial joint was painful from osteoarthritis. Fusion with disk of iliac bone inserted after excision of joint surfaces.

SURGERY OF SPECIAL JOINTS

Wrist Joint. A wrist damaged by infection or injury will be found to be ankylosed in flexion, a position of nonfunction. This is because the flexor tendons and other tissues on the volar aspect of the wrist shorten, producing flexion contracture. The radio-ulnar joint always shares in the infection, so that the motions of pronation and supination will be lost. For such an ankylosed wrist the surgeon should change the position to one of dorsiflexion and either solidify the wrist by arthrodesis or, on rarer occasions, give it motion through arthroplasty. In either case, the motions of pronation and supination should be restored by disconnecting the lower end of the ulna from its attachment in the wrist, by re-

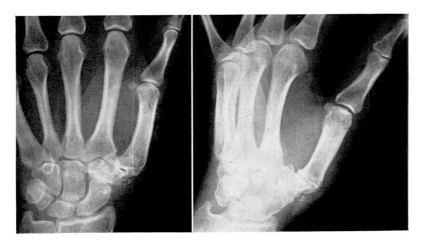

FIG. 372. Reconstruction of ligaments of metacarpotrapezial joint for persistent dislocation according to method shown in Figure 373. Roentgenograms 10 years after operation. Joint painless and with about 70 per cent of normal range of motion.

moving the head of the ulna or a short segment of its neck. The repair of such a wrist is usually only part of an extensive repair involving all the tissues.

Arthrodesis may be indicated when, following injury, the wrist is deformed from any of the various types of dislocation or from loss of some of the carpal bones, making an irregular surface to articulate with the radius and the ulna. Also, it should be done when the wrist becomes progressively involved with arthritis resulting from degenerative disease of the lunate (Kienböck's disease) or of the scaphoid (Preiser's disease) or from old nonunion of a fractured scaphoid.

For old dislocation through the carpus, the wrist should be opened through a lateral incision or a transverse or L-shaped dorsal incision; all restraining ligaments should be freed, traction applied on the fingers, and the dislocation reduced with a skidlike instrument. Usually, it will remain so. If necessary, the bones may be pinned in place readily by 2 Kirschner wires cut subcutaneously and removed after a month. If the articular surface of the carpus is irregular and one-sided from loss of some of the carpal bones, the remainder of the proximal row of carpal bones should also be removed or chiseled through, together with the head of the capitate, so that a properly shaped articular surface will present against the radius and the ulna.

In planning a wrist joint operation the surgeon should keep in mind that the muscle balance of the fingers depends on the position of the wrist—the farther away the position,

from between 20° and 30° of dorsiflexion, the more the digits are off balance.

A dislocation through the carpus backward or forward so upsets the muscle balance or relative tension of the tendons that there is resulting deformity of angulation in each successive joint distally. This can be corrected only by placing the bones back in their normal alignment.

Often in paralytics the motion of the digits is automatic, depending on the movement of the wrist, and will be lost with an arthrodesis. In choosing between arthrodesis and arthroplasty the following considerations may be of assistance:

Following arthrodesis in 20° dorsiflexion and provided that pronation and supination are free, there is excellent function with very little disability. Such a wrist is especially adapted to heavy work. For people who do fine work, such as musicians or women, and also for those desiring good cosmetic appearance, a movable wrist by arthroplasty is desirable. This is especially true when there are ample tendons in good condition to move both the wrist and the digits. If a wrist is ankylosed in an incorrect position, correction by either arthrodesis or arthroplasty is desirable. For spastic cases, arthrodesis is better than arthroplasty, but one should test the effect first by placing a cast on the wrist, as some useful movements may be lost or there may be bad substitution movements. Arthrodesis is indicated in flail wrist and any hands and wrists where there are not enough tendons to move both the wrist and the digits. It makes available for use on the digits the 5 or 6 tendons that normally move the wrist. When 2 of the 3 hand nerves are paralyzed above their branches to the forearm muscles, arthrodesis may furnish enough muscles to move the digits. However, when the number of available tendons is few, one should choose carefully between arthrodesis or the use of the few available tendons to move the wrist. With a movable wrist, automatic digit motion may be obtained by tenodesing their extensor and flexor tendons to the forearm bones. For extreme cases of clubhand, severe malunion about the wrist or severe arthritis, arthrodesis is desirable.

ARTHRODESIS should not be done before the age of eight or, better, 10 years, because of distortion and interference with growth. The optimal position to be obtained is from 15° to 30° dorsiflexion, preferably 20°. Too much dorsiflexion is unsightly and inefficient. The correct amount of dorsiflexion will place the cleft between the opposed thumb and fingers in line with the radius for grasping. Also, the wrist should be in slight ulnar flexion, so that the index metacarpal will be in the line of the radius, and the tendons crossing the wrist will be in their normal line of function. More dorsiflexion than this greatly decreases the efficiency of the hand.

Two types of operation are available: one by the dorsal route and one by the lateral route as described by Smith-Petersen. There is better exposure in the former route, and often a normal radio-ulnar joint may be preserved for pronation and supination. If this is not possible, the head of the ulna is removed through the same incision. It is advisable to retract the tendons gently and to restore their gliding surfaces, since tendon mobilization and transfer often may be necessary at a later operation. When the radio-ulnar joint is involved and the tendons must glide over the carpus, the latter approach will be found to be useful.

For the dorsal route the incision should be curved, with the broad pedicle on the radial side to preserve the branches of the radial nerve. This is preferable to the bayonet incision across the wrist, because it places the suture line remote from, instead of over, the bone graft. The soft parts of the wrist broaden as they shorten, needing more skin circumferentially. Therefore, this wound may be closed as a T-juncture, the V-Y principle being used. It has been suggested that the incision be a Y, the fork embracing the wrist, with the stem distal. This is closed as a V, thus taking from the length and giving to the circumference. Entering between the extensor pollicis

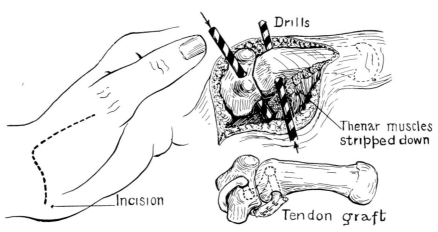

FIG. 373. Operation for correction of chronic dislocation of the 1st metacarpal on the greater multangular. The former is drilled laterally and the latter antero-posteriorly, and the tendon graft from the palmaris longus is threaded through the holes as shown, looping it under the ridge, lashing the metacarpal down so that it cannot displace backward. Fusion is better if arthritis is present.

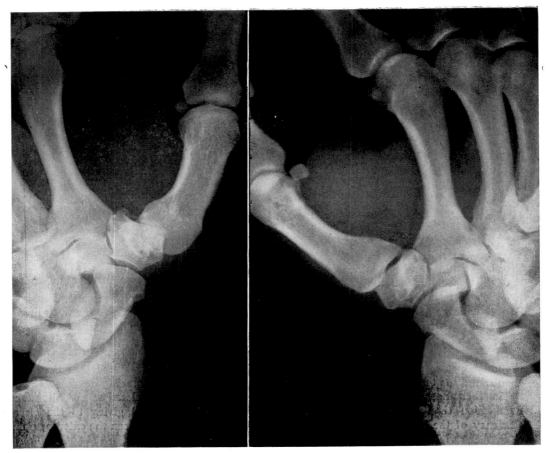

FIG. 374. (*Left*) Old dislocation of the first metacarpal forward on the greater multangular. (*Right*) A stable thumb was obtained by open operation. The debris was removed from between the 2 bones, and the bases of the first 2 metacarpals were lashed together with palmaris longus tendon through drillholes.

longus and the extensor tendons of the fingers, which are retracted to each side, the capsule of the wrist is exposed. A wedge is cut out across and including the radiocarpal joint so that the bones will fit free from cartilage at 20° dorsiflexion. With a broad chisel or a Stryker saw, a transverse slot is made into both the radius and the carpus. Usually, this cut does not quite reach the carpometacarpal joints, but when extra stability is desired, it is extended into the metacarpals. When carpometacarpal joints share in the fusion, some resiliency is lost, and there is risk of breaking. Cartilage from the midcarpal joints is removed where it is accessible.

A semiflexible graft from the iliac crest can be shaped to fit and excels in bone growth properties. Other sources for bone graft are the thin slice cut off the end of the radius or a piece taken from the end of the ulna. The wrist is fixed firmly by 2 strong crossed Kirschner wires cut off beneath the skin. Too large a graft will stretch the limited circumference of the wrist. The work should all be done distal to the epiphysial plate before full growth is attained, the greater part of the wedge being taken from the carpus.

In the lateral approach, through an incision jogged slightly dorsally as it crosses the wrist, the posterior branch of the ulnar nerve is preserved by retracting it volarward. The head of the ulna is freed subligamentously and removed with a short segment of the shaft, exposing the wrist joint. The extensor tendons

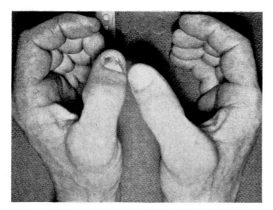

FIG. 375. Radial subluxation of the proximal thumb joint, so-called game-keeper's thumb. If much pain is present and the deformity is of long duration, arthrodesis is indicated.

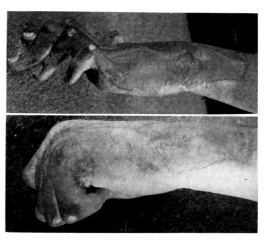

FIG. 376. (*Top*) Dorsal burn from an airplane fire, leaving stiff recurved proximal finger joints. (*Bottom*) Capsulectomy through a split skin graft allowed flexion. The central tendon slips of the middle joints have been burned, necessitating arthrodeses. (L. D. Howard, M.D.)

are stripped and retracted dorsally. The wedge is chiseled from the radius and the carpus. A broad slot to receive the graft is chiseled across the radius and the carpus by the methods described under the dorsal approach. For a graft, the removed head and neck of the ulna or the tibia or the iliac crest are available.

If the arthrodesis is done for a wrist that has been solidified by infection, it is not necessary to place a bone graft; but one is essential if the intercarpal joints are free. The cartilage should be chiseled from the midcarpal joint. If there is marked laxity of the proximal ulna, a tendon sling can be placed around it and the flexor carpi ulnaris. The arm and the hand are put up in plaster of Paris for 2 or 3 months. The first cast should be bivalved during the period when swelling can be expected and should reach to the axilla with the elbow at a right angle to control pronation and supination. There is so much postoperative swelling and the skin about the wrist yields so little that there may be some necrosis of the skin. Should the skin be tight, freeing incisions with skin grafting should be done. It is not wise to combine the arthrodesis with other operations, such as extensive tendon transfers, because of the danger of increasing the swelling and jeopardizing the tendons. On subsidence of the swelling, sutures are removed, and a nonpadded plaster cast is applied.

ARTHROPLASTY. True arthroplasty is seldom indicated in the wrist. Here the operation usually consists of removing either the proximal row or both rows of carpal bones. Enough articular cartilage generally remains to allow motion. However, if, after excising the necessary $\frac{1}{2}$ inch of bone to furnish motion, both of the surfaces are raw, so that granulations will grow across and rejoin the bones, a double or a single layer of free graft of fascia lata should be interposed.

The usual procedure is to remove the proximal row of carpal bones. This should be accompanied by chiseling off the projecting head of the capitate bone, so as to provide a properly curved articulating surface of the carpus. In some cases where there is greater joint destruction it will be necessary to remove both rows of carpal bones. This leaves a rather broad, flat surface which articulates well with the radius and the ulna, with the thumb articulating on the radiostyloid. It does not allow for any lateral movement of the wrist and only 20° or 30° of anteroposterior movement. This motion will be weaker than that in the case in which only the proximal row of carpal bones was removed. In the latter case the joint surface of the carpus is better adapted for both anteroposterior and lateral movement,

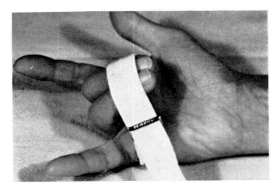

FIG. 377. A web strap with a buckle can provide a most efficient steady force to gain flexion of the middle finger joints.

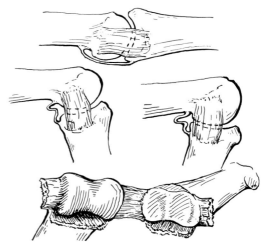

FIG. 378. Middle joint of a finger showing collateral ligaments and close-fitting joint surfaces on which lateral stability depends. Snug-fitting joints are stiffened easily.

and the length of lever arm for action of the tendons that move the wrist will be much greater. If both rows of carpal bones must be removed, arthrodesis is better. With arthrodesis there is a little wrist motion at the carpometacarpal joints which allows a springiness that is very useful.

In producing a movable wrist one should not forget to furnish pronation and supination as well. If the head of the ulna is ankylosed to the carpus it should be excised, but if it is ankylosed to the radius, the distal segment of the shaft of the ulna should be excised.

The incision for arthroplasty depends on whether the head of the ulna or a segment of shaft is to be removed. In the former, the lateral incision is used, removing the head and opening the joint in abduction. Otherwise, one should use a bayonet incision, running down the dorsum of the ulna, then across the wrist with the wrinkles, and then on down a little farther. This allows removal of a segment of the neck of the ulna and, when the extensor tendons of the fingers are retracted en masse radially, exposes the carpus.

The result after these 3 types of operations to mobilize the wrist varies according to the conditions found. Though motion is quite limited after removal of the whole carpus, one can expect about 40° to 50° of motion in good functioning range after true arthroplasty or after removal of the proximal carpal row. Where the cartilages are fairly well preserved, the motion after removal of the proximal car-

pal row may even be a little greater. There are so many tendons about the circumference of the wrist that one can afford to leave a ½ inch space between the bone ends without fear of instability. If arthritis should develop at a later date, arthrodesis always can be done.

PRONATION AND SUPINATION. Normally, when the elbow is held fixed at a right angle at the side, the hand rotates through 180° from palm-up to palm-down position, though the wrist itself moves only about 150°. The motion takes place equally in both the upper and the lower radio-ulnar joints. Anything limiting the motion of either one of these joints limits both. The range of pronation and supination may also be limited by angulation of the shafts of the radius and the ulna in malunion following fractures or can be stopped entirely by synostosis between the shafts of these bones. With the elbow fixed at the side, the midposition is with the thumb pointed vertically. From this position both supination and pronation are to 90°. Voluntary supination is much more useful than pronation. The tendency is for gravity and the muscles of pronation, which are stronger, to cause fixation of the forearm in pronation when motion becomes limited. When limitation of pronation and supination is imminent, the wrist should be near the midposition. In certain types of bench work the slightly pronated position may be desirable.

The distal radio-ulnar joint always becomes involved when the wrist joint is infected, though academically the articular disk, unless perforated, separates these 2 synovial cavities. The head of the ulna becomes fused to either the radius or the carpus or both. In performing an arthrodesis in either case, a segment from the lower end of the shaft of the ulna should be removed; but in performing an arthroplasty, the head of the ulna should be removed if it is fused to the carpus, and a segment of the shaft if the head is fused to the radius. This will free the wrist for practically the complete range of motion of pronation and supination. However, it is often found that people with loose tissues complain of pain from displacement of the end of the ulna backward on pronation. Therefore, when severed above the pronator quadratus, a free graft of tendon, usually from the palmaris longus, is made to encircle both the ulna and the tendon of the flexor carpi ulnaris muscle. The graft can be placed quickly with a Deschamps carrier and a curved hemostat through a short lateral incision over the lower end of the shaft. The tendon may be passed around once or twice and joined to itself by a removable running stainless steel wire. Then the ulna will not displace backward on pronation, because the patient will have the power through the flexor carpi ulnaris muscle to hold it forward.

For proper function at the wrist the radius should be longer than the ulna, and the ulnar collateral and articular disk ligaments which control the radius in its arc about the ulnar head should be intact. When the radius becomes relatively shorter from compression as in Colles' fracture, retarded growth in Madelung's deformity, or damage to a radial epiphysis, the ulna is overprominent on the dorsum of the wrist and protrudes into the carpus, causing disability.

For this longitudinal dislocation, the ulna either can be shortened or a good result may be obtained by the Darrach operation. This consists of excising the head of the ulna interligamentously but not subperiosteally, leaving the styloid process with its 2 ligaments. The shaft is trimmed obliquely to avoid a corner.

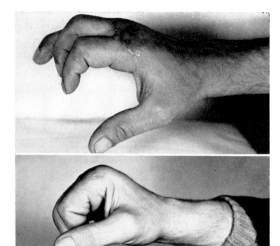

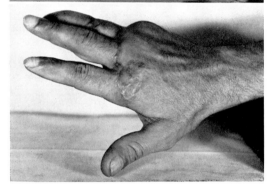

Fig. 379. Case J. T. (*Top*) A circular saw cut across the dorsum of the fingers through the proximal joints. Both extensors and flexors were much limited. (*Center and bottom*) The middle joint of the ring finger was arthrodesed. Capsulectomy was done on the proximal joint of the index finger, and arthroplasty on that of the long and the ring fingers. The little finger was amputated. Fascia from the thigh was placed beneath the extensor tendons. Good function resulted.

A new short ulnar head may form, held in place by its ligamentous attachments.

When the lower end of the radius is fractured, the ulnar head remains fixed, though relatively dislocating on the radius. Thus, in Colles' fracture it is fixed forward and distalward. The mechanism is similar to that of dislocation of the radial head in fracture of the upper end of the ulna. Also, forced supination dislocates the ulnar head forward without fracture unless the fracture is of the styloid process. Once dislocated, there is free to-and-fro movement between the ulnar head and the radius, and the former is prominent dorsally on pronation, displacing with a click on each motion of pronation or supination. The click may be caused by the tendon of the extensor carpi ulnaris jumping back and forth over the ulnar styloid. In supination, when the wrist is flexed, the tendon displaces volarward, and when the wrist is dorsiflexed the displacement is dorsalward, each time with a snap. Pain, tenderness and weakness are noticed, especially when lifting in pronation.

Several corrective procedures are available, some of which are as follows:

1. A tendon or fascial graft encircles (close to the head of the ulna), crosses and is attached to the radius at the dorsal and the ulnar borders of the radio-ulnar joint.

Another strip substituting for the stylotriquetrum ligament but advantageously oblique is half of the tendon of the flexor carpi ulnaris split down and left attached to the pisiform. It then penetrates the head of the ulna at the base of the styloid and is made fast.

A third tendon graft checks the tendon of the extensor carpi ulnaris from jumping over the ulnar styloid by looping around this tendon and fastening to the dorsal ligament of the wrist. This method has been used successfully by the author.

2. Half of the tendon of the extensor carpi ulnaris is split off down to its insertion, brought back through the head of the ulna through a drill hole and fastened to the bone (Taylor).

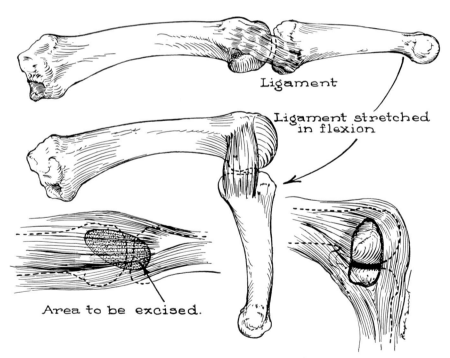

Fig. 380. Capsulectomy of the proximal finger joint. Normally, the collateral ligaments are slack in extension but tight in flexion. If these ligaments, because of edema and immobility, become short and thick, the joint will no longer flex.

Through a short longitudinal incision on each side of the knuckle, the joint capsule is exposed between tendons of the long extensor and the interosseus muscles, and, on excising the collateral ligament from each side, the joint easily can be placed in flexion.

3. In a case with accompanying arthritis, the head of the ulna is fused to the radius, and a segment of the neck of the shaft is excised.

To check rotary movements postoperatively in any of the above procedures, the cast should include the upper arm, and the elbow should be at a right angle.

Surgery of Special Joints
Finger Joints

The proximal finger joints usually stiffen in extension or hyperextension, and the middle and the distal joints in flexion. Several procedures are available to restore motion and overcome the contracture of the ligaments and the capsule.

In mild cases, splinting will result in increased range of motion. A steady firm pressure by traction with web strap and buckle or an elastic or spring splint of proper tension may restore a useful range of motion. As when dealing with the problem of hand deformities the wrist is the key joint, so in correcting the clawed finger the proximal joint is the key. As the wrist is brought into dorsiflexion. thus bringing the digital movers into

balance, the proximal finger joints should be corrected before the middle and the distal joints are attacked.

A fixed extension contracture of the proximal joint which does not respond to purposeful splinting can be relieved by capsulectomy or arthroplasty. Arthrodesis of the proximal joint is seldom indicated, since gross bony irregularities can be overcome and arthroplasty performed.

Proximal Finger Joints. Excision of the collateral ligaments, mistakenly called capsulectomy or capsulotomy, is the commonest operation performed on this joint. It is indicated when there is limited flexion, good joint surfaces and functioning intrinsic muscles. The common extensor tendons on the dorsum of the hand should be free. It usually results in 60° to 70° of flexion.

Through 3 longitudinal incisions between the knuckles, or a single transverse incision, the proximal joints are approached, the interosseus tendons located, and a longitudinal incision made at the dorsal border of the interosseus tendon. This incision may extend a short way into the hood. Retracting the

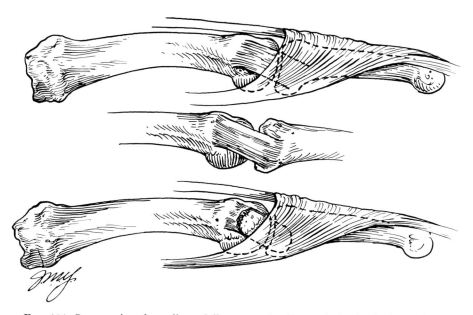

Fig. 381. In exposing the collateral ligament, the fibers of the intrinsic mechanism should be preserved. The incision in the capsule can be short; the distal hood fibers are retracted out of the way. Only the true collateral ligament is excised.

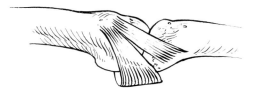

FIG. 382. The lateral ligaments blend into a "fan" ligament which becomes an integral part of the volar plate. Here, the 2 components are shown diagrammatically. For relieving extension contracture, the collateral ligament is excised. When a proximal joint has become contracted in extreme flexion, the fan ligament shortens, holding the volar plate snugly against the metacarpal neck. This can be released at its origin.

fascia, the collateral ligament is defined and excised in a wide ellipse. It is not necessary to cut any of the volar capsular ligament, but all portions of the collateral must be removed. When this is done, the proximal phalanx is pushed into flexion, following the curve of

the metacarpal head. If this motion does not come easily, a blunt probe or a flat curved elevator is used to sweep around the head and free the volar capsular pouch. When excision is complete, the fingers should fall into 50° to 60° of flexion without strain. If not, further ligamentous tissue usually will be found. It is seldom necessary to excise the collateral ligament on the radial side of the index finger or that on the ulnar side of the little finger, since flexion in these digits can be obtained and maintained easily by postoperative splinting. Leaving these 2 marginal ligaments provides some lateral stability to the fingers, and there is less danger of subluxation of the long extensor tendons.

If the joints have been in hyperextension for some time, it may be necessary to strip the extensor tendon and the capsule from the metacarpal head to gain enough flexion. L. D. Howard's alternate approach of splitting the extensor tendon longitudinally, excising the collateral ligaments, and closing the tendon rent with a running wire removable suture is

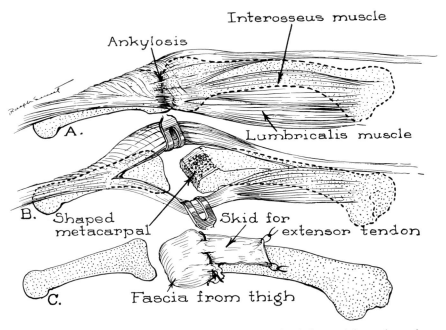

FIG. 383. Arthroplasty for ankylosis of the proximal finger joint; gives about 70° of motion. The proximal prolongation of the fascial hood is used if the extensor tendon is found to be adherent to the bone.

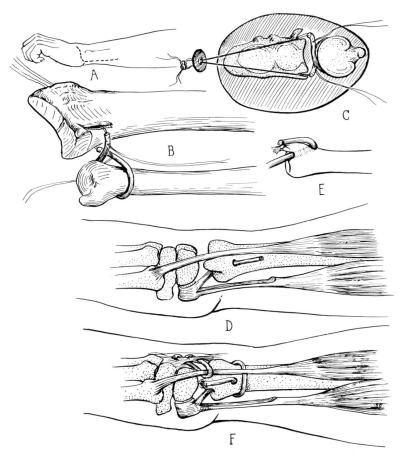

Fɪɢ. 384. Operation for chronic dislocation at the lower radio-ulnar joint.

(A) Incision. The dorsal branch of the ulnar nerve is spared.

(B) Tendon graft, such as palmaris longus, is placed around the neck of the ulna, crossed and embedded in the radius in slits just above and below the socket for articulating with the ulna. This substituted for the radio-ulnar ligament.

(C) End view showing the method of attaching tendon ends in slits. Stainless-steel wire No. 34 is attached to a tendon end, and both strands are passed through a drill hole in the radius and out the other side of the limb. They are tied there over a button. The wire is withdrawn backward after 3 weeks by the pull-out wire.

(D, E) A half-thickness strip of tendon of flexor carpi ulnaris is split off, retaining its attachment to the pisiform bone. It substitutes for the stylotriquetrum ligament by passing through an oblique drill hole in the head of the ulna. There it is turned back and sutured to a ligament. The pull of this ligament is distal and volar, checking dorsal dislocation.

(F) To prevent the tendon of the extensor ulnaris from snapping over the styloid process in flexion of the wrist, a small tendon or fascial graft loops about it and is fastened to the dorsal ligament of the wrist joint.

useful where the extensor apparatus is not shortened or adherent.

It is important to be certain that the base of the proximal phalanx actually slides around the metacarpal head in full contact all the time. Unless it does, the joint merely opens like a book, hinging on its volar lip. Occasionally, a groove in the metacarpal head can be seen from the effect of this prolonged pressure.

If the operation is done in the absence of good periarticular supporting tissues such as the long extensor hood mechanism, the interossei and a good volar capsular ligament, volar subluxation of the joint may occur, and the common extensor tendons may slip off their normal prominences into the ulnar gutters.

The skin over the knuckles may be tight and not allow flexion. If so, a transverse skin incision proximally should be used instead of the 3 longitudinal incisions, the flap being elevated and pushed distally, and, when the joints are flexed, the gap covered with a split-skin graft.

The operation to excise the collateral ligaments frequently can be done at the same time that a malunited metacarpal is corrected.

It is not enough to strip the collateral ligaments from their origin or simply to divide them. Lasting results are seen only when the ligament is excised.

Postoperatively, the joints are immobilized in plaster in full flexion for a period of 3 weeks. The wrist should be in dorsiflexion, and the 2 distal finger joints free for active motion. After 3 weeks, an elastic-powered knuckle-bender splint is used for an additional 3 weeks.

Arthroplasty. Through a dorsolateral incision 1½ inches long the proximal finger joint is exposed, entering it between the tendon of the interosseus muscle and the dorsal aponeurosis which caps the joint. The phalanx and the metacarpal are stripped of their surrounding capsular ligament and separated or even chiseled across if necessary. Usually, there are some remains of articular cartilage on the phalanx. Enough of the head of the metacarpal is excised to make a space between the 2 bones of about 1 cm., and the tissues about the metacarpal end are freed completely for ¾ inch, including the volar capsular pouch. Next, the head of the metacarpal is shaped to receive the phalanx, so that its end is almost flat in the lateral plane but is rather sharply rounded and faces slightly volarward in the anteroposterior plane. Over this is fitted a small hood of thin, deep fascia taken from the lower part of the thigh, forward from the region of the fascia lata or else a sheet of paratenon from over the fascia lata. This is made to fit over the metacarpal head and clasp about its neck

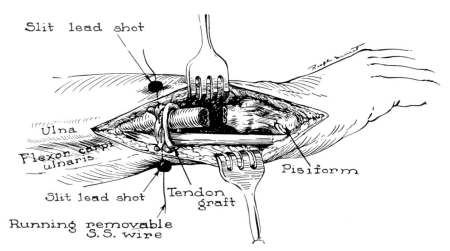

FIG. 385. Restoration of pronation and supination by excising the head of the ulna or a segment from its neck. A sling of free tendon graft (palmaris longus or fascia) looped about the ulna and the tendon of the flexor ulnaris prevents dorsal displacement of the ulna on supination.

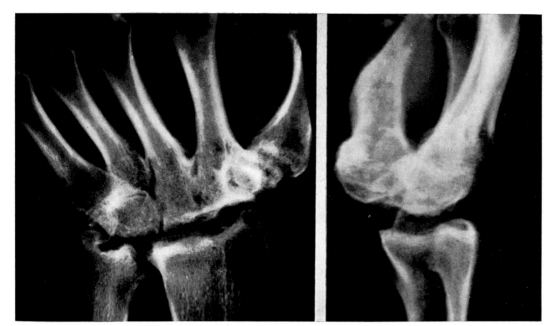

Fig. 386. Case A. F. From a wrist-joint infection starting in the ring finger, the wrist had only 14° of painful motion. The proximal row of carpals and the head of the capitate were removed. These roentgenograms were taken a year later. The wrist was strong and painless and had 30° of voluntary dorsiflexion and 30° of flexion, amounting to 60° of motion.

with a purse-string suture of fine catgut. Sometimes 2 additional side sutures are necessary to hold the graft proximally.

If the extensor tendon is adherent for a distance on the back of the metacarpal, it is best to prolong the dorsal portion of the cap far enough backward to prevent readherence. The cap should separate from the metacarpal all of the tendons on the 4 sides so that they will glide. A dorsal plaster with the joint well flexed to a near right angle is worn for 2 weeks. After that, elastic traction is used. At the end of the first week, while still in the plaster and when the danger of clot formation between the bones is past, longitudinal skin traction may be used, pulling from a wire outrigger.

The plaster keeps the joint flexed, and the traction separates the bone ends. Following these first 2 weeks, the plaster is discarded, and flexion is maintained by leather cuffs looped over the proximal phalanges and pulled by rubber bands to an outrigger. The outrigger of wire is fastened either to a volar plaster slab or a metal cockup splint. Another

means of maintaining the flexion is the knuckle-bender splint. After either capsulectomy or arthroplasty it may be necessary to use elastic splinting for as long as 2 months.

The usual degree of flexion gained is 70°, though it may be somewhat less if the tissues are very cicatricial. One cannot expect to produce a sliding joint like the original, but it is possible to achieve a rocker effect of the phalanx on the narrow edge of the metacarpal. Passive flexion may be greater than voluntary because the intrinsic muscles may be too loose until they have taken up the slack.

To maintain the motion required by excision of the collateral ligaments or by arthroplasty, some intrinsic muscle function must be present or must be restored. Slitting the proximal pulleys holding the flexor tendons to the metacarpal heads and thus changing the angle of approach may give some proximal joint flexor action. Tendon transfers, such as superficialis through the lumbrical canal to the extensor apparatus, may be necessary. (See Chap. 11.)

Another requirement for successful arthro-

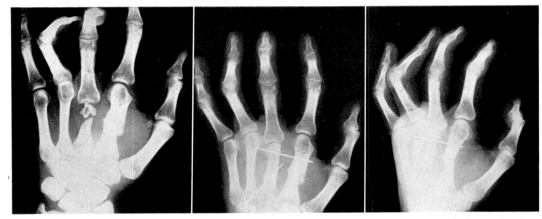

Fig. 387. Metatarsal grafted into metacarpal. To replace loss of the head and the neck of the 3rd metacarpal, which had been injured by a shell fragment, a graft was used from the 5th metatarsal. This consisted of part of the shaft, the head, the proximal articular surface of the joint and the joint capsule. Later, an extensor tendon graft was placed. The result when last checked (9 months later) was good, smooth motion. (W. C. Graham, M.D.)

plasty is proper muscle balance. This may be upset from angulation of the forearm bones, the wrist or the metacarpals that tightens the extensors, causing hyperextension of the proximal finger joints, and the flexors, causing clawing. In such cases, proper bony alignment must be re-established first.

Partial and Whole Joint Grafts. When a metacarpal head is missing, the shaft and the head of a metatarsal may be transplanted, bringing the joint capsule with the graft to fasten around the base of the phalanx. Many of these were done for gunshot wounds in World War II. Early results were promising. Whole joints have been transplanted, Lexer being one of the pioneers in this type of surgery. Joints from toes or other fingers have been used. Some grafted joints, using the pedicle method, regained good motion. Graham and Stephenson grafted the metatarsophalangeal joint of the second toe to the proximal thumb joint for a wringer injury in a 3-year-old child. A tendon graft to the extensor was inserted later. At 10 years there was good appearance and function. The epiphysis apparently remained viable, closing at the age of 13.

Entin has transplanted joints experimentally in dogs, with varying results. In some good function was retained, although considerable degeneration took place, as viewed in the roentgenogram.

H. Wolff reported the first half-joint graft in 1910, replacing a spina ventosa with a toe phalanx. Other pioneers were Lexer, who also grafted a whole joint, Kuettner, Goebel and Roux.

A joint transplanted with its blood and nerve supply intact, as in the pollicization operations, does not change its appearance or function. Even without the overlying skin and tendons, such neurovascular pedicled transfers remain viable and maintain their normal configuration. It is the free half-joint and whole-joint grafts that, in many of the reported cases, have shown absorption and degeneration of the transplanted bone and cartilage. The role of the synovia in joint transfers is very important. Apparently, there is some nutritive element in synovial fluid that helps the articular cartilage to survive. Graham has much experience in this field and feels that, if possible, in half-joint transplants the synovia of the recipient part should be retained and utilized as a sleeve over the graft. In a case in which this was done, Francis McKeever was able to determine at a later operation that the cartilage was normal; a biopsy of the synovia showed no abnormal changes. In whole-joint transfers, it has been suggested that the periarticular tissues of the graft be excised except for the stabilizing collateral and volar capsular ligaments, in order to allow a new blood supply to enter the graft quickly.

All such transplants require firm fixation, preferably with crossed Kirschner wire and immobilization of the part until healed.

Joint Prostheses. Many attempts have been made to provide an artificial joint surface or a hingelike mechanism as a substitute for the whole joint. Caps of metal or plastic for the head of a metacarpal or a phalanx have not been satisfactory, usually due to lateral instability. Brannon used a stainless steel hinge in cases of traumatic fracture-dislocation of the middle joints. There was excellent motion, but with time there was a tendency for the prosthesis to settle into the bone and restrict motion. A modification in design aimed at preventing this complication was developed, but

no reports are available on the long-term results. Flatt has reported its use in the replacement of joints in rheumatoid arthritis but stresses the fact that the procedure is still in the experimental stage. A modification of the design of the intramedullary portions of the apparatus allows more nearly accurate fitting and better stability in preventing rotation of the stem.

Bone is a living substance, and a metallic insert will always settle or work its way into the bone if pressure is maintained long enough. The available prostheses all depend on an intramedullary arm or some modification of it to fix the apparatus in place. Force is applied to these projections on any motion of the joint, so that sometimes the shaft works its way through the cortex of the phalanx. If because of the underlying disease there is relatively little use of the hand and forceful activity is not carried out, a long period of freedom from this complication can be expected. The direct settling of the central portion of the prosthesis into the bone occurs because of the constant axial pressure from the flexor and the extensor mechanisms. If the base of the prosthesis resting on the cut surfaces of the bone is wedge-shaped, this settling will be more pronounced. A simple hinge which has approximately 110° of motion is connected by a hollow rivet pin and has a square shoulder where it joins the intramedullary pin to prevent this wedging effect. In addition, a washer of suitable diameter to cover the cut surface of the bone completely allows a broad area of pressure over the entire bony surface. In a few

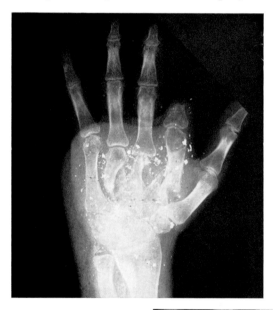

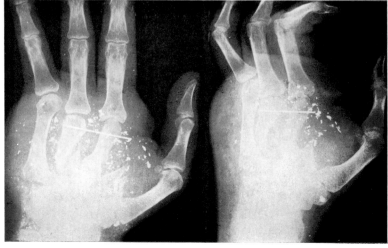

Fig. 388. Metatarsal grafted into metacarpal. (*Left*) This hand held TNT which exploded. The index finger was discarded. (*Bottom*) To replace the metacarpophalangeal joint of the long finger, the distal part of the 5th metatarsal, together with its head and joint capsule, was grafted in. The metacarpophalangeal joint of the long finger moved 70°. (W. C. Graham, M.D.)

carefully selected cases where normal tendon function is present, a middle finger joint has been replaced with this hinge. Some settling of the metal into the bone soon takes place.

MIDDLE FINGER JOINTS. Capsulectomy is only moderately successful, and arthroplasty may give lateral instability. Arthrodesis in moderate flexion, together with shortening of the finger, is a useful procedure. It is done for destruction of the middle joint, for flexion contracture, and in sharp flexion contracture after burns when the central extensor tendon slip has been lost. Union of the bones can be assured if they are either pinned together by 2 fine Kirschner wires made to cross each other or, in addition, are joined, using a small flat key bone graft. When placed, the bones should be pressed together firmly so that the crossed Kirschner wires will not cause distraction and hence nonunion.

A broad bony contact is essential. The joint can be excised and the 2 surfaces approximated and held with crossed Kirschner wire, but a broader surface contact with more lateral stability can be obtained by making the head of the proximal phalanx wedge-shaped and fitting this into its counterpart, a V-shaped slot in the base of the middle phalanx. Using the Stryker sagittal saw, an adjustment of the angles allows shortening and angulation of any desired degree.

Curtis reported some successful cases after capsulectomy for stiff, straight fingers. He attempted to preserve lateral stability by raising and retracting the aponeurosis. The collateral ligaments were excised. Flexion was maintained first by a Kirschner wire and then by rubber traction for 6 weeks.

In selected cases with good surrounding soft tissues, this collateral ligament excision fol-

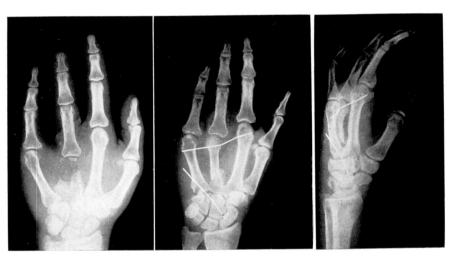

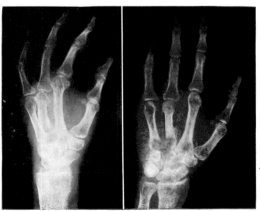

FIG. 389. Case R. E. J. Metatarsal grafted into metacarpal. (*Top, left*) From a gunshot wound, most of the 3rd and the 4th metacarpals were lost. (*Top, right*) The distal two thirds of the 5th metatarsal, together with the head and the joint capsule, were pinned in place on the stub of the 3rd metacarpal. The 5th metacarpal was dislocated over and pinned to take the place of the 4th, narrowing and loosening the hand. (*Bottom*) Good union; joint structures preserved; 70° of flexion.

Fig. 390. Case S. H. (A, B.) Transfer of the metacarpophalangeal joint. Gunshot wound of hand. The proximal joint of the long finger was destroyed and the index finger was badly damaged, except for its skin and proximal joint. Therefore, this joint was transferred over on its pedicle with a blood and a nerve supply and pinned in place of the proximal joint of the long finger. (C) The index finger was filleted and used to cap the end of the thumb. (D, E) A year later, flexion of this joint was 60°. The hand functioned well, the thumb touched all fingers, and the patient had a useful hand.

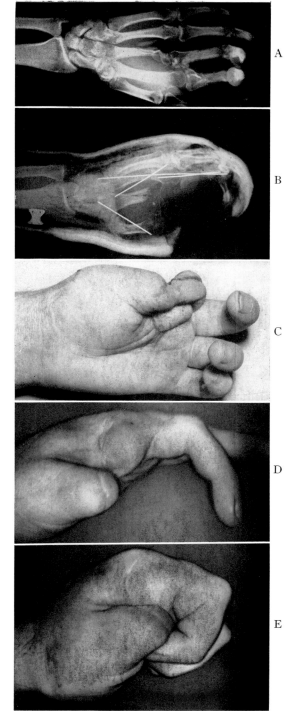

lowed by prolonged elastic splinting has given good results.

Arthroplasty on the middle finger joint should be done only when all other tissues in the vicinity are normal. The incision should be lateral and away from the lateral bands of the *dossiére*. There should be a space of at least 1 cm. between the ends of the bones, and flexion and traction should be maintained postoperatively. The operation is actually an excision of half of the joint. As mentioned above, the operation is only moderately successful. Usually only moderate motion is obtained, and the joint is unstable laterally except when under the strain of gripping. Carroll reported 30 cases, the majority of which he claimed were successful. He removed ½ inch of the end of the proximal phalanx and continued skeletal traction for 6 weeks. The lateral stability was present only while grasping.

Flexion contracture of the middle finger joint is common; when long-lasting, it involves the volar capsular ligament, together with the 2 anterolateral bands which are the collateral ligaments. These must all be severed before the joint will straighten.

A not uncommon injury is rupture of the volar plate of the middle joint of a finger. Sudden hyperextension detaches the distal attachment at the base of the middle phalanx, and the joint space is open. Unless the injury has been compounded or accompanied by tendon damage, the joint usually will remain

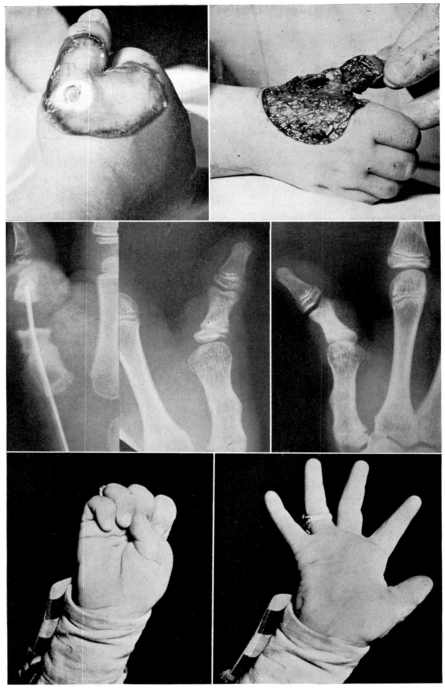

FIG. 391. Free graft of joint and epiphysis. Dr. W. C. Graham's case. (*Top, left*) November 18, 1950, 7 days after a wringer injury in a 3-year-old boy. Débridement and split-skin graft 2 days later. (*Top, right*) The temporary skin graft and the necrotic proximal thumb joint were excised 3 weeks later and an abdominal flap applied. (*Center, left*) November 5, 1951; a metatarsophalangeal joint with the epiphysis of the proximal phalanx was transplanted. Two and a half months later an extensor tendon graft was placed. (*Center, middle*) Roentgenogram taken in 1960, 9 years after joint and epiphysis transfer. (*Center, right*) Roentgenogram taken in 1962, 11 years after joint transfer; patient now 14 years old. (*Bottom, left* and *right*) Extension and flexion of thumb.

FIG. 392. Joint prosthesis. (*Top*) Limited flexion and appearance of middle finger joint after fracture dislocation. (*Bottom*) Roentgenograms taken 1, 2 and 3 years after insertion of prosthesis. Bony overgrowth around edge of prosthesis.

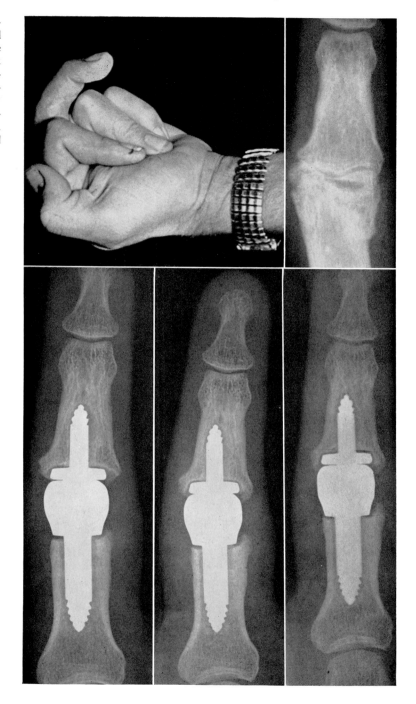

mobile but go into hyperextension; the finger locks in this position.

The torn edge of the volar capsule seals over just as a tendon end does when severed in a sheath, and on opening the flexor tendon sheath there is seen to be a direct connection into the joint. Reconstruction is accomplished by suturing the freshened edge of the volar capsule to a transverse slot made in the base of the phalanx just beyond the articular sur-

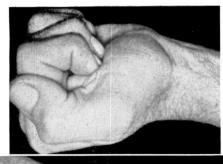

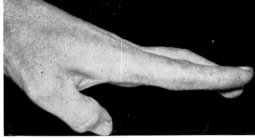

FIG. 393. Same patient shown in Figure 392. Flexion of finger 4½ years after joint prosthesis. Extension is slightly limited. Motion is painless, and the patient performs heavy manual work.

face. Pull-out wires are used, removed after 3 weeks and a protective splint worn for an additional 3 weeks.

If, from injury, the middle joint heals in considerable flexion, not much improvement can be gained from dividing or excising the volar contracted tissues.

Arthrodesis of the middle joints, shortening the finger some, is useful for sharp flexion contractures after burns of the dorsal capsule or for painful and disrupted joints. Arthrodesis of the middle joint leaves a useful finger, but arthrodesis of the proximal joint should be used only in special cases because it prevents the finger from flexing into the palm. In cases of paralysis it may prevent certain substitute compensatory movements.

DISTAL FINGER JOINTS. These are like the middle joints, but surgery seldom is helpful, except to fuse them in slight flexion. This is useful in hyperextension from burns and also after a flexor profundus tendon alone has been severed. Tenodesis of the distal stub of the profundus will prevent hyperextension. Painful distal joints with hypertrophic arthritis are treated most satisfactorily by arthrodesis.

DISLOCATIONS OF FINGER JOINTS. Most interphalangeal as well as metacarpophalangeal dislocations can be reduced easily, with little residual disability. Occasionally, the distal bone remains displaced dorsally. Open reduction shows the head of the proximal bone protruding through a rent in the capsule. When this capsule is removed from between the bones, reduction is maintained easily. If reduced late, there will be considerable impairment of motion.

Joints of the Thumb. Either the distal or the metacarpophalangeal joint of the thumb may be arthrodesed in semiflexion. This will give a useful thumb with very little disability. If the carpometacarpal joint of the thumb is hopelessly stiffened with the thumb in a backward position, due to infection or injury, it is best to resort to a rotary angulating osteotomy of the metacarpal of the thumb so as to place the thumb in the functional position of opposition.

The dorsolateral ligament of the metacarpophalangeal joint of the thumb frequently suffers a transverse rupture when a boxer delivers a swinging blow without clasping his thumb over his fist. If the thumb is at once put up in plaster in full extension and abduction, there will be little impairment. In a neglected case, however, it will be necessary to repair it with a tendon or a fascial graft.

A chronic subluxation radialward of this joint occurs without specific trauma in some manual workers, but, because of its more common appearance in a particular occupation, it has been given the name "gamekeeper's thumb." Because of the way in which hares are killed, the thumb is continually forced into radial deviation at the proximal joint; this stretches the collateral ligament and capsule, and the long and the short extensor tendons displace. An operative procedure to correct the deformity has been described by Kaplan. Arthrodesis of the joint assures correction and provides a stable thumb.

Irreducible dislocation of the metacarpophalangeal joint of the thumb is similar to that seen in the middle and the distal joints of the fingers, though here the head of the metacarpal protrudes through the base of the anterior capsule of the joint and becomes entangled between the 2 heads of the short

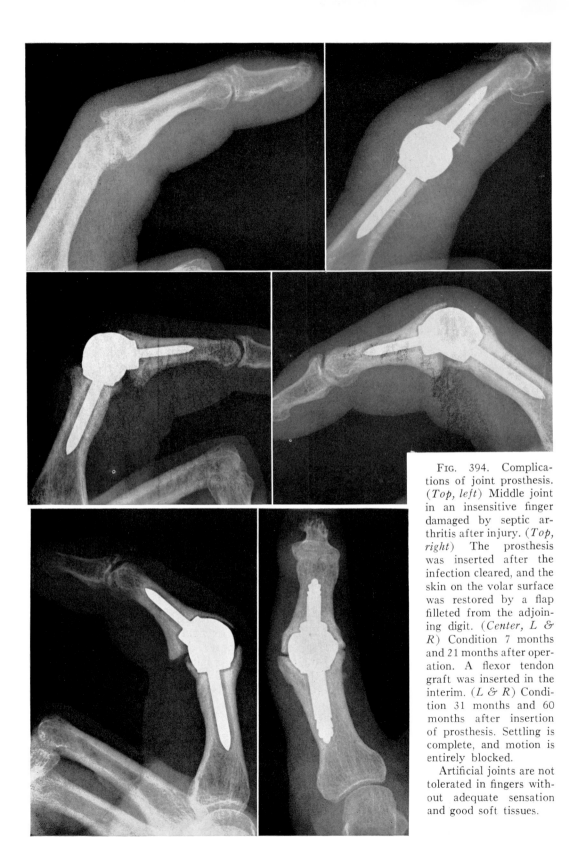

Fig. 394. Complications of joint prosthesis. (*Top, left*) Middle joint in an insensitive finger damaged by septic arthritis after injury. (*Top, right*) The prosthesis was inserted after the infection cleared, and the skin on the volar surface was restored by a flap filleted from the adjoining digit. (*Center, L & R*) Condition 7 months and 21 months after operation. A flexor tendon graft was inserted in the interim. (*L & R*) Condition 31 months and 60 months after insertion of prosthesis. Settling is complete, and motion is entirely blocked.

Artificial joints are not tolerated in fingers without adequate sensation and good soft tissues.

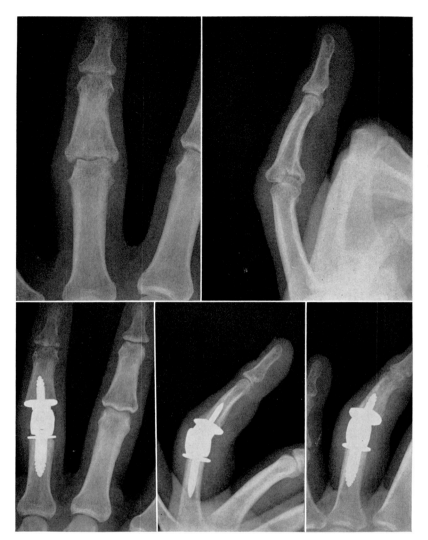

FIG. 395. A washer which fits the cut surfaces of the phalanges should aid in preventing the settling of the prosthesis. This patient has normal soft tissues and tendinous structures. A longer stem of the intramedullary portion is available.

flexor muscle of the thumb. If closed reduction by manipulating the phalanx over the head of the metacarpal is unsuccessful, open reduction is necessary; drawing the tendon of the flexor brevis muscle and the volar part of the capsule away from between the 2 bones will allow easy reduction. The joint is put up in moderate flexion for 2 weeks.

METACARPOTRAPEZIAL JOINT. In case of ankylosis of this joint with the thumb in the lateral position or of painful motion from arthritis, considerable motion of the thumb and good function can be obtained by arthrodesing the joint in the functioning position of opposition, provided that the scaphoid is free to move. For pain from arthritis from a chronic dislocation or from an old Bennett's

fracture, arthrodesis is best. For arthritis of this joint, removal of the trapezium has been used. However, the results are uncertain, and the thumb is left more or less free floating on the scaphoid without the best joint leverage.

In arthrodesis, the joint is uncovered through an L-shaped incision, one arm of which is along the dorsum of the metacarpal, the other following the flexion crease around the thenar eminence retracting the thenar muscles from the bone. After excising the joint, there will be some distraction. Therefore, for compression, a disk of cancellous bone from the ilium is interposed, and all is held firmly together in correct position by 2 crossed Kirschner wires.

Chronic dislocation backward of the meta-

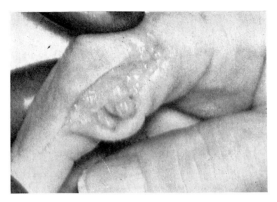

FIG. 396. Tenosynovitis of flexor sheath of index finger in rheumatoid arthritis. (From L. Ramsey Straub, M.D.)

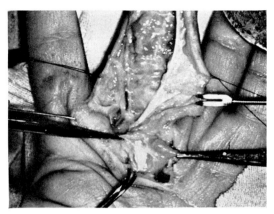

FIG. 397. Diffuse synovitis of flexor tendon sheath in rheumatoid arthritis. (From L. Ramsey Straub, M.D.)

carpotrapezial joint of the thumb occurs as a direct result of injury rupturing the capsular ligament and as a secondary effect of the malunited Bennett's fracture. Normally, the projecting process of the volar edge of the base of the metacarpal hooks around the trapezium, preventing backward dislocation. In a Bennett's fracture the metacarpal displaces backward and proximalward so that malunion occurs, leaving the metacarpal without a hook to hold it forward on the trapezium. Then, each time the patient grasps with the thumb, the metacarpal dislocates backward. This is accompanied by pain, weakness and disability.

Backward dislocation of this joint may be corrected by performing a wedge osteotomy on the base of the metacarpal of the thumb, the wide part of the wedge being dorsal, so that when the bone ends are forced together, the articular surface of the metacarpal will form the necessary forward projecting hook around the trapezium to prevent the dislocation. At the same time, some fascial grafts can be applied to the dorsum and the radial side of the joint to reinforce the torn ligaments. One method is lashing the metacarpal to the trapezium with a strip of tendon or fascia through drill holes. Another method used by Slocum is to place a tendon through a central drill hole through the 2 bones as in the Nicola operation on the shoulder. Others using this method give conflicting reports regarding results—some good, some with pain from arthritis and some with shearing of the tendon. Eggers, after slitting down a strip of

tendon of the extensor carpi radialis longus and anchoring it to the trapezium, reports a satisfactory result.

Following plastic repairs of this joint, some cases in which arthritis has been present continue to be painful. A more reliable cure is achieved by means of arthrodesis. By this, almost full thumb motion may be gained with the single exception of the ability to place the thumb behind the hand.

RHEUMATOID ARTHRITIS

Rheumatoid arthritis is a systemic disease of unknown etiology, often beginning with symptoms in the hands and the feet. The principal tissues affected are the synovial linings of tendon sheaths and joints, though histologic changes can be found also in muscles and nerves. Major deformities in the hands occur in at least one quarter of all patients with rheumatoid disease and most often in women. They follow not only direct damage to supporting ligaments, tendons and bones, which upsets the mechanical balance, but also the spasm or contracture of intrinsic muscles, which alters the dynamic balance.

Because of the many mechanisms involved and the different forces acting on the various structures, no fixed pattern of deformity occurs in an individual patient. The disease may have exacerbations or remissions and often is held in check by prolonged steroid administration.

Some of the deformities seen in rheumatoid

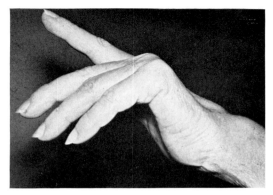

FIG. 398. Synovitis involving extensor tendons with rupture of all finger extensors except extensor indicis.

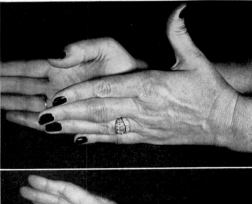

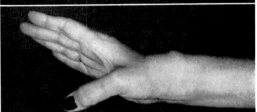

FIG. 399. Synovitis of the dorsoradial aspect of the wrist with rupture of the extensor pollicis longus tendon. (From L. D. Howard, M.D.; from Dr. Bunnell's files)

arthritis can occur in allied syndromes such as systemic lupus erythematosis or scleroderma. Some patients with marked prolonged intrinsic spasm such as parkinsonism and cerebral palsy also may develop deformities which are similar in many ways to those of rheumatoid arthritis.

TENDON LESIONS

The most common lesion of rheumatoid arthritis in the hand involves the tendons. Brewerton found that 64 per cent of 300 patients had tendon lesions. One third of these were "trigger" fingers, and 9 per cent had involvement to such extent that flexion of the finger was blocked. In 17 patients there were 23 tendon ruptures. Laine, Sairanen and Vaino found that 288 of 305 patients with rheumatoid arthritis had some involvement of the hand. Nodules in the flexor tendons occurred in 47, on the extensors in 14; there were 16 trigger fingers and 2 ruptures of the extensor pollicis longus tendon.

The common nonrheumatic trigger finger is usually the result of some thickening of the flexor superficialis or the profundus tendon which interferes with smooth gliding of the tendons through the pulley over the metacarpal head. A similar lesion is found in rheumatoid arthritis, but there has also been reported a nodular thickening of the profundus, which prevents the gliding of this tendon through the bifurcation of the flexor superficialis. This blocks the finger and limits flexion. In rheumatoid disease, there may also

be a diffuse synovitis of the flexor sheath, which interferes with motion. Hydrocortisone injections may help the latter, though synovectomy is best for persistent symptoms.

SYNOVITIS

Tendon Sheaths. Any of the synovial tissues may be involved in the disease. If the flexor tendon sheaths in the fingers are thickened, there may be interference with voluntary flexion and some limitation of extension. At the wrist level, thickening around the flexor tendons compresses the median nerve against the volar carpal ligament, resulting in the carpal tunnel syndrome. When joint synovia become affected, there is softening and distention of the capsules, which then stretch under tension, and subluxations and dislocations occur. On the extensor surface, involvement of the sheaths of the wrist and the digital extensors at the wrist is seen commonly. Synovial disease may invade the tendons directly so that they become frayed and elongate or rupture. Usually, however, other factors are present to precipitate the actual separation of the tendon.

Wrist Joint. According to Brewerton, synovitis involves the wrist joint in 23 per cent of cases. If the wrist involvement results in a flexion deformity, then an imbalance of long extensors, long flexors and intrinsics can occur, and a "clawhand" can develop. Steindler pointed out that the hand is usually pronated in relation to the forearm. A subluxation of the radiocarpal joint may be a prime factor in deformities in the fingers. The wrist is the key joint in the hand, and prevention of wrist flexion deformity is the essential feature of prophylactic splinting.

When the distal radio-ulnar joint is affected, there is loss of ligamentous stability of the lower end of the ulna with dorsal dislocation. Not only is there pain on motion, but the dorsally placed ulna is a factor in the cause of rupture of the extensor tendons.

Metacarpophalangeal Joints. Just as the wrist is the key joint for the hand, the proximal finger joint is the key to finger motions. The joint has 3 motions: flexion-extension, lateral deviation and exorotation-endorotation, all held in check by the normally strong collateral ligaments and hood mechanisms. An important stabilizing factor is the proximal shift of this aponeurotic sleeve resulting from long extensor and interosseus muscle pull. The transverse fibers from the long extensor on the dorsum, extending around each side to attach to the transverse metacarpal ligament or the volar plate, act as a tendon of insertion and provide the lift to hold the proximal phalanx in position. The collateral ligaments alone are not necessary to maintain the phalanx in position, since subluxation following their excision does not occur. However, if the synovia becomes thickened and the fascial aponeurotic hood is attenuated, some loss of collateral ligaments necessarily accompanies the synovitis. Subluxation occurs because of the pull of the flexor components. Though the most common deformity of the proximal joint is volar or anterior subluxation, hyperextension or the clawhand can occur. If with wrist damage a volar displacement and subluxation takes place and the wrist is in palmar flexion, the increased tension on the long extensors may draw the proximal phalanges into hyperextension. Similarly, if disease at the middle joint results in attenuation of the middle extensor slip, the buttonhole deformity occurs,

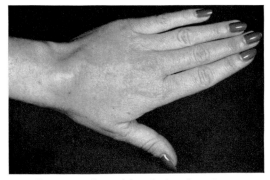

FIG. 400. Synovitis of sheaths of common digital extensors as practically the only indication of rheumatoid disease. (From L. D. Howard, M.D.; from Dr. Bunnell's files.)

with flexion of the middle phalanx and extension of the proximal phalanx.

The Middle Finger Joints. Synovitis of one of these joints results in attenuation and stretching of the middle slip insertion of the extensor aponeurosis which here is an intimate part of the dorsal capsule. With intact lateral slips, the triangular ligament is stretched, and the buttonhole deformity occurs, with flexion of the middle joint and extension of the distal joint. Laine *et al.* found it present in 111 of 305 patients, and Pulkki found it in 32 per cent of 500 patients.

Hyperextension of the middle joint, euphemistically called the swan-neck deformity, is similar to that which results from overactive intrinsic muscles. The proximal joint is usually flexed, the middle joint hyperextended, and the distal joint dropped in some flexion. Laine *et al.* believe it to be a deformity of the more advanced stages of the disease, occurring in their study 44 times in 305 patients. Pulkki noted it in 14 per cent and states that it always follows proximal joint subluxation; he believes that it is due to displacement of the dorsal ligament. Brewerton believed it to be due to intrinsic contracture, but Laine *et al.* disagreed. They described a dorsal shift of the line of pull of the extensor due to volar displacement of the proximal phalanx. When the subluxation was reduced, the deformity of the middle joint disappeared.

The typical deformity can occur without disease of the joint and is seen commonly in spastics, occasionally in Parkinson's disease and usually in severe local Volkmann's ischemia of the hand described by Bunnell. It can occur in the normal finger after removal of the flexor superficialis tendon. There seems to be no doubt that it is due to overactive intrinsic muscles, and that it becomes exaggerated when flexion contracture or subluxation of the proximal joint is present, or when laxness or stretching of the volar capsule allows the middle joint to hyperextend.

The Distal Joint. A flexion deformity of the distal joint, comparable with that following

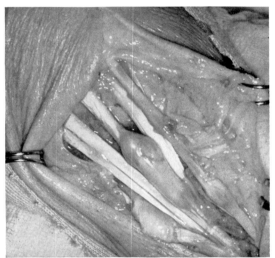

extensor tendon avulsions and ruptures, occurred in 2 per cent of Pulkki's series and in 10 of 305 patients of Laine *et al.* A compensatory flexion is usually present as part of the middle joint hyperextension deformity. By itself the so-called mallet finger is not particularly disabling.

The Thumb Joints. The base of the first metacarpal of the thumb usually drops when this joint becomes involved with the disease, since there is no strong ligament to check this motion. Synovitis of the proximal joint results in a deformity similar to that of the fingers. The proximal phalanx is flexed on the metacarpal and subluxates volarward because of the pull of the flexing muscles. The distal joint is usually hyperextended, sometimes grotesquely, and is often the site of marked bone destruction.

Ankylosis of the carpometacarpal joint usually is reported to accompany wrist ankylosis.

RUPTURE OF TENDONS

Any of the extrinsic extensor or flexor tendons can rupture in rheumatoid arthritis. The

FIG. 401. (*Top*) Direct involvement of extensor tendons on dorsum of wrist without involvement of underlying joint. (*Bottom*) Degeneration within the tendon substance in rheumatoid arthritis. (From L. Ramsey Straub, M.D.)

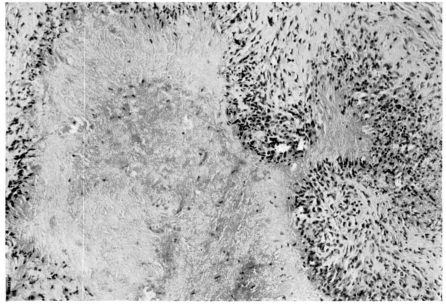

extensor pollicis longus is found to be separated most frequently, but the extensors of the middle, the ring and the little fingers also are commonly affected. Synovial inflammation combined with friction around Lister's tubercle is claimed to be the cause in the former, while the finger extensor ruptures usually are seen in patients with involvement of the distal radio-ulnar joint and dorsal subluxation of the ulna. A bare bony spicule has been described in the base of the synovial mass where the extensors have ruptured. Tendon reconstruction by graft or transfer always should be accompanied by synovectomy and usually by removal of the lower end of the ulna as well.

Flexor tendons also rupture, the flexor pollicis longus most frequently, and usually in the carpal tunnel.

ULNAR DRIFT

This term describes the deformity wherein the fingers are deviated ulnarward at the proximal joint level. It occurs in over 25 per cent of patients with rheumatoid arthritis but can also occur in other diseases. In patients with rheumatoid disease, Brewerton found it in 27 per cent, and Pulkki in 28 per cent. It was 3 times more common in females. Vaino and Oka found it in 28.6 per cent of females and 14.6 per cent of males. Ulnar deviation of the fingers can occur without volar subluxation or dislocation of the joints in nonrheumatoid diseases and even in rheumatoid disease. Brewerton found volar dislocation in only 44 of 82 patients with ulnar drift.

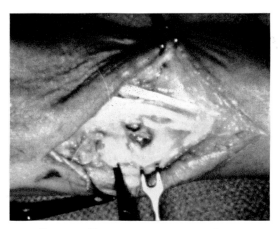

FIG. 402. Damage to extensor tendons on the dorsum of the wrist as a result of synovitis involving the distal radio-ulnar joint. The ulna lies exposed in the base of this mass of granulation tissue, and the tendons wear away from friction on the bony spicule.

In its most exaggerated form in rheumatoid disease, 3 components are usually present: the ulnar deviation of the fingers, a volar subluxation of the proximal phalanges on the metacarpals and a dislocation of the long extensor tendons so that they lie in the trough between the metacarpal heads. Completing the picture, there is usually hyperextension of the middle finger joint and flexion of the distal joint.

Many theories have been proposed to explain this interesting deformity. The force of gravity, pressure on the fingers in daily activ-

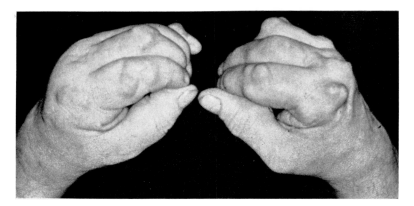

FIG. 403. Rheumatoid nodules. (From L. Ramsey Straub, M.D.)

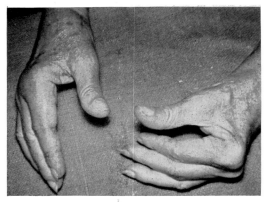

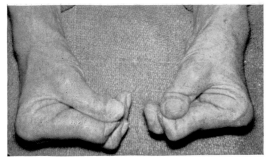

FIG. 405. Grasp and pinch mechanisms with severe deformity of the intrinsic-plus type and the usual lack of stability in the distal joint of the thumb.

FIG. 404. Bilateral rupture of extensor tendons of fingers. Reconstruction has been done on the right hand.

ity, loss of controlling influence of the first interosseus as an abductor, damage to collateral ligaments, synovial changes resulting in swelling and looseness of the proximal joint and the fact that ulnar deviation normally is of greater degree than radial deviation have been proposed as etiologic factors.

It is difficult to determine whether a factor is the cause of the deformity or the result of something else. It would seem that the previously mentioned factors are not usually the primary causes. Ulnar drift can occur in the absence of synovitis, as in Parkinson's disease and some cases of arthrogryposis. It does not follow radial palsy and therefore is not the result of weakness of the long extensors; it does not occur with ulnar palsy. Removal of the collateral ligaments without damaging the hood and the intrinsic tendon mechanism does not cause it, nor does this operation properly done result in anterior subluxation of the joint. Damage to the proximal joint is not a prerequisite of the deformity.

Fearnley in 1951 suggested that the deformity was produced by the use of the hand in an abnormal manner determined by inability to flex the middle finger joints. However, he postulated an abnormal lateral mobility of the fingers with the proximal joints in flexion and assumed that the little finger was "pivotal" in preventing or allowing the deformity.

An interesting phenomenon occurs in patients with ulnar drift whose joints still can be realigned passively. If the flexed and ulnar deviated finger is brought back to the neutral position of alignment, if the subluxation is corrected passively, and if the finger is extended at the proximal joint, the middle joint will extend strongly or hyperextend if the volar capsular structures are lax. This tendency toward middle joint extension can be increased by radial deviation of the finger and decreased by ulnar deviation, without altering the proximal joint position or allowing the proximal joint to subluxate. Thus there is an intrinsic "plus" when the finger is straight or radially deviated, with release of the "plus" when the finger is ulnar flexed. In such a hand grasping an object which prevents proximal joint flexion can be accomplished only by flexing the middle and the distal joints, and this can be accomplished only if the fingers are allowed to deviate ulnarward at the proximal joints. This may be the abnormal type of middle joint activity which Fearnley was describing.

An attempt at thumb-to-index pinch demonstrates the same action. To bring the pulp of the index to the level of the thumb requires some middle joint flexion to compensate for the difference in length of the 2 digits. Thus, patients with an intrinsic plus of the ulnar side of the index finger find that they must deviate the index finger ulnarward at the proximal joint to accomplish the act of pinching.

If this ulnar deviation of the fingers persists, the long extensors are gradually forced ulnarward and drop into the groove between the metacarpal heads. Once this happens, the

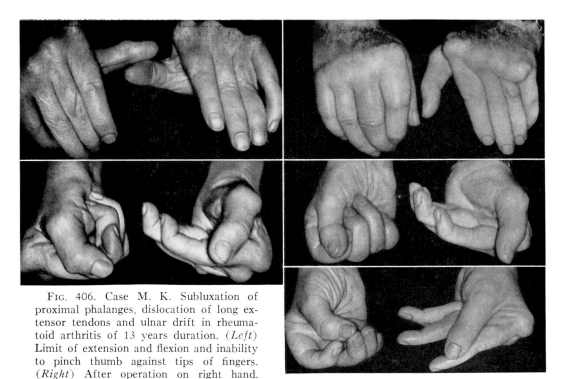

Fig. 406. Case M. K. Subluxation of proximal phalanges, dislocation of long extensor tendons and ulnar drift in rheumatoid arthritis of 13 years duration. (*Left*) Limit of extension and flexion and inability to pinch thumb against tips of fingers. (*Right*) After operation on right hand. Metacarpal heads excised and proximal phalanges temporarily pinned in position. Extensor tendons transposed to the radial side of each joint. Shortening the metacarpophalangeal unit by excising the heads relieved the intrinsic shortening so that the middle joints now flex. Will need arthrodesis of the distal joint of the thumb for more stability.

force producing ulnar deviation is increased, and a vicious circle is set up. The dislocation of the extensor tendons is the result of the primary deforming force and not the principal causative factor in the deformity. Both the intrinsic plus on the ulnar side and the ulnar dislocation of the extensor tendons can occur without synovitis of the joint and swelling of the joint capsule. If, however, there is a synovitis of the joint and subluxation occurs, the deformity is exaggerated, for now the proximal joint subluxates and there is increased tension on the long extensors.

Therefore, the finding commonly present in ulnar drift is the intrinsic plus on the ulnar side of the finger. This phenomenon must be related to the intrinsic extensors, for, if present, it can be relieved by tenotomy of the distally inserted interossei, that is, those which have their maximal insertion into the ulnar wing of the extensor aponeurosis. These are the 1st volar interosseus, the 3rd dorsal, the 4th dorsal and the abductor minimi digiti.

The 1st volar and the 3rd dorsal, according to Salisbury, Eyler and Markee and Landsmeer, are quite consistently inserted into the wing. The 1st dorsal interosseus has been demonstrated to have only a bony insertion on the radial side of the index. Landsmeer feels that the 2nd dorsal also is primarily inserted into the bone or in such a way as to have little or no effect on middle joint extension. This would explain the finding that ulnar intrinsic plus is demonstrated readily and found commonly in these 2 fingers in cases of ulnar drift, whether from rheumatoid disease or from prolonged spasm. In contrast with Fearnley's assumption that the little finger is "pivotal" in preventing or allowing the deformity to develop, the index and the middle fingers appear to be the prime movers.

The spasticity of the muscles inserting into the wings of the extensor assembly is probably the primary cause of ulnar drift, but a secondary factor is the tension of an intact long extensor mechanism. In patients with rupture

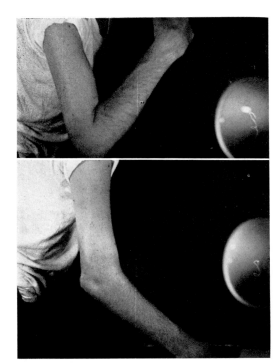

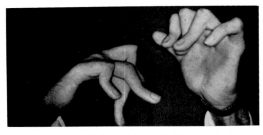

FIG. 407. Arthroplasty of elbow showing range of flexion and extension. Hands also involved with flexion deformities of the middle joints (boutonnière type).

of the long extensors, no ulnar drift was seen. This would conform with Sunderland's views that actions of the intrinsic and the extrinsic extensors are unified and that the function of neither set can be considered to be isolated phenomena.

That there are abnormal changes in the muscles in rheumatoid disease is accepted. Parry and Steinberg found electromyographic changes in the small muscles of the hand as well as the larger limb muscles in 79 of 93 patients with rheumatoid arthritis. Spasm of these intrinsic muscles could account for the abnormal action of the middle joints. When the fully extended index or middle finger is flexed at the middle joint, and the proximal joint remains extended, the ulnar-placed interosseus with the wing insertion must relax. If this interosseus is in spasm, this flexion can be achieved only by shortening the course, and this is accomplished by ulnar deviation at the proximal joint.

A contracture of all the interossei, as in local Volkmann's, does not result in ulnar deviation of the fingers, because this ischemic type of contracture comes on rapidly and is progressive, and the proximal joints are held in flexion. In diseases in which spasm is the principal factor, attempted use results in such strong ulnar deviation that the 2 dorsoradial interossei are overpowered, the radial collateral ligaments become elongated, and the deformity increases.

TREATMENT OF THE RHEUMATOID HAND

SPLINTING AND PROPHYLACTIC TREATMENT

Much can be done to prevent deformity by splinting, relief of spasm and removal of involved synovia. Splinting is indicated in acute episodes of pain and spasm, and, as in other hand conditions requiring immobilization, the wrist is the key to the position of the hand. Light plaster or epoxy resin splints should maintain the hand in the position of function, with the wrist dorsiflexed, the thumb in opposition and the fingers semiflexed and in line with the metacarpals. Slow traction by splints with elastic or light springs can help to correct position and overcome spastic muscle contracture. A reverse knuckle-bender may aid in correcting a flexion contracture of the proximal joints. Hydrocortisone injected locally into the involved synovial sheaths and joints reduces swelling and spasm of the adjoining muscles.

SURGICAL TREATMENT

General Principles. Improvement in function is the primary aim of surgical treatment of the rheumatoid hand. Nonoperative procedures such as splinting may help to prevent or forestall greater disability by preventing deformity and contractures; relatively simple operative procedures to allow better tendon

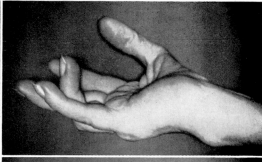

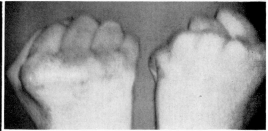

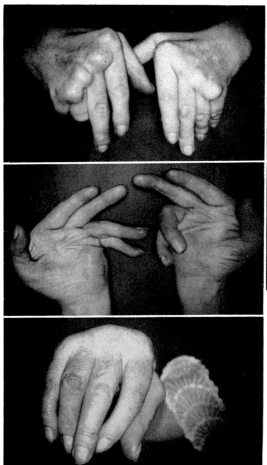

FIG. 408. Case L. O'L. Rheumatoid arthritis 20 years ago. The rheumatic attacks stopped 17 years ago, but deformities have been progressively worse. (*Left, top* and *center*) Fingers show 40° of ulnar drift. All proximal phalanges have dislocated to the front of the metacarpals and cannot be reduced. The extensor tendons have luxated into the interknuckle grooves and so act to ulnar flex the fingers instead of acting as extensors.

Operation on Right Hand: The heads of the metacarpals were resected for about 1 inch. Kirschner wires then pinned the phalanges in place on the metacarpals and were removed later. All extensor tendons were freed from the dorsal aponeurosis, displaced radialward and sutured in a slit of the dorsal aponeurosis. The extensor proprius tendon of the index finger was inserted into the radial lateral band of the proximal phalanx of the index finger. (*Left, bottom,* and *Right*) There was much improvement in function. The patient typed with 4 fingers instead of 1 and had much more use of her hand. (J. Bone Joint Surg. *37-A*:762-763)

action, release nerve compression and intrinsic contractures should be done early before gross deformities result.

Deformity itself, even such grotesque ulnar drifts and subluxations as are seen in chronic arthritics, is not the sole indication for major operative procedures. In some patients function is very good despite the deformity, since the disease progresses slowly over a period of years, and adaptation to the slowly developing changes in the joints and the tendons takes place. If in these instances the surgeon concentrates on the appearance of the hand, there may be a loss of some essential function.

Synovectomy and Release of Constriction. For trigger finger, slitting of the pulley over the metacarpal head may suffice, but if the tendon sheath is thickened or if there is a nodular thickening of the profundus, a more radical excision of the involved tissues is indicated. Compression of the median nerve in the carpal tunnel is relieved by division of the

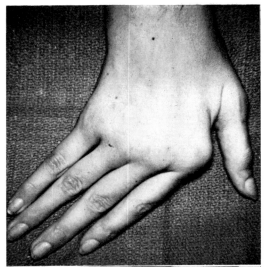

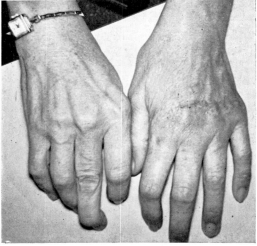

FIG. 409. Ulnar drift. (*Top*) Marked ulnar deviation in a young woman with proximal joint synovitis and intrinsic plus. All common extensors are dislocated ulnarward. (*Bottom*) In the right hand there is ulnar drift, and some extensors are dislocated; the middle finger shows hyperextension at the middle joint. There is no subluxation and no synovitis. The left hand shows results of operative correction by tenotomy of wing-inserted ulnar intrinsics and relocation of extensor tendons. Patient with long-standing parkinsonism, relieved of tremor and rigidity by bilateral chemopallidectomy but left with the deformity of intrinsic contracture and ulnar drift.

even before the late deformities appear, has been recommended to prevent the attenuation and the destruction of the hood and the collateral ligaments. Riordan and Flatt have reported encouraging results from the use of thio-tepa or nitrogen mustard for chemical synovectomy.

Arthrodesis. This procedure is used commonly for the wrist, the thumb joints and the middle finger joints. If the wrist is painful with restricted mobility or fixed in palmar flexion, fusion in the optimal position of slight dorsiflexion is indicated. Radiocarpal arthrodesis brings the extrinsic flexors and extensors back into balance and may even correct digital deformity by correcting this imbalance. If both wrists are involved, one should be placed in a few degrees of palmar flexion.

volar carpal ligament, but the thickened synovia of the flexors should be removed at the same time.

Persistent synovial thickening of the sheaths of the extensors at the wrist should be excised carefully, and the dorsal retinaculum divided or transposed beneath the tendons to protect them from the underlying bony prominences. If the lower end of the ulna is displaced dorsally and there is excessive motion at the radio-ulnar joint, excision of the lower end will improve pronation and supination.

Thick boggy synovia in the proximal joints is excised when the subluxated joints are reduced and the dislocated extensor tendons replaced. Early synovectomy of these joints,

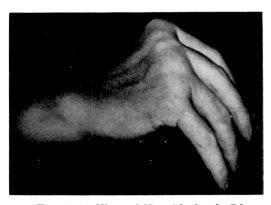

FIG. 410. Ulnar drift with irreducible subluxation of the proximal joints and dislocated extensors. Needs shortening of metacarpals by resection of heads and relocation of extensors.

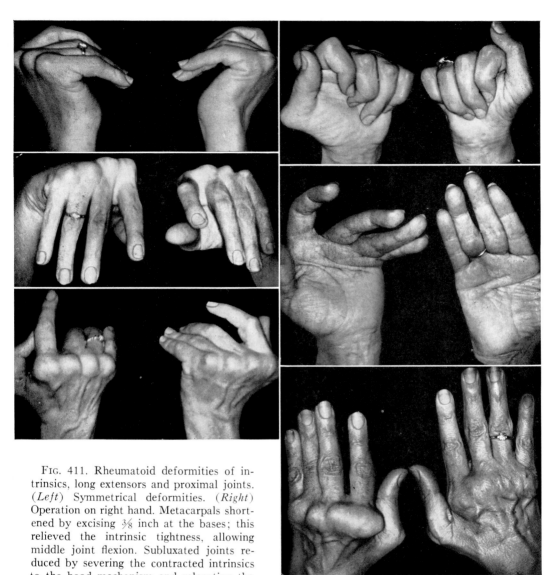

FIG. 411. Rheumatoid deformities of intrinsics, long extensors and proximal joints. (*Left*) Symmetrical deformities. (*Right*) Operation on right hand. Metacarpals shortened by excising ⅜ inch at the bases; this relieved the intrinsic tightness, allowing middle joint flexion. Subluxated joints reduced by severing the contracted intrinsics to the hood mechanism and relocating the long extensors to the radial side of the hood. (J. Bone Joint Surg. *37-A*:764)

Deformity of the thumb joints is common, especially a volar subluxation of the metacarpophalangeal joint. If there is also lateral instability, synovectomy combined with arthrodesis is indicated. The distal thumb joint is often markedly deformed and should be arthrodesed in a good pinching position. Fusion of this joint is accepted treatment for rupture of the flexor pollicis longus tendon.

For long-standing deformities of the middle finger joints, arthrodesis in the optimal position is the best solution. When from attritional changes in the dorsal apparatus a flexion deformity occurs and the lateral slips remain intact so that the distal joint is hyperextended, the deformity is termed the "buttonhole" type. Attempts to reconstruct the middle slip mechanism have not been satisfactory; and, especially when the flexion contracture is irreversible, arthrodesis is indicated. The reverse or "swan-neck" deformity usually accompanies a subluxated flexion contracture of the proximal joint. Reconstructing this proximal joint, the lesion of which is the primary factor in this deformity, may correct the hyperextension of the middle joint, though with overstretched volar capsular tissues it may be unstable. A tenodesis, using the superficialis as Swanson does for spastic deformities, will help to prevent recurrence. When the joint surfaces are damaged, arthrodesis is necessary.

Arthrodesis of the proximal finger joints is seldom indicated except as a last resort. The

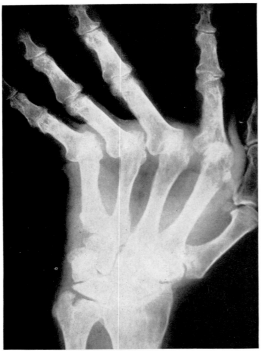

function of a finger is so dependent on motion in this joint that fusion should be avoided at all costs. Even gross bony deformities at this level usually can be corrected by other means. Fusion of the proximal joint of the little finger, once advocated to prevent ulnar drift, is no longer used. Instead, an artificial syndactylia with a bone graft between the proximal phalanges of the middle and the ring fingers is recommended by Bäckdahl.

Arthroplasty. The type of joint reconstruction used in rheumatoid hand deformities and only in the proximal joints is actually an excision of the metacarpal heads; interposition of other tissues as in the standard arthroplasty is not necessary or advisable. Cutting back the deformed head of the metacarpal and shaping the bone end into a blunt wedge tilted radialward results in a shortening of the skeleton and a relative lengthening of the short intrinsics. The operation is done when dislocation of the phalanx is present and often

Fig. 412. Roentgenograms taken before operation and immediately after reconstruction of proximal joints by excision of metacarpal heads. Note level of resection and radial slope to resection line. The little finger proximal joint has been fused. (From L. Ramsey Straub, M.D.)

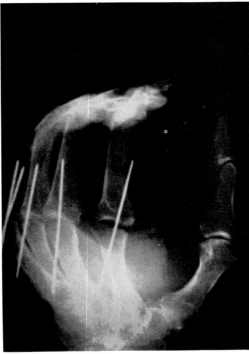
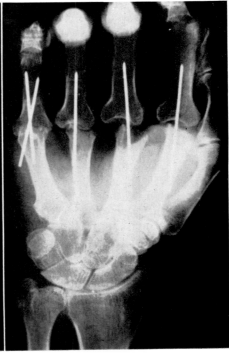

for ulnar deviation. Removing the metacarpal head allows the phalanx to be repositioned and the dislocated long extensors to be relocated. The intrinsic contracture is relieved. The bones should be held with Kirschner wire for several weeks until fibrosis of the surrounding tissues provides some support. Synovectomy is an important part of the procedure. Arthroplasty in the other joints of the hand is usually not advisable.

Arthroplasty of the proximal finger joints is indicated when subluxation cannot be reduced passively and deformity of the metacarpal head is present. If the head is reasonably normal in shape and the subluxation can be reduced passively, synovectomy with release of the intrinsic contracture and relocation of the extensors may correct the malalignment and retain some useful motion in the joint.

Prostheses. Flatt has used a modification of the hinged metallic prosthesis that Brannon and Klein developed for use in the middle finger joints and has reported its use to be particularly advantageous in proximal joint

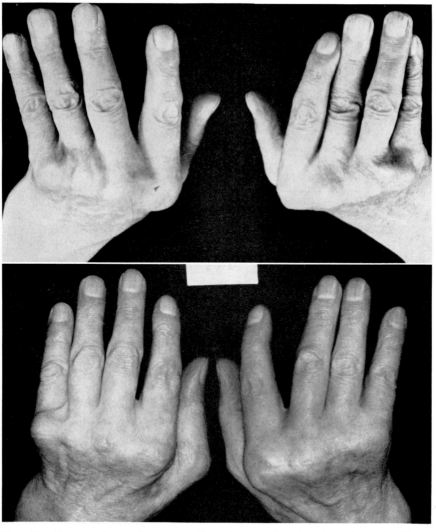

Fig. 413. Preoperative and postoperative photographs of patient shown in Figure 412. (From L. Ramsey Straub, M.D.)

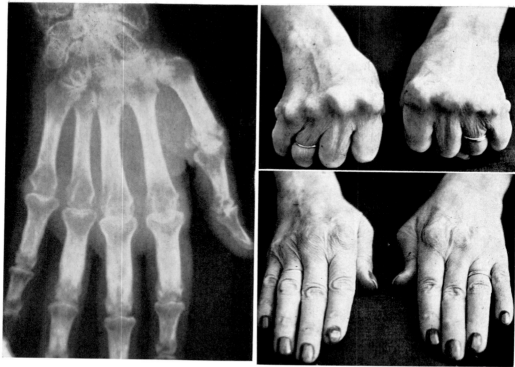

FIG. 414. When subluxation of the proximal joints is reducible and there is minimal bony deformity, joints may be repositioned, dislocated extensors rerouted, and the metacarpal heads preserved. The tight and spastic interossei must be released to maintain the correction. (*Left*) Postoperative roentgenogram of the right hand. (*Right*) Photograph of both hands in flexion and extension 2 years later.

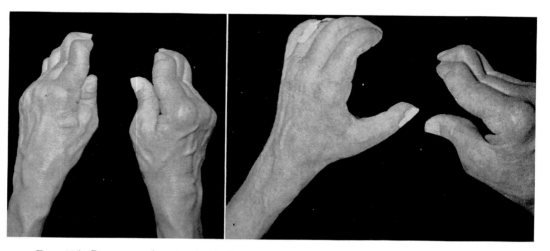

FIG. 415. Reconstruction for intrinsic-plus type of rheumatoid deformity. (*Left*) Typical flexed and subluxated proximal joints, "swan-neck" deformity of middle joints and dislocated long extensors. (*Right*) After operation on left hand. The proximal joints were repositioned after releasing all contracted ulnar-attached interosseus insertions and abductor minimi digiti; the long extensors were relocated into a new slit on the radial side of the joint, and the middle joints were tenodesed in flexion with the sublimis tendon slips as recommended by Swanson,

PLATE 6

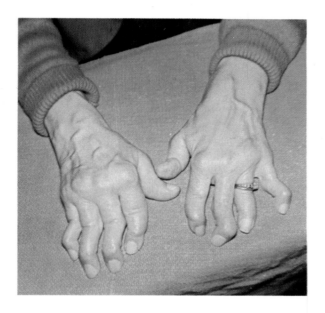

Rheumatoid arthritis with characteristic deformities of fingers.

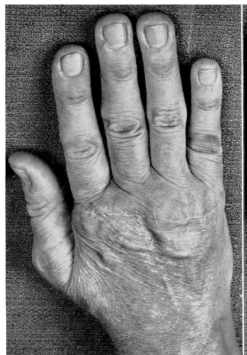
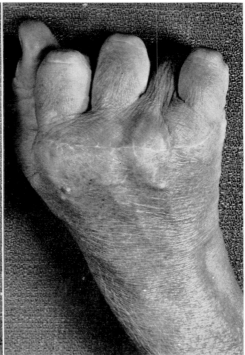

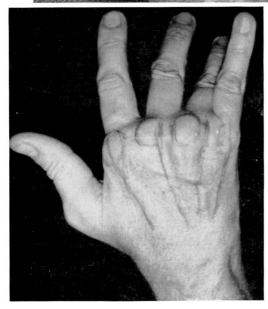

Fig. 416. Recurrence of ulnar drift and dislocation of extensor tendons in spite of fusion of 5th metacarpophalangeal joint. (*Top*) Two years after reconstruction. (*Bottom*) Four years after operation. The ring finger ulnar deviates beneath the arthrodesed little finger. The course of the extensor tendons is indicated. (From L. Ramsey Straub, M.D.)

Release of Intrinsic Contractures. The intrinsics and apparently particularly the distally inserted interossei are in spastic contracture first and then become fibrous and fixed. When the proximal phalanx subluxates, the skeletal-attached interossei also shorten, preventing relocation of the phalanx.

A spastic muscle can be stretched, so that splinting is indicated in the early stages and as a means of preventing deformity. Later, release of the contracture involves either shortening of the skeleton, as by excision of a segment at the base of the metacarpal or of the metacarpal head as in the arthroplasties, or dividing the intrinsic tendons.

Bunnell showed that when the subluxated proximal phalanx could be reduced passively, shortening of the metacarpal at its base re-

deformities. Stability is maintained by the appliance, and the metal has been well tolerated thus far. He advises against its use in long-standing flexion deformities of the middle joint of the "buttonhole" type and in Still's disease.

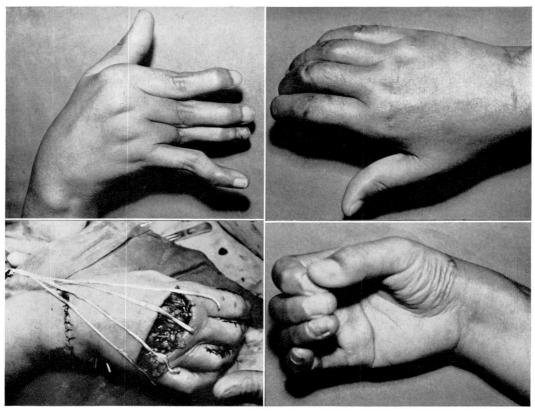

Fig. 417. Tsuge's method of tenodesis for correction of swan-neck and ulnar drift. (*Bottom, left*) The brachioradialis tendon is split into 4 strands, inserting 1 to the radial side of the extensor tendon of each finger at the level of the hood. The middle joints were forced into flexion and held with Kirschner wire. A Swanson tenodesis was performed in the other hand which had a similar deformity. (From Kenya Tsuge, M.D., Okayama University)

lieved the intrinsic pull and the deforming force and allowed the intrinsics to again act as extensors of the middle and the distal joints. The long extensors were relocated radialward. Release of the intrinsic contracture without bony shortening was accomplished by sliding the muscles distalward or by dividing the musculotendinous junction. When tenotomies are done, it is imperative that the long extensor function or there will be no force to extend the middle and the distal joints.

To extend the middle or the distal joints, either the long extensors or the intrinsics which insert into the hood must be functioning. If in arthroplasty the long extensor is tenodesed to the base of the proximal phalanx as recommended by Fowler, the intrinsic attachments must be left intact. Similarly, if

the intrinsic contracture is relieved by tenotomy of the interossei—and both the skeletal and the wing tendons must be cut to obtain full correction when the proximal joint is subluxated—then the long extensor mechanism must be reconstructed in such a way that the common extensor lifts the proximal phalanx and also acts through the aponeurosis to extend the middle and the distal joints. Intrinsic release and tenodesis of the long extensor must not be combined.

In the early stages of intrinsic contracture before proximal joint subluxation has occurred and before the long extensors have dislocated ulnarward, simple division of the wing-inserted tendons or of the wing itself will relieve the intrinsic plus. However, the latter is not indicated if the proximal joint is in flexion con-

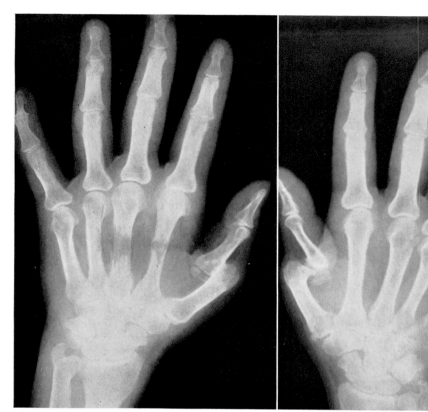

Fig. 418. Rheumatoid arthritis with marked change in the proximal joint of the thumb. Arthrodesis in the functioning position is the best solution for this deformity. (From L. Ramsey Straub, M.D.)

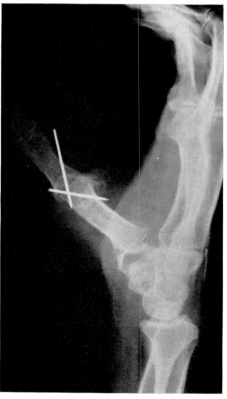

tracture. In this case the musculotendinous junction should be divided, making certain to cut all the fibers of insertion to the hood, the volar transverse capitular ligament and the joint capsule. The hood itself, that is, the sheet of transverse fibers from the long extensor to the volar plate, must be left intact, for this is the "tendon of insertion" of the long extensor and the only means by which the common extensor tendon can maintain the position of the proximal phalanx.

Relocation of the Dislocated Common Extensor Tendons. When the proximal joint subluxation has been reduced and the intrinsic contracture relieved, the long digital extensor tendons which are displaced ulnarward should be brought back to their proper position or even a little to the radial side of their normal location. Several methods have been described for maintaining the new position, such as

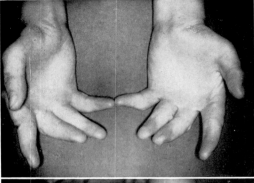

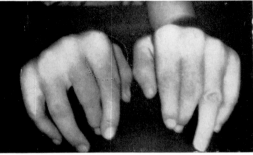

Fig. 419. Case J. H., age 7. Congenital flexion contracture of palm and digits (same as mother). Proximal joints lack 53° of extension. Hollow palm webbed with fingers. Needs zigzags, new skin across the palm, and thumb clefts and webs attended to.

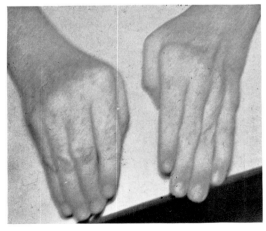

Fig. 420. Congenital flexion-ulnar deformity of fingers. Long extensors dislocate as in rheumatoids. Needs release of ulnar-inserted interossei and relocation of long extensors. Father and one brother have a similar deformity.

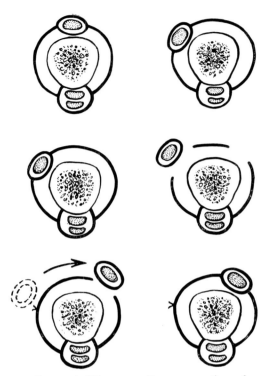

Fig. 421. Diagrammatic cross section of metacarpal head to demonstrate extensor tendons inserted into new location in hood. (Top, left) Normal location of extensor tendon in hood; (right) as it appears in ulnar dislocation. (Center) An incision on each side of the tendon allows it to be lifted, while an incision on the radial side permits shift of the central segment of hood ulnarward. (Bottom) The edges of the hood are closed with a running wire suture, and the tendon is sutured into its new location with running removable wire sutures.

incising the hood longitudinally on the radial side and imbricating it, dividing the ulnar side to allow the extensor tendon to slide over, and reinforcing this by suturing the lumbrical tendon to the "dorsal aponeurosis" (Henderson and Lipscomb); turning a flap of the hood tissues from the ulnar side over the extensor tendon and fastening it to the radial side to act as a sling (Fowler); and moving the tendons to the radial side and "reconstructing the radial collateral ligaments" (Pulkki). Bunnell used a different method which he found to be successful in repairing traumatic dislocations. The extensor tendon is lifted out of its bed by incising the fascia

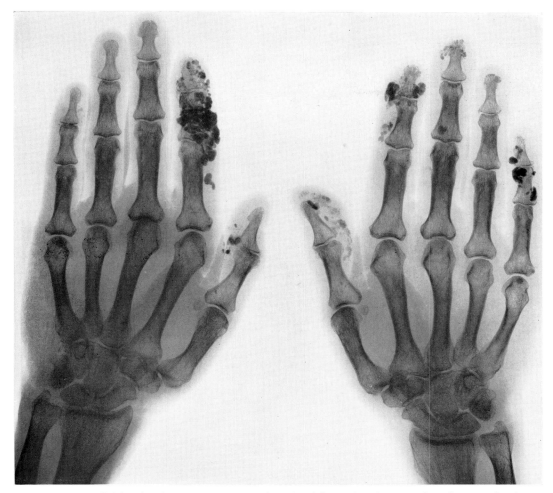

Fɪɢ. 422. Calcinosis circumscripta. Deposits of calcium phosphates and carbonates in the tissues are often accompanied by vascular changes with Raynaud-like syndromes or sclerodermatous changes.

Fɪɢ. 423. Calcification in periarticular tissues, but with destruction of joints, especially the distal joint of the right thumb and the middle joint of the left middle finger. This patient had a clinical diagnosis of scleroderma.

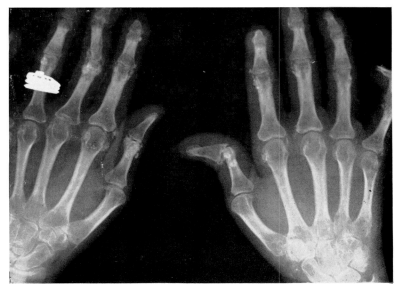

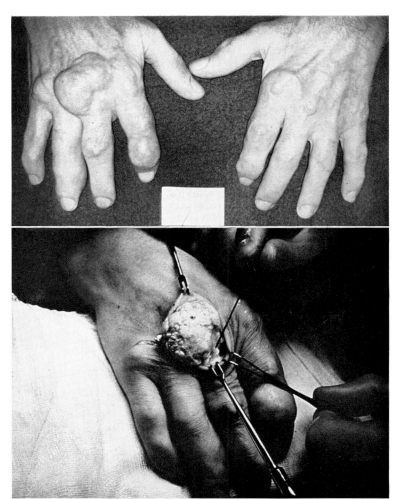

FIG. 424. Tophaceous gout may produce immense swellings. Function and appearance can be improved by removal of most of the urate deposits. (From L. Ramsey Straub, M.D.)

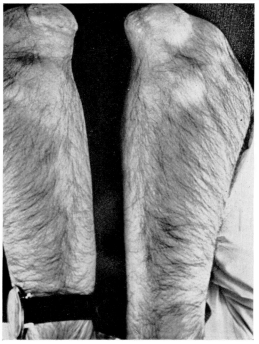

along each side and the hood to its distal edge. This longitudinal slit is closed with a running wire suture after a longitudinal incision has been made on the radial side of the hood and the intertendinous fascial layer. Closure of the gap left by lifting the extensor tendon away pulls the central segment ulnarward and opens up a space on the radial side in the encircling hood fibers and fascia. The extensor is sutured into this space by 2 running wire sutures. The tendon is held in its place without strain, the hood mechanism, with its intact circle of fibers, is maintained, and the tendons are prevented from going ulnarward.

Repair of Tendon Ruptures. For the common rupture of the extensor pollicis longus tendon, transfer of the extensor indicis (old term proprius) is more satisfactory than attempted repair or graft. When the common extensors are ruptured, the thickened synovia at the wrist should be excised, and, if the lower radio-ulnar joint is involved and there is dorsal subluxation, the distal 2 to 3 cm. of the ulna should be removed. Usually a wrist extensor is transferred to the finger extensors to provide this motion.

Flexor tendon ruptures may occur in the carpal canal or in the thumb at the level of either joint. For flexor pollicis longus rupture, arthrodesis of the distal joint is advised. Sublimis ruptures do not require replacement, and profundus ruptures in the palm or at the wrist level should be repaired by graft or transfer along with thorough synovectomy.

Operation for Ulnar Drift. When this deformity is seen early before there is gross destruction of the bones of the proximal joint and when the proximal phalanx can be replaced passively in its normal position with ease, surgical reconstruction can offer much improvement in appearance and function. Each element of the deformity is corrected— the intrinsic contracture, the volar subluxation and the dislocation of the long extensors.

A transverse incision 2.5 to 3 cm. proximal to the metacarpophalangeal joints is made through the skin only, the distal flap is elevated, and the subcutaneous tissues with the longitudinally placed veins are carefully left in place. The veins pass between the joints and over the falx of the intertendinous fascia beneath which the dorsal vessels pass. The intrinsic contracture is released by exposing the interosseus tendons deep in the interdigital space on the ulnar side of the index, the middle and the ring fingers and identifying the tendons inserting into the wing. These are usually more flattened in appearance and can be seen passing over the transverse fibers of the hood proper. They are divided at the musculotendinous junction with the finger held in extension and radial deviation at the proximal joint and with the middle joint forced into flexion. This tenses the fibers that are causing the contracture, and when they are divided, the position of the finger is released suddenly. The middle joint drops into flexion easily, and the finger can be held in radial deviation at the proximal joint without causing an "intrinsic plus." The procedure is repeated on the ulnar side of the middle finger where the 3rd dorsal interosseus usually inserts more into the wing like a volar interosseus. This is divided along with any other fibers which remain taut as the finger is held as described above.

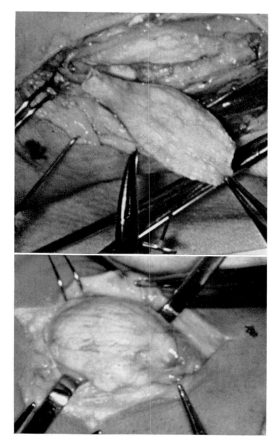

FIG. 425. A large deposit of gouty material in both tendons of the middle finger blocked extension by impinging on the transverse carpal ligament. The superficialis was excised, and the enlarged profundus shaved down to normal size. (From L. Ramsey Straub, M.D.)

A double lumbrical with one belly to the ulnar side of the middle finger is not a rare finding. In similar fashion the ulnar side of the ring finger is released, and, on the ulnar side of the little finger, the tendon of the abductor minimi digiti and any fibers extending into the extensor aponeurosis are divided. It is not necessary to sever the wing insertions on the radial side.

When the intrinsic contracture has been released, the previously subluxated proximal phalanx stays in position easily, unless some of the interosseus insertions into the more volar aspect of the hood are still tight. If the interosseus tendon is divided at the musculotendinous junction, that is, proximal to the hood mechanism, this flexor component will be removed. If, however, an attempt is made to release the wing insertion only, other fibers of these same muscles will still provide a flexing force. It must be emphasized that simple incision or excision of the wing will not remove the force causing the flexion and subluxation. Such releases are suitable only in the earliest phases of the intrinsic contracture and in the mild ischemic contractures. When the proximal joint is flexed and fixed in flexion and especially when subluxated, the division of the interosseus tendons should be proximal to the joint. If the flexion contracture has become firmly fixed as in severe ischemic contracture of the intrinsics, it is often necessary to cut the fan portion of the joint ligaments as well.

In theory, a muscle slide, in which the origins of the interossei are stripped from the metacarpals and allowed to reattach more distally, would be indicated in these flexed and subluxated fingers. Of course, shortening of the metacarpals, at the bases or by excision of the heads, results in relative lengthening of the contracted intrinsics. A tenotomy of the ulnar wing-inserted interossei selects only the muscles causing the deformity and, if the metacarpal heads are reasonably well preserved, is the operation of choice.

The dislocated long extensor tendons are replaced over the knuckles, and slightly overcorrected, that is, slightly to the radial side of the metacarpal head, by the method previously described. The long extensor must not be tenodesed to the proximal phalanx, for it is now the sole extensor of the middle and the distal joints. If a method of relocating the long extensors which results in loss of the encircling hood fibers is used, or if the metacarpal heads are excised and the long extensors are tenodesed to the proximal phalanx to prevent subluxation, it is imperative that the intrinsic wing insertions be left intact to provide middle and distal joint extension. Either the wing intrinsics or the long extensors can extend the middle joints as long as the proximal joint is not hyperextended. Therefore, no matter what procedure is used, one of these systems must be retained.

GOUT

In spite of the development of better means of control of this disease through drugs, some patients with gout still develop large tophi and gross deformities in the hands. Surgical removal of large masses can improve function, and drainage for infection will prevent further damage.

In 1943 Linton and Talbott reported excising 49 tophi from the upper extremities, and, in 1958, Larmon and Kurtz recorded not only excision of the tophi but also joint resections, an amputation and 3 carpal tunnel decompressions. In 1961 Straub *et al.* reported the treatment of 21 patients requiring the removal of 67 deposits in the upper extremities.

In the hand, tophi occur on the dorsum near the proximal joints where they may involve skin, tendon, joint, ligaments and bone, and on the volar surface involve the pulps of the fingers. The flexor tendon may be involved, especially at the wrist level.

Straub emphasizes the necessity of using a tourniquet, identifying and preserving the neurovascular bundles and preserving the tendinous structures, at the expense of leaving some urate material behind. Where the skin is grossly involved he prefers to preserve the skin and avoid skin grafting.

When tophi have been opened and continue to drain, a judicious curettement of the remaining material may allow collapse of the surrounding tissues and early healing. Some tophi act as sequestra, provoking persistent drainage.

In general, the surgery of gout is conservative; it aims to preserve all possible function and to remove mechanically the heavy deposits of urate material. Major reconstructive procedures should be avoided.

Gout may recur in an acute attack following a surgical procedure, as it did in 10 of 36 operations by Straub. This occurred in spite of colchicine therapy. Penicillin administration has been reported to trigger an acute attack of gout.

BIBLIOGRAPHY

GENERAL

Abbott, L. C., Saunders, J. B. deC. M., and Bost, F. C.: Arthrodesis of wrist with use of grafts of cancellous bone (from ilium), J. Bone Joint Surg. *24*:883, 1942.

Albee, F. H.: Principles of arthroplasty, J.A.M.A. *96*:245, 1931.

Astow, J. N.: Locked middle finger, J. Bone Joint Surg. *42-B*:1, 1960.

Bate, J. T.: An operation for the correction of locking of the proximal interphalangeal joint of finger in hyperextension, J. Bone Joint Surg. 27:142, 1945.

Brannon, E. W., and Klein, G.: Experiences with a finger-joint prosthesis, J. Bone Joint Surg. 41-A:1, 1959.

Bruner, J. M.: Recurrent locking of the index finger due to internal derangement of the metacarpophalangeal joint, J. Bone Joint Surg. 43-A:450, 1961.

Bunnell, S.: Occupational therapy of hands, Am. J. Occup. Ther. 4:1, 1950.

Burman, M. S.: Vitallium cap arthroplasty of metacarpophalangeal and interphalangeal joints of fingers, Bull. Hosp. Joint Dis. 1:79, 1940.

Campbell, W. C.: Operative Orthopedics, St. Louis, Mosby, 1939.

Carroll, R. E., and Taber, T. H.: Digital arthroplasty of the proximal interphalangeal joint, J. Bone Joint Surg. 36-A:912, 1954.

Coleman, H. M.: Injuries of the articular disc at the wrist, J. Bone Joint Surg. 42-B:522, 1960.

Curtis, R. M.: Capsulectomy of the interphalangeal joints of the fingers, J. Bone Joint Surg. 36:1219, 1954.

Eggers, G. W. N.: Chronic dislocation of the base of the metacarpal of the thumb, J. Bone Joint Surg. 27:500, 1945.

Flatt, A. E.: Recurrent locking of the index finger, J. Bone Joint Surg. 40-A:1128, 1958.

Forrester, C. R. G.: Author's method of repair of ankylosed joint of hand, Am. J. Surg. 33:101, 1936.

Gervis, W. H.: Excision of the trapezium for osteoarthritis of the trapezio-metacarpal joint, J. Bone Joint Surg. 31-B:537, 1949.

Goldner, J. L., and Clippinger, F. W.: Excision of the greater multangular bone as an adjunct to mobilization of the thumb, J. Bone Joint Surg. 41-A: 609, 1958.

Goodfellow, J. W., and Weaver, J. P. A.: Locking of the metacarpophalangeal joints, J. Bone Joint Surg. 43-B:772, 1961.

Graham, W. C.: Transplantation of joints to replace diseased or damaged articulations in the hands, Am. J. Surg. 88:136, 1954.

Graham, W. C., and Riordan, D. C.: Reconstruction of a metacarpophalangeal joint with a metatarsal transplant, J. Bone Joint Surg. 30-A:848, 1948.

Hucherson, D. C.: Darrach operation for lower radio-ulnar derangement, Am. J. Surg. 53:237, 1941.

Kaplan, E. B.: Dorsal dislocation of the metacarpophalangeal joint of the index finger, J. Bone Joint Surg. 39-A:1085, 1957.

Knutsson, F.: Skeletal changes in sarcoidosis, Acta radiol. (Stockh.) 51:429, 1959.

Koch, S. L.: Disabilities of hand from loss of joint function, J.A.M.A. 104:30, 1935.

Larmon, W. A., and Kurtz, J. F.: The surgical management of chronic tophaceous gout, J. Bone Joint Surg. 40-A:743, 1958.

Linton, R. R., and Talbott, J. H.: The surgical treatment of tophaceous gout, Am. Surg. 117:161, 1943.

Lowman, C. L.: Use of fascia lata in repair of disability at wrist, J. Bone Joint Surg. 12:400, 1930.

MacConaill, M. A.: Mechanical anatomy of carpus and its bearing on some surgical problems, J. Anat. 75:166, 1941.

McKeever, D. C.: The use of cellophane as an interposition membrane in synovectomy, J. Bone Joint Surg. 25:576, 1943.

Manual of Occupational Therapy, Council on Physiotherapy of A.M.A., 1943.

Michaelis, L. L.: Locking wrist, Lancet 2:229, 1940.

Milch, H.: So-called dislocation of lower end of ulna, Ann. Surg. 116:282, 1942.

Muller, G. M.: Arthrodesis of the trapezio-metacarpal joint for osteoarthritis, J. Bone Joint Surg. 31-B:540, 1949.

Murley, A. H. G.: Excision of the trapezium in osteoarthritis of the first carpo-metacarpal joint, J. Bone Joint Surg. 42-B:502, 1960.

Omer, G. E., and Conger, C. W.: Osteochondrosis of the capitulum humeri (Panner's disease), U.S. Armed Forces M. J. 10:1235, 1959.

Patterson, R.: Carpometacarpal arthroplasty of thumb, J. Bone Joint Surg. 15:240, 1933.

Portis, R. B.: Hyperextensibility of the proximal interphalangeal joint of the finger following trauma, J. Bone Joint Surg. 36:1141, 1954.

Schoolfield, B. L.: Injuries about carpometacarpal joint and thumb, South. M. J. 33:354, 1940.

Slocum, D. B.: Stabilization of articulation of greater multangular and first metacarpal, J. Bone Joint Surg. 25:626, 1943.

Smith-Petersen, M. N.: A new approach to the wrist joint, J. Bone Joint Surg. 22:122, 1940.

Sokoloff, L., and Bunim, J. J.: Clinical and pathological studies of joint involvement in sarcoidosis, New Engl. J. Med. 260:841, 1959.

Stamm, T. T.: Excision of proximal row of carpus, Proc. Roy. Soc. Med. 38:74, 1944.

Steindler, A.: Orthopedic Operations, Springfield, Ill., Thomas, 1940.

Straub, L. R., Smith, J. W., Carpenter, G. K., and Dietz, G. H.: The surgery of gout in the upper extremity, J. Bone Joint Surg. 43-A:731, 1961.

Watson-Jones, R.: Fractures and Other Bone and Joint Injuries, Baltimore, Williams & Wilkins, 1940.

Woughter, H. W.: Surgery of tophaceous gout,

a case report, J. Bone Joint Surg. *41-A*:116, 1959.

RHEUMATOID ARTHRITIS

Bäckdahl, M., and Myrin, S. O.: Ulnar deviation of the fingers in rheumatoid arthritis and its surgical correction, Acta chir. scand. *122*: 158, 1961.

Bodenham, D. C.: Control of ulnar deviation of fingers in rheumatoid arthritis, Lancet *2*:354, 1943.

Brewerton, D. A.: Hand deformities in rheumatoid disease, Ann. Rheum. Dis. *16*:183, 1957.

Bunnell, S.: Surgery of the rheumatic hand, J. Bone Joint Surg. *37-A*:759, 1955.

Cregan, J. C. F.: Indications for surgical intervention in rheumatoid arthritis of the wrist and hand, Ann. Rheum. Dis. *18*:29, 1959.

Duthie, J. J.: Arthritis of the hands and feet, Practitioner *186*:729, 1961.

Fearnley, G. R.: Ulnar deviation of the fingers, Ann. Rheum. Dis. *10*:176, 1951.

Flatt, A. E.: Surgical rehabilitation of the arthritic hand, Arthritis Rheum. *2*:278, 1959.

———: The prosthetic replacement of rheumatoid finger joints, Rheumatism *16*:90, 1960.

———: Restoration of rheumatoid finger-joint function; interim report on trial of prosthetic replacement, J. Bone Joint Surg. *43-A*:753, 1961.

———: Salvage of the rheumatoid hand, Clin. Orthop. *23*:207, 1962.

Henderson, E. W., and Lipscomb, P. R.: Surgical treatment of the rheumatoid hand, J.A.M.A. *175*:431, 1961.

Kestler, O. C.: Reconstruction of the deformed arthritic hand, Ann. Surg. *131*:218, 1950.

Kodama, T.: Some clinical aspects of rheumatoid arthritis, Acta Med. Okayama *13*:1, 1959.

Laine, V. A., Sairanen, E., and Vaino, K.: Finger deformities caused by rheumatoid arthritis, J. Bone Joint Surg. *39-A*:527, 1957.

Lush, B.: Ulnar deviation of the fingers, Ann. Rheum. Dis. *11*:219, 1952.

Pulkki, T.: Rheumatoid deformities of the hand, Acta rheum. scand. *7*:85, 1961.

Rose, D. L., and Kendell, H. W.: Rehabilitation of hand function in rheumatoid arthritis, J.A.M.A. *148*:1408, 1952.

Steindler, A.: Arthritic deformities of wrist and fingers, J. Bone Joint Surg. *33-A*:849, 1951.

Straub, L. R.: The rheumatoid hand, Clin. Orthop. *15*:127, 1959.

———: Etiology of finger deformities, Bull. Hosp. Joint Dis. *21*:322, 1960.

Swanson, A. B.: Need for early treatment of the rheumatoid hand, J. Mich. Med. Soc. *60*:348, 1961.

Vaino, K., and Oka, M.: Ulnar deviation of the fingers, Ann. Rheum. Dis. *12*:122, 1953.

Wells, R. M., and Johnson, E. W.: Study of conduction delay in median nerve of patients with rheumatoid arthritis, Arch. Phys. Med. *43*:244, 1962.

Chapter 10

Nerves

IMPORTANCE OF NERVE FUNCTION IN THE UPPER EXTREMITY

The hand is an organ of grasp and of sensation, its movements and sensibilities depending on a functioning nerve system extending from the opposite cerebral cortex through the cord, the brachial plexus and the nerves of the arm. Injuries to this system at any place along the pathway may cripple the hand as much or more than injury to the hand itself. Proper diagnosis and adequate treatment of nerve injuries are a major part of reconstructive surgery of the hand.

Nerves can be damaged directly in lacerations or indirectly in explosions and crushing wounds, stretched in traction injuries or strangled by scar from infection or traumatized tissues.

SYMPTOMS AND SIGNS OF NERVE INJURY

When a pure sensory nerve is severed, there will be loss of tactile sensation, stereognosis and joint-position sense in the part supplied by that nerve. If a motor nerve is severed, there will be loss of certain voluntary motions, atrophy of the muscles, and deformity from unopposed pull of the antagonistic muscles. Trophic changes also occur in all the tissues from skin to bone.

At the cut end of the nerve a multiplication of axons by branching takes place; these new fibers grow down seeking out the distal part of the nerve trunk. Scar tissue blocks their path, and the axons wind and curl into a bulblike neuroma. Some escape into the surrounding tissues. The portion of the nerve trunk distal to the division swells and undergoes Wallerian degeneration, which is complete within a month. Its end may enlarge slightly from a glioma of the fibrous elements of the sheath. If the nerve ends lie close together in a fascial envelope, as in the finger, there is a natural attempt to rejoin. If the gap is small and there is minimal scar, considerable repair takes place. In repairing a nerve the aim should be to close the gap and, by refinement of technic, to provoke minimal scarring. It is almost an axiom that the quality of regeneration of a peripheral nerve is directly proportional to the accuracy of the suture and indirectly to the amount of scar tissue at the junction.

Sensory Changes. Sensibility is highly developed in the hand and especially in the median nerve area supplying the skin of the thumb, the index and the middle finger pulps. Here the dermal network is highly developed, and fine discrimination of qualities of objects is possible through these terminal portions of the nerves.

For practical diagnostic purposes it is sufficient to map out areas of loss of sensibility to light touch and pinprick. Starting in an anesthetic area, a light stroke with a cotton wisp is repeated over widening circles until the patient, with eyes closed, responds each time he feels the cotton. The area of lack of feeling is outlined. Similar tests with a sharp pinpoint verify the loss of light touch. In questionable areas a useful method is to place the test object, cotton or pin, alternately on an adjoining area of normal innervation and on the suspected area. The patient is asked to say whether the feeling is more or less perceptible or the same in the two areas. When a nerve has been injured many months before and some spontaneous regeneration has occurred or if after repair some return has taken place, an evaluation of the state of recovery becomes most difficult. Here the use of more refined tests such as the coin test, 2-point discrimination and the ninhydrin paper test are useful. Details are given in Chapter 4.

Changes in Motor Function. A muscle becomes completely paralyzed when its nerve supply is interrupted. Atrophy begins and may be marked in a month. It is progressive, and

351

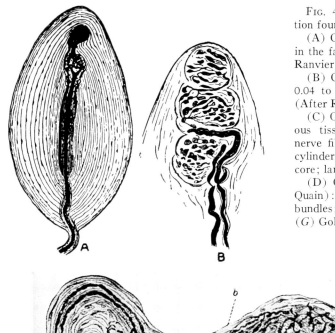

Fig. 426. Special end organs for sensation found in the hand.

(A) Corpuscles of Pacini are conspicuous in the fat; yellow; 2 or 3 mm. long. (After Ranvier)

(B) Corpuscles of Wagner and Meissner, 0.04 to 0.15 mm. long; plentiful in hand. (After Ranvier)

(C) Organ of Ruffini from the subcutaneous tissue. (After Quain): (a) entering nerve fibers; (b, d) endings of their axis-cylinders; (e, c) capsule or organ; (c') core; large.

(D) Organ of Golgi in a tendon. (After Quain): (m) muscular fibers; (t) tendon bundles; (n) 2 nerve fibers passing into (G) Golgi's organ.

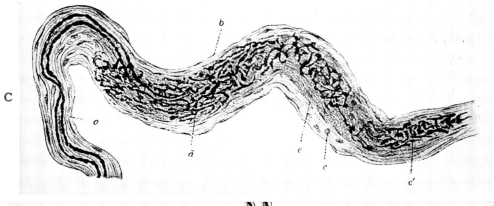

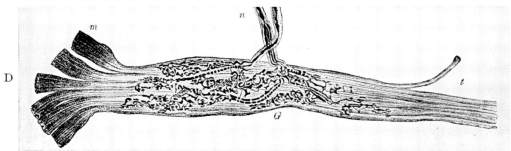

eventually the muscle undergoes fibrous degeneration. This process requires a year or more, but after 2 years fibrosis is so far advanced that even if the nerve regenerates, there is seldom enough muscle tissue available to function effectively. The opposing still-active muscles draw the limb into deformity and thus stretch out the paralyzed muscle, increasing the damage to its fibers.

Some muscles are supplied by more than one nerve, or a lesion of part of the nerve trunk may have spared some of the motor axons. A partially paralyzed muscle may be unable to move the part normally or to overcome the effect of gravity. Careful testing by isolating the muscle function and especially by palpating the muscle as it contracts will aid in diagnosis. Gravity is eliminated by posi-

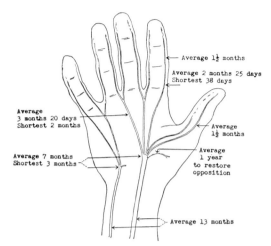

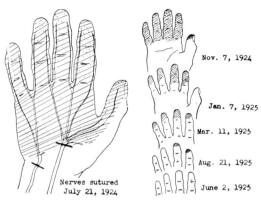

Fig. 427. Diagram showing the average time and the shortest time taken, in this series, to restore sensibility to cotton wool and pinprick over the entire area formerly anesthetic, including the fingertips. The arrows indicate the points at which the nerves were sutured. (Surg., Gynec. Obstet. *44*:145)

Fig. 428. Case A. L., age 54. Five months previously, a forest bit had entered the front of the wrist. This and subsequent infection destroyed all tendons and nerves in the front of the wrist. The ends of the ulnar nerve were separated by 1 inch and the median by 3 inches. Nutrition of the hand was poor. The 2 nerves were sutured where indicated, and 9 tendon grafts from the extensors of the toes were used to bridge the tendons. Anesthesia to cotton wool (*shaded*) and analgesia to pinprick (*dotted*) receded, as shown by the dates on the diagrams. The power of opposition returned to the thumb, as it does in about 66 per cent of repairs by suture of the median nerve. (Surg., Gynec. Obstet. *44*: 145)

tioning, e.g., holding the arm outward with the elbow flexed and the forearm horizontal to test the elbow movers. Limited activity of a muscle is shown by lessened power, amplitude and endurance.

A standard system of recording muscle activity is as follows:

0—complete paralysis
1—flicker of contraction
2—visible and palpable contraction with gravity eliminated
3—contraction against gravity
4—contraction against gravity and some resistance
5—normal power

Testing muscle function requires a thorough knowledge of anatomy and of the motions that can be performed by each muscle. It is important not to test a motion but rather to test an isolated muscle. Paralysis of all 3 wrist flexors is possible, yet wrist flexion is easily accomplished by using the digital flexors. The examiner should position the various parts so as to isolate the muscle being tested. Palpation with the fingertip during attempted contraction is extremely useful in identifying muscle activity. A patient with ulnar nerve

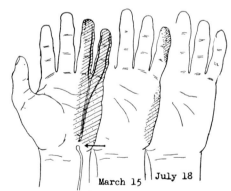

Fig. 429. Case F. R. S., age 44. Twenty-one months previously, the ulnar nerve had been severed on a bottle just proximal to its branches; it was sutured on April 2. The dates on the diagram show how the anesthesia to cotton wool (*shaded*) and analgesia to pinprick (*dotted*) receded. (Surg., Gynec. Obstet. *44*:145)

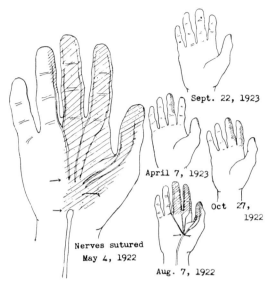

FIG. 430. Case E. C., age 25. While a bottle was being corked, the glass neck broke and severed 2 tendons and the median nerve where it branched. One month later, on May 4, each of the 6 branches was sutured to the end of the median nerve. Anesthesia to cotton wool (*shaded*) and analgesia to pinprick (*dotted*) receded, as shown by the dates on the diagram. Full ability to oppose the thumb was regained after 11 months through suture of the motor thenar nerve. (Surg., Gynec. Obstet. *44*:145)

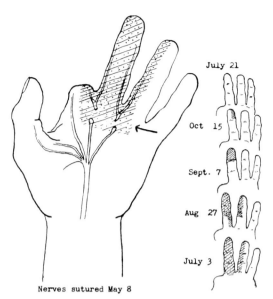

FIG. 431. Case D. B., age 47. Seven months previously, a buzz saw had cut across the distal part of the palm. Two volar digital nerves in the palm were sutured, and anesthesia to cotton wool (*shaded*) and analgesia to pinprick (*dotted*) receded, as shown by the dates on the diagrams. (Surg., Gynec. Obstet. *44*:145)

damage can spread his extended fingers by using the common digital extensors and thus mimic the abducting effect of the interossei; but by isolating each finger and palpating the first interosseus muscle, one can easily determine the state of the ulnar nerve.

Electrical Reactions. Normally, a muscle reacts to stimulation with a faradic or a galvanic current. Four to 7 days after severance of the nerve supply, the response to faradic current is lost, and galvanic stimulation produces a sluggish long amplitude contraction which relaxes slowly. This is the reaction of degeneration which remains in the paralyzed muscle as long as muscle fibers are present.

Electromyography is the recording of electrical muscle potentials by inserting an electrode into the muscle substance. Properly done, this is a very delicate test with a high degree of accuracy. Electromyography can aid in the diagnosis of complete nerve severance 2 weeks or more after injury and distinguish partial nerve lesions as well as evidence of regeneration. It is a most useful tool in peripheral nerve surgery.

Trophic Signs. Changes in the skin include lack of sweat gland action, resulting in a dry, smooth, satinlike feel and appearance. There may be color changes from paralysis of sympathetic fibers to the vessels of the paralyzed part and redness or cyanosis. A partial nerve lesion, especially with irritative phenomena, may produce severe atrophy and a glossy red skin. The fingernails thicken and become brittle, curve excessively—either transversely or longitudinally—and grow slowly. Muscles first lose their tone and then atrophy, leaving conspicuous deformities. Osteoporosis of the bones, thinning of the articular cartilages and loss of elasticity in the ligaments and the joint capsules result from loss of nerve supply.

Vascular changes such as vasospasm or dilatation may result from a nerve lesion and

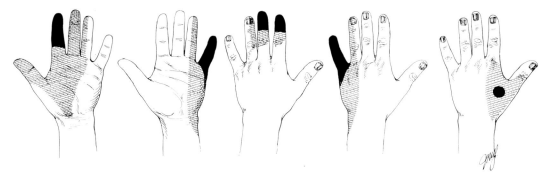

FIG. 432. The areas of sensory disturbance following severance of each of the 3 main nerves in the hand. Though some variations are noted, these patterns are seen commonly. (*Left to right*) Median nerve, ulnar nerve, median (dorsal aspect), ulnar nerve, radial nerve. (*Shaded*) Loss of touch; (*dotted*) analgesia to pinprick.

compound the trophic effects on the hand. It is likely that the same injuring force also directly damaged the major vessels to the extremity. Such injuries to the vessels can cause trophic changes in the hand by lowering the nutrition. There may be ischemic contractures of the paralyzed muscle with extreme deformity from contracture.

Location of the Nerve Lesion

Since a lesion in the nerve pathway from brain to arm exerts its effects on the motions and the sensibility of the hand, a differential diagnosis to locate the level of disturbance is required. Some aid may be obtained from the history, the onset and the progress of the disablement, but a few localizing diagnostic points will help.

Cerebral Lesions. Spastic rather than flaccid paralysis, absence of sensory changes, normal electrical reactions and lack of muscle atrophy indicate a central nervous system lesion.

Cord Lesions. A flaccid paralysis at the level of and spastic changes below the lesion, with involvement of the long sensory and motor tracts of the cords, are found in cord lesions. Changes in the upper extremity will be segmental in pattern instead of by nerve. Sensory patterns from cord segments as well as peripheral nerves are illustrated. From the segments these areas parallel each other longitudinally down the limb starting with the 5th cervical on the radial upper arm and ending with the 2nd dorsal on the ulnar border of the upper arm. Because of overlap, the upper limit in a cord or spinal nerve lesion

is always one segment higher than the sensory loss would indicate. For quick orientation segmental muscle innervations can be grouped roughly as follows:

C-5—shoulder
C-6—upper arm
C-7—wrist, forearm
C-8—fingers
D-1—intrinsics

Reflex changes may aid in verifying a level of injury. Reflexes in the upper extremity are listed according to Bing.

Segmental lesions show characteristic patterns as compared with peripheral nerve injuries. Paralysis from C-7, C-8 and D-1 will involve all the flexor forearm muscles except the flexor carpi radialis and the pronator teres which arise from C-6. If median and ulnar nerves are involved, these 2 muscles are paralyzed along with the other flexors. In radial nerve palsy, all extensors, including the brachioradialis, are paralyzed; but in segmental lesions, this muscle, supplied by C-5, is spared.

Injury to the lower roots of spinal nerves C-8, D-1 and D-2 causes paralysis of the involved muscles but is accompanied by Horner's syndrome—a narrowing of the palpebral fissure, contraction of the pupil and recession of the eye.

Brachial Plexus Lesions. The plexus is formed by the 5 spinal nerves C-5 to D-1 fusing into 3 trunks at the level of the scalenus medius muscle. Before this, the posterior thoracic and the long thoracic nerves supplying the scapular muscles have branched off. The 3 trunks

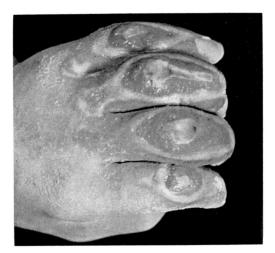

FIG. 433. Accidental burn by a heat lamp in a case of high nerve paralysis.

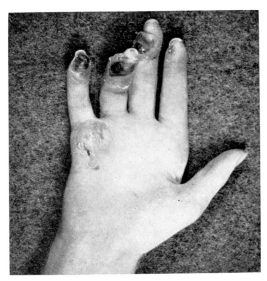

FIG. 434. Frostbite of fingers. The median and the ulnar nerves have been severed.

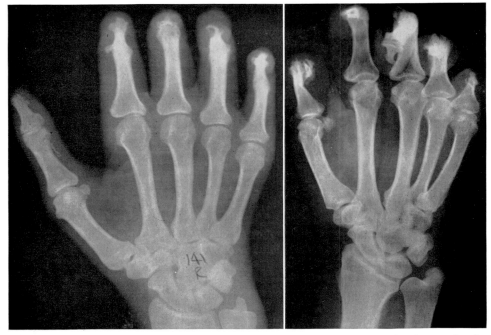

FIG. 435. (*Left*) Leprosy. Loss of the ends of fingers and neurotrophic changes in the stumps. A number of other conditions can cause similar changes. (*Right*) Syringomyelia. Adult female with neurotrophic changes in the ends of the phalanges. Loss of pain sensation results in repetitive trauma with no protection of the injured part. (From R. R. Schreiber, M.D., Los Angeles Orthopedic Hospital)

REFLEXES IN UPPER EXTREMITY

TENDON AND BONE REFLEXES	SKIN REFLEXES	METHOD OF STARTING	EFFECT	LOCALIZATION
—	Scapular reflex	Stimulation of the skin over the scapula	Contraction of shoulder-blade muscles	C-5—D-1
Biceps reflex	—	A blow on the biceps tendon	Flexion of forearm	C-5—C-6
Triceps reflex	—	A blow on the triceps tendon	Extension of forearm	C-6—C-7
Scapulohumeral reflex	—	A blow on the inner side of the lower angle of the scapula	Adduction of arm	C-6—C-7
Radius reflex	—	A blow on the styloid process of the radius	Supination of forearm	C-7—C-8
—	Palmar reflex	Irritation of the palm	Flexion of fingers	C-8—D-1

SEGMENTAL MOTOR INNERVATION—UPPER EXTREMITY

	C$_4$	C$_5$	C$_6$	C$_7$	C$_8$	Th$_1$
Shoulder	-----Supraspinatus---------- ---------Teres minor--------- ---------Deltoid------- ---------Infraspinatus------- ---------Subscapularis------- ---------Teres major-------					
Arm	---------Biceps--------------- ---------Brachialis---------- ------------Coracobrachialis---------------					
Forearm	--------------Triceps brachialis--------------- --------------Anconeus----------- ------Supinator longus------- ------------Supinator brevis--------- ------Extensor carpi radialis---------- ------Pronator teres--------- ------Flexor carpi radialis---- --------Flexor pollicis longus------------- ---------Abductor pollicis longus-------- ----Extensor pollicis brevis------ --Extensor pollicis longus----------------- ----Extensor digitorum longus----------- ----Extensor indicis proprius------------- ----Extensor carpi ulnaris------------- ----Extensor digiti quinti-------------					
Hand	-------Flexor digitorum sublimis------------- -------Flexor digitorum profundus------------- ---------Pronator quadratus-- ---------Flexor carpi ulnaris-- ------Palmaris longus---- ---------Abductor pollicis brevis------------- --------------Flexor pollicis brevis------------- ------Opponens pollicis---------- --------Flexor digiti quinti-- ------Opponens digiti quinti--------- --Adductor pollicis--------------- --Palmaris brevis------------- --Abductor digiti quinti--------- -------Lumbricales---------------- ---------Interossei-------------					

(This table after McDonald, J. J., and Chusid, J. G.: Correlative Neuroanatomy and Functional Neurology, ed. 7, Lange Medical Publications, Los Altos, Calif.)

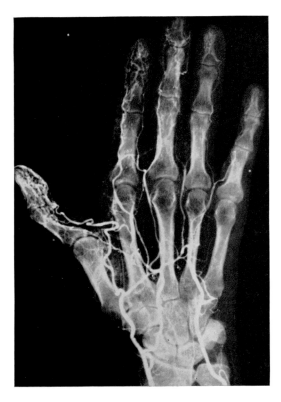

FIG. 436. Neurotrophic changes in vascular system. Arteriogram of hand with ulnar palsy due to leprosy. (From Professor A. Hodgson, Hongkong University)

split, each into an anterior and a posterior division, behind the middle third of the clavicle. The 3 posterior divisions group themselves into a posterior cord carrying all the extensor muscle control. The 3 cords surround the subclavian artery. The lateral or outer cord carries flexor and pronator fibers, and the inner or medial supplies the flexor muscles of the forearm and the intrinsic muscles of the hand. The 3 cords divide into the peripheral nerves.

Injuries to trunks simulate segmental injuries, while brachial plexus cord lesions resemble peripheral nerve lesions. A quick check of the longitudinal level of injury can be made by noting involvement of nerves which usually come off the plexus at certain levels. If in upper plexus injuries the rhomboids and the levator anguli scapulae and the serratus anterior are not functioning, then the nerves are torn near the foramina or in the cord. If the supra spinatus and the infraspinatus muscles are not paralyzed, the lesion is below the trunks. The internal rotators of the shoulder arise from the posterior cord at the next distal level. Thus, the serial motions of shrugging the shoulder, rotating the arm externally, flexing it forward, rotating it internally and abducting it will test for the nerves as they leave the plexus at different levels.

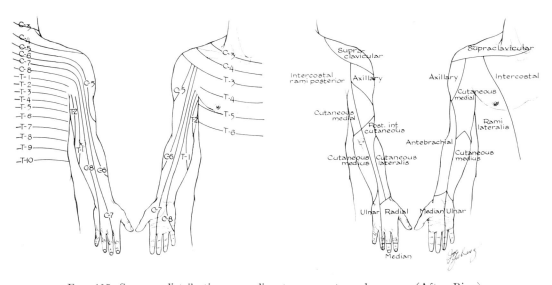

FIG. 437. Sensory distribution according to segments and nerves. (After Bing)

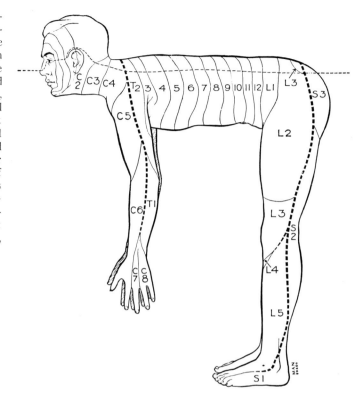

FIG. 438. The alignment of dermatomes in the quadruped position. The horizontal broken line extending from the sacral region to the tip of the nose marks the boundary between the dorsal and the ventral portions of trunk, neck, head and face. The vertical heavy lines on the limbs represent the dorsal axial lines. The facial segments (after Kraus), unlabeled because of variation of their boundaries, are the expression of lamination of the spinal nucleus of the trigeminal nerve. The dermatomic fields are after Foerster. (Haymaker and Woodhall: Peripheral Nerve Injuries, ed. 2, p. 30, Philadelphia, Saunders)

In outer or lateral cord lesions the shoulder muscles are spared, but the pronator teres and the flexor carpi radialis are paralyzed. The deltoid and the teres major are paralyzed, but if the lesion is in the C-7 root, they are spared. Lesions of C-8 and D-1 result in paralysis of all the intrinsic muscles and flexors of the digits, but if the inner or medial cord is involved, the flexors and the thenar eminence muscles supplied by the median nerve still will function.

Most brachial plexus injuries result from traction. This type of force disrupts the nerves, may avulse the roots from the spinal cord or damage the cords, the divisions or the trunks. In the upper plexus type resulting from distraction injury at birth or in adults, called Erb-Duchenne, the arm hangs at the side and is rotated internally; often there is a dislocation backward of the humerus on the scapula. In the lower type, Duchenne-Aran or Klumpke type, the forearm and the hand muscles are paralyzed. The flexor carpi radialis, the pro-nator teres and the flexor pollicis longus may be spared.

Treatment of brachial plexus injuries and reconstructive procedures for the residual of these injuries are described in Chapter 14.

Peripheral Nerves. Assuming that cerebral, spinal cord and plexus lesions have been ruled out, the site of the lesion in a nerve can be determined from the history, the location of the scar and Tinel's sign. This last, a tingling sensation felt when one taps over the severed or injured nerve, is reliable in locating the level. When a nerve is regenerating, this sign can be elicited over the down-growing axons in the distal trunk.

INDIVIDUAL NERVES

MEDIAN NERVE

The median nerve arises from the anterior divisions of the 5th, the 6th and the 7th cervical nerves which carry the sensory fibers and activate the muscles of flexion of the wrist and of pronation, and from the anterior divisions

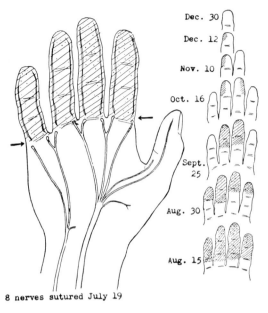

Dec. 30

Dec. 12

Nov. 10

Oct. 16

Sept. 25

Aug. 30

Aug. 15

8 nerves sutured July 19

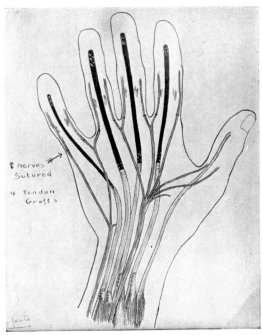

8 nerves Sutured

4 Tendon Grafts

FIG. 439. Case J. T., age 25. Forty-two days previously, the hand had been caught under the sharp edge of a large rotating pipe and every flexor tendon and every volar nerve severed at the base of each finger and the fingers rendered useless. The 8 volar nerves were sutured on July 19. Their ends were approximated by flexing the fingers. Anesthesia to cotton wool (*shaded*) and analgesia to pinprick (*dotted*) receded, as shown by the dates on the diagrams (*left*).

(*Left*) On December 15, the remains of all the flexor tendons were removed from the 4 fingers and in their places free grafts of the sublimis tendons were used to extend the profundus tendons to the ends of the fingers. (Surg., Gynec. Obstet. *44*:145)

(*Right*) This operation had to be delayed until the nerves had regenerated or else it would have failed from lack of trophic supply. Good sensation and motion were obtained in each finger. Eventually, the fingers could flex almost to the palm. (J. Bone Joint Surg. *10*:1)

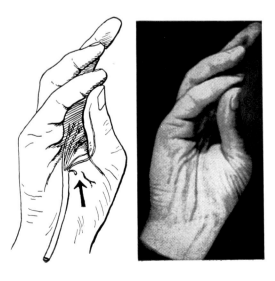

FIG. 440. Case S. P. Six months previously, a laceration in the index finger had resulted in tenosynovitis and an abscess in the thenar space. The latter was drained through an incision in the palm at the base of the thenar eminence. As the thenar branch of the median nerve was severed, the opponens pollicis and the abductor pollicis muscles were paralyzed and became atrophied, so that the thumb could no longer oppose the fingers. On August 4, this tiny nerve was sutured at the point shown in the left-hand drawing, with full recovery of the power of opposition 13 months later. (*Right*) The photograph shows that the thenar muscles are functioning well and that their atrophy has gone. (J. Bone Joint Surg., Jan., 1928)

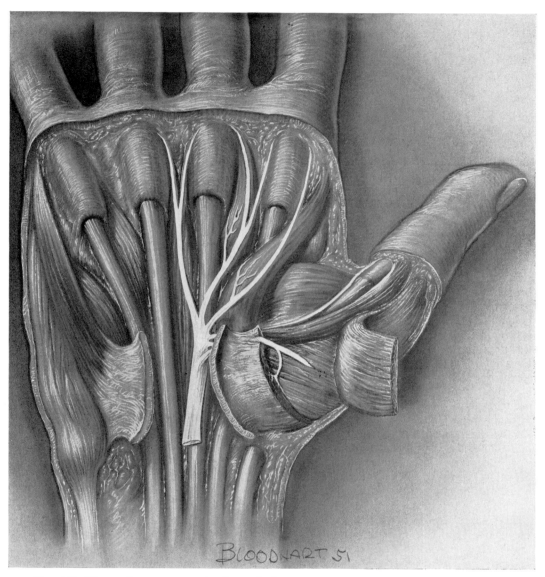

Fig. 441. The median nerve passing beneath the transverse carpal ligament gives off a recurrent motor branch to thenar muscles before separating into divisions to the various digits. These separate bundles may vary, but the motor branch quite constantly arises from the volar aspect of the nerve and pierces the ligamentous fibers and the origins of the short abductor muscle and the palmar fascia.

of the 8th cervical and the 1st thoracic which innervate the flexors of the digits and the muscles in the radial half of the thenar eminence. At the elbow it leaves the blood vessels as it passes between the small ulnar and the larger humeral head of the pronator teres muscle and travels down the median part of the forearm between the superficial and the deep flexor muscles, riding on the profundus tendon to the index finger, until above the wrist it is radial to the superficialis and directly under the palmaris longus tendon. At the distal border of the transverse carpal ligament, where it gives off the motor thenar branch, it branches to the first 4 digits in a plane superficial to the tendons and deep to the superficial ves-

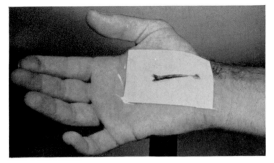

FIG. 442. A large persistent median artery may be present. In this case, trauma resulted in thrombosis, and the perivascular inflammatory swelling caused compression of the median nerve in the so-called carpal-tunnel syndrome.

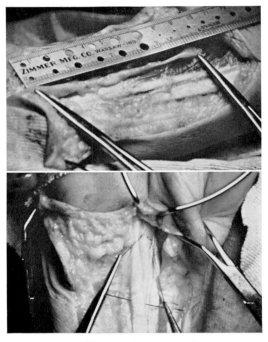

FIG. 443. Cheirogenic loss of substance of median nerve. (*Top*) A segment of median nerve was mistaken for the palmaris longus tendon. The gap is over 9 cm. (*Bottom*) By flexing the elbow, mobilizing the nerve in the forearm and flexing the wrist, approximation was possible at this point just proximal to the wrist. Protective sensibility returned in 12 months, and sufficient return of thenar muscles in 18 months to allow adequate thumb-to-finger pinch.

sels. Just above the elbow its first muscular branches go to the humeral head of the pronator teres. From in front of the elbow to just below the pronator teres there arise, more or less in order, the branches to the remainder of the pronator teres, the flexor carpi radialis, the palmaris longus and the flexor digitorum superficialis. The anterior interosseous nerve branches from it at the upper border of the pronator teres. Passing through the 2 heads, after giving branches to the deep forearm flexors, the flexor of the thumb and the radial half of the flexor profundus, it travels down the interosseous membrane to supply the pronator quadratus. The superficial sensory branch to the palm leaves the nerve above the wrist on the radial side.

The musculature in the hand is supplied by the median and the ulnar nerves. Normally, the division between these nerve supplies runs between the 2 heads of the short flexor of the thumb. The usual division of the sensory supply is a line down the ulnar third of the palm and down the center of the ring finger. The first 2 lumbricales usually are supplied by the median, and all of the interossei by the ulnar. In a small minority of cases, this line of division may shift either way. Either nerve may supply the profundus of the middle or the ring fingers. In the thenar eminence the median nerve may even extend to supply the adductors and the first 2 interosseus muscles, or the ulnar supply may include the opponens pollicis. The division of the nerve supply of the lumbricales may shift 1 or 2 muscles either

way. Of the sensory area, the median may supply all of the ring or the ulnar half of the middle finger along their volar surfaces.

These variations are uncommon, and in examining and treating injuries of the nerves of the hand, the standard pattern is seen most often. Explaining a lesion on the basis of "aberrant" nerves or "congenital abnormalities" usually means inaccurate observation and lack of understanding of substitute motions. Injuries to the median nerve in the upper arm or near the elbow may result in paralysis of an ulnar intrinsic muscle in the hand because of an atavistic communication between the nerves in the forearm.

Entrapment or Compression Syndromes. Pressure on the median nerve causing sensory and motor changes in its peripheral distribution has been reported, especially at 2 levels.

The upper lesion occurs where the nerve passes through the 2 heads of the pronator teres muscle, and the distal site is beneath the volar carpal ligament. This, the so-called carpal tunnel syndrome, is a common cause of tingling and paresthesia in the thumb and the index and the middle fingers. It may occur when there is any radical change in the boundaries of the carpal canal, as after Colles' fracture, or when any deformity occurs to produce pressure in the unyielding tunnel, as from a dislocated semilunar bone or from synovitis accompanying rheumatoid disease or the menopause. Symptoms have been produced by an abnormally low muscle belly of a flexor superficialis or by a ganglion encroaching on the tunnel space or a thrombosis of the aberrant median artery.

The syndrome of compression in the carpal tunnel occurs most commonly in middle-aged and elderly women, in or past the menopause, and is not a sequel to injury. A thickening of the peritendinous synovia accounts for the compression force, and the symptoms are usually pain and/or paresthesia in the median area, worse at night and relieved by activity. It is a frequent finding in rheumatoid arthritis.

In the study of a large series Lipscomb found that 72 per cent were caused by a non-specific tenosynovitis of the flexor synovia. In addition to the 20 per cent with rheumatoid synovitis, the most common accompanying conditions were diabetes, myxedema and pregnancy.

Relief is obtained by division of the volar carpal ligament; this must be complete and include all the fibers. In some cases a gross narrowing of the nerve is seen, with a pseudo-neuromatous enlargement just proximal to the constriction. Paralysis of thenar muscles with loss of opposition occurs in only a small number of cases, but careful examination may disclose relative weakness of the muscles. An electromyogram showing changes in the thenar muscles with normal reactions in the forearm flexors and the ulnar intrinsics helps to differentiate this syndrome from that of compression or traction on the lower cords of the plexus.

Signs of Median Nerve Damage. The area of isolated sensory supply of the median nerve includes only the distal and part of the middle segments of the index and the middle fingers, both volar and dorsal. Though some variations occur in the standard pattern, for lesions at or below the wrist one can depend on the accepted normal distribution of the nerves to the hand. In lesions of the upper arm, variations in the area of sensory loss are seen more often. On the thumb, the superficial radial may supply enough of each side to confuse the careless examiner.

Lesions above the elbow result in loss of flexion of the thumb and the index and the middle fingers, though the last may flex to some degree through its interdigitations with the profundi in the palm. The flexor carpi radialis and the pronator teres will be paralyzed, and the wrist will tend to flex ulnarward. Atrophy of the involved forearm muscles is apparent, and the thumb lies at the side of the hand, the thenar eminence is flat or concave, and the thumb cannot be brought forward into opposition.

In some median palsies opposition of the thumb is not entirely lost, due to extension of ulnar nerve supply. Even so, it is rare to be able to place the thumb as far forward from the base of the middle finger as in the other hand and with the nail parallel with the palm. Often burns are seen in the pulps of some of the first 3 digits. Loss of tactile sense in this area supplied by the median nerve, the main nerve of feeling, greatly handicaps the manual worker. The injured median nerve is more frequently the cause of pain than are the other nerves in the arm, not only during recovery from major injuries but often from minor injuries as well. It is the usual nerve of causalgia. Most frequently, this nerve is severed just above the wrist or in the palm and the digits but often is also injured in the upper arm and in the brachial plexus.

SURGICAL REPAIR. A severed nerve tends to retract, and during the repair procedure, after excising the neuroma and the glioma, there is a gap between the ends. In the palm 2 cm. can be gained by flexing the proximal finger joint. To overcome a gap in the nerve at or near the wrist, 5 cm. can be gained by flexion of the wrist. However, it is better to gain some length by using the elbow also. This can be accomplished simply by gripping the nerve with a piece of gauze and drawing on it gently while the elbow is flexed. This must be done with a sympathetic feel to avoid overpulling.

The investments of the nerve will be found to yield almost 5 cm. without breaking any of the muscular branches or the accompanying vessels in the upper part of the forearm. By flexing the wrist and the elbow, an 8-cm. gap in the nerve can be overcome. A wide gap in the palm is overcome by freeing the nerve as far upward as necessary and, after flexing the wrist and the elbow, drawing the nerve down. If the motor thenar branch is intact, it may be teased upward from the main nerve until it will not be pulled on. If the gap is greater than 8 cm., more radical means can be used such as dissecting out the nerve in the upper arm, rerouting it superficially at the elbow, and flexing the elbow. For this, it is necessary to strip up the various muscular nerve branches with the back of a pointed scalpel to well above the elbow and, by temporarily detaching the origin of the humeral head of the pronator teres, to plant the nerve anterior to that muscle. If still more length is needed, the nerve can be exposed and freed high in the upper arm and then the shoulder can be flexed. Plaster of Paris maintains flexion in these 3 joints for a month before gradual extension over the period of another month is allowed.

By the above radical means a gap of 10 cm. can be overcome. If a nerve graft is resorted to, one should use the sural nerve in a 3-strand cable graft. When the nerve is irreparable, muscle transfers are in order.

The function of opposition of the thumb returned in two thirds of 108 cases of median nerve suture that were tabulated. If this function does not return in 1½ or 2 years, or if the injury occurred more than 2 years previously, the pulley operation of tendon transfer will furnish the desired opposition (Chap. 12). This transfer operation may be done simultaneously with the nerve suture in sutures of the median nerve at the higher levels and when the nerve has been severed for a long time.

RADIAL NERVE

The radial nerve arises from the posterior cord and supplies the extensor muscles of the arm and the hand. The radial nerve furnishes all of the extension of the elbow, the wrist and the digits, with the exception of the distal 2 joints of the fingers which can also be extended by the intrinsic muscles in the hand.

The axillary nerve, which is from the 5th and the 6th cervical nerves, rides along with the radial nerve on the subscapular muscle to as far as its outer border. It then turns backward and rounds the neck of the humerus to the deltoid, the teres minor and a patch of sensory area back of the deltoid. This nerve may be reached from either the front or the back of the latissimus. In the latter instance, the arm is raised upright, and the approach is through the hollow of the axilla. This is also a good approach for the radial nerve from the subscapulars to the upper part of the arm.

The radial nerve proper then travels along the anterior surface of the tendons of the teres major and the latissimus dorsi, to follow down the humerus, hugging it closely as it curves around it in the musculospiral groove, exactly along the line of maximal convexity of the outer head of the triceps.

Passing forward through the intermuscular septum, the nerve, following along under the brachioradialis muscle, divides at the elbow into its sensory and motor branches, the superficial radial and the posterior interosseous nerves. The superficial radial continues under the brachioradialis muscle until it perforates the insertion of this muscle, travels to the subcutaneous layer over the dorsum of the radius and fans out in numerous branches down the dorsum of the first 3 digits. The posterior interosseous nerve dives through the substance of the supinator brevis muscle supplying it, to emerge in the dorsum of the forearm between the superficial and the deep muscle layers, dividing at once into 2 portions; one of these enters the undersurface of the extensor digitorum communis, the extensor minimi digiti and the extensor carpi ulnaris, and the other runs on down the forearm to enter the superficial surfaces of the 2 extensors of the thumb, the abductor pollicis longus and the extensor indicis.

By visualizing where each branch, sensory and motor, leaves the radial nerve, the level of the lesion can be determined. At the lower border of the tendon of the latissimus dorsi, branches are given off in turn to the inner, the long and the outer heads of the triceps muscle in the musculospiral groove, there being an additional branch to the anconeus and the lower part of the middle head of the triceps between the 2 latter. The posterior cutaneous branch comes halfway down the arm, dividing in 2, one to supply a strip in the back of the upper arm and one down the dorsum of the forearm, until it reaches the area supplied by the superficial radial. When the nerve is between the brachioradialis and the brachialis anticus it supplies both, and also the extensors of the wrist. The brachialis anticus had a dual supply because that muscle resulted from the fusion of the anterior and the posterior primary muscle divisions.

The radial nerve is injured more often than any other, and, because of its close proximity to the shaft of the humerus; the same force that produces a fracture damages the nerve, or it becomes involved in the callus. The axillary nerve may be injured in dislocations of the humerus, and in the axilla it is affected in crutch and drunkard's palsy, the latter from hanging the arm over the back of a chair. If traction for a fractured humerus is applied over the radial surface of the forearm, the posterior interosseous nerve may become paralyzed. This nerve may be injured surgically where it rounds the neck of the radius, and it and the lower part of the superficial radial may be severed in lacerations.

The radial nerve may become involved in callus in a healing fracture of the humerus or may be caught between the fragments. An opening through the bone may be seen on roentgen examination. Duthie reported such a case, and Roaf described the same thing occurring to the median nerve when caught in a fracture dislocation of the elbow.

Symptoms of Radial Nerve Injury. The area of anesthesia after severance of the radial nerve is not of much practical importance; it includes a strip down the back of the lower half of the upper arm, the forearm, and a triangular area on the back of the hand, bounded by the first 2 metacarpals and extending down the back of the thumb, the proximal segment of the index and half that of the middle finger. The area in the hand is quite variable in both size and shape and is not especially useful for tactile purpose. The isolated area, if any at all, may be only a small spot over the first interosseus muscle.

The radial nerve is rarely the seat of painful lesions, as is the median, though an injury to or a terminal neuroma in the superficial radial or its branches is often exquisitely painful,

troublesome and difficult to remedy. Any touch of the region, even to the coat sleeve, causes stinging pain and necessitates either surgical treatment of the neuroma by severance of the nerve at a higher level or suture of the nerve at the site.

Motor paralysis from radial nerve lesions is characterized by pronation of the forearm and lack of voluntary extension of wrist, thumb and fingers. The thumb tends to be adducted, so that it may interfere with flexion of the fingers. Flexion of the fingers is limited in this position because of the flexed position, but if the patient throws his arm in supination, the wrist falls into dorsiflexion, and he can make a fist.

In testing the triceps, gravity should be eliminated by placing the upper arm in a horizontal position with the forearm hanging vertically. In this position one can also test supination and extension of the wrist. Action of the extensors of the wrist can also be determined by palpation over their muscle bellies and their tendinous insertions, and by placing the styloid process of the radius at the top so as to eliminate gravity when testing for ability to dorsiflex the wrist. Here finger extension is judged only in the proximal joints. For thumb and finger extension, the tendons and the muscles are watched and palpated. In the thumb, voluntary action of all 3 of the extensors should be sought for, that of the longus being easiest to determine, since it affects all thumb joints. In loss of abductor pollicis longus the thenar eminence rides forward, and the thumb is useless because of loss of stability in its basal joint.

In testing for motions in the hand one should guard against misinterpretation of automatic movements. Normally, the abductor and the flexor pollicis brevis can extend the distal joint of the thumb. All other movements should be eliminated when one is testing for any particular movement, for if the patient is allowed to move either digits or wrist or even pronate or supinate his forearm, he will be able to extend his wrist or fingers by these automatic movements.

In radial palsy, lateral movements of the wrist are very poor because of loss of the long thumb abductor, the long extensor and the extensor carpi ulnaris. The grip is weak from inability to stabilize the wrist in dorsiflexion.

The styloradial reflex, which is entirely through the radial nerve, is absent. The atrophy on the dorsum of the forearm is conspicuous, whereas instead there should be the prominent bellies of the extensors of the wrist and the extensors of the fingers.

Surgical Repair. The results of repair of the radial nerve are superior to those of the median or the ulnar nerve, probably because the nerve is more nearly pure, having only a minority of sensory bundles. The superficial radial and the posterior interosseus are pure nerves. To expose the radial nerve throughout its length in the upper arm requires 3 separate incisions, corresponding to the nerve's locations about the humerus. In exposing it in front of the elbow, due consideration must be given the flexion crease by using a transverse or L-shaped incision to avoid keloid flexion contracture. The nerve is injured easily where it rounds the neck of the radius 2 cm. below the head. To expose it in the supinator brevis, this muscle either must be split in places or severed and rejoined. The approach in the forearm is between the extensors of the wrist and those of the fingers.

A gap of 7.5 cm. in the middle upper arm can be overcome by freeing the nerve downward and upward and strongly flexing the elbow; for greater gaps the nerve can be transferred to an anterior position, but not much is gained by this.

If the nerve is irreparable or if too long an interval has elapsed since the accident (as shown by loss of reaction or degeneration), tendon transfers should be made in the forearm. This operation is preferable to shortening the humerus to approximate the nerve ends. There is no satisfactory transfer for paralysis of the triceps, but here gravity compensates somewhat for disability.

Splinting the limb so that the paralyzed muscles remain in continuous relaxation is especially necessary in radial palsy. The airplane splint is used for the deltoid. A splint is not necessary for the triceps, since gravity keeps it in relaxation. Splinting is necessary to keep the wrist in mild dorsiflexion, the proximal finger joints straight, and the base of the thumb in moderate extension. All other joints and movements should be free. The Oppenheimer and the Thomas are satisfactory splints.

The return of muscle function after nerve repair usually occurs serially down the nerve as the respective branches come off, returning in most cases in the order of extensors of wrist, fingers and thumb. Usually, all muscle groups regain function, but if one happens to be left out, it is likely to be the thumb. Frequently, after radial nerve repair, in contrast with median and ulnar repair, function returns almost to normal.

ULNAR NERVE

The ulnar nerve arises from the inner cord which comes from the 8th cervical and the 1st thoracic nerves. In its course down the arm it leaves the artery in the lower third and passes to the rear of the intermuscular septum, along the inner head of the triceps, to pass through the angle formed by the epicondyle and the olecranon under the dense fascia which bridges these two. Here the first branches go to the humeral and the ulnar heads of the flexor ulnaris muscle, and 2 branches go to the ulnar part of the flexor digitorum profundus. Coursing between these 2 muscles it is joined in the upper part of the forearm by the ulnar artery on its outer side; the 2 then pass on together, the nerve giving a lower branch to the flexor carpi ulnaris muscle.

At the wrist the ulnar nerve detours with the artery forward through an opening in the transverse carpal ligament, leaving the sensory branch at the lower border of this ligament and diving deeply between the abductor and the flexor muscles of the little finger, again to become deep and travel across the palm with and beneath the deep transverse arch. While in front of the transverse carpal ligament, it supplies the palmaris brevis and grooves the radial side of the pisiform bone; there, separating from the sensory branch, it supplies the hypothenar muscles and, as it dips into the palm, loops around the ulnar aspect of the hook of the hamate. In crossing the depth of the palm it supplies the inner 2 lumbricales in front of it and the interossei behind it, passing between the interossei and the adductor of the thumb, both of which it supplies.

In the forearm the ulnar nerve sends a second branch to the lower part of the flexor ulnaris muscle, and then a dorsal sensory branch leaves it, passing under the tendon of the flexor ulnaris to the side of the head of

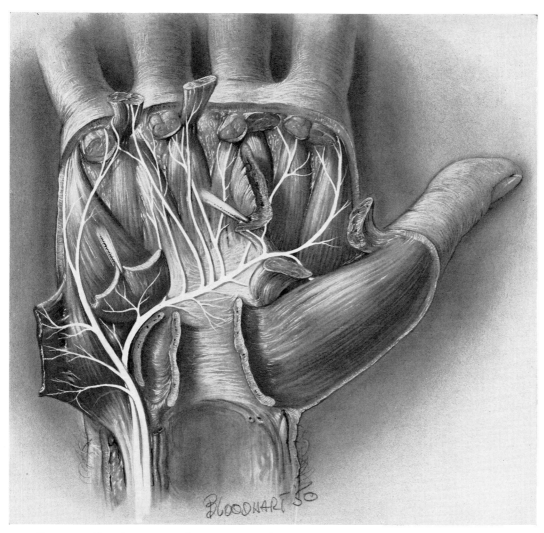

FIG. 444. The ulnar nerve, showing its multiple branches in the palm. The branches of the deep motor portion of the nerve are remarkably constant. Note the tiny twigs from the superficial ulnar nerve that supply the palmaris brevis muscle, the definite branch from the deep portion going to the abductor minimi and the location of the nerve supply to the transverse adductor pollicis, the oblique adductor and the first interosseus muscle. (J. Bone Joint Surg. 37-A:920)

the ulna and over the tendon of the extensor ulnaris to supply the dorsum of the ulnar part of the hand, the dorsum of the little and the ring fingers to the root of the nails and the ulnar half of the dorsum of the proximal segment of the middle finger. The 2 volar sensory branches supply the ulnar part of the palm and the volar surface of the little finger and half of the ring finger. These volar branches do not supply the dorsum of the last 2 finger

segments as they do in the case of the median nerve.

Symptoms When Damaged. The ulnar border of the hand and the little and the ring fingers, both on the palmar and the dorsal surfaces, constitute the area of anesthesia to light touch and pin prick commonly resulting from severance of the ulnar nerve. Occasionally, the anesthesia may run a few inches up the inner side of the arm due to a low sensory branch of the nerve, but if it runs higher along the ulnar border of the forearm, thus showing involvement of the internal cutaneous nerve, a higher lesion must be suspected. The isolated sensory supply is limited to the little finger. Trophic changes are seen in the skin of the anesthetic areas and often burns in the pulp of the little or the ring fingers.

In severance of the ulnar nerve above the elbow there is paralysis of the flexor carpi ul-

naris and the ulnar third of the flexor profundus muscles, resulting in a conspicuous hollow over these muscles from atrophy and loss of ulnar flexion of the wrist and of flexion of the distal joint of the little finger. All the hypothenar and the interosseus muscles and 2 lumbricalis muscles on the ulnar side, the adductors of the thumb and the inner head of the flexor pollicis brevis are paralyzed. This results in atrophy of these muscles of the hand,

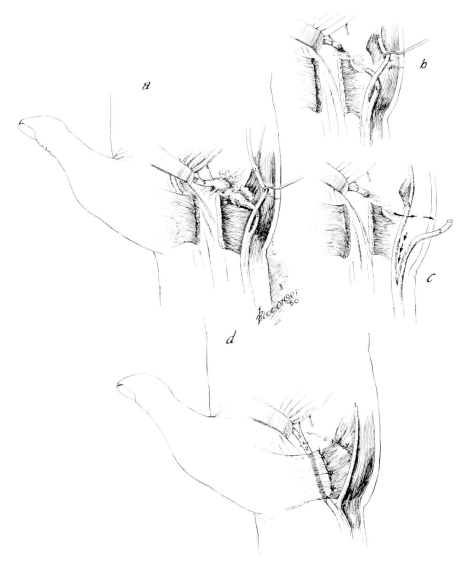

Fig. 445. Method of rerouting the motor branch of the ulnar nerve through the carpal tunnel to allow suturing where loss of substance is present. (J. Bone Joint Surg. *37-A*:920)

shown by conspicuous concavities over the first interosseus muscle and the hypothenar eminence and between the metacarpals.

There is also deformity of the hand in that there is some clawing of the ring and the little fingers. However, this clawing is less conspicuous when the ulnar nerve is severed above the elbow. It is greater when severance occurs below the nerve supply of the ulnar part of the flexor digitorum profundus muscle. This muscle, now unopposed by the intrinsic muscles in the hand, draws the distal 2 joints of the ring and the little fingers into flexion, while the proximal joints become extended. If the profundus is strong, clawing is great, but the flexion is greatest if the flexor tendons are adherent in the forearm. The clawing may involve the middle finger to some extent but is most prominent in the little finger. The 2 radial lumbricales, which are supplied by the median nerve, prevent the deformity in the index and the middle fingers. The ring and the little fingers can no longer be flexed simultaneously in the proximal joints and extended at the distal 2 joints. Clawing is much influenced by the amount of cocking back of the fingers, depending on the degree of laxness of the volar capsules of the proximal finger joints. If the ligaments are tight, hyperextension cannot

occur. In high ulnar palsy the little and the ring fingers do not flex well in making a fist.

In ulnar paralysis, lateral motion of the fingers is largely lost. The index and the middle fingers deviate ulnarward, but there still may be some weak radial flexion from their lumbricales, and, because fingers diverge on extension, the long extensors may spread the fingers moderately, especially the little finger. The first interosseus muscle is conspicuously atrophied. By testing each finger individually for lateral motion, including spreading the fingers, pinching between the fingers and adducting the little finger, the paralysis will be apparent. If the straight fingers cannot pinch together on the examiner's finger, the 3 volar interossei and the 2 dorsal interossei of the middle finger are not working. In this, it helps to place the hand palm down on a flat surface or to flatten the metacarpal arch, or to test lateral motion when the proximal joints are in slight flexion. With the fingers partially extended, it is impossible to converge their tips.

Because of loss of the adductors, the thumb no longer pinches against the index finger to make a good circle or against the little finger to make an ellipse. The pinch is weak, the metacarpophalangeal joint may drop into hyperextension and the distal joint of the thumb

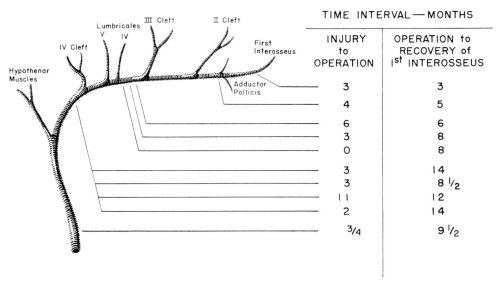

FIG. 446. Rate of regeneration of the motor branch of the ulnar nerve after repair in the palm at various levels and as evidenced by visible and palpable activity in the first interosseus muscle. (J. Bone Joint Surg. *37-A*:920)

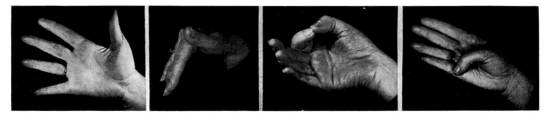

FIG. 447. Restoration of complete function after suture of the ulnar nerve at the wrist, severed on a window 7 months previously.

These photographs, taken 2 years after the nerve was sutured, show 4 tests for ulnar-nerve function. From left to right: the spread of the fingers; flexing the proximal joints and at same time extending the distal 2 joints; the ability to pinch firmly, making a good O and arch of the thumb without the metacarpophalangeal joint dropping into extension (adductor test); the ability to scrape the extended thumb across the fingers and the palm (adductor test).

into excessive flexion. In other words, the arch of the thumb is lost because there is loss of ability to stabilize the metacarpophalangeal joint in flexion. A paper held between the thumb and the index finger can be withdrawn easily. It should be noted that loss of the stabilizing action of the abductor pollicis longus in holding the carpometacarpal joint in extension will give the same deformity and weak pinch as will contracture between the first 2

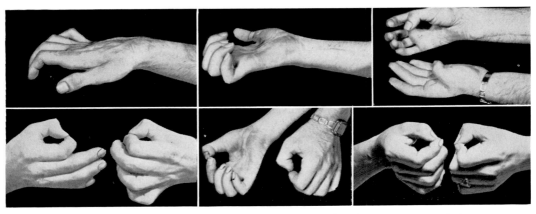

FIG. 448. Signs of paralysis of ulnar nerve. Case R. C. Ulnar nerve severed above wrist.

(Top, left and center) Atrophy of the intrinsic muscles supplied by the ulnar nerve. The hypothenar and the first interosseous concavities are conspicuous. Claw-hand is greatest toward the ulnar side and more pronounced when the nerve is severed below its supply to the flexor digitorum profundus, as in this case.

(Top, right) Scrape test. With loss of the adductors of the thumb, the extended thumb cannot scrape across the extended fingers and the palm but leaves the palm at the radial side of the index finger, as in the upper hand.

(Bottom) Pinch test to show loss of action of the adductors of the thumb. The normal thumb makes a good O with the index finger and pinches firmly with a good arch to the thumb (left). In ulnar paralysis, the O is faulty, the distal joint over-flexes, the metacarpophalangeal joint drops into extension, and the pinch is weak. A paper can be easily pulled from between. A similar deformity occurs when the tendon of the abductor pollicis longus is severed. For proper muscle balance in the pinch, the adductors of the thumb should stabilize the proximal joint in flexion and the long abductor of the carpometacarpal joint in extension.

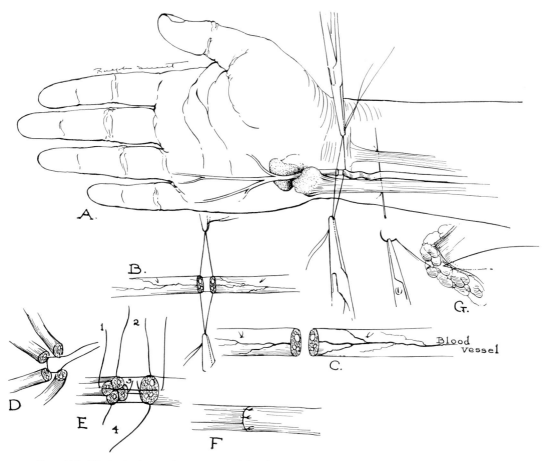

FIG. 449. Method of suturing a nerve (ulnar).

(A) During suturing, the proximal end may be held free from tension by impaling it on a needle. The ulnar nerve is anterior to the carpal tunnel lying on the transverse carpal ligament. Its relationship to the pisiform and the hook of the hamate and its motor branch are shown.

(B, C) Exact rotation is determined by marking the midline of each nerve by a knot of silk, by the flatness of the nerve, by matching the nerve bundles, by the striations of the nerve and by the blood vessels. Two guide sutures are placed.

(D, E, F) Method of suturing a main nerve to its several branches or suturing a cable graft. First, one stitch groups the branches into one, and then the suturing proceeds as usual.

(G) Greasing the thread before using, by passing it through subcutaneous fat.

metacarpals. To make a firm pinch, the index finger should abduct and the thumb adduct. This action of both the first interosseus muscle and the adductor of the thumb is lost in ulnar palsy (Chap. 12).

The grip in ulnar palsy is markedly decreased because of the loss of intrinsic flexors of the proximal joints and the adductors of the thumb, which in gripping should work against each other.

In ulnar paralysis, the extended thumb can no longer scrape across the bases of the fingers and the distal part of the palm. Instead, it leaves the palm and comes forward at the radial border of the index finger. As the adductors are recovering, it may leave the palm at various points farther ulnarward. Atrophy and loss of voluntary motion of the adductor muscle of the thumb can be felt by through-and-through pinching of this muscle when the

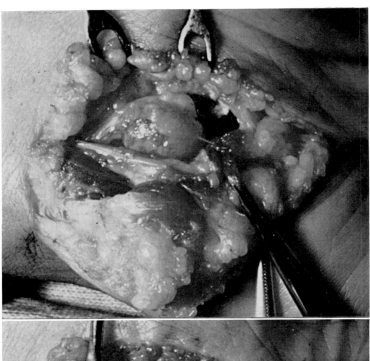

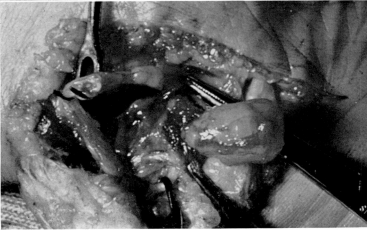

FIG. 450. Ganglia from the carpus may displace, stretch and paralyze the motor branch of the ulnar nerve. The association may be so intimate that the mass resembles a tumor of the nerve itself. See Figure 451.

thumb attempts to adduct against resistance. Normally, the thumb adducts—though somewhat dorsally—also through the action of the extensor pollicis longus muscle. In ulnar paralysis the muscle balance in the hand will be so upset from loss of action of the intrinsic muscles that the hand will have lost its skill and be awkward at work. Lesions of the cord or the lower 2 nerves of the brachial plexus need not be confused with ulnar nerve palsy if the nerve examination is sufficiently extensive; for in poliomyelitis there will be absence of sensory symptoms, in syringomyelia a dissociation of temperature and pain from touch, and in other cord lesions signs of involvement of the long sensory or motor tracts. When the lower 2 nerves of the brachial plexus are involved, there is paralysis of the muscles of flexion of the fingers and of opposition of the thumb, combined with anesthesia of the internal cutaneous nerve.

Surgical Repair. The results of repair of the ulnar nerve are not as good as those of the median or the radial nerve. The ulnar is a mixed nerve with many motor and sensory fibers. Therefore, the results of repair depend

PLATE 7

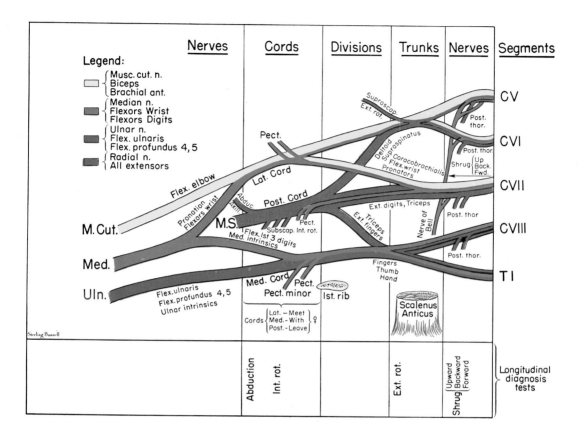

SCHEMATIC BRACHIAL PLEXUS AS A GUIDE IN DIAGNOSIS

The order and the level of the parts of the plexus are indicated. Thus, *trunks* are under the scalenus anticus muscle; *divisions* are in the neck behind the middle third of the clavicle and down to the first rib; *cords* start at the far edge of the first rib. The distribution of nerve fibers from segments to nerves is shown in color.

To diagnose the longitudinal level, see the bottom brackets. Have the patient, in order, (1) shrug his shoulder upward, backward and forward for the posterior thoracic nerve, the first to leave the plexus; (2) externally rotate for the suprascapular nerve at the trunks; (3) internally rotate for the subscapular and the pectoral nerves at the cords; and (4) abduct for the axillary nerve at the end of the cords.

The musculocutaneous nerve goes to the arm but the median and the ulnar nerves go to the forearm and the hand. The musculospiral (radial) supplies muscles in the arm and the forearm.

PLATE 8

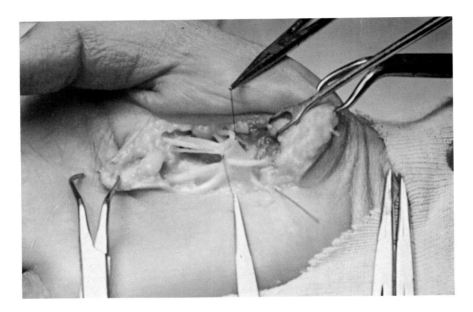

Secondary repair of median nerve in palm. The motor branch and the ulnar component going to second and third clefts are intact. Guide sutures 180° apart facilitate handling of nerve. Note that the proximal trunk has been mobilized in the carpal tunnel and the nerve drawn distally with the wrist flexed. A slender needle through the transverse carpal ligament impales the nerve for temporary fixation.

on accurate approximation of the nerve ends. Low in the forearm the median is almost purely sensory, but low in the upper arm the radial is almost purely motor; this accounts for good results from suturing these, even with inaccuracy in rotation. Suture of either the motor or the sensory branches of the ulnar nerve in the hand gives excellent results. In suturing the deep motor branch of the ulnar nerve, about 1.5 or 2 cm. can be gained by slitting the carpal ligament and stripping up the motor branch so as to pass it along the hypotenuse of the triangle. Also, either the median or the ulnar nerve may be drawn down until the motor branch can be sutured.

At the wrist a gap can be overcome by flexing the wrist. For longer defects one must transplant the nerve from the back to the front of the elbow and then flex both elbow and wrist. More can be gained by freeing the nerve high and flexing the shoulder. To transplant the nerve at the elbow, a midlateral incision is made paralleling the nerve, and the large triangular flap of skin is dissected forward from the deep fascia. The length of the nerve is uncovered by slitting the fascial bridge at the condyle and on down through the flexor ulnaris muscle between its 2 heads. Then the nerve can be lifted out of its groove and is held only by its motor branches. These are slit up with the back of a pointed knife to well above the elbow, so that they may remain in place without holding back the nerve when it is transplanted forward.

In women, or in persons with weak muscles, the nerve may be left between the deep and the superficial fascia, suturing these together to keep the nerve from displacing backward;

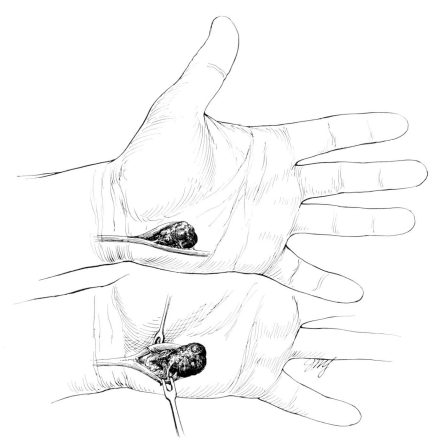

Fig. 451. Artist's conception of ganglion involving the motor branch of the ulnar nerve.

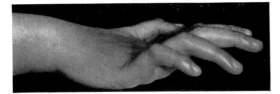

FIG. 452. Median and ulnar palsy, with clawing of all digits, thumb at the side of the hand and secondary wrist flexion. With paralysis of the intrinsic muscles, the long extensors are unopposed, and hyperextension of the proximal joints occurs if the volar capsular tissues are lax.

but in muscular individuals it will be found that the prominence of the flexor muscles is so hard that the nerve will be subject to injury from pressure on it by outside objects. Some surgeons have recommended placing the nerve in the deep fascia and muscles, but it is better to reroute the nerve between the flexor profundus behind and the flexor superficialis and the pronator teres in front. This can be done by disconnecting the origins on the epicondyle and reconnecting them again, or, if the nerve has been divided, the intermuscular passageway can be tunneled and the nerve end drawn through. If a nerve is placed through a muscle, the paramysium will penetrate and strangle the nerve. Therefore, the nerve should be laid in the cleavage plane between the epicondylar and the deeper muscles.

The ulnar nerve regenerates in serial fashion, first the forearm muscles, then the sensory components. Muscles within the hand rarely show much return in less than a year. Voluntary action is noticed first in the hypothenar muscles. Later the clawing lessens, and finally come lateral motion of the fingers and adduction of the thumb. Occasionally, one or several of these intrinsic muscles does not recover. Early signs of recovery are pain when the hypothenar muscles are pinched and a hypothenar reflex when the nerve is pressed on just proximal to the pisiform. Sensibility usually returns throughout the whole anesthetic area, though good quality returns last in the little finger.

Patients with ulnar palsy differ much in their functional impairment, but furnishing abduction to the index finger, thus resorting the scissor action of the pinch of the thumb, helps all these cases. In only a few cases of cocked-back fingers is the muscle balance operation for clawing needed. These tendon transfers are discussed in Chapter 12.

Splinting in ulnar palsy is not necessary unless the clawing is pronounced. It should consist of holding the proximal joints of the ring and the little fingers in flexion lest the finger joints become organized and stiff. A simple contrivance for this is 2 light rubber bands stretching from in front of the wrist from a wrist band to 2 soft leather loops over the dorsum of the proximal segments of the ring and the little fingers. If stronger action is needed, a splint of sheet aluminum, held to the dorsum of the hand with a web belt, and

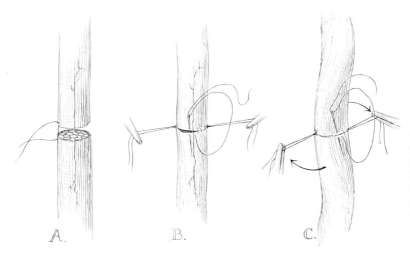

A.   B.   C.

FIG. 453. Technic of nerve repair. First, fine suture material through the sheath is placed as 2 guide sutures 180° apart. Then the remaining sheath is approximated carefully with a continuous or an interrupted stitch.

an extension to hold the proximal joints of the ring and the little fingers in flexion will suffice. Clawing is greatest when the flexor muscles are adherent in the forearm. In hands inclined to stiffen, clawing may become a fixed deformity. Transferring the extensor indicis proprius to act as an abductor of the index may be done in a late case at the time of the nerve suture. When the little finger is permanently clawed and anesthetic it should be amputated, especially if the patient works with machinery. Usually it is not necessary to restore adduction to the thumb in ulnar paralysis, but in combined ulnar and median paralysis, the tendon T operation will be of much benefit (Chap. 12).

COMBINED NERVE LESIONS

In combined nerve lesions the area of anesthesia is greater than one would expect, because the overlap is equivalent to an isolated nerve supply. The loss of motion from paralysis of the 2 sets of muscles is very disabling.

COMBINED LESIONS OF MEDIAN AND ULNAR NERVES

This combination results from lesions in the forearm and the upper arm. The area of anesthesia covers the whole palm and the volar surface of all the digits and, on the dorsum, the last 2 segments of the middle and the index fingers the last segment of the thumb, and all segments of the ring and the little

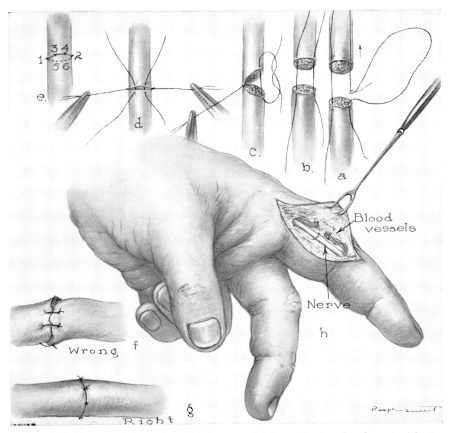

FIG. 454. Suture of the volar digital nerve joining only the sheath and with the finest silk. Accurate approximation ensures good regeneration. Nerves can be sutured to as far as the distal digital crease. The motor thenar branch of the median can be sutured readily. (a to e) Order of procedure. (f) Careless repair gives poor result. (g) Accurate repair. (h) Nerve sutured.

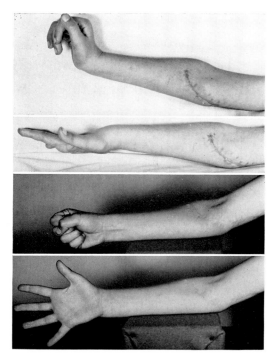

FIG. 455. Case G. M., age 5. A glass door had lacerated the arm across the elbow, severing the brachial artery and the median and the ulnar nerves (*see top 2 illustrations*). A 2-inch gap in each nerve was overcome by advancing the nerve at the elbow and suturing. Good sensation returned, including stereognosis, as well as excellent function of the intrinsic muscles (*see the bottom 2 pictures*).

fingers. From overlap of the radial and the internal cutaneous nerves there may be a little feeling left in the palm at the cleft of the thumb and over the thenar eminence. Deep joint sense may be lacking, and deformity and contractures occur quickly.

Deformity is conspicuous. The wrist bends slightly backward and ulnarward unless there is flexion contracture and the hand inclines toward supination. Because of loss of the intrinsic muscles of the hand, the carpal and the metacarpal arches straighten so that the hand is flat. The thumb is at the side of the hand and has no power of opposition or adduction. The amount of clawing of the fingers and of flexion of the thumb depends on whether the lesion in the nerves is above or below the nerve supply of the flexor muscles in the fore-

arm. If above, these deformities are not so great. If below, and the flexors in the forearm are activated, clawing of all fingers is extreme, there being hyperextension of the proximal joints and sharp flexion of the distal two, the long flexors being unopposed by the paralyzed intrinsic muscles. Clawing is greatest when the flexor muscles are adherent in the forearm. If the lesion is above the nerve supply of the forearm muscles, the long flexor of the thumb, as well as the thenar muscles, will be paralyzed, and the thumb will assume a position back of the plane of the hand, drawn there by its long extensors. If the lesion is below the forearm muscles, the thumb will be able to flex, but it will be at a position at the side of the hand, devoid of opposition and adduction. If the nerves are irreparable in combined median and ulnar palsy, muscle balance in the fingers, abduction of the index finger and adduction and opposition of the thumb may be given by tendon transfers as outlined in Chapter 12. In severe rigid clawing of long standing, the middle finger joints may be arthrodesed in mild flexion and, similarly, the distal joint of the thumb if this is overflexed. A great variation in deformities of the hand from positions assumed occurs from combined lesions high up the arm and in the brachial plexus, depending on which muscles are paralyzed or spared.

Active treatment should be given to the hand from the time of injury to the resumption of employment. It should consist of keeping the hand in the position of function, keeping the joints mobile and encouraging whatever movements are present. The patient should be taught how to move the joints of his injured hand with his other hand and instructed to move them gently but regularly until function returns. This is the best form of physiotherapy, and it should be carried out conscientiously. Some patients will need arthrodeses and tendon transplants. Precautions should be taken not to burn or injure the anesthetic parts. The surgical repair of the nerve requires only a short time, but attention to the hand must be continuous.

Splinting is necessary in combined median and ulnar nerve paralysis to hold the proximal finger joints in flexion, the metacarpal arch curved and the thumb in opposition. (See Chap. 6, Splints.)

Nerves in the Hand Itself

The branches of the median and the ulnar nerves, both motor and sensory, which supply the hand, are frequently injured. Repair is accomplished satisfactorily and easily. Function of the nerves is important, for a hand that is unable to feel is a blind club.

In 1925 Bunnell tabulated the results of 105 nerve repairs in the hand, stressing the importance of accurate approximation of the freshened ends of the nerves to obtain the maximal regeneration.

In the hand itself, the nerves are essentially no longer a mixture of motor and sensory fibers but are purely one or the other. Regeneration after repair of a pure sensory or a pure motor nerve is always better than that in a mixed nerve, for exact rotation of the nerve ends is less important.

Since they are closer to the periphery, the nerves in the hand regenerate to their end organs more quickly, and thus the habit patterns and the trophic changes set up by long disuse are not so likely to occur—the closer the lesion is to the periphery, the greater the regenerative power of a peripheral nerve.

Importance of Function in Hand Nerves. The hand is a motor organ for grasp, but it is also

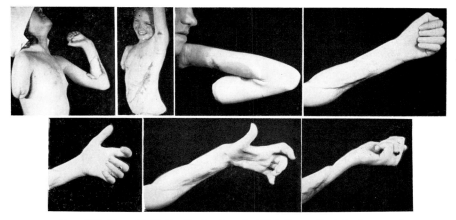

Fig. 456. Case H. T. On September 4, 1938, the patient had grasped a high-voltage transformer with the right hand; the left forearm touched a ground wire. The right arm was amputated. In the left arm, the flexor muscles and the median and the ulnar nerves were destroyed.

(*Top, left*) Condition when brought for repair. All intrinsic muscles are paralyzed. No flexor to the digits is functioning. Anesthesia covers the hand and the lower forearm with the exception of the area supplied by the radial nerve.

(*Top, 2nd picture*) Vertical pedicles leave unsightly scars, later excised and zigzagged.

Operation: June 12, 1939. It was imperative to repair the nerves, especially to restore the intrinsic muscles in the hand. Much scar was excised from the forearm and the elbow and the keloid borders of the pedicle. A 4-inch gap in the ulnar nerve and a 3-inch gap in the median were overcome by transplanting each and flexing the elbow. The only remaining muscle tissue was dissected out with a long strip of scar tissue and connected up to the tendon of the thumb. Two plastic procedures were done later to eliminate the contractures and the keloid borders of the pedicle.

By January 30, 1940, 8 months later, sensation had returned throughout, and by July 18, 1942, 3 years after nerve suture, all intrinsic muscles of the hand were working.

The 5 remaining pictures show relief of contracture of the elbow and of clawhand, as well as return of automatic movements by flexing and dorsiflexing the wrist, the flexors of the fingers acting as tenodeses.

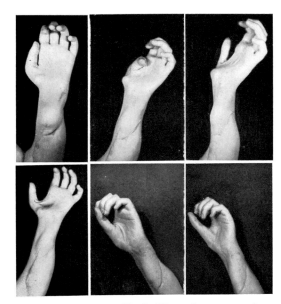

Fig. 457. Case N. G. The volar aspect of the forearm had been gouged out in an automobile wreck, including all of the muscles, except at the extreme top of the forearm. A pedicle graft had been applied to the forearm.

(*Top*) Showing condition when coming for repair. Flat hand, thumb at side, absence of opposition (shown at extreme right) and limit of extension and flexion of fingers as shown in first 2 pictures.

Operation: A 5-inch gap in the median nerve and a 4-inch gap in the ulnar nerve were overcome by freeing, transplanting and flexing. A strand of scar was used for a thumb flexor. A pulley operation for the thumb was done, looping the tendon about the tendon of the flexor ulnaris. The distal parts of tendons were freed but left adherent in the forearm to act in moving the fingers by automatic movements.

(*Bottom*) Condition a year later, showing motion of fingers, opposition of thumb and curve of hand. Sensation had returned throughout; motion in the intrinsic muscles was just starting.

an organ for sensation. These 2 functions are of equal importance. Lacking the ability to feel, and especially that exquisite sense of touch known as tactilegnosis, a manual worker is greatly handicapped. For fine work and an extreme delicacy of touch the pulps of the thumb and the index and the middle fingers are the most important areas. In the thumb the ulnar side is more important, but in the index and the middle fingers the radial side of the pulp is more useful.

Severance of a volar nerve at the base of the finger results in anesthesia of that half on the volar surface, and division of the common digital nerve in the palm results in anesthesia of the contiguous sides of the fingers on each side of the cleft. Division of the major branches of the median nerve also results in loss of joint and position sense in the important index and middle fingers.

If the motor components of the median nerve are damaged, opposition of the thumb is lacking; damage to the deep motor branch of the ulnar nerve results in a clawhand deformity, lack of spread and control of lateral motions, and weakness of grip and pinch.

Trophic changes in the skin and the joints follow, and when nerve injury is combined with damage to other structures, an insensitive hook may result. A finger in this condition is sometimes a handicap to the rest of the hand. Amputation of such a digit saves the remaining function of the hand.

When nerve injury accompanies damage to other structures, the ideal treatment would be to repair the nerves first, wait for regeneration and then complete the reconstruction. Economically, this is not usually feasible, and nerve repair and tendon reconstruction commonly are carried out at the same time.

Rate of Regeneration. A study of the rate of recovery of protective sensibility, that is, the ability to distinguish light touch and pin prick and some temperature change, showed that regeneration took place at the rate of one finger segment each month. There was no appreciable difference between median and ulnar nerves or between thumb and fingers.

Regeneration of nerves sutured above the wrist required an average of 13 months, in the proximal palm 7 months, and the distal palm 3 months. Regeneration from the proximal segment of a finger required 2 to 3 months and from the middle segment 1½ months.

Speed of regeneration was not influenced by the length of time from injury to repair, though in the series this averaged only 4 months and exceeded 1 year in only 6 patients.

Age seemed to be a factor in that rapid regeneration took place more often in the younger groups. Later studies showed this to be particularly true in repair of major nerve trunks in the forearm and the upper arm.

FIG. 458. Case A. V. The top 2 pictures show severe laceration across the front of the elbow by a glass window, severing the median and the ulnar nerves and resulting in paralysis of all intrinsic muscles and many flexors in the forearm. There was a typical paralytic hand without sensation or function. Position of nonfunction and clawed.

Operation: Sutured the median and the ulnar nerves. In 2½ years, there was excellent return of nerve function as shown in the 3 remaining pictures. The forearm filled out, and the position of the hand was corrected. All intrinsic-muscle functions returned except opposition.

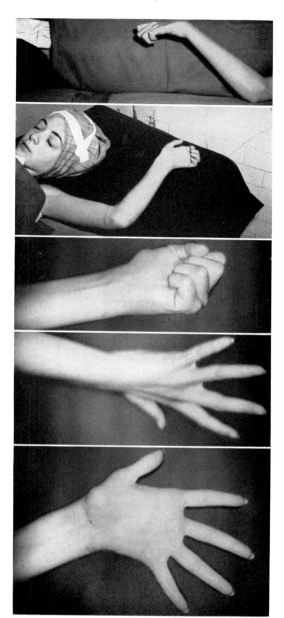

The most important factor was the state of nutrition of the hand. A hand filled with scar from past infection or severe crushing with poor circulation from damage to the blood vessels is not the ideal location for regenerating nerves.

Quality and Order of Regeneration. Recovery of sensibility after repair of the digital nerves is usually progressive down the finger. Coarse touch is felt first, then pin prick and light touch. The last is often more like a paresthesia with a tingling feeling in response to the stimulus. This abnormal response tends to disappear slowly over 1 or 2 years with recovery of some ability to distinguish form and texture after the 2nd year. This stereognostic sense or, as Moberg defines it, tactilegnosis may never return to normal. In children or in adults with good soft tissues and with constant re-education, the quality of return may approach the normal.

Trophic disturbances diminish gradually as the nerves regenerate, so that eventually form and contour are restored and the skin, instead of being smooth, dry, and satiny, again is moist and resistant.

Motor function returns to the intrinsic muscles when the recurrent branch of the median or the deep volar branch of the ulnar are repaired.

TREATMENT OF INJURED NERVES

The object of repairing a severed nerve in a limb is to restore function to the hand; but, if attention is directed to the nerves only, the hand will become fixed with the joints stiff and in deformed positions. Such a hand, if not exercised, will atrophy from disuse until it is only a useless claw.

SPLINT TO KEEP PARALYZED MUSCLES RELAXED

After every injury with motor nerve involvement the limb should be splinted so that

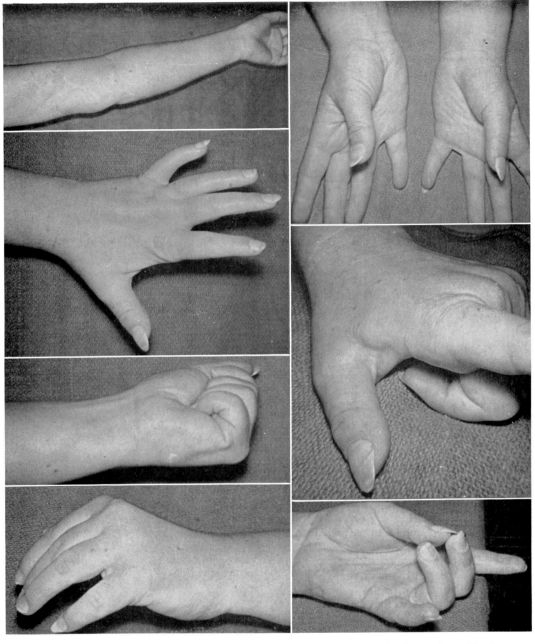

FIG. 459. Recovery of median and ulnar nerve function after nerve repair. Laceration of both nerves above elbow at age 6. Repair of median nerve by flexing the elbow; the distal portion of the ulnar nerve was passed through the flexor origins to shortcut across the flexor surface of the elbow. The medial cutaneous was also repaired. Operation 8 weeks after injury. All photographs were taken 13¼ years after operation, showing scars, lack of clawing, full flexion of fingers, ability to flex the proximal and extend the 2 distal joints, return of thenar opposing muscles, individual flexor tendon action and activity of first interosseus muscle. Only the superficialii of the index and the little fingers and the interossei of the fourth cleft failed to recover. Two-point discrimination is 2.5 mm. compared with the normal 1 mm. on index pulp, 4 mm. compared with 2 mm. on middle finger and 6 mm. compared with 2 mm. on thumb. The forearm is ¼ inch less in circumference, and she wears a left glove ½ size smaller than the right. She plays the piano and the accordian and is training to be a nurse.

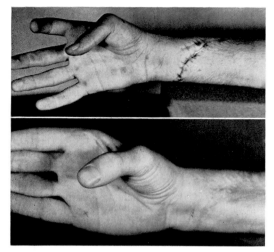

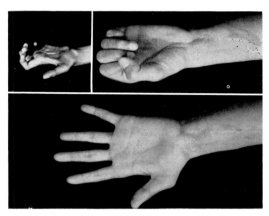

FIG. 460. Case R. R. The arm had gone through a windshield, lacerating the volar aspect. (*Top*) Drained 2 months. Median nerve severed. Flexion of the first 3 fingers limited. Thumb flexor out.

Operation: Sublimis of the ring finger transferred to the thumb flexor; distal sublimis attached to the sublimis of the long finger; median nerve sutured. (*Bottom*) Two years later, good opposition and thenar eminence from nerve suture. The thumb flexed well.

FIG. 461. Case V. P. (*Top, left*) Hand had gone through a glass window, lacerating the arm across the wrist and cutting the median and the ulnar nerves and all the flexor tendons. Primary suture had been done, using silk.

Operation: Excised the scar, exposing the contents of the wrist. Tendons were joined but adherent. Removed much silk which had formed silkomata. Repaired some tendons and used the sublimis tendons for opposition. Placed a free graft of deep fascia beneath the tendons and repaired the median and the ulnar nerves. There was excellent recovery, even of the intrinsic muscles, restoring balance, as shown in the remaining 2 pictures.

the paralyzed muscles will be kept in relaxation for as long a time as is necessary for their recovery.

When a muscle is paralyzed, its antagonist, now unopposed, draws the limb into deformity so that the paralyzed muscle becomes too long. When the nerve finally regenerates, the elongated muscle is at such a disadvantage in trying to work against the resistance of the healthy muscle that recovery will be limited or greatly delayed until the muscle finally shortens. Therefore, splinting is necessary to prevent overstretching. The splint need not hold the limb overcorrected to the opposite deformity; it should merely hold it in the position of balance. Rigid overcorrection by splints stiffens and wrecks hands. The fault is in the type of splint. The splint should be light and minimal in size and should not interfere with the continual use of the hand. It should be elastic or springy, not rigid, for full use of the hand so that the hand will stay active and limber. The strength of the spring

should just counterbalance the loss of muscle power and should not support any joints except those involved. Ulnar palsy should be splinted only when the long flexors are strong enough to produce clawing. Radial palsy and combined median and ulnar palsy require splinting as described in the section on those nerves.

WHEN TO OPERATE

Whenever possible, nerves should be repaired before tendons; in a paralyzed limb tissues do not thrive, tendons become adherent, and joints stiffen. How soon following an injury should one repair the nerves? Primary suture gives better results than secondary suture, but only when surgical conditions are optimal and one can make a perfect nerve juncture. Immediate primary suture in ideal situations yields the best results. In wounds from explosives, the nerves may have been injured further back than appears. Allowance could be made for that, but because of the character of the wound it is better to postpone the neurorrhaphy until a clean suture can be made. The nerve should never be sutured in the presence of infection or an open granulating wound, because the junction will not be perfect. Nerve repair should be postponed in the presence of an infected wound until the danger of latent infection is past. When healing is complete and the local tissue reaction has gone, secondary repair can be done.

In war wounds, half the cases with nerve injury recovered spontaneously. Of course, this included many minor cases and those in which the nerve was physiologically blocked because of injury to adjacent structures caused by the passage of a missile. Sensation returns after nerve repair, even though this is done 6 years after the injury; but motor nerves should be repaired as early as possible, because the steadily progressing fibrous degeneration of the nerve and the muscle will prevent return of function if the nerve is repaired too late. Many good results are

obtained by repairing the nerve a year after the accident. A motor nerve can be repaired even 2 or 3 years after injury, though 2 is usually considered to be the maximal time. If the muscle still reacts to galvanic current, it will react to the repaired nerve. This is the best guide.

If the type of wound is such that the nerve is probably severed, operation is indicated. Most nerves show at least some signs of recovery in 5 months. Absence of any of these signs is an indication for exploration. An exploratory operation, carefully done with due consideration for the other structures in the limb, does no harm and in many cases will give the patient the opportunity to have his nerve repaired early. As regards motor function at least, the earlier the repair the sooner and better the recovery.

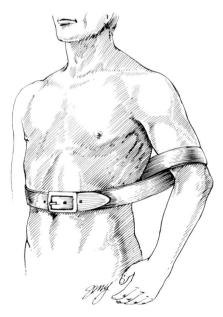

FIG. 462. A strap applied as a figure-of-eight around the trunk and the arm restrains abduction when such motion would strain a nerve suture line in the upper arm.

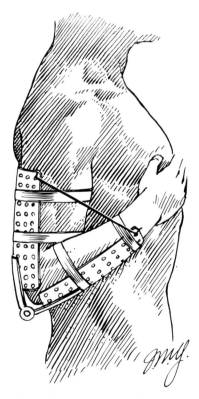

FIG. 463. A posterior elbow splint with a hinge can be used to facilitate the gradual extension of the elbow after nerve suture. The "snubbing" cord allows flexion at all times but limits extension to a predetermined angle.

The proper functioning of the hand is so dependent on the arm nerves that as soon as the wounds have healed, repair of the nerves of the arm should have priority, considering the hand as the important part of the arm. These nerves should be repaired at the same time or even before the bones are repaired. This work should not be postponed for many months while one waits for the bones to unite. Also, soon after an injury, joints may be flexed, thus allowing nerve ends to be approximated. It is impossible to approximate nerve ends if the adjoining joints have stiffened in extension. If the elbow is stiff, it may be necessary to bend the arm at the fracture or to separate a fused joint to permit approximation of the nerve ends. The median and the ulnar nerves are the most important for the preservation of the hand. The loss of the radial nerve can be easily compensated for by tendon transfer.

Primary vs. Secondary Suture

Following repair of any nonsurgical wound the surface scar in the skin is usually coarse and thick. For cosmetic purposes it is often excised and resutured. The same is true of the junction of the severed nerve repaired primarily. A repair done at the time the tissue was traumatized and potentially infected, even though primary healing occurred, usually will result in a very crude union of the nerve ends just as is seen in surface scars. Considering that the degree of recovery after nerve suture is in direct proportion to the accuracy of the juncture, the patients who are not re-operated on after the usual primary nerve repair are denied the chance of obtaining as good a result as that to which they are entitled. In many such cases a secondary operation reveals a very cicatricial, inaccurate juncture. In these cases, by following the rule to resuture nerves that have been repaired in a primary operation, the findings have fully justified the procedure.

As a primary procedure it is advisable to join the 2 nerve ends together with 1 stitch of stainless steel wire to keep them from retracting.

However, this does not apply to fresh incised wounds treated in the best surgical surroundings, by complete excision of every particle of the wound and in conformance with the surgical principles described in Chapter 15. This converts a traumatized, potentially infected wound into a clean surgical wound, and here primary suture is advisable and gives excellent results, even better than does secondary suture.

Frequently, a patient who had a primary suture a year previously has obtained a partial or mediocre recovery. Should one resuture the nerve, destroying the precious function that he has already regained in hope of obtaining better function later? When resuture is done routinely soon after an injury, such a predicament will not arise, and in the long run the result will be far superior.

Technic of Nerve Repair

In dissecting a nerve out from a scar one should not approach it within the scar where it is relatively easy to damage the nerve, but should approach from above and below, following the nerve into the scar. It is preferable always to dissect the nerve downward,

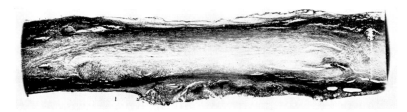

Fig. 464. Low-power photomicrograph of a fresh autogenous nerve graft in the sciatic nerve of a cat 4 weeks after the operation. To the left is the proximal nerve, to the right the distal nerve. Between the two bits of sutures lies the graft. The new axons stain black. The gradually decreasing number as one approaches the distal end is apparent. (Am. J. Surg. *44*:64-75)

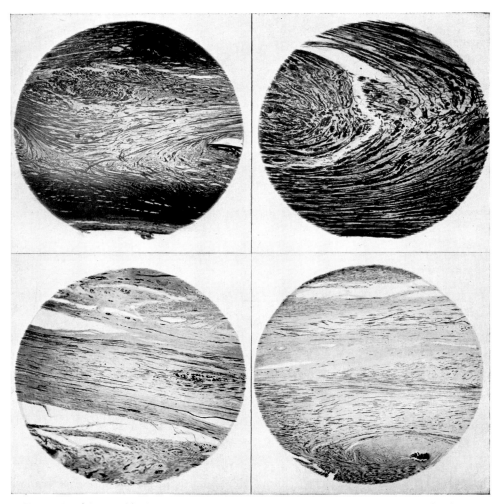

Fig. 465. (*Top, left*) A higher magnification of Fig. 464, showing the proximal suture line. A bit of suture appears at 3 o'clock.

(*Top, right*) A section of the proximal suture line of a fresh autogenous graft in the sciatic nerve of a cat 6 weeks after operation. At the lower edge are seen the coarse fibers of the proximal nerve; nearer the center, the fibers have become turned back in their course, and at the left center some have reversed direction completely. The many spiral tubes called Perroncito apparati are an indication of obstructed growth, in this case due to folding back of nerve tracts; an example of poor approximation.

(*Bottom, left*) A section through the midportion of a degenerated nerve graft in the sciatic nerve of a cat 4 weeks after operation. The proximal nerve is to the left. Note that the central core has fewer fibers and that it still contains necrotic products because the graft has not yet developed a good blood supply in the central portion. This explains the failure of grafts of large diameter.

(*Bottom, right*) A section of the distal suture line of a degenerated nerve graft in the sciatic nerve of a cat 4 weeks after operation, showing nerve fibers crossing the scar joining the nerve graft to the peripheral nerve. A bit of suture at 5 o'clock marks the level of the anastomosis.

(Am. J. Surg. *44*:64-75)

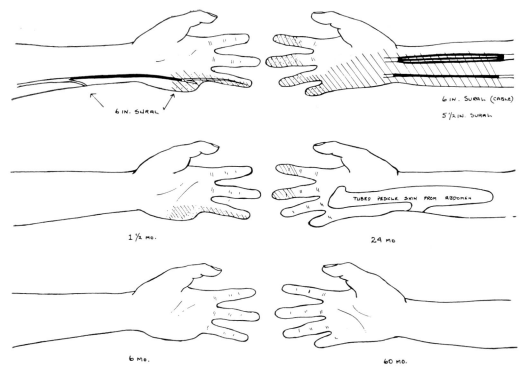

FIG. 466. (*Left*) Case J. B. K. Eight months after laceration of the wrist from a broken windshield and subsequent infection had resulted in amputation of the little finger and loss of the ulnar nerve, a 6-inch sural graft was placed in the nerve, as shown in the diagram. In 5 months, sensation to touch and pinprick could be felt throughout. The ulnar motor branch had not been sutured.

(*Right*) Case S. T. Eleven months after a blast from a shotgun and subsequent infection had gutted the right forearm of tendons and nerves, and after good skin had been supplied by a tubular pedicle from the abdomen, the median nerve was repaired by a 3-ply 6-inch graft from the sural nerve, and the ulnar nerve was united by a single strand 5½ inches long. Five months later, flexor tendons were supplied to all digits, a "pulley" operation for opposition of the thumb was performed, and the radial nerve was sutured. Five years after the first operation, sensation was present throughout.

(Am. J. Surg. *44*:64-75)

because of the danger of tearing off its branches. It is imperative to have a dry field. A tourniquet should be used wherever possible, and if the location does not permit a tourniquet, one should stop and tie or fulgurate every tiny vessel so that one may progress always in a dry field.

As soon as each nerve end is uncovered, a single suture should be placed to mark the proper rotation. The oblong shape of the cross section of the nerve as it lies in its bed away from the site of trauma, and striations along it, as from funiculi or blood vessels, can be matched in each nerve end. On cross section, the pattern of the funiculi should be studied in each end and matched as accurately as possible. For instance, in a median nerve above the wrist there is one special bundle destined for opposition of the thumb; if this is not matched properly, this function will not return. Usually, the funiculus for any particular nerve is found on the side of the main nerve from which that nerve arises. Eventual recovery is proportionate to exactness of rotation and accuracy of coaptation of the nerve ends. In this exacting work adequate exposure, a dry field, controlled lighting and the use of visual aids such as the operating microscope all aid in obtaining accurate apposition.

Each nerve end is cut off boldly until a perfect pattern of funiculi is seen, with the axon bundles projecting like the wires from the cross section of a cable. To do this, it is usually necessary to cut through the soft neck of the neuroma. The nerve ends should be crisp and free from any intervening cicatrix and, by delicate handling, should be kept firm and unfrayed. The end of the nerve should be free of scar so that the sheath will slip back when it is grasped with a fine forceps, thus allowing the bundles to project. To do this, the sheath must be soft and free of scar. Seddon calls this the prepuce test.

Suturing is done with fine silk on a tiny curved cutting needle. Ethicon 7-0 silk with a G-5 needle is preferred. First, the silk is drawn through some adjoining fat to grease it. Petrolatum is not advisable, since it produces a tissue reaction. First, a guide suture is placed, one on each side, and held with clamps. In this way the exact rotation is controlled, and sheath edges are approximated. Then the entire circumference is sutured with interrupted sutures in the sheath.

After suturing one side, one of the guide sutures is passed under the nerve, and the nerve is turned over for suture of the other side. Extreme accuracy is needed for a good result.

In repairing the tiny nerves in the hand, a hand lens or a magnifying mechanism is useful in determining whether or not there are good axon bundles. The motor branch of the ulnar, the motor thenar branch of the median nerve, and the digital nerves as far distally as the pulp of the finger can be sutured with proper instruments and care.

Tantalum wire No. 40 has been used to lessen reaction, but accuracy in axon approximation and sheath closure seem to be the true essentials. A single tantalum wire can be tied into the sheath on each side of the juncture in order that one may determine later, by x-ray, whether the nerve has pulled apart. Otherwise, there is no advantage in the wire as a suture over the 7-0 silk, since it is located in the sheath. Also, there is the disadvantage

of mechanical irritation by the stiff and pointed metal in movable tissue, and for the latter reason, wire never should be used in small hand nerves, subject as they are to repeated trauma.

The task of suturing nerves in the wrist, the elbow or the bases of the fingers when these joints must be flexed in order to allow the nerve ends to come together is often very awkward, and one must work off balance; however, it can be done. After suturing the nerve, the juncture is rolled a little between the finger and the handle of a scalpel so as to arrange the bundles properly, and then is placed in a good bed of normal tissue. For this, first the surrounding cicatrix is dissected out. A space between 2 muscles or in good, soft fat is excellent for a bed. Occasionally, one must swing a pedicle of fat from a nearby location or lay over a piece of smooth fascia to separate a nerve juncture from scar tissue. If the juncture is placed in scar, that scar will generate more scar, which will encase the nerve and jeopardize the result.

Certain practices in nerve suture are mentioned only to be condemned. Intubation of the nerve juncture with various membranes. blood vessels or even foreign bodies only creates more cicatrix, and if any regeneration occurs, it is in spite of them.

To envelop a nerve juncture in a sheath of tantalum foil is to build about it an effective fence that prevents the ingrowth of blood supply so necessary for healing. Nerves frequently are free for a long distance. If, then, their central intrinsic blood vessels thrombose, as they very likely will, the segment of nerve walled off by the tantalum will necrose. The real essential for a nerve juncture is not a smooth exterior but accuracy of sheath suture and placing the nerve in a good vascular bed of normal tissue. It is better to excise the surrounding cicatrix en bloc and displace the nerve laterally to a good bed, or swing fat or or fascia under it, than to expect foil to prevent strangulation by surrounding scar.

Tantalum may be inert chemically, but like any other metal, it is irritating mechanically in the ever-moving tissue, especially opposite a joint. From this, the tantalum is often found to be fragmented and surrounded within and without by cicatrix. Many nerves have regenerated in spite of it, but too many have not. There has been found strangulation,

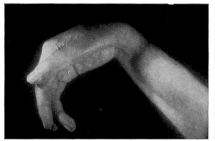 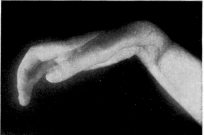

FIG. 467. Case E. B., age 23. Four years previously, a buzz saw had passed two thirds through the carpus from the radial side, and a considerable length of the median and the radial nerves and most of the tendons had sloughed out. The hand was totally useless. Atrophy and absence of sensation were present except in the ulnar area. There were no pronation and no supination and practically no motion, as shown in the 2 top pictures, which show the hand and the wrist in full flexion and full extension, respectively.

Operation (in 2 stages 6 months apart): (the 2

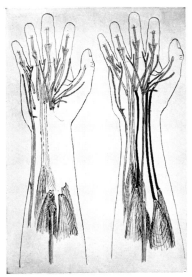 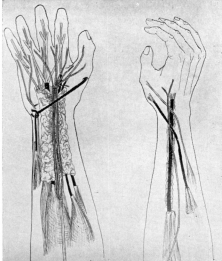

lower drawings): Superficial and deep scar tissue were excised from both the front and the back. A segment of ulna was removed to give pronation and supination, and the joints were placed in functioning positions. The only tendons remaining were the extensors of the fingers, the long extensor of the thumb and 2 roughened strands of flexors to the long and the ring fingers. The deficiencies of the other tendons were made up by free grafts from the extensor tendons of the foot with their paratenon.

(*Bottom, right*) The graft into the extensors of the wrist is shown to be surrounded with its paratenon. Another free graft was joined to the flexor ulnaris muscle in constructing a pulley operation for opposition of the thumb. A wide sheet of paratenon fat was grafted from over the triceps tendon and interwoven about the flexor tendons to furnish mobility. A 6-inch, 3-ply nerve graft was used to bridge the gap in the median and another graft was placed to bridge that in the radial nerve. (J. Bone Joint Surg. *10*:1-25)

white necrosis, a palpable lump from excess of cicatrix and free fluid. In some, function returned on removal of the foil. In others, resuture was necessary, this time very late. Diathermy applied 2 cm. away will burn the nerve.

If opposition of the thumb or muscle balance of fingers has not recovered 18 months after nerve suture, as happens in one third of the cases, tendon transfer is indicated.

SPECIAL PROCEDURES

Overcoming a Gap. Frequently, it appears that the nerve ends cannot be brought together easily. A normal nerve has a certain amount of slack and by dissecting back along the nerve in the surrounding tissues, the nerve ends will yield several millimeters. A nerve never should be stretched beyond a certain degree because axons will break, and there will be internal hemorrhage followed by a scar reaction and loss of function. Frequently, considerable length can be gained by flexing the joint above and exerting just enough traction to drag the nerve through the tissues until its normal tension is reached in the new position of flexion. The yield will not be enough to disrupt the motor branches, which are slackened by this maneuver. This is especially useful for the median nerve in the forearm. If there is still insufficient slack to bring the ends together, each joint above is bent until all of the joints up to the shoulder are in flexion.

A nerve will not strip that length through the tissues, so that one must make incisions along the length of the nerve to free it in the vicinity of each joint.

If too long a length of nerve is freed from its surrounding tissues, that portion of the nerve must act somewhat as a nerve graft. It has only its own internal blood vessels, which may be insufficient. Return of function in it may be delayed for 3 to 4 months. Therefore, enough tissue should be left along the length of a nerve to provide an adequate blood supply.

In drawing a nerve along to gain slack one should be careful to protect its branches. Often it will be necessary to dissect these up and out of the nerve trunk for varying distances with the back of a pointed scalpel. Nerve ends brought together by flexing joints should be protected from being pulled apart by partially encasing the limb in plaster of Paris. Flexion of the shoulder can be maintained by tying the hand to the opposite shoulder and the elbow to the side. To gain length high in the nerve the clavicle or a segment of it may be removed, and the scalenus anticus may be severed so that when the arm is flexed across the chest the nerves will take a short cut. Flexion of the neck is maintained by a strap from a plaster band about the head and around under the axilla. Flexion of the joints should be maintained for 1 month, after which the

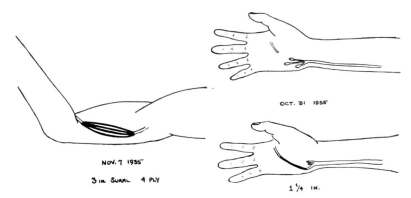

FIG. 468. (Left) Case F. L. H. Twenty-two and a half months after a compound fracture of the humerus, received when an oil drum exploded and wrapped its ends around the patient's left arm, and 5½ months after all osteomyelitis had healed, the musculospiral nerve was bridged by a 4-ply cable graft 3 inches long from the right sural nerve. Only an inner slip of the triceps had remained innervated. Eighteen months later, anesthesia had disappeared from the hand, and voluntary motion was present in the extensors of the wrist and the extensor pollicis longus. Examination 3 years after operation showed absence of anesthesia and good power to extend the fingers and the thumb, even with the wrist passively held dorsiflexed, but only a little of voluntary dorsiflexion of the wrist. The nerve pathway for dorsiflexion of the wrist evidently was missed mechanically by the down-growing axons, since it is the only nerve branch that did not regenerate and since this branch of the radial nerve is usually the first to regain function.

(Right) Case T. S. Four years before, the patient had fallen on a glass, severing the ulnar nerve and the flexor tendons to the ring and the little fingers and opening the wrist joint. Infection followed an attempted primary repair and lasted 2 months. At operation on October 31, 1935 (performed at a meeting of the American College of Surgeons), the little finger was amputated, including its metacarpal. Its extensor tendon was transferred to the adductor of the thumb, its flexor to the interossei of the ring finger and a 1¼-inch gap in the deep motor branch of the ulnar nerve was closed with a graft from one of the sensory branches of the ulnar. Twenty months later, the interossei recovered, and their atrophy had disappeared. He could adduct the straight thumb to the same degree as in the opposite hand. (Am. J. Surg. 44:64-75)

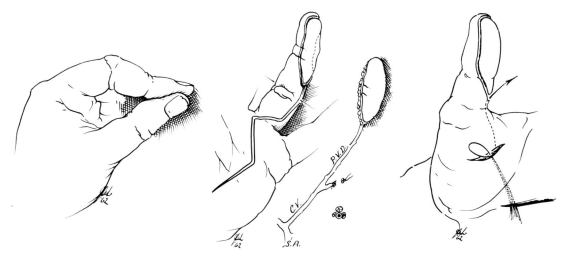

Fig. 469. Neurovascular pedicle or "island transfer." (*Left*) The surfaces of the thumb and the index finger as used for ordinary pinch. (*Center*) The volar and ulnar aspect of the insensitive pulp of the thumb is replaced by a flap of similar size from a digit. (*Right*) The ulnar side of the ring finger is removed on its own vascular and nerve pedicle and transposed beneath the palmar skin to the defect in the thumb. (From J. William Littler, M.D.)

joints should be extended gradually, each time adjusting a restricting splint so that the nerve will have time to grow long enough instead of being stretched. In the usual case of moderate flexion, 2 weeks is sufficient time to extend the limb gradually, but when multiple joints have been strongly flexed, a month or more should be taken. It will be found that other tissues will have contracted and will act as a natural checkrein to extension, yielding by degrees. The tension produced in drawing out a nerve does not all come on its juncture, for it has also become attached to the surrounding tissues. If a nerve is sutured at the wrist, it is better to overcome the gap by flexing the elbow instead of the wrist, as then the traction, on gradual extension, will come less on the suture line. Traction steadily applied to a nerve results in paralysis, so that this should be avoided when using splints.

Another method of gaining slack in a nerve is to transplant it to a place where it can make a shortcut across a joint, e.g., the median and the ulnar nerves at the elbow.

If a nerve is kept stretched to its maximum, it will, like skin, be white from ischemia and become reduced to a fibrous cord. When kept overstretched, the distal portion of the nerve shows more degeneration than does the proximal portion. As a joint is allowed to extend

gradually, it should not be kept on an extension strain by a turnbuckle, since that would cause ischemia of the nerve. Instead, a checkrein should be used which allows the degree of extension desired and also gives freedom to flex intermittently, so as to flush the nerve tissues with blood supply. For this snubbing effect malleable splints are used for the elbow and the wrist; there is no restricting bandage to prevent voluntary flexion of the limb.

If there is more of a gap in a nerve than can be overcome readily, free nerve grafting offers a good chance for success. In the small nerves of a hand these work splendidly; but for the larger nerves in the forearm, cable grafts should be used so that the nerve strands will be nourished through and through. Details of nerve grafting are described at the end of this chapter.

Another method of overcoming a gap in a nerve is to free the nerve well, flex the joints, and suture the neuroma and the glioma together, or bring the neuroma as far distally as possible and suture it to some fixed structure. This so-called bulb-suture technic has proved to be of value especially in children. After a month, the limb is extended gradually, drawing out the nerve; then, when the operation is repeated, there will be found to be sufficient slack for suturing.

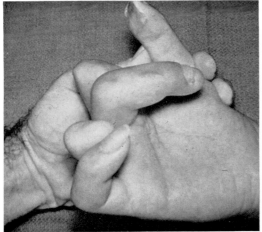

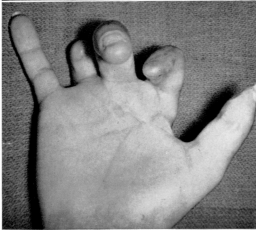

FIG. 470. Here the very important ulnar side of the thumb pulp has been destroyed, but only the middle finger is uninjured. The index is irreparable but has some skin that can be used for the island transfer.

Freeing Nerves. A nerve encased in cicatrix or callus on being dissected free shows a narrowing from strangulation. Its sheath should be slit longitudinally in several places so that it can expand. First, however, some surgeons inject the nerve with salt solution until it is tight in order to balloon out the fibers in the sheath and break up internal adhesions. If the region of the nerve is cicatricial, it can be inspected by making a longitudinal cut in it. Several such cuts can be made, preferably using the back edge of a pointed knife, but if much cicatrix is present it is better to excise it all and suture the nerve end-to-end. If the nerve has

merely compressed, function may return at once. However, if the constriction is extreme, the nerve will have undergone wallerian degeneration, and it will take just as long for return of function as if the nerve had been cut and sutured, for the axons of the proximal end must grow all the way down.

Partial Nerve Injuries. A nerve that has been near the course of a missile, but not hit, may show a fusiform swelling called pseudoneuroma of attrition. If it is from thickening of the connective tissue between the nerve bundles, recovery usually occurs without excision and suture.

A nerve may show a notch with a nodule above and below. This indicates partial severance and separation of the severed fibers. First, the nerve fibers should be split, preserving those that are still intact. Those terminating in the nodules should be trimmed off until good fibers present, and then sutured together. This will necessitate splitting up and down the nerve and buckling the fibers which have remained unhurt. The same procedure is followed when a nerve shows a neruoma on one side, though here it is more likely that some fibers have found their way through the neuroma.

Nerve Transfers. By this is meant suturing end-to-end one nerve or part of a nerve to another. Of course, it would be absurd merely to implant the end of a nerve between the fibers of another. End-to-end transfers are just as successful as are nerve sutures and are occasionally useful. If too great a length in an important nerve is lost for repair, its distal segment can be transplanted into an adjoining nerve. However, this is practical only when it is done high in the adjoining nerve before the nerve bundles have become arranged into funiculi, each having a special function. Part of the nerve should be cut squarely across and sutured to the distal segment of the paralyzed nerve. An excellent result was obtained from nerve transfer done by Bunnell for paralysis when a man's shoulder had been hit by a falling tree, avulsing various nerves about the shoulder and resulting in amputation above the elbow. The 3 useless nerves in the amputation stump were drawn out, split and attached to the distal segments of the circumflex, the supraspinatus and the long and the middle subscapular nerves. Function returned to all their respective muscles, so that now

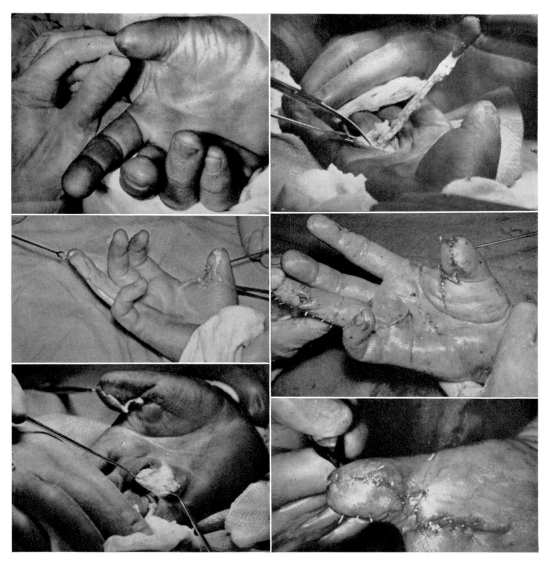

FIG. 471. To remove scar from the thumb stump and provide good sensible skin without further loss of length, an island transfer is used, and a Z-plasty improves extension and abduction. (*Left*) The scarred area of the thumb is excised, and a flap of similar size is cut on the ulnar side of the ring finger. The neurovascular bundle is dissected free through a midlateral finger incision and separate incisions in the palm, all placed to avoid crossing flexion creases. (*Right*) The pedicle and the flap from the finger. The donor area is covered with a thick split graft. Note that the flap is more to the ulnar side of the pulp.

he efficiently manipulates an artificial arm. Seddon utilizes nerve transfer in the reconstruction of damage from Volkmann's ischemia by suturing the ulnar to the median nerve.

Nerve Grafts. There is now no doubt that under certain conditions free nerve grafts live

and function. Sufficient evidence, both clinical and experimental, shows that small-caliber autogenous grafts are particularly useful in the hand. When larger nerves are involved, the use of multiple-strand cable grafts has proved to be successful. The pessimism in the past, based on the results from illogical methods such as end-to-side implants, turning down nerve flaps, suture at a distance with catgut strands and interposition of blood vessel segments, was justified. It is difficult to explain why the example of the poor results gained from wrapping the suture lines with materials varying from cargile membrane to petrolatum gauze did not prevent the recent erroneous use of tantalum foil. The use of nerve grafts demands the same exacting technic as nerve suture with accurate approximation and the provision of a succulent scar-free bed to allow the graft to regain its nutrition.

Nerve grafts are used only when all other possible means of repair have been exhausted.

In 1878 Albert described the first use of a nerve graft. Platt in 1919 reported 20 cases, all failures. These were large-diameter single nerves instead of cabled grafts and were enclosed in fascia or vein. Huber proved regeneration through grafts experimentally, and Balance and Duel reported using grafts in facial nerve lesions. Bentley and Hill and Bunnell and Boyes proved that predegenerated grafts had no advantage over fresh autogenous grafts. Bunnell, whose series reached over 100 cases, reported a detailed follow-up study of 26 autografts in 15 patients. Seddon found that 67.3 per cent of 52 nerve grafts yielded a useful return, and in 38.5 per cent that the result was as good as that after direct nerve suture. Grafts have been used in the facial nerve by Kettel, Bunnell and Martin.

The sural nerve in the calf is the donor area of choice. Sensory loss usually is not noticed by the patient, and 25 to 40 cm. are available. It is not necessary or justifiable to sacrifice function to obtain a nerve graft. The small size of the graft allows it to be nourished quickly, and, just as a thin skin graft or a small-caliber tendon graft lives and gets a new blood supply quickly, so does the small-caliber nerve. If a thick-skin or large-caliber tendon graft is used, its central portion dies before it can obtain a blood supply.

Conclusive proof of return of function has been provided by blocking the involved nerve or other adjoining nerves in the hand and by return of voluntary action in previously paralyzed muscles.

Grafting Large-Caliber Nerves. A large-central diameter nerve grafted intact will undergo necrosis, but if split into several small strands it will live. In certain instances a large nerve may be transplanted as a pedicled graft. When there is a major defect in both median and ulnar nerves, the median innervated area of the hand can be supplied by first dividing the ulnar nerve high in the upper arm and suturing the 2 nerves together at the elbow. When Tinel's sign progresses up the ulnar nerve—evidencing growth of axons—the ulnar nerve is swung down and sutured to the distal median nerve. In such a patient (referred by Captain Selverstone), Bunnell found sensibility in the palm which remained when the radial nerve was blocked. Strange has reported convincing regeneration from a similar procedure.

Success in nerve grafts depends on avoiding infection, liberal excision of scar, especially at the nerve ends, accurate approximation and a good vascular bed for the graft.

Painful Neuromata. A neuromata in an amputation stump is the result of the natural healing process of the cut nerve end. Most are painless, and many stumps that are tender at first eventually become painless. When a simple guillotine amputation was done followed by a re-amputation through clean tissue, as in war amputations, painful neuromata were rare. Neuromata caught in scar or in poorly nourished tissue or so placed that they are subject to constant trauma may remain painful. For most cases, if the scar is excised, the neuroma removed and the divided end of the nerve placed in good tissue away from trauma, the results are as good as any following more elaborate methods of treatment. Injecting with alcohol, capping the end with plastics or other foreign bodies, crushing and tying and embedding the nerve end in bone— all have been discarded.

Irreparable Nerves. If a motor nerve cannot be repaired or if the lesion is central as in poliomyelitis, useful motion can be restored by substitutes such as muscle or tendon transfers. Combinations of arthrodeses, tenodeses and tendon transfers are described in Chapter 11.

ISLAND TRANSFER FOR PULP SENSATION. When the loss involves the sensory components and especially the important pinching and grasping areas of the thumb and the fingers, other methods of substitution can be used. The pulp of the thumb consists of specialized skin and subcutaneous tissue. When lost, it may be restored cosmetically as far as size and contour are concerned by pedicled skin and fat. Such a substitute will not have the quality of sensibility needed to provide normal tactilegnosis, and function will be impaired. It is necessary that tissue of comparable characteristics be transplanted with nerve and vascular supply intact if the area is to be used normally. Such a transfer on a neurovascular pedicle is the so-called island transfer. Based on the Esser flap and developed as an extension of the pollicization procedure, where a whole digit is transposed on its neurovascular pedicle, these transfers provide a sentient area for precision pinch and grasp. They are useful in restoring function to an area where tissues are poorly nourished, to replace scarred pulp areas and to improve the sensibility of these areas when regeneration of the nerves is incomplete. Many refinements in this technic have been reported by Moberg, Littler, Tubiana, Böhler and Frackelton.

Loss of tactile skin on the thumb, and particularly its ulnar side, is the primary indication for operation. If the thumb has been resurfaced by pedicle graft, or if a thumb post has been reconstructed of pedicle and bone, transfer of normal skin in a neurovascular pedicle to its pinching surface will improve the function greatly.

The radial side of the pulp of the ring finger normally innervated by the median nerve is the donor area of choice, though any other normally innervated area can be used. The radial side of the index and the middle fingers is left intact, since they are used to oppose the thumb.

Approximately half the pulp of the donor finger is removed, and, through a midlateral incision proximally on the finger, the complete neurovascular bundle is dissected free. The incision can be extended onto the palm by jogging across the base of the finger, or a separate palmar incision may be made. When the island with its intact neurovascular bundle is completely free, it is put through a tunneled passage under the skin to the base of the thumb or located directly through a separate midlateral incision in the thumb. The skin area to be replaced is excised, and either it or a comparable-sized piece of skin graft is sutured into the donor area. Great care must be taken to avoid kinking or pressure on the pedicle. It is neither necessary nor advisable to take both digital vessels and nerves in the pedicle. Patients usually learn to localize the touch sensation to the thumb quickly, especially in handling objects, since the motions involved transmit impulses through the deep tendons and the joints. An interesting finding is the regeneration of some protective sensa-

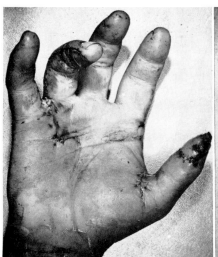 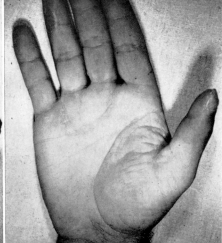

Fig. 472. Island transfer from ring finger to thumb. Note carefully placed incisions and minimal scars resulting (From Wm. H. Frackelton, M.D.)

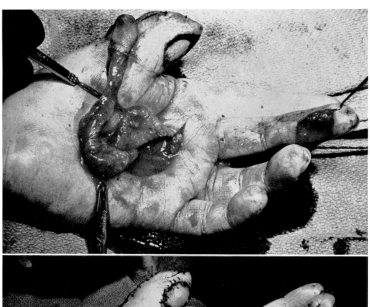

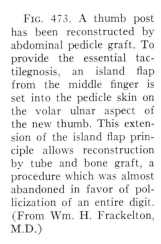

Fig. 473. A thumb post has been reconstructed by abdominal pedicle graft. To provide the essential tactilegnosis, an island flap from the middle finger is set into the pedicle skin on the volar ulnar aspect of the new thumb. This extension of the island flap principle allows reconstruction by tube and bone graft, a procedure which was almost abandoned in favor of pollicization of an entire digit. (From Wm. H. Frackelton, M.D.)

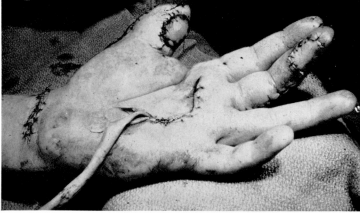

tion in the recipient area at the edges of the transplanted island of normal skin.

CEREBRAL PALSY

In a few patients with cerebral palsy, surgery can help to improve function of the hand. The works of Steindler, Goldner and Swanson illustrate the proper approach to surgical treatment of impairment of the hand.

SELECTION OF PATIENTS

Evaluation of the whole patient, not simply his hand, is important. From a group of 800 patients Goldner selected only 300 for treatment, and of this number in only 12 (4%) was any surgical procedure performed on the hand. From 300 spastic children Swanson selected 12 for treatment of the hand.

There is agreement on the contraindications for surgical treatment. Insufficient trial of conservative therapy, generalized muscle weakness, lack of voluntary control, athetosis, sensory disorders, emotional instability, an I.Q. below 70 and age below 7—all are adequate reasons for not recommending surgical reconstruction of the hand. In addition, the presence of adequate grasp and release mechanisms and a reasonably good thumb should be a signal to avoid doing anything that would destroy these most important functions.

COMMON DEFORMITIES IN CEREBRAL PALSY

The principle problems encountered in the hand are pronation of the forearm, a flexed wrist, the thumb-in-palm position and the lack of extension of the fingers at their proximal joints, sometimes with hyperextension at the middle joints.

Pronation of the Forearm. Tenotomy of the

pronator teres is usually insufficient and should be combined with various tendon transfers.

Mayer advises that the pronator teres and the flexor carpi ulnaris muscles be united and transferred subcutaneously about the dorsum of the forearm to the radius. Similarly, according to the method of Steindler, the flexor carpi ulnaris is passed subcutaneously across the dorsum of the forearm to insert on the radius. To extend the wrist, the pronator teres and the flexor carpi radialis can be transferred to the extensor carpi radialis and the flexor ulnaris to the extensor ulnaris.

Green passes the tendon of the flexor carpi ulnaris deep to the digital extensors, attaches it to the radius and uses plaster fixation for several months. Osteotomy of the radius to place the forearm in more supination has been used.

Flexion Deformity of the Wrist. Arthrodesis should be a last resort. If the transfer to wrist extensors is not sufficient, it is important that a trial of plaster immobilization be carried out to determine the feasibility of and the proper position for arthrodesis.

Thumb in Palm. This deformity of the

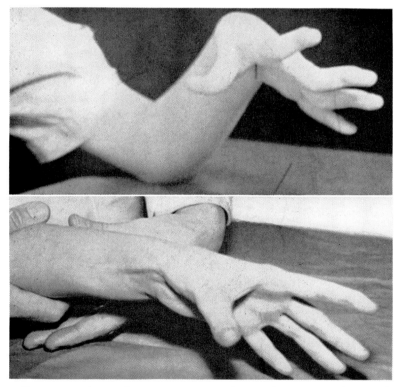

FIG. 474. Print made from a preoperative movie, showing the spastic hand of a 16-year-old girl with spastic hemiplegia, while she was attempting to open her hand. Note the flexion of the wrist, the flexion of the distal interphalangeal joints, and the hyperextension of the proximal interphalangeal joints. The same hand 3 years after tenodeses of the sublimis tendons at the proximal interphalangeal joints of the fingers, transfer of the flexor carpi radialis tendon to the rerouted long extensor of the thumb, and fusion of the metacarpophalangeal joint of the thumb. The patient is now able to open her hand without flexion of the wrist, and there is no hyperextension of the proximal interphalangeal joints, even when the wrist is flexed. (Swanson, A. B.: J. Bone Joint Surg. *42-A*:958)

strongly adducted and flexed thumb as been overcome by several methods. If the wrist is held in strong ulnar deviation, the thumb may open, so that a preliminary splinting of the wrist should be tried. Other means are stripping the thenar intrinsic muscles, neurectomy or bone block of the first 2 metacarpals. Goldner transferred the flexor carpi radialis to the rerouted extensor pollicis longus and fused the proximal thumb joint or, after release of the spastic muscles, provided opposition by tendon transfer and stabilized the proximal thumb joint. The flexor pollicis longus may require lengthening. All the thumb joints can be fused and the thumb converted to a fixed post.

Lack of Finger Extension. For the flexion deformity of the fingers, a general weakening by tenotomy may aid in the release but destroy much of the grasp. For this deformity Swanson transfers the superficial flexors to the common digital extensors and tenodeses the distal part of the superficialis across the middle finger joint to overcome the hyperextension deform-ity. However, if flexion of the fingers is weak, the proximal tendons can be tapped into the profundi above the wrist. If instead of the hyperextension deformity of the middle joint there is a flexion deformity, the Bunnell transfer of superficialis tendons through the lumbrical canals may help.

NEURECTOMY FOR SPASTIC PARALYSIS

Of the various types of spastic paralysis, only those lesions of the pyramidal tract in which only the upper neuron is involved, not the various coordinating nuclei and tracts of the brain, are suitable for neurectomy. This eliminates cases of Little's disease, athetosis, ataxia, chorea, progressive spastic paralysis and hemiplegia. Its use is limited to cases ranging from definite deformity to mild contracture and caused by loss of the inhibitory action of the upper neuron, thus resulting in hyperactivation of the muscles by the lower neuron. There should be some muscle action in the opposing group. The upper neuron cor-

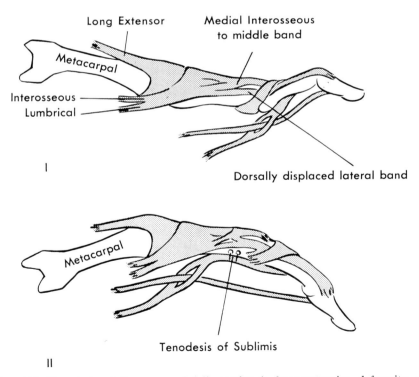

FIG. 475. Tenodesis of flexor superficialis tendon in hyperextension deformity of middle joint. (Swanson, A. B.: J. Bone Joint Surg. *42-A*:958)

tical pattern overrules any peripheral muscle attack.

In addition to the tendon transplants, tenotomies, tendon lengthenings and arthrodeses which often can improve function, there are the neurectomy methods developed by Stoffel. His first plan was to resect the portions of the nerve trunk which controlled the spastic muscles. It was found that in ascending the nerves these bundles soon lost their pattern, due to various plexuses within the nerve itself. Faradic stimulation of certain bundles aided in identification, but this was not sufficient. Therefore, Stoffel's second operation—tracing the nerve to the muscle and there locally reducing or removing the nerve supply—became the operation of choice.

The object is to correct the muscle imbalance, but if too much nerve supply is removed, the opposite deformity will be produced.

In the upper extremity, in contrast with the lower, the flexor muscles are more powerful than are the extensor. In spasticity they overpull their antagonists, resulting in flexion and pronation. At the shoulder there is adduction and internal rotation. The elbow becomes flexed, and the forearm is drawn into pronation. The wrist and the fingers are flexed, and the thumb is adducted or opposed.

Neurectomy is rarely used at the shoulder, and in the elbow it is not needed, since some degree of flexion is not objectionable in the use of the arm. The usual neurectomy procedures are performed on the median and the ulnar nerves.

Median Nerve. Here is the aim to correct excessive pronation, flexion of the wrist and the fingers and of the thumb. The nerve is uncovered just below the elbow where its muscular branches come off in the order noted above. Enough are severed, depending on the severity of the case, to restore balance in the forearm muscles. Usually, more nerve supply must be removed from the pronator and the flexor carpi radialis than from the flexors of the fingers. It may be necessary to arthrodese the metacarpotrapezial joint of the thumb and perhaps the metacarpophalangeal joint also.

Ulnar Nerve. The nerve is exposed just below the elbow, taking most of the supply from the flexor carpi ulnaris and a little from the flexor digitorum profundus. In the hand,

to decrease adduction of the thumb, the deep motor branch of the ulnar nerve is exposed deep in the palm, and its terminal branches are severed.

Muscle transfers and tenotomies are resorted to for spastic paralysis in the upper extremity more frequently than is neurectomy, the latter being used supplementarily.

PROGNOSIS IN NERVE INJURIES

Including all injuries involving nerves, such as contusions, fractures and dislocations as well as open wounds, spontaneous regeneration or recovery of nerve function takes place in the majority of cases. A severed nerve will bridge a gap of some distance, and a contused nerve, if in continuity, will recover. A nerve stretched by prolonged positioning or splinting usually recovers in 3 months.

The degree of recovery varies directly with the accuracy of coaptation of the divided axons and indirectly with the amount of scar and the nutrition of the parts.

A most important factor is the technic of the surgeon. The best results are achieved by excising scar, approximating the nerve ends with the finest suture, maintaining exact rotation and avoiding tension. Errors in rotation probably account for the poor results seen in ulnar nerve repair, since this same nerve, repaired after its branching in the palm, can be repaired in either the motor or the sensory division with good results. This rotation error is not easy to overcome. In secondary repairs, scarring interferes with the form and the location of the nerve and its fascicular pattern so that rotational landmarks are missing.

It is only at the time of the original laceration that the epineural vessel configuration and the fascicular pattern are well defined. It is at this step in the reconstruction that a careful alignment of the nerve and its approximation with one wire suture will allow the formal suture later to be done with maximal accuracy.

Suturing a nerve should be done with the finest silk on atraumatic needles. The stitch is placed through the sheath only. Any tension on the suture line is relieved by positioning the nearby joints and not by using retention sutures or heavy suture material.

Given ideal conditions and accurate repair,

the nerve should regenerate 1 or 2 mm. a day. Some muscles may not recover from suture in the upper arm because the axons do not grow down the correct pathways or because the muscle itself is incapable of recovery from fibrosis. Because of the distance the nerve has to regrow, injuries of the major nerves in upper arm, the axilla or the shoulder should be repaired early. Some sensory recovery can take place from repair as long as 5 or 6 years after injury, but after 2 years hardly any motor recovery can be expected.

A motor nerve should be repaired as soon as possible, because muscles undergo progressive atrophy and fibrosis as long as they are denervated. Bowden and Guttman studied biopsies of muscle in various stages. They found atrophy to be slight after 3 months, moderate between 3 and 12 months and extreme after 3 years.

The distal portion of a severed nerve also undergoes a progressive change. Wallerian degeneration is complete in about 3 weeks, but there is further degeneration with increase in fibrous tissue.

Seddon classifies nerve injury as (1) neurotomesis, or disruption of the nerve, (2) axonotemesis, or disruption of axons within the intact sheath, and (3) neuropraxia, a physiologic blocking without interruption of the axon.

Perfect regeneration of a sutured nerve never takes place. Careful detailed examinations of both motor and sensory functions will disclose failure of some muscles to regain size, strength or coordination or the finer degrees of sensibility may be lacking, and there may be paresthesias or abnormal responses to normal stimuli.

Nerves which are incised sharply and repaired primarily achieve the best recovery, those which are torn by traction injuries the poorest. Like a rope under stretch, a few fibers break at one level and others at other levels until finally the continuity is broken. Surgical repair requires excision of as much of the damaged area as possible.

SIGNS OF RECOVERY OF NERVE FUNCTION

When a damaged nerve is repaired or a block of the axon transmission system is released, signs of recovery usually appear in an orderly way.

Sensation returns before voluntary muscle activity and from proximal to distal areas. Recovery of deep sensation and coarse touch precedes light touch and pinprick. A sign preceding actual sensibility to touch is an uncomfortable or painful reaction to pinching the anesthetic skin or the paralyzed muscle. Tinel's sign, a tingling sensation felt when one taps over the regenerating axons, is a reliable guide to the level of growth of the new fibers. To avoid misinterpretation, one hand presses on the skin between the nerve juncture and the point being tapped.

At first there will be some shrinking in the area of anesthesia due to overlap from adjoining normal nerves. This does not occur in the isolated supply areas such as the distal segment of the little finger for the ulnar nerve. Anesthetizing the normal nerve shows the extent of this phenomenon. In overlap areas pinprick will be localized accurately, whereas in regenerating areas it will not.

Axons growing down the nerves to a different finger may result in a mixing up of the impulse registration in the cerebrum. Re-education and association usually correct this in a short time.

Motor function recovers more slowly than sensory reception. Not only must the nerve regenerate to the muscle, but enough recovery of the muscle must take place to make a motion perceptible to the examiner. After repair of a posterior interosseus nerve there may be visible muscle action in 3 months; but from an ulnar nerve repair at the elbow, it may be a year before any signs are seen in the intrinsic muscles. When first recovering, a muscle may show only a flicker of activity, be unable to move the part against gravity or it may tire easily.

Electromyography can show signs of recovery of the muscle long before they are seen clinically. Performed by a competent operator who must be well versed in anatomy, an electromyogram is the best laboratory aid available in diagnosing and determining the prognosis of injuries of the motor nerves.

Trophic changes are progressive until some signs of sensory recovery occur. In a pure motor nerve, a slight increase in muscle size appears before voluntary activity is seen. The severe atrophy of a denervated muscle may be lessened by splinting to avoid overstretching.

Jackson and Seddon claim that galvanic stimulations repeated many times daily and started early will prevent severe atrophy. From a practical standpoint in clinical practice this is not used. The use of electrical stimulation as commonly performed, without regard to overuse or done for a few minutes once or twice a week, is useless if not detrimental.

Sometimes in areas of recovering sensibility or following a partial nerve injury, particularly to the median nerve, a peculiar painful state develops. Termed causalgia by Weir Mitchell, its cause and treatment are perplexing. Further discussion will be found in Chapter 18.

BIBLIOGRAPHY

Abreau, L. B. de, and Moreira, R. G.: Median nerve compression at the wrist, J. Bone Joint Surg. *40-A*:1426, 1958.

Agassiz, C. D. S.: Cerebral palsy, Med. Press *228*:581, 1952.

Aschan, W., and Moberg, E.: The ninhydrin finger printing test used to map out partial lesions to hand nerves, Acta chir. scand. *123*:365, 1962.

Atlas, L. N.: Further observations on etiology of vasomotor disturbances following peripheral nerve section, Surgery *10*:318, 1941.

Babcock, W.: Standard technique for operation of peripheral nerves with especial reference to closure of large gaps, Surg., Gynec. Obstet. *45*:364, 1927.

Bang-Rasmussen, K.: Peripheral nerve lesions in the upper extremity, J. Bone Joint Surg. *44-B*:443, 1962.

Barnes, R., Bacsich, P., and Wyburn, G. M.: A histological study of a predegenerated nerve autograft, Brit. J. Surg. *33*:130, 1945.

Bateman, J. E.: Peripheral nerve injuries, Instruct. Course Lect., Am. Acad. Orth. Surg. *13*:85, 1956.

Bauwens, P.: Electro-diagnosis and electro-therapy in peripheral nerve lesions, Proc. Roy. Soc. Med. *34*:459, 1941.

Benisty, A.: Clinical Forms of Lesions of Nerves; Medical and Surgical Therapy, New York, Appleton, 1918.

Bennett, M. D.: Care of severely paralyzed upper extremities, J.A.M.A. *149*:105, 1952.

Bentley, F. H., and Hill, M.: Possibilities of nerve grafting, Brit. M. J. *2*:352, 1940.

Bowden, R. E. M.: The factors influencing functional recovery of peripheral nerve injury in man, Ann. Roy. Coll. Surg. Eng. *8*:366, 1951.

Bowden, R. E. M., and Gutman, E.: Denervation and re-innervation of human voluntary muscle, Brain *67*:273, 1944.

Bowden, R. E. M., and Napier, J. R.: Assessment of hand function after peripheral nerve injuries, J. Bone Joint Surg. *43-B*:481, 1961.

Boyes, J. H.: Repair of the motor branch of the ulnar nerve in the palm, J. Bone Joint Surg. *37-A*:920, 1955.

Brand, P. W.: The reconstruction of the hand in leprosy, Ann. Roy. Coll. Surg. Eng. *11*:350, 1952.

————: Deformity in leprosy; orthopaedic principles and practical methods of relief *in* Cochrane, R. G. (ed.): Leprosy in Theory and Practice, p. 265, Bristol, John Wright & Sons, 1959.

Bristow, R., and Elkington, J. St. C.: Discussion on injuries to peripheral nerves, Proc. Roy. Soc. Med. *34*:513, 1941.

Bristow, W. R.: Injuries of peripheral nerves in two world wars, Brit. J. Surg. *34*:333, 1947.

Brooks, D. M.: Open wounds of the brachial plexus, J. Bone Joint Surg. *31-B*:17, 1949.

Buck-Gramcko, D.: Restoration of sensitivity in partial loss of the thumb, Langenbeck arch. klin. Chir. *299*:99, 1961.

Bunnell, S.: Surgery of nerves of the hand, Surg., Gynec. Obstet. *44*:145, 1927.

————: Repair of nerves and tendons of the hand, J. Bone Joint Surg. *10*:1, 1928.

————: Surgical repair of the facial nerve, Arch. Otol. *25*:235, 1937.

————: Hand surgery: The surgery of nerves of the upper extremity, Instr. Course Lect., Am. Acad. Orth. Surg. *13*:101, 1956.

Bunnell, S., and Boyes, J. H.: Nerve grafts, Am. J. Surg. *44*:64, 1939.

Bunten, W. A.: Diagnosis and management of peripheral nerve lesions, Colorado Med. *28*:134, 1931.

Burman, M. S.: The spastic hand, J. Bone Joint Surg. *20*:133, 1938.

Cairns, H., and Young, J. Z.: Treatment of gunshot wounds of peripheral nerves, Lancet *2*:123, 1940.

Cameron, B. M.: Occlusion of the ulnar artery with impending gangrene of the fingers relieved by section of the carpal ligament, J. Bone Joint Surg. *36-A*:406, 1954.

Cannon, B. W., and Love, J. G.: Tardy median palsy; median neuritis; median thenar neuritis amenable to surgery, Surgery *20*:210, 1946.

Childress, H. M.: Recurrent ulnar nerve dislocation at the elbow, J. Bone Joint Surg. *38-A*:978, 1956.

Chusid, F. G., and McDonald, J. J.: Correlative Neuroanatomy and Functional Neurology, ed. 7, Los Altos, Calif., Lange Med. Pub., 1954.

Clippinger, F. W., Goldner, J. L., and Roberts, J. M.: Use of the electromyogram in evaluating upper extremity peripheral nerve lesions, J. Bone Joint Surg. 44-A:1047, 1962.

Coleman, C. C.: Surgical treatment of peripheral nerve injuries, Surg., Gynec. Obstet. 78:113, 1944.

Davis, L.: Peripheral nerve surgery, Surg., Gynec. Obstet. 80:444, 1945.

Davis, L., and Cleveland, D. A.: Experimental studies in nerve transplants, Ann. Surg. 99:271, 1934.

Davis, L., Perret, G., and Carroll, W.: Surgical principles underlying the use of grafts in the repair of peripheral nerve injuries, Ann. Surg. 121:686, 1945.

Deery, E. M.: Injuries to peripheral nerves, Surg. Clin. N. Amer. 21:469, 1941.

Duel, A. B.: History and development of surgical treatment of facial palsy, Surg., Gynec. Obstet. 560:384, 1933.

Dunn, G. R.: Symposium on fractures and other trauma; peripheral nerve injury, Minnesota Med. 23:748, 1940.

Duthie, H. L.: Radial nerve in osseous tunnel at humeral fracture site diagnosed radiographically, J. Bone Joint Surg. 39-B:746, 1957.

Eccles, J. C.: Changes in muscles produced by nerve degeneration, Med. J. Aust. 1:573, 1941.

Esser, J. F. S.: Island flaps, New York M. J. 106:264, 1917.

Fontaine, R., and Bertrand, P.: Pathogenesis and treatment of reflex functional disturbances in paralysis of radial nerves, Presse méd. 49:380, 1941.

Forrester, C. R. G.: Peripheral nerve injuries with results of early and delayed suture, Am. J. Surg. 47:555, 1940.

Forrester-Brown, M.: Peripheral nerve injuries in civil practice, Med. Press 203:246, 1940.

Frackelton, W. H., and Teasley, J. L.: Neurovascular island pedicle—extension in usage, J. Bone Joint Surg. 44-A:1069, 1962.

Flynn, J. E.: Reconstruction of the hand after median nerve palsy, New Engl. J. Med. 256:676, 1957.

Goldner, J. L.: Reconstructive surgery of hand in cerebral palsy and spastic paralysis resulting from injury to spinal cord, J. Bone Joint Surg. 37-A:1141, 1205, 1955.

————: Upper extremity reconstructive surgery in cerebral palsy or similar conditions, Instr. Course Lect., Am. Acad. Orth. Surg. 18:169, 1961.

Grant, B. D., and Rowe, C. R.: Motor paralyses of extremities in herpes zoster, J. Bone Joint Surg. 43-A:885, 1961.

Green, W. T.: Tendon transplantation of the flexor carpi ulnaris for pronation-flexion deformity of the wrist, Surg., Gynec. Obstet. 75:337, 1942.

Green, W. T., and Banks, H. H.: The flexor carpi ulnaris transplant and its use in cerebral palsy, J. Bone Joint Surg. 44-A:1343, 1962.

Harley, H. R.: Notes on peripheral nerve injuries, Guy's Hosp. Gaz. 54:262, 288, 338, 1940.

Harmer, T. W.: Traumatic lesions of nerves of wrist and hand, Am. J. Surg. 47:517, 1940.

Harris, W.: The Morphology of the Brachial Plexus, London, Oxford Univ. Press, 1939.

Haymaker, W., and Woodhall, B.: Peripheral Nerve Injuries; Principles of Diagnosis, Philadelphia, Saunders, 1945.

Henderson, W. R., and Taverner, D.: Some therapeutic and neurological aspects of peripheral nerve injuries, Lancet 256:1084, 1949.

Highet, W. B., and Sanders, F. K.: Effects of stretching nerves after suture, Brit. J. Surg. 30:355, 1943.

Holmes, W.: Histological observations on the repair of nerves by autografts, Brit. J. Surg. 35:167, 1947.

————: The problem of nerve homografts, Med. Illustr., London 6:556, 1952.

Huber, G. C.: Transplantation of peripheral nerve, Arch. Neurol. Psychiat. 2:466, 1919.

————: Repair of peripheral nerve injuries, Surg., Gynec. Obstet. 30:464, 1920.

Hunt, J. R.: Thenar and hypothenar types of neural atrophy of hand, Brit. M. J. 2:642, 1930.

Hyman, I., and Beswick, W. F.: Measurement of skin resistance in peripheral nerve injuries, War Med. 8:258, 1945.

Kaplan, E. B.: Surgical anatomy of the flexor tendons of the wrist, J. Bone Joint Surg. 27:368, 1945.

Kilvington, B.: Some experiences on nerve regeneration, Aust. New Zeal. J. Surg. 10:266, 1941.

King, T.: Treatment of traumatic ulnar neuritis, Aust. New Zeal. J. Surg. 20:33, 1950.

Kirklin, F. W., et al.: Suture of peripheral nerves, Surg. Gynec. Obstet. 88:719, 1949.

Kirsten, J.: The experimental use of a muscle graft in the regeneration of a peripheral nerve; discussion, J. Bone Joint Surg. 43-B:401, 1961.

Koch, S. L.: Injuries of nerves and tendons of the hand, J. Oklahoma M. A. 26:323, 1933.

————: Injuries of nerves and tendons of the hand, Penn. M. J. 37:555, 1934.

————: Injuries of nerves and tendons of hand, Wisconsin M. J. 33:655, 1934.

————: Some surgical principles in repair of divided nerves and tendons, Quart. Bull. Northwestern Univ. Med. School 14:1, 1940.

Koch, S. L., and Mason, M. L.: Division of

nerves and tendons of hand, with discussion on surgical treatment and its results, Surg., Gynec. Obstet. *56*:1, 1933.

Kopell, H. P., and Thompson, W. A. L.: Pronator syndrome, a confirmed case and its diagnosis, New Engl. J. Med. *259*:713, 1958.

Kune, G. A.: Ganglia causing ulnar nerve palsy, Aust. New Zeal. J. Surg. *31*:322, 1962.

Larsen, R. D., and Posch, J. L.: Nerve injuries in the upper extremity, Arch. Surg. *77*:469, 1958.

Lewin, P.: Delayed or tardy ulnar palsy, Surg. Clin. N. Amer. *5*:1077, 1925.

Lexer, E.: Muscular incision and muscular neurotization, Beitr. klin. Chir. *141*:436, 1927.

Littler, J. W.: Neurovascular skin island transfer in reconstructive hand surgery *in* Wallace, A. B. (ed.): Trans. Internat. Soc. Plast. Surg., Second Congress, London, p. 175, Edinburgh, Livingstone, 1959.

Lyons, W. R., and Woodhall, B.: Atlas of Peripheral Nerves, Philadelphia, Saunders, 1949.

MacKenzie, I. G., and Woods, C. G.: Causes of failure after repair of the median nerve, J. Bone Joint Surg. *43-B*:465, 1961.

McMurray, T. P.: Use and abuse of splints and other instruments in treatment of nerve lesions, Brit. J. Phys. Med. *5*:20, 1942.

Manzini, V.: Some remarks on the etiology of the carpal tunnel compression of the median nerve, Bull. Hosp. Joint Dis. *22*:56, 1961.

Mannerfelt, L.: Evaluation of functional sensation of skin grafts in the hand area, Brit. J. Plast. Surg. *15*:136, 1962.

Mason, M. L.: Injuries to nerves and tendons of hands, J.A.M.A. *116*:1375, 1941.

Meadoff, N.: Median nerve injuries in fractures in the region of the wrist, Calif. Med. *70*:252, 1949.

Merle d'Aubigné, R.: Symposium on reconstructive surgery of paralysed upper limb; treatment of residual paralysis after injuries of main nerves (upper extremity), Proc. Roy. Soc. Med. *42*:249, 1949.

Moberg, E.: Objective methods for determining the functional value of sensibility in the hand, J. Bone Joint Surg. *40-B*:3, 1958.

————: Examination of sensory loss by the ninhydrin printing test in Volkmann's contracture, Bull. Hosp. Joint Dis. *21*:296, 1960.

————: Peripheral nerves and hand function, editorial, J. Bone Joint Surg. *43-B*:423, 1961.

Muller, A., and Muller, R.: Principles and rules for preliminary and after-treatment in trauma of motor system, Arch. klin. Chir. *201*:775, 1941.

Murphey, F., Kirklin, J. W., and Finlayson, A. I.:

Anomalous innervation of the intrinsic muscles of the hand, Surg., Gynec. Obstet. *83*:15, 1946.

Napier, J. R.: Use of splints in peripheral nerve injuries, Brit. J. Phys. Med. *14*:1, 1951

Ney, K. W.: Treatment of nerve injuries, Mil. Surgeon *49*:277, 1921.

Nissen, K. I.: Pain in the arm and the carpal tunnel syndrome, Postgrad. M. J. *35*:379, 1959.

Önne, L.: Recovery of sensibility and sudomotor activity in the hand after nerve suture, Acta chir. scand., Supp. 300, 1962.

Peacock, E. E., Jr.: Reconstruction of the hand by the local transfer of composite tissue island flaps, Plast. Reconstr. Surg. *25*:298, 1960.

Peer, L.: Transplantation of Tissues, vol. 1, Baltimore, Williams & Wilkins, 1955.

Perret, G.: Experimental and clinical investigations of peripheral nerve injuries of the upper extremities, J.A.M.A. *146*:556, 1951.

Phalen, G. S.: Spontaneous compression of the median nerve at the wrist, J.A.M.A. *145*:1128, 1951.

Phalen, G. S., *et al.*: Neuropathy of the median nerve due to compression beneath the transverse carpal ligament, J. Bone Joint Surg. *32-A*:109, 1950.

Phelps, W. M.: Orthopedic surgery in cerebral palsy, J. Bone Joint Surg. *39-A*:53, 1957.

Platt, H.: Results of bridging gaps in injured nerve trunks by autogenous fascial tubulization and autogenous nerve grafts, Brit. J. Surg. *7*:384, 1920.

————: Discussion on injuries of peripheral nerves, Proc. Roy. Soc. Med. *30*:863, 1937.

Platt, H., and Bristow, W. R.: Operation for injuries of peripheral nerves, Brit. J. Surg. *11*: 535, 1924.

Pollock, L. J.: Supplementary muscle movements in peripheral nerve lesions, Arch. Neurol. Psychiat. *2*:518, 1919.

————: Peripheral Nerve Injuries, New York, Hoeber, 1933.

Pollock, L. J., and Davis, L.: Peripheral Nerve Injuries, Am. J. Surg., Serial of 12 from 1932, Vol. 15 to Vol. 18.

Ranson, S. W.: Degeneration and regeneration of nerve fibers, J. Comp. Neurol. Psychiat. *22*: 487, 1912.

Raymon y Cajal, S.: Degeneration and Regeneration of the Nervous System (translated by R. M. May), London, Oxford Univ. Press, 1928.

Riordan, D. C.: The hand in leprosy, a seven-year clinical study, J. Bone Joint Surg. *42-A*: 661, 1960.

————: The hand in leprosy, a seven-year clinical study; Part II, orthopaedic aspects of leprosy, J. Bone Joint Surg. *42-A*:683, 1960.

Roaf, R.: Foramen in the humerus carved by the median nerve, J. Bone Joint Surg. *39-B*:748, 1957.

Rosenthal, A. M.: Electrodiagnostic testing in neuromuscular disease, J.A.M.A. *177*:829, 1961.

Sanders, F. K.: The repair of large gaps in the peripheral nerves, Brain *65*:281, 1942.

————: The fate of nerve homografts in the rabbit, J. Anat. *83*:80, 1949.

————: The preservation of nerve grafts *in* Preservation and transplantation of normal tissues, p. 175, CIBA Foundation Symposium, London, Churchill, 1954.

Sanders, F. K., and Young, J. Z.: Degeneration and re-innervation of grafted nerves, J. Anat. *76*:143, 1942.

Seddon, H. J.: The use of autogenous grafts for the repair of large gaps in peripheral nerves, Brit. J. Surg. *35*:151, 1947.

————: Nerve lesions complicating certain closed bone injuries, J.A.M.A. *135*:691, 1947.

————: War injuries of peripheral nerves, Brit. J. Surg. (Suppl.) *36*:325, 1949.

————: Peripheral nerve injuries in Great Britain during World War II, Arch. Neurol. & Psychiat. *63*:171, 1950.

Seddon, H. J. (ed.): Peripheral Nerve Injuries, Medical Research Council Report 282, H. M. Stationery Office, 1954.

Seddon, H. J., and Holmes, W.: Late condition of nerve homografts in man, Surg., Gynec. Obstet. *79*:342, 1944.

————: Ischaemic damage in the peripheral stump of a divided nerve, Brit. J. Surg. *32*:389, 1945.

Seddon, H. J., and Medawar, P. B.: Fibrin suture of human nerves, Lancet *143*:87, 1942.

Seddon, H. J., Young, J. Z., and Holmes, W.: Histologic condition of a nerve autograft in man, Brit. J. Surg. *29*:378, 1942.

Seletz, E.: Surgery of Peripheral Nerves, Springfield, Ill., Thomas, 1951.

Shaffer, J. M., and Cleveland, F.: Delayed suture of sensory nerves of the hand, Ann. Surg. *131*:556, 1950.

Solnitzky, O.: Pronator syndrome; compression neuropathy of the median nerve at level of pronator teres muscle, Georgetown M. Bull. *13*:232, 1960.

Spurling, R. G.: Peripheral nerve injuries, J.A.M.A. *129*:1011, 1945.

Stein, A. H., Jr., and Morgan, H. C.: Compression of the ulnar nerve at the level of the wrist, Am. Pract. *13*:195, 1962.

Steindler, A.: Pathokinetics of cerebral palsy, Inst. Course Lect., Am. Acad. Orth. Surg. *9*:118, 1952.

Stiles, H. J., and Forrester-Brown, M. F.: Treatment of Injuries of Peripheral Spinal Nerves. New York, Oxford Univ. Press, 1922.

Stookey, B.: Surgical and Mechanical Treatment of Peripheral Nerves, Philadelphia, Saunders, 1922.

Strange, F. G. St. C.: An operation for nerve pedicle grafting, preliminary communication, Brit. J. Surg. *34*:423, 1947.

————: Case report on pedicled nerve graft, Brit. J. Surg. *37*:331, 1950.

Stromberg, W. B., McFarlane, R. M., Bell, J. L., Koch, S. L., and Mason, M. L.: Injury of the median and ulnar nerves, J. Bone Joint Surg. *43-A*:717, 1961.

Sunderland, S.: Blood supply of nerves of upper limb in man, Arch. Neurol. Psychiat. *53*:91, 1945.

Swan, J., and Worster-Drought, C.: Discussion on injuries to peripheral nerves, Proc. Roy. Soc. Med. *34*:521, 1941.

Swanson, A. B.: Surgery of the hand in cerebral palsy and the swan neck deformity, J. Bone Joint Surg. *42-A*:951, 1959.

Tachdjian, M.: Sensory disturbances in the hands of children with cerebral palsy, J. Bone Joint Surg. *40-A*:85, 1958.

Tajima, T., and Morohashi, M.: Result of nerve repair in the upper extremity with special reference to the recovering process, J. Jap. Orthop. Surg. Soc. *32*:1136, 1959.

Tanzer, R.: The carpal tunnel syndrome, J. Bone Joint Surg. *41-A*:626, 1959.

Tarlov, I. M., and Benjamin, B.: Autologous plasma clot suture of nerves, Science *95*:258, 1942.

Tarlov, I. M., and Epstein, J.: Nerve grafts; importance of adequate blood supply, J. Neurosurg. *2*:49, 1945.

Tarlov, I. M., Hoffman, W., and Hayner, J. C.: Source of nerve autografts in clinical surgery, Am. J. Surg. *72*:700, 1946.

Thompson, I. M.: Diagnostic application of our knowledge of normal variability of cutaneous nerve areas, exemplified by median and ulnar nerves, J. Anat. *69*:159, 1935.

Thompson, W. A. L., and Kopell, H. P.: Peripheral entrapment neuropathies of the upper extremity, New Engl. J. Med. *260*:1261, 1959.

Thornburn, W.: End results of injuries to peripheral nerves treated by operation, Brit. M. J. *2*:462, 1920.

Tinker, M. B., and Tinker, M. B., Jr.: Repair of peripheral nerve injuries, Ann. Surg. *106*:943, 1937.

Tubiana, R., and Dupare, J.: Restoration of sensibility in the hand by neurovascular skin island transfer, J. Bone Joint Surg. *43-B*:474, 1961.

Tubiana, R., Dupare, J., and Moreau, C.: Restoration of sensation to the hand by transplant of heterodigital skin as neurovascular pedicle, Rev. chir. orth. *46*:163, 1960.

Von Muralt: Neurophysiology, Lancet *266*:473, 1954.

Ward, L. E., Bickel, W. H., and Corbin, K. B.: Median neuritis (carpal tunnel syndrome) caused by gouty tophi, J.A.M.A. *167*:844, 1958.

Wartenberg, R.: Sign of ulnar palsy, J.A.M.A. *112*:1688, 1939.

Watkins, A. L., and Brazier, M. A. B.: Studies on muscle innervation in poliomyelitis and nerve injuries, Arch. Phys. Med. *26*:69, 1945.

Woodhall, B., and Lyons, W. R.: Peripheral nerve injuries, Surgery *19*:757, 1946.

Woods, A. H.: Misleading motor symptoms in diagnosis of nerve wounds, Arch. Neurol. Psychiat. *2*:532, 1919.

Young, J. Z., Holmes, W., and Sanders, F. K.: Nerve regeneration; importance of peripheral stump and value of nerve grafts, Lancet *2*:128, 1940.

Young, J. Z., and Medawar, P. B.: Fibrin suture of peripheral nerves; measurement of rate of regeneration, Lancet *2*:126, 1940.

Zachary, R. B.: Thenar palsy due to compression of the median nerve in the carpal tunnel, Surg., Gynec. Obstet. *81*:213, 1945.

Zachary, R. B., and Holmes, W.: Primary suture of nerves, Surg., Gynec. Obstet. *82*:632, 1946.

Zrubecky, G.: On the restoration of sensation to the tip of an insensitive thumb formed from abdominal skin; further study on the use of the sensory replacement operation, Zbl. Chir. *85*:1671, 1960.

Zrubecky, G., and Kreuz, L.: Die Hand, Das Tastorgan des Menschen, Stuttgart, Ferdinand Enke, 1960.

Chapter 11

Tendons

The restoration of tendon function in a disabled hand is difficult. While it is easy to suture a tendon and maintain apposition of the ends until union takes place, it is difficult to restore a mechanism which enables the tendon to glide smoothly in the tissues and through its full amplitude of motion.

Principles of primary care of tendon injuries are discussed in Chapter 15.

MORPHOLOGY

A tendon glides in the tissues by one of two mechanisms, in a sheath or in paratenon. Wherever a tendon passes across the concavity of a joint, a sheath and a pulley mechanism will be present. If the tendon pulls in a straight line or acts only to bring a joint to a straight line, it is surrounded by paratenon. These two mechanisms differ in their structure, respond in characteristic ways to trauma and differ in the reparative process. Extensor tendons on the back of the hand distal to the wrist provide typical examples of the paratenon mechanism. The digital flexor tendons illustrate a sheath mechanism.

PARATENON

Paratenon is a specialized loose tissue which fills the space between a tendon and the immovable fascial compartment through which the tendon moves. It is elastic and pliable with long fibers, allowing the tendon to move back and forth in either direction. Paratenon is not a true gliding mechanism; the tendon is not free, as in a sheath, but is intimately attached to the paratenon. The loose tissue is simply dragged with the tendon, its other end being attached to fascia or some fixed structure. In the forearm proximal to the radial and the ulnar bursae the tendons lie in paratenon, and even in the palm a small area of the flexor tendons of the index and the middle fingers and sometimes the ring finger is covered with paratenon.

TENDON SHEATH STRUCTURE

A tendon sheath mechanism consists of 2 layers of synovia: a visceral layer covering the tendon and a parietal layer lining the fascial tunnel through which the tendon glides. Just like the enveloping peritoneum, the parietal joins the visceral layer in a double layer, the mesotenon. This mesenterylike structure is loose and filmy and does not limit motion of the tendon. It is located on the convex side of the tendon away from friction and carries the blood vessels to the tendon. On the concave side, the friction-bearing tendon surface is compact and relatively avascular.

In its sheath formation the tendon is like a piston in a cylinder, gliding on a thin film of synovial fluid between the 2 surfaces just as the metal surfaces do on a film of oil.

As a tendon in a sheath glides back and forth, the ends of the sheath form invaginating folds. In a sagittal section one end or the other of these loose folds pulls out straight to allow the normal excursion. The visceral layer enveloping the tendon is called epitenon, and the outer layer is called the sheath. Fibrous septa running from the epitenon and dividing the tendon into bundles are called endotenon.

The mesotenon carries the blood vessels and is a thin transparent membrane. In the finger this mesotenon is reduced to 2 vincula, the longus and the brevis, carrying the vessels.

A pulley mechanism is necessary wherever a tendon spans the concavity of a joint. These annular ligaments are tough and fibrous, lined with the parietal synovia, and act to prevent bowstringing of the tendon which would destroy its mechanical efficiency. These pulleys or thickened parts of the fascial sheath are not opposite the joints but between them. They are essential to proper tendon function and should be preserved or reconstructed. At the wrist the volar and the dorsal retinacular ligaments represent a similar mechanism.

The blood supply of a tendon is from both ends—its origin and its insertion and through the vincula. The profundus tendons in the palm also gain some blood supply through the lumbricals. Vessels enter the tendon on the mesotenon side, run longitudinally in the epitenon on the nonfriction side and send branches at right angles along the endotenon septa.

RESPONSE OF TENDONS TO INJURY AND INFECTION

When a tendon is cleanly severed in a sheath, its ends round over and lie free in the synovial cavity. If a tendon is severed in para-tenon, a proliferation of the paratenon covering and the endotenon takes place, sending out fibrous projections which adhere to the surrounding structures and contract. This healing process is so pronounced that many extensor tendon repairs occur without formal suturing of the ends if the severed parts are prevented from retracting.

If infection occurs when a tendon is severed in a sheath or if the sheath itself is damaged as from a crush, the tendon end will attach to the surrounding cicatrix. Infection in para-tenon likewise increases the scar formation.

Tendons lying in the firm tunnels of the pulley mechanisms, e.g., in the finger or under the volar carpal ligament, suffer great damage when swelling from trauma or infection occurs. Because they are lying in a closed space, swelling results in ischemia and then necrosis. A sloughing tendon is replaced by scar which joins that in the sheath, contracting and flexing the joints. The result is a firm fibrous cord which cannot be drawn out by splints or physiotherapy.

When a tendon is severed and the end is free, the muscle contracts. As long as 2 months after injury direct approximation usually can be made, but after that the muscle contracture cannot be overcome.

Tendons become soft and thick from disuse and are too friable for grafts. If the tendon end has been adherent so that some muscle activity has kept it on tension, it will maintain some texture.

A tendon severed in paratenon will attempt to link its severed ends by reaching out with new fibrous processes. Sometimes, a thick cordlike mass even larger than the tendon is formed, as in unrepaired wrist flexors, or sometimes, as in the palm, a thin gray jellylike tube. This process is so efficient that in lacerations of the wrist where multiple structures are severed, most experienced surgeons concentrate their efforts on the digital tendons and do not suture either the flexor carpi radialis or the flexor carpi ulnaris tendons. In other areas, this ordinarily useful and functional activity of the tendon is detrimental, but steps can be taken to prevent its harmful effects.

If the "unsatisfied" end of a tendon should attach to some fixed part, then that tendon's function is impaired. A tendon of a common muscle such as the profundus, if severed in the palmar area where it lies in paratenon, will

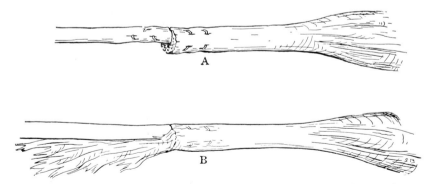

Fig. 476. If there is left an "unsatisfied" end of a tendon, or if, in suturing together a small and a large tendon, part of the latter end is left exposed or "unsatisfied" (A), that part will grow, principally from its epitenon, a pseudopodium (B) which will reach out and attach itself to the surrounding tissues and contract, so that the motion of the tendon will be checked. (J. Bone Joint Surg. *14*:31)

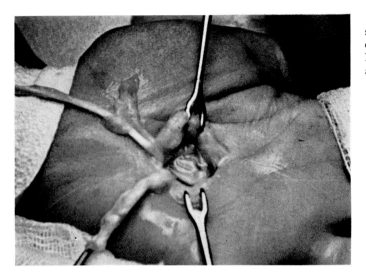

Fig. 477. Both flexor tendons severed in a finger have been withdrawn through a palmar incision. Note the hypertrophied paratenon around the superficialis.

attach itself and hold back the other tendons of their common muscle. The same thing may result if, in an amputation, the tendon adheres to or is sutured to the stump. Holding the ring finger in extension while attempting to flex the remaining fingers illustrates this hold-back effect.

When a small diameter tendon is sutured end-to-end to one of larger caliber, some means of enclosing the unsatisfied end is necessary, or it will reach out, attach to surrounding tissues and limit motion. In tendon transfers where an active tendon is used as a donor and attached to one or more recipient tendons,

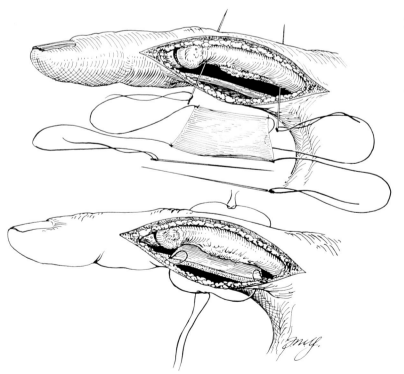

Fig. 478. When an adherent tendon is freed from bone or a fixed fascial structure, it will attach promptly unless some gliding material is interposed. Illustrated is a method of placing a thin layer of paratenon or a patch of polyethylene film. Fine catgut sutures passed through the skin remain long enough to allow fixation of the graft.

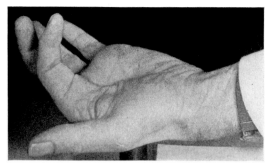

FIG. 479. Loss of the pulley at the base of the finger results in spanning of the flexor tendon and decreases the efficiency of the flexor mechanism.

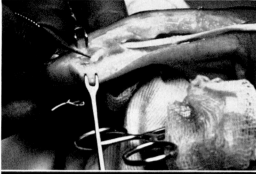

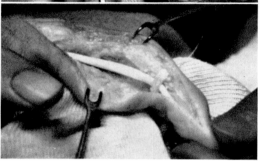

the loose free end of the donor should be buried within the substance of a tendon. If the distal end of a cut tendon is left free in the finger and there is infection, hematoma or sheath damage, it will attach and contract and draw the finger into contracture.

When a tendon is partially severed or is crushed and bruised from a closed injury, it swells and softens. Such healing tendons often rupture from ordinary muscle pull several days to 3 weeks later.

A healing tendon requires rest, but whenever possible all other uninjured parts are allowed and encouraged to move. A hand that remains swollen and edematous is the ideal setting for the development of fibrosis in and around tendons, ligaments and joint capsules. Early movement as soon as the healing of the tissues allows it is the best means of preventing stiffness. Dynamic splinting to help correct position allows motion while correction is taking place.

through the middle segment pulley which
FIG. 480. (*Top*) A tendon graft is passed has been preserved carefully. (*Bottom*) The normal pulley has been damaged irreparably, but a slip of the flexor superficialis has been left attached at its normal insertion on the ulnar side and its proximal end swung across to be attached to the phalanx on the radial side.

HEALING OF TENDONS

When cut tendon ends are held together by appropriate suture methods, the healing process is a progressive fibrosis and reconstitution of the tendon.

FIG. 481. Repairing an annular ligament or pulley using removable stainless-steel wire tied over a bolster to minimize the tissue reaction compared with that from silk or catgut.

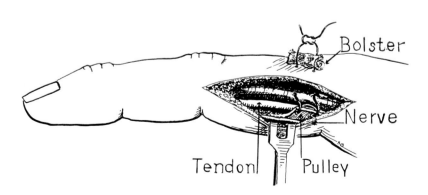

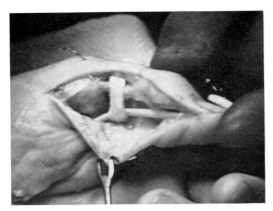

FIG. 482. A pulley mechanism for the thumb flexor can be provided by a tendon graft attached to the phalanx on each side. A completely encircling pulley at this location, even though it passes subcutaneously on the dorsum, tends to interfere with extensor function.

FIRST WEEK

In this week the fibroblastic splint is formed. A translucent jellylike substance joins the 2 ends in a soft fusiform swelling, and connective tissue cells start to grow into this. The tendon ends become red and swollen for about ½ inch due to increased vascularity and connective tissue proliferation. The connective tissue elements in and about the tendon contribute to this early repair by growing out as fibroblasts into the homogeneous jellylike substance and soon converting to connective tissue fibers. This process comes not from the tendon cells but from the epitenon, the tendon sheath, the paratenon and the endotenon. During the first week the tendon ends become joined by this swollen fibroblastic splint, formidable looking but devoid of strength. Proliferation of the cells within the tendon commences only after the 4th or the 5th day.

SECOND WEEK

During this week connective tissue proliferates. Swelling of the tendon increases to its maximum, and there is much redness, vascularity, edema and, especially, proliferation of the connective tissue elements which bridge the gap between the tendon ends but do not furnish strength. Through this connective tissue and jellylike mass the ingrowth of tendon fibers and cells begins to be conspicuous by the 8th day and bridges the gap between the 10th and the 14th days. Until the ends of the tendon are bridged by tendon fibers and collagen, the juncture can be ruptured easily. The fusiform mass of tendon juncture is continuous with the surrounding tissues, which aid the 2 tendon ends in furnishing vascularity.

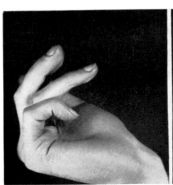
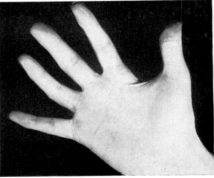
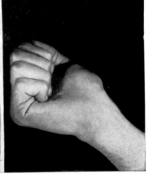

FIG. 483. Case M. S. (*Left*) Limitation of flexion of the fingers from an automobile accident. There was a laceration across the palm, fracturing the metacarpals, and followed by infection. At operation, the tendons were freed from dense adhesions to the metacarpals, and a sheet of paratenon fat from over the triceps tendon was grafted beneath them. The sublimis tendons to the long and the ring fingers were so rough that they were removed from the palm and the fingers and their proximal ends sutured into the profundus tendon. Two severed nerves were sutured. (*Center* and *right*) Full range of motion and sensation returned 4 months later.

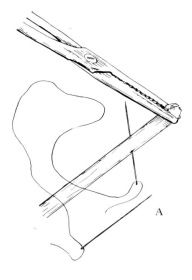

A

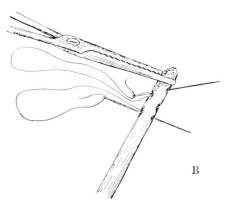

B

Fig. 484. Showing the former method of uniting tendons end-to-end with silk. The delicate epitenon is not traumatized.

As shown in (A), with the tendon held taut by a Kocher hemostat, 1 of the 2 needles is passed through it diagonally, starting about 1 cm. back. Three similar stitches in all are taken with this needle. At each, the needle re-enters the tendon a short transverse distance from where it emerged, and finally the needle emerges 2 or 3 mm. from the hemostat, but on the opposite side of the tendon from where it first entered.

In (B) is shown the other needle starting its first stitch transversely across the tendon, entering only a few fibers transversely away from where the first needle entered (reversed in the diagram). With this needle, 3 diagonal stitches are taken, just as with the first needle, emerging from the tendon directly opposite where the first needle emerged.

The traumatized cicatricial tip of the tendon is snipped off, as in (C), and in the inset the stitch is shown as it will be when finally placed.

In (D), while the tendon is held taut over the finger by one suture, the other suture is passed back through the point where it emerged and is made to emerge from the end of the tendon on that same side.

Then each suture is pulled firmly to remove all slack and is tied to the suture opposite it, which emerges from the end of the other tendon, and the result is as shown in the inset.

(J. Bone Joint Surg. *10*:10)

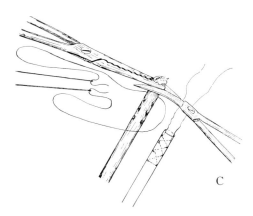

C

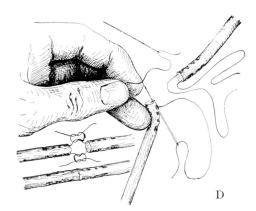

D

THIRD WEEK

During this week production of tendon collagen fibers takes place. The juncture is still swollen and vascular but is firmer and a little less red. Tendon fibers have formed across the gap, and increased mitosis of the cells between them can be seen extending from 1 cm. back into each tendon end. The juncture, which was quite soft during the first 4 days and firmer in the 2nd week, now has a definitely firm feeling, since the soft edematous tissue is being

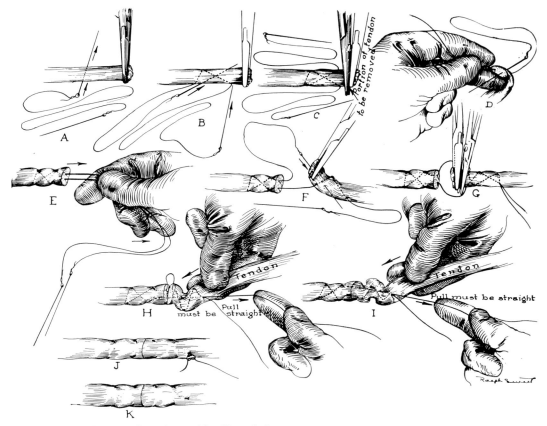

FIG. 485. Suture of tendons with silk technic.

(A to D) With a thread and 2 needles, the sutures are placed traversing the tendon with each needle from 2 to 4 times and emerging through the end.

(E) All slack is drawn out.

(F, G) The suture is continued similarly up the other tendon. Both ends are brought out at the same spot. In placing the last strand in the second tendon end, the needle must not spear the other thread or they will not slip. By keeping the needles on separate sides of the tendon this is avoided, or better, both needles may be thrust through the tendon simultaneously.

(H, I) To prevent the tendon ends from separating under strain, the slack is removed from the second tendon. To do this, one suture is pulled at a time as the tendon is shoved along it to snug against the other tendon end.

(J, K) There is only one knot; when tied, it sinks into the tendon at a place where it receives the least strain, since knots are the weakest parts of a tendon suture.

replaced by connective tissue and tendon fibers. Already, at the juncture between the tendon and the surrounding tissue a cleavage or separation is taking place to allow for movement of the tendon. By the end of the 3rd week there is a fair degree of strength present, largely from formation of the strong tendon collagen fibers themselves. Nelson Howard suggested that the long spindle-shaped cells within a tendon are flat oval endothelial cells in the walls of longitudinal canals throughout the tendon. The strong cords of collagen composing the bulk of the tendon are the products of connective tissue cells and are arranged parallel and longitudinally in response to stress of tension.

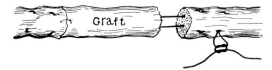

FIG. 486. Bridging a tendon by a short tendon graft, using a silk suture. The silk is fastened to one tendon end and threaded through the graft, while the latter is held taut by 2 hemostats, and then braided through the distal tendon end. To slide the tendon ends together, each silk strand is tightened alternately, not at the same time. A tiny suture may be used to keep the graft from sliding away from a tendon end.

FOURTH WEEK

It is during this week that resolution takes place. The swelling and the vascularity decrease, and the loosening of the tendon from the surrounding tissues already allows some degree of gliding. By the end of the 4th week there is good strength in the juncture, though not quite equal to normal.

The process of repair in paratenon formation takes place faster and more luxuriantly than in sheath formation, since the vascularity from the surrounding tissues is greater, and the proliferation of the paratenon itself adds strength.

Repair of a tendon sutured within a sheath is dependent on the blood supply from the

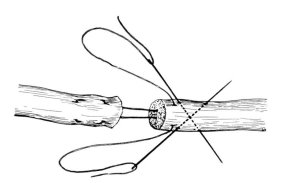

FIG. 487. In suturing tendons with silk, if a needle penetrates a silk strand, the tendon cannot be slid down the suture against the other tendon end. To avoid this, both needles are thrust through the second tendon end simultaneously.

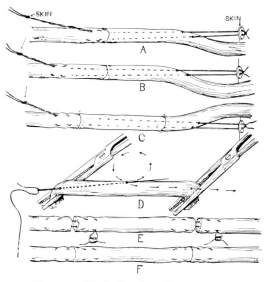

FIG. 488. Methods of tendon suture.

(A, B, C) Stainless-steel pull-out sutures.

(A) Threading the suture through the distal tendon end holds the tendon ends in good approximation. The pull-out wire is twisted to prevent tissue growing between and hindering withdrawal.

(B) Placing the splicing part of the suture at a distance to lessen adhesions at the important place, the junction.

(C) A short graft may be threaded on the suture wires. A tiny stitch of the finest silk keeps each end of the graft opposed to the tendon end.

(D) Method of threading the sutures longitudinally through a tendon.

(E, F) Inserting a graft between tendon ends, using a silk suture. Short grafts may be threaded on the silk as in (C).

damaged sheath or from the surrounding soft tissues. If a tendon within a sheath is completely blocked, as with polythene, the new blood vessels are prevented from entering into the healing process, and healing is delayed. This granulation tissue from the soft tissues carrying the blood supply to the repaired tendon turns to scar. If this scar is adherent to a fixed point such as a fascial plane or a pulley, motion will be limited. If the scar is soft and elastic and in paratenon, it will not interfere with the gliding of the tendon. For this reason Mason recommended excision of the

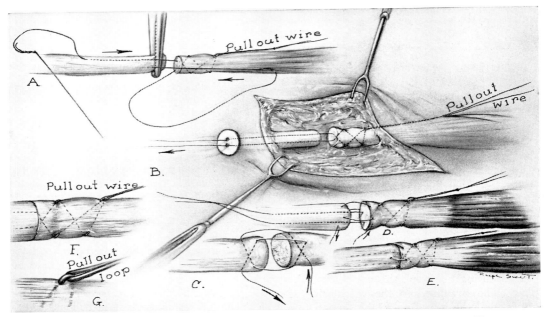

Fig. 489. Suturing a tendon with removable stainless-steel wire. After 3 weeks, a silk suture has fulfilled its mission and, if it remains, is merely an irritating foreign body. Only one tendon end pulls, the other being passive. (B) The button on the skin spares the juncture from muscle pull. (B, G) A pull-out wire is brought out through the skin to withdraw the suture in 3 weeks. (Inset C and E) Showing the double right-angle suture of finest silk used merely for approximation and rarely necessary.

sheath or the pulley at the level of the tendon junction.

ACTIVITY AND TENDON HEALING

The experiments of Mason and Allen on the effect of function on healing of tendons showed that comparing the process in mobilized tendons with that in immobilized tendons there was no difference in the strength of the union up to the 15th day, but the mobilized tendon was more swollen and more adherent. From 15 to 21 days both improved in strength, but after that only the exercised tendon continued to improve in strength. The immobilized tendon showed the least reaction to its surroundings and the best appearance.

Since excessive activity during the first 15 days is apparently detrimental, it seems to be best to allow the tendon to rest and then use graded activity up to 21 days. After that some increased activity is desirable but not maximal pull until the end of the 4th week.

In exercising to pull the flexor tendon through the finger, the proximal segment should be held to move the tendon past the middle joint and then the middle segment to move it through the distal joint.

A tendon completely freed from its surrounding blood supply or a free tendon graft requires the same staged control of its activity. Freeing a damaged tendon of dense enveloping scar and then demanding constant daily activity is the best way to cause rupture of the tendon.

TECHNIC OF TENDON REPAIR

It is easy to repair a tendon but difficult to obtain a good gliding tendon when healing is complete. Scar tissue binds the tendon in its bed, limiting its excursion. The surgeon's problem is to expose the tendon and suture it in such a way that this scarring is minimal and yet to maintain apposition of the tendon ends until new tendon fibers grow across the gap.

In a primary repair, additional exposure will be required to locate the retracted tendon ends. This surgical trauma added to that of

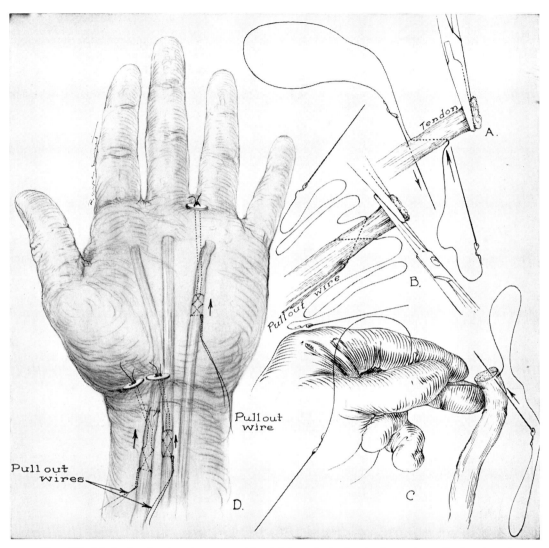

FIG. 490. Methods of using the removable stainless-steel wire tendon suture. Each suture has a pull-out wire for use after 3 weeks. The suture is placed in the muscled tendon end only and fastened outside the skin to a button. In the hand are 3 types of suture, the first being called "suture at a distance" because it is made remote from the juncture to avoid causing adhesions. The pull-out wire may be twisted to avoid catching tissue in its loop.

the injury must be minimized by careful atraumatic technic, gentleness in handling of tissues, hemostasis and prevention of infection. For principles of primary tendon repair see Chapter 15, Wounds.

In secondary repairs and reconstructions the problem is to restore tendon function by repair, graft or transfer in a part already damaged and scarred. Dissecting out damaged tendons and nerves from a mass of scar requires skill, patience, a knowledge of anatomy and a plan. Starting in good tissues away from the scar and identifying the structures, one works toward the damaged area from each end. Sharp dissection with the knife is preferable to scissors technic, and the use of a tendon stripper is reserved for removal of irreparable tendon masses.

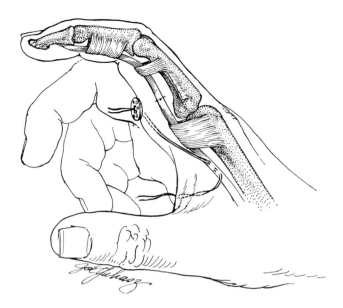

FIG. 491. When a tendon severed in the sheath is repaired by a pull-out suture in the palm and simple approximating sutures in the finger, the sheath and any part of the pulley mechanism lying directly over the junction should be excised rather than incised.

All proliferating paratenon should be excised, and the scar surrounding a tendon as well as the damaged tendon itself should be removed. To dissect out a tendon from a mass of scar and then place a tendon graft on this cicatricial bed or against raw bone or a cut edge of a fascial compartment is to court failure. Deep cicatrix should be excised back to normal tissue and bone or to fascia covered with an interposed layer of paratenon or a local flap of gliding material.

In a reconstructive procedure involving many tendons, the decision regarding restoration of the most useful function is made after all the dissection has been completed. Ade-

quate motors and sufficient tendons to provide the needed motion are obtained by grafts or transfers and a gliding mechanism restored. A fundamental rule is a minimal number of moving parts and a maximal amount of gliding material.

SUTURING TECHNIC

Principle. In joining a tendon end-to-end by suture the object is to hold the ends together firmly until physiologic union occurs. After 3 weeks the suture material is superfluous. The amount of suture material or foreign body should be kept to a minimum. It is better to have 2 strong strands than multiple weak

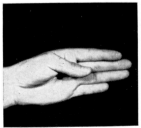 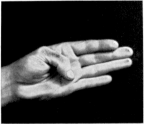 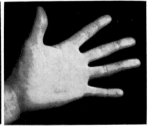

FIG. 492. Case M. B. The flexor pollicis longus had been severed by a knife puncture wound through the thenar eminence 10 days previously. (*Left*) The scar and loss of flexion of the distal joint of the thumb are shown. The tendon was recovered at the base of the thenar eminence and was fastened to its distal end by a removable stainless-steel wire suture which passed on down the thumb to be fastened outside the skin to a button. (*Center* and *right*) Taken 6 months later, these 2 pictures show complete recovery.

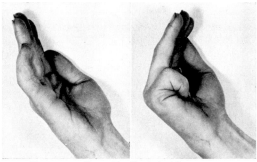

FIG. 493. Case T. C. A knife cut across the base of the little finger had severed both flexor tendons and one nerve of the little finger. Primary débridement and suture of the profundus tendon by pull-out and volar digital nerve in the little finger. These pictures show the result in the little finger. Sensation returned.

strands. The suture should be braided or spliced into a length of tendon to give adequate strength and not placed in such a way as to strangle the tendon tissue. A core suture is preferable to a surface suture. The latter produces adhesions on the surface of the tendon where they are least wanted. All the slack should be taken up before the tendon ends are approximated. Otherwise, this will be worked out later, and the tendon ends will separate. The

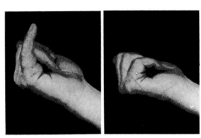

FIG. 494. Case M. S. While the patient was skinning a deer, the knife had lacerated across the base of the little finger. The wound healed per primam, and a month later, while lifting a sheep, he could no longer flex his finger. (*Left*) Showing lack of flexion after secondary tendon rupture. At operation, both flexors were found to be severed at the proximal pulley. The sublimis tendon was removed, but the profundus tendon was united directly, using removable stainless-steel wire and fastening it to a button down the side of the finger. (*Right*) Degree of flexion obtained 3 months later.

part of the tendon in the bite of the suture will undergo necrosis, but this will be followed by gradual substitution of good tendon tissue.

Formerly, silk was spliced in each tendon end so that 2 strands emerged from the cut end of each tendon. The slack was pulled out, and the opposing silk strands tied to each other, leaving 2 knots between the tendon ends. Now the silk, after being placed in one tendon end and the slack drawn out, is continued, splicing it up the other tendon end where its slack is also drawn out. Pulling 1 strand at a time to slide the tendon end down over this straightened strand snugs the tendon ends together. Then a single knot is tied and allowed to sink into the tendon. The advantages are 1 knot instead of 2, no knots between the tendon ends, and the knot, which is the vulnerable part, placed where it will be subject to the least strain. This technic, with stainless steel wire instead of silk, is now preferred wherever the suture material is to be left in place. Whenever possible the removal "pullout wire" technic is used.

Buried-Wire Technic. Because silk is prone to produce foreign body reactions, 34-gauge stainless steel Halliday suture wire is recommended for flexor tendons. For a flexor tendon of a finger the smallest size that will withstand a 3-pound pull should be used.

A piece of wire 30 cm. long is threaded at each end with a spear-point Bunnell needle. Each tendon end to be joined is grasped at

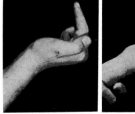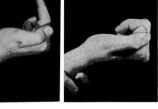

FIG. 495. Case J. B., age 11. (*Left*) Six weeks previously, the flexor tendons of the index finger opposite the metacarpal head had been severed by a glass bottle. The tendons were sutured with removable stainless-steel wire, and the volar digital nerve was also sutured. (*Right*) Four months later, the tip lacked only ⅜ inch of touching the distal crease in the palm. Sensation returned.

its very tip by a hemostat and held taut. Commencing 1.5 cm. back, each needle is passed back and forth through the tendon 3 or 4 times in opposite directions progressively down the tendon, to exit just above the clamp on the tendon end. Then the crushed portion of the tendon is cut off, and each needle is passed through the cut end of the tendon. After drawing them taut to remove the slack, the sutures are passed on up the opposite tendon end in the same way and brought out about 1.5 cm. up. One of the strands is pulled straight and taut, and one tendon end is slid down over it until it pushes against the other. Then the second strand is drawn straight and taut. The 2 strands are tied, sinking the knot into the depth of the tendon. At a 5-pound pull the tendon begins to separate. Where a tendon glides freely, as in the forearm or the base of the palm or does not turn a corner, this buried wire suture is satisfactory. A strong, fine, flexible twisted stainless steel wire, "Fagersta" or its equivalent sizes in Surgaloy, can be used. It has less tendency to kink than monofilament wire.

SUTURING TENDON GRAFTS. The same technic is used in suturing a tendon graft to a tendon end; but when a short graft of 2 or 3 cm. is simply spliced in a tendon, the graft is merely threaded over the 2 strands of wire and held in this position between the tendon ends. It may be attached to each tendon end by a fine approximation suture of nerve silk but only if necessary. To pass the 2 sutures longitudinally through a short segment of tendon graft, the graft is held taut at each end

by a hemostat. Then the hemostats are rolled away from each other slightly, and the long, straight needles are thrust longitudinally through the length of the graft, drawing the suture after them. The ends of the graft are clipped off.

Technic of Removable Stainless Steel Wire Tendon Suture. PRINCIPLE. Suture material for tendon repair must be nonabsorbable to hold for 3 weeks. Most materials act as foreign bodies and provoke fibrous, proliferative reactions. Stainless steel wire, chosen because it is the least irritating suture, is smooth and strong. A tendon sutured with wire shows less tissue reaction than with silk, which formerly was the choice for tendon suture. Tantalum is inert in tissues, but its tensile strength is low and it does not tie smoothly.

When a tendon junction sutured with wire is subjected to constant angulation, as when opposite a wrist or other joint, inspection later reveals either that the wire has fragmented into many pieces and is embedded in the tendon but doing no harm or that some tissue reaction from mechanical irritation is present. At insertions and where tendons pull straight without angulating, the wire suture remains inert in the tissues. The removable-wire technic eliminates any mechanical irritation and holds the tendon in place for the necessary 3 weeks, at which time physiologic union has taken place; then the suture is withdrawn.

The tension or pull on a tendon suture is from one end only, that to which the muscle is attached; the other end of the tendon remains passive. Therefore, the wire suture is

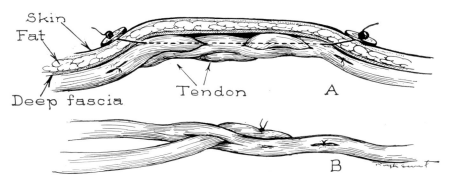

FIG. 496. Method of interweaving tendons, using withdrawable stainless-steel wire. One tendon entwines through the other. Free tendon ends are buried.

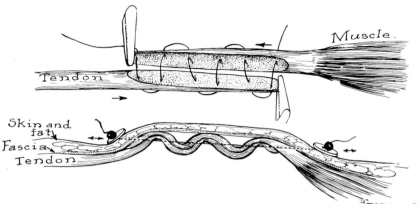

FIG. 497. Running suture of removable stainless-steel wire for use in joining tendons side-to-side. The wire is tightened and fastened by 2 shot. This straightens the wire but makes the tendon undulate. Wire withdrawn without resistance.

spliced into the proximal end only, is passed on down the limb through the other tendon and brought out through the skin, there to be fastened firmly over a button or to the fingernail. Thus, the proximal end of the tendon is held distalward against the passive distal tendon end.

Placing a pull-out wire under the proximal loop of the stitch makes it possible to remove the suture. Both ends of this wire are threaded on a needle and brought out through the skin proximal to the tendon juncture and left there. In 3 weeks the sutures are clipped off where they emerge at the button, and the pull-out wire is pulled gently; this withdraws the wire suture. If there is any resistance, a small rubber band is fastened to the pull-out wire and to adhesive plaster up the limb; within 24 hours the suture will be out. The "pull-out wire" technic is used primarily at the insertion

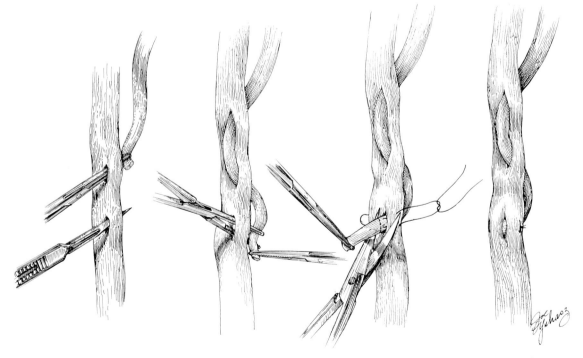

FIG. 498. The tendon of an active muscle can be woven into one or more recipient tendons in tendon-transfer operations. No free exposed tendons remain to become attached to surrounding tissues.

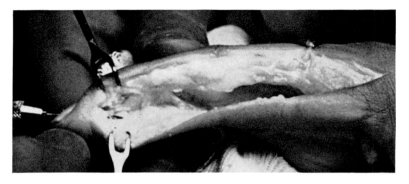

FIG. 499. Fastening tendon to bone. A drill passed through nail and phalanx to the opening in the volar cortex leaves a tract through which the 2 wires of the tendon suture are brought and tied over a button.

or whenever a tendon is fastened into bone.

In placing stainless steel wire great care should be taken never to allow it to kink, or the wire will break. As the loop of each bite is pulled, the assistant follows it with a probe to prevent kinking.

The following are various applications in the use of the removable stainless steel tendon suture.

END-TO END. The suture, doubly armed with straight needles, is passed back and forth through the tendon, each time crossing just a few tendon fibers and always progressing until it emerges from the tendon end. Before commencing with the second needle, a strand of similar wire is laid across the suture to be used as a "pull-out." Then the second needle is passed back and forth through the tendon to emerge from its distal end, just as did the first, the second needle having passed through the tendon 3 and the first 4 times.

The ends of the suture are pulled to remove

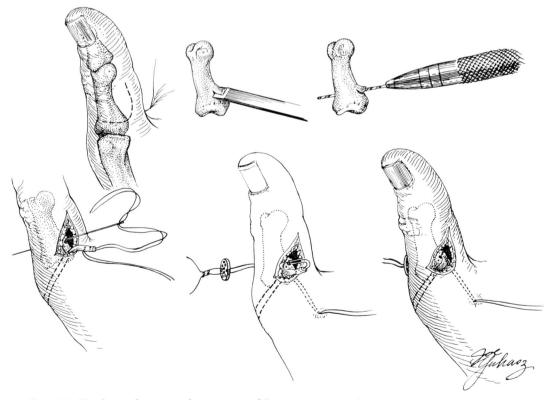

FIG. 500. Tendon to bone attachment as used in opponens transfer operation. The tendon is held in place for 3 weeks, after which the suture is withdrawn with the pull-out loop.

FIG. 501. The steps in proper attachment of flexor tendon to distal phalanx, using the pull-out wire technic. (*Top*) A flap of cortex is elevated at the site of proposed insertion, and the drill is aimed from the dorsum of the midportion of the nail to the exposed bone. (*Center*) A loop of wire is passed through nail and phalanx as a guide wire. Both ends of the tendon suture wire are passed through the loop of the guide wire. (*Bottom*) The raw cut end of the tendon is brought snugly up against the raw surface of the bone, and the suture is tied over a button on the nail. The pull-out loop is passed through the skin of the volar surface in the midline and at such a point proximally that the entire suture course is a straight line.

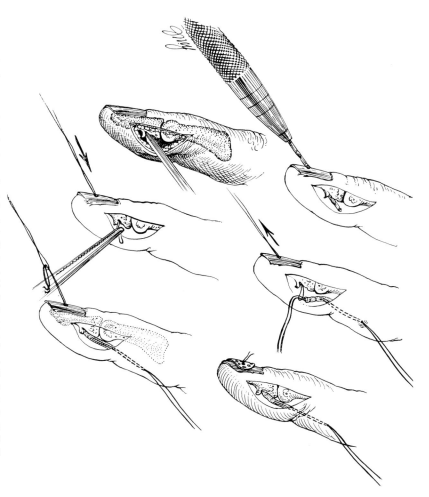

all the slack from the tendon, and the ends of the pull-out wire are drawn up to narrow its loop so that it will not catch tissue when it is withdrawn. The loop should not be squeezed closed with forceps because it may kink and be weakened. Before removing the forceps from the tendon end, the pull-out wire and the suture should be pulled back and forth through the tendon just as with a subcuticular suture so that it will withdraw easily. Next,

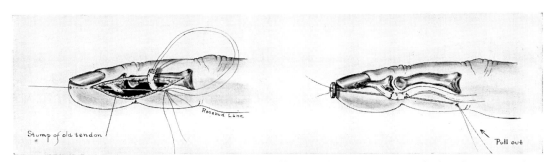

FIG. 502. Method of attaching a tendon to the distal phalanx in a finger, utilizing the stump of the old tendon and using removable stainless-steel wire.

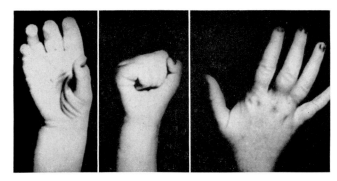

Fig. 503. Primary repair of all structures on volar aspect of wrist. Recovery of full motion and all intrinsics 1 year later. Child age 6.

both ends of the pull-out wire are threaded on a curved skin needle which is passed along the tendon and out through the skin. Then the 2 suture ends are passed on their needles longitudinally down the center of the distal part of the tendon for 2 or 3 cm. The tendon is held at its tip with a hemostat which is rotated a little and draws the tendon taut while the needles are inserted. The part of the tendon held by the hemostat is cut off. The sutures pass on up the sheath a little and then diagonally out through the skin to be anchored over a button or to the nail. If suturing is done in the forearm, the sutures are brought out through the annular ligament and fastened by a button outside the heel of the palm.

END-TO-END SUTURE AT A DISTANCE. The object is to utilize the wire and the pull-out feature to overcome the muscle pull but have only a minimal amount of material at the suture line. The suture is placed exactly as in the end-to-end type but proximal to the juncture and then is passed down the tendon sheath and out the skin and anchored at such tension that the tendon ends will be in approximation. These ends may be approximated with a simple double right-angle stitch of the finest nerve silk. Usually, the tendon ends will lie together without the necessity of any approximation suture. The suture "at a distance" is advisable when the tendon juncture is in a narrow tunnel, as in a finger, where adhesions caused by the presence of a suture would be detrimental. The pull-out wire is placed as above.

TENDON-TO-BONE. In fastening a tendon to a bone, a simple method is first to chip up an osteoperiosteal flap from the surface of the bone and then to drill and pass a straight needle with the tendon suture ends through

the hole in the bone and out the skin on the opposite side of the limb. The tendon end is drawn snugly against the raw bone as the wires are passed through 2 holes of a button and tied. A pull-out stitch is placed as usual. To facilitate withdrawal, the hole in the bone

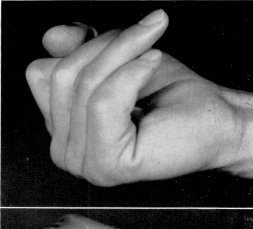

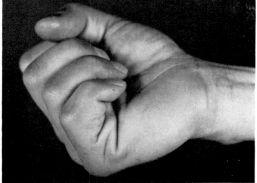

Fig. 504. Case H. G. (*Top*) The hand had gone through a window, being lacerated across the bases of the last 3 fingers, injuring the flexor tendons. (*Bottom*) Freeing the tendons gave an excellent result.

should be drilled obliquely in the line of the pull-out wire instead of at a right angle to it. A fine Kirschner wire can be used instead of a drill. There should be intimate tendon-to-bone approximation free from interposed tissue. This method is suitable for joining tendons or ligaments to bone anywhere in the body.

ATTACHING FLEXOR TENDON TO DISTAL PHALANX IN A FINGER. Through the mid-lateral incision the volar cortex of the distal phalanx is penetrated with a small chisel. A hole is made diagonally, penetrating the dorsum of the nail and the phalanx, emerging where the latter was bared. A pin vise with a No. 60 twist drill is used. A loop of fine wire is passed through the drill hole into the finger, and the ends of the tendon suture are passed through the loop and drawn out through the phalanx, there to be tied over a button on the surface of the fingernail. This holds the tendon end snugly against the bare bone. A pull-out wire should be placed so that the suture can be withdrawn after 3 weeks. If the tendon is attached too far distally on the phalanx, it will have too much leverage, and the distal joint will stay flexed.

Another method is to preserve the stump of the flexor tendon cut squarely off at its insertion. The needles and the tendon suture are passed through this and on out the tip of the finger and tied over a button. A pull-out wire is placed as usual. This junction is not as strong as that of tendon to bone.

SIDE-TO-SIDE UNION. This type of suture is useful only where the tendon ends can be overlapped, as in the forearm. It is used in lengthening and in shortening tendons. The steel wire enters the limb through the skin proximal to the tendon juncture and then is made to pass back and forth through the overlapping tendon ends through the length of their overlapping and then brought out through the skin distal to the tendon juncture. On pulling taut the ends of the wire, which are then outside the skin, the wire straightens and can be drawn freely back and forth. A split lead shot is placed on each wire where it emerges from the skin. The wire is straight, but the tendon is zigzag. At the end of 3 weeks one end of the wire under the shot is cut off; the wire is withdrawn easily by pulling on its other end. The tendon will be firmly united and free from suture material.

SIDE-TO-SIDE SUTURE BY INTERWEAVING THE TENDONS. Where tendon ends are joined by overlapping, one tendon can be passed back and forth through slits made in the other tendon to give intimate contact and a splicing effect. The removable running stitch is placed just as in the side-to-side stitch.

END-TO-SIDE JUNCTURE. This is useful in

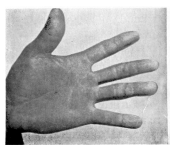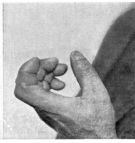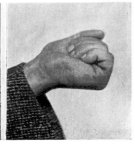

FIG. 505. Case D. B. (*Left*) The flexor tendons of the index, the long and the ring fingers were cut across at the middle phalanges. The distal joints hyperextended so that the fingers were useless to the patient in his sheet-metal work. Operation 1 month later consisted in uniting the severed ends of the tendons, using tendon clamps and lateral incisions, and planting a sleeve of free fat about each sutured tendon. The photograph shows the degree of voluntary extension and flexion of the distal interphalangeal joints. (*Center*) Showing good voluntary flexion in each distal interphalangeal joint after the repair of the flexor tendons in the first 3 fingers. (*Right*) Showing the normal amount of flexion obtained in the repaired fingers. (Surg., Gynec. Obstet. *26*:108)

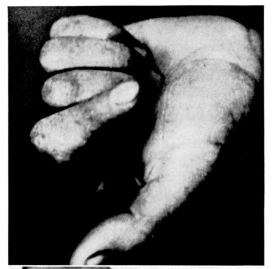

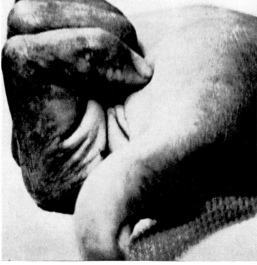

FIG. 506. When the profundus has been severed near the insertion, the cut end is advanced and inserted into the distal phalanx by a pull-out wire suture. Photographs show the condition before and after the advancement operation.

transferring one tendon to another or in embedding a tendon end in an adjoining tendon so as not to leave any free, unsatisfied tendon end. A pointed scalpel thrust through the recipient tendon is followed by a mosquito hemostat which draws back the end of the donor tendon. This is repeated once farther distally. Then the cut end is embedded in the host tendon with a core suture of wire. Next, the projecting end of the tendon so embedded is tucked in, and the slit in the latter is closed with a stitch of No. 00000 catgut, which will disappear in a couple of days. The union takes place not where the tendons are woven but at the unsatisfied end of the tendon which is embedded.

Tension for Suturing Tendons. Mayer's rule states that when the origin and the insertion of the muscle are made to approach as near to each other as possible the tension should be zero. This is the ideal tension for tendon transfers but does not hold for late repairs, since the muscle will have contracted. If the accident took place less than 2 months previously, the cut tendon ends usually can be sutured together. The tendon will be a little taut for full extension, but as soon as it is healed, the muscle will elongate to the normal degree. When more than 2 months have elapsed since injury, a tendon graft or transfer will have to be resorted to because, with few exceptions, the tension will be too great for the tendon ends to be sutured directly. If the transfer is done to several of the digital tendons, the tension should be adjusted so that the fingers, under the same muscle pull, will each be flexed to the normal position, with increasing flexion from index to little finger.

A means of estimating tension when using a graft is to place the wrist straight and adjust the length of the graft to bring the digit into the same degree of flexion as the adjoining normal ones, remembering that there is more flexion as one progresses to the little finger side of the hand.

If a large-caliber graft is used, there will be some shrinkage which must be allowed for.

When the muscle has limited amplitude, the tendons should be joined under that tension which will place the limited range of motion where it will be most useful. When a muscle has been relaxed for a long time due to severance of its tendon, allowance should be made for some limitation of amplitude from its normal excursion. The tension should be adjusted for the most useful range of motion. A little tension on the tendon will encourage the muscle to elongate to some degree. When a muscle retracts half its length, its strength is gone. If drawn to the limit of its normal length, its strength is greatest. Beyond that it loses strength as its sarcolemma stretches. If placed under too much tension, it loses strength, and if under too little tension, it

FIG. 507. Sources of tendon and paratenon grafts. (*Left*) The long extensors of the 4 lateral toes can be removed through 3 incisions. The extensor brevis tendons are kept intact to provide extension. (*Left center*) An incision to expose the tendon of the plantaris muscle. If present, its proximal portion may be removed with a Brand stripper or through an incision in the upper mid calf. (*Right center*) The palmaris longus can be removed even with all its paratenon through transverse incisions. (*Right*) The smaller area is the site for removal of fascia, and the larger oval represents the area for removal of the layer of paratenon which lies over the fascia lata.

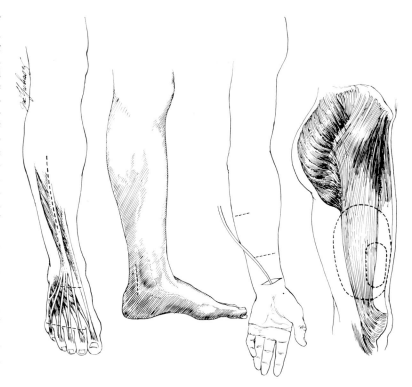

will have no power to contract. A profundus tendon severed in the palm retracts very little because of the interdigitations with the other profundus tendons in the palm. The strength of a muscle is in proportion to its cross-section area, but excursion is in proportion to its fiber length.

Splinting After Tendon Suture. After repairing a flexor tendon anywhere in its course from wrist to fingertip, the same splinting can be used; namely, a slab of plaster of Paris placed over the dorsum of the wrist, the hand and the forearm and ending at the proximal knuckles. This should keep the wrist in flexion but should not hold the fingers flexed. With the wrist in flexion, the flexor muscles will be robbed of strength but still can move a little. The wrist joint should not be fixed in forced flexion, because such a strain injures the joint. One should flex the wrist to the full degree and then back off slightly as the plaster hardens. A gauze bandage holds the plaster in place. If fingers are splinted in a flexed position, they cannot be extended; also, tendons adhere in this position.

In splinting for repaired extensor tendons of the wrist, the plaster slab is laid on the flexor

surface of the forearm and the hand and reaches to the distal creases of the palm. The wrist is held in dorsiflexion. If it is the long digital extensor tendons that are sutured on

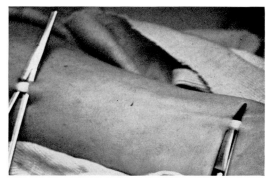

FIG. 508. The palmaris longus tendon, if exposed at the wrist (right edge of photograph) and made tense by passing an instrument beneath it, can be found easily in the forearm. Here an opening in the fascia allows passage of a clamp beneath the tendon and the muscle. When divided at the distal incision, the tendon can be withdrawn easily with its smooth epitenon layer intact.

the dorsum of the hand or the forearm, the splinting need not extend beyond the middle finger joints. This will keep the distal 2 joints of the fingers mobile and prevent stiffness.

PROBLEM OF GLIDING

Tendons will not glide through cicatrix or poorly nourished tissues, and the restoration of this gliding function is a common problem in the surgery of tendons. It may be necessary to excise the surface cicatrix and to replace it with skin and subcutaneous tissue of good quality by pedicle graft. At the same time the surrounding skin around the complete wound margin should be undercut from the deep fascia, allowing it to retract. Then the skin of the full circumference of the limb will be slack enough to permit good nutrition.

In addition to this one must also excise the deep cicatrix en bloc to mobilize the parts further, to free the nerves and the blood vessels for better nutrition and to furnish for the tendons a bed which is not cicatricial. Of course, any cicatrix left in place will heal with cicatrix and bind the tendon. Thus the first prerequisite is to provide the tendon with a soft bed of healthy tissue, preferably of loose, pliable texture of the paratenon variety.

If a tendon attached by a single light adhesion is freed and motion is begun early, the tendon will remain mobile. If, however, a tendon is released from cicatrix until it moves freely and then is dropped back into its cicatricial bed, it will adhere and in 2 weeks will be as immobile as ever. After freeing a tendon from cicatrix, if all the cicatrix cannot be excised, it will be necessary to interpose some paratenon or smooth deep fascia between the tendon and the immobile cicatrix. Paratenon or specialized fat can be obtained from other tendons. A convenient source is that thin layer covering the broad triceps tendon. A large, thin, veil-like piece can be taken

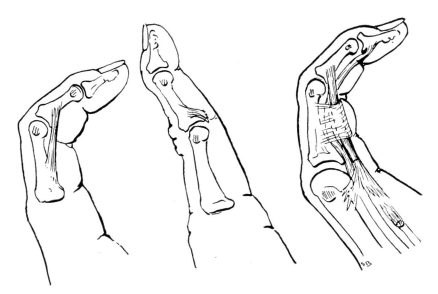

Fig. 509. In reconstructing tendons in a finger, usually the sublimis tendon must be removed in order to prevent inevitable adhesions between the sublimis and the profundus tendons. The sublimis tendon flexes the middle joint, and the profundus tendon the distal joint. Therefore, adhesions joining the 2 tendons will prevent action of the profundus tendon on the distal joint. (*Left*) If the sublimis tendon is cut off too long, the distal end will attach itself to the proximal segment of the finger and draw the middle joint into flexion contracture. (*Center*) If the sublimis tendon is cut off too short, the middle finger joint will overextend. (*Right*) If the sublimis tendon is severed in the palm or the base of a finger, the end of its distal portion will proliferate, attach and contract, producing a flexion contracture of the finger. (J. Bone Joint Surg. *14*:32)

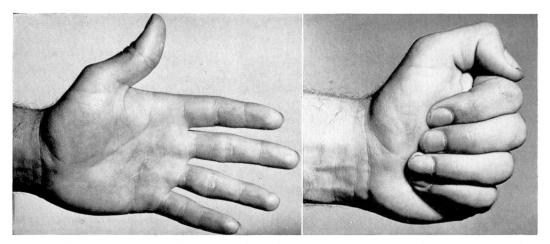

FIG. 510. One year after the flexor tendons of the middle, the ring and the little fingers had been severed and unsuccessfully repaired, a toe extensor was used as a graft in the middle finger, and the palmaris longus in the ring finger; in the little finger the intact superficialis was advanced to the profundus stump. Photographs show extension and flexion 1 year after the operation.

from the outer surface of the lower two thirds of the thigh. This is the thin layer immediately overlying the fascia lata. It is of somewhat better quality in the posterior half of this area. This furnishes ample material to spread over, under or between multiple tendons in the forearm. However, care should be used not to exclude the tendons too completely, since this blocks the blood supply. Peer found that transplanted fat loses 45 per cent of its weight. A tendon should be exercised if the slippery surface of the paratenon is to be maintained; if the tendon is not exercised, the paratenon changes to scar tissue.

Thin deep fascia makes excellent gliding material. A small piece can be obtained from the front or the back of the forearm or from over the peroneus longus tendons in the regions where these tendons glide; a larger piece is available from over the quadriceps

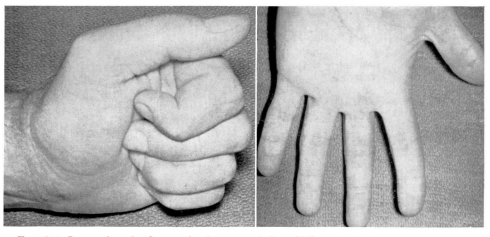

FIG. 511. Lacerations in the proximal crease of the middle and the ring fingers resulted in loss of function of flexor tendons. A reconstruction using as grafts the palmaris longus tendon in the ring finger and the proximal portion of a superficialis in the middle finger gave this result as seen 5 months later.

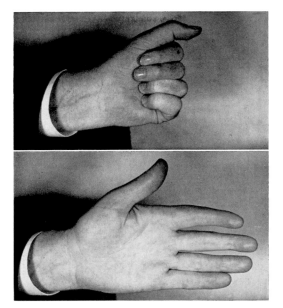

FIG. 512. Case H. L. A tin can had cut across the bases of the index and the long fingers, severing 4 nerves and 4 tendons. Twenty-four hours later, staphylococci and streptococci were present, so that operation was postponed. Four months later, the 4 nerves were sutured, and the profundus tendons in the fingers from the base of the palm were replaced by free grafts of the flexor sublimis tendons. Sensation and, gradually, motion returned. These pictures show motion of the hand 27 years after operation.

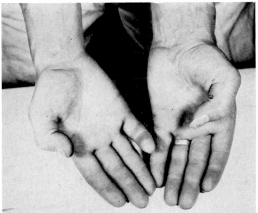

FIG. 513. Case L. de L. Laceration of the palm by a porcelain faucet, causing loss of flexion of the thumb and anesthesia of the thumb and the index finger. Sutured the 3 nerves and took a tendon graft plus paratenon from the foot for the flexor of the thumb. An excellent result in sensation and motion was obtained.

muscle anterior to the fascia lata. If after removing a patch of this the fascia cannot be closed by suture, it is advisable to slit it longitudinally, both up and down, so that a small circular muscle hernia will not develop and cause complaint. The fascia is placed slippery side toward the tendon, and its cut edges are turned away from the tendon to prevent their adhering to it. The best fascia is in the lower part of a limb segment where it is slippery for gliding of tendons rather than higher over the muscles where gliding is minimal.

Small pieces of fat or fascia are difficult to suture in place. The following method is useful.

A strand of 4-0 catgut threaded on a needle is tied to each of the 4 corners of the piece. Then the 2 strands from one side of the piece are passed by their needles under the tendon

and out through the skin on the opposite side of the finger or the limb and are drawn on through until the fat or the fascia is in place between the tendon and its underlying bed. These 2 catgut strands are tied together outside the skin. Similarly, the 2 near strands are brought out through the skin on the near side and tied together. In this way the piece is anchored in place by its 4 corners, and any additional part of its edges may be held by extra stitches placed through the skin and tied outside. In a few days these stitches brush off, leaving the piece in place.

Tendons that have become adherent following injury or repair often can be made mobile in this way. The method is especially useful for freeing flexor or extensor tendons over the site of fracture of a phalanx or a metacarpal.

When withdrawn, most tendons have a thin, slippery, gliding layer over the epitenon which can be slid back and forth along the tendon. This often furnishes enough insulation against adhesions to allow such a tendon to glide when transferred or grafted. In other cases, when the bed is too cicatricial, one can graft a tendon and its paratenon as a complete gliding assembly. Such a structure is obtained readily from the palmaris longus or the ex-

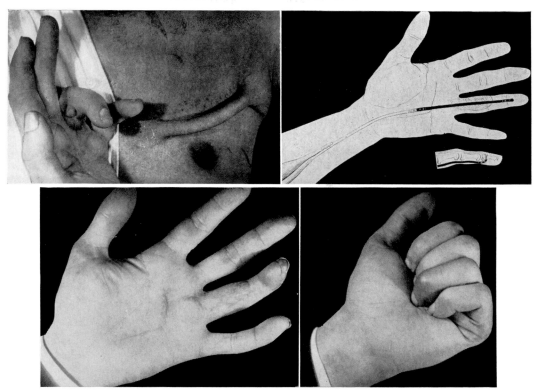

Fig. 514. Case C. J. J. An infection 5 months previously in the sheath of the flexor tendons of the ring finger, which was drained through a median longitudinal incision in the base of the finger, resulted in loss of the flexor tendons and in the scar contracture of the finger which limits the extension, as shown in the top left-hand picture.

Operation: The scar was removed from the volar surface of the finger together with the remains of the flexor tendons, the finger was straightened on a splint, and the denuded area was covered by a skin graft from the tubular pedicle in the pectoral region shown in the top left-hand picture. Four months after good skin was supplied, a new flexor tendon was transplanted into the finger from the flexor sublimis of the same digit, which was removed from the forearm. In the palm, it was sutured to the tendon of the flexor profundus, and distally it was fastened through a drillhole in the distal phalanx to the insertion of the extensor tendon, as shown in the top right-hand picture. (*Bottom*) Taken 3 months later, these 2 pictures show the result. (Surg., Gynec. Obstet. *39*:267)

tensors of the toes on the dorsum of the foot. In the palm the lumbrical muscle can be used to surround a tendon juncture, usually with good results, though in some there follows a proliferation of the perimysium of the muscle, with some tendency to adhere. The lumbrical has a function contrary to that of the profundus, in that it contracts to pull the profundus distalward as the extensors tighten. If, when a lumbrical is wrapped about a profundus juncture, the lumbrical does not have sufficient slack, it will snub or check the profundus tendon, keeping it from flexing the distal 2 joints. Therefore, if the lumbrical is contracted and cicatricial, it should not be allowed to adhere to the profundus. If in good

condition, it should be pulled distalward first to allow full motion of the profundus. This may be tested readily by determining that a pull on the profundus completely flexes the finger. When the bed within the finger is cicatricial, palmaris longus and paratenon or the equivalent will give more voluntary action of the finger than will a graft of the flexor sublimis tendon with its epitenon.

A tendon juncture should not be made at a place where it will adhere, such as in the firm fascial tunnel in a wrist or in the narrow firm sheath in a finger. Whenever possible, one should place tendon junctures where adhesions formed by them will do the least harm, as at the insertion of a tendon or in a place where

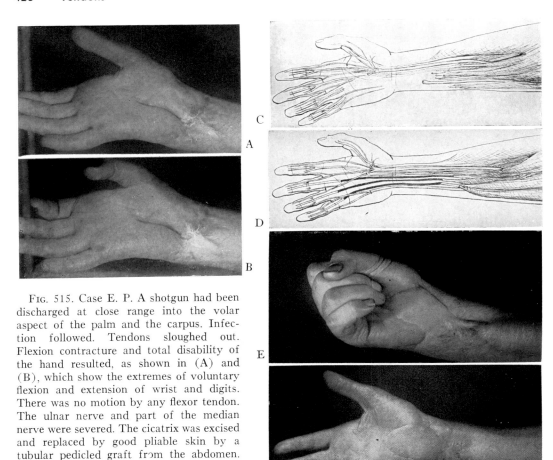

FIG. 515. Case E. P. A shotgun had been discharged at close range into the volar aspect of the palm and the carpus. Infection followed. Tendons sloughed out. Flexion contracture and total disability of the hand resulted, as shown in (A) and (B), which show the extremes of voluntary flexion and extension of wrist and digits. There was no motion by any flexor tendon. The ulnar nerve and part of the median nerve were severed. The cicatrix was excised and replaced by good pliable skin by a tubular pedicled graft from the abdomen. The deep cicatrix was also excised. The improvement in nutrition is shown in (E) and (F). (C) Shows the condition of the tendons and the nerves found at operation. (D) Shows the repair of the tendons by freeing some, by placing tendon grafts in others, and by suturing the nerves. Sensation throughout, good nutrition, excellent motion, and ability to work resulted, as shown in (E) and (F). (J. Bone Joint Surg. *14*:35)

the limb is thick and the tendon is surrounded by soft, movable tissue, as in the palm and the forearm. In the distal part of the palm there seems to be a special tendency for the formation of adhesions to the edges of the fascial septa which go to the sides of the metacarpals and to the edges of the annular sheath ligaments over the heads of the metacarpals. These are the special areas where proliferation of fascia occurs in Dupuytren's contracture. By choosing a site well proximal in the palm, this region is avoided. Here the tendon juncture may be wrapped around by the lumbrical muscle which normally moves with the ten-

don, thus preventing adhesions. For the thumb flexor, the junctures of a graft should be at the distal phalanx, in the thenar eminence or above the annular ligament in the wrist. A juncture at the base of the thumb will adhere.

It is necessary to keep skin incisions remote from tendons and especially tendon junctures. They may cross a tendon at a point but should not parallel it, or a long line of adhesions to the tendon may form. Delicate handling of the tissues by atraumatic technic, as described in Chapter 5, is compulsory in the vicinity of tendons. Rough handling of the tissues or marring of the epitenon is sure to be followed

FIG. 516. Case S. T. While this man was drawing a shotgun toward him, the charge entered the palm and the forearm. Infection followed, and the flexor tendons of the palm and the forearm and 6 inches of the median and the ulnar nerves sloughed out. The illustration shows the contracted and totally disabled hand after healing, and also the tubular pedicle of abdominal skin ready for grafting. There was no motion or sensation in the hand except from the radial nerve and the extensor tendons. (J. Bone Joint Surg. *14*:36)

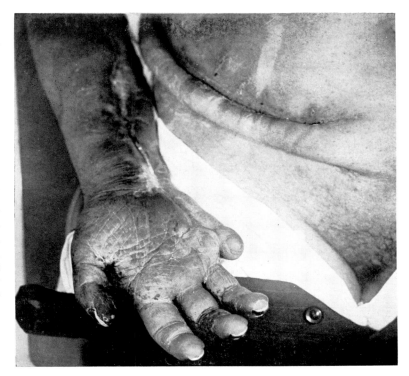

by tissue reaction and adhesions. Postoperative hematoma formation similarly prevents gliding.

In general, in tendon repairs, one should aim to have a minimum of moving parts but a maximum of gliding material. It is far better to let one branched tendon do the work of several and to have ample room for gliding than to attempt to reproduce the normal number of tendons packed closely in a cicatricial channel where they will adhere to one another and to their surroundings.

METHOD OF MAKING AN ARTIFICIAL TENDON SHEATH

Leo Mayer used a celluloid tube, and Thatcher used one of stainless steel for implantation into the finger to form a synovial-lined sheath. Microscopically, such a sheath was demonstrated. Straight rods which did not conform to the natural undulating course of the tendon in the finger were used, so that no accommodation was made for the annular sheaths or pulleys. At the end of 3 weeks the rod was withdrawn, and a tendon graft was placed through the channel. There was a tendency for the tendon juncture in the distal

part of the palm to become adherent, but the principle of producing a synovial-lined sheath may have its applications.

J. E. Milgrim inserted steel ribbons in the hand, about the forearm and the lower leg, making them about 10 times wider than the tendon and suturing the tendon within this artificial sheath. He states that the metal should be removed within 3 weeks to prevent excessive cicatrix about it. D. C. McKeever used a special cellophane (No. 300 PUT 71 DuPont), which he claims is nonirritating, to intervene between tendon and scar and to separate the bones in arthroplasty. He states that the cellophane fragments and collects in wads, but that good cleavage is established. Farmer determined that if cellophane is wrapped around the tendon the result is not so good. Polythene film 0.001 inch thick has been used beneath the tendons in the forearm, the hand and the fingers as an interposed film in the same manner as paratenon. It may be withdrawn later if there is any reaction.

MAKING PULLEYS

When the volar carpal or the dorsal carpal ligament is destroyed, the flexor and the ex-

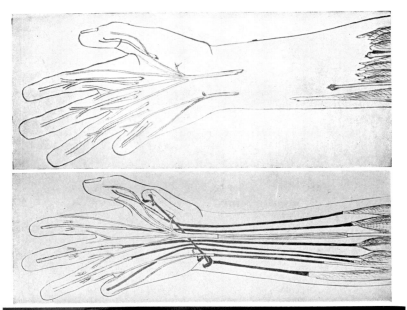

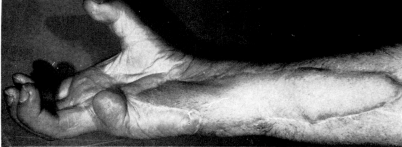

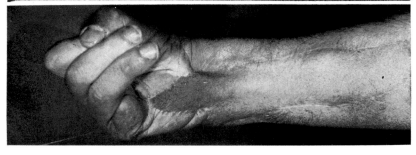

FIG. 517. Case S. T. (*Continued*). Showing the condition found at operation after dissecting cut the cicatricial tissue. There are wide gaps in all the flexor tendons and in the median and the ulnar nerves. The pedicled skin graft was applied, and later tendon grafts from the extensors of the toes and nerve grafts from the sural nerves were placed, as shown in the second illustration. A pulley operation was also done, as shown, to regain opposition of the thumb. Good function resulted, as shown in the bottom 2 illustrations, and the patient was able to return to work as a welder. (J. Bone Joint Surg. *14*: 36)

tensor tendons will bow across the wrist on flexion and dorsiflexion, respectively. A new ligament is constructed readily, using either a band of fascia lata or a tendon graft and contacting it at the sides of the wrist to ligament or bone.

The 2 pulleys in the flexor aspect of a finger are important. The proximal pulley, really of 2 parts separated at the proximal joint, extends about 3 cm. from the head of the metacarpal to just beyond the middle of the proximal phalanx. The distal pulley, which is opposite the center of the middle phalanx, is about 1.5 cm. long. Either of these can be reconstructed quite simply with a free tendon graft made to loop around the flexor tendons and either the metacarpal or the middle phalanx. To do this, a curved mosquito hemostat is passed through part of the circumference and out a stab wound on the opposite side. As it is withdrawn, the tendon graft is dragged after it. It is sutured to itself with 2 interrupted buried

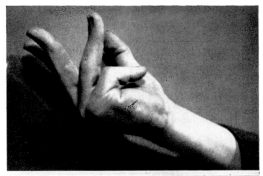

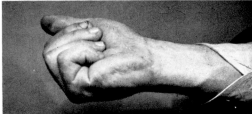

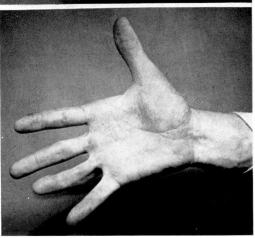

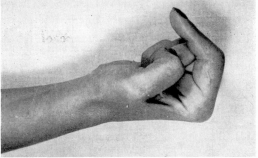

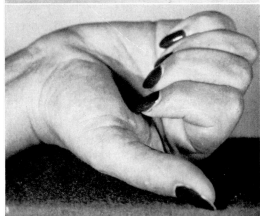

FIG. 519. Case J. R. W. (*Top*) Laceration across the middle flexion crease by a milk bottle, severing both flexor tendons. The tendons had been sutured but adhered. Removed the flexor tendons from the finger and grafted into the profundus tendon, from the base of the palm to insertion in the finger, a free tendon graft of palmaris longus plus paratenon. (*Bottom*) An excellent result was obtained.

FIG. 518. Case E. L. Every finger had been lacerated across its proximal segment 3 months previously by a sheet of tin, severing all the flexor tendons of all the fingers except a portion of the sublimis in the little finger. The wound healed per primam. (*Top*) Limit of flexion preoperatively. At operation, all flexor tendons were removed from all the fingers. The 4 flexor sublimis tendons were withdrawn in the forearm, and each was used as a free graft to extend its respective profundus tendon from palm to distal phalanx. Each stump of sublimis in the forearm was sutured to its profundus tendon for added strength. (*Center* and *bottom*) Function 10 months later. Distal joints tested separately flexed for the index to the little finger 45°, 42°, 42° and 50°, respectively.

sutures, and this juncture is swung around to the side. For a middle segment pulley, one slip of sublimis may be spared and looped over the profundus tendon to be sutured to the other side of the finger or a circumferential graft is used.

If one side of the pulley has been incised, it may be sutured by the pull-out wire technic, thus preventing any foreign body reaction from buried catgut or silk. This principle of using withdrawable stainless steel wire in order to avoid leaving suture material has many applications, e.g., closing dead spaces, fascial incisions and in tendon work throughout the limbs.

FREE TENDON GRAFTS

Free tendon grafts are usually required in secondary reconstruction because of muscle contracture, loss of tendon substance or the necessity of making the new tendon junction at a different level.

After 2 months, with few exceptions, the muscle becomes contracted. After a tendon is severed, each end is usually damaged for at least ½ inch back, so that some tendon length must be sacrificed. After a tendon has been nonfunctioning for several months, the degeneration of disuse sets in and renders it unfit for repair. This applies especially to the distal end of a tendon and to the curled-up proximal end. Where a tendon is found to be quite rough and adherent, rather than attempt to repair it and have it readhere it is better to excise it completely and substitute in its place a normal tendon. Slippery epitenon is always transplanted with a graft, but where the bed is too cicatricial, paratenon fat should accompany the tendon as a gliding assembly or should be placed about it later.

Grafts are used to place junctures at strategic sites. A graft is so placed that its 2 junctures are never in a finger, a carpal tunnel or the distal half of the palm, since they will adhere. One is made at the terminal phalanx where it does not have to glide and the other where it can glide in the base of the palm or above the carpal tunnel. In the palm, the lumbrical is wrapped about the juncture at its natural attachment. In the thumb, a graft from the distal phalanx reaches to above the carpal ligament, thus avoiding a juncture within the thumb. A graft of gliding assembly, namely, tendon and paratenon as from the palmaris longus or the long extensors of toes, yields more motion than will a graft of a tendon alone, such as the sublimis. Small caliber tendon is preferable, because its volume, being smaller, gains a blood supply more quickly and is less prone to adhere.

Fate of Tendon Grafts

A free tendon graft receives its nourishment from the surrounding tissues until it finally becomes vascularized. Therefore, its surface lives, but in the center of the tendon there occur patches of necrosis, most apparent at the end of the 1st week. Growing cells in tendons can be seen in grafts after 11 days, and eventually these patches of necrosis are replaced by regular tendon cells and fibers. During the first 2 or 3 weeks the tendon graft is considerably swollen and is surrounded by newly formed vessels. Its repair lags behind the repair of a normal tendon by only about a week, so that after a month a tendon graft is fairly strong, and by the end of 5 weeks the danger of breaking is over. Even at 3 weeks, when cells are still actively proliferating in these grafts, there is enough strength for guarded exercise. During the stage of swelling the appearance of the graft is somewhat pink and translucent, but eventually it contracts to

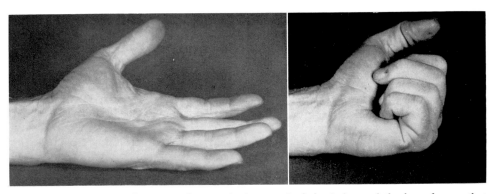

Fig. 520. Case R. P. A pneumatic press had so crushed the index and the long fingers that the flexor tendons were severed. The tendons were sutured, but the patient had no flexor action in the long finger. A free tendon graft of palmaris longus plus paratenon was placed in the long finger. Six weeks later, while gardening, he ruptured the graft at the metacarpal head. A new similar graft was placed from the other forearm. This man worked conscientiously to rehabilitate his hand, and excellent function resulted.

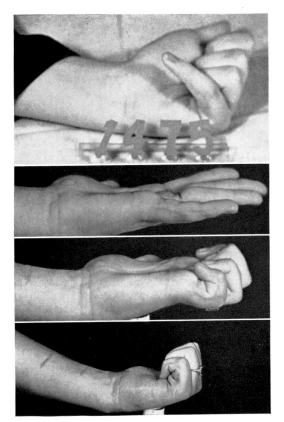

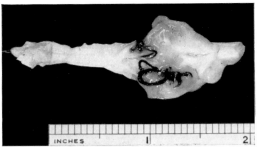

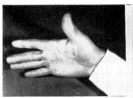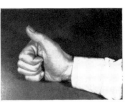

Fig. 522. Silk suture versus removable stainless-steel wire suture.

Case A. T. Six months previously, after laceration on a bottle, a primary suture of the severed flexor tendons of the index finger had been done in the proximal segment. It was ascertained that the wound had healed per primam, but he had only a trace of voluntary movement of the middle joint and none in the distal joint. The ulnar side was anesthetic. (*Top*) Appearance of tendon which had been primarily sutured with silk and healed without infection. The cicatricial reaction bound them solidly in their bed. Tendon ends had separated half an inch. This argues for the use of removable stainless-steel wire. The tendons and the cicatrix were removed, the volar nerve was repaired, and a free tendon graft of flexor sublimis was placed with removable stainless-steel wire. (*Bottom*) Taken 2 years later, these pictures show complete motion. Sensation returned in 3 months.

Fig. 521. Tendon graft of palmaris longus plus paratenon. (*Top*) Both flexors had been severed in the proximal segment of the left little finger in this violinist. An ill-advised median incision had been made extending into the palm, and both tendons repaired with silk. The scar was excised, all tendon remnants removed from the finger, and Z-plasties done. Pictured is the amount of voluntary flexion before insertion of the graft. The 3 lower photographs show the range of extension and flexion 3 months after a full-length graft of palmaris longus with its paratenon. The transverse scars in the forearm mark the incisions used to excise the graft.

normal size, takes on a pearly sheen and can scarcely be distinguished from normal tendon. Microscopically, it is the same as normal tendon.

Only tendons of moderate size, such as those in the forearm, can be grafted; the larger tendons are so thick that much of their centers must undergo necrosis and substitu-

tion. A tubular graft of fascia lata used in repairing large tendons acts similarly, because the inner surface of the tube does not become nourished. It is better to use a flat piece of thick fascia lata and refrain from tubularizing it in order to give it nourishment through each surface.

In placing tendon grafts one should make them slightly longer than they normally should be, because in healing there is some tendency to contract. Tendon grafts which become infected usually slough. Tendon grafts that live hypertrophy to fulfill the demand

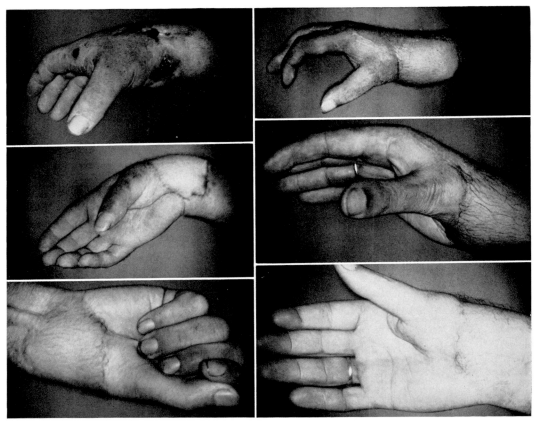

Fig. 523. Case D. M. This 23-year-old man who early had lost one arm, one leg and part of the other foot, lost all the function of his remaining hand from a shotgun injury through the carpus. The wound had almost healed. (*Left, top*) When the wound healed, first sutured the median nerve, overcoming a 2-inch gap. (*Left, center*) A month later, a pedicle was applied over the wrist. Two months later, the flexor and the extensor tendons to the thumb and the index and those that extended and flexed the wrist were dissected out and replaced by free tendon grafts from both the palmaris longus and the sublimis of the long finger. The metacarpal of the thumb was mounted on an iliac graft on the carpus. Excellent function was restored, as shown in the 4 remaining pictures. Good sensation returned.

put upon them. Tendon grafts placed in infancy grow with the child. Lowman's fascial transplants for paralysis of the abdominal wall show marked hypertrophy in response to use. If not used, they atrophy. Whether a tendon graft lives and survives as a graft or is replaced by cells from the recipient tissues is still a point of argument. The question is academic because from a practical standpoint these grafts are successful and function in every way like tendons.

SOURCES OF TENDON GRAFTS

The palmaris longus tendon is the most common source of tendon for use in the hand. It is 12 or 15 cm. in length and adequate in caliber and is present in about 80 per cent of the population. Its presence is shown by opposing the thumb or, better, by flexing the wrist against resistance. After exposing the tendon at each end through a ¼-inch transverse cut in the skin, it can be withdrawn readily from its bed if drawn distalward. It can be drawn out proximalward but less readily. There will be a thin layer of slippery material on the epitenon, but if paratenon is desired with the tendon, it is best to make 3 transverse incisions and, by lifting the skin, to dissect out the tendon with its surrounding

FIG. 524. Case F. E. (*Top*) Charge from a shotgun entered the palm, emerging dorsally and shattering the carpus and the lower radius and severing many tendons, the extensors of the thumb, the fingers, and the wrist and the median nerve. Débrided, filleted the index finger, and skin-grafted. Considerable infection followed.

First Operation: Excised scar and placed a pedicle.

Second Operation: Furnished tendon grafts plus paratenon to extend the thumb, the fingers and the wrist. Freed the flexor tendon of the thumb and did a pulley operation for opposition of the thumb. Sutured the median nerve to its 4 branches. The wrist became fused. Sensation and motion and opposition returned, so that he had a very useful hand, as shown in the 5 remaining pictures.

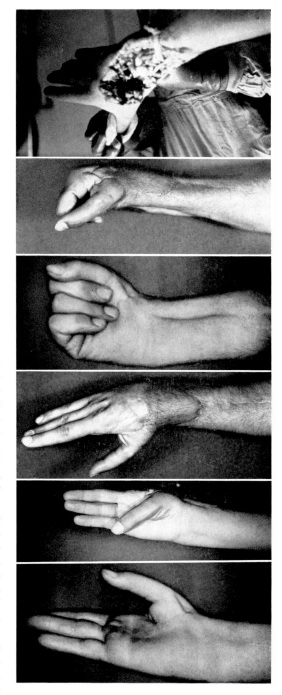

tissues in 1 block. A longitudinal incision or a long wavy line leaves an ugly scar.

The tendon of the flexor superficialis (old term, sublimis) is often used as a graft to prolong the tendon of the flexor profundus from the base of the palm to its insertion in the distal phalanx. The graft can be withdrawn through a short transverse incision on the volar aspect of the forearm a little above the wrist. The superficial flexor tendons do not interdigitate as do the profundi and, therefore, can be withdrawn without resistance. In some cases these tendons may be too short. If one or more digits have been amputated, there are available both flexor and extensor tendons of these digits.

One or 2 of the digital extensor tendons can be taken from the dorsum of the hand and the forearm for grafts provided that the distal stumps are joined to the adjacent tendons, so that the loss will not be noticed. The grafts are obtained through 2 small transverse incisions, one in the middle of the dorsum of the hand just proximal to the tendon interdigitation and another in the forearm 2½ inches above the wrist. By pulling on the tendon to the middle or the ring finger, one ascertains which tendon moves both fingers. Then the other tendon may be removed without disability.

When several grafts are needed, the long extensor tendons of the toes are available. Function is not impaired provided that the tendons of the extensor digitorum brevis which extend the toes are spared.

Four tendons or 1 tendon with 4 tails can be obtained in each foot. The long extensor tendon of the great toe, because of its useful function, usually is not taken. There is no extensor digitorum brevis tendon for the little toe. Therefore, if one takes the little toe ex-

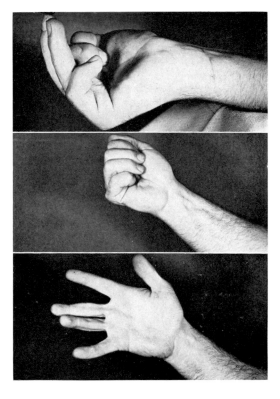

FIG. 525. Case W. V. (*Top*) A heavy edge of steel dropped across the volar aspect of the proximal segments of the long and the ring fingers, severing the long flexor tendons. Had operation of tendon grafts elsewhere and then another of freeing. The flexors did not act on the distal 2 finger joints. (*Center* and *bottom*) Removed graft from the finger, which was adherent throughout, and used a graft of the left palmaris longus plus paratenon. Good function resulted.

by running a tendon stripper down them from above, thus allowing the tendons to be drawn out through this upper incision. If paratenon is to be used with the graft, a long curved incision is made, and the whole unit is dissected free. Another incision is made longitudinally in the lower leg just external to the tibialis anticus. On picking up the tendons of the extensor digitorum communis it will not be possible to withdraw them from the foot, because they branch to the peroneus tertius tendon. Therefore, with a probe, a strand of suture material is passed up the tendon sheath. Its lower end is looped about the tendons distally, drawn up and out through the incision in the lower leg, stripping off the tendon of the peroneus tertius.

If it is available, the plantaris tendon can be used. It is small in caliber, strong and quite long. An incision on the inner side of the ankle behind the malleolus and just over the anterior edge of the Achilles tendon shows it lying next to the latter. A long stripper, de-

tensor tendon, its distal stump should be embedded into the adjoining short extensor tendon of the 4th toe. To obtain the long extensor tendons, each tendon is severed at the base of the toe through a transverse incision, sparing the brevis. Through a short transverse incision high on the dorsum of the foot these tendons are freed from their paratenon

FIG. 526. Case H. H. (*Left*) From a porcelain faucet injury, which severed the tendons, the patient could not flex the last 3 fingers nor feel over the ring finger. (*Right*) Four months later, the 2-inch gaps in the tendons were repaired by grafts from the palmaris longus, and the nerves were su-

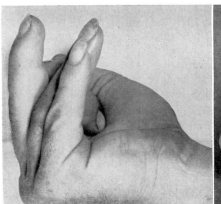

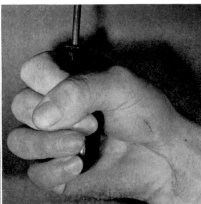

tured. Sensation and fairly good flexion returned. Extension was complete.

signed by Brand, facilitates its removal, but its upper part can be reached through a calf incision.

If grafts are still needed from another source, one can use strips of fascia lata or of triceps tendon with or without a thin encirclement of paratenon tissue. With the conventional pipelike fascia stripper one can obtain a long strip of fascia lata through a small incision above the knee. Fascial strips for tendon grafts are satisfactory in the volar or the dorsal aspect of the forearm; but due to their raw edges, which have a tendency to proliferate and attach, they are not so suitable for use in the digits.

Preserved Tendon or Fascia for Grafts

Much has been written about the use of homografts of fascia or of tendon preserved in alcohol or other chemicals, and experiments have shown that the eventual result is a tendon that looks fairly like the normal tendon, both grossly and microscopically. The preserved graft as such does not live but in the course of a month and a half, by the process of gradual substitution, is replaced by live tendon tissue. The result is not as satisfactory as that obtained from a live autograft. It becomes more adherent; its appearance is yellowish; there is more foreign body reaction about it; and it stains more like fixed tissue.

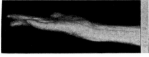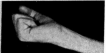

FIG. 527. Case M. T., age 17. Six months previously, the patient had tripped and fallen, striking his hand on a broken stump, lacerating across the base of the little finger and severing the flexor tendons. He had good flexion of the proximal joint of the finger but no voluntary flexion in either the middle or the distal finger joint, the finger inflexion extending straight forward.

At operation, the distal ends were recovered at the middle joint and removed, and the proximal ends in the palm. The tendon of the palmaris longus was used as a free graft to prolong the profundus tendon, the suturing being in the base of the palm and to the distal phalanx. Also, a 2-ply pulley over the metacarpal head was constructed of the sublimis tendon. Removable stainless-steel wire was used. Complete range of motion was obtained, as shown in the photographs, taken 2½ months later.

For these reasons, and because an adequate number of autografts are available, homografts are not recommended for use in the hand.

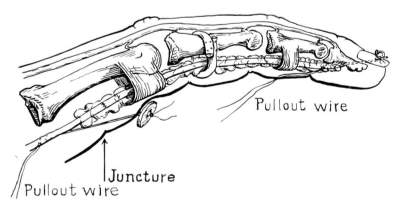

FIG. 528. Diagram of reconstruction of a tendon in a finger which is quite cicatricial. A free tendon graft plus its paratenon has been threaded through 3 pulleys (2 natural and 1 reconstructed). The graft is sutured to the profundus in the palm and to the distal phalanx where adhesions will do the least harm. The distal phalanx is first scraped for bony contact. Suturing is with removable stainless-steel wire, the proximal one being a "suture at a distance."

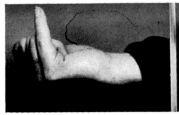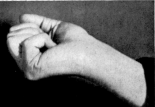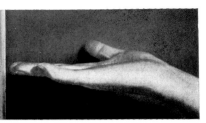

Fig. 529. Case E. Y. A spike of glass had severed both flexor tendons and the nerve to the radial side of the base of the little finger. The wound healed without drainage. (*Left*) There is no ability to flex the distal 2 joints. The intrinsic muscles flex the proximal joint. The radial side is anesthetic. Three weeks from the accident, the small nerve was sutured. The flexor profundus tendon was not sutured in the proximal pulley where it might adhere. Instead, a free graft from the flexor sublimis was used, removing the old tendon and suturing the graft to the distal phalanx and to the profundus in the palm. (*Center* and *right*) Showing the amount of flexion regained. Sensation returned in 2 months.

TENDON TRANSFERS

PRINCIPLES

A tendon transfer is that procedure in which the tendon of insertion or of origin of a functioning muscle is mobilized, detached or divided and reinserted into a bony part or into another tendon to supplement or substitute for the action of the recipient tendon. The term transfer is used in this context, as opposed to the term transplantation which will be used to mean a free tendon graft. A transferred tendon remains attached to its muscle with blood and nerve supply intact, while a transplanted tendon is free of all connections. A tendon transfer may be prolonged by a tendon transplant.

Tendon transfers are used primarily to improve function following damage to the major nerve trunks, the brachial plexus or the cord and the brain and to substitute for motions lost through trauma to muscles in the forearm and the hand. The function provided by the transfer may be a stabilizing one to enable remaining muscles to function, or, by a combination of arthrodeses and tenodeses, stability may be gained, releasing some of the active muscles for other uses.

Stabilization is an essential part of a functioning upper extremity. Unless there is control through shoulder, elbow and wrist, the hand cannot function efficiently. Wrist stability, controlled if possible or fixed by arthrodesis if necessary, is essential to digital function. To make a firm power grasp the

wrist should be able to be maintained in dorsiflexion or fixed there. To pinch, the base of the thumb must be stabilized. For good finger motion a complex system of extrinsic and intrinsic mechanisms comes into action, each stabilizing while the other moves.

The wrist is the key joint of the hand. Ideally, it should have controlled dorsiflexion and palmar flexion. Since the major axis of wrist motion is from dorsoradial to ulnovolar, the 2 radial wrist extensors and their antagonist, the flexor carpi ulnaris, always should be preserved or their action restored. Next in importance is the proximal finger joint. Control or stability of this joint is essential to functioning of the digital flexors and extensors.

FIVE ESSENTIALS IN TENDON TRANSFERS

Tendon transfer is one of the oldest of orthopedic operations. Vulpius is said to have performed over 100 in the foot alone, the first before 1900. The names of Codivilla, Tubby, Sir Robert Jones, Anhavsau, Perthes, Mayer, Bielsalski, Stoffel, Putti, Starr, Stiles, Steindler and Abbott all appear in writings on this phase of tendon surgery.

From these, and especially from the writings of Mayer and Steindler, the essential principles of the tendon transfer operation have been summarized.

1. **Correction of Contracture.** When a muscle group has been paralyzed for some time and the part is unsupported, deformity occurs. This may become fixed through contracture of the soft parts from scarring or fibrosis; or, if

Requirements in Radial Palsy

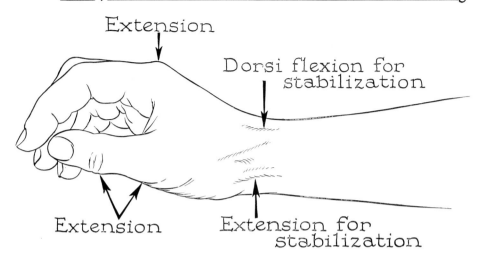

Extension

Dorsi flexion for stabilization

Extension

Extension for stabilization

Available for radial palsy

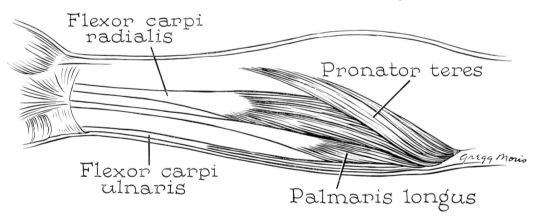

Flexor carpi radialis

Pronator teres

Flexor carpi ulnaris

Palmaris longus

FIG. 530. The upper diagram shows the 4 requirements and the lower diagram 4 muscles which are available for transfer.

during a growing period, by an adaptive shortening of the structures. A contracture of skin may necessitate pedicle grafts to bring in additional tissue; capsular and joint ligaments may require release through excision or capsulectomy; and osteotomy be necessary to correct bony deformity. A tendon transfer cannot overcome a contracture and can function only when the deformity has been cor-

rected and the limb can assume the desired position without resistance. (See Chap. 7, Skin Contractures, and Chap. 9, Joint Contractures.)

2. **There must be adequate power** in the transferred muscle. If the muscle is weak, the deformity will recur. Transferring a muscle cannot increase its power, for this is a fixed value, determined by the cross-section area

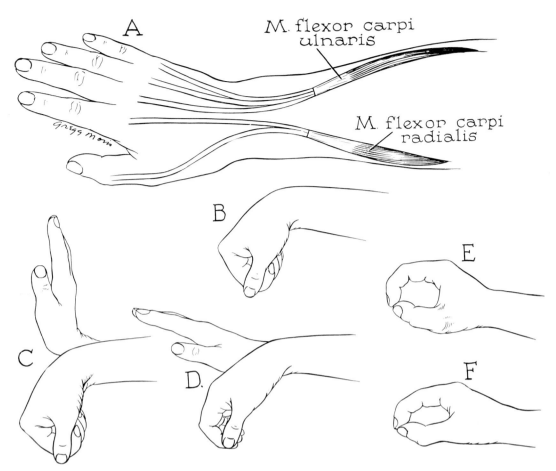

FIG. 531. (A) Shows the simplest tendon transfer for radial palsy; (B, D, F) show the fallacies. (B) On making a fist, the wrist flexes unless a tendon is provided to dorsiflex the wrist. (C, D) Normal range of motion of wrist and digits and the range gained by transferring wrist movers with their limited excursion to move the digits which require a longer range of excursion. (E) Normal pinch in the form of a circle. (F) Poor pinch is the shape of an ellipse unless the stabilizing action of the abductor pollicis longus is furnished.

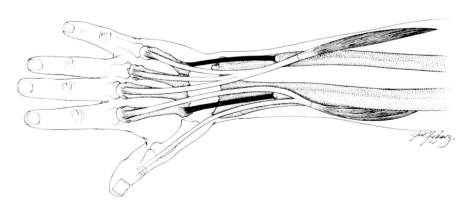

FIG. 532. The simplest transfer for radial palsy combined with tenodeses to maintain wrist dorsiflexion. Usually called the Perthes transfer.

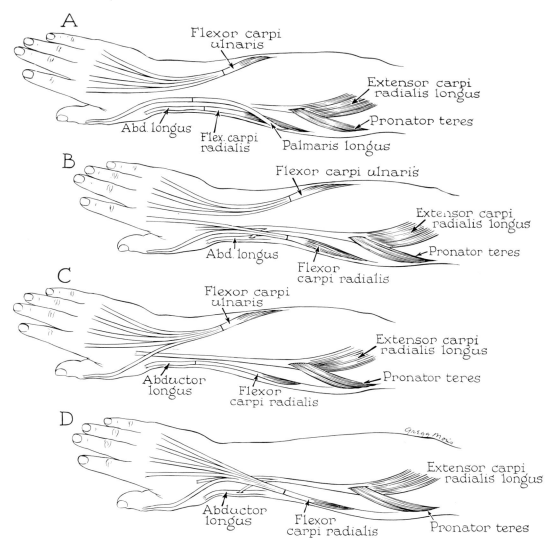

Fig. 533. Methods of tendon transfer for radial palsy in all of which provision is made for stabilizing the wrist in dorsiflexion and the metacarpotrapezial joint in extension.

of the muscle. Its leverage may be altered, but its absolute power remains unchanged. Steindler accepts the value of 3.65 Kg. times the physiologic cross section as the absolute power of the muscle. If a muscle of too much power is used, the opposite deformity may result. The work capacity of the muscle is the product of its power and amplitude.

3. **There must be sufficient amplitude of motion** in the transferred muscle tendon unit to carry out the desired motion. Normal amplitudes have been determined for most of the muscles of the hand and the forearm. (see Chap. 1). Amplitude of tendon movement can be limited by scarring and adhesions and lack of gliding material through which the tendon passes. The normal amplitude, which is related to the length of the muscle fiber, will never be regained completely after transfer; therefore, one should choose a muscle of

more than adequate amplitude for the donor.

As a working rule it can be estimated that wrist movers will have an average of 33 mm. in amplitude; the digital extensors and the flexor of the thumb an average of 50 mm.; and the finger flexors 70 mm. A compromise position, adjusting the tension of the transfer so that the available limited amplitude is in the best functioning range will be required whenever a short-amplitude donor is transferred to a tendon of normally longer excursion.

The measurements of amplitude and the figures referred to above are based on normal structures and the usual motions. Several factors may alter these figures. From trauma to the muscle or damage to the tendons some loss of both power and amplitude may have resulted and this will have to be considered in the choice of motors. Sometimes the amplitude of a muscle may be increased, not by altering its fiber length, but by liberating it from surrounding fascial attachments. This is particularly true of the brachioradialis, the amplitude of which can be doubled by a release of the binding forearm fascia and its broad tendon of insertion on the radius. Another way in which the effective amplitude of a muscle can be altered is by changing it from a mono-articular to a bi-articular or multi-articular muscle. An example of this is a wrist extensor transferred to a digital flexor. In its normal location, acting to dorsiflex the wrist, its amplitude would be 50 mm., but when transferred to a digital flexor it is now possible for this same muscle to flex the fingers completely and yet allow the fingers to open completely in extension. Something has increased the effective amplitude from 50 to 70 mm. It is the intercalated segments and the movement of those that provide the increase in effective amplitude. Choice of motors thus depends on a careful evaluation of many factors.

4. **A straight line of pull is desirable** when any muscle tendon unit is transferred. Maximal efficiency and strength are maintained when the tendon and the muscle remain in a straight line and are not forced to take a devious course through the tissues. In forearm transfers, this direct route is sometimes through the interosseus membrane rather than around the radius or the ulna. In some transfers, to cause the tendon pull in the right direction, it will be necessary to violate this precept. Here the pulley or the T-Y principle is used, as exemplified in the opponens and other transfers for the thumb (see Chap. 12). If a pulley mechanism is used, a muscle of adequate strength is required to overcome the additional friction.

Transferred tendons should be placed in good gliding tissues, away from bare bone, raw surfaces of cut fascial planes or a hole in the fascia. The junction of donor to recipient tendon should not be in a carpal tunnel or on the dorsum under the retinaculum.

5. **The integrity of the muscle should be maintained** so that it can provide one motion essential to function. A muscle tendon unit cannot provide 2 different degrees of power and amplitude by acting on 2 recipients of differing excursion. A tendon attached to the short and the long extensors of the thumb will pull effectively only through the amplitude of the lesser of the two. One cannot split the triceps and make one part a flexor of the elbow.

However, it is possible to maintain some of the original function of a donor and yet allow it to perform another action. Pronator teres transferred to extensor carpi radialis longus and brevis still acts as a pronator of the forearm because of the direction of pull. Brachioradialis transferred to flexor digitorum profundus still acts as an elbow flexor. It is now a pluri-articular instead of a mono-articular muscle.

Timing of Tendon Transfer Operations

A tendon transfer is an elective operation and should be done at the optimal time. After trauma, tissues react with swelling, edema and induration. When this process has subsided and the tissue equilibrium (Steindler) has been restored, and when deformities and contractures have been relieved, then transfer can be done. After peripheral nerve lesions or polio it is not necessary to wait for long periods if the lesion can be defined accurately. A transfer done before contractures occur or before bad habit patterns are set up will be more successful. Electromyography can be a definite help in shortening the time between onset of paralysis and operative correction. When from nerve damage or from direct loss of a muscle it is certain that function cannot be restored, operation can be done as soon as the local tissue reaction has disappeared. In poliomyelitis, with adequate care, 50 per cent of the ultimate strength of a muscle is recovered in 3 months, 75 per cent in 6 months. If after 3 months there is only a trace of activity, there is no need to waste time expecting physiotherapy to restore an adequate functioning muscle.

Synergists and Antagonists

When the fingers are strongly flexed, the wrist extensors tighten, stabilizing the wrist in dorsiflexion and making the grasp more efficient and more powerful; thus the wrist extensors are synergists to the digital flexors. In the same way, the wrist flexors, especially the flexor carpi radialis and the palmaris longus, tense when the fingers are extended. When the digital flexors tighten, the digital extensors must relax to allow the joints to move. This synergistic action of wrist motion and finger motion is automatic and was once considered to be an unbreakable reflex act. It is no longer necessary to consider this action in choosing donors for transfer. Experience has shown that in the hand and the forearm any muscle and tendon when transferred (provided that the 5 essentials are present) can

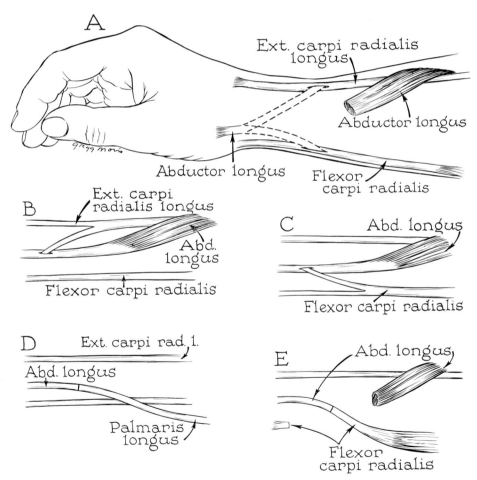

Fig. 534. Methods of activating the abductor pollicis longus to stabilize the metacarpotrapezial joint in extension for a proper pinch between the thumb and the index finger. When the tendon of the abductor pollicis longus is liberated by slitting its tunnel over the radial styloid, the transferred flexors, palmaris longus or flexor carpi radialis retain their action of flexing the wrist,

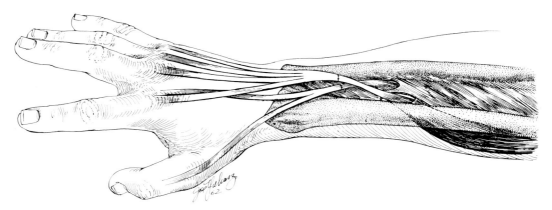

Fig. 535. Diagram showing transfer of flexor superficialis of middle and ring fingers through the interosseus membrane to provide extension of thumb and fingers. Not shown but of necessity included in the operation are transfer of the pronator teres to the wrist extensors and of the flexor carpi radialis to the abductor pollicis longus.

carry out any desired motion. Thus a wrist extensor can act as a digital extensor, a digital flexor, a wrist flexor or a motor for opposition and adduction of the thumb. A most dramatic example is seen in the use of a superficial digital flexor, normally flexing the middle finger joint, used as an extensor of this same joint by rerouting it to the dorsum of the finger. One possible exception to this general rule is the flexor carpi ulnaris when used as a digital flexor. In the instances in which this transfer was done, the range and the power have been so poor that other donors are preferred.

Movements of the hand are patterned in the brain as motions, not as specific muscle actions; as Steindler describes it, there is no motion in the hand that a transferred muscle enters into with which it is not already familiar.

ARTHRODESES, TENODESES AND AUTOMATIC MOTIONS

Stability of the proximal parts to allow better control of the distal ones is a fundamental part of the reconstructive plan. One or many joints may be arthrodesed or the action stabilized by tenodesis or bone block. One should think of the hand as a complex mechanism of moving parts, based on a fundamental unit of wrist extension, thumb opposition and finger motion, with higher and more refined actions superimposed. In formulating a plan for reconstruction one must determine

how much of this basic unit can be restored and then which of the refined motions can be added. Usually, it is necessary to settle for a lower degree of functional action.

It is here that arthrodeses of the principal joints provide the basic foundation on which to build the specific motions needed.

Arthrodesis of the wrist is a useful procedure; it fixes the wrist in the most useful position for the most function and releases any previously active wrist motors to supply digital motion. However, it should be used primarily for painful wrists and for correction of bony deformities, while for paralytic problems tenodeses and transfers are better designed to utilize the wrist motions. A little wrist motion, even if purely automatic, makes many digital transfers more efficient.

Flexion and extension of the wrist are used by many paralytics to extend and flex the digits automatically. Fusing the wrist robs them of these motions which in many cases could not be supplied in any other way. An extreme case is the paraplegic with only an active wrist dorsiflexor. Tenodeses of the digital movers to the forearm allow some grasp when he dorsiflexes the wrist, and grasp is released when the wrist is palmar flexed by gravity. If there is strong supination of the forearm, tenodeses of the digital flexors to the ulna allow some grasp.

Thus, in most complicated reconstructions, tendon transfers cannot be planned arbitrarily. It is necessary to consider each problem individually, determining which functions are required and what muscle power is available and then, by judicious use of arthrodeses, tenodeses and transfers, give to the hand its basic functions of power and precision grasp and as many of the more refined motions as possible.

In all problems involving loss of the motor function of the hand, it is important that the surgeon not focus his attention so much on the loss and the restoration of motion that he forgets that the hand is also an organ of sensation. A hand devoid of feeling, especially in the median nerve area, the pulps of the thumb and the index and the middle fingers, is severely impaired. Restoration of some sensibility to these critical areas is just as important as restoration of motion.

Major Nerve Paralyses

The history of tendon transfers begins with attempts to restore motion in irreparable lesions of the major nerve trunks. The nerve most commonly involved was apparently the radial, and the literature on operative procedures to restore lost extensor power is extensive. The problem of radial palsy illustrates well the principles involved in tendon transfer operations.

Radial Palsy. In this there is loss of voluntary extension of the wrist, the thumb and the proximal finger joints and the action of the long thumb abductor. If the lesion is below the elbow, the brachioradialis still will function, and if lower in the supinator, the radial

wrist extensors remain and the paralysis is only of the digital extensors and the extensor carpi ulnaris.

Wrist stabilization in dorsiflexion is of prime importance, and transfer of the pronator teres to the 2 paralyzed radial wrist extensors, as done by Robert Jones, is the accepted procedure. Schreigg and later Perthes tenodesed the paralyzed extensors to the forearm bones, and Pennell used a fascial graft between the middle and the ring metacarpals and the radius to hold the wrist in dorsiflexion. During this period the finger extensors were motored by transfers of the 2 wrist flexors, 1 around each side of the forearm; however, as early as 1899, both Franke and Cappeler are reported to have passed the flexor carpi ulnaris through the interosseus membrane to obtain a more direct line of pull. The importance of obtaining stability or some action in the abductor pollicis longus was recognized by Fischer in 1915 though he combined it with the extensor pollicis longus, which has a different amplitude. Stoffel used a superficial finger flexor transferred to the long thumb abductor, but most reports describe it as being activated by either the flexor carpi radialis or the palmaris longus and combined with the extensor pollicis longus or brevis or both. The flexor carpi ulnaris was transferred to all the finger extensors or sometimes only to those of the middle, the ring and the little fingers, the index being included with the thumb extensor.

In 1946 Zachary surveyed the results of many transfer operations and emphasized what

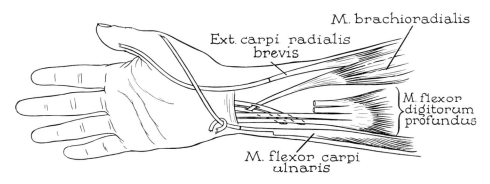

Transfers for median palsy

Fig. 536. Tendon transfers for median palsy. The flexor ulnaris furnishes opposition to the thumb. The flexor digitorum profundus supplied by the ulnar nerve is made to activate all the profundi and is reinforced by the supinator longus. The extensor carpi radialis brevis is transferred to the long flexor of the thumb.

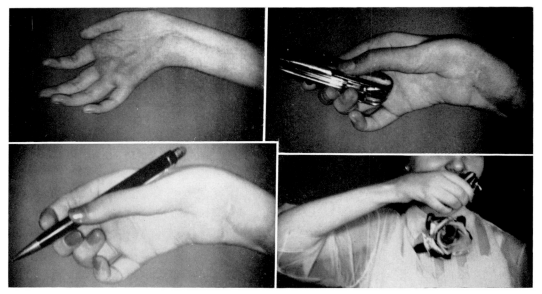

FIG. 537. Case L. M. W. Poliomyelitis resulted in flail shoulder and no flexors in the hand. Arthrodesed the shoulder and the wrist simultaneously so that the patient could place the hand. The only available muscles for transfer were the supinator longus, the extensor carpi ulnaris and the palmaris longus. The extensors of the digits were working. Used the extensor carpi ulnaris to flex the 5 digits, the long extensor of the ring finger for opposition. Slit the proximal pulleys to flex the proximal joints by the long flexors. Used the palmaris longus to abduct the thumb. The patient gained much use of the hand and grasped objects ranging from a sheet of paper to an object 4½ inches in diameter. She could place her hand well by her shoulder and held a position in a bank.

Starr had pointed out in 1922—that retention of 1 wrist flexor is essential. The palmaris longus is sufficient, but he suggested leaving the flexor carpi radialis. Starr had retained the flexor carpi ulnaris, as had Jones in some cases. When all wrist flexors had been used, Luckey and McPherson attached a finger flexor to the volar carpal ligament to act as a substitute.

With wrist extension supplied by the pronator teres to radial wrist extensors it seems more logical to retain the flexor carpi ulnaris, since this is the direct antagonist of the extensors acting in the major axis of wrist motion.

Junctions of the transferred tendons should not be made under the dorsal retinaculum but higher up the forearm. A natural tenodesis or deliberately attaching the digital extensors to the radius so that as the wrist palmar flexes the fingers extend is useful when no muscles

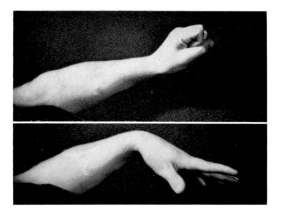

FIG. 538. Case L. K. A wringer injury had avulsed the extensors of the forearm. Fractures of the radius and the ulna healed with synostosis, stopping pronation and supination. Applied pedicle to dorsum. Bridged ulna with double onlay. Excised the synostosis, wrapping each bone two thirds around with polythene. Patient obtained 28° of supination and 35° of pronation. The hand shows excellent flexion and extension from tenodeses on the forearm, using automatic motions.

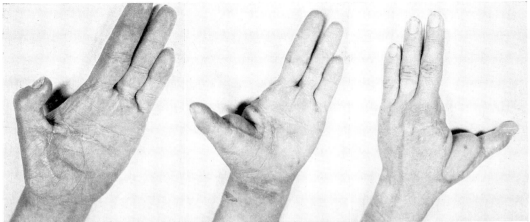

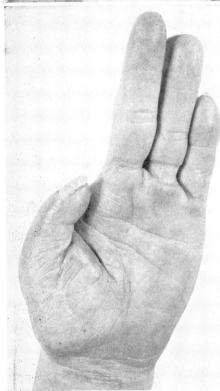

FIG. 539. (*Top, left*) From the explosion of a 20 mm. shell, this patient lost the index finger and had a flexion contracture of the first cleft with destruction of the adductor muscles and ankylosis of the distal thumb joint in excessive flexion. (*Top, center* and *right*) A thumb cleft was established by removing the remains of the second metacarpal and placing a pedicle skin graft, but the thumb could not adduct. The sublimis tendon of the missing finger was threaded through a pulley of tendon made in the palm and fastened to the ulnar side of the first metacarpal. (*Bottom*) The thumb adducts to the hand. (W. C. Graham, M.D.)

are available. Fusion of the wrist is contra-indicated in radial palsy.

There are many methods of stabilizing the base of the thumb or providing action of the long thumb abductor. Arthrodesis of the meta-carpotrapezial joint will prevent drop of the first metacarpal if tendons are not available for transfer. When tendons are available, sev-eral methods, using various motors or a slip from one of the transferred tendons, can be employed.

Examples of Some Procedures for Radial Palsy. Flexor carpi ulnaris to extensors of mid-dle, ring and little fingers. Here the muscle must be freed well up the forearm to allow a straight course. Flexor carpi radialis to ex-tensor of index and long extensor of thumb. Pronator teres to extensor carpi radialis lon-gus and brevis. The palmaris longus can be transferred to the abductor pollicis longus and the extensor pollicis brevis. This method fails to leave a wrist flexor, which is essential. If the palmaris longus is left to act as a wrist flexor, then abduction of the thumb can be ob-tained by various methods such as a slip from the extensor carpi radialis longus activated by the pronator teres transfer. If the flexor carpi radialis has been retained as a wrist flexor, it can be transferred to the abductor of the

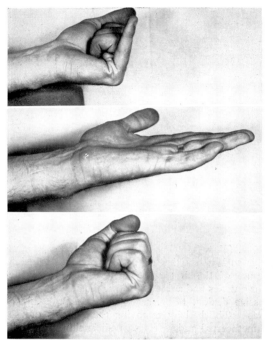

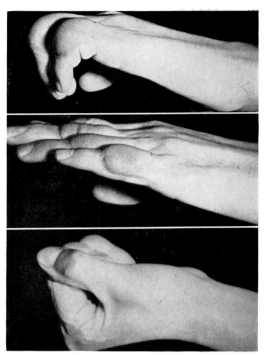

Fig. 540. Case P. S. (*Top*) A milk bottle had lacerated the hand at the proximal flexor crease in the little finger, severing both flexors. (*Center* and *bottom*) Transferred the flexor sublimis of the ring finger to the profundus insertion in the little finger 1½ years later. Perfect result.

Fig. 541. A burn destroyed the dorsal extensor apparatus over each middle joint. After a flap was applied, the superficialis flexor of each finger was withdrawn in the palm, extended by a graft from toe extensors and placed as a crisscross graft on the dorsum. Result is full extension and practically complete flexion.

thumb, slitting the latter's sheath, so that it still acts as a wrist flexor, or the long extensor tendon of the thumb can be lifted out of its normal recess behind Lister's tubercle, passed to the volar radial side of the wrist and attached to the palmaris longus (Riordan). This provides some abduction as well as extension.

A PROCEDURE FOR RADIAL PALSY. Since the usual transfers for radial palsy cannot restore the normal degree of motion—the wrist motors as used for digits do not have enough amplitude to provide wrist and finger motion together—there is a need for a procedure that will give wrist motion, thumb abduction, full finger extension and, if possible, separate thumb and index extension and yet preserve a wrist flexor, preferably the flexor carpi ulnaris.

The following procedure has been used since 1959 with satisfactory results. The pronator teres is divided at its insertion and attached to both the radial wrist extensors. The flexor carpi radialis is divided at the wrist and sutured into the abductor pollicis longus and the extensor pollicis brevis distal to the fibrous tunnel enclosing these tendons over the distal end of the radius. Thus some flexor component remains, while a strong abduction component is given to the thumb. The flexor superficialis tendons of the middle and the ring fingers are divided at the level of the proximal finger segment through short transverse incisions. Their distal ends will remain free in the sheath. The proximal end of each tendon is withdrawn through a forearm incision, usually an extension of that used to expose the pronator teres. The tendon of the middle finger is passed between the profundus mass and the flexor pollicis longus muscle, and that of the ring finger to the ulnar side of the profundi. At

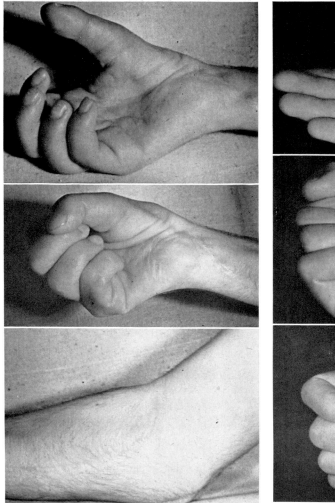

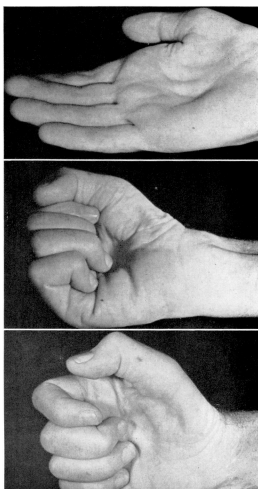

FIG. 542. For loss of all flexion of the fingers from some unidentifiable peripheral nerve disease, the biceps tendon was extended and inserted into the profundi. The lacertus fibrosus was swung across the elbow as a pulley. Photos show range of extension and flexion and absence of spanning at the elbow.

FIG. 543. Poliomyelitis resulted in loss of all flexor power in fingers and thumb. The brachioradialis was transferred to the profundi, and the flexor carpi radialis to the flexor pollicis longus. (*Top*) Postoperative extension. (*Center* and *bottom*) Full flexion. The brachioradialis has adequate amplitude for finger flexion if its muscle is well mobilized.

the proximal edge of the pronator quadratus, 2 large openings are made in the interosseus membrane by excising the fascia, and not simply by forcing an opening with a clamp. The 2 superficial flexor tendons are passed through to the dorsal compartment, that of the middle finger is woven into the extensor digitorum communis and that of the ring finger into the tendons of the extensor pollicis longus and the extensor indicis. By mobilizing the muscles well, making the openings at this level and suturing to the recipients in the middle forearm, as straight a line of pull as possible is obtained, and the muscle, rather than the tendon, is in the interosseus opening. All junc-

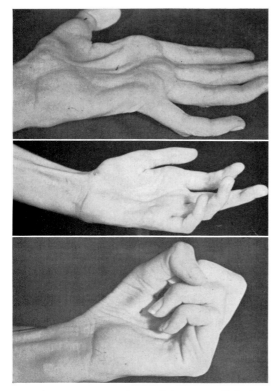

FIG. 544. Postpoliomyelitis loss of digital flexors. (*Top*) Preoperative inability to flex. (*Center*) Extension after transfer. (*Bottom*) Flexion of thumb by flexor carpi radialis and of fingers by brachioradialis.

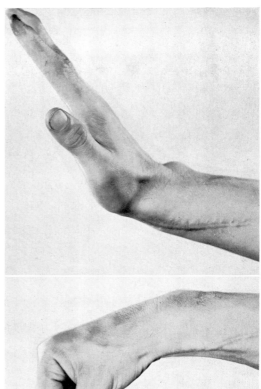

FIG. 545. Radial palsy after transfer of superficialii to extensors. With wrist dorsiflexed, the thumb and the fingers can be extended, and (*bottom*) flexion is possible even with the wrist in palmar flexion. This voluntary reversal of the usual automatic motions illustrates that the transferred superficial digital flexors are not acting as tenodeses.

tions are made with buried stainless steel wire sutures and under moderate tension. The digital flexor tendons are used as motors because they have sufficient amplitude and power to extend the fingers, even with the wrist extended, and to allow some flexion even with the wrist flexed. The flexor carpi ulnaris is retained as a wrist flexor, and some individual action between thumb and fingers is possible.

In patients with posterior interosseus nerve palsy, the pronator transfer is not necessary unless, as in one patient, the lesion is such that only the extensor carpi radialis longus remains active. In this case, there was marked radial deviation of the wrist; to compensate for this, the pronator teres was transferred to the extensor carpi radialis brevis, and the distal end of this tendon was shifted to the extensor carpi ulnaris.

Prior to the development of this transfer of digital flexors through the interosseus membrane, posterior interosseus palsy was treated by transfer of the extensor carpi radialis brevis to the extensor digitorum communis and the palmaris longus to the extensor pollicis longus.

Median Nerve Palsy. For lesions of the nerve in the upper forearm, flexion of the fingers, flexion of the thumb and opposition of the thumb are needed. The flexor carpi ulnaris and the profundi of the ring and the little fingers function as well as the muscles supplied by the radial nerve.

A satisfactory combination is to attach the profundi of the index and the middle fingers to the active profundi of the ring and the little fingers high in the forearm, and to insert the brachioradialis below this point into all 4 profundus tendons to give additional strength. Flexion of the thumb is obtained through transfer of the extensor carpi radialis, either longus or brevis, into the flexor pollicis longus.

Opposition is restored by transfer, prolonged with a graft of flexor carpi ulnaris or extensor carpi ulnaris. If the lesion is in the mid-forearm but the pronator teres has been spared, this is an ideal motor for opposition. Lesions of the median nerve at the wrist or the base of the palm cause loss of opposition only. (For these transfers, see Chap. 12, Intrinsic Muscles.)

Median nerve lesions result in loss of sensibility in the most important surface areas of the hand. Restoration of this function may be as important as return of motion.

Ulnar Palsy. Lesions of the ulnar nerve in the forearm result in loss of most of the intrinsic muscle function and in weakness or loss of profundus action in the ring and the little fingers. The principal effects are clawing from muscle imbalance, weakness of pinch from lack of stability of the proximal thumb joint by the adductor pollicis and the first interosseus and loss of the finer motions of the fingers. Clawing may be absent or only slight, depending on the amount of "cock-back" of the proximal phalanges, and thumb function may be only moderately impaired in some individuals with restricted joints and a median

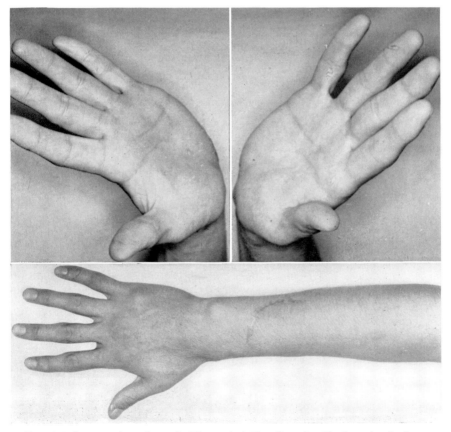

FIG. 546. Same patient shown in Figure 545. Excellent dorsiflexion of wrist by pronator teres transfer and abduction of thumb by flexor carpi radialis. In lower photograph note that the hand does not deviate radially because the flexor carpi ulnaris remains as the primary wrist flexor.

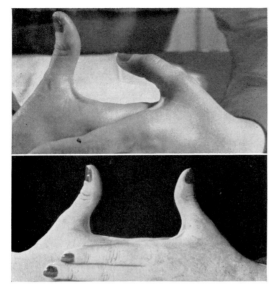

Fig. 547. Latent rupture of extensor pollicis longus tendon reconstructed by transfer of extensor indicis.

innervated strong flexor pollicis brevis. If the flexion of the ring and the little fingers in these high ulnar lesions is restored by transfer or by tapping them into the remaining flexors, clawing may be increased.

Transfer for adduction of the thumb and a procedure for relief of clawing are discussed in Chapter 12, Intrinsic Muscles.

Combined Median and Ulnar Paralysis. If severed above the branches to the forearm muscles, it is best to ankylose the wrist in dorsiflexion, thus making available the 3 extensors of the wrist. The extensor carpi radialis longus can be attached to the profundus tendons for flexion of the fingers, and the extensor carpi radialis brevis to the long flexor of the thumb. Then opposition may be restored to the thumb by using the brachioradialis, prolonged by a tendon graft, looped around the flexor ulnaris tendon and passed subcutaneously across the thenar eminence to insert on the ulnar side of the base of the dorsum of the proximal phalanx of the thumb. Since the flexor ulnaris is paralyzed, the muscle will yield. Therefore, the tendon should be tenodesed to the ulna just above the part used for a pulley, allowing enough slack to extend the wrist or a piece of the tendon turned back to

make a loop for the pulley. As an alternative, the tendon of the extensor carpi ulnaris can be passed around the wrist and prolonged subcutaneously by a graft to the ulnar side of the base and the dorsum of the proximal phalanx of the thumb. To restore muscle balance of the fingers, curvature of the arch and adduction of the thumb, see Chapter 12.

If the nerves are severed low in the forearm, only the transfers for paralysis of the intrinsic muscles will be necessary.

If arthrodesis of the wrist is not desirable, a tenodesis above the wrist can be made of the flexor profundus and the flexor pollicis longus tendons. Then the 5 digits will flex automatically when the wrist is dorsiflexed. In such a case, fixed opposition of the thumb may be furnished by a bone block or strut procedure between the first 2 metacarpals or by a pulley operation with tenodesis to the ulna.

Combined Radial and Ulnar Paralysis. For this the wrist is fused, the flexor carpi radialis is transferred to the extensors of the thumb and the index finger, and the pronator teres is prolonged with a tendon graft to the extensors of the middle, the ring and the little fingers. The palmaris longus can be used to abduct the thumb, and, if clawing is a problem, either a transfer of a superficialis flexor or a tenodesis can be done.

BRACHIAL PLEXUS PALSIES

In lesions of the peripheral nerves the pattern of paralysis is usually uniform, and, as a consequence, the standard transfers discussed above were designed; experience over many years has proved their value.

In lesions of the brachial plexus or the cord that accompany fracture dislocations of the cervical spine, there is also a pattern, but some variation is found, and it is necessary to study each extremity, carefully testing the individual muscles before outlining a plan of reconstruction.

For lower plexus palsies, the basic needs are opposition of the thumb, intrinsic finger-muscle action and digital flexion. Usually, there will be available the flexor carpi radialis, the 2 radial wrist extensors, the brachioradialis and the pronator teres. The basic grasp can be restored by using the brachioradialis to flex the fingers, the pronator teres for flexion

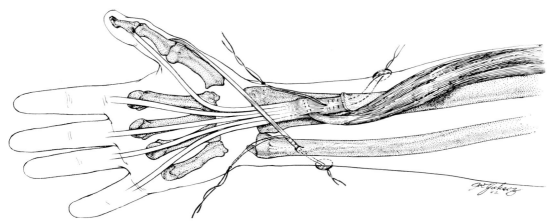

FIG. 548. For paraplegia from lesions between C-6 and C-7, tenodeses combined with transfer of the still functioning brachioradialis can utilize the active dorsiflexion of the wrist to provide some grasp. All digital flexors are tenodesed to the radius, and a graft is used to tenodese the thumb to the ulna as in the pulley operation for loss of opposition. The brachioradialis is inserted into the digital flexors below the tenodesis, potentiating the automatic flexion which results when the wrist is dorsiflexed.

of the thumb and the flexor carpi ulnaris for opposition. Adductor power to the thumb and intrinsic transfer for clawing can be powered by a superficial flexor, or a tenodesis can be done. If the individual long extensors of the index and the little fingers are functioning, each can be divided at the insertion and split, 1 strand being passed deep to the transverse metacarpal ligament and attached to the intrinsic aponeurosis.

PARAPLEGIA

Fracture dislocations with injury to the cord result in varying paralyses, but with careful planning, a combination of tenodeses and transfers will restore considerable function.

Paraplegias With Cord Lesion Between C-6 and C-7. Here the only voluntary motion present may be dorsiflexion of the wrist through the extensor carpi radialis longus. The brachioradialis may be spared, since it is supplied from C-5. If the wrist extensor is strong, the automatic function is utilized, and grasp is obtained by tenodesing the digital flexors to the radius so that the fingers will close when the wrist is dorsiflexed. The thumb can be made to oppose by tenodesing a graft to the ulna, where, by acting as a fixed checkrein, it pulls the thumb into opposition as the wrist is dorsiflexed. Flexion of the fingers can be supplemented by attaching the brachioradialis

into the flexors distal to the tenodesis, or if the wrist extensor is weak, by transferring the brachioradialis to provide dorsiflexion of the wrist.

Paraplegias From Fracture Dislocation of Cervical Vertebrae. Fracture dislocations of C-5 and C-6 vertebrae may result in loss of all but one wrist extensor and the brachioradialis, or there may be recovery of the pronator teres and the flexor carpi radialis. Fracture dislocations of C-6 or C-7 usually have a good pronator teres and flexor carpi radialis and occasionally a trace of activity in the digital flexors. In lower lesions, the long extensors of the digits will be active.

For the upper lesions, when the muscles are available, Lipscomb and Henderson used a 2-stage procedure. The first stage included transfer of the extensor carpi radialis longus to the extensor digitorum communis and the extensor pollicis longus, the latter being lifted out of the groove behind Lister's tubercle, and a slip from the extensor carpi radialis brevis to the abductor pollicis longus. A tenodesis was done for clawing, passing a strip of tendon on the radial side of each finger, from the extensor aponeurosis at its lumbrical insertion, along the lumbrical canal, beneath the transverse metacarpal ligament and to the dorsum of the wrist. It was attached here to the radius or to the dorsal retinaculum. The

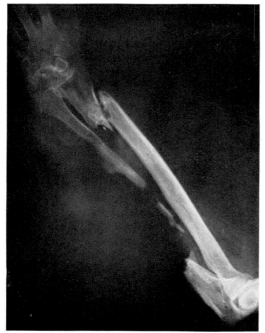

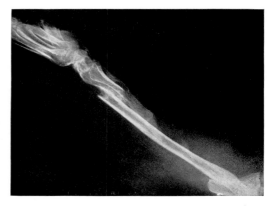

FIG. 549. From a gunshot wound, much of the ulna, the ulnar nerve and all the muscles in the forearm, except the extensors and the flexor of the thumb, were blown off. (*Top*) After replacing the cicatrix with a large skin flap, the wrist was ankylosed in dorsiflexion. (*Bottom, left*) The extensor carpi radialis longus and brevis were transferred to give useful flexion to thumb and fingers as shown in the bottom right-hand pictures. (W. C. Graham, M.D.)

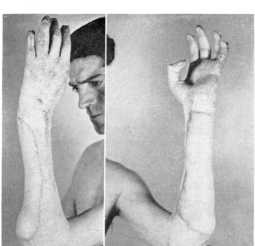

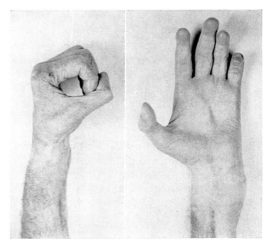

second stage included use of the flexor carpi radialis for opposition and transfer of the pronator teres to the profundi and of the brachioradialis to the flexor pollicis longus. Since the brachioradialis is more powerful than the pronator teres and, when mobilized well, has sufficient amplitude for the digital flexors, it is probably better to use it for finger flexion and the pronator teres for the thumb.

Pronation Deformity. In cerebral palsies of spastic type, some birth palsies and Volkmann's ischemic contracture the forearm is kept in marked pronation. Correction is difficult, and the Tubby procedure is not efficient. Mayer stripped the pronator teres and transferred it and the flexor carpi radialis subcutaneously around the ulnar side of the forearm to insert low on the radius. Steindler used the flexor carpi ulnaris, passing it around the forearm to insert low on the radius. Green re-

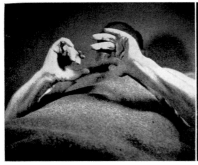 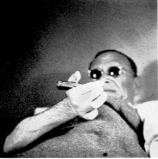 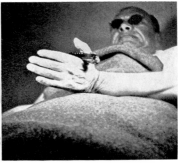

FIG. 550. (*Top*) Paraplegia between C-6 and C-7. The only active motion of the hand is dorsiflexion of the wrist. The patient was unable to hold objects other than by the method shown. (*Bottom*) The flexor profundus tendons and the long flexor of the thumb were tenodesed to the radius, and, for opposition of the thumb, a sublimis tendon was tenodesed to the ulna 1½ inches above the wrist. Dorsiflexion of the wrist caused fingers and thumb to flex and the thumb to oppose. Some voluntary flexion of digits was given by transferring the brachioradialis into the flexors below the point of tenodesis. The patient could pick up objects, help himself and be free of complete dependence on nurses.

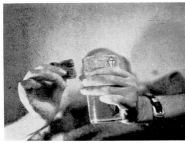 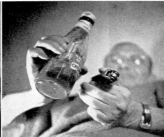 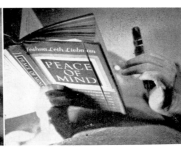

ported good results from this procedure in a long follow-up of patients with cerebral palsy. The insertion was into a radial wrist extensor, and plaster correction was maintained for several months. He felt that it made wrist fusions unnecessary.

In old extreme cases, a rotary osteotomy of the ulna or fusion of the lower ulnoradial joint will maintain correction.

OTHER TENDON TRANSFERS

In reconstruction following trauma, there is not the fixed pattern of muscle loss seen following major nerve injuries; usually, there is much scarring, and tendon transfers become only one aspect of the restoration of function. In these cases a study of the function required and of the motors available usually will lead to one best choice.

Extension of the Wrist. A wrist extensor must be strong, and, if it is available, the brachioradialis, the strongest of the forearm muscles, should be used. In spastic paralysis, it will often be under good control and, when used as a motor for wrist extension, can provide the motion for automatic finger flexion. For ulnar flexion deformity, transfer of the flexor ulnaris to the extensor carpi radialis not only takes away one of the deforming forces but brings the wrist up into functioning position.

Extension of Fingers. Radial palsy is the commonest cause of loss of finger extension, but traumatic avulsion of the muscles, irreparable posterior interosseus nerve lesions and tendon ruptures in rheumatoid arthritis are other causes. Often, one of the wrist extensors has been used, but if the tissues are relatively normal, the use of a superficial flexor tendon, as described under radial palsy, is recommended. Intrinsic extension of the fingers properly belongs to the problem of intrinsic muscle reconstruction discussed in Chapter 12, but for direct loss of the extensor apparatus

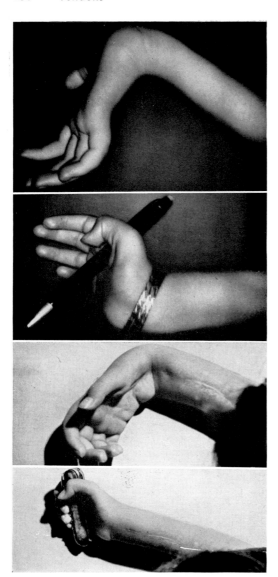

FIG. 551. Case J. L., age 8. (*Top*) Automatic movements. From poliomyelitis there were no flexors of the wrist or of any of the 5 digits. The second picture shows that the only function was a weak pinch between the side of the hand and the thumb by the long extensor of the thumb. Transferred the brachialis anticus to the flexor carpi radialis to give flexion to the wrist. Then tenodesed the long flexor profundus and the flexor of the thumb to the radius with the wrist in flexion so that grasping could be carried out by dorsiflexing the wrist. She had a small muscle in the thenar eminence that gave opposition of the thumb. Extension of the digits and grasping by automatic motion are shown in the 2 bottom illustrations.

flexion is to be achieved. The extensor carpi radialis longus works well when the wrist is movable and can be controlled, in spite of a relatively short amplitude. The brachioradialis, often thought to be a poor choice because of limited amplitude, is the most powerful muscle in the forearm and, if liberated thoroughly from its enveloping fascia, has sufficient effective amplitude to allow full extension and flexion of the fingers. However, when the intrinsics are paralyzed, the clawing from muscle imbalance will often be increased if a strong muscle is used to provide finger flexion. One means of avoiding this is to tap the motor into the superficialis as well as the profundi tendons, adjusting the attachment so that flexion starts with the middle joint. If this is not done, the tips flex first, then the middle and finally the proximal joints, so that the fingers roll into the palm, pushing out the object to be grasped. If an intrinsic transfer can be used to overcome this, or if, with the proximal joints blocked, the fingers can be extended voluntarily, a simple tenodesis of the proximal joint or advancement of its volar capsule will correct the clawing. The flexor carpi ulnaris is a poor motor for flexion of the fingers unless the wrist is fused. In spite of its power, next to the strongest in the forearm, its amplitude is so short that it permits flexion through only a small part of the normal arc of motion. When flexion of only 1 digit is needed, the superficialis of the adjoining finger can be transferred; this is particularly valuable for loss of profundus action of the little finger.

over the dorsum of the middle joints, commonly from burns, a useful transfer is available. Assuming that the skin is soft and pliable or can be made so by a pedicle flap, a long strand of tendon graft, attached at its center to the middle phalanx is crisscrossed over the joint, each end being passed proximally along each side of the proximal segment into the palm and attached to the divided superficialis tendon.

Flexion of the Fingers. A strong muscle with long amplitude is necessary if maximal finger

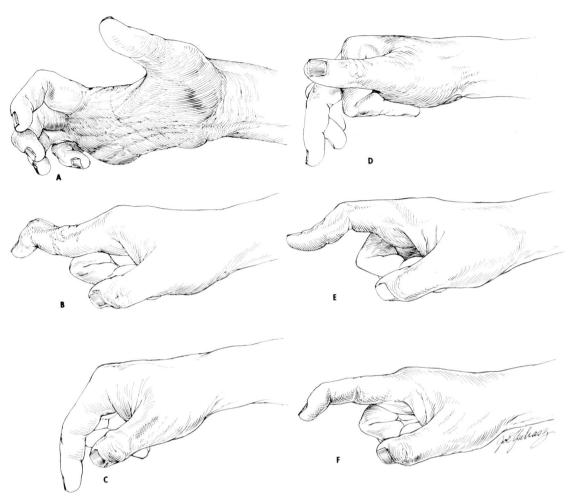

Fig. 552. Common finger deformities. (A) Clawhand from intrinsic muscle paralysis. (B) Hyperextension of middle joint or "swan neck" from rupture of volar plate of middle joint or long-standing intrinsic contracture. (C) Severance of extensor at proximal joint. (D) Severance of profundus tendon with superficialis intact. (E) Damage to middle slip and triangular ligament at middle joint. (F) "Mallet" or drop finger from disruption of extensor tendon at or near insertion.

Flexion of the Thumb. Almost any of the flexor muscles of the wrist or the other digits may be used to supply this motion. One of the flexor superficialis tendons, usually that of the ring finger, can be used and functions well, but the flexor carpi radialis is an excellent choice if the junction can be made in the forearm. The palmaris longus is strong enough to provide a stable pinch if the other thumb muscles are normal. In many cases, loss of flexion of the distal joint of the thumb is only one of the problems. If the proximal joint is unstable or if there is a dropping of the arch because of loss of adductors, the best function of the thumb as a whole unit may be obtained by fusing the distal joint in the optimal position and concentrating reconstructive efforts on restoring control to the more proximal portions. The pronator teres, prolonged with a tendon graft, can provide good flexion of the thumb, as can either one of the radial wrist extensors.

Extension of the Thumb. Loss of function of the long extensor tendon of the thumb is often

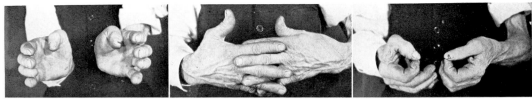

FIG. 553. Case O. V. J. Deformity from severance of the thumb stabilizer, the tendon of the abductor pollicis longus, left hand. (*Left*) The thenar eminence rides forward. Note the thenar crease. (*Center*) Extension of the thumb is limited in the carpometacarpal joint. (*Right*) Pinch against the index finger is weak and makes an ellipse instead of a good O, since the carpometacarpal joint cannot be stabilized in extension to give a good arch of the thumb.

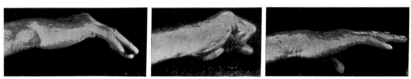

FIG. 554. Case H. B. The right hand and wrist were caught under a cave-in, the dorsum of the wrist and a distance up the forearm becoming gangrenous. The extensor tendons to the digits and the extensor ulnaris sloughed, and, as the head of the ulna was exposed, the wrist joint became infected. The head of the ulna was excised, and, after severing the tendon of the flexor ulnaris, the wrist was drained widely open. All healed in 2 months.

(*Left*) Preoperative condition.

First Operation: After excising the 3½ by 1½ inch cicatrix, a flap of skin from the dorsum was swung to cover the area, and the part left denuded on the radial side was covered by skin graft. The tendon of the flexor ulnaris was seen to be reunited.

Second Operation: Three months later. New tendons were supplied to the fingers by 5-inch grafts of fascia lata, joining the muscles to the tendons at the center of the dorsum of the hand, and one to the extensor carpi ulnaris.

(*Center* and *right*) Taken 4 months later, showing good function of the fingers. The wrist has 30° of motion, and there is full pronation and supination. Adduction is strong. He works steadily.

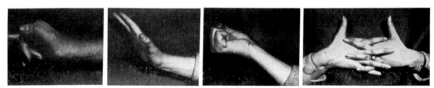

FIG. 555. Case S. A. A laceration across the wrist had severed the extensor tendons of the first 3 fingers and the extensor carpi radialis brevis. Ten days later, as the patient grasped a telephone, the extensor pollicis longus ruptured. (*Far left*) Preoperative inability to extend the thumb and the first 3 fingers. Grafts of several inches of fascia lata, extensor indicis and palmaris longus were used to restore the continuity of the severed tendons. The 3 remaining pictures show that good function returned to the hand.

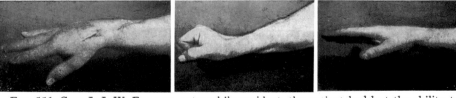

FIG. 556. Case J. J. W. From an automobile accident, the patient had lost the ability to extend either wrist or digits due to a laceration on the dorsum of the wrist which severed all tendons. Their distal ends were adherent at the wrist, checking flexion. (*Left*) Preoperative inability to flex or extend wrist or digits. (*Center* and *right*) Five grafts 5 inches long of fascia lata and proprius tendons were placed after removing cicatrix. He resumed his occupation, working well as a machinist.

Fig. 557. Case C. M. S. (*Left*) Six months previously, the two short extensor tendons of the thumb and the radial nerve had been severed by a knife. Considerable disability of the hand resulted, in that the thenar eminence rode forward. Abduction of the thumb was limited ½ inch, and

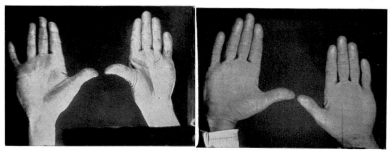

the thumb lost much of its function. The patient grasped either without the thumb or on the dorsal surface of the flexed thumb. The pinch of the thumb was weak, in that the arch of the thumb was gone. As the metacarpal lacked extension, the metacarpophalangeal joint dropped forward in pinching. The radial nerve was sutured, and, as the muscles had retracted, a 2-inch tendon graft from the palmaris longus, plus its paratenon, was used to bridge each of the short extensor tendons of the thumb. (*Right*) In 3 months, sensation returned, and he had normal function of the thumb. (J. Bone Joint Surg. *10*:6)

due to direct injury and not uncommonly to a latent rupture. In polio there may be marked weakness together with the paralysis of the intrinsic muscles. In these cases, a modification of the opponens transfer, inserting the transferred tendon into the long extensor instead of into the proximal phalanx will provide the needed extension.

The most commonly used transfer is that of extensor indicis to extensor pollicis longus. This transfer fulfills almost all of the requirements of an ideal tendon-transfer operation. The donor and the recipient are of practically the same size, of equal amplitude, parallel

each other in the forearm and have a common nerve supply. Their actions are often combined in ordinary activities of the hand. Suturing must be done under proper tension, and protection must be given to the suture line against the strong pull of the opposing flexors. The extensor digiti minimi can be used, simply passing it under or over the common extensors. To provide some abduction component as well as extension to the thumb, the long extensor tendon can be rerouted to the volar aspect of the wrist and motored by the palmaris longus.

Abduction of the Thumb. This is a very

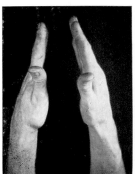
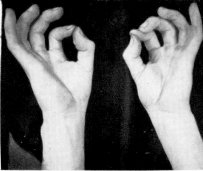
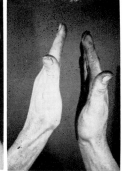

Fig. 558. Case R. R. Three months previously, the tendon of the abductor longus pollicis had been severed with a knife. (*Left*) The thenar eminence rides forward. The thumb is drawn backward on spreading by its long extensor and lacks ½ inch of full extension measured at its tip. (*Center*) In pinching, the arch of the thumb is lost because the metacarpophalangeal joint drops from lack of the abductor, thus making a poor O and a weak pinch. (*Right*) At operation, the tendon had retracted so far that it was necessary to use a 3-inch graft of 2-ply palmaris longus to bridge the gap. The graft and the corrected position of the thenar eminence show clearly in the photograph.

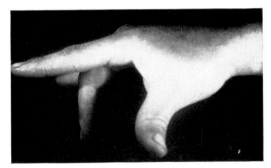

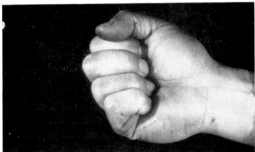

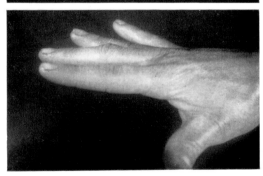

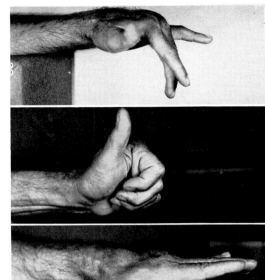

FIG. 560. Case F. W. (*Top*) From an auto accident, skin and tendons were avulsed from the dorsum of the hand, resulting in loss of power to extend the first 3 fingers. (*Center* and *bottom*) A pedicle was applied to the dorsum, and grafts from the palmaris longus were threaded through the fat. Excellent function resulted.

FIG. 559. Case F. S. (*Top*) Drop finger at the proximal joint from an exploding bottle severing the extensor tendon at the joint. (*Center* and *bottom*) Simple suture restored the hand to normal.

important function. Loss of the long abductor action allows the first metacarpal to drop, breaking the longitudinal arch of the thumb and causing an imbalance of the proximal and the distal joints. The pinch is greatly weakened, and opposition is impaired because of the instability at the metacarpotrapezial joint. If, from injury or as in polio this long abductor function should be impaired along with loss of opposition, it is imperative that abduction be restored, or the opponens transfer will not function properly. If available, the flexor carpi radialis is an ideal motor. By re-

moving the abductor from its sheath over the radial styloid a straight line of pull is obtained, and abduction of the thumb will be restored, yet the wrist flexor function will be retained. Either one of the radial wrist extensors or the palmaris longus can also be used.

For other transfers involving the intrinsics, see Chapter 12.

POSTOPERATIVE TREATMENT

After tendon suture, graft or transfer, the repair must be protected for 3 weeks and excessive strain prevented for an additional 2 weeks. Extensor tendons require protection for a longer period than flexor tendons.

After flexor tendon repair, the wrist is placed in palmar flexion, not at the extreme range but slightly less to avoid straining the joint. The fingers are not held in flexion by splinting but are allowed to extend with the wrist flexed. Extensor tendon repairs are protected by volar splints.

Dressings are of fluffed gauze. Dead spaces, if needed, are drained with a small rubber tube drain for 24 hours. Firm even compression is applied, using steel wool pads for uniform gentle pressure, and the whole dressing is held with bias-cut stockinette bandage. Splints for immobilization are used, usually a slab of plaster on the volar or the dorsal surface over the stockinette. A layer of sheet wadding beneath the plaster facilitates changes of dressings later.

Care must be used in applying a compression bandage and any circular binding of the hand. Venous obstruction can result from tight bandaging over the dorsum of hand and the wrist, and the hand may be pulled out of shape in making the turns of the bandage. The normal metacarpal arch should be maintained, and the thumb should be in the forward opposed position. Unless there is some specific contraindication, all bandaging is done with the forearm in supination. The purpose of a bandage and a splint is to provide rest of the part, restrict activity and relieve strain on sutured parts. The tips of the fingers should be visible so that one can check the circulation. Elevation is maintained for a few days, and any constricting bandage relieved as soon as possible. If a drain is used, a long strand of wire attached to a safety pin through the drain is brought out under the edge of the dressing so that the drain can be removed without disturbing the compression. The elbow is often included in the immobilization, especially in children.

The purpose of a splint after tendon surgery is not to immobilize the part as for a fracture but rather to restrict certain motors. Therefore, plaster splints rather than complete encircling casts are used.

The protection should be maintained for at least 3 weeks. Skin sutures usually are removed after 10 to 12 days, though in small children a plain catgut skin suture is used to ease the handling of these patients. A pull-out wire suture or a running wire is removed after 3 weeks, and cautious active motion is started. At this stage patients are instructed to remove the splint and wash the hand and the forearm in lukewarm soapy water once or twice a day and to try to flex the fingers vol-

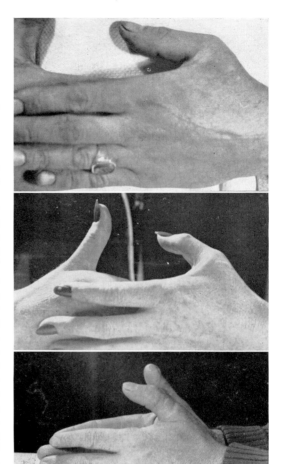

Fig. 561. Three examples of rupture of tendon of extensor pollicis longus to show variation in deformity resulting from loss of function of this tendon.

untarily. Detailed instructions by the surgeon with personal demonstration of the motion to be strived for are necessary. After 4 weeks all splints are discarded, though in some extensor tendon injuries a 6-week period of some protection is advisable.

When active flexion is begun and the danger of rupture of the graft or the suture line is past, some specific exercises for flexor tendon action are often useful. The patient should be shown how, with his other hand, he can hold the proximal finger joint in extension, while trying to flex the middle joint. This makes the flexor tendon glide through the finger instead of using up all its restricted amplitude to flex the proximal joint. Similarly, when the middle

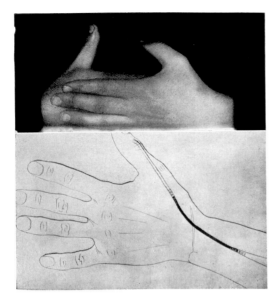
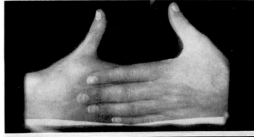
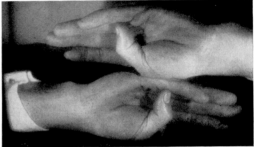

FIG. 562. Case E. L. J. Three months previously, the tendon of the extensor longus pollicis had been severed in a laceration from a broken bottle across the dorsum of the wrist. An infection resulted, and about 2½ inches of the above tendon sloughed out. The resulting inability to extend the thumb is shown in the top left-hand picture.

Operation: A 2½-inch length of the palmaris longus tendon was used as a free graft, as in the second diagram. The resulting function 3 months later is shown in the 2 right-hand pictures. (Surg., Gynec. Obstet. *39*:268)

segment is held, motion is stimulated at the distal joint. Another exercise is to have the patient hold the involved finger in full flexion passively, while trying to flex and slide the tendon through the palm and the finger.

Use of a rubber ball is of no value in mak-

ing a tendon glide through the finger but can help to exercise the muscle and increase its strength. Gripping a soft piece of rubber sponge or a thin wooden block shaped to fit the hand so that a fulcrum is provided over which the finger flexes is of more value. A

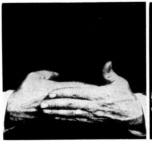
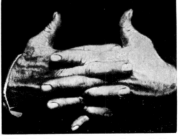

FIG. 563. Case T. L. B. (*Left*) Loss of extension of the thumb from rupture of the tendon of the extensor pollicis longus on a spicule of bone 3 months following a Colles's fracture. It had been present for 3 years. (*Right*) Extension was restored by transferring the tendon of the extensor digitorum communis from the base of the index finger to the distal portion of the extensor tendon to the thumb. The tendon stump of the extensor communis was sutured to the extensor indicis proprius to prevent rotary deformity.

silicone compound called "bouncing putty" provides an interesting diversion along with the exercise.

Patients must be willing to work, exercising vigorously and often if a good result is to be obtained.

In some patients in whom fear of pain is a factor, a temporary local block with lidocaine (Xylocaine) of the median or the ulnar nerve at the wrist may allow enough motion to enable them to continue when the anesthesia wears off.

Repeated encouragement and stimulation are necessary, and visits at weekly intervals during the 4th to the 8th weeks are usually necessary.

Physiotherapy, as too commonly performed with bubble baths, "magic" lights and passive manipulations called massage, is a waste of time, effort and money. An experienced physiotherapist can aid the patient by advice, example and encouragement. As Moberg so aptly put it, in this type of work the best physiotherapist is a bilateral above-elbow amputee.

In our experience there has been no benefit from microwave diathermy or ultrasound.

The prevalent idea that stiff joints can be mobilized by passive "stretching" has no basis in fact; "stretching" usually aggravates the joint stiffness, each "treatment" resulting in tears of the fibrosed structures and additional swelling and hemorrhage.

Excessive use of heat results in swelling, edema and redness, the syndrome of "the cooked hand." Return to useful work as soon as possible is one of the best therapeutic measures possible. If a cooperative employer or labor representative will allow return to work even with some restrictions, motion and strength will improve, and the costs of injuries will be greatly reduced.

After 1 month there is usually only a little motion present; this increases gradually, but the maximal result is not obtained until at least 6 months have passed. Some patients continue to improve even up to 1 year after surgery.

After all methods of obtaining motion are used and progress seems to stop, a tenolysis may be considered. If the juncture was in the distal palm near a fascial septum, there may be a dense adhesion holding the tendon in its bed. It may be necessary to interpose some paratenon gliding material or even to replace the tendon with a graft.

EVALUATION OF RESULTS AFTER TENDON RECONSTRUCTION

It is almost impossible to evaluate the results of tendon reconstruction operations by any statistical method. There are so many variables—e.g., the type and the extent of the injury, the age of the patient, the accompanying injuries to nerves and vascular structures, and the procedures used—that only general conceptions, based on experience, can be used. In some cases, where the only resulting function is a weak pinch and some protective sensation, one might consider the result as being satisfactory because the previous condition is known, but in others one could consider the operation to have been a failure if the digit does not move through at least half its normal range.

After tendon repair, in the forearm or the palm, and in the presence of good nutrition and nerve supply, one should expect a result

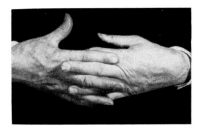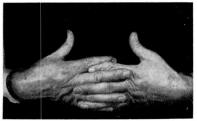

Fig. 564. Case H. E. C. (*Left*) Inability to extend the left thumb due to severance of the tendon of the extensor pollicis longus at the wrist with a knife 6 months previously. (*Right*) Repair was made by a 3½-inch tendon graft from the palmaris longus.

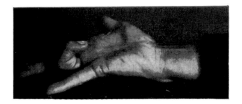

Fig. 565. Case T. G. M. Trigger finger trapped in flexion following gardening. At operation, the ligamentous sheath was found to be thickened, and a fusiform swelling of the tendons was present where the sublimis straddled the profundus. Simple lateral slitting through the annular ligament effected a cure.

approaching normal. In certain areas, as in "no man's land" or under the most ideal conditions, there will be many complete failures and only a few satisfactory results.

Nerve damage influences the results of tendon repair, and people whose joints stiffen easily will never have a perfect result. All of these factors must be taken into consideration in determining the aim of reconstruction, in choosing the type of procedure to be done and in evaluating the results. As a surgeon, one evaluates impairment of function of the hand from the standpoint of the basic functions common to all humans, but in planning procedures one must consider the other aspects of the patient's life, his specific work, his hobbies, his economic status and his future employability.

Other factors being equal, the best results from tendon repair are those following severance of the wrist tendons and, in descending order, the abductor pollicis longus, the digital extensors and flexors in the forearm and the finger extensors on the back of the hand.

Tendons in the fingers are the most difficult to repair and especially the flexors between the distal crease of the palm and the middle joint of the finger. In this area, it is considered advisable in most cases not to attempt a primary suture but to reconstruct the flexor mechanism by a free tendon graft as an elective secondary procedure.

This is one procedure for which statistical studies have shown the effect of selected variables. Four factors—age, scarring and cicatrix, nerve damage and joint stiffness—were studied, as well as the effect of damage to multiple tendons and the effect that certain technical changes have had on results.

In 138 consecutive grafts done in 118 patients, all for damaged flexors in "no man's land," the factor of age was found to have little effect. Scarring from the original injury or ill-advised primary repairs were detrimental, as was the presence of joint stiffness which had to be treated and relieved before tendon grafting was attempted. In these digital flexor reconstructions, damage to one nerve did not have much effect, but if both nerves were damaged, and especially if there were trophic changes from damage to nerves and vessels, the results were poorer than those in the ideal cases. Technical factors, such as a change from silk to wire suture material and careful excision of all remaining sheath tissue in the finger, definitely affected the results.

With ideal conditions it was shown that with the technic described here, 1 in 4 patients flexed the finger to the distal crease of the palm, and in half the patients the tip came to the palm or within ½ inch of touching it.

SPECIAL SITUATIONS AFFECTING TENDONS

RUPTURE OF TENDONS

A normal tendon seldom ruptures, but the insertion may give way, sometimes avulsing a fragment of bone. The musculotendinous junction or the belly of the muscle will part when strong distracting force is applied, though seldom will the origin be torn. It is

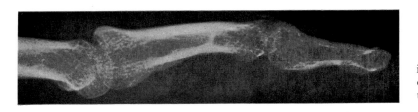

Fig. 566. Avulsion of insertion of extensor tendon. Treatment is for tendon disruption.

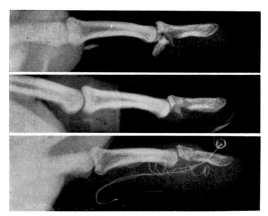

Fig. 567. Case F. M. T. Avulsion of the flexor profundus insertion in a surgeon from a fall on the finger, with loss of voluntary flexion of the distal joint. (*Top* and *center*) Unfortunately, the distal broken fragment had been removed. The end of the retracted profundus tendon is shown at the proximal flake of bone. (*Bottom*) Operative repair. Through a lateral incision, the profundus end was drawn by a stainless-steel suture to the distal phalanx. The wires penetrated phalanx and nail to be tied to a wire ring. The pull-out wire can be seen in place, and also the suture closing the incision. Three months later, he had 35° of voluntary flexion in the distal joint.

only when a tendon is diseased, its nutrition impaired from recent trauma, or when its structure has been worn away that the rupture occurs within the tendon substance. A tendon crushed against a bone by a hard object swells and softens and if strain is applied it may rupture at any time from 1 to 4 weeks after the initial injury. Tuberculous tenosynovitis and rheumatoid tenosynovitis weaken tendons so that they rupture easily.

McMaster, Fink and Wyss showed experimentally that a normal tendon is the strongest link in the musculotendinous chain. Fingers caught in machinery have been torn free, pulling the profundus tendon along with some of its muscle from the forearm. If half the fibers of a tendon are divided, it still requires extreme stress to rupture the tendon. Even a few fibers left intact in a lacerated wound are enough to allow action and lull the unsuspecting surgeon into making a false diagnosis. A

few days later these fibers swell, soften and lose their tensile strength. The tendon now parts on ordinary use, and function is lost.

A partially severed tendon should be approximated by suture and protected through the healing period.

Common tendon ruptures, avulsions of the insertion or breaks in continuity some place in the chain take place at the insertion of the extensors into the dorsum of the distal phalanx, producing the so-called mallet finger deformity, or at the insertion of the middle slip of the extensor mechanism at the base of the dorsum of the middle phalanx, the boutonnière finger. Either the profundus of the superficialis insertions may be avulsed in the fingers.

Tendons become attenuated and weakened from disease, particularly tenosynovitis from rheumatoid disease or tuberculosis or from direct trauma due to bony abnormalities (as after a Colles' fracture or carpal deformities) and occasionally from chronic synovitis caused by occupational overuse. The term "drummer boy's palsy" or rupture of the extensor pollicis longus tendon at Lister's tubercule was coined for this entity reported during the Franco-Prussian War. Senility is not an important factor inasmuch as most ruptures occur in young healthy adults.

Rupture of Extensor Tendons. The most common extensor tendon rupture occurs at the insertion into the distal phalanx, but the middle slip insertion to the middle phalanx may

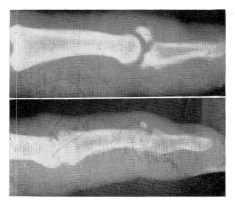

Fig. 568. (*Top*) An intra-articular fracture requiring reduction and immobilization; not a tendon injury. (*Bottom*) Avulsion of bony fragment with tendon insertion. Treat as tendon injury. (J. Bone Joint Surg. *44-A*:1061)

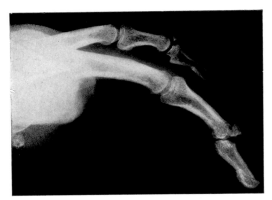

FIG. 569. Double avulsion of bone fragment at the insertion of the extensor tendons, from stubbing the fingers. Can be held in place by 1 stainless-steel wire looped through the tendon about the piece and passed through the phalanx and the skin to be tied over a button on the pulp. If not held firmly, the bone absorbs.

also rupture, though not in the same finger. Ruptures of the common finger extensors occur at the wrist, particularly in rheumatoid arthritis involving the distal ulnoradial joint, and rupture of the extensor pollicis longus can result from the same disease or occur as a "spontaneous" lesion long after trauma to the distal radius.

RUPTURE OF EXTENSOR AT DISTAL PHALANX. If a finger is suddenly overflexed, especially with a taut extensor as in catching a ball, striking an object with the extended finger or stubbing the finger as in making a bed, the insertion of the extensor tendon or with it

a small piece of bone is avulsed from the distal phalanx. The dorsal joint capsule, which is intimately attached to the tendon, may rupture. The finger drops into flexion at the distal joint, and the middle joint may hyperextend—resulting in the aptly named mallet finger. A similar deformity results from fracture of that portion of the base of the terminal phalanx with the extensor insertion; the rest of the phalanx subluxates volarward. This lesion requires open reduction and fixation, whereas the tendon rupture should be treated by splinting. Exact diagnosis is required.

Tendon ruptures occur most often in men, though more in women in the older age groups. The middle finger is involved most often, the little finger next, the index seldom, and the thumb rarely. Two thirds occur in the dominant hand, and in 1 in 4 a chip of bone is avulsed with the tendon. Trivial trauma accounts for over 40 per cent of the deformities. The deformity may not occur immediately, especially after crushing injuries.

Treatment should be conservative. All manner of splints, sutures, internal wire and various operative procedures have been recommended. Some studies indicate that even without treatment many recover to within a few degrees of normal extension. Even if there is some loss of extension, disability is not great, and treatment often magnifies the impairment, since it may result in loss of middle joint flexion, or, if an open form is used, there may be infection requiring subsequent amputation.

Conservative treatment consists of splinting the finger with the distal joint in hyperexten-

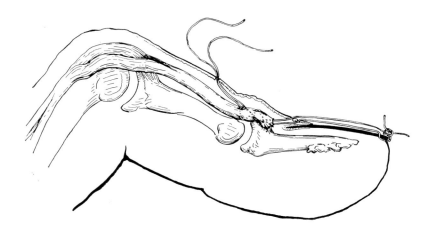

FIG. 570. Method of using stainless-steel wire for late repair of insertion of the extensor tendon, fastening the suture wire to the fingernail and later removing it by the pull-out wire. (Am. J. Surg. 47:505)

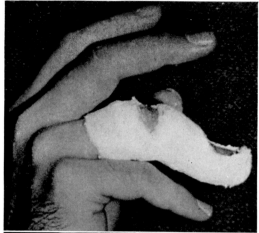

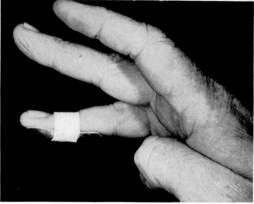

FIG. 571. (*Top*) Plaster dressing for rupture of extensor insertion; the middle joint is in slight flexion. (*Bottom*) For incomplete rupture or following plaster removal, a volar aluminum splint protects the healing tendon. (J. Bone Joint Surg. *44-A*: 1064)

sion and the middle joint in moderate flexion. This relaxes the ruptured tendon and approximates the torn areas, and, if the position is maintained for 5 weeks, healing will take place. The best splint is of plaster, leaving the nail exposed as well as the dorsum of the middle joint. The distal joint should not be strained in hyperextension, since this compresses the skin on the dorsum, making it ischemic and resulting in necrosis under the plaster.

Other forms of splints of aluminum or plastic may be used, and in some instances only the distal joint need be immobilized.

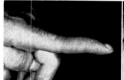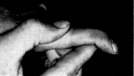

FIG. 572. Case C. B. A heavy plate had dropped on the dorsum of the distal joint of the ring finger, resulting in dropfinger. The finger was splinted straight and eventually lacked 40° of extension in the distal joint. At operation, the tendon was found to be stuck to the head of the middle phalanx. It was freed and did not seem to be too long. A piece of polythene was placed between the tendon and the bone and removed 2 months later. Fairly good function resulted.

Treatment depends on several factors:

1. *Time Since Injury.* If seen within 10 days of injury, plaster including the middle joint is worn for 5 weeks. This is followed by wearing a splint for the distal joint only for 4 weeks. If seen from 10 to 30 days after injury and without prior treatment, a short metal distal joint splint is worn for 2 months. If the finger has been splinted since injury, such as on a tongue blade, the plaster dressing is applied for 4 weeks and followed by a short splint for a month. If the injury is 1 to 2 months old, a short splint to the distal joint for 2 months will improve extension. After 2 months, treatment is only for pain and soreness and consists of temporary splinting of the distal joint.

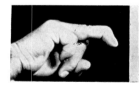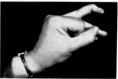

FIG. 573. Drop finger from loss of insertion of the extensor tendon by severance, rupture or evulsion of a piece of bone, often from stubbing the finger. There is complaint of the finger getting in the way.

The illustrations show drop finger, one from stubbing, the other from laceration by glassware. Good function was restored to both by repairing with removable stainless-steel wire.

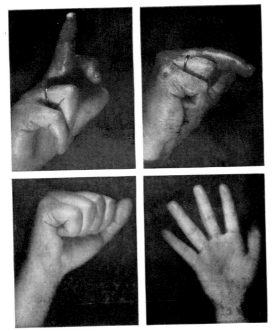

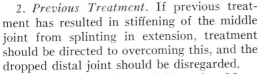

FIG. 574. Case A. E. Two months previously, on striking a basketball with the fingers, the long finger would no longer flex. The tendon had torn from the muscle in the forearm. (*Top*) Position and limit of flexion of the long finger. Through the 2 transverse incisions shown, the flexor tendons to the long finger were shortened. (*Bottom*) Full motion resulted.

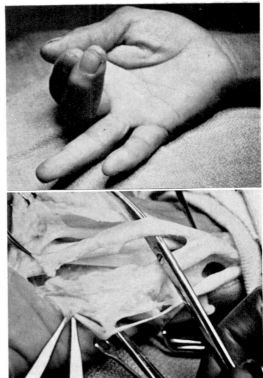

FIG. 575. Rupture of flexors of ring and little fingers in thickened ulnar bursa in patient with syringomyelia.

2. *Previous Treatment.* If previous treatment has resulted in stiffening of the middle joint from splinting in extension, treatment should be directed to overcoming this, and the dropped distal joint should be disregarded.

3. *The Degree of Loss of Extension.* Many ruptures are partial in that the tendon is stretched or too long. Some voluntary extension from the flexed position is possible. In these, a short splint for 2 months will improve the extension. In these incomplete ruptures spontaneous recovery to a considerable degree may occur.

4. *The Degree of Functional Disability.* If the patient is seen 2 months after injury and is unable to work, surgical repair or arthrodesis of the distal joint is indicated. If the patient is able to work, no treatment is recommended.

5. *The Age of the Patient.* In patients over 60 years of age, treatment should be simple,

i.e., a short splint for a few weeks; immobilization of the middle joint should be avoided.

Operative Treatment. If operative treatment is undertaken, great care is necessary in handling the delicate tissues to avoid further damage and scarring which will make the tendon adhere and checkrein the flexor action. Operation is aimed at freshening and approximating the edges of the tear; splinting is used to maintain the position until healing takes place. The same complete plaster as in the closed treatment is used. If the tendon is adherent to the middle phalanx and is freed, a sheet of polythene film can be interposed and removed after 6 weeks. A bone fragment of any size is reattached with a pull-out wire but if small may be excised and the tendon reinserted by a pull-out wire through tiny drill holes.

In selected cases Pratt uses a Kirschner wire passed through the finger and into the proximal phalanx. Stark, Boyes and Wilson re-

PLATE 9

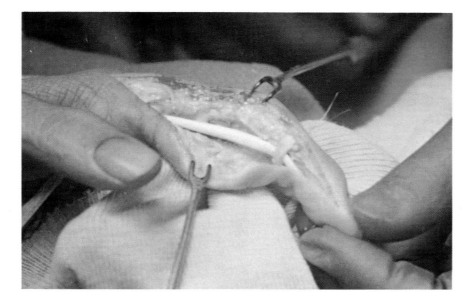

A pulley in the middle segment of the finger can be reconstructed by retaining one slip of the superficial flexor insertion and swinging the free proximal end across the flexor tendon to insert into the side of the phalanx.

PLATE 10

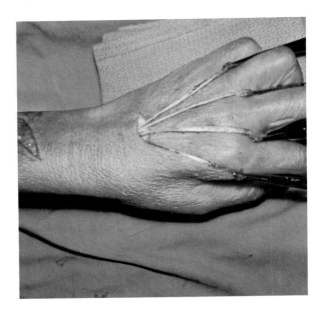

A four-tailed tendon graft from the brachioradialis is used to overcome clawing in median and ulnar palsy as in this patient with leprosy. The motor power is the flexor carpi radialis passed through the interosseus membrane. Each graft is passed through the interossei, beneath the transverse metacarpal ligament and inserted alongside the lumbrical tendon into the extensor aponeurosis.

ported 163 mallet fingers with only 4 treated by open operation and none with Kirschner wire.

RUPTURE OF EXTENSOR TENDON AT MIDDLE JOINT. The insertion of the middle slip of the extensor assembly on the dorsum of the finger may be avulsed from its insertion into the dorsal lip of the middle phalanx, with or without a chip of bone; or, from a blow or crushing injury, softening takes place and the tendon attenuates and stretches. If now the middle point is flexed strongly, the triangular ligament tears, and the result is impaired extension of the middle joint; and, because the lateral slips that remain intact shift volarward, and since their tension is increased when the central slip attachment gives way, the distal joint is drawn into extension or hyperextension. The deformity, erroneously named boutonnière or buttonhole, is exactly contrary to that of a mallet finger. The strong pull of the superficialis insertion flexes the middle joint and prevents the tendon from uniting except by intervening scar, and all attempts to extend the finger voluntarily simply aggravate the condition by exerting more force on the lateral slips which displace below the axis of the middle joint and become a flexing force. A similar result takes place from lacerations across the dorsum of the joint which damage or sever the middle slip and the triangular ligament.

When seen immediately following injury there is usually swelling and even joint effusion, the whole digit is painful, and voluntary motions are much restricted. The diagnosis is often missed, the injury called a sprain, and the finger, if splinted at all, placed in semiflexion. This keeps the ruptured surfaces apart and prevents healing. Most patients are seen some days after the injury, at which time the findings are characteristic. The middle joint is swollen, there is tenderness on the dorsum, and the finger is held in semiflexion. Full flexion of the finger in both middle and distal joints is possible, but extension of the middle joint lacks 30° to 50°. If the middle joint can be extended to a straight line passively, then it will be found that the distal joint is limited in flexion, both voluntarily and passively, and can be freed from this limitation only by flexing the middle joint. This is a form of intrinsic plus as seen in contractures of the interossei, but here it involves only the middle and the

distal joints and is the result of the imbalance between the middle and the lateral slips. It might be called an "intrinsic intrinsic plus." Holding the middle joint in full extension or, if it has become passively limited, drawing it into complete extension on a "safety pin" splint, the range of flexion of the distal joint should be measured carefully and compared with that of the same finger on the other hand, held in the same position. If the injury is a few weeks old, there may be only 5° to 10° of voluntary flexion possible at this time.

Treatment consists of splinting the middle joint in extension but leaving the distal joint free. If the middle joint cannot be fully extended passively, it must be brought to full extension by splinting, using the solid safety pin and a nonelastic strap. The distal crossbar of the splint must end at the distal finger crease, to leave the distal joint free. The patient is instructed to wear the splint constantly and to practice strong voluntary flexion of the distal joint. The splint is worn for 5 weeks, when, if the exercises for the distal joint flexion have been done correctly, it usually will be found that the distal joint will flex to the same degree as that on the other hand. If not, then the splint must be replaced and the exercises repeated until the distal joint flexion is obtained. Once the distal joint can be fully flexed with the middle joint extended, the 2 components of the extensor apparatus are back in balance, and the splint can be removed.

If the tendon is lacerated in an open wound, repair of the tendon consists of simple approximation by a figure-of-eight or running stainless steel wire suture to maintain apposition of the tendon. The splint described above is used postoperatively for 5 weeks; the distal joint is left free, and the patient is instructed to flex it.

Operative repair of this rupture has been done for only 2 conditions. (Since 1957 the splint treatment has been used in all other conditions with complete satisfaction.) If a bony fragment of the insertion has been avulsed and is lying free over the dorsum of the joint, it should be replaced or excised and the tendon reattached with a pull-out wire. The other condition requiring operative excision and repair is a long-standing deformity in a young person. Here the scar between the tendon ends is excised, and the lateral slips are freed completely, both proximal and distal to the joint level. The middle slip is sutured with the middle joint in extension, and the lateral slips are tacked to the sides of the central portion, while the distal joint is held in flexion. At the time of operation it must be possible to hold the middle joint fully extended and simultaneously flex the distal joint completely. If not, then a diagonal cut through the conjoined lateral slips on the dorsum of the middle segment lengthens this part of the extensor apparatus.

If all of the extensor apparatus at the middle joint level is destroyed from an avulsion or a burn, either fusion of the joint is necessary, or, if the soft tissues permit, a tendon transfer can be done.

RUPTURE OF EXTENSOR POLLICIS LONGUS. This tendon turns a corner behind Lister's tubercle and runs in a bony groove in its own separate sheath. It passes over the radial wrist extensors and to the thumb, the diagonal course giving it a strong adduction effect on the latter. Because of this constant rubbing at the point of angulation it may wear and rupture. Latent ruptures following trauma, particularly Colles' fracture, have been reported many times. The average interval between fracture and rupture is 3 months, but it varies from 1 week to 10 years. Rupture results in loss of extension of the distal joint and occasionally some loss of extension at the proximal joint. Examination for loss of function of this tendon is done with the wrist extended and the thumb abducted while the examiner palpates for the tendon in the tissues. Some extension of the distal joint is provided through the abductor brevis and the adductor pollicis, which may confuse the examiner.

Treatment. It is impossible to suture the frayed ends of the ruptured tendon without placing too much tension on the thumb. Either a graft from a point proximal to the dorsal retinaculum to the dorsum of the metacarpal or a tendon transfer will be needed. A graft is used if the muscle has not contracted and become fibrosed. The ideal transfer is extensor indicis, divided just proximal to its insertion and sutured to the extensor pollicis longus over the first metacarpal. Splinting should be maintained for at least a month.

Rupture of Flexor Tendons. The first recorded tendon rupture in the hand was that of the flexor pollicis longus reported by Von Zander in 1891. Like tendon ruptures in other areas, pre-existing disease or damage to the tendon predisposes to rupture. In a series of 80 flexor tendon ruptures in the hand, 16 gave no history of trauma, but in 13 there was evidence of pathologic changes.

Half of all ruptures seen were in the profundus tendons, the ring finger most commonly, the middle finger, the thumb, the little finger and the index finger following in that order. One patient ruptured all 4 profundi. In 21 per cent both the profundus and the superficialis ruptured, and 19 per cent involved the thumb. Only 2.5 per cent occurred in patients over 60 years of age, the average age being 40 years; 8.8 per cent occurred in patients under 21 years of age.

Sudden hyperextension of the finger was the cause of rupture in 41 per cent, and flexion against resistance the cause in 14 per cent. In 25 patients rupture took place within the tendon substance, but in only 3 was there absence of some pathologic change. Various causes were rheumatoid arthritis, congenital abnormality in the carpal bones, fracture of the radius and a previous crushing injury. A roughened hook of the hamate and a bipartite capitate accounted for ruptures of the profundus and the superficialis.

The hyperextension injuries most often produced ruptures at the insertion. When rupture accompanied or followed a crushing or lacerating wound, the rupture was frequently at the insertion also. Flexion against resistance ruptured the insertion except where the tendon tensile strength was decreased by pathologic changes. Reduced tensile strength was apparent in 20 per cent, and the pathologic changes usually caused rupture to occur in the palm, the carpal tunnel or the wrist.

TREATMENT. The loss of function from rupture of a flexor tendon may be slight. Treatment depends on the location of the rupture, the underlying disease and the amount of impaired function. Many cases should be left untreated.

LUXATION OF TENDONS

Dislocations of tendons occur in several locations in the hand.

The extensor carpi ulnaris may dislocate over the head of the ulna when the forearm is pronated. It usually follows a dislocation of the lower ulnoradial joint rather than fractures of the lower radius. Such fractures may result in shortening of the radius, leaving the ulnar head prominent or even somewhat lax, with excessive movement, but true tendon dislocation is not common unless the fascial tunnel for the ulnaris has been torn.

The lateral bands of the extensor apparatus dislocate volarward in ruptures of the middle slip, as described above. In old tears of the distal insertion of the extensor, the middle slips tend to slip dorsally toward each other in the midline when the middle joint hyperextends.

When the pulley mechanism of the digital flexors is destroyed, the tendons span the flexing angle, and efficiency is impaired.

The common extensor tendons over the prominent proximal finger joints can dislocate following trauma, persistent spasm of the intrinsics or in rheumatoid arthritis. Trauma to the radial side of the joint may weaken the capsule, allowing the tendon to be pulled ulnarward. Since the finger joint has more angular motion ulnarward than radially, and because the whole activity of flexion and extension, combined with the anatomic arrangement of the interossei, tends to pull the fingers in this direction, practically all dislocations will be into the groove on the ulnar side. Only after a compound injury to the joint area have radial dislocations been seen. In 2 cases, a sudden forcing of the fingers ulnarward while flexed, resulted in dislocation of the extensor of the middle finger. One of the patients was a young woman who was grasping a steering wheel tightly when it spun, pushing the fingers ulnarward. The tendon snapped over into the ulnar groove. The other was a gynecologic surgeon whose middle finger extensor slipped ulnarward as he reached deep into the pelvis and, with the wrist palmar and ulnar flexed, attempted to close a heavy forceps; the middle finger in the ring of the handle was pushed forcefully into ulnar deviation. Both were treated by splinting the finger and preventing the ulnar displacement of the tendon by a local pressure pad. Immobilization was continued for 5 weeks. Dislocation of the tendon limits extension and pulls the finger ulnarward.

Ulnar dislocation of the tendons is common in rheumatoid disease and is part of the ulnar-drift phenomenon discussed in Chapter 9.

In congenital deformities, ulnar luxation has

been found in arthrogryposis, producing the deformity called windmill hands.

Treatment. If seen immediately, the traumatic closed dislocations can be treated as described above. Later, operative reconstruction will be necessary. Various methods have been reported. Habermen turned a transverse flap from the ulnar to the radial side over the tendon, a method still used by Fowler in rheumatoids; and Fitzgerald used a strip of fascia lata across all the tendons, suturing it to each side of the capsular ligament. Bunnell wove a palmaris longus tendon through each extensor and its capsule and fastened it to the 2nd and the 5th metacarpal heads. A better method is to lift the dislocated tendon out of the extensor apparatus through an incision on each side of it and transpose it to the radial side where it is inserted into a slit cut in the aponeurosis. This method is extremely useful in rheumatoid dislocations, if done before synovial disease has destroyed the ligaments.

TRAUMATIC TENOSYNOVITIS

Unaccustomed use or excessive, repetitive motions cause changes in the tendon sheaths or the epitenon covering the tendon, resulting in swelling, redness and, usually, crepitation. A single traumatism may also set the stage for later development by producing edema or ecchymosis. Common sites are the radial extensors of the wrist or the extensor ulnaris over a malunited styloid, the long abductor and the short extensor of the thumb (DeQuervain's disease) and the flexor tendons of the thumb and the fingers at the proximal joint levels.

Changes consist of edema and inflammation of the sheath, the epitenon and the paratenon. The changes extend up to and may involve the muscle and seem to be most apparent at the musculotendinous junction. Crepitus is from the thickened folds of synovia and fibrin deposits rolling over each other. Various causative factors have been described, such as muscle fatigue and excess lactic acid.

Symptoms are pain on any activation of the involved tendon, swelling and crepitation. Immobilization, if complete, relieves the pain, but symptoms may persist for many months.

Treatment. In mild cases the process may be self-limited. In others, strapping the part and maintaining the activity may result in relief; this is particularly true in well-motivated athletes or workmen.

In most cases, rest is indicated, and plaster fixation gives relief. The fixation is applied so that all motion of the tendon is prevented. Unaffected parts are left free to move to prevent stagnation and edema. Complete immobilization should not be prolonged, but after the acute symptoms have subsided, intermittent release from the splint is started with increasing active motion as tolerated.

Cortisone preparations injected into the sheath give dramatic and often lasting relief, though temporary exacerbation of the symptoms may occur during the first 24 hours. A poor response demands a review as to correct diagnosis and, if necessary, aspiration and culture. Gonorrheal tenosynovitis and tuberculous tenosynovitis still occur and require specific treatment.

DeQuervain's Disease or Stenosing Tenosynovitis at the radial Styloid

In 1895 DeQuervain first described this condition in the abductor pollicis longus tendon over the lower end of the radius. It is more common in women.

Etiology. The tendon of the abductor pollicis longus, accompanied by that of the extensor pollicis brevis, runs through a synovial-lined sheath over the prominence of the radial styloid. Here it is in a shallow bony groove with a ligamentous covering. At the styloid process the tendon is subject to an unusual degree of sharp angulation in the various motions of the wrist. The thenar eminence moves on the forearm much more than does the hypothenar, and this exaggerates the angulation of the tendon as it passes from the radius to the first metacarpal, so that in many of these cases the angle equals 105°. The joints in women angulate farther than in men, suggesting an explanation for the preponderance of these cases in women. Evidently, it is the friction between the tendon, the tendon sheaths and the bony prominence incurred in holding the tendon in its bed through its great range of angulation that results in tenosynovitis which eventually becomes stenosing. It is most frequent in manual workers, particularly those who pinch with the thumb while moving the wrist. The abductor pollicis longus is a strong stabilizer essential for a hard pinch

with the thumb. The onset is usually gradual but in many patients starts acutely following a blow or sudden strain of gripping or lifting; or it may follow a hard day's work of typewriting, piano playing, twisting a drill, drafting or gripping books.

Symptoms. Whether the onset is gradual or acute, the symptoms persist and may not be relieved by splinting. The main complaint is of aching above the styloid, radiating down the hand and up the arm to the shoulder. This is increased by use of the hand and especially by motions of the wrist and the thumb. When the thumb is strained in extension against resistance, or especially when the wrist is ulnar flexed and the thumb adducted, pain is produced and is exaggerated by local digital pressure. Passive tensing of the tendon by flexing the wrist and the thumb may elicit pain. Tenderness and swelling are present along the tendon. Motions of the wrist and the thumb may be normal or slightly limited. There is complaint of weakness of the thumb and actual diminution of grip. Occasionally, a nodule can be felt at the site of pain and may move with the tendon. Crepitation is not common.

Pathology. In mild cases the changes may be inconspicuous, but in severe ones they may be quite marked. On exposing the outer surface of the sheath one may notice reddening from increased vascularity and some edema over a distance of 2 to 3 cm. opposite the prominence of the lower end of the radius. A small probe can be inserted in the tendon sheath from above and below to locate the region of the stricture which is usually present.

On opening the sheath the synovial fluid may be increased and may be yellowish. Spider-web-like adhesions may extend between the tendon and the sheath. The ligamentous sheath which normally is about 0.75 mm. in thickness may be from 2 to 4 times as thick. The tendon and the sheath may be less lustrous, and over the tendon itself the epitenon is inflamed, ranging from a slightly edematous to a reddish or brownish congested, scumlike dull covering of the tendon. Occasionally, one finds a constriction and bulbous enlargement of the tendon. Microscopically, the sheath is thickened and vascular and shows cellular infiltration. The synovia may be eroded in places.

Treatment. Conservative treatment consists of immobilizing the tendon in a nonpadded half cast of plaster of Paris, including the volar two thirds of the forearm, the palm and the thumb to its distal crease. The wrist should be in slight dorsiflexion and the thumb in its normal position. Local cortisone injections must be made directly into the sheath and not into the subcutaneous tissue. One or 2 injections usually give prompt relief. If symptoms persist in spite of local injection or splinting for 1 month, operative treatment is indicated.

It is not necessary just because the tendon runs longitudinally to make the customary longitudinal incision which so often forms a conspicuous scar or even a keloid. A short transverse incision will suffice and later becomes invisible. As soon as the skin is cut it should be undermined upward and downward for the required distance. Then a longitudinal incision should be made through the superficial fascia from above downward so as not to injure any twig of the superficial radial nerve. The branches of this nerve diverge from each other in the deep part of the superficial fascia. On retracting this layer the tendon sheath is inspected. The sheath is slit open for its length and left open. It is important that the abductor and the short extensor tendons each be identified with certainty, for if by chance they lie in separate compartments and one is not released, symptoms will persist.

Aberrant Tendon Thumb

Of 22 cases treated surgically for symptoms of DeQuervain's disease, Bunnell described 12 in which there was an extra tendon in the sheath.

Most of the aberrant tendons had a separate muscle slip which fused higher into the muscle of the abductor pollicis longus. In one, the tendon forked at the tendon-muscle juncture, and in another case it was bilateral. The tendons lay along the volar aspect of the tendon of the abductor. None of them inserted into the thumb metacarpal, nor did any of them move the thumb when pulled; instead, they radial-flexed and palmar-flexed the wrist. They were inserted variously into the scaphoid or the trapezium, or both, or into the transverse carpal ligament or the fascia over the thenar eminence. In one, the aberrant tendon had been

rolled by the other tendons, producing a snap. In another case the synovial fluid was yellow.

These aberrant tendons should not be confused with a multiple-tendoned abductor, that is, a single muscle having several strands of tendon all inserting on the same point. There was no essential difference in the symptomatology or the findings in cases with and without the true aberrant tendon.

It is not difficult to understand how a true aberrant tendon can produce symptoms considering that so often pain, cramps, weakness and even tenderness are produced when 1 of 2 tendons pulled by a common muscle are held from moving, i.e., if a person holds 1 of his fingers, such as the little or the ring finger, in full extension and strongly flexes the others, or in full flexion and strongly extends the others, he feels sharp pain and cramps. Apparently, it is due to longitudinal strain of one part of the muscle on the other. The amplitude of motion of the aberrant tendon, which has a shorter lever arm, is shorter than that of the tendon of the abductor pollicis longus, so that when they are pulled by a common muscle the mechanics are not right. Slitting the sheath affects the long tendon more than the short, thus tending to equalize their amplitude and explaining cures achieved when the sheath was split and the aberrant tendon not removed.

Many authors have described variations in the extensor tendons of the thumb and their sheaths. The extensor pollicis brevis may be absent, or it may extend the distal point of the thumb. The sheath of the abductor pollicis longus may contain from 1 to 5 tendons, and it or several tendons may have separate sheaths. It is only when a common muscle has different amplitudes of tendon action that the aberrant tendon will produce symptoms and should be removed.

Trigger Thumb

This snapping or catching of the thumb as it is flexed is due to a thickening of the sheath and the tendon at the level of the metacarpal head. Sometimes, more often in infants, the thumb remains locked in flexion because the nodule on the tendon cannot be forced back through the tight pulley. Operative release is simple through a transverse incision along the flexion crease, carefully avoiding the nerves and excising the thickened annular sheath. In adults local cortisone injection may give temporary relief.

Grob and Stockmann claim that a congenitally enlarged sesamoid bone is the cause of trigger thumb in infants.

Trigger Finger

The trigger phenomenon, or sudden snapping movement of a finger, may be from a number of causes: flexor tendons slipping over each other in the forearm, the long extensor slipping on and off the proximal knuckle, 2 lateral bands slipping volarward or back at the middle joint, or from a nodule in the flexor tendons catching at a constriction in the annular sheath opposite the metacarpal head.

The last, which is the usual type, is from a single or multiple direct trauma usually incurred in grasping and affects the middle and the ring fingers especially. The ligamentous sheath and the flexor tendon are pinched between the object and the head of the metacarpal until, from local tenosynovitis, a thickening forms in the sheath with local swelling in the tendons.

When the finger is two-thirds flexed, the motion is held up until, on more force, the nodule pulls through, and the finger snaps into the palm in flexion. A similar phenomenon occurs at the same place on extending the finger. A nodule moving with the tendon can be felt under the examining finger. Finally, due to this increased irritation, the nodule no longer slips through the constriction, and the finger is caught in either extension or flexion. If the distal joint is extended first, the thickenings of the 2 tendons will not coincide, thus allowing the tendon to slip through.

The ligamentous sheath shows a whitish, cicatricial collarlike thickening. In the tendons there is a fusiform enlargement at the bifurcation of the superficialis and some enlargement of the profundus, too. The enlargement is due to edema and inflammatory proliferation of epitenon and a homogeneous, bluish or yellowish expansion of the tendon from thickening of endotenon between the tendon bundles. Some giant cells may be present.

Treatment. The condition may subside with rest or cortisone injection but otherwise is easily cured surgically. Through a short transverse incision in the palm proximal to the nodule, the tendon and the annular band are exposed. With pointed scissors, the annular band is slit through, taking care to avoid cutting the volar digital nerve.

It is impossible to excise any discrete nodule or to slice a wedge from the tendon, for a new lump would form as a reaction to any incision in the tendon itself. Slitting the sheath alone will suffice.

Rupture of one slip of the superficialis tendon may leave a nodular thickening on the proximal end. It should not be excised locally, because this will be followed by a similar nodule; the ruptured end should be stripped up into the palm and cut off there.

Calcification in Tendons

Calcification in tendons as seen in the shoulder area can occur in and about the tendons in the wrist or the hand. The commonest location is in the flexor ulnaris at the pisiform. Special views may be necessary to identify it on the roentgenogram. Other areas of involvement are in the flexor carpi radialis, at the base of the thumb, near the triceps insertion and at the origin of the wrist extensors where symptoms are those of "tennis elbow."

Another form of calcification in the tissues, the calcareous material lying in normal fascial planes rather than in traumatized or degenerated tendon, is seen in the fingers of women with scleroderma or Raynaud's phenomenon. Called calcinosis circumscripta to distinguish it from the generalized universalis type seen more commonly in children, it usually does not require treatment.

The acute calcareous tendinitis mentioned above as occurring at the wrist may have a sudden onset with extreme pain, local redness, heat and swelling. It responds to rest by splinting the involved tendon in a relaxed position and responds promptly to needling, injection of local anesthesia or cortisone preparations. It may subside spontaneously. When seen near the flexor tendon insertions of the fingers or in the vicinity of the interphalangeal joints, conservative therapy, rest and local aspiration or injection usually will cure the condition. Operative treatment is seldom necessary.

BIBLIOGRAPHY

Tendons, General

Adamson, J. E., and Wilson, J. N.: The history of flexor-tendon grafting, J. Bone Joint Surg. *43-A*:709, 1961.

Akamatsu, H.: Clinical studies on the secondary repair of flexor-tendon injuries of the hands; evaluation and analysis of their end-results as influenced by various factors, J. Jap. Orthop. Assn. *35*:1059, 1962.

Ashley, F. L., Stone, R. S., Edwards, J. W., and Sloan, R.: Further studies on the application of monomolecular cellulose filter tubes to create artificial tendon sheaths in the hand and wrist, West. J. Surg. *68*:156, 1960.

Babcock, W. W.: Ligatures and sutures of alloy steel wire, J.A.M.A. *102*:1756, 1934.

Ball, J., Mason, M. L., Koch, S. L., and Stromberg, W. B.: Injuries to flexor tendons of the hand in children, J. Bone Joint Surg. *40-A*:1220, 1958.

Batty-Smith, C. G.: An operation for increasing the range of independent extension of the ring finger for pianists, Brit. J. Surg. *29*:397, 1942.

Blum, L.: Use of myotomy in repair of divided flexor tendons, Ann. Surg. *116*:461, 1942.

Bove, C.: Suturing of flexor tendons of hand (transfixation), Med. Rec. *153*:94, 1941.

Boyes, J. H.: Immediate vs. delayed repair of the digital flexor tendons, Ann. West. Med. & Surg. *1*:145, 1947.

Brockis, J. G.: The blood supply of the flexor and extensor tendons of the fingers in man, J. Bone Joint Surg. *35-B*:131, 1953.

Bunnell, S.: Repair of tendons in the fingers and description of two new instruments, Surg., Gynec. Obstet. *26*:103, 1918.

———: Repair of tendons in the fingers, Surg., Gynec. Obstet. *35*:88, 1922.

———: Surgery of tendons *in* Lewis, D. (ed.): Practice of Surgery, vol. 3, Hagerstown, Md., W. F. Prior Co., 1927.

———: Repair of nerves and tendons of the hand, J. Bone Joint Surg. *10*:1, 1928.

———: Reconstruction of the injured hand, Rocky Mount. M. J. *20*:269, 1938.

———: Treatment of tendons in compound injuries of the hand, J. Bone Joint Surg. *23*:240, 1941.

———: Suturing tendons, Am. Acad. Orth. Surg. Lect., p. 1, 1943.

———: Primary and secondary repair of flexor tendons of hand, J. Am. Soc. Plast. Reconstr. Surg. *12*:65, 1943.

———: Surgery of tendons, Proc. Kessler Inst. Rehab. *1*:1, 1955.

Burnett, C. H., *et al.*: Hypercalcemia without hypercalcuria or hypophosphatemia, calcinosis and renal insufficiency, New Engl. J. Med. *240*:787, 1949.

Carroll, R. E., Sinton, W., and Garcia, A.: Acute calcium deposits in the hand, J.A.M.A. *157*:422, 1955.

Carstam, N.: Effect of cortisone on the formation of tendon adhesions and on tendon healing, Acta. chir. scand., suppl. 182, 1953.

Cooper, W.: Calcareous tendinitis in the metacarpophalangeal region, J. Bone Joint Surg. *24*:114, 1942.

Couch, J. H.: Principles of tendon suture in hands, Canad. M. A. J. *41*:27, 1939.

Cowan, I., and Stone, J. R.: Painful periarticular calcifications at wrist and elbow; diagnosis and treatment, J.A.M.A. *149*:530, 1952.

Eccles, J. C.: Muscle atrophies arising from disuse and tenotomy, J. Physiol. *103*:253, 1944.

Edwards, D. A. W.: The blood supply and lymphatic drainage of tendons, J. Anat. *80*:147, 1946.

Edwards, H. C.: Injuries of tendons and muscles, Lancet *1*:65, 1932.

Fitzgerald, R. R.: Habitual dislocation of digital extensor tendons, Ann. Surg. *110*:81, 1939.

Garlock, J. H.: Symposium: Industrial diseases and accidents to hand; management of injuries of tendons and nerves of hand, New York J. Med. *36*:1740, 1936.

Gonzalez, R. I.: Experimental tendon repair within the flexor tunnels: Use of polyethylene tubes for improvement of functional results in the dog, Halsted Experimental Surgical Laboratory, Dept. of Surgery, Univ. of Colorado Medical Center, 1949.

Gratz, C. M.: History of tendon suture, Med. J. Rec. *127*:156, 1928; *127*:213, 1928.

Grayson, J.: Cutaneous ligaments of digits, J. Anat. *75*:164, 1941.

Haines, R. W.: Laws of muscle and tendon growth, J. Anat. *66*:578, 1932.

Harmer, T. W.: Tendon and nerve repair, Boston Med. & Surg. J. *194*:739, 1926.

Hart, D.: Tendon suture and plastic repair *in* Nelson Loose Leaf Surgery, Vol. 3, Chap. 5-A, New York, Thomas Nelson & Sons, 1927.

Hesse F.: Healing processes in synovial sheaths after suture of tendons; experimental study in transplantation, Arch. klin. Chir. *169*:252, 1932.

———: Treatment of injured tendons, Ergebn. Chir. Orthop. *26*:174, 1933.

Hill, A. V.: Mechanics of voluntary muscle, Lancet *261*:947, 1951.

Huber, H. S.: Application of general principles in tendon suture, Surg. Clin. N. Amer. *19*:499, 1939.

Iselin, M.: Note sur l'reparation des tendons fléchisseurs des doigts d'apres 24 observations, Bull. mém. Soc. nat. chir. *57*:1227, 1931.

Kaplan, E. B.: Pathology and correction of finger deformities due to injuries and contractions of extensor digitorum tendon, Surgery *6*:35, 1939.

———: Correction of a disabling flexion contracture of the thumb, Bull. Hosp. Joint Dis. *3*: No. 2, 1942.

Kaufman, L. R., Johnson, W. W., and Wesser, A.: Clinical study of alloy steel wire sutures in hernia repair, Surg., Gynec. Obstet. 69:684, 1939.

Kernwein, G. A.: A study of tendon implantations into bone, Surg., Gynec. Obstet. 75:794, 1942.

Key, J. A.: Fixation of tendons, ligaments and bone by Bunnell's pull-out suture, Ann. Surg. 123:656, 1946.

Koch, S. L.: Suturing tendons, Indust. Med. 11:327, 1942.

————: Tendon and nerve injuries, New York J. Med. 42:1819, 1942.

————: Nerve and tendon injuries, Bull. Am. Coll. Surg. 28:125, 1943.

————: Division of flexor tendons within digital sheath, Surg., Gynec. Obstet. 78:9, 1944.

Konig, F.: Plastic surgery of muscle defects and use of muscle loops, Zbl. Chir. 62:2531, 1935.

Kyle, J. B., and Eyre, B.: The surgical treatment of flexor tendon injuries in the hand, Brit. J. Surg. 41:502, 1954.

Large, O. P.: Comparison of tissue reactions from new sutures, Am. J. Surg. 50:415, 1943.

Latarjet, A., and Etienne-Martin, M.: Serous sheaths of extensor tendons of fingers and toes on back of hands and feet, Ann. anat. path. 9:605, 1932.

Lindsay, W. K., and McDougall, E. P.: Digital flexor tendons: An experimental study, Part III, Brit. J. Plast. Surg. 13:293, 1961.

Lomas, J. J. P.: Peritendinitis calcarea affecting the hand, case report, Ann. Phys. Med. 5:94, 1959.

McCash, C. R.: The immediate repair of flexor tendons, Brit. J. Plast. Surg. 14:53, 1961.

MacKenzie, C.: The Action of Muscles, Including Muscle Rest and Muscle Re-education, New York, Hoeber, 1930.

Martin, J. F., and Brogdon, B. G.: Peritendonitis calcarea, (x-ray) of the hand and wrist, Am. J. Roentgenol. 78:74, 1957.

Mason, M. L.: Immediate and delayed tendon repair, Surg., Gynec. Obstet. 62:449, 1936.

————: Principles of management of tendon injuries to the hand, Physiother. Rev. 18:119, 1938.

————: Primary and secondary tendon suture; discussion of significance of technique in tendon surgery, Surg., Gynec. Obstet. 70:392, 1940.

————: Nerve and tendon injuries, Indust. Med. 11:61, 1942.

Mason, M. L., and Allen, H. S.: Rate of healing of tendons; experimental study of tensile strength, Ann. Surg. 113:424, 1941.

Mason, M. L., and Shearon, C. G.: Process of tendon repair; experimental study of tendon suture and tendon graft, Arch. Surg. 25:615, 1932.

Mayer, L.: Reconstruction of digital tendon sheaths; contribution to physiologic method of repair of damaged finger tendons, J. Bone Joint Surg. 18:607, 1936.

————: Repair of severed tendons, Am. J. Surg. 42:714, 1938.

————: Celloidin tube reconstruction of extensor digitorum communis sheath, Bull. Hosp. Joint Dis. 1:39, 1940.

Milch, H., and Green, H. H.: Calcification about the flexor carpi ulnaris tendon, Arch. Surg. 36:660, 1938.

Miller, H.: Repair of severed tendons of hand and wrist; statistical analysis of 300 cases, Surg., Gynec. Obstet. 75:693, 1942.

Moberg, E.: Experiences with Bunnell's pull-out wire sutures, Brit. J. Plast. Surg. 3:249, 1951.

Napier, J. R.: The attachments and function of the abductor pollicis brevis, J. Anat. 86: Part 4, 1952.

Nikolaev, G. F.: Significance of early resumption of function following plastic repair of tendons according to Bunnell, Novy khir. arkhiv. 45:327, 1940.

O'Shea, M. C.: Severed tendons and nerves of hand and forearm, Ann. Surg. 105:228, 1937.

Peacock, E. E., Jr.: Some problems in flexor tendon healing, Surgery 45:415, 1959.

————: Antigenicity of tendon, Surg., Gynec. Obstet. 110:187, 1960.

Phalen, G. S.: Use of physical therapy in postoperative management of transfers and grafts in hand, Arch. Phys. Med. 29:77, 1948.

————: Calcification adjacent to the pisiform bone, J. Bone Joint Surg. 34-A:579, 1952.

Pinkerton, M. C.: Amnioplastin for adherent digital flexor tendons, Lancet 1:70, 1942.

Posch, J. L.: Injuries to the hand in children, Am. J. Surg. 89:784, 1955.

Pratt, G. H.: Nine years' experience with steel wire as a suture material, Surg., Gynec. Obstet. 74:845, 1942.

Preston, D. J.: Effects of sutures on strength of healing wounds with notes on clinical use of annealed stainless steel wire sutures, Am. J. Surg. 49:56, 1940.

————: Mechanical superiority of annealed stainless steel wire sutures and ligatures, Surgery 9:896, 1941.

Pulvertaft, R. G.: Repair of tendon injuries in the hand, Ann. Roy. Coll. Surg., p. 3, 1948.

Reimann, A. F., Daseler, E. H., Anson, B. J., and Beaton, L. E.: Palmaris longus muscle and tendon; study of 1,600 extremities, Anat. Rec. 89:495, 1944.

Salsbury, C. R.: Consideration of tendons in hand injuries, Am. J. Surg. *21*:354, 1933.

Schink, W., and Gersbach, R.: An experimental study of tensile strength of tendons sutured by different methods, Arch. klin. Chir. *297*:191, 1961.

Schorcher, F.: Snapping of finger joints due to injuries of tendons, Zbl. Chir. *67*:627, 1940.

Shephard, E.: Deposit of calcium salts at the wrist, J. Bone Joint Surg. *37-B*:453, 1955.

Stahel, W.: Injury of tendons of the hand, Schweiz. med. Wchr. *67*:51, 1937.

Steindler, A.: Mechanics of muscular contractions in wrist and fingers, J. Bone Joint Surg. *14*:1, 1932.

Stewart, D.: Experimental study of return of function after tendon section, Brit. J. Surg. *24*:388, 1936.

Stilwell, D. L., Jr.: The innervation of tendons and aponeuroses, Am. J. Anat. *100*:289, 1957.

Stoffel, A.: The treatment of spastic contracture, Am. J. Orthop. Surg. *10*:611, 1912-1913.

Straus, F. H.: Luxation of tendons of hand, Ann. Surg. *111*:135, 1940.

Thatcher, H. V.: Use of stainless steel rods to canalize flexor tendon sheaths, South. M. J. *32*:13, 1939.

Venable, C. S.: Factors in choice of material for bone plates and screws, Surg., Gynec. Obstet. *74*:541, 1942.

Venable, C. S., and Stuck, W. G.: Use of vitallium appliances on compound fractures, Am. J. Surg. *51*:757, 1941.

————: Three years' experience with vitallium in bone surgery, Ann. Surg. *114*:309, 1941.

Venable, C. S., Stuck, W. G., and Beach, A.: Effects on bone of presence of metals; based upon electrolysis; experimental study, Ann. Surg. *105*:917, 1937.

Verdan, C., and Michon, J.: Tendolysis of flexor tendons; indications in cicatricial blocking, Rev. Med. Nancy *81*:69, 1956.

Verdan, C. E.: Primary repair of flexor tendons, J. Bone Joint Surg. *42-A*:647, 1960.

Von Baeyer, H.: Translocation of tendons, Z. orthop. Chir. *56*:552, 1932.

Wagner, C. J.: Delayed advancement in the repair of lacerated flexor profundus tendons, J. Bone Joint Surg. *40-A*:1241, 1958.

Walkingshaw, R.: Ossification in tendon sheath, J. Malaya Br., Brit. Med. Assn. *2*:252, 1939.

Weckesser, E. C.: Tendolysis within digit using hydrocortisone locally and early postoperative motion, Am. J. Surg. *91*:682, 1956.

Wheeldon, T. F.: Use of cellophane as permanent tendon sheath, J. Bone Joint Surg. *21*:393, 1939.

Wilmoth, C. L.: Tendinoplasty of flexor tendons of hand; use of tunica vaginalis in reconstructing tendon sheaths, J. Bone Joint Surg. *19*:152, 1937.

Zancolli, E.: Surgery of the tendons; anatomy and physiology of the flexor tendons, Prensa med. argent. *48*:1249, 1961.

TENDON TRANSFER

Bauer, K. H.: Wesentliche Vereinfachung der "Perthesplastik" bei Radialislähmung, Chirurg *17*:1, 1946.

Bonola, A.: Tendon transplantation in treatment of inveterate radial paralysis; physiologic aims, technic and results, Chir. org. movimento *22*:239, 1936.

Boyes, J. H.: Tendon transfers in the hand, Proc. of Fifteenth General Assembly of The Japan Medical Congress, Tokyo, Vol. 5, p. 958, 1959.

————: Tendon transfers for radial palsy, Bull. Hosp. Joint Dis. *21*:97, 1960.

————: Tendon transfer in the hand, Manitoba Med. Rev. *42*:422, 1962.

————: Selection of a donor muscle for tendon transfer, J. Hosp. Joint Dis. *23*:1, 1962.

Bruner, J. M.: Tendon transfer to restore abduction of the index finger using the extensor pollicis brevis, Plast. Reconstr. Surg. *3*:197, 1948.

Clark, H. M. P.: An appraisal of muscle and tendon transfers, discussion, J. Bone Joint Surg. *43-B*:172, 1961.

Clippinger, F. W., Jr., and Irwin, C. E.: The opponens transfer; analysis of end results, South. M. J. *55*:33, 1962.

Dunn, N.: Surgery of muscle and tendon in relation to paralysis and injury, Post-Grad. M. J. *13*:374, 1937.

Farill, J.: Reconstructive surgery of paralysis of upper extremity, Medicina, Mexico *13*:284, 1933.

Gallie, W. E.: Further experiences with transplantation of tendons and fascia, Trans. West. Surg. Assn. *46*:47, 1937.

Ghormley, R. K., and Cameron, D. M.: Tendon transfer for paralysis of radial nerve, Proc. Mayo Clin. *15*:537, 1940.

Graham, W. C., and Riordan, D.: Sublimis transplant to restore abduction of index finger, Plast. Reconstr. Surg. *2*:459, 1947.

Green, W. T.: Transplantation of flexor carpi ulnaris for pronation-flexion deformity of wrist, Surg., Gynec. Obstet. *75*:337, 1942.

Henderson, E. D.: Transfer of wrist extensors and brachioradialis to restore opposition of the thumb, J. Bone Joint Surg. *44-A*:513, 1962.

Irwin, C. E.: Surgical rehabilitation of hand and forearm disabled by polio, J. Bone Joint Surg. *34-A*:825, 1951.

Krida, A.: Tendon transplantation for irreparable musculospiral injury, Am. J. Surg. 9:331, 1930.

Lipscomb, P. R., Elkins, E. C., and Henderson, E. D.: Tendon transfers to restore function of hands in tetraplegia, especially after fracture-dislocation of the sixth cervical vertebra on the seventh, J. Bone Joint Surg. 40-A:1071, 1958.

Littler, J. W.: Tendon transfers and arthrodeses in combined median and ulnar nerve paralysis, J. Bone Joint Surg. 31-A:225, 1949.

Luckey, C. A., and McPherson, S. R.: Tendinous reconstruction of the hand following irreparable injury to the peripheral nerves and brachial plexus, J. Bone Joint Surg. 29:560, 1947.

Mayer, L.: The physiological method of tendon transplantation, Surg., Gynec. Obstet. 22:182, 1916.

————: Operative reconstruction of paralyzed upper extremity, J. Bone Joint Surg. 21:377, 1939.

Merle d'Aubigne, R.: Palliative treatment of traumatic paralyses, J. Pract., Par. 62:25, 1948. Abst: Excerp. Med. IX, 3:1298.

Merle d'Aubigne, R., and Lance, P.: Tendon transplantation in treatment of posttraumatic radial paralysis, Semaine hôp., Par. 22:1666, 1946.

Merrill, W. J.: Tendon substitution to restore function of extensor muscles of fingers and thumb, J.A.M.A. 78:425, 1922.

Milgram, J. E.: Of biceps and triceps to paralyzed fingers through artificially created tendon sheaths, Bull. Hosp. Joint Dis. 15:45, 1954.

————: Transplantation of tendons through preformed gliding channels, Bull. Hosp. Joint Dis. 21:250, 1960.

Phalen, G. S., and Miller, R. C.: The transfer of wrist extensor muscles to restore or reinforce flexion power of the fingers and opposition of the thumb, J. Bone Joint Surg. 29:993, 1947.

Riordan, D. C.: Tendon transplantations in median nerve and ulnar nerve paralysis, J. Bone Joint Surg. 35-A:312, 1953.

————: Surgery of the paralytic hand, Am. Acad. Orth. Surg. Instr. Course Lect. 16:79, 1959.

Scherb, R.: Biological and technical considerations in tendon transplants in poliomyelitis, Z. orthop. Chir. 61:303, 1934.

Schottstaedt, E. R., Larsen, L. J., and Bost, F. C.: Complete muscle transposition, J. Bone Joint Surg. 37-A:897, 1955.

Scuderi, C.: For irreparable radial nerve paralysis, Indust. Med. 23:258, 1954.

Sharrard, W. T.: Muscle recovery in poliomyelitis, J. Bone Joint Surg. 37-B:63, 1955.

Sorokina: Transplantation of tendons in therapy of sequels of infantile paralysis, Ortop. travmatol. 9:130, 1935.

Stamm, T. T.: Surgical treatment of paralysis, Guy's Hosp. Gaz. 53:312, 1939.

Starr, C. L.: Army experience with tendon transference, J. Bone Joint Surg. 4:3, 1922.

Steindler, A.: Tendon transplantation in upper extremity, Am. J. Surg. 44:260, 1939.

————: Tendon transplantation in upper extremity, Am. J. Surg. 44:534, 1939.

Swart, H. A., and Henderson, M. S.: Transplantation of tendons for paralytic wrist-drop, Proc. Mayo Clin. 9:377, 1934.

White, W. L.: Restoration of function and balance of the wrist and hand by tendon transfers, Surg. Clin. N. Amer. 40:427, 1960.

Wilson, J. N.: Providing automatic grasp by flexor tenodesis (wrist mobility in paralytic hands), J. Bone Joint Surg. 38-A:1019, 1956.

Young, H. H.: Tendon transplantation for radial nerve paralysis, Proc. Mayo Clin. 15:26, 1940.

Young, H. H., and Lowe, G. H.: Tendon transfer operations for irreparable paralysis of the radial nerve, Surg., Gynec. Obstet. 84:1101, 1947.

Zachary, R. B.: Tendon transplantation for radial paralysis, Brit. J. Surg. 33:358, 1946.

TENDON GRAFTS

Bastos, A. M.: Successful and unsuccessful transplantations of tendon, Cir. ortop. y traumatol., Madrid 1:5, 1936.

Beykirch, A., and Meyer, H.: Transplantation of fixed tendon tissue in animals, Beitr. klin. Chir. 148:630, 1930.

Biesalski, K., and Mayer, L.: Physiological Tendon Transplantation, Berlin, Springer, 1916.

Boyes, J. H.: Flexor tendon grafts in the fingers and thumb, an evaluation of end results, J. Bone Joint Surg. 32-A:489, 1950.

————: Hand surgery; operative technique of digital flexor tendon grafts, Am. Acad. Orth. Surg. Instr. Course Lect. 10:263, 1953.

————: Evaluation of results of digital flexor tendon grafts, Am. J. Surg. 89:116, 1955.

Brand, P. W.: Tendon grafting, J. Bone Joint Surg. 43-B:444, 1961.

Bunnell, S.: Greffes nerveuses et tendieuses de la main, Arch. francobelges de chir., No. 2, 1927.

Burman, M. S., and Umansky, M.: Experimental study of periosteal transplants wrapped around tendon, with review of the literature, J. Bone Joint Surg. 12:579, 1930.

Carpenter, A. R.: Tendon transplantation; end result study of 458 transplantations, J. Bone Joint Surg. 21:921, 1939.

Cleveland, M.: Restoration of digital portion of flexor tendon and sheath in hand, J. Bone Joint Surg. 15:762, 1933.

Flynn, J. E.: Flexor tendon grafts in the hand, New Engl. J. Med. *241*:807, 1949.

Flynn, J. E., Wilson, J. T., Child, C. G., and Graham, J. H.: Heterogenous and autogenous tendon transplants, J. Bone Joint Surg. *42-A*: 91, 1960.

Graham, W. C.: Flexor-tendon grafts to the finger and thumb, J. Bone Joint Surg. *29*:553, 1947.

————: Use of frozen stored tendons for grafting; an experimental study; presented at meeting of Orth. Research Soc., Jan. 29, 1955.

Haas, S. L.: The union of grafts of live and of preserved fascia with muscle, Arch. Surg. *23*: 571, 1931.

Harrison, S. H.: Primary flexor tendon grafts, Brit. J. Plast. Surg. *11*:106, 1958.

Kaplan, E. B.: Device for measuring length of tendon graft in flexor tendon surgery of the hand, Bull. Hosp. Joint Dis. *3*:No. 3, 1942.

Koch, S. L.: The use of tendon grafts in injuries of the flexor tendons of the hand, South. Surgeon *13*:449, 1947.

Koontz, A. R., and Shackelford, R. T.: Comparative results in use of living and preserved fascia as suture material in bone, Surgery *9*: 493, 1941.

Littler, J. W.: Free tendon grafts in secondary flexor tendon repair, Am. J. Surg. *74*:315, 1947.

McCormack, R. M., Demuth, R. J., and Kindling, P. H.: Flexor tendon grafts in the less-than-optimum situation, J. Bone Joint Surg. *44-A*: 1360, 1962.

May, H.: Tendon transplantation in the hand, Surg., Gynec. Obstet. *83*:631, 1946.

Peacock, E. E., Jr.: Morphology of homologous and heterologous tendon grafts, Surg., Gynec. Obstet. *109*:735, 1959.

————: Homologous composite tissue grafts of the digital flexor mechanism in human beings, Transplant Bull. *7*:418, 1960.

————: Restoration of finger flexion with homologous composite tissue tendon grafts, Am. Surg. *26*:564, 1960.

Posch, J. L.: Secondary tenorrhaphies and tendon grafts in injuries to the hand, Am. J. Surg. *85*:306, 1953.

Pulvertaft, R. G.: Repair of tendon injuries in the hand with special reference to flexor tendons, Postgrad. Med. Eng. *8*:81, 1950.

————: Tendon graft for flexor tendon injuries in fingers and thumb; technic and results, J. Bone Joint Surg. *38-B*:175, 1956.

————: Experiences in secondary flexor tendon grafting in the hand, Acta orthop. belg. *24*:62, 1958. Abst: Excerp. Med. IX, *13*:7008.

————: The results of tendon grafting for flexor tendon injuries in fingers and thumb after long delay, Bull. Hosp. Joint Dis. *21*:317, 1960.

————: The treatment of profundus division by free tendon graft, J. Bone Joint Surg. *42-A*: 1363, 1960.

————: Treatment of flexor tendon injuries in the hand; discussion, J. Bone Joint Surg. *43-B*: 403, 1961.

Rank, B. K., and Wakefield, A. R.: Flexor tendon repair in the hand, Aust. New Zeal. J. Surg. *19*:232, 1950.

Strandell, G.: Tendon grafts in injuries of flexor tendons in fingers and thumb; end results in consecutive series of 74 cases, Acta chir. scand. *111*:124, 1956.

Tsuge, K., Akamatsu, H., and Matsushita, M.: The tendon grafting in finger and our method, Acta med. Okayama *12*:174, 1958. Abst: Excerp. Med. IX, *13*:5528.

Tubiana, R.: Grafts of the flexor tendons of the fingers and of the thumb; technic and results, Rev. chir. orthop. *46*:191, 1960.

Van't, Hof, A., and Heiple, K. G.: Flexor tendon injuries of the fingers and thumb, J. Bone Joint Surg. *40-A*:256, 1958.

Wakefield, A. R.: Late flexor tendon grafts, Surg. Clin. N. Amer. *40*:399, 1960.

Webster, G. V.: Late repair of tendons in the hand, Am. J. Surg. *72*:171, 1946.

Weinberg, E. D.: Dead (ox) fascia grafts in tendon defects, Arch. Surg. *37*:570, 1938.

White, W. L.: Secondary restoration of finger flexion by digital tendon grafts; evaluation of 76 cases, Am. J. Surg. *91*:662, 1956.

————: Tendon grafts: A consideration of their source, procurement and suitability, Surg. Clin. N. Amer. *40*:403, 1960.

TENDON RUPTURE

Backdahl, M.: Ruptures of extensor aponeurosis at distal joints, Acta chir. scand. *111*:151, 1956.

Boyes, J. H.: Rupture of tendons; report of four cases of latent rupture of tendon of extensor pollicis longus, West. J. Surg. *43*:442, 1935.

Boyes, J. H., Wilson, J. N., and Smith, J. W.: Flexor-tendon ruptures in the forearm and hand, J. Bone Joint Surg. *42-A*:637, 1960.

Brickner, W. M., and Milch, H.: Ruptures of muscles and tendons, Internat. Clinics *2*:94, 1928.

Broder, H.: Rupture of flexor tendons associated with malunited Colles's fracture, J. Bone Joint Surg. *36-A*:404, 1954.

Christophe, K.: Rupture of the extensor pollicis longus tendon following Colles' fracture, J. Bone Joint Surg. *35-A*:1003, 1955.

Eilers: Subcutaneous rupture of extensor tendons of finger with special reference to button-hole dislocation of first interphalangeal joint, Deutsche Z. Chir. *223*:317, 1930.

Ehrlich, G. E., Peterson, L. T., Sokoloff, L., and Bunim, J. J.: Pathogenesis of rupture of extensor tendons at the wrist in rheumatoid arthritis, Arth. Rheum. *2*:332, 1959.

Ewald, P.: Treatment of rupture of extensor tendons of terminal phalanx of finger, Zbl. Chir. *57*:714, 1930.

de Francesco, F.: "Spontaneous rupture" of tendons (contribution to normal and pathologic anatomy and mechanism of pathogenesis), Arch. ortop. *49*:625, 1933.

Gilcreest, E. L., and Albi, P.: Rupture of muscles and tendons, particularly subcutaneous rupture of biceps flexor cubiti, J.A.M.A. *84*:1819, 1925.

Golla, F.: Bilateral rupture of extensor aponeurosis of terminal phalanx; treatment, Beitr. klin. Chir. *162*:594, 1935.

Gunter, G. S.: Traumatic avulsion of the insertion of flexor digitorum profundus, Aust. New Zeal. J. Surg. *30*:1, 1960.

Haldeman, K. O., and Soto-Hall, R.: Injuries to muscles and tendons, J.A.M.A. *104*:2319, 1935.

Hallberg, D., and Lindholm, A.: Subcutaneous rupture of the extensor tendon of the distal phalanx of the finger; "mallet finger"; brief review of the literature and report on 127 cases treated conservatively, Acta chir. scand. *119*:260, 1960.

Hauck, G.: Operation for rupture of thumb tendon and fracture of radius, Arch. klin. Chir. *124*:81, 1923.

Horwitz, A.: Surgical and non-surgical treatment of ruptured extensor tendon of terminal phalanx of finger, Deutsche med. Wchr. *57*:445, 1931.

James, J. I. P.: A case of rupture of flexor tendons secondary to Kienbock's disease, J. Bone Joint Surg. *31-B*:521, 1949.

Kallius, H. U.: Buttonhole rupture of extensor tendon at terminal phalanx of finger, Zbl. Chir. *57*:2432, 1930.

Kantala, J.: Treatment of subcutaneous rupture of extensor tendons of terminal phalanges of fingers, Duodecim *52*:31, 1936.

Kaplan, E. B.: Mallet or baseball finger, Surgery *7*:784, 1940.

————: Anatomy, injuries and treatment of the extensor apparatus of the hand, Clin. Orthop. *13*:24, 1959.

Kwedar, A. T., and Mitchell, C. L.: Late rupture of extensor pollicis longus following Colles' fracture, J. Bone Joint Surg. *22*:429, 1940.

Lipshutz, H.: Spontaneous rupture of flexor tendons, Brit. J. Plast. Surg. *14*:50, 1961.

McMaster, P. E.: Tendon and muscle ruptures; clinical and experimental studies on causes and location of subcutaneous ruptures, J. Bone Joint Surg. *15*:705, 1933.

————: Late ruptures of extensor and flexor pollicis longus tendons following Colles' fracture, J. Bone Joint Surg. *14*:93, 1932.

Mason, M. L.: Rupture of tendons of the hand, with study of extensor tendon insertions in fingers, Surg., Gynec. Obstet. *50*:611, 1930.

Milch, H.: Buttonhole rupture of extensor tendon of finger, Am. J. Surg. *13*:244, 1931.

Moore, T.: Spontaneous rupture extensor pollicis longus tendon associated with Colles' fracture, Brit. J. Surg. *23*:721, 1936.

Nichols, H. M.: Repair of extensor tendon insertion in the fingers, J. Bone Joint Surg. *33-A*:836, 1951.

Platt, H.: Observations on some tendon ruptures, Brit. M. J. *1*:611, 1931.

Posch, J. L., Walker, P. J., and Miller, H.: Treatment of ruptured tendons of hand and wrist, Am. J. Surg. *91*:669, 1956.

Pratt, D. R., Bunnell, S., and Howard, L. D., Jr.: Mallet finger; classification and methods of treatment, Am. J. Surg. *93*:573, 1957.

Selig, S., and Schein, A. J.: Irreducible buttonhole dislocations of fingers, J. Bone Joint Surg. *22*:436, 1940.

Smillie, I. S.: Mallet finger, Brit. J. Surg. *24*:439, 1937.

Smith, F. M.: Late rupture of extensor pollicis longus tendon following Colles' fracture, J. Bone Joint Surg. *28*:49, 1946.

Stark, H. H., Boyes, J. H., and Wilson, J. N.: Mallet finger, J. Bone Joint Surg. *44-A*:1061, 1962.

Stewart, I. M.: Boutonniere finger, Clin. Orthop. *23*:220, 1962.

Stracker, O.: Treatment of rupture of extensor tendon of terminal phalanx of finger, Zbl. Chir. *58*:727, 1931.

Van Ree, A.: Treatment of subcutaneous rupture of extensor tendons of distal phalanges of fingers, Nederl. tijdschr. geneesk. *80*:1999, 1936.

Stenosing Tenosynovitis

Cormio, C., and Picchio, A.: Snapping finger, Reumatismo *13*:156, 1961.

Diack, A. W., and Trommal, J. P.: de Quervain's disease; frequently missed diagnosis, West. J. Surg. *47*:629, 1939.

Fahey, J. J., et al.: Trigger finger in adults and children, J. Bone Joint Surg. *36*:1200, 1954.

Forcella, I. G.: Acquired snapping finger, Minerva ortop. *7*:31, 1956.

————: Stenosing tendovaginitis (de Quervain type); relation to snapping fingers and radial styloiditis, Chir. org. movimento *43*:289, 1956.

————: Snapping finger, Chir. org. movimento 43:478, 1956.

Giles, K. W.: Anatomical variations affecting the surgery of de Quervain's disease, J. Bone Joint Surg. 42-B:353, 1960.

Grob, M., and Steckman, M.: Stenosing tenovaginosis, a typical affection of early childhood, Helvet. paediat. acta 6:112, 1951.

Hart, G. M.: Trigger thumb, J. Lancet 80:436, 1960.

Hauck, G.: Tendovaginitis and snapping finger, Arch. klin. Chir. 123:233, 1923.

Hodgins, T. E., and Lipscomb, P. R.: Bilateral trigger fingers in child; case, Proc. Mayo Clin. 31:279, 1956.

Howard, N. J.: New concept of tenosynovitis and pathology of physiologic effort, Am. J. Surg. 42:723, 1938.

————: Pathological changes induced in tendons through trauma and their accompanying clinical phenomena, Am. J. Surg. 51:689, 1941.

James, T.: Bilateral trigger thumb in infants, Arch. Dis. Child. 35:302, 1960.

Kladosek, K.: Subcutaneous surgery of the snapping finger, Z. Orthop. 93:589, 1960.

Kneppler, A.: Crepitant tenovaginitis, Novy chir. arkhiv. 20:347, 1930.

Lamphier, T. A.: de Quervain's disease, Ann. Surg. 138:833, 1953.

Lapidus, P. W., and Fenton, R.: Stenosing tenovaginitis at the wrist and fingers, Arch. Surg. 64:475, 1952.

Leão, L.: de Quervain's disease, J. Bone Joint Surg. 40-A:1063, 1958.

Lipscomb, P. R.: Stenosing tenosynovitis at the radial styloid process, Ann. Surg. 134:110, 1951.

Lorthioir, J.: Surgical therapy of trigger fingers by subcutaneous route, Acta chir. belg. 55:246, 1956.

————: Surgical treatment of trigger finger by subcutaneous method, J. Bone Joint Surg. 40-A: 793, 1958.

MacDonald, J. E., and Stuart, F. A.: Stenosing tenovaginitis at radial styloid process, J. Bone Joint Surg. 21:1035, 1939.

Patterson, D. C., and Jones, E. K.: de Quervain's disease; stenosing tendovaginitis at radial styloid, Am. J. Surg. 67:296, 1945.

Potter, P. C.: Stenosing tendovaginitis at radial styloid (de Quervain's disease), Ann. Surg. 117: 290, 1943.

Reid, S. F.: Tenovaginitis stenosans at carpal tunnel, Aust. New Zeal. J. Surg. 25:204, 1956.

Rhodes, R. L.: Tenosynovitis of the forearm, Am. J. Surg. 73:248, 1947.

Schneider, C. C.: Stenosing fibrous tenovaginitis over radial styloid, Surg., Gynec. Obst. 46:846, 1928.

Schneider, H.: Stenosing tendovaginitis (de Quervain) and styloiditis of radius, Wien. med. Wchr. 106:523, 1956.

Wilber, M. C.: Trigger finger in children involving digits other than the thumb, Med. Ann. D. C. 31:95, 1962.

Winterstein, O.: Relations between stenosing tenovaginitis and deforming arthritis, Zbl. Chir. 57:1347, 1930.

Zadek, I.: Stenosing tenovaginitis of thumb in infants, J. Bone Joint Surg. 24:326, 1942.

Zelle, O. L., and Schnepp, K. H.: Snapping thumb; tendovaginitis stenosans, Am. J. Surg. 33:321, 1936.

Chapter 12

Intrinsic Muscles of the Hand

INTRINSIC MUSCLES
OF THE FINGERS

The intrinsic muscles provide the balance of forces between the long flexors and the long extensors of the fingers. When they are interacting normally with the extrinsic motors, the whole hand is in balance; and, if the wrist is in the optimal functioning position, the fingers (when relaxed) are semiflexed in all their joints, the degree of flexion increasing from the index to the little finger. The transverse metacarpal arch is maintained by their activity; with paralysis, the hand is flat and the fingers clawed; with contracture, the curve is accentuated and the fingers are in the "accoucheur's" position. Loss of function of the intrinsic finger muscles results from paralysis due to damage to the nerve supply, principally the ulnar (C-8 to T-1) or from spasm or contracture due to overactive nerve stimulation as in spastic conditions or parkinsonism, local con-

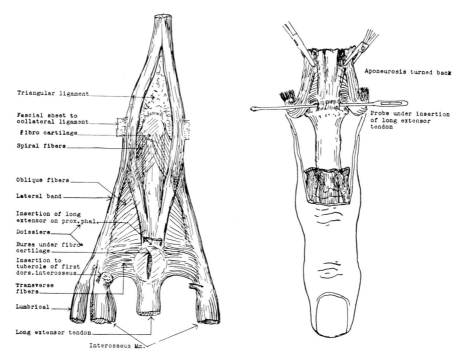

Triangular ligament

Fascial sheet to collateral ligament

Fibro cartilage

Spiral fibers

Oblique fibers

Lateral band

Insertion of long extensor on prox. phal.

Doissiere

Bursa under fibro cartilage

Insertion to tuberole of first dors. interosseus

Transverse fibers

Lumbrical

Long extensor tendon

Interosseus Mm.

Aponeurosis turned back

Probe under insertion of long extensor tendon

FIG. 576. (*Left*) View of the undersurface of the dorsal aponeurosis of the left index finger. This complicated aponeurosis coordinates the muscle action of the long extensor, the interossei and the lumbricales. (*Right*) The *dossière* ("cloth over the back of a throne") is turned back to show the insertion in the capsule of the proximal joint. (J. Bone Joint Surg. *24*:8)

tracture as in rheumatoid arthritis or loss of muscle substance and fibrosis from crushing wounds or ischemic contracture.

ANATOMY AND FUNCTION

It is customary to describe the anatomy and the function of the intrinsic muscles by isolating each one, observing what happens if it is paralyzed or stimulated, and then deducing a function related to it alone. This may be an incomplete picture, for the entire mechanism acts and functions as a unit. Rank and Wakefield describe such attempts as achieving "only a rationalization of a subdivision of movements which does not exist in reality."

Most of our understanding of the functions of these structures has been gained by observations of paralyzed hands—the motions that are lost are assumed to be related to the function of the paralyzed part. However, Sunderland pointed out that consideration must be given to the interdependence of muscles in executing a particular movement.

Lumbricales. Four small wormlike muscles, one to the radial side of each finger, are unique in that they originate on the flexor profundus tendon of the digit on which they act. The muscles arising from one tendon, as in the index, or from 2 adjoining profundi, as in the other fingers, lie between the profundi and the superficialis tendons and wrap around the latter. Distalward, the tendinous portion passes volar to the transverse metacarpal ligament, which separates it from the interossei. Their course is then dorsalward to join the outermost fibers of the expansion of the dorsal aponeurosis. Because of their large angle of approach they have a great potential flexing power.

The action of the lumbrical muscle as judged from its anatomic position and attachments would be to flex the proximal finger joint or extend the middle and the distal finger joints, either simultaneously or separately, depending on the state of contraction of the extrinsic flexors and extensors. Thus, if the proximal phalanx is held in extension either passively or by action of the long extensor, a pull on the lumbrical should extend the 2 distal joints and tend to deviate radially and rotate the finger. This motion has been demonstrated repeatedly during operative procedures. When

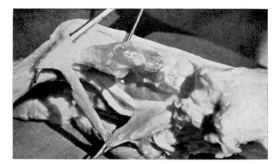
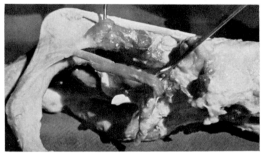
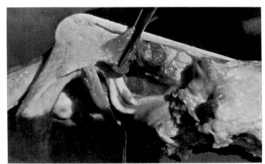

FIG. 577. (*Top*) Insertion of the lumbricalis and the interosseus into the aponeurosis. A pull on either flexes the proximal joint by the transverse fibers, which form a sling over the dorsum of the proximal phalanx. (*Center*) The lumbricalis is pulled. (*Bottom*) The interosseus is pulled. (J. Bone Joint Surg. *24*:11)

the proximal finger joint is fully flexed, the action is no longer possible.

The origin of the lumbrical is on the profundus tendon, which makes possible a variation in its action, depending on the activity of the profundus muscle.

Backhouse and Catton studied the action of the second lumbrical muscle by electromyography and found it to be active during extension of the middle and the distal joints, re-

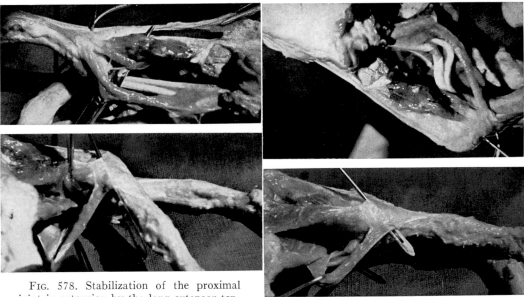

FIG. 578. Stabilization of the proximal joint in extension by the long extensor tendon pulls the aponeurotic sleeve proximally until it is over the joint (*Top, left*). Then the intrinsic muscles pull on the lateral band and extend the distal 2 joints (*Bottom, right*). A shift of the aponeurotic sleeve distalward changes their function to flexors of the proximal joint (*Top, right*) and (*Bottom, left*). In (*Top, left*) and (*Top, right*) a probe marks the joint, and a hemostat on the aponeurosis shows the shift. (J. Bone Joint Surg. *24*:11)

gardless of the position of the proximal joint, but more active when the proximal joint was being flexed simultaneously. When both the proximal and the middle joints were flexed voluntarily, no lumbrical action was noted. Stimulation of the lumbrical caused extension of the middle joint, with added flexion of the proximal finger joint if strong stimulation was used. No radial deviation could be produced. From their observation they concluded that the lumbrical was the major extensor of the middle joint and confirmed Sunderland's claim that its action was to prevent hyperextension of the proximal joint.

Long and Brown studied the lumbrical in a similar way but with simultaneous readings on the interossei and the extrinsics. The lumbrical activity was found to be present on extending the finger in all its joints; this motion was accompanied by action in the long extensor but not in the interossei. Flexion of the proximal joint with extension of the middle joint showed marked lumbrical action, with lessened activity in the long extensor and some activity of the profundus and the superficialis in a few of the subjects. With fingers extended, flexion at the proximal joint showed both lumbrical and interosseus activity and, in some subjects, long flexor activity, usually in the superficialis. Extension of the proximal joints from this position showed activity in the long extensors and the lumbricals, with superficialis flexor action in half the subjects. With the proximal joints passively held in flexion, voluntary extension of the middle joint showed activity principally in the interossei, with variable activity of the long extensor.

Kaplan has observed the lumbrical muscle during operations under local anesthesia and states that there is no contraction on voluntary flexion of a digit but that the muscle consistently contracts when the finger is extended voluntarily, thus acting to pull the profundus distally and allow the finger to extend.

Loss of lumbrical action as an isolated lesion cannot be determined clinically, and its function, except as a weak supplementary force, has been overrated.

The index and the middle finger lumbricals are supplied by the median nerve through branches from the common digital trunks. The ulnar lumbricals are supplied by branches from the deep volar division of the ulnar nerve.

There may be considerable variation in the lumbrical muscles in the hand. Mehta and Gardner found only 1 of 38 cadavers in which the lumbrical origins and insertions followed the textbook ideal plan. The 1st lumbrical was most uniform but varied in having occasional added origins from the superficialis tendon or the metacarpal or even tendon attachments to the bellies of the flexor muscles in the forearm. The 2nd lumbrical was abnormal about one third of the time, mainly by variations of insertion, either to the phalanx or the transverse metacarpal ligament. The 3rd lumbrical was "normal" in less than half the hands. A split insertion was most common, going to both the middle and the ring fingers and into the phalanx or the metacarpal ligament as well as the extensor expansion. The 4th lumbrical was absent in over 5 per cent and had a bony insertion in 72 per cent. They found the true insertion in extensor apparatus in only 4 hands.

Interossei. Traditionally, the 7 interosseus muscles are divided into 4 dorsal and 3 volar. Albinus (in 1734) is considered to be the first to have made the distinction between the 2 types. He also described the position of the 1st interosseus and its insertion only into bone and the insertion of the volar or palmar interossei only into the extensor tendon expansions.

Duchenne considered variations to be present in bony and tendinous insertions, but most authors of anatomy texts have assumed that each interosseus muscle had both a skeletal insertion into the phalanx and a tendinous insertion into the dorsal aponeurosis. In 1937 Salsbury carefully investigated the interossei and, in 28 cadavers, found the 1st dorsal to be inserted exclusively on the phalanx. This has been verified by Bunnell and Landsmeer. The 2nd dorsal had a bony insertion in 22 cases, and a tendon insertion as well in 20. The 3rd dorsal always had a tendinous insertion, and in only 6 was there also a bony insertion. The 4th dorsal in 10 cases inserted only into the extensor apparatus, the other 18 having both a skeletal and a tendinous insertion. In dissecting more than 30 hands, Eyler and Markee found that the 1st and the 2nd volar interossei exhibited the same pattern of insertion as those studied by Salsbury, but for the

3rd volar interosseus their findings indicated a higher percentage of insertion into the tendon. For the dorsal interossei, they found a slightly higher percentage of bony attachments in the 2nd and the 4th, but a lower percentage for the 3rd.

Landsmeer has made an extensive study of the interossei, the extensor aponeurosis and the proximal and the middle finger joints. He agrees with Salsbury, Bunnell and Eyler and Markee, though he feels that the variation in interosseus insertions is not as great as Salsbury's figures would indicate. He points out also that the 2-point insertion of a dorsal interosseus into bone and tendon is a division of the whole muscle. Eyler and Markee state that this can be demonstrated by microdissection and quote Duchenne's electric experiments to illustrate it. Landsmeer credits Bouvier with this finding.

From these studies, the traditional division of dorsal and volar interossei, based on the location of the muscle bellies in relation to each other, must give way to a division based on their function and differentiated by their insertions. Two types of insertion occur—phalangeal or skeletal and wing or tendinous.

The wing insertions of the interossei and the lumbricals are symmetrical, whereas the skeletal or bony insertions are not. Using this classification, and with an understanding of the dorsal aponeurotic mechanism, a clearer view of the intricate action of the fingers as well as some possible explanation for the deformities of paralysis or contracture can be obtained.

A typical idealized dorsal interosseus muscle has 2 parts. The more dorsal belly, called the superficial, arises from the 2 adjacent metacarpals, while the deeper and more volar part arises from the metacarpal of the digit on which it acts. The superficial usually passes to the phalanx to insert into the tubercle, while the deep belly passes the joint slightly more volarly and swings dorsalward to insert into the wing. The first dorsal is unusual in that the deep part coming from the radial side of the 2nd metacarpal rolls over the 2-bellied superficial part, as occurs in the pectoralis major muscle, and tendons of both then insert into the transverse lamina and bone. There is no action of the 1st dorsal interosseus on the extensor wing and therefore no possibility of extension of the middle and the distal joints

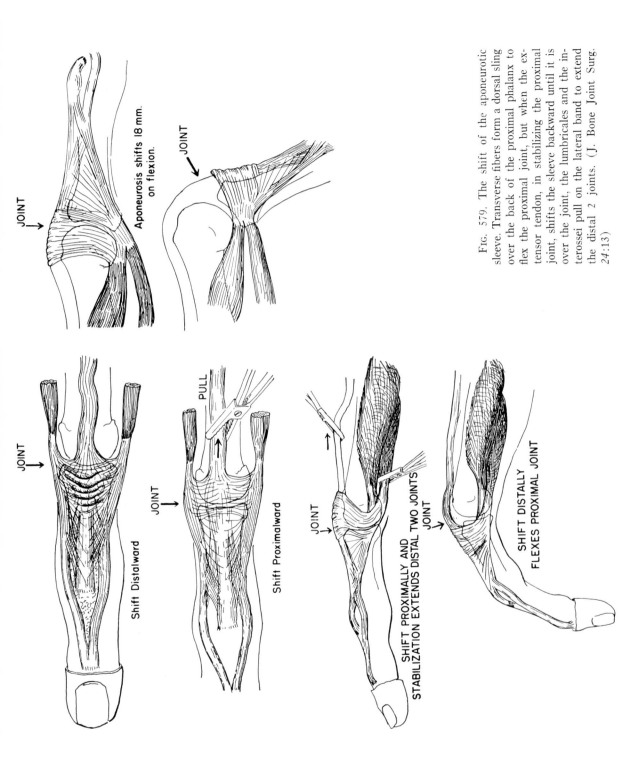

JOINT

Aponeurosis shifts 18 mm. on flexion.

JOINT

JOINT

Shift Distalward

JOINT

PULL

Shift Proximalward

JOINT

SHIFT PROXIMALLY AND
STABILIZATION EXTENDS DISTAL TWO JOINTS

JOINT

SHIFT DISTALLY
FLEXES PROXIMAL JOINT

Fig. 579. The shift of the aponeurotic sleeve. Transverse fibers form a dorsal sling over the back of the proximal phalanx to flex the proximal joint, but when the extensor tendon, in stabilizing the proximal joint, shifts the sleeve backward until it is over the joint, the lumbricales and the interossei pull on the lateral band to extend the distal 2 joints. (J. Bone Joint Surg. 24:13)

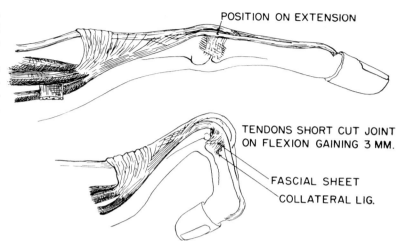

FIG. 580. The volar shift of the 2 lateral bands at the middle joint. On flexion, the 2 lateral sheets automatically displace the tendons, so that they shortcut across the joint. (J. Bone Joint Surg. 24:17)

POSITION ON EXTENSION

TENDONS SHORT CUT JOINT ON FLEXION GAINING 3 MM.

FASCIAL SHEET
COLLATERAL LIG.

of the index finger by the 1st dorsal interosseus. The lumbrical on the radial side and the 1st volar interosseus on the ulnar side carry out this motion.

According to Landsmeer, the 3rd dorsal is also exceptional in that all 3 muscle bellies fuse to form 1 central tendon which has its principal action on the extensor wing; or, if there are 2 tendons, both insert into the wing. Thus, from a functional standpoint, the 3rd dorsal is similar to a volar interosseus.

The volar interossei arise from the metacarpal by a single belly, more deeply or volar than the dorsal interossei and, consequently, with a greater angle of approach, and never insert into the bone. Because of their insertion into the extensor apparatus they can extend the middle joint of the finger.

The Dorsal Aponeurosis or Extensor Apparatus. This thin sliding assembly of transverse, oblique and longitudinal fibers is a continuation of the long extensor tendon, and into it the interossei and, on the radial side and more distally, the lumbricals send fibers to join

those from the long extensor. It can be palpated over the dorsum of the proximal joint and phalanx and its to-and-fro motion visualized beneath the thin dorsal skin.

A band of transverse fibers forms a sling around the proximal phalanx. From the long extensor on the dorsum, this sling extends around each side of the proximal joint, as the "transverse lamina" (Landsmeer) or the "perforating fibers" (Poirer) and volarly is attached to the transverse capitular ligament.

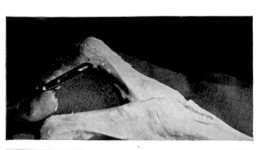

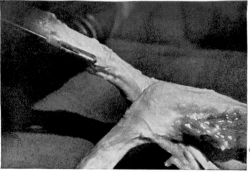

FIG. 581. (*Top*) Showing the volar shift of the lateral bands on flexing the middle joint. (*Bottom*) Showing the resumption of the dorsal position of the bands on extension. A probe passes under the lateral sheet, which is attached to the collateral ligament and the middle phalanx, and automatically causes the volar shift. (J. Bone Joint Surg. 24:18)

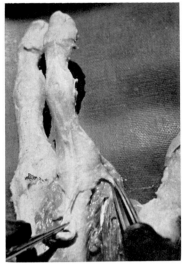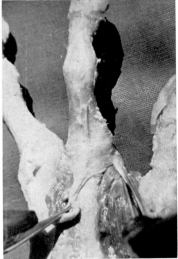

Fig. 582. When the proximal joint is stabilized in extension by the long extensor tendon, the lumbricales and the interossei impart lateral motion to the finger. In both pictures the long extensor is taut; in the left-hand picture the interosseus is relaxed, while in the right-hand one it is pulled upon, imparting lateral motion. (J. Bone Joint Surg. *24*:16)

According to Landsmeer, this transverse lamina is the continuation of the intertendinous fascia from the dorsum of the hand. The fascia does not extend distally into the web, but instead a falx here allows a space through which the dorsal vessels pass to the subcutaneous tissues of the finger.

Thus, this encircling band of transverse fibers has a more or less fixed point volarly at the attachment of the transverse capitular ligament but is movable in its dorsal part, being pulled proximally by the contraction of the long extensor or distally by the middle band of the extensor made taut by flexion of the middle joint.

While the proximal border of this transverse lamina is rather well defined, distally it blends into the aponeurosis proper into which the lumbricals, the volar interossei and the tendinous insertions of the dorsal interossei all join with the various divisions of the long extensor to make up the complex mechanism of the extensor assembly.

On the under side of the extensor tendon just as it reaches the area of the transverse fibers, Kaplan found (in 38.5% of cases) a deep ribbon thought to act as a tendon of insertion and to provide for extension of the proximal phalanx by the long extensor. Sunderland thinks that this slip is of little importance as an extensor attachment. The transverse lamina with its volar attachment to the transverse capitular ligament provides a more effective anchor than a capsular attachment. Tension on the long extensor makes it possible to lift the proximal phalanx by the sling insertion of the transverse fibers. As the long extensor reaches the proximal joint level, it divides into a middle and 2 lateral slips, these latter then joining with the lateral band extensions of the lumbrical muscle and the interossei to pass across the middle joint and fuse to make the terminal tendon. At both the middle joint and the distal joint, the extensor tendon and the joint capsule are inseparable.

SHIFT OF APONEUROTIC SLEEVE. The tendons of the long extensor, the interossei and the lumbricals join in a sheet of fibers making a continuous hoodlike covering over the proximal joint, extending by the transverse fibers well around the sides and, distally, running out to a narrower band at the middle joint level. There is really one fixed point where the transverse fibers on the volar surface are attached to the transverse ligament. The dorsal part shifts proximally or distally depending on the position of the joint and the tension of the various tendons passing into it. Thus, when the long extensor pulls the sleeve proximally and stabilizes the proximal joint, the interossei are in a position to exert their maximal effect as extensors of the middle and the distal joints or as lateral movers, but if the long extensor is relaxed or the aponeurosis is shifted distally by flexion of the middle joint, the lateral tendons act more as flexors of the

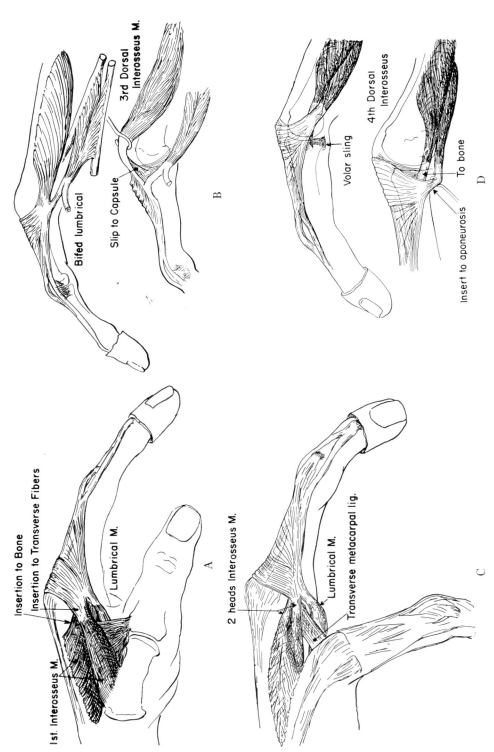

Fig. 583. Showing types of insertions. Lumbricales insert into the dorsal aponeurosis; interossei by several heads from fairly distinct muscle bellies insert variously into the phalangeal tubercle (A), (B), (C) and (D), into the capsule of the joint (B), and into the aponeurosis (A), (B) and (C). (J. Bone Joint Surg. 24·9)

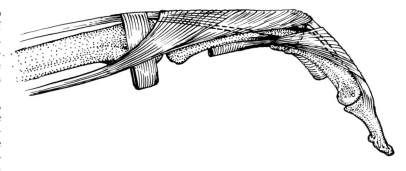

Fig. 584. Diagram to illustrate components of extensor aponeurosis. From the common extensor where it joins the transverse hood fibers there is a division into 1 central and 2 lateral slips, here represented by the dotted lines in the aponeurosis. Distal to the middle joint is the retinacular ligament with transverse and oblique components originating on the tendon sheath and the proximal phalanx and inserting into the terminal tendon. (Redrawn from Landsmeer, Anat. Rec. *104*:31)

proximal joint. In this position, with the intrinsics holding the proximal joint in flexion, the long extensor works through the aponeurosis and exerts its maximal effect to extend the 2 distal joints. If the intrinsics cannot function as from median or ulnar palsy, then the long extensors pull the sleeve proximally, and, if the joint is lax, there will be hyperextension or the claw position.

SHIFT OF THE EXTENSOR TENDON (LATERAL SLIPS) AT MIDDLE FINGER JOINT. The 2 lateral bands of the extensor mechanism which lie dorsal to the axis of motion of the middle finger joint shift volarward whenever

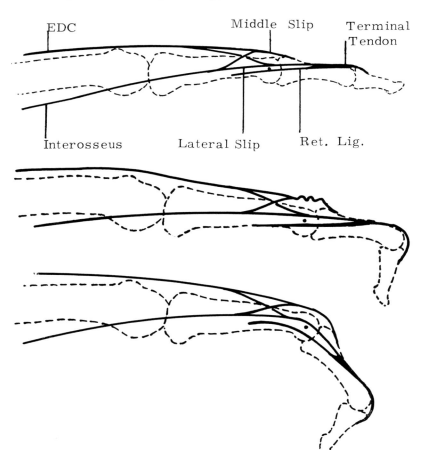

Fig. 585. Schematic drawing of dorsal aponeurosis. (*Top*) The finger in extended position. (*Center*) Forced flexion of terminal phalanx while middle phalanx is forcibly held in extension. Aponeurosis shifts distally from pull on lateral bands relaxing the middle slip. Oblique (retinacular) ligament is tense. (*Bottom*) The middle joint has flexed in response to forces on the oblique ligament; the lateral slip has displaced volarward, releasing the distal joint. Further flexion drawing the middle slip distally allows further slack in lateral slips so that the distal joint will flex. (Landsmeer: Anat. Rec. *104*:31)

the joint flexes. They are prevented from slipping completely over the side, in which case they would become flexors, by interconnecting fibers of the triangular ligament. If they did not cut across the flexed joint, it would be impossible to flex the distal joint at the same time as the middle joint. When the finger is in extension, each of these lateral slips lies in a groove between the central tubercle attachment of the middle slip and 2 lateral prominences of the base of the middle phalanx. As soon as the middle phalanx is flexed, this lateral support for the tendons disappears, and then they displace to slacken the pull on the terminal tendon. They are directed in this motion by a fascial sheet joining the tendon to the side of the base of the middle phalanx.

FUNCTION OF INTEROSSEI. The interossei flex the proximal joints and, except for the 1st dorsal which has purely a bony insertion, also extend the 2 distal joints. If the proximal joint is held in extension passively or is stabilized in this position by the pull of the long extensor on the encircling sling, then they not only extend the middle and the distal joints but also provide lateral motion. The interossei are more powerful than the lumbricals, but they have a shorter excursion and a lesser angle of approach in starting flexion. With intrinsic paralysis, the fingers curl when one attempts to flex them, starting at the distal joint so that objects are pushed out of the hand by the advancing fingertips instead of being grasped by the coordinated uniform flexion of all 3 joints as seen in the normal hand.

Extension of the 2 distal joints by the interossei is most effective when the proximal joints are straight or slightly flexed and least effective when the proximal joints are sharply flexed. The long extensor tendon is most effective when the proximal joints are flexed and least effective when they are extended; it has very little or no effect when they are hyperextended. It should be understood that either the extrinsics or the intrinsics can extend the middle and the distal joints if the other is paralyzed, except that the long extensors cannot extend the 2 distal joints if the wrist and the proximal joints are passively hyperextended to the maximum.

The gradation in activity between the long

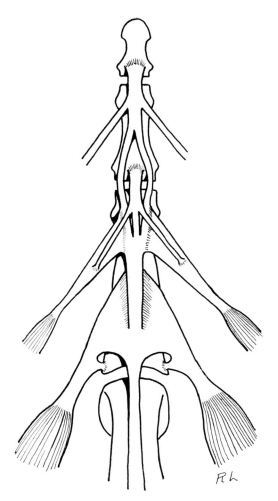

FIG. 586. Schematic drawing of extensor apparatus with 3 paired systems, proximal or skeletal interossei, distal or winged intrinsics and oblique retinacular ligaments. (Stack, H. G.: J. Bone Joint Surg. *44-B*: 899)

extensor and the intrinsics is an overlapping and relative affair. There are variations in the intrinsic muscles, as well as a difference in joint laxity, so that some individuals can voluntarily hyperextend the middle joints and flex the distal joints, locking their fingers in the intrinsic-plus position.

Hypothenar Muscles. The abductor minimi digiti inserts on the lateral tubercle of the proximal phalanx and the joint capsule and has fibers of insertion into the transverse as well as the lateral bands resembling those of

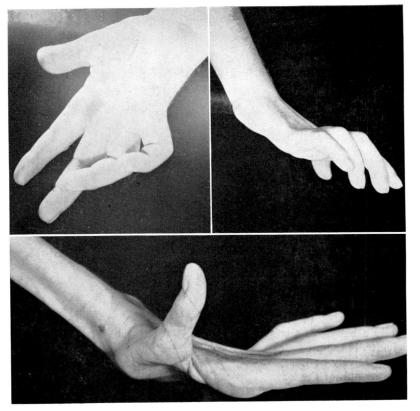

FIG. 587. (*Upper Left*) Paralysis of interossei and of ring and little finger lumbricales from ulnar palsy. The index and the middle fingers do not claw, because lumbrical action with functioning flexor tendons maintains balance. (*Upper Right*) Poliomyelitis with loss of function of all intrinsics. (*Bottom*) Polio with loss of all intrinsics and all digital flexors.

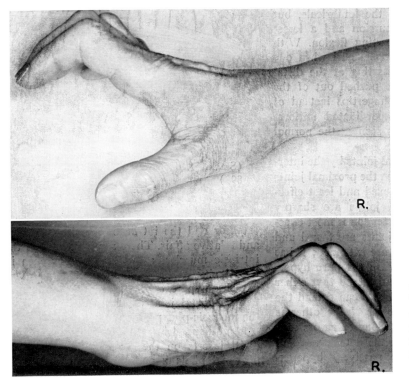

FIG. 588. Median and ulnar palsy from leprosy. The profundi of the ring and the little fingers are not functioning, but the intact superficialii cause flexion of the middle joints.

the interossei. However, it does not extend the distal 2 joints. It flexes the proximal joint when the long extensor tendon is slack and abducts the finger when the proximal joint is stabilized. The opponens digiti minimi rotates the little finger to some extent, similar to opposition in the thumb. The short flexor and the opponens help to maintain the carpal arches.

Movements of Hand in General. Lateral movement of the fingers is possible only when the proximal joints are straight or nearly so. Absence of side motion when in flexion is desirable, since it gives firmness to the grasp. When the joint is straight, the proximal phalanx has free lateral motion on the narrow vertical saddlelike end of the metacarpal. This lateral motion is not true abduction and ad-duction, but a rotary component is present. Ulnar deviation is accomplished by exorotation, radial deviation by endorotation. In flexion the phalanx slides volarward on an ever-widening articular surface. The lateral ligaments now become true collateral ligaments, and lateral motion is prevented.

One should not mistake the spread of the fingers, when fully extended by the long extensors, for the action of intrinsic muscles, because this spreading is due to the divergence of the line of pull on the long extensors and some flattening of the metacarpal arch. Lateral movement by intrinsic muscles should be checked by determining the individual lateral motion of the fingers when the proximal joints are in slight flexion. This can be tested by

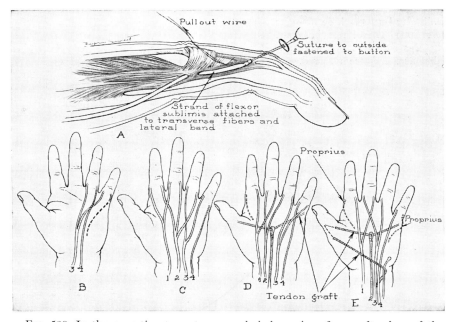

FIG. 589. In the operation to restore muscle balance in a finger after loss of the intrinsic muscles, the tendon, or a strip thereof, follows a straight course through the lumbricalis canal and is inserted into the transverse fibers and the lateral band of the dorsal aponeurosis, by a simple stitch of stainless-steel wire No. 35 which passes on out through the skin to a button. The wire is removed by the pullout wire after 3 weeks. The tendon and the dorsal surface of the lateral band have been scraped for better attachment. (B, C, D and E) show combinations for placing tendons, so that the lateral motion supplied by each single tendon to several fingers will be in the same direction. The small numbers indicate which tendon is used. In (D) is shown a combination with a tendon T operation for adduction of the thumb and restoration of the arches, and also an index long extensor used for abduction of the index finger. In (E) is shown the same with the addition of a tendon for opposition of the thumb and another for abduction of the little finger.

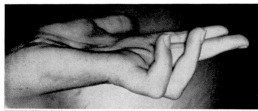

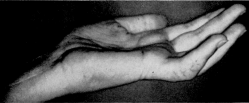

Fig. 590. Case B. D. (*Top*) Ulnar paralysis from a cyst along the motor branch of the ulnar nerve in the palm. The cyst was resected and the motor branch sutured, bringing return of function to the intrinsic muscles distally but not those opposite the cyst. (*Bottom*) Therefore, the clawhand deformity was corrected by 2 transfers for muscle balance. Balance restored.

noting the ability or the inability to move each finger alone and also by having the patient pinch the examiner's finger with each pair of adjoining fingers with the fingers extended, noting the strength of the pinch.

LOSS OF INTRINSIC MUSCLE FUNCTION IN THE FINGERS DUE TO PARALYSIS —THE INTRINSIC-MINUS HAND

When the nerve supply of an intrinsic muscle is interrupted any place from the ventral horn to the muscle end plate, a flaccid paralysis results, the muscle loses its power of contraction, and, if placed under tension, it stretches. When the intrinsics are paralyzed, the balance of the hand is destroyed, and the extrinsic muscles place the digits in characteristic positions. The proximal finger joints are extended or, if the volar capsule is lax, go into hyperextension from the unopposed pull of the long extensors. The middle and the distal joints remain in semiflexion, and "clawing" of the fingers results. If only the ulnar nerve is involved, the deformity is limited to

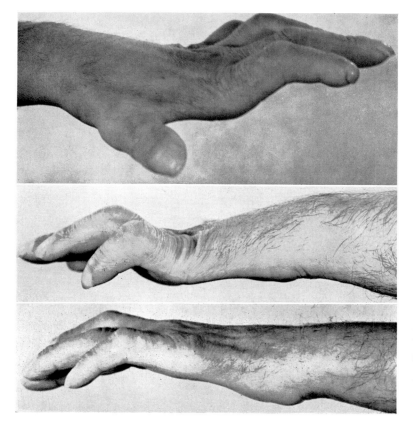

Fig. 591. Clawhand from leprosy, corrected by transfer of flexor superficialis tendons through lumbrical canals to extensor aponeuroses. (From D. C. Riordan, M.D.)

the ring and the little fingers, since the lumbricals of the index and the middle fingers are supplied by the median nerve, and this lumbrical action is sufficient to maintain the position of the proximal joints so that the long extensor can functon as an extensor.

The metacarpal arch flattens with loss of the hypothenar muscles, and lateral movements of the fingers are lacking. The index cannot be stabilized for a good pinch with the thumb and tends to swing ulnarward from lack of support from the 1st interosseus muscle.

If the clawed position is maintained, structural changes follow with capsular and ligamentous contractures; these must be corrected before restoring motion.

For ulnar paralysis it is necessary to correct the clawing of the ring and the little fingers and to restore the metacarpal arch. Combined median and ulnar paralysis requires restora-

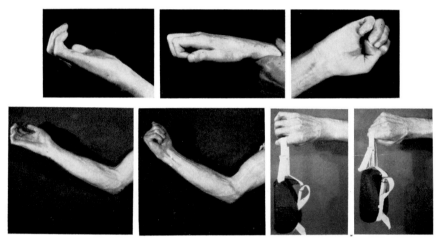

Fig. 592. Case J. A. C. Restoration of muscle balance to the intrinsic muscles in the hand. The right arm had been pulled between a belt and a pulley, fracturing the humerus and crushing off the median, the ulnar and the internal cutaneous nerves high in the arm. These were sutured. Between the ends of the musculocutaneous there was a 3-inch gap, of the ulnar one of 4 inches and of the median one of 5 inches. These were overcome by flexing neck, shoulder and elbow, and transplanting the ulnar nerve at the elbow. In 1 year, the flexors in the forearm worked well, but not the intrinsic muscles, and sensation returned throughout except beyond the middle finger joints. By 1½ years, sensation had returned completely throughout, though not yet to a normal degree in the fingertips. The intrinsic muscles did not recover except slightly in the 2 eminences, but, as the flexors in the forearm became strong, and he had not worn his splint, there had become established strong clawhand with thumb at the side.

(*Top*) Showing clawing, flathand, limits of extension and flexion of the fingers and of opposition of the thumb. Because of his useless hand, he was not able to find occupation. Operation was done for muscle balance in the fingers. Also, for opposition of the thumb, he had a pulley operation and, for adduction of the thumb and curvature of the arches, a tendon T operation.

(*Bottom*) Taken 2 years later, the 2 left-hand pictures show fairly good muscle balance in the fingers and a practical opening and closing for grasp. The thumb now adducts to the ulnar side of the ring finger and opposes to 2 inches in front of the long finger; the patient has curvature of both carpal and metacarpal arches. There is good sensation throughout, and stereognosis has returned. He works well as a welder. The 2 right-hand illustrations show strong lateral motion of the index finger lifting a heavy metal cellophane-tape dispenser. In the operation for muscle balance, the sublimis of this finger was transferred to the lateral band of the dorsal aponeurosis to act as an interosseus muscle.

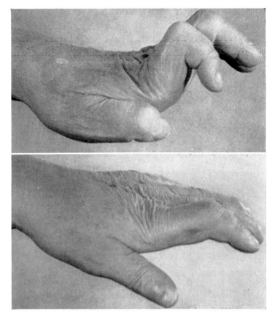

FIG. 593. Good correction of claw deformity in leprosy by Bunnell's superficialis transfer to fingers and opponens transfer for thumb, in which the tendon is inserted into the extensor pollicis longus to overcome the flexion deformity of the distal joint. (From D. C. Riordan, M.D.)

tion of thumb motions as well. For details of thumb paralysis see the following section of this chapter.

Poliomyelitis may involve the nerves to all the intrinsics, or there may be a selective paralysis of some, while others are normal or simply weakened.

Leprosy involves the ulnar nerve most often, but commonly both the median and the ulnar nerves are affected.

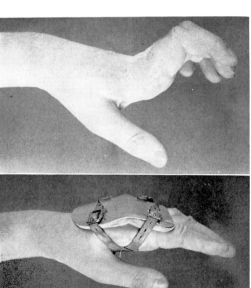

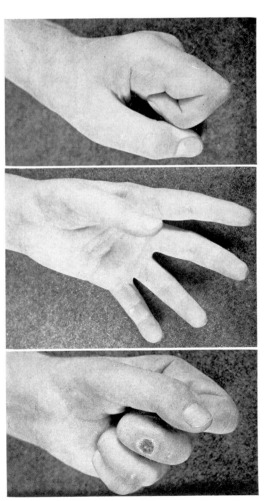

FIG. 594. (Left, top) Deformity from paralysis of the intrinsic muscles resulting in clawed fingers. (Left, bottom) Splint used to flex the proximal finger joints. The knuckle-bender splint is better. (Right) Muscle balance operation has been done in the fingers: the sublimis tendons have been transferred from the palm down the lumbrical canals to insert into lateral bands in the fingers. Note flexion of proximal joints, extension of distal 2: also, ability to spread fingers. (W. H. Frackelton, M.D.)

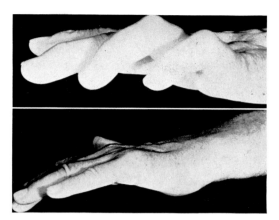

FIG. 595. Clawing of ring and little fingers in ulnar palsy can be relieved in some cases by preventing hyperextension of the proximal joints. Lower photograph shows postoperative condition after advancing the volar capsules proximally on the metacarpals and slitting the proximal pulleys.

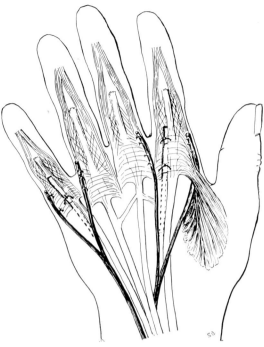

FIG. 597. For paralysis of the interossei and the lumbricali (paralytic clawhand), the 2 extensor proprius tendons each may be split and transferred to a lateral band of each finger to furnish spreading of the fingers and correction of muscle balance by extending the distal 2 finger joints. The proprius indicis and the minimi digiti (*shaded*) are first dissected from their beds well down the fingers. The bordering aponeurosis is sutured as shown, so that the extensor tendons will not extend the joints in rotation. The action is not so strong as when sublimi are used, and to flex the proximal finger joints the proximal pulleys must be advanced in addition.

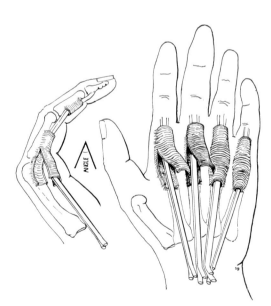

FIG. 596. Pulley advancement operation to increase voluntary flexion of the proximal finger joints in clawhand. The proximal pulley is slit through on each side, avoiding the nerves, until there is a sufficient angle of approach for the long flexor tendons to act well on the proximal joints.

LOSS OF INTRINSIC MUSCLE FUNCTION IN THE FINGERS DUE TO SPASM OR CONTRACTURE—THE INTRINSIC-PLUS HAND

Lesions of the central nervous system such as Parkinson's disease and cerebral palsy, systemic alterations such as tetany, and local irritative lesions such as rheumatoid arthritis can produce spasm and overactivity in the intrinsic muscles of the fingers. Such hyperactivity upsets the balance as does paralysis, but the deformity is that of accentuation of the metacarpal arch, flexion of the proximal joints and extension of the middle and the distal joints.

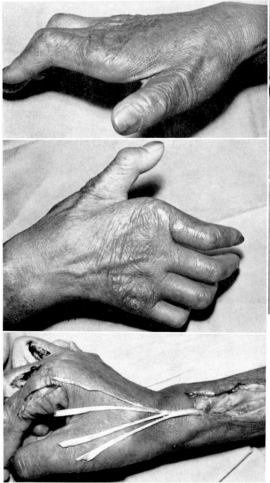

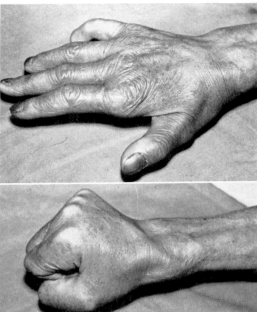

FIG. 598. Tenodeses to overcome clawing and ulnar deviation at proximal joints. The brachioradialis tendon is dissected off the muscle but left attached at its insertion. The broad sheet of tendon is split into 4 strands, each then passed below the transverse metacarpal ligament and inserted into the extensor aponeurosis on the radial side of the fingers. (*Right*) Postoperative extension and flexion. When the wrist is dorsiflexed, the tenodesis is relaxed and the middle joints can be flexed. (From K. Tsuge, M.D., Okayama University)

Scarring and fibrosis from injury and especially ischemic contracture produce the same deformity. See Chapter 7, Local Ischemic Contracture in the Hand for diagnostic test and pathologic physiology.

TREATMENT OF DYSFUNCTION OF INTRINSIC MUSCLES OF FINGERS

Paralysis. If the cause of loss of function is a lesion of the peripheral nerve, nerve suture should be done wherever it is technically possible. If the lesion is of such long standing that the muscles have degenerated and become fibrosed, then tendon transfers are indicated. If a motor nerve has been severed for more than 2 years, recovery of the involved muscles probably will not take place except in the very young. Technically it is possible to repair the small, almost terminal branches of the motor nerves in the palm. Tendon transfers to provide a substitute motion can be successful only if the joints are movable and the soft tissues suitable. If there is also damage to the extrinsic muscles, the plan should be to provide by arthrodeses and transfers a fundamental grasp or hooklike function and not to attempt to reconstruct a normally balanced mechanism.

Operations to Restore Balance in Clawing of the Fingers. In 1922 Sir Harold Stiles transferred the superficialis tendon, taking one slip of the insertion around each side of the finger and suturing each to the extensor tendon on the dorsum of the proximal phalanx. The results in this case are not known, but the operation in other hands was not successful.

BUNNELL'S TRANSFER FOR CLAWING OF THE FINGERS. To provide a more direct line of approach for the tendon through a region less liable to provoke adhesions and with an insertion comparable with the lumbrical, Bunnell devised the operation of passing the transferred tendons through lumbrical canals to the lateral bands of the extensor apparatus. The operation is designed to restore muscle balance, promote flexion of the proximal finger joints, aid in extension of the middle and the distal joints and provide for the lateral motion normally provided by the interossei.

Through a midlateral incision in the finger, the length of the proximal segment, the superficialis tendon is cut off in the sheath opposite the joint. If cut too long, the stumps attach, producing flexion contracture of the middle joint. The tendon is withdrawn enough to split it an inch or more and then, through an incision in the palm paralleling the creases, is withdrawn and split its length. If desired, it may be split into 4 strands.

A stainless steel wire with a needle on each end is sewed into the end of each strand of superficialis tendon, as in the pull-out wire

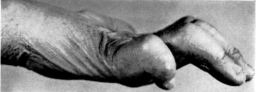
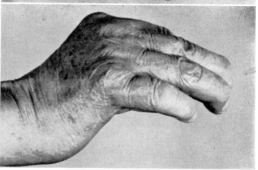

FIG. 599. Tendon grafts passed through the interosseus spaces below the transverse metacarpal ligament and into the aponeuroses for clawhand of leprosy. The motor force here is the flexor carpi radialis passed subcutaneously around the radial border of the forearm. (From D. C. Riordan, M.D.)

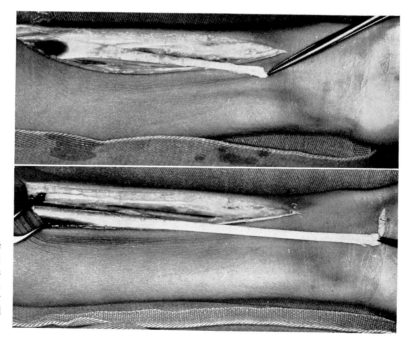

FIG. 600. (Top) The brachioradialis tendon; the upper portion can be split into 4 strands. (Bottom) The flexor carpi radialis is freed and mobilized.

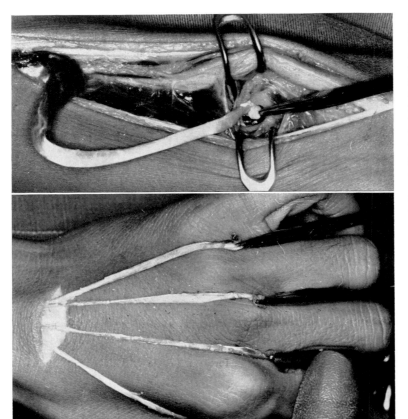

FIG. 601. (*Top*) Passing the flexor carpi radialis through a large opening in the interosseus membrane. (*Bottom*) Through an incision in the lower forearm, not shown here, the flexor carpi radialis tendon is retrieved, extended with the 4-tailed graft of the brachioradialis tendon and passed to the dorsum of the hand. From here each strand will pass through an interosseus space, volar to the transverse metacarpal ligament, and insert in the extensor aponeurosis. (From Prof. A. Hodgson, Orthopedic Department, Hong Kong University)

technic. Then the 2 end wires are threaded on 1 needle, which is passed down the lumbrical canal and on out the lateral incision in the finger and over the lateral band, the top surface of which is scraped to receive it. Next, the wires are passed out through the dorsal skin, where they are fastened to a button. Both ends of the pull-out wire are threaded on 1 needle and passed out through the skin proximally, where they are left for use in pulling out the stitch 3 weeks later. To remove it, the ends are cut off close to the skin under the button, and the stitch is withdrawn backward by the pull-out wire. The running wire suture can also be used.

From the one lumbrical canal 2 tendon strands will pass, 1 to each side of the cleft. The bed of the tendon is in soft gliding tissue all the way. The tendon should be threaded in and out the aponeurosis so that it will both flex the proximal finger joint and extend the distal 2 joints. The adjoining tendon surfaces should be scraped clean for better union. The tendon is the right length, reaching to within a centimeter of the middle joint on the dorsum of the finger.

The split strands from any one tendon motor should go to the radial sides of the fingers. It is possible to plan that some tendons will abduct or spread from the middle finger and others will adduct or converge to the middle finger, but for practical purposes, it will suffice to supply each finger with a tendon on the radial side and the little finger with one on the ulnar side.

One may plan to use to the best advantage whatever tendons are available. Each finger should have at least 1 strand, so that the distal 2 joints will extend and the proximal joint will flex well. The extensor proprius tendons can be used for this purpose if desired. The tendon to the radial side of the index finger should go to the lateral band instead of the tubercule, if it is expected to extend the distal 2 joints. Theoretically, it is advisable to transfer tendons to each side of each finger, but one must be sure to have enough tendons for also furnishing adduction and perhaps opposition to the thumb. There are available in certain instances the 2 extensor proprius tendons, the palmaris longus, and even free tendon grafts from the palmaris longus or extensors of the small toes. These can be motored by a wrist extensor or flexor. In a case of ulnar palsy in which the nerve is severed above the elbow, use of the superficialis, which is supplied by the median nerve, would rob the little finger of flexion unless its profundus tendon could be joined to the other profundus tendons in the forearm.

The hand and the fingers are splinted for 3 weeks with the wrist in flexion and the fingers in the intrinsic-plus position, followed by light exercise for a week; the hand should not be used for hard work for 2 months.

This operation to restore muscle balance is the basic operation for restoring intrinsic muscle function to the fingers and was designed primarily for those hands with normal long flexors, both superficialis and profundi. Failure to note this and use of this procedure in cases of high ulnar palsy and in leprosy has resulted in overcorrection of the deformity.

ARTHRODESIS OF FINGER JOINTS. In some cases, fusion of the middle joints in a functioning position and operative restoration of the long-flexor action on the proximal joints provides better function. Extreme clawing with structural changes that do not respond to splinting requires middle joint fusion in moderate flexion. When volar advancement of the proximal pulleys and proximal advancement of the volar capsules of the metacarpophalangeal joints is added, there will result better flexion of the fingers and a more efficient grasping mechanism.

The proximal joints should not be fused except as a last resort, because this joint is the key in the finger mechanism.

THE RELATION OF PROXIMAL JOINT CONDITION TO CLAWING. In most intrinsic paralyses, as Beevor showed, slight pressure on the dorsum of the proximal finger segment, just enough to prevent hyperextension, corrects the balance and allows the long extensor to extend the distal 2 joints. For this reason, patients with tight volar capsules and intrinsic paralysis may show no clawing of the fingers. Extension of the 2 distal joints may not be powerful, but the claw deformity will not be present. Similarly, Forrester-Brown and Wright both noted that clawing did not occur when the long flexors are paralyzed.

If this cockback of the proximal joint is present and the long flexors are active, the fingers are curled, and the tips are so close to the proximal finger segments that the hand cannot be opened well for grasp. People with this condition attempt to compensate by flexing the wrist, thus putting more tension on the long extensors and exaggerating the cockback. This flexion deformity of the wrist is common in long-standing intrinsic paralyses.

If the cockback can be prevented by splinting during the early paralytic period, this late development can be prevented.

Static Measures Used To Prevent Cockback. Such "splinting" can be internal as by a tenodesis of the proximal joint or a proximal advancement of the capsule. Zancolli, who has written extensively on this procedure, tests before operation to determine the optimal angle of flexion in which to place the joint. Dividing the metacarpal attachment of the volar capsule and slitting it up each side, advancing it proximally and inserting the cut edge into a slit in the cortex of the metacarpal with fixation by a pull-out wire has been most successful. Advancement volarward of the proximal pulley at the same time helps to give a better angle of approach for the flexor tendons.

Similarly, a tenodesis prevents cockback, but if the tenodesis is attached proximal to the wrist or to the transverse carpal ligament and distally to the lateral slips, there can be some automatic intrinsic action. Riordan uses a strip of tendon peeled off a wrist extensor, passed through the interosseus spaces, then volar to the transverse metacarpal ligament and out the lumbrical canal to the lateral band. For the clawhand of leprosy, Tsuge uses the brachioradialis tendon, splits the proximal broad portion into 4 strands and, leaving the insertion on the radius intact, passes 1 strand down to each finger through the interosseus, under the transverse metacarpal ligament and into the lateral band. Thus, dropping the wrist

Rupture middle slip
long extensor – primary

Longitudinal tear allowing
dislocation of lateral bands–

–secondary

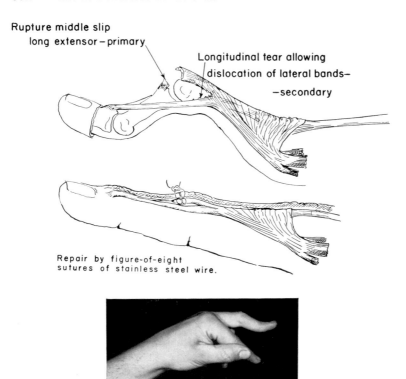

Repair by figure-of-eight
sutures of stainless steel wire.

FIG. 602. (*Top*) The *boutonnière* deformity is caused by rupture of the central extensor tendon slip at the middle joint and a subsequent tear of the aponeurosis. The lateral bands then flex the middle joint and extend the distal joint. A simple figure-of-eight removable stitch of stainless-steel wire, together with splinting, is sufficient to cure a recent case. In a long-standing case, the slit also should be closed by a removable figure-of-eight suture through skin and tendon. (J. Bone Joint Surg. *24*: 20) (*Bottom*) The deformity.

into palmar flexion tends to prevent the proximal joints from extending and, if the transplanted tendon slides, to extend the 2 distal finger joints.

TRANSFER OF PROPRIUS TENDONS. The extensor indicis and the extensor minimus can be used as active transfers. Each is split into 2 strands. One strand is looped around the 1st interosseus tendon and into the lateral band on the radial side of the index finger; another is passed beneath the transverse metacarpal ligament and to the radial side of the middle finger. Similarly, the little finger proprius is used. One strand is passed around the tendon of the abductor digiti minimi and the other to the ulnar side of the ring finger. These 2 proprius muscles are not very powerful, but a strong tenodesis effect is obtained even if the transfer becomes adherent.

OTHER TRANSFERS FOR INTRINSIC PARALYSIS. Brand, in India, used the Bunnell modification of Stiles' operation, the transfer of superficialis through lumbrical canal to lateral bands, for the clawing caused by leprosy. Because of the laxity of the middle finger joints in these patients, who normally have the ability to hyperextend their fingers to an extreme degree, removal of the flexor power of the middle joint by dividing the superficialis and transferring it to the extensor apparatus resulted in an overcorrection and the production of the intrinsic-plus deformity. Therefore, he employed the proprius transfer operation principle but used tendon grafts, usually from the plantaris; he passed them along the same line used in Riordan's active tenodeses but attached them at the wrist to the divided extensor carpi radialis brevis tendon. Since the primary flexor of the middle joint was left undisturbed, overcorrection did not occur.

Riordan, feeling that the compensatory flexion of the wrist which occurs in long-standing clawhands exaggerated the clawing, describes the use of the flexor carpi radialis tendon as the motor; it is passed around the radial side of the forearm and elongated with the many-

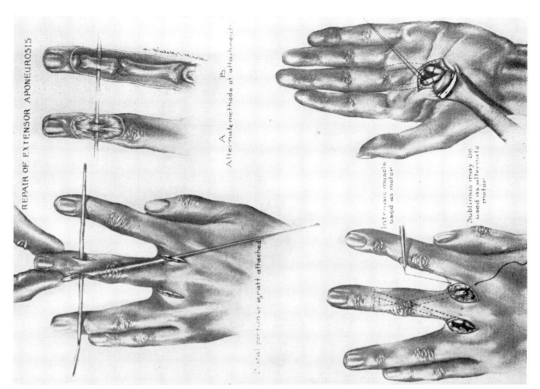

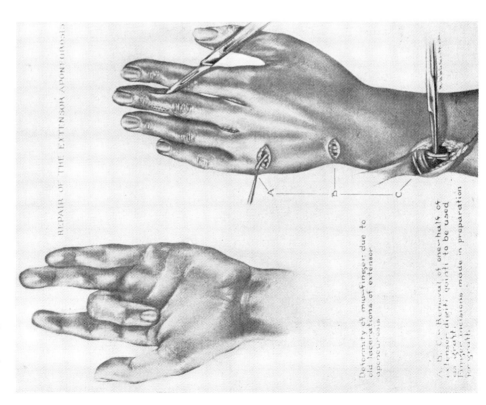

Fig. 603. Supplying a new extensor tendon for the middle finger joint, using a slender tendon as a graft and crossing it over the middle finger joint. It is motored by the interossei muscles or, if they are paralyzed or more strength is desired, by the sublimis tendon. (From S. Benjamin Fowler, M.D.)

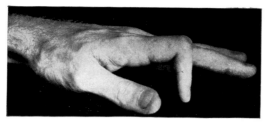

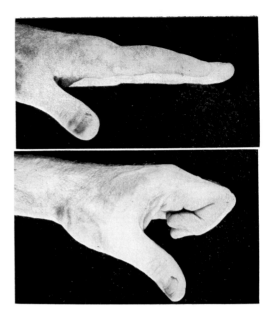

Fig. 604. (*Top*) Limit of extension of the middle joint because its extensor tendon had been severed by a shell fragment. (*Right*) Result after repair by the method of Fowler, using as a graft an extensor tendon from the little finger, passing it transversely through a drill hole in the middle phalanx, crossing the ends over the dorsum of the middle joint and fastening them to the interosseus tendon on each side. (S. Benjamin Fowler, M.D.)

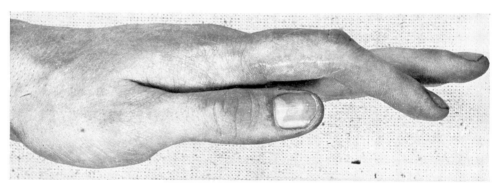

Fig. 605. (*Top*) Due to an open fracture of the proximal phalanx, the extensor tendon had been ruptured. The position of the phalanx was first corrected by osteotomy. The patient cannot extend the middle finger joint. (*Right*) Excellent movement of the middle finger joint was by the cross-tendon graft method of Fowler, using the extensor tendon of the little finger and fastening it into the interossei. (S. Benjamin Fowler, M.D.)

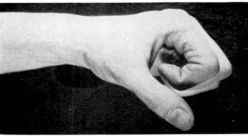

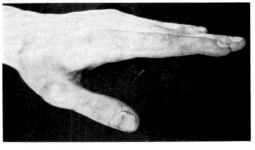

tailed graft, thus removing some of the deforming power and transposing it to the extensor side.

A tendon transfer passing through a fascial sheet is prone to adhere to the opening, and in all the dorsal transfers based on the proprius principle the tendon or tendon graft passes through the interosseus fascia and

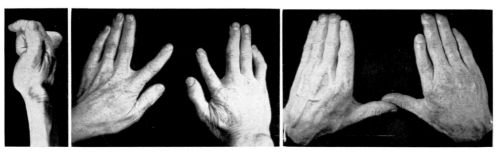

FIG. 606. Case C. M. Q. Repair of interosseus tendon by tendon graft. Following striking a man in the teeth and immediate suture, infection occurred, resulting in ankylosis of the proximal joint of the index finger. Six months later, an arthroplasty was done. At this time, the tendon of the palmaris longus was used to fill a 1½ inch gap in each of the long extensor tendons and the tendon of the first interosseus muscle, where they had sloughed from infection.

(*Left*) Flexion in the proximal joint from arthroplasty. (*Center*) Abduction of the index finger (*right*) through the tendon graft in the interosseus tendon compared with that in other hand. (*Right*) Adduction of the index finger compared with the other hand.

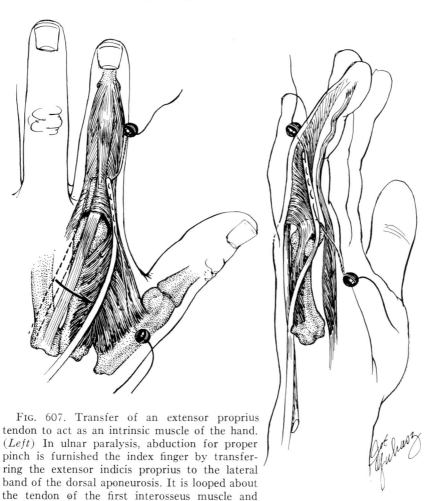

FIG. 607. Transfer of an extensor proprius tendon to act as an intrinsic muscle of the hand. (*Left*) In ulnar paralysis, abduction for proper pinch is furnished the index finger by transferring the extensor indicis proprius to the lateral band of the dorsal aponeurosis. It is looped about the tendon of the first interosseus muscle and fastened to the lateral band (after scraping each) by a removable running suture of stainless-steel wire. (*Right*) When a flexion component is needed, an extensor proprius of the index or the little finger may be transferred to the lateral band after passing it volar to the transverse metacarpal ligament.

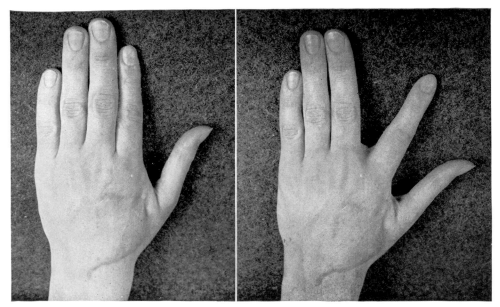

FIG. 608. The first interosseus muscle is paralyzed. Ability to abduct is given the index finger by transferring the tendon of the extensor proprius indicis to the tubercle on the outer side of the base of the proximal phalanx. The 2 pictures show the motion gained. Note the pedicle graft over the bullet wound that severed the motor nerve. (L. D. Howard, M.D.)

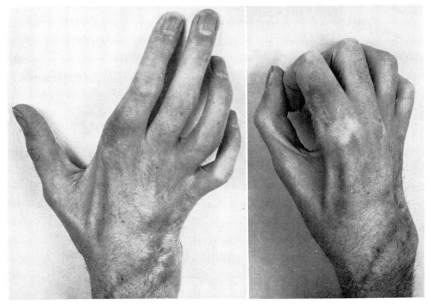

FIG. 609. (*Left*) The index finger fell into adduction from ulnar palsy and could not be abducted. (*Right*) The sublimis tendon of the finger was detached, drawn out at the wrist and passed over the back of the thumb to attach to the lateral band on the radial side of the proximal segment of the index finger (Graham). Showing tendon beneath the skin and voluntary abduction gained. (Walter C. Graham, M.D.)

sometimes pierces the intertendinous fascia of the common extensors.

The flexor carpi radialis can be brought through a wide excised opening in the interosseus membrane and elongated with a many-tailed graft under the common extensors and then through the interosseus fascia with perhaps less tendency to adhere. The straight-line approach of the flexor to the extensor surface of the forearm is also more efficient. If the brachioradialis tendon is used as the graft, all the procedure is done in one operative field. This procedure was introduced at the Queen Mary Hospital, Hong Kong, on the University service of Professor A. Hodgson, and was found to be most satisfactory.

Restoration of Abduction of Index Finger. The ability to abduct the index finger is an essential part of the pinching mechanism. Function of the first interosseus muscle is often lost in poliomyelitis and commonly accompanies thenar palsy. It can result from local lesions of the deep motor branch of the ulnar nerve in the palm or from direct injury to the first-cleft structures. Abduction of the index finger can be restored by transfer of the extensor indicis to the first interosseus tendon. If the middle joint of the index finger can be extended either by an active first volar interosseus or through the action of the long exten-

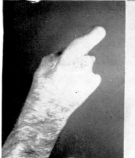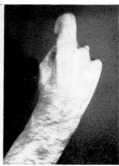

FIG. 610. Case H. F. The first interosseus and the lumbricalis muscles are irreparable, producing the deformity of ulnar flexion in the proximal joint of the index finger. The extensor tendon of the amputated ring finger was transferred to that of the first interosseus muscle. The illustrations show the strong lateral motion restored to the finger.

sors or an intact lumbrical, it is not necessary to place the transfer into the lateral band. The tendon is divided over the proximal joint, withdrawn at the wrist through a short transverse incision and passed distally around the radial border of the second metacarpal to insert into the first interosseus tendon below the axis of motion of the proximal joint. Bruner transferred the extensor brevis of the thumb, and

FIG. 611. Tendon transfers to give abduction to the index finger. (*Left*) The flexor sublimis tendon, detached at its insertion, is withdrawn in the palm, passed down the lumbrical canal and attached to the lateral band by a running stitch of withdrawable stainless steel. This flexes the proximal finger joint, extends the distal two and abducts the finger. (*Center*) In special cases, in order to give

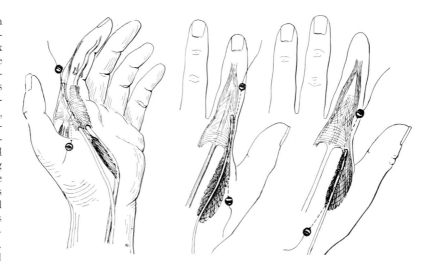

more of an extension component, the sublimis tendon is withdrawn at the wrist, passing it over the dorsum of the thenar eminence to gain the lateral band (Graham). (*Right*) The extensor pollicis brevis is transferred to act as the first interosseus band (Bruner). It reaches only to the tendon.

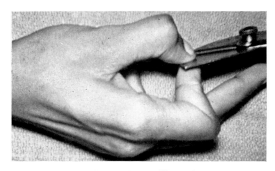

FIG. 612. Loss of stability of 1st meta-carpal and abduction of index finger in ulnar palsy. The distal thumb joint must be flexed sharply to tense the extensor policis longus and allow it to act as an accessory adductor, and the index must be "backed up" by the other fingers.

Graham passed a superficialis subcutaneously from the wrist back of the thumb to insert in the lateral band of the index finger.

This abduction power of the digit against which the thumb can pinch is necessary and important. In amputations of the index ray, it is best to preserve the 1st dorsal interosseus and insert its tendon into that of the 2nd dorsal interosseus. This makes a better-appearing cleft and also provides more abduction power for grasping.

Reconstruction of Extensor Apparatus at Middle Joint. Direct injury to the dorsum of the middle joint area often results in loss of skin and tendon. Direct repair is impossible, but if adequate skin can be supplied and the joint action preserved, a tendon graft attached transversely across the middle phalanx or looped through the conjoined extensor tendon can be crisscrossed over the middle joint and an end on each side passed proximally and sutured to the interossei. Fowler reported this as well as a modification in which the proximal ends were passed into the palm and sutured to a divided flexor superficialis tendon.

Treatment of Dysfunction From Contracture of Intrinsic Muscles of the Fingers. (See also Chap. 7, Ischemic Contracture in the Hand.) This intrinsic-plus phenomenon in the fingers is disabling because it makes it impossible to open the hand for grasp or, in mild forms, to flex the middle and the distal joints of the fingers around an object which holds the proximal joints extended.

Theoretically, if an intrinsic contracture is released completely, one would expect the opposite deformity of clawing to occur. This seldom happens because there usually is enough fibrosis in the proximal joint area to prevent the cockback of these joints. If the release should result in cockback and, therefore, clawing, an advancement of the volar capsules and the proximal pulleys can be done.

The proximal joint is the key joint in the finger, as the wrist is the key joint for the hand. Therefore, efforts to relieve an intrinsic contracture should be directed toward achieving extension of the proximal joint and a balanced effect of the long flexors and the long extensors.

INTRINSIC MUSCLES OF THE THUMB

ANATOMY AND FUNCTION

Thumb motions can be described as 3 paired and opposite actions: extension—flexion, ab-

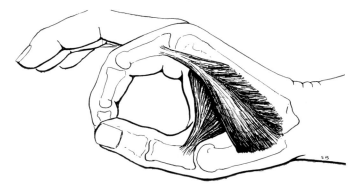

FIG. 613. Illustrating the reason for the weak pinch in ulnar palsy: the inability to make an O with the thumb and the index finger and to scrape the extended thumb across the palm. The abductor (1st interosseus) of the index finger and the adductor of the thumb are necessary antagonists to give a firm pinch.

Fig. 614. Case C. S. Restoration of action of the intrinsic muscle. Two years previously, the hand had been crushed in a press and the palm lacerated, resulting in loss of

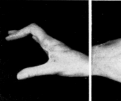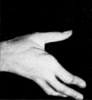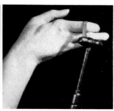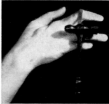

the index finger, the intrinsic muscle of the long finger and flexion contracture of that finger. There was complaint of inability to work because the long finger was drawn into ulnar flexion in its proximal joint and flexion in its middle joint.

The 2 left-hand pictures show that the proximal joint of the long finger cannot abduct and that the middle joint is in flexion contracture of 62°.

The flexor sublimis tendon was detached from its insertion, brought out in the palm and made to fuse to the lateral band of the dorsal aponeurosis, to act for the interosseus muscle. The scar was so dense and adherent to the bone at the knuckle that a graft of deep forearm fascia was placed between tendon and bone. The 2 right-hand illustrations, taken 6 months later, show the flexion contracture better by 22° and good ability to abduct the proximal joint against the weight of a hammer. The patient then used the hand without complaint.

duction—adduction and opposition—reposition. All are combinations of motions. For example, extension of the thumb, i.e., spreading it in the plane of the metacarpals, may be called lateral abduction and involves activity of the abductor pollicis longus as well as the long and the short extensors. If the thumb is brought away from the hand at right angles to the metacarpal plane in what is called palmar abduction, the short abductor acts with the long to provide the motion. The opposite motion, adduction, though carried out primarily by the strong adductor pollicis, is aided by the first interosseus belly arising from the

first metacarpal and by the oblique line of pull of the extensor pollicis longus. Opposition and reposition are actions requiring the use of many muscles. Therefore, one should not let the name of a muscle imply that its action is that movement only.

The stability of the thumb is provided by the action of the abductor pollicis longus (radial nerve) which lifts the first metacarpal at the trapeziometacarpal joint. The adductor pollicis (ulnar nerve), by its insertion on the proximal phalanx, counterbalances the long abductor, and the thumb is kept arched longitudinally. If the long abductor is severed or

Fig. 615. Case J. R. Restoration of action of the intrinsic muscle. From a buzzsaw injury a year previously, the patient had little use of the little finger. He could not flex or radioflex its proximal joint and lacked 55° of extension of its middle joint. Capsulectomy increased the flexion of the proximal joint to 88°, and severing the insertion of the flexor sublimis allowed the middle joint to straighten. The sublimis was passed from the palm through the lumbrical canal to the lateral band, substituting for the interosseus muscle.

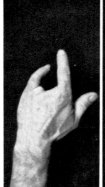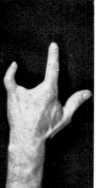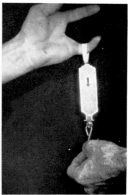

(Left and center) Showing good lateral control of the little finger, its tip moving through an amplitude of 1⅞ inches. (Right) Restored power of abduction of the little finger registers 6 pounds as compared with only 1 pound in his normal hand.

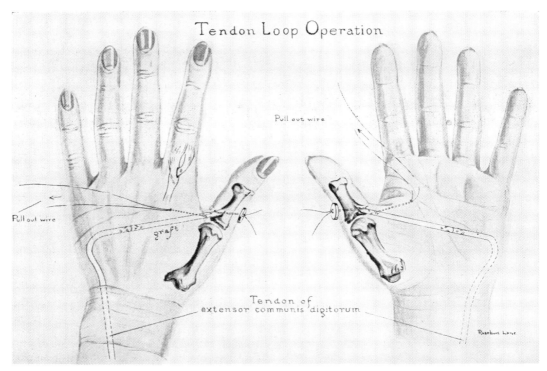

Tendon Loop Operation

FIG. 616. In the tendon loop operation to restore adduction to the thumb, the extensor communis tendon from the index finger is extended with a tendon graft and then passed subcutaneously around the ulnar border of the hand and across the palm under the flexor tendons to act as an adductor of the thumb. Attachment to the thumb is by fine stainless-steel wire through a drillhole to a button outside the skin. A flake of bone is chipped up at the insertion. A pull-out wire is placed so that the suture may be removed in 3 weeks. The stump of the extensor communis of the index finger is attached to the extensor indicis proprius to prevent rotation deformity.

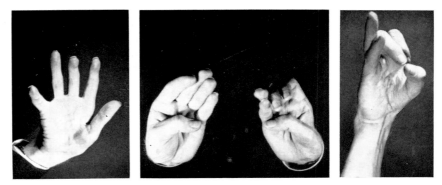

FIG. 617. Case E. W. Loss of both adduction and opposition of the thumb from severance of both the motor branch of the ulnar and the motor thenar branch of the median nerves, there being too great a gap in each of them for suture. (*Left*) Limit of adduction and opposition of the thumb. A pulley operation was done for opposition, using the palmaris longus as motor and the extensor pollicis brevis as tendon and looping about the flexor ulnaris as a pulley. A tendon loop operation was done for adduction, looping the tendon of the extensor digitorum communis of the index finger around the ulnar border of the hand and to the adductor tubercle in the proximal phalanx of the thumb. The median nerve was sutured to 5 of its sensory branches. (*Center* and *right*) These 2 photographs, taken 1 year later, show excellent ability to adduct and oppose the thumb. Sensation returned throughout by the 8th month.

paralyzed, the first metacarpal drops, pinch is severely impaired because now the strong adductor pulls the proximal phalanx toward the palm, and the proximal thumb joint goes into hyperextension. If the adductor is paralyzed, the same deformity occurs because the proximal joint cannot be flexed.

Function of the long abductor or provision for stabilization of the carpometacarpal joint is essential for good thumb function. In planning operations for the restoration of opposition or adduction it may be necessary to provide this abductor component first or the subsequent transfers will fail.

The intrinsic thenar muscles are analogous to the interossei of the fingers. The abductor pollicis brevis sends fibers of insertion into the base of the proximal phalanx on the radial side and also fibers into the extensor aponeurosis over the dorsum of the proximal phalanx. On the ulnar side, the adductor pollicis similarly has a double insertion, so that spasm or contracture of these muscles flexes the proximal and extends the distal thumb joint. This deformity is seen commonly in rheumatoid arthritis, Parkinson's disease and the ischemic contractures. The ability to extend the distal joint of the thumb by means of these intrinsic insertions varies, and the resulting motions may cause confusion when division of the long extensor tendon is suspected.

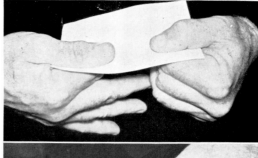

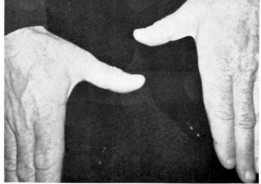

Fig. 618. Ten years after tendon loop operation for loss of adductor of thumb. Pinch is improved, and there is no loss of abduction of the thumb.

PARALYSIS OF ADDUCTORS OF THUMB

When the ulnar nerve is severed, there is loss of function in the adductor pollicis and a variable portion of the flexor pollicis brevis. The longitudinal arch of the thumb cannot be maintained in attempts to pinch against the index finger, and a compensatory hyperflexion of the distal joint takes place. There is atrophy of the first cleft. Froment's sign, a dropping of this arch and excessive flexion of the distal joint, is best shown by having the patient grasp a folded newspaper between the thumb and the index finger. The excessive flexion of the distal joint in this test is not due to loss of extensor power from paralysis of the thenar muscles but is a compensatory means of increasing the tension on the extensor pollicis longus, which is acting as a supplementary adductor of the thumb.

Paralysis of the adductor pollicis results in inability to scrape the thumb across the palm, since the abductors and short flexor are no longer opposed. The adductor muscle, if functioning, can be palpated in the first cleft.

Since the commonest cause of adductor paralysis is interruption of the ulnar nerve, the interossei are also lacking in action, which further interferes with pinch and grasp and means that measures to restore their action, especially that of the first interosseus, should be planned.

Restoring Adduction of the Thumb. As in all paralyses from peripheral nerve lesions, repair of the nerve should be done if possible and when reasonably favorable conditions are present. Repair of the deep motor branch of the ulnar nerve has been done with good results. When nerves are irreparable, tendon transfers are available. Not all patients with loss of adductor pollicis will need a transfer, but when median and ulnar palsies are combined or for restoration of pinch after pedicle reconstruction of first cleft contractures, some added power in this motion will greatly improve function.

TENDON TRANSFERS FOR ADDUCTION OF THUMB. Several methods are available: the tendon loop operation, the tendon T, the superficialis transfer and the brachioradialis transfer.

Tendon Loop Operation. The tendon of the extensor digitorum communis to the index finger is detached, just before it spreads out over the proximal joint of the index finger, and is withdrawn at the base of the back of the hand. It is elongated by a free graft from the palmaris longus or some other tendon, then passed subcutaneously around the ulnar border of the hand and across the palm deep to the flexor tendons, to be inserted on the ulnar side

of the base of the proximal phalanx of the thumb at the adductor tubercle.

The communis tendon is selected instead of the proprius because its muscle is stronger. It is essential to attach its stump in the finger to the proprius tendon, or the index finger will show deformity of rotation and adduction. A short transverse incision is used there, and also on the dorsum of the hand at the distal edge of the annular ligament. The incisions at the ulnar border of the hand and the ulnar side of the thumb are midlateral.

In passing the tendon around the ulnar side of the hand, it was found to be better not to pass it under the hypothenar muscles, because their perimysium adhered to it. The tendon is attached to the bone in the thumb by the pull-

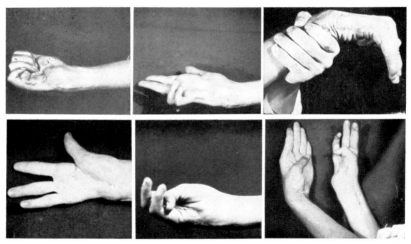

FIG. 619. Case T. S., age 11. (*Top, left* and *center*) Four years previously, the patient had lacerated the ulnar border of the hand, the ulnar nerve and the flexor tendons to the ring and the little fingers, followed by infection, ulnar palsy, clawhand and a thumb that could not adduct.

Operation: Removed a wedge of carpus to adduct the wrist. Amputated the little finger, using its skin. To correct the claw, used the flexor profundus prolonged by the flexor superficialis of the little finger to attach to each paralyzed interosseus to the ring finger. To give adduction to the thumb, passed the extensor tendon of the little finger across the palm under the tendons to attach to the adductor tubercle on the proximal phalanx of the thumb, as in the tendon loop operation. There was a defect in the motor branch of the ulnar nerve; this was filled by a 1¼-inch graft from one of the sensory branches. Two years later, the tendons were freed, and some paratenon from the fascia lata was grafted beneath them. Examination 2 years later showed excellent function of the hand.

(*Top, right*) The ring finger could flex in its proximal joint and at the same time extend in its distal 2 joints.

(*Bottom*) The thumb could adduct as well as could the other thumb, and the arches of the hand were well curved. The transferred tendon for adduction could be felt moving about the ulnar border of the hand, and because of the nerve graft the adductor muscles of the thumb could be felt to move.

out wire technic, the tendon being placed into the bone proper and not simply attached to the adductor tendon. This results in better stability of the arch, but all other intrinsic and extrinsic tendons of the thumb must be functioning well if this transfer is to work.

Tendon T Operation. The tendon T operation gives adduction to the thumb and the little finger and cups of the hand, restoring the metacarpal arch. A free tendon graft spans the palm behind the flexor tendons from the base of the proximal phalanx of the thumb to the neck of the metacarpal of the little finger. One of the long flexor tendons of the forearm, such as a superficialis, is attached by a loop to the center of this cross tendon, forming a T. On contraction of the muscle in the

forearm, the T is drawn to a Y, the thumb and the 5th metacarpal are drawn toward each other, and the arch is restored. The cross member lies in soft, movable tissue back of the profundus tendons and can be drawn proximalward without resistance. It does not press or pull against the deep branch of the ulnar nerve which is behind it. The cross part of the T comes in full flexion as far proximally as the carpus, and the angle of the Y thus formed is 40°.

The 5th metacarpal is exposed in its ulnar and volar aspects. One end of the cross tendon is fastened to the bone by a pull-out wire. The palm is opened by an incision paralleling the creases, and the tendon is passed across and through the palm behind the flexor tendons

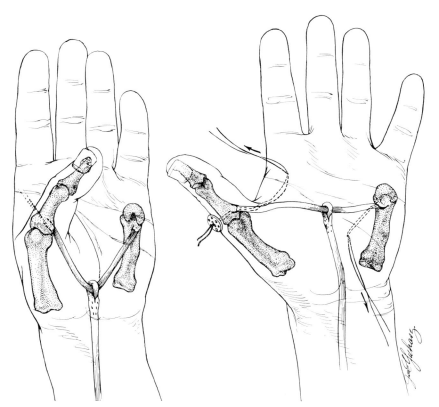

Fig. 620. In the tendon T operation to restore adduction to the thumb and curvature to the carpal and the metacarpal arches, a tendon graft spans the distance between the little finger metacarpal and the adductor insertion in the proximal phalanx of the thumb. A long flexor tendon of the forearm (a sublimis or the palmaris longus prolonged by a strip of its palmar fascia) is looped over its center to form the T. This, when in action, changes to a Y, adducting the thumb and curving the arches.

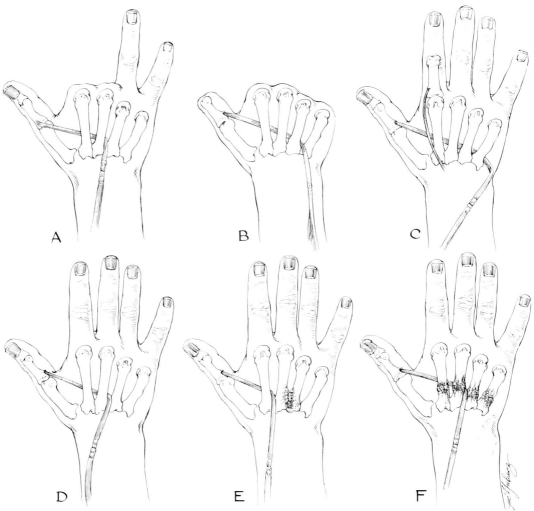

Fig. 621. Transfers for adductor paralysis. (A) A finger extensor to the rerouted extensor pollicis brevis in 3rd cleft. (B) Extensor carpi ulnaris as a motor, extended with tendon graft through 4th cleft. (C) Brachioradialis plus tendon graft around ulnar border. Index proprius to 1st interosseus. (D) Extensor of wrist plus graft. (E) Brachioradialis plus graft through 2nd cleft to avoid area of scar from injury. (F) Brachioradialis plus graft through site of injury should have been rerouted around the ulnar border of the palm.

and brought through a small lateral incision over the ulnar aspect of the base of the proximal phalanx of the thumb. Here it is attached to the phalanx with a pull-out wire. The tendon should be slack when the hand is fully spread, since grafts shrink a little. For the cross member, the tendon of the extensor pollicis brevis, which is already attached to the thumb, may be used. The flexor tendon used

as a motor is looped around the center of the cross tendon, embedding it into itself.

Any motor from the forearm can be used, though a flexor superficialis is preferred because it can be spared more easily and because it has a long amplitude.

The Flexor Superficialis Transfer or Y-V Transfer. Littler took a superficial flexor, divided it at its insertion and withdrew it in the

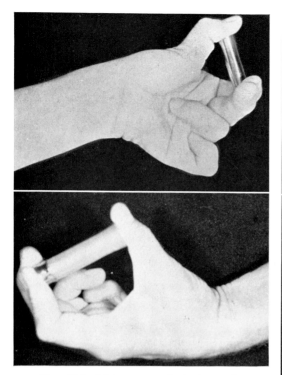

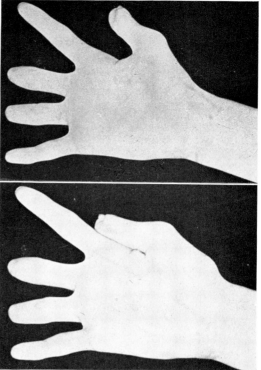

Fig. 622. Adductor paralysis from ulnar palsy. Lower photograph shows improved stability after transfer of brachioradialis plus tendon graft through 3rd interspace to adductor insertion.

Fig. 623. An exploding bomb blew off the tips of some fingers and penetrated the palm, irreparably damaging the nerve to the adductor pollicis. Good power of adduction was restored by transfer of brachioradialis extended by a tendon graft through the 3rd interosseus space and to the adductor insertion.

palm. One slip was sutured to the adductor tubercle and the other to the lateral slip of the index or to the 5th metacarpal. The result is that the 2 points of attachment are drawn toward each other whenever the muscle is activated.

The Brachioradialis Transfer. When all the structures of the first cleft have been destroyed and a pedicle graft has been applied to overcome the adduction contracture, a thumb may stand out in good position and be capable of being opposed and flexed. Without a strong adductor, pinch and grasp are lacking; and though the cosmetic result is good, function is poor. Also, in some ulnar paralyses, where the short flexor is also impaired, the thumb is markedly limited in providing the firm base for the fingers to pinch or grasp against. A strong adductor is needed, and its direction of pull should parallel the fibers of the transverse adductor, from 3rd metacarpal to adductor tubercle. Such a transfer has maximal power because it pulls at a right angle to the axis of the thumb.

A tendon graft is attached by pull-out wire suture to the proximal phalanx on the ulnar volar border at the adductor tubercle. Then this graft is passed along the volar surface of the paralyzed adductor to the ulnar side of the 3rd metacarpal, around which it is brought through the paralyzed interossei of the 3rd cleft and out to the dorsum. Here, under the extensor tendons, it is turned toward the radial side of the hand and passed into the subcutaneous tissues. A donor is chosen from one of the extensors of the fingers, a radial wrist extensor or the brachioradialis. The last is preferred, since it is strong, and, if the muscle is

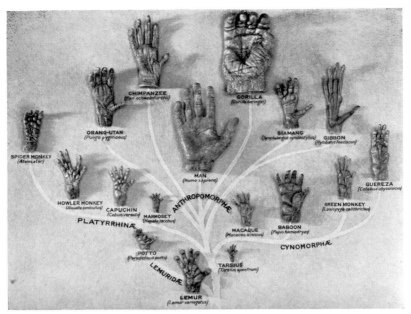

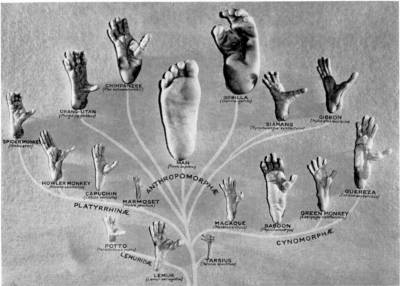

FIG. 624. (*Top*) Hands of man and monkeys. Those with the most opposable thumbs are, in order: man, gorilla, baboon, chimpanzee, orangutan. The more ground-dwelling the monkey, the better developed the opposable thumb; the more arboreal, the less thumb. The more prehensile the tail, as in new-world monkeys, the less use the animal has for a thumb, i.e., the spider monkey has none at all.

(*Bottom*) Feet of man and monkeys. In man, the feet are used entirely for locomotion, so that the hallux has entirely lost the power of opposition and the pollex has developed it. All monkeys have a far better developed opposable hallux, with the exception of the gorilla and the baboon, than pollex. (American Museum of Natural History, New York City, and J. Bone Joint Surg.)

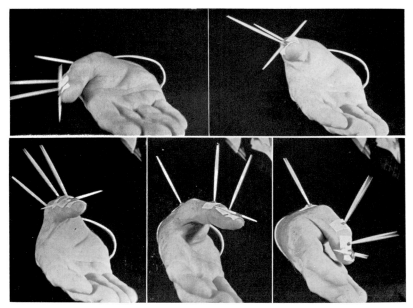

FIG. 625. The successive positions assumed by the thumb in transcribing its normal forward arc of opposition. The toothpicks—one placed crosswise and parallel with the nail and 3 each vertical to a separate segment of the thumb—are to show more graphically the angulatory and the pronatory thumb movements. (*Top, left*) The thumb starts at the side of the hand. The nail is at a right angle with the palm, and the vertical toothpicks are in line with each other. (*Top, right*) After the first third of the arc has been traversed, the thumb commences to pronate. (*Bottom, left*) The greatest pronation is between the 2 positions illustrated (*top, right* and *bottom, left*). (*Bottom, center*) Position of full opposition with the thumb well forward from and opposite the base of the long finger, angulated toward the ulna, and with the nail parallel with the palm. Note the degree of pronation shown in the relative positions of all 4 toothpicks. (*Bottom, right*) The thumb, now past the position of opposition, is completing its arc and approaching the base of the little finger. (J. Bone Joint Surg. *20*:272)

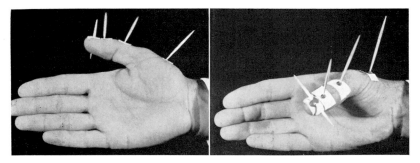

FIG. 626. Views from the front with the thumb at the side of the hand and in full opposition. Note the degree of pronation of the segments of the thumb made graphic by toothpicks. The nail rotates through 90°. The greatest pronation occurs at the metacarpophalangeal joint. (J. Bone Joint Surg. *20*:273)

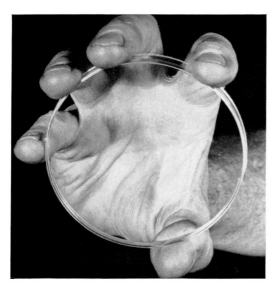

Fig. 627. The thumb in the motion of opposition-reposition moves through an arc from the side of the index to the tip of the little finger.

mobilized properly by dividing its overlying fascia, the amplitude of motion is sufficient to allow action of the transfer whether the wrist is flexed or extended.

OPPOSITION OF THE THUMB

The term "opposite" implies being set in position apart from another object. In astronomy, planets 180° apart in their orbits are said to be in opposition. Thus, touching the thumb to a fingertip is not necessarily opposition, but if the thumb is brought forward and its pulp turned toward a finger, it is said to be opposed.

True opposition of the thumb is a composite action involving many muscles and motion in all 3 thumb joints. The opponens pollicis muscle is only a minor factor in the completed motion. The act of opposition implies motion of the tip of the thumb through a large arc. What happens during this movement starting from the position of reposition illustrates well the mechanism of the thumb.

At the start, the thumb and the thenar eminence form a cone protruding laterally from the hand. The thumb is extended and abducted. When midway in the path of the arc, this cone projects forward from the hand, and

the thenar crease is folded to a right angle. At the start the nail is at a right angle to the plane of the palm, and the bones are in a straight line as seen from behind. These relations are maintained as the thumb is lifted away from the hand and brought forward, but as the first third of the motion is completed, the nail starts to rotate in pronation, and the proximal phalanx angulates radially on the metacarpal. As this occurs, the muscles in the radial half of the thenar eminence conspicuously spring into action and continue the motion. A strain occurs when the adductors are fully stretched by the long extensors of the thumb. The adductors insert on the ulnar side of the proximal phalanx and, when under tension, tend to supinate but are opposed by the muscles attached to the radial side of the phalanx—principally the outer head of the short flexor. The latter pronates and, after pronation is started, also angulates the phalanx radially. The strain is relieved just as the adductors are relaxed, and the short flexors have their way. Throughout the arc, the long extensors maintain the necessary stabilization in extension of the 3 joints of the thumb until the thenars have exhausted their amplitude; then the long flexor bends the distal joint, and the nail is pronated further.

The motion of opposition takes place in the carpometacarpal and the metacarpophalangeal joints. This motion is of 2 types—angulatory and rotary. The carpometacarpal joint furnishes most of the angulatory motion, and the metacarpophalangeal joint most of the pronatory motion. The sum of the angulatory movement in opposition is shown in the distal segment of the thumb, which angulates through an arc of about 120°; and the sum of the pronatory movement is shown in the plane of the thumbnail, which rotates 90° from a position at a right angle to the palm to one parallel with it. The abductor pollicis brevis angulates and rotates the proximal phalanx at the metacarpophalangeal joint.

When the thumb opposes, there is no perceptible change in the position of the scaphoid and only a questionable shift in the trapezium, provided that the wrist is held immobile.

With the wrist dorsiflexed and the thumb in opposition, the cleft open for grasp between the thumb and the palm is in a direct line with the forearm. Opposition between the

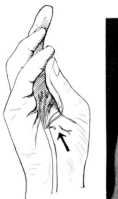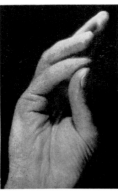

FIG. 628. Case S. P. Restoration of opposition of the thumb by suture of the tiny motor thenar branch of the median nerve. (*Left*) In this case, the nerve had been severed, by surgical incision for drainage of the thenar space, which resulted in atrophy of the muscles and loss of opposition. (*Right*) The photograph, taken 13 months later, shows the well-restored thenar eminence and ability to oppose the thumb. (J. Bone Joint Surg. *24*:275)

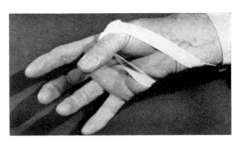

FIG. 629. A splint of adhesive plaster to hold the thumb in the position of opposition. A small pad protects the skin. The resultant of pull by the 2 arms of adhesive is in the direction of the pisiform bone. This splint is useful in protecting paralyzed thenar muscles and newly placed tendons and in bending stiffened joints into this functioning position, including increasing the carpal arch. (J. Bone Joint Surg. *24*: 275)

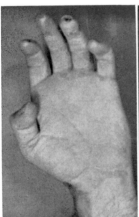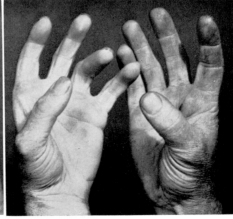

FIG. 630. Case E. S. Restoration of opposition of the thumb by suture of the median nerve at the wrist. (*Left*) From laceration at the wrist, both the median and the ulnar nerves and several tendons had been severed, resulting in clawhand with atrophy of the thenar muscles and complete loss of opposition and adduction of the thumb. (*Right*) Two years later, function of the intrinsic muscles had been restored by suture of the median and the ulnar nerves. The thenar eminence and the other intrinsic muscles, as well as the ability to oppose the thumb, had been restored so that the patient was able to resume the practice of dentistry. (J. Bone Joint Surg. *20*:276)

thumb and the index finger forms a circle, that between the thumb and the little finger an ellipse.

The degree of opposition may be expressed by the distance which the pulp of the thumb reaches in front of the base of the middle finger and also by the angle of the plane that the nail makes with the palm. Thus, opposition in the injured hand may be expressed as 2.5 cm. and 45° of angle, compared with 7.5 cm. and an angle of zero in the normal hand.

Causes of Loss of Opposition. Lack of function of the median nerve or the loss of the thenar muscles supplied by the median nerve deprives a thumb of opposition. Cord lesions, as in poliomyelitis, or displaced disk between C-6 and C-7 may often result in loss of opposition. Other causes are flexion contractures from cicatrix on the dorsum of the hand or

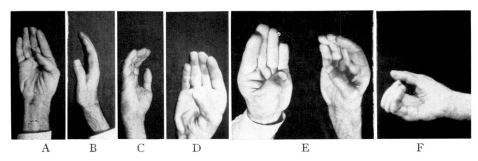

| A | B | C | D | E | F |

Fig. 631. Case S. L. Median palsy and loss of the flexor tendons of the digits resulting from a severe infection starting in the thumb.

(A) Limit of opposition of the thumb. (B, C) Limits of extension and flexion of the digits. The median nerve was sutured to all its branches, including the motor thenar. Four-inch tendon grafts from the extensors of the toes were used to join up the flexor tendons of the thumb and the fingers. (D) Return of opposition from suture of the median nerve to its motor thenar nerve 2 years previously. (E) Return of flexion of the thumb and extension of the fingers. (F) Degree of flexion of the fingers.

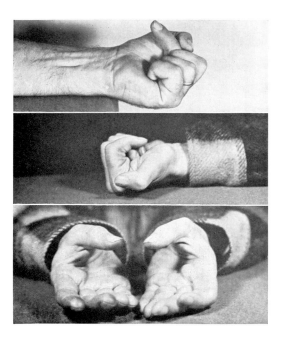

Fig. 632. Case P. S. (*Top*) Crushing injury across the volar aspect of the index finger at the middle joint. A tendon graft had been done elsewhere, using the median nerve for a graft! Sensation in the median area and opposition of the thumb were lost, and the index did not flex.

Operation: Sutured the median nerve, overcoming a 4-inch gap by transposing the nerve at the elbow and flexing the joints. Did a pulley operation for opposition of the thumb and grafted the palmaris longus plus paratenon to act as a profundus tendon in the index.

(*Center* and *bottom*) Showing the degree of flexion of the index and opposition of the thumb obtained. Sensation returned.

between the first 2 metacarpals, adhesions holding the tendon of the extensor pollicis longus, flathand from flat splinting, and injury of the joints or arthritis bordering the trapezium. Compression of the median nerve between the lower edge of the carpal ligament and the radius produces atrophy of the thenar muscles as seen after malunion of Colles' fracture, dislocated semilunar or fracture of the scaphoid. Long-standing synovitis around the flexor tendons producing a carpal tunnel syndrome can result in thenar atrophy. Local ischemic contracture of adductor muscles prevents opposition.

Methods of Restoring Opposition. Often opposition may be restored, depending on its cause, by nerve suture, by excision of the cicatrix binding the 1st and the 2nd metacarpals, of dorsal skin or adhesions of the extensor pollicis longus tendon, or by a tendon transfer or a bone or joint operation such as rotary angulatory osteotomy of the metacar-

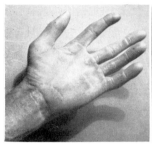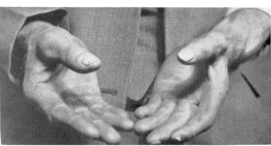

FIG. 633. Case A. H. (*Left*) The median nerve had been severed at the wrist and sutured 3 years previously, but without return of the thenar eminence or ability to oppose the thumb. (*Right*) A tendon transfer pulley operation promptly restored ability to oppose the thumb as shown in the hand with the atrophied thenar eminence and the sleeve rolled up. The flexor carpi ulnaris tendon was split in two near its insertion. One half was used to make a pulley, and the other was detached at its insertion and extended by a free graft from the tendon of the palmaris longus. This was passed through the pulley, across the thenar eminence subcutaneously, over the dorsum of the proximal joint of the thumb and attached by a drillhole to the base of the proximal phalanx at its dorso-ulnar aspect. (J. Bone Joint Surg. *20:279*)

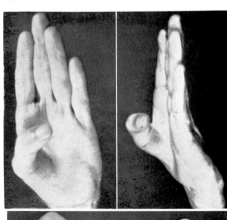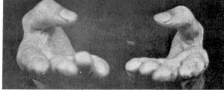

FIG. 634. Case P. C. A burn from a bottling machine had destroyed the thenar eminence. This was covered by a pedicle skin graft. The ability to oppose the thumb was restored by a tendon transfer pulley operation, The tendon of the extensor pollicis brevis was detached at its muscle, withdrawn through an incision at its insertion, and then passed subcutaneously across the thenar eminence toward the pisiform bone. The tendon of the palmaris longus was detached at its insertion, looped about the tendon of the flexor carpi ulnaris for a pulley and then sutured to the tendon of the extensor pollicis brevis. (*Top*) Good opposition restored. The tendon pulling beneath the skin is apparent. (*Bottom*) Showing loss of the thenar eminence. (J. Bone Joint Surg. *20:279*)

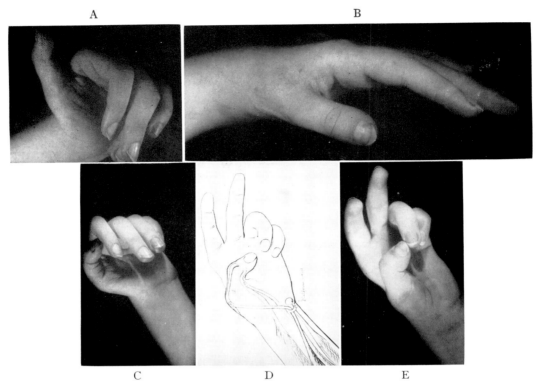

Fig. 635. Case M. V., age 20. Infantile paralysis at the age of 4 had left the patient with paralysis of the extensors of the fingers and of the thenar muscles. She had no power of extending the fingers, as shown in (A, *top, left*), and no ability to oppose the thumb against the fingers, (C, *bottom, left*) and (A). Flexion of the thumb was very weak.

Operation: The tendon of the extensor carpi radialis brevis was transferred to pull on the tendons of the extensor communis digitorum, thus restoring the power of extension of the fingers, as shown in (B, *top, right*). The tendon of the flexor sublimis digitorum of the ring finger was transferred in its insertion to the tendon of the flexor longus pollicis, thus giving strength to the motion of flexion of the thumb. The tendon of the palmaris longus, together with its extension, the palmar fascia, was passed through a pulley at the pisiform bone, made by a free tendon graft from an extensor tendon of the toe, and passed on subcutaneously and inserted into the tendon of the extensor longus pollicis. (D, *bottom, center*) Good power of opposition was obtained, as shown in (E, *bottom, right*). (Surg., Gynec. Obstet. *39*:273)

pal, carpal-wedge osteotomy in case of ankylosis of the carpus, and bone-graft bridging of the first 2 metacarpals. Suture of the motor thenar branch of the median nerve was done in 35 cases to restore opposition. The motion returns in about 13 months. In a series of 108 repairs of the median nerve by suture, opposition was restored in 66 per cent.

Tendon transfers or muscle transfers are the most commonly used methods of restoring opposition. The joints and all restraining structures must be free so that the thumb will assume the required position without any strain.

In choosing the type of tendon transfer operation for restoring loss of opposition of the thumb, it is essential that the condition of the other intrinsics of the thumb as well as the function of the extrinsic extensors and flexors be known. The loss of opposition is one thing, but the condition of the rest of the thumb movers is equally important. When the median

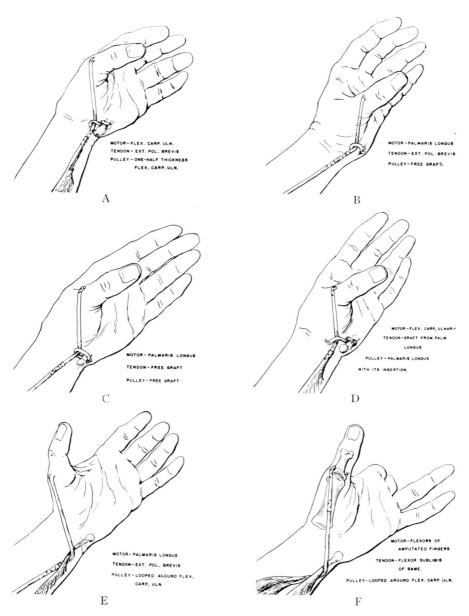

MOTOR—FLEX. CARP. ULN.
TENDON—EXT. POL. BREVIS
PULLEY—ONE-HALF THICKNESS
FLEX. CARP. ULN.

A

MOTOR—PALMARIS LONGUS
TENDON—EXT. POL. BREVIS
PULLEY—FREE GRAFT.

B

MOTOR—PALMARIS LONGUS
TENDON—FREE GRAFT
PULLEY—FREE GRAFT

C

MOTOR—FLEX. CARP. ULNARIS
TENDON—GRAFT FROM PALM LONGUS
PULLEY—PALMARIS LONGUS WITH ITS INSERTION.

D

MOTOR—PALMARIS LONGUS
TENDON—EXT. POL. BREVIS
PULLEY—LOOPED AROUND FLEX. CARP. ULN.

E

MOTOR—FLEXORS OF AMPUTATED FINGERS.
TENDON—FLEXOR SUBLIMIS OF SAME.
PULLEY—LOOPED AROUND FLEX. CARP. ULN.

F

Fig. 636. Operation advised to restore ability to oppose the thumb. The 2 essential principles are: (1) the tendon should pull in the right direction; namely, subcutaneously diagonally across the thenar eminence toward the pisiform bone to angulate the thumb forward and toward the ulna; (2) the insertion of this tendon should be into the dorso-ulnar aspect of the base of the proximal phalanx, so as to pronate the thumb. Then one may use whatever seems to be best in the individual case for motor power, tendon and pulley. These drawings illustrate what muscle and tendon material may be used, and ways of constructing the pulley. (J. Bone Joint Surg. 20:274, No. 2)

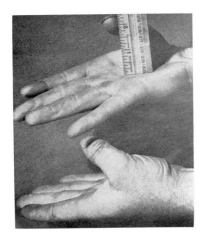

FIG. 637. Case R. F. A porcelain faucet had lacerated the thenar eminence, damaging the motor thenar branch of the median nerve beyond repair and thus paralyzing the abductor and opponens, pollicis muscles, so that the patient could not oppose the thumb. The flexor tendon and the 2 volar nerves of the thumb were also severed. Four months later, the flexor pollicis longus tendon was repaired by a free graft from the palmaris longus tendon, and the 2 sensory nerves were sutured. A tendon transfer pulley operation was done to restore opposition. The tendon of the extensor pollicis brevis was detached at its muscle, withdrawn near its insertion, and then passed subcutaneously across the thenar eminence. Here it was passed through a pulley made from a free graft of the palmaris longus and was sutured to the tendon of the flexor carpi ulnaris which was detached from its insertion for the purpose. (*Top*) Showing the ability to oppose the thumb to 2 inches in front of the base of the ring finger and 2½ inches in front of that of the long finger. (*Bottom, left*) The pronation and forward position gained. (*Bottom, right*) Atrophy of the thenar eminence. The original function of the flexor carpi ulnaris muscle has not been lost. (J. Bone Joint Surg. *20:* 280)

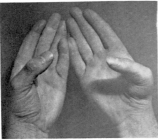

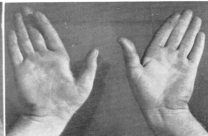

nerve is cut at the wrist, the abductor pollicis brevis, the opponens pollicis and a variable part of the flexor pollicis brevis are paralyzed. All others are normal and maintain their power and action. Of extreme importance is the recognition of the normal state of the adductor pollicis and the long abductor and the long flexor and extensor. To provide a thumb with opposition under these conditions requires a strong motor, the proper direction of pull and a secure attachment at the insertion. The pulley operation reported in 1924 was designed for this loss from this lesion. It is obviously a different problem when opposition is lost and there is also paralysis of the first interosseus, the adductor pollicis, the entire flexor brevis and sometimes the long abductor or the long extensor. Such losses are common following poliomyelitis. In these a weaker motor will suffice, since most of the antagonists are paralyzed. The course and the direction of the transfer can be varied by shifting the location of the pulley to give a greater abduction component, and the insertion can be into the abductor brevis. This insertion will give some pronatory effect if there are no strong antagonists. It can even be into or around the long extensor, as reported in 1924, to provide extension of the distal segment if the extensor pollicis longus is weak.

Depending then on the specific conditions, any transfer that takes into account the 2 basic considerations of direction of pull and site of attachment will provide opposition or a close approximation of it in a specific case. The best operation for loss of opposition is the one that, considering the condition of the other muscles of the thumb, is able to restore to the thumb the ability to sweep through a normal arc, away from the fingertips, and to pronate the proximal phalanx and the metacarpal, abduct the thumb and approximate the direction of the plane of the nail to that of the palm. Thus opposition, not apposition, is obtained.

Two Basic Considerations in Tendon Transfer for Opposition. A motor of sufficient strength and amplitude must pull from the ulnar aspect of the wrist somewhere in the vicinity of the pisiform to provide the major component of force needed for opposition. If the line of pull is too far distal the abduction

FIG. 638. Case T. T. Ability to oppose the thumb was lost by a wide excavation of a dado saw through the thenar eminence, which destroyed beyond repair the muscles and the motor thenar branch of the median nerve.

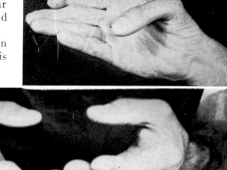

Ability to oppose the thumb was regained by a tendon transfer pulley operation, using the flexor carpi ulnaris muscle for the motor power. The tendon of the extensor pollicis brevis, which had been withdrawn from above, was passed subcutaneously across the thenar eminence and through a pulley at the pisiform bone. This pulley was constructed from a free tendon graft of the palmaris longus and was sutured to the tendon of the flexor carpi ulnaris. The latter was detached from its insertion at the pisiform for the purpose but did not lose its function, as is shown in the bottom illustration. Opposition of the thumb was restored as shown in the top and center illustrations. The atrophy of the thenar

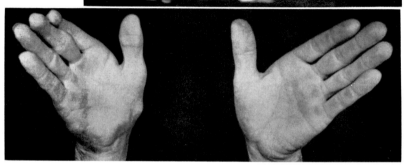

eminence shows in all 3 pictures. (J. Bone Joint Surg. *20*:281)

component will be insufficient; if too proximal, there will be inadequate force to bring the thumb opposite the fingers. In simple median nerve paralysis when all other muscles are normal, a line from the proximal joint of the thumb to the pisiform is correct. In more extensive paralyses, if there is irreparable weakness of the long abductor, more abduction from the transfer can be obtained by placing the pulley or the loop higher up the forearm proximal to the pisiform. As an extreme position, a tendon (for radial palsy Riordan uses the extensor pollicis longus, divided at the musculotendinous junction and withdrawn on the dorsum of the proximal joint) can be passed up the volar surface of the forearm and attached directly to the palmaris longus without a pulley. Here it becomes almost entirely an abductor.

If the tendon is placed distal to the pisiform or especially if radial to it, there will be too much force pulling the thumb toward the palm into a flexed and adducted position

instead of an extended and abducted position as in true opposition.

The second consideration in tendon transfers for opposition is the proper attachment of the tendon to give the abduction effect at the proximal thumb joint, and the rotary effect on both the metacarpal and the proximal phalanx. In the normal thumb, these 2 motions are provided by the abductor pollicis brevis and the opponens pollicis and are opposed by the adductor pollicis, the extensor pollicis longus and a part of the first interosseus. If these antagonistic muscles are paralyzed also, only a weak rotary force is needed, and a transfer attached to the abductor pollicis brevis tendon through its insertion into the hood can provide the motion. But if all the antagonists are normal, as they are in simple median nerve palsy, it is necessary to insert the transfer on the dorsum and the ulnar aspect of the proximal phalanx to obtain the rotary component.

Krukenberg split the flexor superficialis ten-

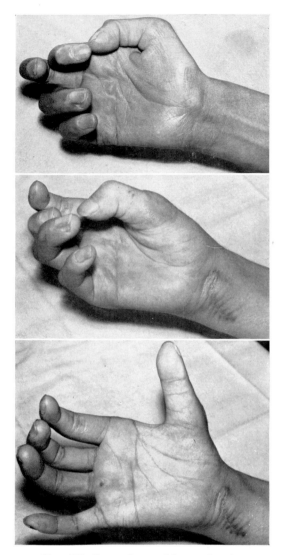

FIG. 639. Loss of opposition and restoration of motion by transfer of ring finger superficialis. The transfer was inserted into the extensor pollicis longus to aid extension of distal thumb joint. (From K. Tsuge, Okayama University)

don of the middle finger and inserted it in the radial half of the 1st metacarpal.

Roeren did the same with the flexor superficialis tendon of the ring finger.

Ney used the tendon of the extensor pollicis brevis detached above; after passing it under the transverse carpal ligament, he joined it to either the palmaris longus or the flexor carpi radialis.

Royle transferred the flexor superficialis tendon, still under the carpal ligament, down through the sheath of the thumb flexor, and inserted one branch on the back of the proximal phalanx and the other on that of the metacarpal.

T. C. Thompson modified Royle's method by passing the tendon from the lower border of the carpal ligament to the thumb subcutaneously instead of through the flexor sheath. A pulley mechanism results from the angulation of the tendon around the ulnar border of the palmar aponeurosis.

Lyle employed the same method but, in addition, combined it with Steindler's operation on the flexor pollicis longus tendon.

Steindler split the distal end of the flexor pollicis longus tendon, detached the radial half from its insertion, passed it around the radial side of the thumb and reinserted it at the back of the base of the proximal phalanx.

Silfverskiöld risked the use of the whole flexor tendon of the thumb, transplanted it around the radial side of the thumb and inserted it at the base of the proximal phalanx.

Von Baeyer freed the insertion of the flexor pollicis longus, passed it around the radial side of the thumb and reinserted it at its original insertion.

Jahn passed the extensor tendon of the 3rd digit around the ulnar border to the volar side of the hand and inserted it into the 1st metacarpal. He repaired the defect with a free fascial transplant.

Cook's operation, as described by Taylor, consisted of passing one of the extensor tendons of the little finger around the wrist subcutaneously and inserting it into the 1st metacarpal.

Huber and Nicolaysen independently used the abductor minimi digiti as a muscle transfer on its neurovascular bundle and fastened it to the 1st metacarpal.

Howell severed the flexor pollicis longus tendon at the wrist, slit the thumb from end to end, lifted the tendon from its bed and passed it around the radial side of the thumb. Then it was brought subcutaneously across the thenar eminence and resutured to itself in the radial side of the wrist.

Camitz inserted the tendon of the palmaris

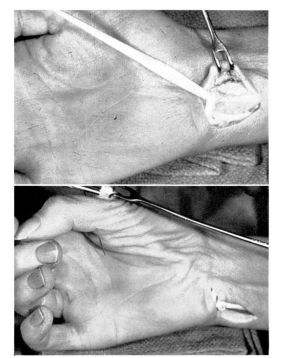

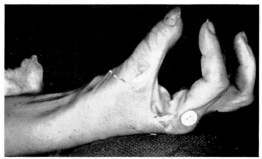

FIG. 641. When abduction of the index finger is weak, transfer of the extensor indicis to the 1st interosseus is done at the same time as the pulley operation for opposition. A button holds the suture in the 1st interosseus. The insertion of the opponens transfer is on the dorso-ulnar aspect of the base of the proximal phalanx to obtain maximal pronation effect.

FIG. 640. Here, a pulley just proximal to the pisiform is made of a tendon graft sutured into the flexor carpi ulnaris tendon. Then the transferred superficial digital flexor is passed subcutaneously across to the thumb.

longus with some of the palmar fascia on the lateral side of the metacarpophalangeal joint of the thumb.

Kortzeborn used a fascial sling to fix the thumb in opposition, did a plastic operation on the palm and lengthened the extensor tendons.

Spitzy, and also Baldwin, performed an arthrodesis on the carpometacarpal joint of the thumb.

Foerster planted a 3-cm. bone graft from the tibia between the first 2 metacarpals.

Technic of the Bunnell Pulley Operation. This operation was designed primarily to restore opposition in cases of loss of thenar muscle activity due to median nerve lesions or of direct loss of the thenar muscles.

FREEDOM FROM CONTRACTURES. The joints and the tissues must be mobile enough to allow the full movement. Flexion contracture on the dorsum or between the 2 metacarpals should be relieved; if necessary, capsulectomy of the carpometacarpal joint may be done, but care should be taken not to cause dislocation. If the deformity is too fixed, a preliminary rotary, angulatory osteotomy can be done on the metacarpal.

TWO ESSENTIAL CONSIDERATIONS. If 2 primary considerations are kept in mind, there is a choice in the selection of muscle and tendon and in the construction of the pulley, depending on which are available or advantageous in the particular case. Each hand is a problem in itself, and, as the injured parts differ, so it is necessary to adapt the procedure to the available material, at the same time remembering 2 simple considerations—namely, direction of pull and correct insertion to give pronation.

The insertion should be into the ulnar side of the base of the proximal phalanx. The tendon should pass subcutaneously directly over the dorsum of the metacarpophalangeal joint (a common error is to cross just distal to the joint), and then should pass subcutaneously across the palm to a pulley just above the pisiform bone.

In certain paralyses, the distal joint of the thumb is in flexion. Then the insertion of the tendon for opposition should be into the dorsal aponeurosis over the metacarpophalangeal joint of the thumb, which serves to extend the distal joint.

To supply a motor, a tendon and a pulley, any of the following may be available:

Motor. One may use the flexor carpi ulnaris, the palmaris longus, the flexor digitorum superficialis of the ring finger or any available long flexor muscle. The excursion needed is small, so that even the palmaris longus may be used. A transfer for opposition should be put up on the tight side. The extensor carpi ulnaris and the extensor carpi radialis brevis are strong and can be elongated with a tendon graft to give good opposition without the need of a pulley if made to cross around the ulnar border of the forearm. The pronator teres and the brachioradialis have been used.

Tendon. The extensor pollicis brevis is

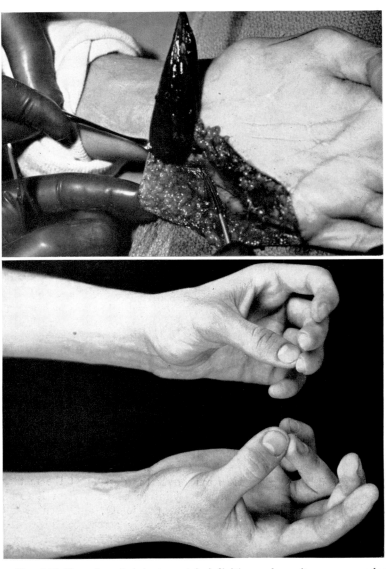

Fig. 642. Transfer of abductor minimi digiti muscle on its neurovascular pedicle according to the method of Huber and Nicolaysen. (*Top*) At operation; note flattened thenar eminence. (*Bottom*) Postoperative appearance of left compared with the normal right hand. Excellent cosmetic as well as functional result. (J. William Littler, M.D.)

excellent, because it already has the correct insertion and can be transposed and sutured to the motor just proximal to the pulley at the pisiform bone. Any tendon desired can be pieced out by a free tendon graft either from the palmaris longus tendon or from any other tendon that may be available.

Pulley. For the construction of a pulley at the pisiform bone, a free tendon graft either from the palmaris longus or from any other available tendon can be looped through the short muscle and tendon attachment to the pisiform bone and sutured to itself so that it forms a circle 2 cm. in diameter. The sutured junction is slipped around until it is within the muscle.

Another method of making a pulley is to use half the thickness of the flexor carpi

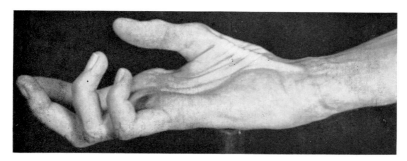

FIG. 643. When first cleft muscles are paralyzed, and all thenars are lacking as in this postpoliomyelitis hand, the opponens transfer can pass across the midline of the wrist and insert into the abductor pollicis brevis tendon. This provides a greater abduction component with less pronatory effect.

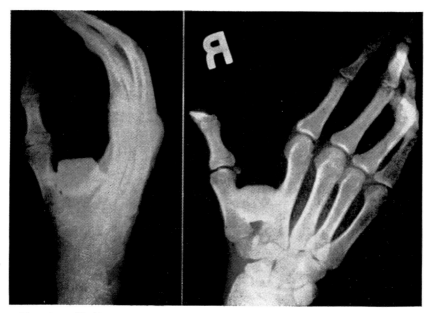

FIG. 644. (*Left*) A flat bone graft from the tibia has been fitted into slots in the metacarpals, with the thumb in position of opposition. (*Right*) Appearance 5 years later. (Thompson, C. F.: J. Bone Joint Surg. *24*:908)

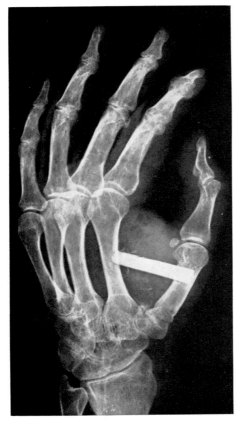

FIG. 645. From a gunshot wound there was a fracture dislocation at the base of the thumb metacarpal, and the thumb was held by cicatrix tight to the side of the hand. The thumb metacarpal was inserted into the trapezium, and, after the mass of intervening cicatrix was excised, the first 2 metacarpals were spread and held so by bone graft. To maintain correct position of opposition, the pulps of the first 3 digits had been sutured together. (J. William Littler, M.D.)

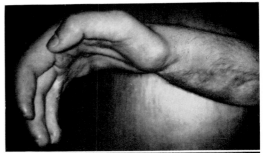

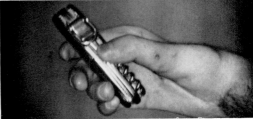

FIG. 646. Case O. C. (*Top*) Electric burn of both hands at age 12. One hand had been amputated; the other was useless. The thumb was at the side of the hand, and the fingers were semiflexed, lacking 2¼ inches of touching the distal crease in the palm. The distal 2 joints had only a trace of motion, and the proximal joints were stiff and straight. The intrinsics were paralyzed. Applied a pedicle to the wrist. Freed the flexor of the thumb and all the profundi. Did web plasties and a Z-plasty on the thumb cleft and a rotary angulatory osteotomy on the thumb, positioning it, and pinned it in place. Slit the proximal pulleys, did a pulley operation for opposition, grafted deep fascia between tendons and bones. (*Bottom*) The patient obtained a good hand with the wrist dorsiflexed, the thumb opposed, and all in a position of function. He grasped 2 to 4 of the examiner's fingers strongly and flexed the proximal joints 62°.

ulnaris tendon, severing one of the halves high and suturing this free end to the ligament of the pisiform bone to complete the loop.

Similarly, the tendon of the palmaris longus can be severed 4 cm. above its insertion and made to act as a loop or pulley by suturing it into the pisiform ligamentous tissue, leaving its original insertion intact.

Instead of constructing a pulley, one can pass the tendon used around the flexor carpi ulnaris tendon and onto its insertion in the phalanx of the thumb. The flexor carpi ulnaris then aids in the opposition. If the flexor carpi ulnaris is also paralyzed, it will yield and bow inward. Therefore, if paralyzed, its tendon should be tenodesed to the ulna just above the pulley site or sutured to the extensor ulnaris.

Opposition by Tenodesis. In some cases of poliomyelitis and in paraplegias of C-6 and C-7, there may be good power of wrist extension but nothing else. In these, instead of passing the tendon through a pulley, it is inserted into the ulna above the wrist. When the wrist dorsiflexes, the thumb is pulled into opposition.

Opposition by Arthrodesis or Bone Block.
The thumb can be placed in the optimal position for pinch or grasp and fixed there by arthrodesis of the metacarpotrapezial joint or by a bone graft bridging the 1st and the 2nd metacarpals.

Sometimes a thumb contracted in poor position can be rotated into a more functional position where its restricted range of motion will be useful. Rotary or angulatory osteotomies of the base of the 1st metacarpal are such procedures; sometimes they are combined with an opponens transfer.

In cases where the entire wrist is fused, a wedge osteotomy in the carpus itself will place the thumb in a better position.

Fixed positions of the thumb such as result from arthrodeses or bone block operations are procedures of final resort. Paralysis without available muscles for transfer, spastic paralysis with adduction contracture and severely scarred first clefts are the main indications. Iliac grafts heal more surely and quickly than tibial grafts. Secure fixation should be obtained by fitting the graft into slots in the 2 metacarpals; a Kirschner wire traversing both bones and the graft helps to maintain position. Positioning of the thumb is very important—if too far forward it interferes with finger flexion, if too far out the tip cannot reach the finger for pinch.

PARALYSIS AND CONTRACTURE OF THE THUMB—INTRINSIC PLUS

As in the fingers, contracture of the intrinsic thumb muscles results in a plus deformity. The thumb may stand out from the palm if the short abductor and the opponens are relatively more contracted, but usually the adductor and the short flexor are contracted also, and the thumb is drawn toward the palm, interfering with opening for grasp, and impairing finger flexion by being fixed in the plane of action of the digits.

Adduction Contracture. Cicatrix following direct damage to the first cleft musculature or ischemic contracture and improper splinting result in a thumb pulled toward the index finger. The skin of the 1st cleft may be shortened. Correction usually involves division or excision of the damaged adductor and the 1st metacarpal belly of the first interosseus or a capsulotomy of the metacarpotrapezial joint. Fixation of the thumb in the cor-

rected position, with a Kirschner wire strut or crossed wires helps to maintain the position during healing. If skin replacement is necessary, the flap or graft must extend from the palm to the dorsum, hinge to hinge, to allow adequate motion. Tubed pedicles, direct patterned flaps or sliding local rotational flaps can be used. (See Chap. 7, Skin and Contractures.) If the index finger has been damaged, its skin can be used as a neurovascular pedicled flap to line the new cleft. When healing is complete, and good abduction has been obtained, consideration must be given either to fixing the thumb in this position, e.g., by an intermetacarpal bone block, or, if the joints are mobile, to restoring adduction by tendon transfer.

Complete Intrinsic Contracture of the Thumb. This entity, which usually accompanies ischemic contracture of the fingers, can result from too tight bandaging or splinting or vascular lesions. Typically, the thumb metacarpal is pulled toward the 3rd metacarpal, the proximal joint is flexed, and the distal joint is hyperextended. When seen in patients with rheumatoid arthritis, there is an accompanying volar subluxation of the proximal phalanx on the metacarpal. If the adduction contracture of the first cleft is predominant, the 1st metacarpal is pulled in tightly, and the proximal joint may be hyperextended.

Release of the contracture of the short abductor, the short flexor and the opponens is accomplished most satisfactorily by shortening the 1st metacarpal. Attempted release of the muscle origins has not been successful. Some benefit has been reported in rheumatoid deformities from division and shifting of the insertions on the proximal phalanx proximally to the metacarpal. In ischemic contractures, with involvement of all the thenars, resection of a segment in the proximal third of the metacarpal will relieve the contracture of all except the adductor. Tenotomy of this structure or stripping its origin from the third metacarpal should be done. (For further discussion see Chap. 7, Ischemic Contracture, and Chap. 9, The Rheumatoid Hand.)

BIBLIOGRAPHY

Backhouse, K. M., and Catton, W. T.: An experimental study of the functions of the lumbrical muscles in the human hand, J. Anat. *88*:133, 1954.

Baldwin, W. I.: Orthopedic surgery of the hand and wrist *in* Jones, Sir Robert (ed.): Orthopedic Surgery of Injuries, vol. 1, p. 277, London, Oxford Univ. Press, 1921.

Basu, S. S., and Hazarg, S.: Variations of the lumbrical muscles of the hand, Anat. Rec. *136*:501, 1960.

Batty-Smith, C. G.: An operation for increasing the range of independent extension of the ring finger for pianists, Brit. J. Surg. *29*:397, 1942.

Benisty, A.: The Clinical Forms of Nerve Lesions, London, Military Med. Manual, Univ. of London Press, 1918.

————: Treatment and Repair of Nerve Lesions, London, Military Med. Manual, Univ. of London Press, 1918.

Bingham, D. L. C., and Jack, E. A.: Buttonholed extensor expansion, Brit. M. J. *2*:701, 1937.

Björkesten, G. Af.: Position of fingers and function deficiency in ulnar paralysis, Acta chir. scand. *93*:99, 1946.

Böhler, J.: Lähmung der Binnenmuskeln der Hand. Ersatz Operation mit superficialis Verlagerung im Opponensplastike, Arch. klin. Chir. *299*:140, 1962.

Borchardt, M.: Schussverletzungen peripherer Nerven, Beitr. klin. Chir. *97*:233, 1915.

Braithwaite, F. *et al.*: The applied anatomy of the lumbrical and interosseous muscles of the hand, Guy's Hosp. Rep., Vol. 97, 185, 1948.

Brand, P. W.: Paralytic claw hand, J. Bone Joint Surg. *40-B*:4, 1958.

Brooks, D. M.: Inter-metacarpal bone graft for thenar paralysis, J. Bone Joint Surg. *31-B*:511, 1949.

Brooks, H. St. J.: Variations in the nerve supply of the flexor brevis pollicis muscle, J. Anat. Physiol. *20*:641, 1886.

————: Morphology of intrinsic muscles of little finger, J. Anat. Physiol. *20*:645, 1886.

————: Variations in the nerve supply of the lumbrical muscles in the hand and foot, with some observations on the innervation of the perforating flexors, J. Anat. Physiol. *21*:575, 1887.

Bruner, J. M.: Tendon transfer to restore abduction of the index finger using extensor pollicis brevis, Plast. Reconstr. Surg. *3*:197, 1948.

Bunnell, S.: Reconstructive surgery of the hand, Surg., Gynec. Obstet. *39*:259, 1924.

————: Opposition of the thumb, J. Bone Joint Surg. *20*:269, 1938.

————: Surgery of intrinsic muscles of hand other than those producing opposition of thumb, J. Bone Joint Surg. *24*:1, 1942.

————: Muscle transplants opposition of thumb, Am. Acad. Orth. Surg. Lect., p. 283, 1944.

————: Reconstruction operations for ulnar paralysis when the nerve is irreparable, Reconst. Surg. Traumatol. *1*:193, 1953.

Burman, M.: Kinetic disabilities of hand and their classification; study in balance and imbalance of hand muscles, Am. J. Surg. *61*:167, 1943.

Calberg, G.: Intrinsic-plus position of the hand caused by contracture of the interosseous muscles, Acta orthop. Belg. *27*:604, 1961.

Camitz, H.: Surgical treatment of paralysis of opponens muscle of thumb, Acta chir. scand. *65*:77, 1929.

Cliffton, E.: Unusual innervation of the intrinsic muscles of the hand by median and ulnar nerves, Surgery *23*:12, 1948.

Coleman, S. S., *et al.*: The insertion of the abductor pollicis longus muscle, Quart. Bull. Northwest. Univ. Med. Sch. *27*:117, 1953.

Duchenne, G. B.: Physiology of Motion, trans. by E. B. Kaplan, Philadelphia, Lippincott, 1949.

Eilers: Über die subkutanen Fingerstrecksehnenrupturen, mit besonderer Berücksichtigung der Knopfloch-luxation am ersten Interphalangealgelenk, Deutsche Z. Chir. *223*:317, 1930.

Ewald, P.: Zur Behandlung des Strecksehnenabrisses der Fingerendglieder, Zbl Chir. *57*:714, 1930.

Eyler, D. L., and Markee, J. E.: The anatomy and function of the intrinsic musculature of the fingers, J. Bone Joint Surg. *36-A*:1, 1954.

Foerster, O.: Value of orthopedic fixation operations in nerve disease; compensation for combined serratus-trapezius paralysis by fixation of scapula to ribs with silver wire; compensation for thenar paralysis by fixation of first metacarpal in flexed position by a bone implant between first and second metacarpals, Acta chir. scand. *67*:351, 1930.

Gobell, R., and Freudenberg, K.: Favorable results of surgical therapy of aplasia of opponens muscle of thumb by transplantation of tendons of flexor digitalis sublimis; survey of methods, Arch. orthop. Unfall-Chir. *35*:675, 1935.

Graham, W. C., Brown, J. B., Cannon, B., and Riordan, D. C.: Transposition of fingers in severe injuries of the hand, J. Bone Joint Surg. *45*:998, 1947.

Grunkorn, J.: Die Daumenopposition, ihre muskelphysiologische Erklärung und die Behandlung des Oppositionsausfalls, Z. orthop. Chir. *57*:517, 1932.

Hames, R. W.: The extensor apparatus of the finger, J. Anat. *85*:251, 1951.

Harris, C., Jr., and Riordan, D. C.: Intrinsic contracture in the hand and its surgical treatment, J. Bone Joint Surg. *36-A*:10, 1954.

Hauck, G.: Die Ruptur der Dorsalaponeurose am ersten Interphalangealgelenk, zugleich ein Beitrag zur Anatomie und Physiologie der Dorsalaponeurose, Arch. klin. Chir. *123*:197, 1923.

————: Über eine Tendovaginitis stenosans der Beugesehnenscheide mit dem Phänomen des schnellenden Fingers, Arch. klin. Chir. *123*:233, 1923.

————: Der Strecksehnenabriss am Fingerendgelenk und sein, Naht. Med. Welt *3*:1657, 1929.

————: Rupture of dorsal aponeurosis, Arch. klin. Chir. *123*:197, 1932.

Hopper, J., Jr.: An inquiry as to the insertion of the extensor digitorum communis, the lumbricales and the interossei. Unpublished thesis.

Howell, B. W.: A new operation for opponens paralysis of the thumb, Lancet *1*:131, 1926.

Huber, E.: Hilfsoperation bei Medianuslahmung, Deutsch. Arch. klin. Med. *136*:271, 1921.

Inclan, A., and Rodriquez, R.: Tendinoplasty for repair of loss of opposition of thumb following infantile paralysis (Bunnell's technic), Cir. ortop. traumatol., Habana *6*:140, 1938.

Irwin, C. E.: Transplants to thumb to restore function of opposition; end results, South. M. J. *35*:257, 1942.

Irwin, C. E., and Eyler, D. L.: Surgical rehabilitation of the hand and forearm disabled by poliomyelitis, J. Bone Joint Surg. *33-A*:825, 1951.

Jacobs, B., and Thompson, T. C.: Opposition of the thumb and its restoration, J. Bone Joint Surg. *42-A*:1015, 1960.

Jahn, A.: Aktiver Ersatz bei Oppositionslahmung des Daumens, Z. orthop. Chir. *51*:100, 1929.

Johner, T.: Joining dorsal aponeurosis and tendons in second and fifth fingers; therapy of injury to extensor tendons of fingers, Schweiz. med. Wchr. *68*:111, 1938.

Jones, F. W.: Voluntary muscular movements in cases of nerve lesions, J. Anat. *54*:41, 1919.

Kallius, H. U.: Knopflochartiger Strecksehnenabriss an Nagelendglied, Zbl. Chir. *57*:2432, 1930.

Kaplan, E. B.: Extension deformities of the proximal interphalangeal joints of the fingers, J. Bone Joint Surg. *18*:781, 1936; correction, *19*:1144, 1937.

————: Pathology and operative correction of finger deformities due to injuries and contractures of the extensor digitorum tendon, Surgery *6*:35, 1939; correction, *6*:451, 1939.

————: Embryological development of the tendinous apparatus of the fingers, J. Bone Joint Surg. *32-A*:820, 1950.

Kelikian, H.: Functional restoration of the thumb, Surg., Gynec. Obstet. *83*:807, 1946.

Kirklin, J. W., and Thomas, C. G.: Opponens transplant: An analysis of the methods employed and results obtained in seventy-five cases, Surg., Gynec. Obstet. *86*:213, 1948.

Koch, S. L.: Plastic surgery for opponens pollicis, Chirurg. *4*:67, 1932.

Kopsch, F.: Die Insertion der Musculi lumbricales an der Hand des Menschen, Monthly Internat. J. Anat. Physiol. *15*:70, 1898.

Kortzeborn, A.: Operativ-Behandlung der sogenannten Affenhand, Arch. klin. Chir. *133*:465, 1924.

Krukenberg, H.: Über Ersatz des M. opponens pollicis, Z. orthop. Chir. *42*:178, 1921-1922.

Landsmeer, J. M. F.: The anatomy of the dorsal aponeurosis of the human finger and its functional significance, Anat. Rec. *104*:31, 1949.

————: A report on the co-ordination of the interphalangeal joints of the human finger and its disturbances, Acta morph. Neerl.-Scand. *2*:59, 1958.

————: Studies in the anatomy of articulation. II. Patterns of movement of bi-muscular, bi-articular systems, Acta morph. Neerl.-Scand. *3*:304, 1960.

Lange, F.: Die epidemische Kinderlähmung *in* Lehmanns medizinische Lehrbücher, vol. 11, Munich, J. F. Lehmann, 1930.

Littler, J. W.: Tendon transfers and arthrodeses in combined median and ulnar nerve paralysis, J. Bone Joint Surg. *31-A*:225, 1949.

Lyle, H. H. M.: The disabilities of the hand and their physiological treatment, Ann. Surg. *78*:816, 1923.

————: Result of an operation for thenar paralysis of the thumb (extensor-flexor-flexor-plasty). Ann. Surg. *79*:933, 1924.

————: The operative treatment of thenar paralysis, Ann. Surg. *84*:288, 1926.

McFarlane, R. M.: Extension of the distal phalanx of the thumb, J. Bone Joint Surg. *42-A*:5, 1960.

Mason, M. L.: Rupture of tendons of the hand with a study of the extensor tendon insertions in the fingers, Surg., Gynec. Obstet. *50*:611, 1930.

Mayer, L.: Loop operation for paralysis of the adductors of the thumb, Am. J. Surg. *2*:456, 1927.

Mehta, H. J., and Gardner, W. V.: A study of lumbrical muscles in the human hand, Am. J. Anat. *109*:227, 1961.

Milch, H.: Buttonhole rupture of the extensor tendon of the finger, Am. J. Surg. *13*:244, 1931.

Montant, R., and Baumann, A.: Recherches anatomiques sur le système tendineux extenseur des doigts de la main, Ann. Anat. Pathol. *14*:311, 1937.

————: Rupture-luxation de l'appareil extenseur des doigts au niveau de la première articulation interphalangienne (physiologie et clinique), Rev. d'orthop. *25*:5, 1938.

Murphey, F., Kirklin, J. W., and Finlayson, A. I.:

Anomalous innervation of the intrinsic muscles of the hand, Surg., Gynec. Obstet. *83*:15, 1946.

Napier, J. R.: The attachments and functions of the abductor pollicis brevis, J. Anat. *86*:335, 1952.

Ney, K. W.: Tendon transplant for intrinsic hand muscle paralysis, Surg., Gynec. Obstet. *33*:342, 1921.

Nicolaysen, J.: Transplantation des M. abductor dig. V. bei fehlender Oppositionsfähigkeit des Daumens, Deutsche Z. Chir. *168*:133, 1922.

Nilsonne, H.: Treatment of paralysis of opponens muscle of thumb, Acta orthop. scand. *1*:66, 1930.

————: Case of bilateral adductor paralysis of thumb, Hygeia *92*:856, 1930.

Pacher, W.: Plastic surgery of flexor tendons of hand, with special reference to paralysis of opponens pollicis, Arch. orthop. Unfall-Chir. *40*:93, 1939.

Pitzen, P.: Plastic operations on great toe and thumb, Z. Orthop. *70*:93, 1939.

Platt, H., and Bristow, W. R.: The remote results of operations for injuries of the peripheral nerves, Brit. J. Surg. *11*:535, 1923-1924.

Rank, B., and Wakefield, A. R.: Surgery of Repair as Applied to Hand Injuries, p. 29, London, Livingstone, 1960.

Reinhardt, F. E.: Insertion of lumbricalis muscle in human hand, Anat. Anz. *20*:129, 1901.

Riordan, D. C.: Tendon transplantations in median nerve and ulnar nerve paralysis, J. Bone Joint Surg. *35-A*:312, 1953.

Rountree, T.: Anomalous innervation of the hand muscles, J. Bone Joint Surg. *31-B*:505, 1949.

Royle, N. D.: Operation for thenar paralysis, Med. J. Austr. *2*:155, 1936.

————: Operation for paralysis of intrinsic muscles of thumb, J.A.M.A. *111*:612, 1938.

Salisbury, C. R.: The interosseus muscles of the hand, J. Anat. *71*:395, 1936.

Scheck, M.: New method for relief of paralysis of opponens pollicis, Indian Med. Gaz. *75*:464, 1940.

Schink, W.: On the surgical treatment of combined median and ulnar nerve paralysis, Langenbeck Arch. klin. Chir. *299*:748, 1962.

Silfverskiöld, N.: Sehnentransplantationsmethode bei Lahmung der Oppositionsfähigkeit des Daumens, Acta chir. scand. *64*:296, 1928.

————: Zur Behandlung der Zerreissung des Streckapparates der Fingerendgleider, Zbl. Chir. *56*:3210, 1929.

Smillie, I. S.: Mallet finger, Brit. J. Surg. *24*:439, 1937.

Spitzy, H.: Die krankhaften Veränderungen der oberen Extremität, Verhandl. deutsch. orthop. Gesellsch., 25th Congress, pp. 76-113, 1931.

Stack, H. G.: Muscle function in the fingers, J. Bone Joint Surg. *44-B*:899, 1962.

Steindler, A.: Orthopedic operations on the hand, J.A.M.A. *71*:1288, 1918.

————: Flexor plasty of thumb in thenar palsy, Surg. Gynec. Obstet. *50*:1005, 1930.

————: Die poliomyelitischen Lähmungen der oberen Extremität, Verhandl. deutsch. orthop. Gesellsch., 25th Congress, p. 113, 1931.

————: Kinesiology, Springfield, Ill., Thomas, 1955.

Stiles, Sir H. J., and Forrester-Brown, M. F.: Treatment of Injuries of the Spinal Peripheral Nerves, p. 166, London, H. Frowde & Hodder & Stoughton, 1922.

Stracker, O.: Zur Behandlung der Fingerstrecksehnenruptur am Endgleid, Zbl. Chir. *58*:727, 1931.

Strasser, H.: Lehrbuch der Muskel-und Gelenkmechanik, Berlin, Julius Springer, 1908-1917.

Sunderland, E.: The action of the extensor digitorum communis, interosseus and lumbrical muscles, Am. J. Anat. *77*:189, 1945.

Taylor, R. T.: Reconstruction of the hand, Surg., Gynec. Obstet. *32*:237, 1921.

Thole: Kriegsverletzungen peripherer Nerven, Beitr. klin. Chir. *98*:131, 1915-1916.

Thompson, C. F.: Fusion of metacarpals of thumb and index finger to maintain functional position of thumb, J. Bone Joint Surg. *24*:632, 1942.

Thompson, T. C.: Modified operation for opponens paralysis, J. Bone Joint Surg. *24*:632, 1942.

Troxell, E. L.: The thumb of man, Scient. Monthly *43*:148, 1936.

Tsuge, K., Tani, T., and Tanaka, S.: Tendon transfers for claw hand, Acta med. Okayama *12*:157, 1958.

VanDemark, R. E.: The Bunnell operation for opponens paralysis, S. Dakota J. Med. Pharm. *3*:362, 1950.

Van Ree, A.: De Behandeling der onder huidsche streckpeesafscheuring aan de eindphalangen der vingers, Nederl. t. geneesk. *80*:1999, 1936.

von Baeyer: Bewegungslehre und Orthopadie, Z. orthop. Chir. *46*:24, 1925.

Weil, S.: Operative Behandlung der sogenannten Opponenslahmung, Klin. Wchr. *5*:650, 1926.

Zancolli, E.: Surgery of intrinsic muscles, Prensa med. argent. *43*:1299, 1956.

————: Claw hand caused by paralysis of the intrinsic muscles, J. Bone Joint Surg. *39-A*:1076, 1957.

Chapter 13

Reconstruction of the Thumb

LOSS OF THE THUMB

A hand without a thumb is severely crippled. Grasp and pinch are almost impossible, and the other hand must be used to pick up and hold objects for the most basic daily needs. To be of some use, a thumb need not have full motion, nor be of normal length.

However, it must be in the optimal position, or be capable of being brought into it by muscular action; it must either be fixed by arthrodesis or bone block or be capable of being stabilized by tendon action, and it must have a surface covering with adequate sensibility. Lacking any of these, it will not be used.

The thumb should stand out from the hand

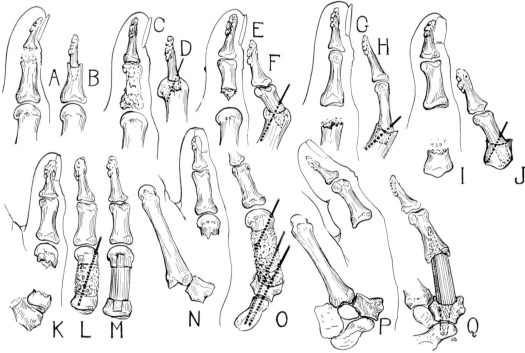

Fig. 647. Stabilizing the thumb by arthrodesis and bone grafting. A short, strong thumb is useful. (A, B) For loss of the distal joint, a distal segment may be fused to the proximal segment. (C, D) After loss of the proximal phalanx, the distal phalanx may be fused to the metacarpal. (E, F) Defect in the proximal phalanx is remedied by fusion, a pin ensuring stability. (G, H) Fusion for loss of the head of the metacarpal. (I, J) Same for the head and the shaft of the metacarpal. (K, L, M) Defect of the shaft of the metacarpal may be filled by iliac or cortical grafts. The shorter immobilization needed for cancellous grafts is that much less time to cause stiffening of the hand. (N, O) Iliac graft pinned to the thumb ray of the carpal bones and the head of the metacarpal to fill large defect of the metacarpal. (P, Q) Defect from loss of the metacarpal bridged by a cortical graft spiked into the proximal phalanx and the thumb ray of the carpal bones, the trapezium and the scaphoid.

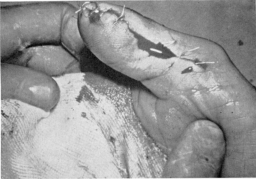

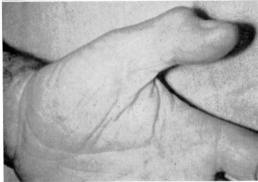

FIG. 648. Advancement of volar skin by extending midlateral incisions on each side of thumb brings normally innervated skin to the tip. Function of the thumb is improved even though a flexion contracture of distal joint may result. (*Top*) Advancement for amputation of portion of distal phalanx. (*Bottom*) Postoperative view of similar problem.

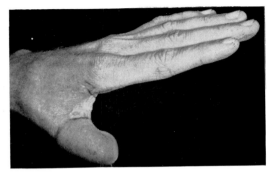

FIG. 649. Good coverage of avulsed wound of thumb. Tactile surface now can be restored by island-flap technic (see Chap. 10).

in the position of opposition so that the fingers can work against it. Too frequently a reconstructed thumb lies in a position outside the zone of action of the fingers. There should be enough motion to enable the thumb to aid in grasping, through either flexor or adductor motion. The sensation should be of the highest quality whenever possible, good tactile skin being applied by local flap, Z-plasty or transfer on a neurovascular pedicle from another digit.

PARTIAL LOSS OF THE THUMB

Amputation of the thumb through the distal segment or as far proximal as the middle of the proximal segment may leave a useful thumb, if the stump is covered with good skin and tenderness is absent. Some patients, even

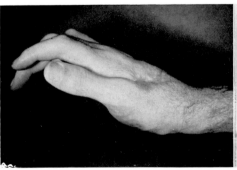

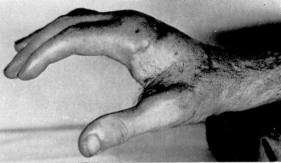

FIG. 650. Case I. S. (*Left*) A crushing injury resulted in a contracture of the cleft, binding the thumb to the hand and leaving stiff straight proximal finger joints and malunited metacarpals. The cicatrix was excised, opening out the cleft. By osteotomies, the metacarpals were realigned, and by capsulectomies the proximal finger joints were flexed. A pedicle graft was laid across the cleft. (*Right*) A useful hand resulted.

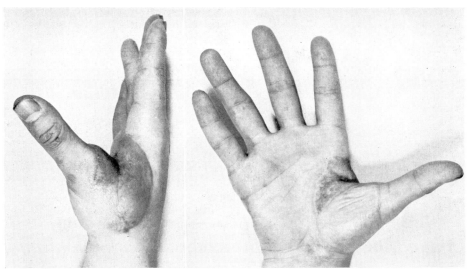

FIG. 651. Case T. H. The patient's hand had been drawn between 2 metal rollers, so lacerating and injuring it that a thumb cleft contracture developed. This was excised, dissecting out much of the fibrous musculature, and the cleft was covered by a long diamond-shaped pedicle graft.

those with amputation at the metacarpophalangeal joint level, learn to use this short stump with great dexterity. As a general rule, if these stumps are covered with good tactile skin and are painless, there is no indication for reconstructive lengthening procedures.

If there is adequate length but poor cover-

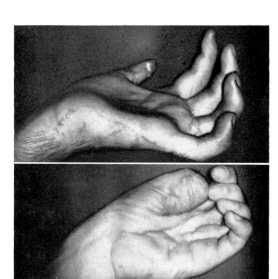

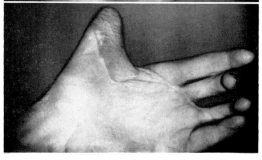

FIG. 652. Case L. G. (*Top*) A power saw had amputated the thumb and cut across the distal part of the palm, severing all nerves to the first 3 fingers; the tendons were damaged and became adherent. There was no sensation or flexion in the first 3 fingers. The 6 volar digital nerves were sutured, drawing the median nerve down the forearm to reach. The flexor tendons to the thumb and the first 3 fingers were freed, and deep fascia plus paratenon was grafted beneath them. A pedicle graft was applied to cover the palm and the thumb. A year later, sensation returned throughout. The fingers extended fairly well, and all touched the palm proximally. The thumb worked well against the fingers. The patient has a very useful hand, though he has some difficulty in manipulating tiny nuts. This will improve with quality of sensation. (*Center* and *bottom*) Showing the recovery when it was partial 2 months later.

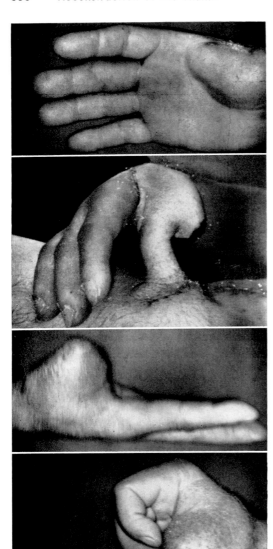

FIG. 653. (*Top*) With a skill saw, the right thumb had been amputated through the base of the metacarpal. In one operation, the cicatrix was excised, an iliac bone graft was pinned onto the stump of the metacarpal, and a tube pedicle in one was applied. This gave the patient a very useful movable stub of a thumb. The natural skin over the thenar eminence was swung up to cover the tactile surface of the thumb for stereognosis.

ing of the tactile surface, a procedure recommended by Moberg can be used to provide a better tactile surface. The volar sensible skin is elevated through bilateral midline incisions and dissected free as far proximally as necessary. With the distal joint in some flexion, this volar skin can be advanced to cover the tip or to replace a scarred or insensitive pulp area. This is particularly useful for those insensitive tips resulting from lacerations across the pulp, where the nerves to the distal part cannot be repaired.

A method of providing cover by utilizing local skin and also providing more length was called the "cocked-hat" method of Gillies. A dorsal curved incision elevates the skin like a cape over the metacarpal end, the volar pedicle carrying the blood and the nerve supply. An iliac bone graft is used to lengthen the bony stump, and the remaining denuded area is covered with a split-skin graft.

Amputation Through the Metacarpal. A relative lengthening of the thumb can be gained by deepening the first cleft, thus aiding the grasp of objects. Simple skin plasty is not enough, for the adductor pollicis and the first interosseus muscles almost fill the web space. These muscles are stripped down from the 1st metacarpal, especially the head of the 1st interosseus arising on the thumb metacarpal. A deep Z-plasty or one combined with a split-skin graft will cover the cleft. A sliding flap can be used from the dorsum of the hand, and a split graft covers this donor area. In cases of severe contracture, a pedicle graft from the abdomen is used. If possible, some adductor muscle power should be preserved.

If the index finger has been amputated or cannot be repaired, it should be removed through the base of the metacarpal. The 1st interosseus tendon is sutured to the 2nd dorsal interosseus, and a good cleft is restored. Any remaining portion of the middle metacarpal should be preserved.

When metacarpals of the index, the middle and the ring fingers have been lost and only the thumb and the little finger remain, it will be necessary to rotate one of them by osteotomy to provide some pinching action. Increased motion in the little finger can be gained by removing the base of the ring metacarpal. In these cases which lack the necessary length and joint action to provide full grasping ac-

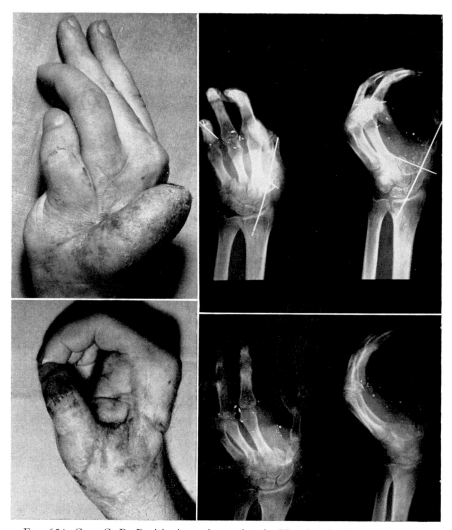

FIG. 654. Case C. R. Positioning a loose thumb. The thumb cleft was gone, and the metacarpals of the thumb and the index finger overlapped. The cleft was opened dorsally and closed by a fillet of the index finger, meanwhile thrusting the pointed proximal end of the thumb metacarpal into the trapezium and the scaphoid and pinning them there. The pedicle on the dorsum was discarded. A 1½-inch graft of a nerve from the index finger was sutured in the radial side of the thumb. The patient obained a useful hand.

tion, one should strive for the function of pinch. Even 2 metacarpals, if covered with good tactile skin and under control of adequate tendons and muscles, can function well as a substitute hand with this precision type of grip.

When all 5 digits have been amputated at the metacarpophalangeal joints, useful function can be restored by phalangization. The 2nd and the 4th metacarpals are removed, the clefts closed by sliding local skin and free split-skin grafts, and a pinching mechanism furnished by rotating the 1st and the 5th metacarpals into position. Additional power

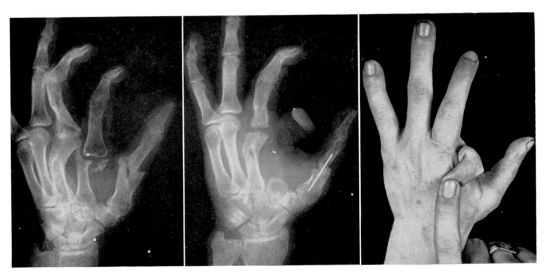

Fig. 655. Arthroplasty of the proximal joint of the long finger. Because of loss of the proximal joint of the thumb, arthrodesis was done by pinning. The useless index finger was filleted and used to cover the dorsum of the hand. (L. D. Howard, M.D.)

may be gained by tendon transfers, on the principle of the tendon T operation.

Increasing Stability of the Thumb. Loss of bony structure may be replaced by grafts to any part of the metacarpal or the phalanges. Iliac bone grafts are used for more rapid healing, and a shorter but more stable thumb is obtained. Adequately nourished soft tissues are essential before such bone grafting operations are done. A circular scar should be released by local transposition flap, distal flaps or Z-plasty. If grafts can be supplied for bone and joint loss and only the carpometacarpal joint remains, a useful motion will result. If the trapezium is missing, the 1st metacarpal base can be lashed to the scaphoid with a tendon graft. If necessary, the 1st metacarpal can be stabilized by joining it to the 2nd with a bone graft. There should be voluntary control of at least 1 joint of the thumb; otherwise, it is a fixed post. In this case, to be useful, it must be placed in the plane of action of the fingers and only pinch restored, the action being obtained through motion of the fingers.

TUBED PEDICLES TO LENGTHEN THE THUMB

A thumb need not be of normal length to be useful, but it should be stable or under voluntary control, and its tactile surface must be covered with well-innervated skin. If the am-

putation is proximal to the metacarpophalangeal joint, one method of adding length is by tubular pedicle skin graft from the abdomen or the chest wall. Bony stability is supplied by grafts from ilium, tibia or rib. Attempts to carry bone with the pedicle, either by inserting it in the tube as it is being formed or making the tube in such a location that an underlying bone can be transferred with it, have been made many times. Albee carried a piece of clavicle with the pedicle. Broadbent and Woolf made tubes incorporating the underlying iliac bone, as well as those involving a rib. It is of no advantage to combine the tube and the bone transfer, but it is preferable first to attach the pedicle to the hand or the base of thumb with the seam of the pedicle dorsal and, 3 weeks later, to detach it from the trunk, leaving a liberal blind end. Sometimes the blind end of a pedicle becomes cyanotic, so that it is better to have a little reserve length. After the new soft thumb has vitality, it is reopened along the scar, and the spike of bone is driven into a hole drilled in the metacarpal, if present, or, if not, the car-

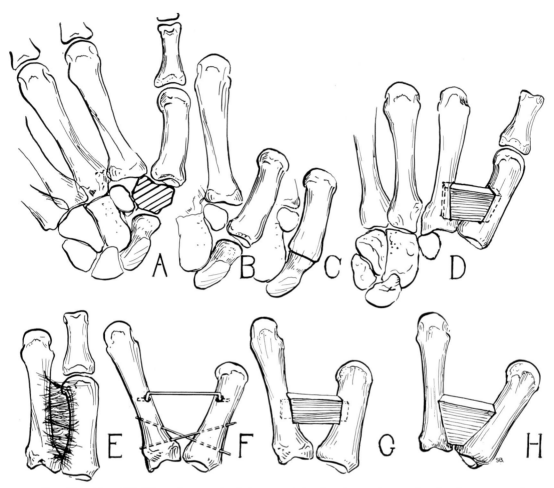

FIG. 656. (A to D) When the carpals that support the thumb are absent, the thumb metacarpal needs stability. (A, B, C) When the trapezium is absent, the thumb metacarpal may be made to articulate with the scaphoid or into an improvised socket in the carpus. Arthrodesis to the scaphoid gives stability without too much loss of motion. (E to H) When cicatrix between the first 2 metacarpals draws the thumb close to the hand, excision of the cicatrix allows spreading. A pedicle skin graft may be necessary. (F) Contracture will recur unless the metacarpals are held apart for a few months, as indicated. The lower is the better method. (G, H) If cicatrix is excessive, a bone block or bridge graft in the position of moderate opposition will ensure permanent spreading.

pus—preferably impaling the trapezium and the scaphoid, since these 2 carpals give some thumb motion when tendons are attached to the thumb. Care should be taken to drive the spike in the correct position of opposition, drilling the hole for it at a forward angle when necessary. If ilium or rib is used, it is pinned in place. Operations by the above methods have been reported by Nicoladoni (1897), Schepelmann, Ritter, Payne, Albee, Pierce, Dial and others. A great number were done during World War II.

Such a thumb is anesthetic at first but gradually acquires a certain degree of sensation to light touch and pinprick which reaches the end of the thumb after about a year; however,

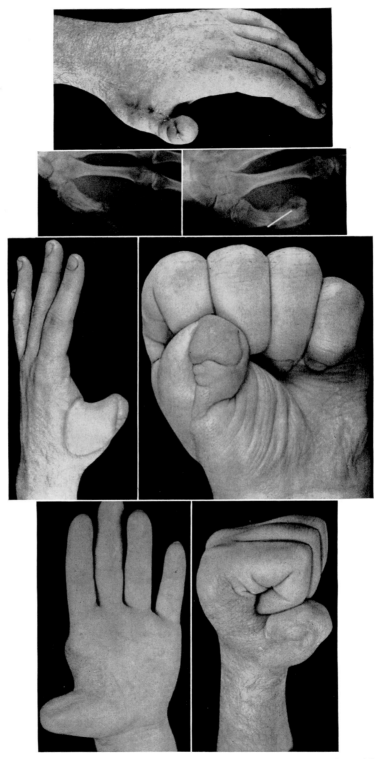

Fig. 657. Elongation of metacarpal by bone graft, phalangization with pedicle flap and preservation of tactile skin on the grasping surface restore function to the thumb. (L. D. Howard, M.D.)

it never acquires stereognosis as a thumb should. If they are in good position of opposition, these thumbs become very useful, but if they are made parallel with the hand or cannot be used, the bone will atrophy from disuse.

A conservative policy is essential in treating injured thumbs, building them out if the end is poor rather than amputating. A tip of thumb can be added by pedicle in one stage. A thumb in the right position is useful even though it is short and several of its joints are fused. A long postlike immobile thumb is in the way in putting the hand in a pocket or in working in tight places, and it may break. A short thick post thumb in a position where the fingers work against it easily is better.

Importance of Sensibility in Reconstructed Thumb

When a new thumb has been reconstructed by the tubed pedicle and bone-graft method, there will be, in time, a recovery of nerve function in the skin which often is sufficient to provide protection. However, the quality of sensibility never can approach that of the normal thumb, and skillful function is impaired. Normal dorsal skin can be transposed to cover the tactile surface, or, by a pedicle, the normally innervated skin of the radial side of the index finger can be used. Ideally, pulp skin with its normal nerve and blood supply should be used. This can be obtained from another finger utilizing the island-flap technic (see Chap. 10). Moberg, Littler, Tubiana and Frackelton all have reported using this technic, usually taking the pulp from the ring finger and keeping its neurovascular pedicle intact, transferring it to the volar and slightly ulnar aspect of the thumb. Use of this procedure has obviated the major difficulty formerly encountered with the tube-pedicle reconstruction and now makes it possible to retain the normal index or middle finger for strength of grasp and yet provide a sentient thumb post.

POLLICIZATION OPERATION

The index or the middle finger, together with a part or the whole of the metacarpal, has been transplanted to the stump of the metacarpal of the thumb or to the trapezium, but this was first done without conservation of

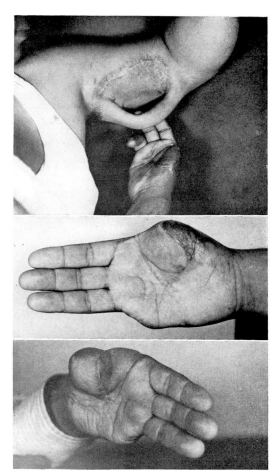

Fig. 658. Case M. T. The patient's hand had been injured in gears, losing much of the thumb and all of the little finger. A thumb cleft was made, and the tube pedicle laid across. A flap of skin with normal sensation was placed on the tactile part of the thumb. He had good function and gripped 26 kilograms.

all nerves, tendons and muscles. In 1903, Luksch pollicized the index finger, but on severing the pedicle he cut off the nerves. In 1921 Perthes pollicized the index finger. He does not state that he carried the nerves with it, and at that time digital nerves were not sutured. Verrall had 2 cases in 1919 but did not join the tendons or the nerves. In 1923, Dunlop used a pedicle from the abdomen for the digits, as did Huguier and Iselin.

A full-length finger is too long and too tapering to make a good thumb, and if the trans-

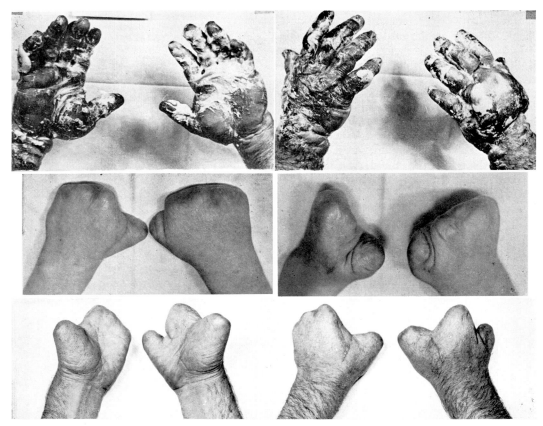

FIG. 659. Case N. R. K. Both hands were frozen from exposure for 2 hours at high altitude. (*Top*) Appearance of hands. (*Center*) Amputation of all digits at proximal joints. (*Bottom*) After operation. Left hand: phalangization of thumb metacarpal and rotary osteotomy of 5th metacarpal to provide pinch. Right hand: phalangization of thumb metacarpal and rotary osteotomy at its base. Excised ring metacarpal. Used hands well.

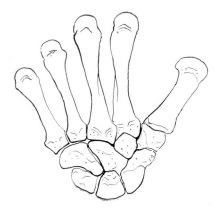

FIG. 660. The 2nd and the 3rd metacarpals are largely fixed to the carpus, since their joints are interlocking. The 4th and especially the 5th metacarpals are attached more loosely to the carpus and are more mobile. They give the transverse metacarpal phalangization, the 5th metacarpal has 2 inches in arch, and, when the 4th metacarpal is deleted, as of motion at its end.

fer is not successful, the sacrifice of a good finger will be lamented by the patient. If the surgeon knows from experience that he will succeed, it is justifiable to transplant a normal index finger to act as a thumb, but only if nerve and blood supply and tendons are brought over intact and the tendons and the muscles of the thumb are added. Amputation at the distal joint leaves a more acceptable-looking digit. Often, however, part of the index finger has already been amputated with the thumb, thus making its remainder available. In 1929 Bunnell reported in detail such an operation with transfer of the index metacarpal and the phalangeal stump to the trapezium, together with all nerves and vessels and establishment of connections of all tendons and muscles, and phalangization. It was the first reconstructed thumb which furnished both movement and normal sensation, including stereognosis.

In 1946, Murray reported 6 cases of thumb reconstruction, including pollicization, digital transfer and the reconstruction of a digit. In 3, attention was paid to the nerves.

Since 1950, a number of surgeons—Marcer, Dehne, Murray and Hilgenfeldt—have reported pollicization, carrying over the nerves and the blood vessels and using a bridge of skin. In 1950, Hilgenfeldt reported many cases of thumb reconstruction, osteotomizing the thumb and pollicizing the index finger, but in most cases he pollicized the middle fin-

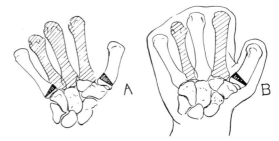

FIG. 661. (A) When all metacarpals except those of the thumb and the little finger are absent, one or both of these should be angulated around by a rotary angulatory wedge osteotomy through the metacarpal base so that the fingers can work against each other. (B) When all the digits have been lost, as from frostbite, the 2nd and the 4th metacarpals should be removed so as to phalangize widely and deeply between the 1st and the 3rd and the 3rd and the 5th. An angulatory rotary wedge osteotomy through the base of the 1st metacarpal will place the phalangized thumb where it will work against the other two phalangized digits more easily.

ger, since he considered the index finger to be more versatile. If the middle finger is used, the index finger ray should be jogged over to the 3rd metacarpal to give a better hand and to widen the thumb cleft.

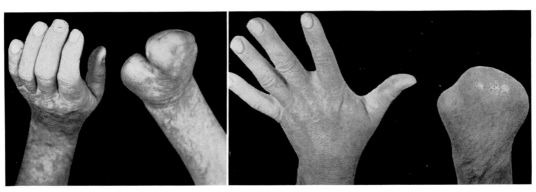

FIG. 662. Case H. G. (*Left*) A power saw had amputated all the digits through the proximal phalanges, leaving a mitten hand with no thumb cleft. By a plastic maneuver removing the index metacarpal, a thumb cleft ¾ inch deep was made. (*Right*) The thumb opened ¾ inch and contacted firmly with the hand for prehension. The patient could write.

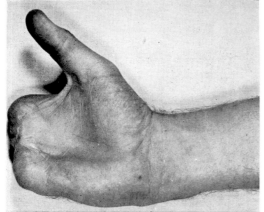

Fig. 663. Case M. S. (*Top*) Fingers lost between a sprocket and a chain. Excised the tender neuromata of the stump, undermined and drew the skin down for better coverage. Excised the metacarpal of the ring finger, covering the sides of the new digits by plastic maneuvers, in order to give more mobility (2 in.) to the metacarpal of the little finger. Deepened the thumb cleft by zig-zag. (*Center* and *bottom*) The patient obtained a strong and useful grasp between the thumb and the phalangized index, the long and the little fingers.

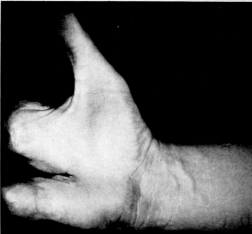

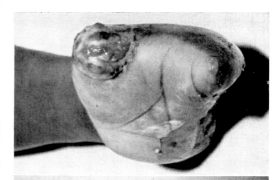

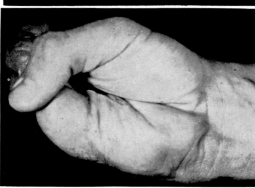

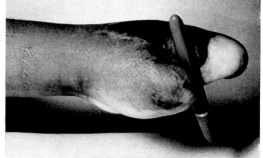

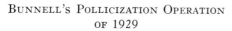

BUNNELL'S POLLICIZATION OPERATION OF 1929

A 40-year-old carpenter amputated the thumb through the metacarpotrapezial joint and the index finger through the proximal phalanx 1 year before operation. The proximal portions of the thenar muscles remained.

Fig. 664. Case W. J. (*Top*) Crushing amputation through all the metacarpals and the thumb and the index finger through the proximal joints. Devoid of function. Excised the stump of the long metacarpal and jogged the index over on it and pinned. By plastic maneuvers, made a thumb cleft. Transferred tendon for motion of the thumb. Did a pulley operation for opposition of the thumb. Placed a long tendon graft of an extensor around the palm to give adduction of the thumb. Placed a pedicle graft. (*Bottom*) The patient obtained prehension and pinched firmly.

At operation a dorsal skin flap was developed and used to cover the thumb, while a volar flap determined the depth of the new cleft.

The index ray with flexor and extensor tendons, as well as volar nerves, was shifted on the 2 pedicles, the articular surface of the index metacarpal being placed on the trapezium to form a new joint. A section of the extensor carpi radialis longus tendon taken with the ray was passed through drill holes in the trapezium to encircle and stabilize the new joint. The thumb extensors and the flexor tendon were united to the transferred digit. The dorsal and the volar interossei were kept intact, and the remnants of the thenar muscles were attached to the new metacarpal. Remaining denuded areas were covered with a full-thickness skin graft.

The new thumb could touch the full length of the middle finger and the base and the tip of the ring finger. It abducted to give a 1½ inch opening for grasp. The new metacarpo-trapezial joint had 25° of motion in a functional range. Sensibility was normal, the skin was of good quality, and the patient pursued his trade as a carpenter for 19 years.

POLLICIZATION ON A NEUROVASCULAR PEDICLE

Early pollicizations were based on the vascular pedicle idea, and the digit was carried

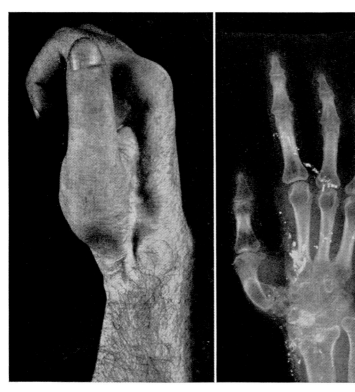

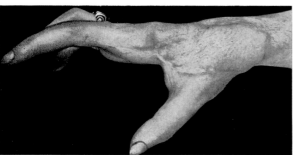

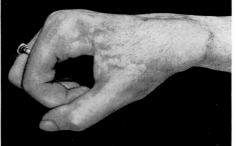

FIG. 665. (*Top*) Gunshot wound with resulting adduction contracture of first cleft. (*Bottom*) Scar excised, osteotomy and pinning thumb metacarpal and application of pedicle graft in one stage. (L. D. Howard, M.D.)

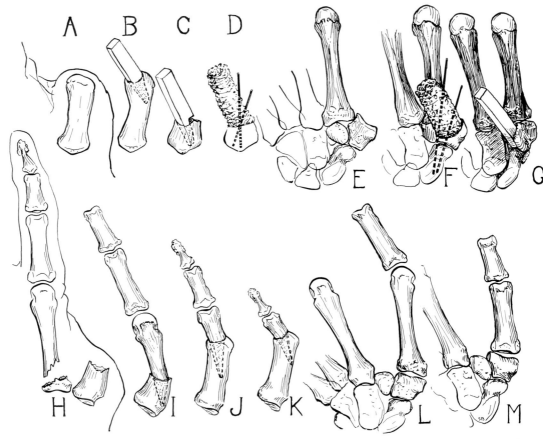

FIG. 666. Reconstructing the thumb after loss. (A, B, C, D) Building out the metacarpal, or part of it, by bone grafts, showing 2 cortical and 1 cancellous graft. (E, F) For complete loss of the thumb, a post of iliac graft is pinned to the trapezium. Thumb posts should be short, thick and just inside the path of movement of the fingers. (G) Cortical bone is thrust through the trapezium and the scaphoid and should project well forward to contact the fingers as they close on it. A tubular pedicle is placed first to receive the graft. (H to M) Pollicization of the index finger. (I) Index metacarpal thrust into that of the thumb. Index shortened by its distal segment. (J, K) Proximal and middle phalanx of the index finger thrust into the metacarpal of the thumb. (L, M) Metacarpal and proximal phalanges of the index finger transferred onto the trapezium. Index shortened.

to its new location with an intact bridge of skin, soft tissues and vessels. The idea of a vascular pedicle without skin is not new, Gersung having described it in 1887, but Esser popularized the procedure, calling it an island flap.

The adaptation of this principle of transfer of tissues solely on a neurovascular pedicle to pollicization operations paved the way for many reports of such procedures since 1948.

The index finger is used most often, being carried on a neurovascular pedicle as an island transfer, that is, without a skin bridge. This simplifies the skin closure and, when the dorsal venous return in the subcutaneous tissues is preserved, it can be done with little risk. If an index finger of normal length is used for loss of the entire thumb metacarpal, the palm is narrowed, and the new thumb is long and slender. To some the appearance is distinctly unpleasant. A good web of pedicle skin and the building of a pseudothenar eminence will improve the appearance.

Littler has described the technic of index transfer in several reports. It is important that the new thumb be in proper position and of adequate length; preferably, the tendon action should be provided by secondary shortening, if necessary, or attachment to the normal thumb motors.

Hilgenfeldt's pollicization of the middle finger is likewise still being done, also without the skin bridge. Under ordinary conditions the index finger is preferred.

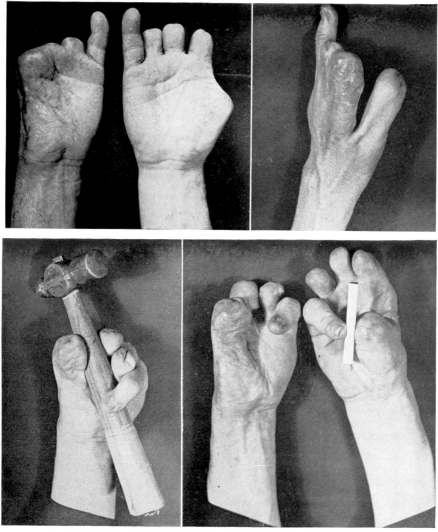

Fig. 667. Reconstruction of the thumb after loss of the digits. (*Top, left*) Preoperative. (*Top, right*) Pollicization and phalangization of the index ray. The 2nd metacarpal was lashed by tendon to the greater multangular. The long tendons of the thumb were transferred to those of the index finger. The sensory nerves were preserved and carried with the finger. The thumb has been phalangized, and an angulatory rotary osteotomy was done on the base of the 5th metacarpal. (*Bottom*) There was good function. (William H. Frackelton, M.D.)

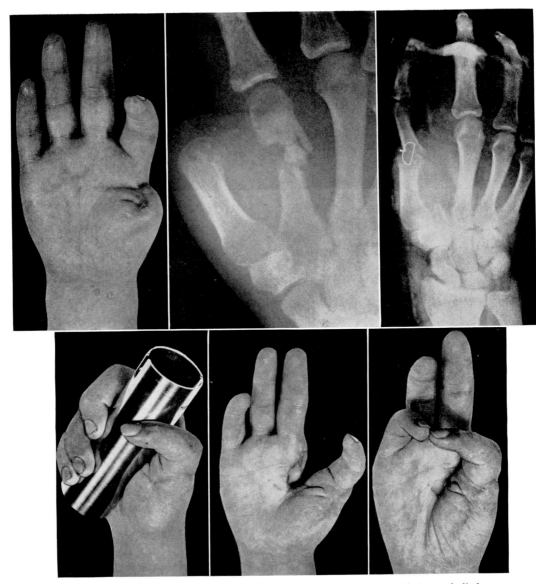

FIG. 668. (*Top, left*) Loss of thumb and damage to index metacarpal from shell fragment. (*Top, right*) Transfer of index phalanges to first metacarpal. (*Bottom*) The cleft was completed and lined with a pedicle graft. Good function resulted. (Walter C. Graham, M.D.)

In some instances, where the little finger has been damaged through its metacarpal, pollicization of this digit can be done. Kelleher and Sullivan pollicized the little finger for losses of the thumb phalanges, with excellent cosmetic and functional results. A transfer of the 5th to the 1st ray, passing the finger with its intact flexor tendons, nerves and vessels under the median nerve, is illustrated. The extensor tendon of the thumb was sutured to the divided extensors of the finger. The flexors were of proper length and functioned well.

Pollicization for Congenital Absence of the Thumb. When the thumb ray is absent, there is often an accompanying absence of the trapezium and the scaphoid. In these instances

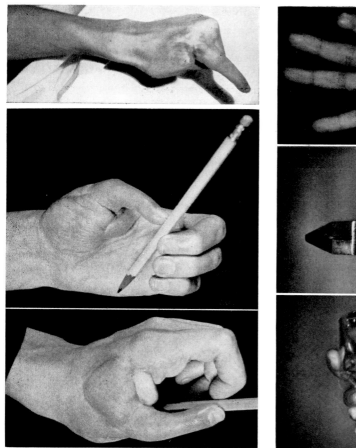

FIG. 669. Pollicization of the index finger, preserving the nerves. The cleft was made by tube pedicle. The tendons were joined, but the joints were stiff. (Ernst Dehne, M.D.)

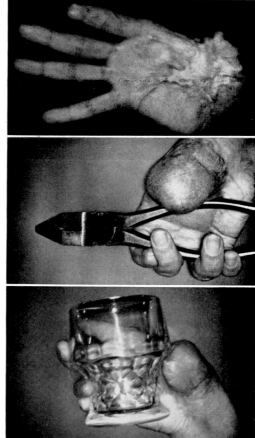

FIG. 670. For loss of thumb and damage to the index finger, a pedicle replaced the scar, and an iliac bone graft gave support. Transfer of index proprius restored abduction of index finger.

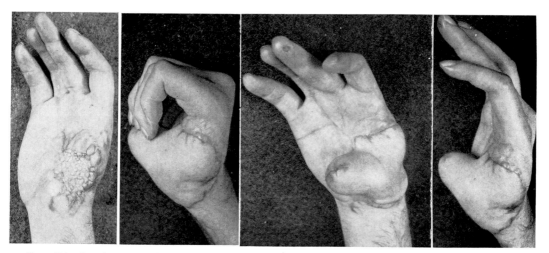

FIG. 671. Gunshot wound with loss of thumb. Reconstruction by pedicle graft and bone graft. A short thick post is more useful. Sensibility can be improved by island transfer.

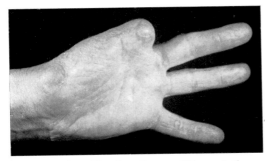

FIG. 672. Showing the condition of the hand before reconstruction. The thumb has been amputated through its carpometacarpal joint and also the index finger, as frequently happens, through its proximal phalanx. The hand is unfit for work. (Surg., Gynec. Obstet. *52*:245)

pollicization consists of shifting the index finger to a position opposite the fingers, stabilizing the new thumb by bone graft to the middle finger metacarpal. Barsky and Matthews describe the technics. Where a "floating thumb" is present, it is tempting to broaden its skin base by Z-plasty and stabilize it by bone grafts. This is feasible only when the thumb is of reasonable size and when it can be shifted proximally to a more functional position. Many of these floating thumbs are tiny projections from the side of the index finger, hanging by a slender thread of skin and lying quite distal as compared with a normal thumb. In these, amputation is indicated, with pollicization of the index finger at the age of 3 or 4 years, if indicated.

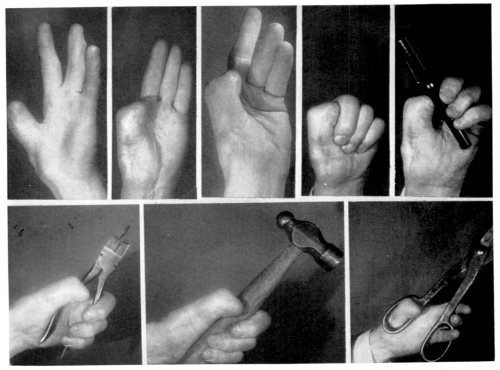

FIG. 673. Same patient as shown in Figure 672. Physiologic reconstruction of thumb by transfer of index metacarpal, preserving normal blood and nerve supply and motor function. Operation by Sterling Bunnell, April, 1929.

DIGITAL TRANSFER

A finger from the other hand or from a foot has been transferred to make a thumb. Nicoladoni pioneered this in 1898, and many authors reported attempted transfers. Little attention was paid to nerve supply, and the results were poor. The new digit was atrophic, stiff and insensitive. In a review of 20 cases, Guellette found only 7 with active movement and 3 with perfect results. Necrosis or ulceration occurred in 5.

H. H. Campbell used a ring finger for transfer in 2 cases, as did Joyce. Clarkson has transplanted the great toe or the forefoot for congenital absence, and Freeman used the second toe. The limber joints of children are more tolerant of the position necessary for toe-to-thumb transfer, and a better quality of sensation returns in the young.

Clarkson feels that pollicization of the index finger narrows the hand and that this is a disadvantage. Only a toe-to-thumb transfer can add substance to the hand. He feels that adequate tendon reconstruction and the use of nerve grafts where necessary help to restore maximal function. A long period of treatment is necessary, with fixation of the hand to the foot for 4 to 6 months. Freeman transplanted the 2nd toe to the thumb in a child, with excellent appearance and function.

RÉSUMÉ OF PRINCIPLES IN THUMB RECONSTRUCTION

A short thumb with controlled movement and a painless skin-covered stump can be of considerable use. A moderate lengthening can be accomplished by the "cocked-hat" technic or the use of a local well-innervated flap and some additional bone. A pedicled flap to give a broad postlike thumb or a tubed pedicle with a bony strut will provide the structural part of a thumb. This technic was abandoned in favor of pollicization of the index finger because of the lack of adequate sensibility and the development of trophic changes. However, the shifting of an island transfer of skin from one of the other digits now makes this method useful when the remaining fingers are normal. Insertion of the skin with its intact

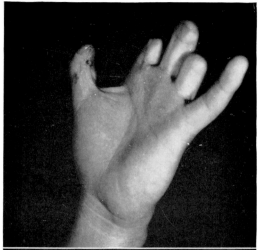

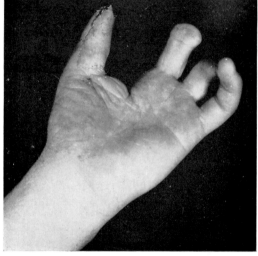

Fig. 674. Case D. G., neurovascular pedicle. (*Top*) A shotgun blast had injured all the digits except the little finger. The thumb was in need of new cover over its volar aspect. The index finger was poor, but it had good skin over its radial side. Dissected this skin off completely and transferred it to the volar aspect of the thumb on a neurovascular pedicle. The skin was passed under a bridge of good skin at the base of the thumb and sutured to cover the distal 2 segments of the thumb. (*Bottom*) This furnished normal sensation and stereognosis to the volar aspect of the thumb. The remains of the index finger at the metacarpal were removed.

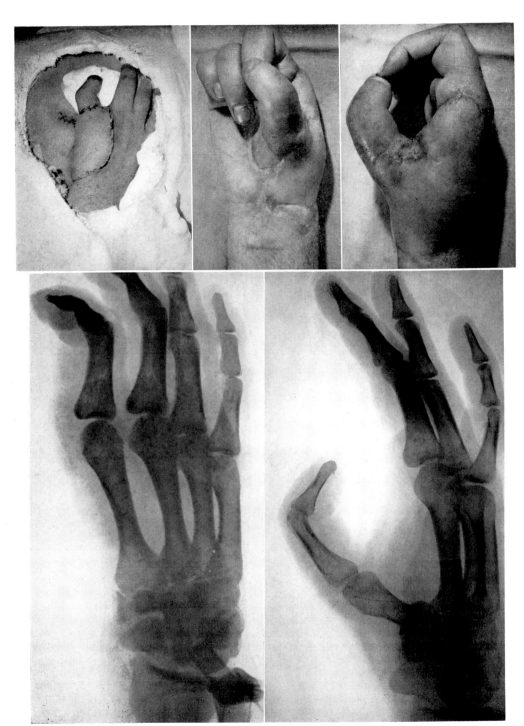

FIG. 675. Case R. W. (*Top, left*) Condition of hand preoperatively. The thumb and the adjoining part of the dorsum of the hand had been lost by gunshot wound, and a pedicle skin flap was applied to the hand. The index finger had been amputated through its distal joint and the thumb through the base of the metacarpal. On October 10, 1951, at Letterman Army Hospital, the index finger was pollicized. The skin at its base was completely circumscribed. The 2 volar digital vessels and nerves were exposed and preserved, and these were used as a neurovascular pedicle by which this finger was transferred to act as the thumb. The nerve to

FIG. 676. Avulsion of thumb and index metacarpal in auto accident. The volar nerves and the flexor tendons of the index were intact. (*Bottom*) A tubed pedicle replaced the proximal scar and, when detached from the abdomen and the index pollicized, the end of the tube was laid into the cleft. Extensor function was restored later.

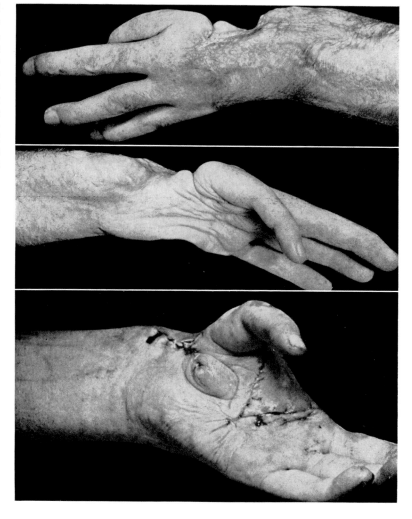

neurovascular pedicle not only provides a tactile gripping surface with normal perception but, by bringing new blood supply to the part, diminishes the trophic changes which usually followed. If the index, the middle or the little fingers have been injured, pollicization of the damaged digit may be the operation of choice.

If the middle finger is used, the index metacarpal should be transected and the whole ray shifted to the base of the 3rd metacarpal, improving the cleft space. If the little finger is used, transfer is made beneath the median nerve distal to the carpal tunnel, and the extensors are sutured to the stumps of the thumb

the 2nd digital cleft was slit back to the base of the palm, and the vessels to the long finger were cut and tied to preserve the blood supply to the index finger. The distal part of the metacarpal of the index finger was thrust into the base of the metacarpal of the thumb and held by 1 Kirschner wire. The long extensor tendon was preserved but shortened and rejoined. (*Top, center* and *right*) Condition after operation. Stereognosis, position of thumb and motion were achieved. (*Bottom*) Roentgenograms made before and after operation. The metacarpal of the index finger has been fused to that of the thumb. (J. Bone Joint Surg. *34-A*, 772-773)

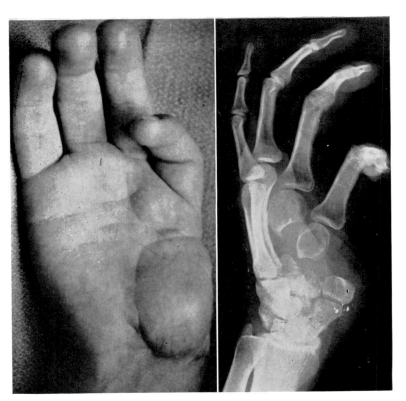

Fig. 677. Loss of thumb including entire metacarpal and most of the shafts of index and middle metacarpals. For reconstruction see Figure 678.

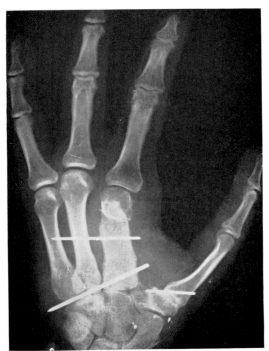

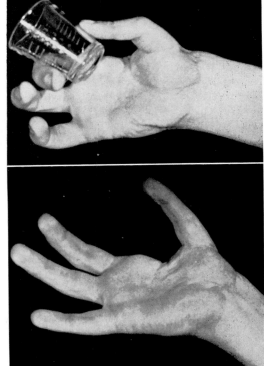

Fig. 678. An iliac graft restored the shaft of the middle metacarpal, and the index was transferred on its neurovascular pedicles. The proximal phalanx was fused to the trapezium. (*Right*) Good extension and flexion. (J. William Littler, M.D.)

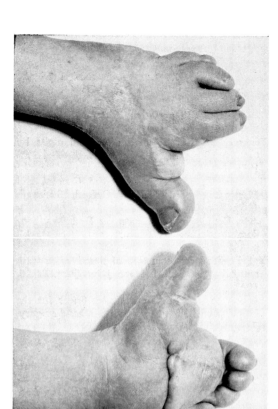

FIG. 679. Transplant of the forepart of a foot to a hand congenitally defective of fingers. Good nourishment, scars inconspicuous, sensation almost throughout. Needs positioning of thumb and tendon action. (Patrick Clarkson, London)

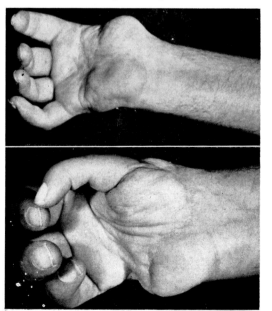

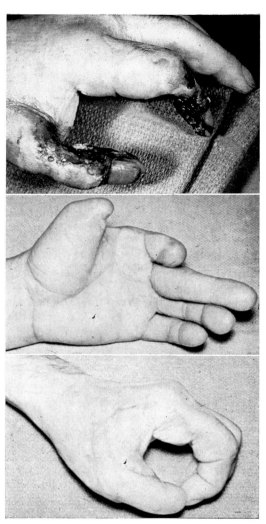

FIG. 681. An electrical burn destroyed portions of the left thumb and index finger. A one-stage pollicization restored good pinching ability and the cleft.

FIG. 680. The thumb was amputated, and the little finger metacarpal and its extensor tendons damaged. Pollicization of the entire digit including part of the metacarpal, with flexor tendons and volar nerves and blood supply, was accomplished by passing it across the palm beneath the median nerve just distal to the transverse carpal ligament. The extensor tendon of the thumb was joined to the finger extensors,

tendons, or the extensor indicis proprius is used.

With these methods available, it is felt that there is little need for the toe-to-thumb transfer operations, except in children with severely disabling congenital deficiencies.

Each case must be studied individually, taking into consideration the factors of age, handedness, occupational skills and economic loss. Function is of prime importance, but appearance must be considered also, lest one leave the patient with what Clarkson calls a "bad biologic tailoring job in need of a proper finish."

BIBLIOGRAPHY

Aguirre, S. C., and Oberlander, H.: Total reconstruction of thumb, Prensa med. argent. *43*: 2360, 1956.

Albee, F.: Orthopedic and Reconstruction Surgery, p. 1015, Philadelphia, Saunders, 1919.

————: Synthetic transplantation of tissue to form a new finger with restoration of the function of the hand, Ann. Surg. *69*:379, 1919.

Almasann, S.: Phalangization of first metacarpal bone, Rev. chir., Bucuresti *43*:807, 1940.

Apetrosyan, K. A.: Plastic reconstruction of fingers by means of transplantation of toes, Ortop. i. travmatol. *13*:74, 1939.

Arana, G. B.: Phalangization of the first metacarpal, Surg., Gynec. Obstet. *40*:859, 1925.

von Arlt, B. R.: Daumenplastik, Wien. klin. Wchr. *30*:15, 1917.

Barsky, A.: Congenital Anomalies of the Hand and Their Surgical Treatment, Springfield, Ill., Thomas, 1958.

Berson, M.: Reconstruction of index finger with nail transplantation, Surgery *27*:594, 1950.

Blair, V. P., and Byars, L. T.: Toe to finger transplant, Ann. Surg. *112*:287, 1940.

Broadbent, T. R., and Woolf, R. M.: Thumb reconstruction with contiguous skin-bone pedicle graft; a case report, Plast. Reconstr. Surg. *26*:494, 1960.

Buck-Gramcke, D.: Wiederherstellung der Sensibilitat bei Teilverlust des Daumens, Arch. klin. Chir. *299*:99, 1961.

Bunnell, S.: Reconstructive surgery of the hand, Surg., Gynec. Obstet. *39*:259, 1924.

————: Physiological reconstruction of a thumb after total loss, Surg., Gynec. Obstet *52*:245, 1931.

————: Digit transfer by neurovascular pedicle, J. Bone Joint Surg. *34-A*:772, 1952.

————: Reconstruction of the thumb, Am. J. Surg. *95*:168, 1958.

Campbell-Reid, D. A.: Reconstruction of the thumb, J. Bone Joint Surg. *42-B*:444, 1960.

Chandler, R., and Clarkson, P.: A toe to thumb transplant with nerve graft, Am. J. Surg. *95*: 315, 1958.

Clarkson, P.: Reconstruction of hand digits by toe transfer, J. Bone Joint Surg. *37-A*:270, 1955.

Clarkson, P., and Pelly, A.: The General and Plastic Surgery of the Hand, Oxford, Blackwell, 1962.

Dehne, E.: Operativer Ersatz des Daumens, Sonderabdruck aus der Chirurg, vol. 23, Part 12, p. 566, 1952.

Dial, D. E.: Reconstruction of thumb after traumatic amputation, J. Bone Joint Surg. *21*:98, 1939.

Dunlop, J.: The use of the index finger for the thumb; some interesting points in hand surgery, J. Bone Joint Surg. *5*:99, 1923.

Esser, J. F. S.: Island flaps, biologic or artery flap, New York Med. J. *106*:264, 1917.

Esser, J. F. S., and Ranschburg, P.: Reconstruction of hand and four fingers by transplantation of middle part of foot and four toes, Ann. Surg. *111*:655, 1940.

Flynn, J. E., and Burden, C. N.: Reconstruction of the thumb, Arch. Surg. *85*:394, 1962.

Frackelton, W., and Teasley, J.: Neurovascular island transfer; extension in usage, J. Bone Joint Surg. *44-A*:1069, 1962.

Freeman, B. S.: Reconstruction of thumb by toe transfer, Plast. Reconstr. Surg. *17*:393, 1956.

Gersung, R.: Plastischer Ersatz der Wangenschleimhaut, Zbl. Chir. *14*:706, 1887.

Gillies, H.: Autograft of amputated digit; suggested operation, Lancet *1*:1002, 1940.

Gordon, S.: Autograft of amputated thumb, Lancet *2*:823, 1944.

Gosset, J.: Le pollicisation de l'index, J. chir. (Par.) *65*:403, 1949.

Graham, W. C., Brown, J. B., and Conover, B.: Elongation and digitalization of the first metacarpal for restoration of function of the hand, Arch. Surg. *61*:17, 1950.

Greeley, P. W.: Reconstruction of the thumb, Ann. Surg. *124*:60, 1946.

Gueullette, R.: Etude critique des procédés de restauration du pouce, J. Chir. *36*:1, 1930.

Haas, S. L.: Plastic restoration for loss of all fingers of both hands, Am. J. Surg. *36*:720, 1937.

Henry, A. K.: Conservation of useful thumb after complete phalangeal necrosis, Lancet *1*: 1123, 1940.

Hilgenfeldt, O.: Operativer Daumenersatz, Stuttgart, Ferdinand Enhiverlag, 1950.

Hueck, H.: Ein Fall von Daumenersatz durch einen unbrauchbaren Finger, Deutsche Z. Chir. *153*:321, 1920.

Iselin, M.: Chirurgie de la Main, Paris, Masson et cie, 1945.

Jeffery, C. C.: A case of pollicisation of the index finger, J. Bone Joint Surg. *39-B*:120, 1957.

Jepson, P. N.: Transformation of middle finger into a thumb, Minnesota Med. *8*:552, 1925.

Joyce, J. L.: A new operation for the substitution of a thumb, Brit. J. Surg. *5*:499, 1918.

————: The results of a new operation for the substitution of a thumb, Brit. J. Surg. *16*:362, 1929.

Kaplan, I., and Plaschkes, J.: One-stage pollicization of little finger, Brit. J. Plast. Surg. *13*:272, 1960.

Kelikian, H., and Bintcliffe, E. W.: Functional restoration of the thumb, Surg., Gynec. Obstet. *83*:807, 1946.

Kirklin, J. W., and Thomas, C. G.: Opponens transplant: An analysis of the methods employed and results obtained in seventy-five cases, Surg., Gynec. Obstet. *86*:213, 1948.

Kleinschmidt, O.: Zum Ersatz des Daumens durch die zweite Zehe, Arch. klin. Chir. *164*:809, 1931.

Koster, K. H.: Plastic operation for loss of thumb, Acta orthop. scand. *9*:115, 1938.

Kuhn, H.: Reconstruction of the thumb by "Hilgenfeldt's flap," Ann. chir. plast. *6*:259, 1961.

Lambert, O.: Résultat éloigné d'une transplantation du gros orteil en remplacement du pouce, Bull. Mém. Soc. Chir. *46*:689, 1920.

Landivar, A. F.: Phalangization of first metacarpal bone, Bol. Soc. cir. B. Air. *23*:637, 1939.

Lenormant, C.: Le traitement des mutilations des doigts et en particulier du pouce par les autoplasties et transplantations, Presse Méd. *28*:223, 1920.

Littler, J. W.: The neurovascular pedicle method of digital transposition for reconstruction of the thumb, Plast. Reconstr. Surg. *12*:303, 1953.

Lyle, H. H. M.: The formation of a new thumb by Klapp's method, Ann. Surg. *59*:767, 1914.

————: Deformity of the hand—formation of a new thumb from stump of first metacarpus, Ann. Surg. *74*:121, 1921.

————: Formation of thumb from first metacarpus, Ann. Surg. *76*:121, 1922.

————: Treatment of disabilities of the hand, Ann. Surg. *78*:816, 1923.

McFarlane, R. M., and Stromberg, W. B.: Resurfacing of the thumb following major skin loss, J. Bone Joint Surg. *44-A*:1365, 1962.

Machol: Die Gelenkbindung, insbesondere die Arthrodese in der Kriegschirurgie, Beitr. klin. Chir. *114*:170, 1919.

Manasse, P.: Vorstellung eines Falles mit Daumenersatz und Fingerauswechselung, Berl. klin. Wchr. *56*:717, 1919.

Marcer, E.: Pollicizazione dell indice e dell secondo metacarpo, Minerva ortop. *2*:42, 1951.

Matthews, D. N.: Congenital absence of functioning thumb, Arch. klin. Chir. *299*:95, 1961.

Meyer, W.: Plastic surgery to restore function after loss of thumb, Helvet. Med. Acta *6*:872, 1940.

Müller, G. M.: Construction of a palmar post, Brit. J. Plast. Surg. *3*:47, 1950.

Müller, W.: Anatomische Studien zur Frage des Daumenersatzes, Beitr. klin. Chir. *120*:595, 1920.

Murray, A. R.: Reconstructive surgery of the hand with special reference to digital transplantation, Brit. J. Surg. *34*:131, 1946.

————: Reconstructive surgery of hand; special reference to digital transplantation *in* Year Book of General Surgery, 1947. Year Book Publishing Co., Chicago. Editor, Evarts A. Graham.

Neuhof, H.: Transplantation of toe for missing finger; end-result, Ann. Surg. *112*:291, 1940.

Nicoladoni, C.: Daumenplastik und organischer Ersatz der Fingerspitze (Anticheiroplastik und Dactylo-plastik), Arch. klin. Chir. *61*:606, 1900.

————: Weitere Erfahrungen über Daumenplastik, Arch. klin. Chir. *69*:695, 1903.

Novitskey, S. T.: Total transplantation of large toe to replace thumb, Vestnik khir. *57*:352, 1939.

Nuzzi, O.: Intermetacarpolisi distali chirurgica, Riforma Med. *37*:248, 1921.

Ombrédanne, M. L.: Constitution autoplastique d'un pouce prenant au moyen du Ier metacarpien, Bull. mém. Soc. chir. Paris *46*:158, 1920.

Perthes, V.: Über plastischen Daumenersatz insbesondere bei Verlust des ganzen Daumenstrahles, Arch. orthop. Unfall-Chir. *19*:198, 1921.

Petersen, N.: Plastic reconstruction of thumb, S. Afr. M. J. *17*:137, 1943.

Pierce, G. W.: Reconstruction of the thumb after total loss, Surg., Gynec. Obstet. *45*:825, 1927.

Pieri, G.: Reconstruction of thumb, Chir. org. movimento *3*:325, 1919.

Pitzler, K.: On the fundamental principles of the recovery of the grasping capacity of the hand, based on a thumb replacement operation, Mschr. Unfallheilk. *64*:285, 1961.

Rapin, M.: Reconstitution d'un pouce (Thesis), Univ. de Lausanne Clinic Chirurgicale, Editions Medecine et Hygiene, Geneve, 1949.

Rogova, K. F.: Phalangization of first metacarpal bone, Khirurgiya *11*:150, 1939.

Saraluce, J. A.: Transplantation of large toe to replace thumb, Semana méd. españ. *3*:81, 1940.

Schepelmann, E.: Das spaetere Schicksal einer Daumenplastik, Z. orthop. Chir. *39*:181, 1919.

Schmiedt, W.: Beitrag zur Daumenplastik, Deutsch. Z. Chir. *145*:420, 1916.

Shirokov, B. A.: Phalangization of first metacarpal bone in plastic restoration of thumb: Anatomic basis of author's method, Khirurgiya *11*: 115, 1939.

Søiland, H.: Lengthening a finger with the "on the top" method, Acta chir. scand. *122*:184, 1961.

Spencer, W. G.: Plastic operations on the thumb, Med. Sc. Abst. & Rev. *3*:29, 1920.

Verrall, P. J.: Three cases of reconstruction of the thumb, Brit. M. J. *2*:775, 1919.

Wittek, A.: Successful substitution of second metacarpal bone for missing thumb, Chirurg *13*:577, 1941.

Young, F.: Transplantation of toes for fingers, Surgery *20*:117, 1946.

Zancolli, E.: Transplantation of the index finger in congenital absence of the thumb, J. Bone Joint Surg. *42-A*:658, 1960.

Zrubecky, G.: Operativer Daumenersatz am beiden handen, Langenbeck Arch. klin. Chir. *299*: 142, 1961.

Zsulyevich, I.: Index finger to replace thumb, Chirurg *10*:433, 1938.

Chapter 14

Shoulder and Elbow

SHOULDER

There is an old saying, "Don't examine the hand through a hole in the blanket." The hand depends on the arm for its nerve and blood supply and for a stable base on which it can move. Placement of the hand for use depends on a functional range of shoulder and elbow motion. Some diseases and some traumatic conditions in the neck, the shoulder or the elbow often cause symptoms in the hand, and these may be the presenting complaints.

This chapter is not meant to be a complete discussion of surgery of these parts but only to point out some conditions affecting the hand. The bibliography lists the standard reference works.

SHOULDER MOTIONS

Moseley has pointed out 6 locations where movement takes place when the arm is normally moved on the trunk. Only the coordinated actions of the muscles of the scapula, the humerus and the clavicle producing motions a these points result in the normal range of motion.

When the arm is brought ahead in forward flexion or lifted at the side in abduction, the scapula is fixed to the trunk by its muscles, and the arm is moved by muscles attached to the humerus. Beginning at about 30° abduction or 60° forward flexion, additional motion is the result of combined action, the scapula providing approximately one third of the range. Thus, a fused shoulder with good scapular control is still capable of a good range of motion.

For full motion, not only must there be free action at the glenohumeral joint, but the humerus must rotate for full elevation. The clavicle enters into the motion by rotating like a crankshaft, and the biceps tendon must move normally through its sheath.

Measurements of function are noted as the angle of forward flexion, backward flexion or extension, both relating to the angular movement between the arm and the trunk in the sagittal plane. Abduction is raising the arm at the side in the coronal plane. External and internal rotation are commonly measured with the arm abducted to the horizontal or adducted to the side. Full elevation of the arm to the vertical has been called the "pivotal" position. To describe accurately the position of the arm in relation to the body one must designate the angle of abduction and the angle of the plane of that movement in reference to the coronal plane of the body and the rotation of the humerus. Thus the "airplane" position is 90° abduction in the coronal plane with zero rotation. This description does not include the scapular motion; therefore, a review committee of the American Orthopedic Association (in 1942) specified the recommended position for arthrodesis in boys as 45° to 50° abduction with reference to the vertebral border of the scapula, not the trunk. Forward flexion and internal rotation each of 15° to 20° completes the exact location with reference to the scapula.

Motion may be limited because of paralysis of muscles caused by polio, brachial plexus lesions or severed nerves. Rupture of muscle attachments or traction injuries on the nerves cause distinctive deformities. Contractures, calcification in tendons and joint diseases are all possible factors in limiting motions.

NERVE LESIONS

Cervical spine lesions may cause pain in the forearm and the hand, depending on the root involvement. Disk lesions most often produce cord symptoms. Pain from the 5th nerve would be felt along the shoulder, the elbow, the dorsum of the forearm, the thumb and the index finger. The 6th and the 7th follow the patterns described in Chapter 10, Nerves. Pain, paresthesias, numbness, limited neck motions and roentgenographic changes indi-

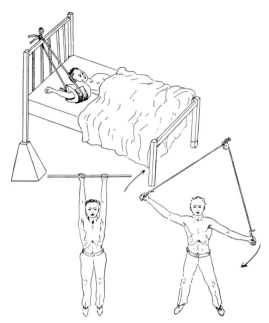

Fig. 682. Method of relieving flexion contracture of the shoulder due to disuse. When an arm is not raised for 2 months or more, from whatever cause, such as an injured hand, then it cannot be raised. Starting with the bed method, the arm is raised steadily by bandage, pillow and piece of cardboard; in the second week, the exercises are added. Two weeks of this is sufficient and far preferable to that of forcing under anesthesia.

cate that the cervical spine is the origin of symptoms.

Brachial Plexus Injuries. Traction from birth trauma or, in adults, sudden jerking of the arm away from the body or falls on the shoulder are the most common causes of brachial plexus injuries. Direct trauma from gunshot wounds or stab wounds is infrequent in peacetime.

The problems of diagnosis are the same regardless of the cause.

LOCATION OF LESION IN THE PLEXUS. In a downward pull on the arm or pushing the head away from the shoulder, the upper portion of the plexus—the 5th and the 6th and sometimes the 7th nerves—is involved. This type of injury is the most common and is the cause of Erb-Duchenne paralysis. An upward pull strains or ruptures the lower nerves, the 8th cervical and the 1st thoracic, and results in Klumpke's paralysis. Direct outward traction can affect all nerves. It is more common to have what appears to be a total lesion at the onset and a residual paralysis of the Erb-Duchenne type.

The site of the lesion depends on the direction of the force and the position of the arm. The more distal nerves are held less firmly in the surrounding fascia, while proximally the cords and the trunks are larger and stronger; near the roots the nerves are again smaller but are snubbed more firmly by the fascial sheaths and attachments to the transverse processes (Stevens). Any level may be disrupted if the forces and the angles are excessive.

Avulsion of the root from the cord is irreparable, and any sign that verifies this is of diagnostic and prognostic value. It is more common in the lower type of lesion and in birth palsies as compared with adult traction injuries.

In the upper lesions, paralysis of the nerves that supply the rhomboids, the levator scapulae and the serratus anterior is an indication of nerve avulsion. In the lower lesions, Horner's syndrome—miosis, enophthalmus and a narrowed palpebral fissure—indicates involvement of sympathetic fibers from root avulsion. It may not appear until 2 or 3 weeks after injury. Bonney states that severe pain with Horner's syndrome indicates a bad prognosis. In lesions proximal to the posterior ganglia he found a positive reaction to the axon flare test, a local vasodilatation and flare reaction to pricking the skin through a drop of 1 per cent histamine acid phosphate. He recommends testing 4 areas on the forearm and 2 on the hand and advises against operation if 2 or more areas show a positive response.

Diagnostic Points. Rupture of the 5th and the 6th cervical nerves often occurs just beyond the foramina. This results in paralysis of the shoulder rotators, the deltoid, the flexors of the elbow and the brachioradialis. Lesions may be present in the nerves distal to the cords.

In upper lesions the arm is rotated inwardly and lacks power of abduction and elbow flexion, and the shoulder muscles show atrophy. In the lower lesions there is a clawhand, with

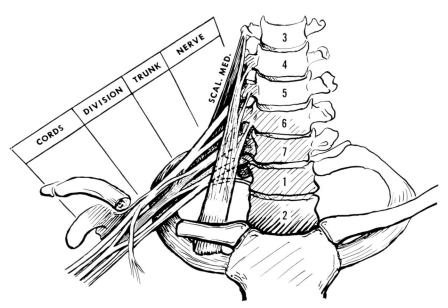

FIG. 683. The parts and the relations of the brachial plexus.

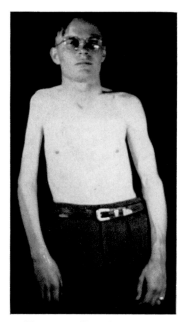

FIG. 684. Complete brachial plexus palsy. Six months previously, while riding a motorcycle, he had rammed a truck, evulsing from the cord C-6, C-7, C-8 and T-1, and reducing C-5 to a ragged cord.

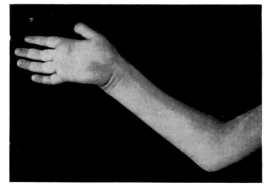

FIG. 685. Case C. G., age 8. Lower brachial plexus palsy. At 13 months the patient had fallen out of an automobile, which left the entire arm limp for 6 months. Now, extensors of the wrist and the fingers work, but of the flexors only the flexor carpi radialis and some of the pronator teres are working. All intrinsic muscles are paralyzed. Anesthesia is over the ulna, two thirds of the hand and a strip of forearm. The lesion includes C-8, T-1 and most of C-7.

FIG. 686. Case P. R., age 16. As determined at operation (see brachial plexus cases), at the age of 4, C-8, T-1 and most of the C-7 nerves were avulsed from the spinal cord, rendering the hand useless, the only functioning muscles being the extensors of the wrist, the flexor carpi radialis and the pronator teres. (*Top, left*) Useless hand at age 16. The arm was useful only to the wrist. The wrist was arthrodesed, sparing the radioulnar joint, and the following tendons were transferred: extensor

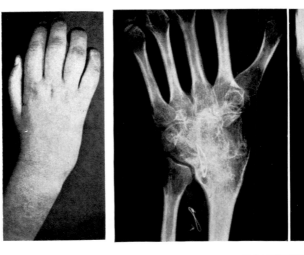
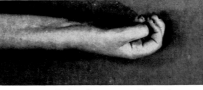
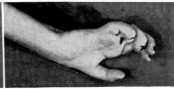
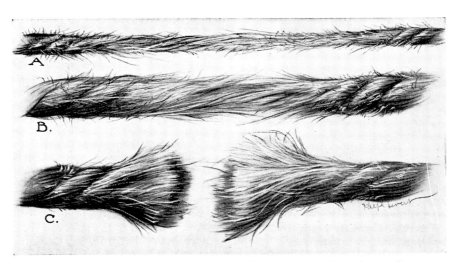

carpi radialis brevis to the extensors of the fingers and the long extensor of the thumb; flexor carpi radialis to the flexor of the thumb; extensor carpi radialis longus to the flexor profundus; supinator longus plus a tendon graft from the palmaris longus looped around the flexor ulnaris to give opposition to the thumb. (*Top, right*) X-ray pictures of arthrodesis. (*Below*) The hand gained strong motion and could pick up and hold objects, becoming very useful.

FIG. 687. A nerve and a rope act alike when under traction. Axons (i.e., rope fibers) break all along for quite a length, until finally one point is weakest, and there the nerve or rope pulls apart. Suture of the ends of such a nerve is useless, since axons have multiple rupture. If, though, the whole enlarged cicatricial segment is excised and the good ends sutured, regeneration follows the same as after suturing a severed nerve. This explains many poor results after suture of a ruptured brachial plexus.

the thumb at the side with intrinsic paralysis and atrophy of the flexors on the ulnar side of the forearm.

See Chapter 10, NERVES, for further diagnostic points.

FINDINGS AT OPERATION. When a nerve is pulled apart it responds as a rope does when overstretched, some fibers breaking at one level, some at other levels over a long distance. Such a nerve is damaged well back of the level of separation of the ends. Because some fibers are torn but bound in place by the surrounding fascias and others are merely stretched and temporarily not functioning, there may be considerable recovery over a period of 1 or 2 years. A long fusiform neuromatous mass is found at delayed operations, and excision of this mass until good fibers can be obtained presents a problem to the surgeon. Operation done early would facilitate exposure, but because of the amount of spontaneous recovery, it has been customary to wait for 6 to 12 months to evaluate this. An electromyogram properly done at the end of 1

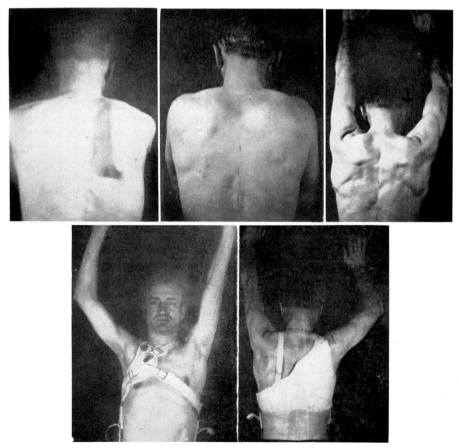

FIG. 688. Case J. S. While shoving on a barrel, the patient felt a tear. He had ruptured his serratus anterior muscle from the scapula, which left him unable to raise his arm more than to just above the horizontal. (*Top, left*) Showing the deformity of winged scapula. Through a posterior incision, the muscle was resutured in place. The 2 photographs show correction of deformity and disability. (*Bottom*) Special brace for winged scapula which holds scapula in place, making it possible to raise arm, used postoperatively in this case. The straps at the sides extend down to the crotch.

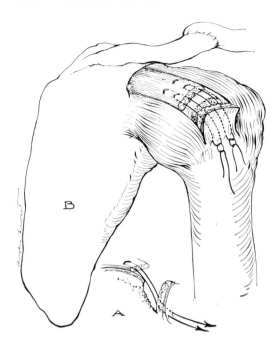

Fig. 689. Repair of ruptured tendon of the supraspinatus. When the ruptured tendon is split well up from the capsule, it can be drawn down freely. Its end is buried in the greater tuberosity, tying the permanent stainless-steel wire as the arm is extended.

month can be of much value. If the muscles show unequivocal signs of denervation activity, operation should be carried out.

Operations on the plexus injured by traction require a high degree of skill, absolute knowledge of detailed anatomy and a willingness to excise the scarred nerves and suture them under extremely difficult conditions. Division of the clavicle greatly enhances the exposure, and the bone may be excised to allow closure of a broad gap in the nerves.

PROGNOSIS. After a traction injury the amount of recovery is never as good as that after direct division by knife. Results in adults are not as good as those in children. Bunnell

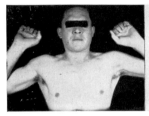
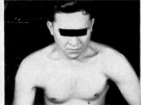
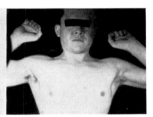

Fig. 690. Case D. S. A truck had rolled over the patient, rupturing from its insertion the left pectoral muscle, resulting in weakness in the motions of the arm that should be supplied by this muscle. (*Left* and *center*) Showing the deformity. (*Right*) Pectoral muscle reattached to its insertion by braiding a broad strip of fascia lata into the muscle and attaching it by removable stainless-steel wire to the humerus.

Fig. 691. (*Left*) From a stab wound in the axilla 12 years previously, the ulnar nerve and much of the median nerve are paralyzed. Tendon transfers are indicated; a pulley operation for opposition; a tendon T operation for adduction of the thumb and curvature of the arches; and a clawhand operation for muscle balance. (*Center* and *right*) Deformity of imbalance of the muscles.

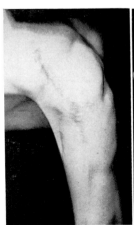
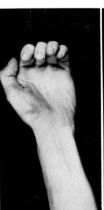
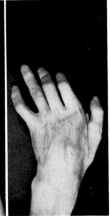

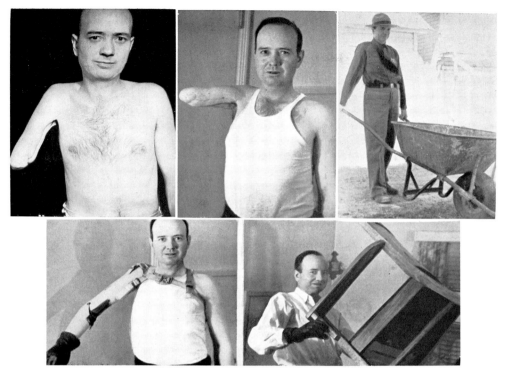

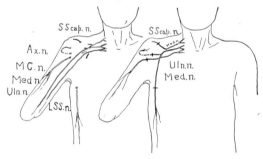

FIG. 692. Case J. E. B. A tree had fallen on the patient's shoulder, resulting in gangrene from tearing off the axillary artery and the following branches of the brachial plexus: suprascapular, circumflex, long subscapular, musculocutaneous, radial.

On June 14, 1934, the flexion contracture at the axilla was relieved, and a nerve supply was furnished to the paralyzed muscles (supraspinatus, infraspinatus, teres minor, deltoid, biceps, latissimus dorsi) by transferring the median and the ulnar nerves to the distal ends of the torn ones. The upper division of the median nerve was transferred to the circumflex. The lower division of the median was split, one half being sutured to the suprascapular at the notch and the other to the long subscapular nerve. The ulnar nerve was transferred to the musculocutaneous, and the intercostohumeral nerve was sutured.

(*Top, left*) Preoperative condition. Could not abduct arm. Could only internally rotate and adduct. Sixteen months later, action had returned to the paralyzed muscles, starting at 8 months. By 16 months, he wore an artificial arm and returned to

work. Function returned to all of the paralyzed muscles. Examination 8 years later showed strong motion at the shoulder in all directions. He wears an artificial arm and with it is able to keep his job in the State Department of Fish and Game.

(*Top, center* and *right; Middle, left* and *right*. Photographs supplied by the patient to demonstrate function. The legs of the chair must be resting on a table.

(*Bottom*) Showing (*left*) the torn nerves and (*right*) the transferred ones.

reported cases of traction injury and 1 of bullet wound, all operated on, with 6 showing some improvement. Sensation returned, and there was enough motion of the shoulder and the elbow to be useful. In only 1 case did any

muscle below the elbow recover. Nerve transfers of the intact median and ulnar nerves, in a patient with above-elbow amputation, were done to activate the shoulder muscles, making it possible to use a prosthesis.

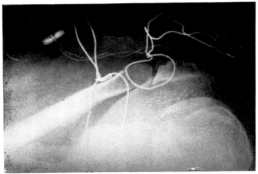

FIG. 693. (*Top*) Repair of dislocation of the acromioclavicular joint, using a long strip of fascia lata so placed as to reproduce the conoid and the trapezoid ligaments. To hold the bones in place while the ligamentous graft is becoming strong, 2 loops of stainless-steel wire are used so placed that they are removable. (*Bottom*) Method of placing stainless-steel wire so that it is removable. This kink is useful in holding fractures and dislocations. To remove after 3 or more weeks, a pull on each wire straightens out the kinks and the wire is withdrawn easily.

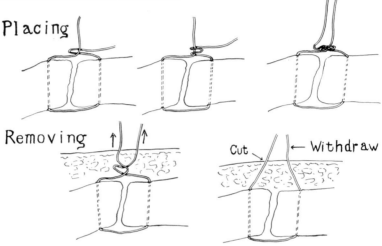

OBSTETRICAL PARALYSES. Most of these are of the upper type and may follow vertex as well as breech presentations. Most appear to be severe, with little or no swelling, but many recover in a few weeks. Most recovery will take place in 6 to 8 months, leaving a residual paralysis of the deltoid, the biceps, the external rotators and sometimes the triceps.

The shoulder may be injured at the time of birth, but most shoulder lesions as seen later are the result of muscle imbalance and inadequate support resulting in growth deformities.

Treatment. From the onset, splinting to relax paralyzed muscles favors return of function and prevents contractures and late deformity. A simple method is to place the hand behind the head, holding it there by a loop of bandage or strap around the wrist and beneath the shoulder.

If the whole plexus is involved and there is no recovery in 3 months, operation is indicated. Taylor, in a large series, proved the value of surgical repair. Delaying operation until the patient was 2 to 3 years old reduced the percentage of good results.

LATE OPERATION FOR DEFORMITY FROM PLEXUS LESIONS. The objectives in reconstructive procedures for deformities from the upper plexus lesions of obstetric type are to relieve the adduction and the internal rotation of the shoulder, the posterior luxation of the humeral head or the torsion of the humerus.

Sever's operation done at 4 or 5 years of age divides the pectoral insertion and the tip of the coracoid and the tendon of the subscapularis. Splinting in the fully corrected position for 6 months is essential. Some loss of motion occurs later, so that L'Episcopo's operation—transferring the latissimus dorsi and the teres major into the back of the humerus to provide more external rotation power —is preferable.

Wickstrom described the results of conservative therapy in 87 patients. The plexus was not explored. Fifty-four were the upper type, 11 the lower type, and 22 involved the whole

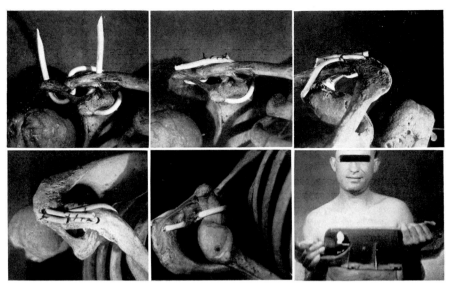

FIG. 694. For dislocation of the acromioclavicular joint: a method of placing a 12-inch graft of fascial lata to reproduce the conoid and the trapezoid ligaments.

(*Top, left*) Showing the anatomy of the conoid and the trapezoid ligaments, the position of the 3 holes in the bones and the fascial graft (indicated by rubber tube) in place but not yet drawn up. (*Top, center*) Showing the fascial graft (indicated by the rubber tube) in place and sutured, as seen from in front. (*Top, right*) Posterior view of same.

(*Bottom, left*) Superior view showing extra reinforcement of the joint capsule. (*Bottom, center*) Inferior view. (*Bottom, right*) Showing patient on whom this operation had been performed 6 months previously. Although he is lifting a heavy anvil, no difference can be detected in his 2 acromioclavicular joints. The original anatomy is reconstructed, and function is normal. (Surg., Gynec. & Obstet. *46*:563)

plexus. For correction of the internal rotation deformity he found the L'Episcopo operation to be better; and when the humerus was subluxated, he modified the Fairbank's reduction by detaching the pectoral and pinning the glenohumeral joint with a Steinmann pin.

When the upper end of the humerus was deformed, rotary osteotomy of the humerus above the deltoid insertion improved abduction as well as rotation.

W. T. Green lengthens the pectoralis major by a Z cut and the subscapularis by a sliding

FIG. 695. Operation for dislocation of the sternoclavicular joint (Bankart's method). The ends of the fascial strip have been brought through holes in the sternum and tied and are being held tight by an assistant while the surgeon sews the joint firmly with linen thread sutures. The firm surface of the joint which has been chiseled and turned down is replaced over the fascia (Bankart, A. S. B.: Brit. J. Surg. *26*:322).

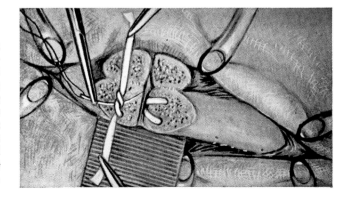

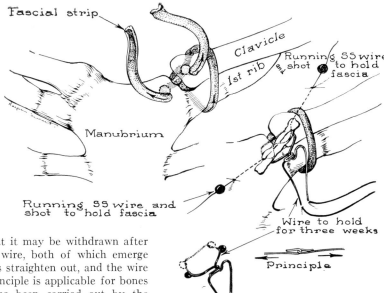

Fig. 696. Operation for dislocation of the sternoclavicular joint. Fascia lata 1 foot long is threaded through 2 holes and around the first costal cartilage in the manner shown and fastened to itself in front with a removable stainless-steel wire fastened outside the skin with 2 shot. The joint is kept from dislocating while the fascial graft is healing by a No. 22 stainless-steel wire placed through the 2 holes and fastened to itself in such a way that it may be withdrawn after 3 weeks. On pulling each wire, both of which emerge through the skin, the bends straighten out, and the wire can be withdrawn. This principle is applicable for bones elsewhere. The method has been carried out by the author with success.

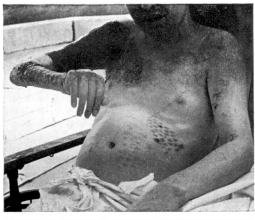

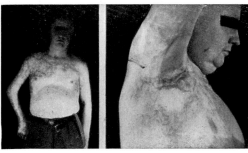

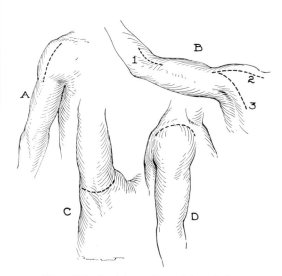

Fig. 697. Case C. B. (*Top*) An electrical flash burn which later caused flexion contracture of the axilla. (*Bottom, left*) Limit of abduction. The keloid was excised, substituting a split-skin graft held in place by a wax stent. (*Bottom, right*) Contracture relieved by skin graft.

Fig. 698. Incisions, harmful and harmless. (A, B) These incisions form broad scars and contractures, because they are in a direction at a right angle to the flexion creases. (C, D) These incisions give ample exposure of either side of the shoulder joint, leaving inconspicuous scars,

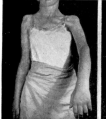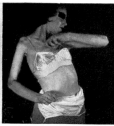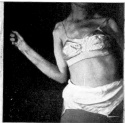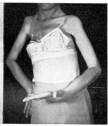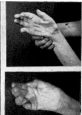

FIG. 699. Case B. H., age 22. From poliomyelitis at the age of 11, neither arm could be abducted and neither elbow flexed. (*Left*) Showing the limit of abduction at the shoulder and flexion at the elbow of either arm. (*Second picture*) Abduction of the left shoulder after arthrodesis. (*Third and fourth pictures*) Showing limit of flexion of each elbow and some supination after transferring the origin of the flexor muscles in the forearm from the internal epicondyle to up the external border of the humerus, using a free graft of fascia lata to span the distance. The object of fastening to the external border is to correct the pronatory tendency present when the internal border of the humerus is used.

FIG. 700. (*Left*) Keloids from burns due to the proliferation of deeper parts of the dermal layer. (*Right*) If the keloids are excised and skin grafts are applied, keloids do not reform. (William H. Frackelton, Lt. Col., M.C., Beaumont General Hospital.

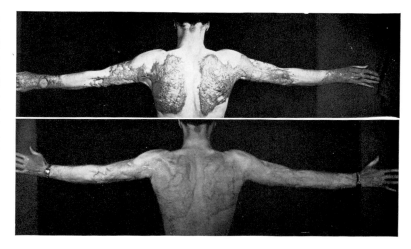

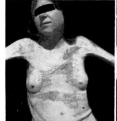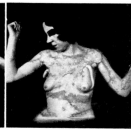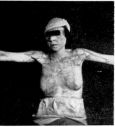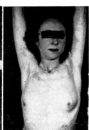

FIG. 701. Case G. M. The patient's dress had caught fire, resulting in disfiguring burns and inability to raise the arms. (*Left*) Flexion contractures of the axillae. Tubular pedicles have been made. (*Second picture*) Pedicles are being waltzed to the axillae. Some keloids have been removed from the arms. (*Third picture*) Intermediate stage Pedicled skin crosses the axillae. (*Fourth picture*) Keloids have been excised in stages, Lines of tension have been broken by pedicled skin,

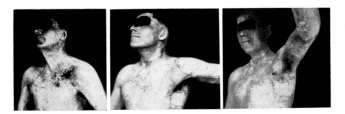

FIG. 702. Case J. S. (*Left*) Flexion contractures from burn. The patient cannot abduct his arm. (*Center* and *right*) Pedicle graft from abdomen to wrist to axilla allows raising of the arm. The neck was zigzagged.

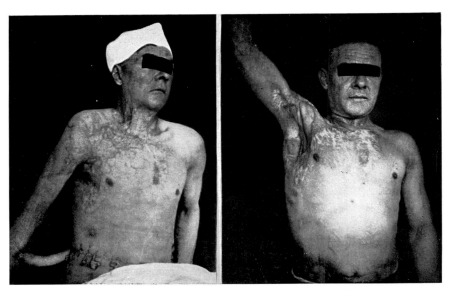

FIG. 703. Case F. C. (*Left*) Flexion contracture of the axilla from burn. An abdominal tubular pedicle has been attached to the wrist for transportation to the axilla. (*Right*) Pedicle skin has been placed across the line of tension of the contracture. Plastic work also was done on the neck.

FIG. 704. Arthrodesis of the shoulder 3 years after the Gill operation. After removing articular cartilage, the acromion is denuded and thrust into a slit in the humerus, suturing the periosteum above the acromion to the joint capsule attached to the humerus. The humerus forms an angle with the vertebral border of the scapula of about 45°, it being slightly greater in males. (Gill, A. B.: J. Bone Joint Surg. *13*:294)

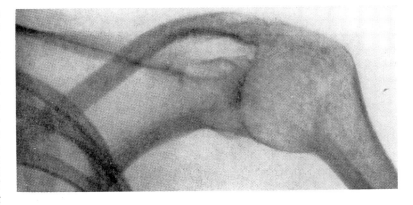

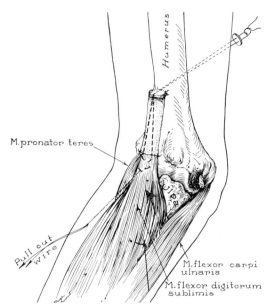

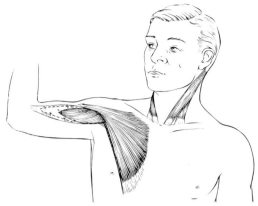

FIG. 707. Clark's operation, transferring the lower 2½-inch strip of pectoralis major down into the biceps, suturing into tendon. (J. Bone Joint Surg. *33-A*:567)

FIG. 705. Bunnell's modification of Steindler's operation for paralysis of the flexors of the elbow to furnish supination as well as flexion. The flexor muscles in the forearm are detached from the internal epicondyle, elongated by a free graft of fascia lata, which in turn is attached to the outer margin of the humerus so as to give not only flexion but also supination. Removable stainless-steel wire is used.

flap and transplants the latissimus dorsi and the teres major to give external rotation. For posterior subluxation, the capsule is reefed, and the triceps is shifted to the spine of the scapula. If necessary, a rotary ostotomy is done in the lower third of the humerus.

Scaglietti combines a rotary osteotomy of the surgical neck with the Sever procedure.

SALVAGE OPERATIONS FOR ADULTS WITH OLD PLEXUS LESIONS. In adults with severe residual paralysis, Yeoman and Seddon recom-

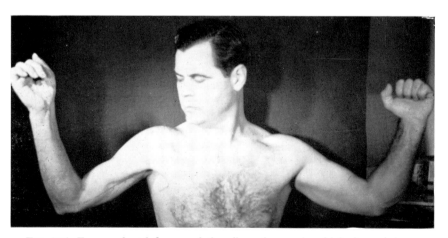

FIG. 706. For paralyzed flexors of the elbow from a brachial plexus injury, a 2½-inch strip from the lower part of the pectoral muscle was detached at its lower end and transferred with its nerve supply into the biceps muscle, restoring useful function.

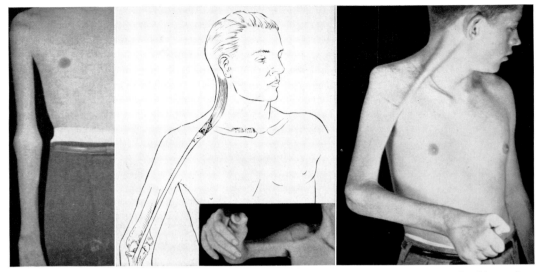

FIG. 708. Postpolio paralysis with flail shoulder and elbow and a few hand motions. Shoulder and wrist arthrodeses were done, and the sternocleidomastoid elongated with fascia lata to biceps to give elbow flexion. Transfers in the hand improved digital motions. (J. Bone Joint Surg. *33-A*:569)

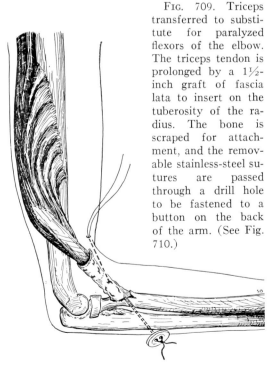

FIG. 709. Triceps transferred to substitute for paralyzed flexors of the elbow. The triceps tendon is prolonged by a 1½-inch graft of fascia lata to insert on the tuberosity of the radius. The bone is scraped for attachment, and the removable stainless-steel sutures are passed through a drill hole to be fastened to a button on the back of the arm. (See Fig. 710.)

mended amputation through the arm, shoulder arthrodesis and the use of a prosthesis. Of 17 patients treated in this way, 5 obtained satisfactory results. Factors acting against a good result were a long period between injury and amputation, osteoporosis of disuse and severe pain. Eight other patients were treated by various reconstructive procedures; none had a satisfactory result. Yeoman and Seddon felt that the prognosis could be determined within 8 weeks of injury and that in addition to a positive axon flare test, spasmodic pain and injuries from high-velocity missiles gave a bad prognosis. The optimal stump was 8 inches long with the shoulder fused in 20° flexion and 25° abduction, as determined by the vertebral borders of the scapula. Only 9 of 15 amputees used the prosthesis.

MUSCULOSKELETAL DISTURBANCES

Symptoms in the hand and the forearm may be the result of various disturbances at the thoracic outlet. Malunion of the clavicle, cervical ribs or poor posture may cause disturbances in the nerves or the vessels leading to

FIG. 710. Case J. M. Triceps elongated by tendon graft to the tuberosity of the radius for paralysis of the flexors of the elbow. This is a case from a series reported of repair of brachial plexus in which all 5 nerves were sutured. (*Left*) Abduction through suture of the brachial plexus. (*Right*) Strong flexion of the elbow

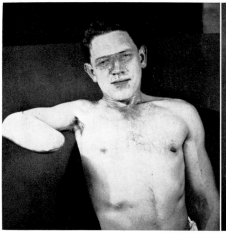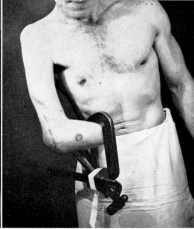

(can lift 20 lb.) through triceps transfer. Note the shadow of the triceps. The triceps was elongated by a 1½-inch tendon graft from an extensor of the wrist. Regenerated condylar flexors were also transferred up the humerus. At first he tensed the entire arm to flex the elbow, but after 5 months the elbow flexed naturally. All motions of the shoulder returned and felt natural, showing that the brain adapts to this degree.

complaints of pain, paresthesias, numbness or trophic changes in the fingers.

The scalenus anticus syndrome, in which the structures of the plexus are compressed behind a hypertrophied muscle or by a cervical rib, accounts for some of the symptoms. Most

discomfort should be in the ulnar nerve area. There may be a vasospasm, coldness or cyanosis, and gangrene of the finger has been reported. Adson's sign is obliteration of the pulse, when the chin is tilted up and turned to the affected side while the patient is sitting

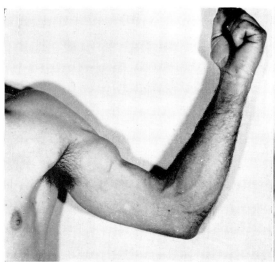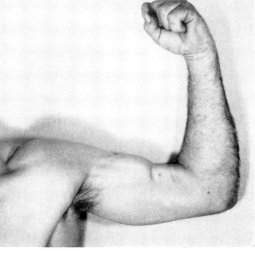

FIG. 711. Case W. E. I. (*Left*) A log the patient was holding fell, rupturing his lower biceps tendon at the insertion. Flexion of the elbow was weak and painful. Seven months later, the biceps was sutured to the bicipital tubercle of the radius through a graft of fascia lata according to the method described in this book. (*Right*) Four months later, there was good contour and strength. His grip was equal in both hands.

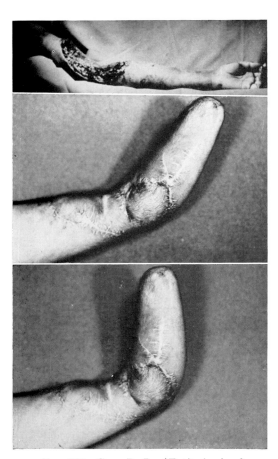

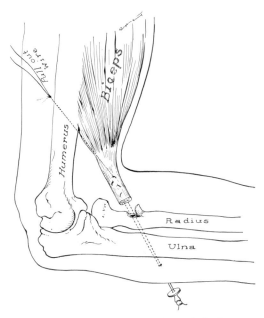

FIG. 713. Repair of evulsion of the lower tendon of the biceps by a simple method. The tuberosity of the radius is exposed by retracting apart the brachioradialis and the pronator teres muscles. After chipping up its surface, the stainless-steel wire sutures in the biceps tendon are passed through a drillhole and out the posterior side of the limb. On flexing the elbow and pulling on the sutures, the tendon is snugged into place and the sutures tied over a button. A pull-out wire is placed to withdraw the suture after 3 weeks.

FIG. 712. Case P. L. (*Top*) A circular saw had gouged out this boy's whole ante-cubital space, including the brachial artery and vein and the radial, the median and the ulnar nerves. A pedicle graft had been applied to the denudation. An attempt was made to overcome the 6½-inch gap in each nerve and unite them by suture. This was done by flexing the joints and shortening the humerus. However, the circulation of the arm proved insufficient, so that amputation was done through the forearm. Later, to give flexion to the elbow, the high stump of the biceps muscle was joined to the radius by a free graft of fascia lata. The 2 bottom illustrations show voluntary motion of the elbow 6 weeks postoperative.

up. Symptoms should be increased when the arm is pulled downward while the head is rotated away and backward. Conservative treatment and postural exercises will relieve the symptoms in most patients. Operation con-

sists of division of the scalenus anticus through an incision paralleling the skin creases. Ordinarily, it is not necessary to remove a cervical rib.

Paralysis of Scapulothoracic Muscles. These muscles stabilize and control the scapula and are the foundation of the kinetic chain that helps the hand to function. Three groups provide the motions. Those of the upper trapezius and the levator scapulae function can be helped by shifting a weak levator to a more lateral position or by transferring the sterno-cleidomastoid to the acromion.

The middle group (trapezius and rhomboids), if weak, can be stripped from the scapula and sutured on its dorsal surface. A fascial strap (Lowman) from the opposite scapular

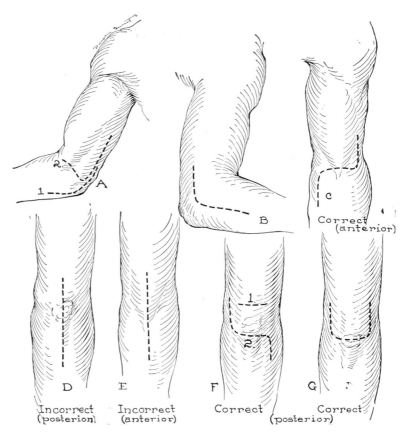

FIG. 714. Incisions for exposure about the elbow. (A) 1 — Exposes ulnar nerve for transplanting.   2 — Exposes front of elbow joint and humerus. (B) External lateral incision. (C) Exposes antecubital space without making a contracture. (D, E) Median longitudinal incisions in front and back of elbow which form keloid contractures and should not be used except for arthrodesis. (F, G) Exposure of back of elbow without causing contractures. 1—Shows incision for obtaining a graft of specialized paratenon fat from over the triceps tendon.

spine is useful, or several strips can be attached to the dorsal spinous processes.

Schottstaedt reported using the latissimus dorsi muscle of the opposite side, which was attached to the scapula and substituted for the rhomboids.

The lower muscle controlling the scapula, preventing winging and acting as a strong stabilizer, is the serratus anticus (anterior). Its insertion on the scapula may pull loose, or the nerve may suffer a stretch palsy. A brace to hold the scapula can be made for use postoperatively.

The scapula can be held to the chest wall

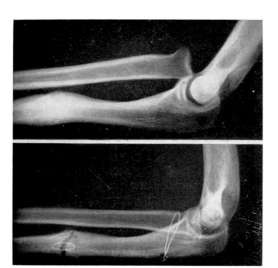

FIG. 715 (*Top*) Case G. P. Dislocation of the head of the radius with angulation of the ulna at fracture, where a horse had kicked the back of the ulna a year previously. (*Bottom*) At operation, the ulna was straightened, allowing the head of the radius to be replaced. Through a drillhole in the ulna, both a stainless-steel wire and a graft of the palmaris longus tendon were looped about the neck of the radius to hold it in place. The wire held until the tendon graft was strong, within a month, and then it was removed.

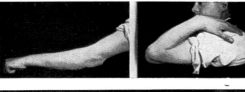

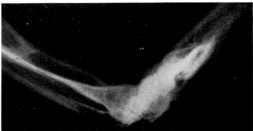

FIG. 716. Case A. E. H. Arthroplasty for stiff elbow from fracture. The tongue of the triceps tendon was turned down, the humerus shaped and capped with fascia lata and the head of the radius removed for rotary motion. (*Top, left*) Postoperative extension and pronation. (*Top, right*) Postoperative flexion and supination. (*Bottom*) Preoperative condition.

by fascial strips to the ribs, or the pectoralis minor can be transferred with good results. The pectoralis major has also been used.

Acromioclavicular Dislocation. Dislocations of the acromioclavicular joint should be treated conservatively, for Rowe showed that in 28 complete dislocations 80 per cent had excellent or good results regardless of the type of treatment. Moseley recommends that in all cases where there is evidence of increased coracoclavicular spacing with traction or weights applied to the arm, the outer end of the clavicle be resected and the upward displacement of the clavicle be prevented by passing a fascial strip around the coracoid and the clavicle. In young adults, Rowe passes Kirschner wires across the joint with direct suture of the ruptured coracoclavicular ligament if possible. Incomplete separations can be treated with sling and bandage with good results, though derangement of the joint often occurs. For late arthritis, resection of the distal end of the clavicle gives satisfactory results.

A reconstruction operation restoring both the coracoid and the trapezoid ligaments consists of using a fascia lata graft passed through the acromion back up through the clavicle, around the back of the clavicle to hook under the coracoid process and back up through the clavicle again. The ends are sutured together over the bone denuded of periosteum. Removable wire sutures aids stabilization until the fascia heals.

Sternoclavicular Separation. If painful and unstable, a fascial graft can be passed through the 2 bones (Lowman) or looped behind the joint exposed by turning back a bone flap (Bankart) or by a strand of fascia through the sternum and the clavicle and looped behind the first costal cartilage. Removable wire holds the bones in place until the fascia has healed.

Deltoid Paralysis. Arthrodesis of the shoulder is the best procedure for complete deltoid paralysis, since tendon transfers require good strong action in all the other shoulder rotators as well as some deltoid activity.

Mayer's operation is a fascial graft to lengthen the detached trapezius insertion to the deltoid insertion. Unless there is good function in the supraspinatus and the infraspinatus and some remaining activity in the deltoid, arthrodesis is advisable.

Ober's operation—transfer of biceps (short head) and triceps (long head) to a slit in the acromion—requires some remaining deltoid activity for satisfactory results.

Harmon, in patients with remaining activity in the posterior third of the deltoid, shifts this active portion anteriorly; he reports good results.

Hildebrandt used two thirds of the pectoral, detaching its origin and swinging it over the acromion.

Schottstaedt, Larson and Bost used the entire muscle, transposing its origin and leaving the insertion in place.

Contractures From Disuse. After a hand injury or operation, patients will try to protect the part by holding the arm at the side, or, from prolonged use of a sling there will develop limited shoulder motions. Demanding a full range of motion every day from the beginning is the best prevention. The shoulder-depressing muscles are much stronger than the abductors and the external rotators, and gravity aids them. Biceps tendonitis or spasm in the biceps muscle causes much shoulder impairment.

TREATMENT. Exercises, active and directed,

such as "climbing the wall," hanging from parallel bars or, if necessary, traction on a sloping bed are all used. Manipulation under anesthesia is seldom necessary or advisable.

Surgical Approaches. Some of the commonly used incisions result in ugly thick keloid scars when they cross the creases. A transverse "saber cut" incision over the top and similarly a transverse incision in the axilla provide excellent exposure and result in minimal scarring.

ARTHRODESIS OF SHOULDER. Gill's operation can be done after the age of 6 if there is good scapular control. The joint surfaces are denuded, and a wedge is cut in the greater tuberosity to receive the denuded acromion. Referring to the vertebral border of the scapula, abduction of 45° and flexion and internal rotation of 15° is recommended for girls; 10° more in abduction and flexion is advised for boys. The worst thing in an arthrodesis is a position of external rotation. If forward flexion is limited, resection of the outer end of the clavicle will improve the position (Milgrim). In females it is important to preserve the conoid and the trapezoid ligaments.

The use of a Steinmann pin as a temporary fixation to determine the optimal position for fusion has been recommended by Davis.

FIG. 717. (*Top*) Cicatrix at elbow. (*Bottom*) Defect at elbow covered by direct pedicle flap. Raw areas were skin grafted. (W. B. Macomber, M.D.)

ROTATOR CUFF TEARS. From a fall, repeated trauma or attrition of age a part of the musculotendinous cuff of the shoulder may tear, producing pain and tenderness over the point of injury and impaired shoulder motion. In tears of the supraspinatus portion there will be apparent atrophy of the muscle. McLaughlin feels that tears are through pathologic tissue and that the results of delayed operation are as good as those done early. Operative reconstruction consists of excision of damaged tissue and closure of the rent in the cuff by approximation of healthy tissues. Removal of a portion of acromion can be done if it blocks abduction.

LONG HEAD OF BICEPS. Rupture of this tendon is frequent; the belly is displaced toward

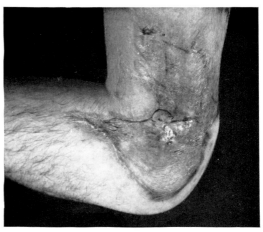

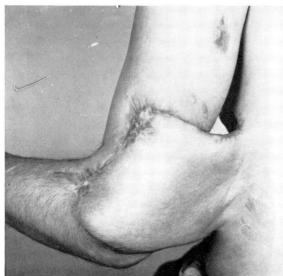

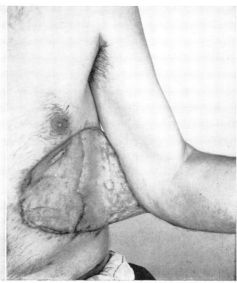

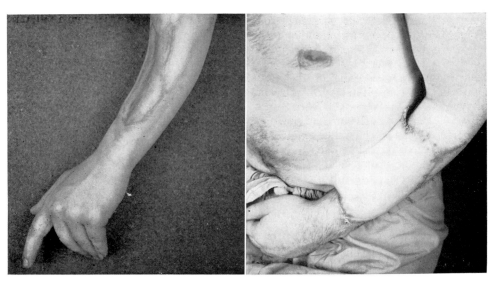

Fig. 718. Cicatrical defect of the radiodorsal aspect of the forearm. Direct flap from the abdomen applied preparatory to tendon grafts and transfers. (L. D. Howard, M.D.)

the elbow, and elbow flexion is slightly weaker. Unless there is a bicipital tendinitis of the intracapsular portion of the tendon or injury to the rotator cuff, shoulder symptoms will be lacking.

Treatment consists of attaching the ruptured distal portion into the bicipital groove or into the tendon of the short head. The former is preferred. If shoulder symptoms are present, the capsule should be exposed to check the cuff tendons and excise the remains of the biceps tendon.

If the biceps tendon dislocates in and out of the bicipital groove, it should be fixed in the groove as described above.

DISLOCATION OF THE SHOULDER. For recurrent shoulder dislocations the Bankart and Putti-Platt operations are most often used. A method utilizing an axillary approach severs only the subscapularis tendon. The plicated capsule and the distal stub of this tendon are sutured to the freshened edge of the glenoid. A pull-out wire suture is used. The subscapularis is used to reinforce the repair.

ELBOW REGION

PARALYSIS OF ELBOW FLEXORS

Paralysis of elbow flexors markedly impairs the function of the hand. This motion is of

major importance in placing the hand, bringing it to the mouth and the head and pulling objects toward the body. If the shoulder is stable or under good control and the hand is not a flail hand, efforts to restore elbow flexion are justified.

Steindler Flexorplasty. This is an advancement of the origin of the flexors and the pronator teres up the humerus, changing the angle of approach and giving ability to flex the elbow. If the flexor muscles are strong, good flexion is obtained with some loss of extension. Unless strong supinators are present, there is a tendency toward pronation. A weak triceps predisposes to flexion contractures. A modification which lengthens the muscles with a fascial graft to reach the lateral aspect of the humerus tends to prevent excessive pronation. A modification by Eyler, leaving the flexor ulnaris intact and transposing the origins of the pronator, the flexor carpi radialis and the superficialis to the midline of the arm results in less pronation deformity. Transfer of the flexor carpi ulnaris around the forearm to insert on the radius aids in supination.

Triceps to Biceps Transfer. The triceps is divided, brought around the humerus under the radial nerve, lengthened with a fascial or tendon graft and inserted into the radius. Strong flexion results, but all extensor power

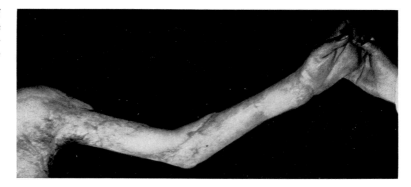

FIG. 719. Relief of flexion contracture at the elbow by a tubular pedicle graft from the abdomen.

is destroyed, since the entire triceps insertion must be used. In patients using crutches, triceps function should be retained and some other means of obtaining flexion found.

Pectoralis Major Transfer. Clark used the lower part of the pectoral muscle; it was separated from its origin, mobilized and swung on its neurovascular pedicle, and passed down the arm to attach to the biceps tendon. Seddon used this method in loss from poliomyelitis and brachial plexus lesions with good results if the shoulder was stable, and later Brooks and Seddon reported a modification in which the long head of the biceps was deliberately devascularized, drawn out at a lower incision and then passed back up through the divided pectoral tendon and returned down the arm to be attached to itself. If the shoulder was stabilized by arthrodesis, results were good.

Bradford in 1910 used the pectoralis minor, and Spira reported a case in which he lengthened it with a fascial graft. The elbow flexed through an arc of 135°.

Schottstaedt, Larson and Bost transferred the muscle origin as in the Clark procedure but also shifted the insertion to the coracoid. They also used the latissimus dorsi, shifting both its origin and insertion.

Sternocleidomastoid to Biceps. For flail shoulder and elbow, the shoulder is arthrodesed, and the sternocleidomastoid elongated by a fascial graft to the radial tubercle. R. Carroll reported its use in 15 patients with resulting satisfactory elbow flexion in 80 per cent. He points out that the attachments are made under maximal tension.

Elbow Flexion by Prosthesis. A lightweight hinged prosthesis can be activated by the other shoulder to provide elbow flexion, or a cable over the shoulder to a spring-powered reel on the shoe can be used as the motor (from Robin's Aids).

RUPTURE OF DISTAL BICEPS TENDON

This injury is less common than rupture of the tendon of the long head in the upper arm and often consists of a tear at the insertion, making repair difficult. Reconstruction should be done by restoring the true action of the biceps as a supinator and not just suturing to the brachialis fascia. Exposure can be obtained through a transverse incision, undermining the skin and opening the deep fascia longitudinally between the pronator teres and the brachioradialis. The tubercle is exposed, and, with the forearm supinated, a flap of bone is raised and a hole drilled through the radius. The tendon, lengthened with a graft if necessary, is attached with a pull-out wire tied to a button on the extensor surface of the forearm. The elbow is splinted in flexion for a month, and the sutures are removed.

PARALYSIS OF TRICEPS

Extension of the elbow is useful in walking on crutches and in pushing up from a bed or a chair. Ober and Barr used the brachioradialis, transferring it behind the condyle to the triceps fascia. Merle d'Aubigne transferred the posterior deltoid to the triceps. Schottstaedt, Larsen and Bost transposed the latissimus dorsi attaching its origin to the triceps tendon and its insertion to acromion.

NERVE INJURIES AT ELBOW

The ulnar nerve is subject to trauma in its course behind the internal condyle and is often

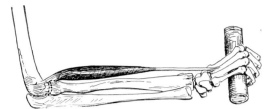

Fig. 720. Mechanism of tennis elbow. Gripping is accomplished by stabilizing the wrist in dorsiflexion by the 3 extensor carpi muscles while the flexors of the digits contract. If done to excess, the origin of the extensor carpi radialis brevis is strained and remains sore (tennis elbow).

stretched and bruised in elbow dislocations and fractures in this area. A tardy ulnar palsy may develop from old injuries and deformities. The nerve can be transposed to the front of the elbow, shortening its course, and large defects in the forearm can be overcome.

Transposition of the nerve should be through a long incision curving anteriorly over the internal condyle, dividing the flexor muscle origins. After careful freeing of the nerve, it is passed on a direct line to the forearm beneath the flexor muscles. The sharp edge of the intermuscular septum extending proximal from the condyle should be excised, and at the distal end the nerve should not be allowed to make a sharp turn into the muscle. The nerve lies in the natural intermuscular plane, not through the muscle bellies. The muscle origins are resutured, and the elbow is splinted in flexion for 3 weeks.

ELBOW JOINT

Surgical Aspects. Incisions in the elbow region as in any area should follow the skin creases. Lateral incisions curve around the condyles. Transverse incisions are used on the volar and the dorsal surfaces, undermining the skin widely to allow access to the longitudinal structures beneath. A lateral extension of the transverse incision up one side and down the other as a bayonet gives wide exposure. Splitting the triceps tendon and muscle exposes the back of the elbow joint and the lower humerus.

The antecubital space should be protected and its venous plexus preserved, and in postoperative dressings and splints all pressure in

this area should be avoided. The skin of this area may be used for a full-thickness graft to the hand, and, especially in children, suturing the edges with the elbow flexed avoids wide undermining and does not permanently limit extension.

Arthrodesis of Elbow. No one position is optimal for this joint, but if both elbows are to be stiff, one should be at such an angle to enable the hand to reach the month. One at 70° and the other at 115° is a good compromise.

Arthroplasty. Except in children and the aged this is a satisfactory operation. Lateral stability is usually good, and a useful range of motion can be obtained. The operations devised by Murphy, MacAusland and Campbell are used. Fascia lata is used for interpositio membrane, and the upper radius is freed for pronation and supination.

Excision of Elbow. For extremely comminuted fractures involving the elbow joint, excision may give a reasonable range of motion and a stable elbow. Intact strong biceps and triceps muscles are necessary for stability, and all ligamentous structures and muscle attachments are maintained.

Osteochondritis of Elbow. Following a minor injury to the elbow roentgenograms may show an irregularity of the capitellum that is difficult to explain on the basis of trauma. Panner's disease or an osteochondritis of this area usually can be distinguished by comparable views disclosing the deformity of the whole articular surface.

TENNIS ELBOW—EPICONDYLITIS

This term is used to describe a painful condition of the region of the external epicondyle or over the radiohumeral joint. Tenderness is usually marked and quite localized over the origin of the extensor carpi radialis brevis, and any action such as dorsiflexing the wrist or strong grasp accentuates the pain. It is often self-limited but usually can be relieved by rest and local injection of hydrocortone into the painful area. Refractory cases may be relieved by operative division of the fibers at the origin, but the results hardly warrant its use routinely. Bosworth described a group of patients with symptoms of pain and tenderness, relieved by sectioning of the orbicular ligament of the upper radioulnar joint.

BIBLIOGRAPHY

Abbott, L. C., and Lucas, D. B.: The tripartite deltoid and its surgical significance in exposure of the scapulohumeral joint, Ann. Surg. *136*: 392, 1952.

Adson, H. W.: The gross pathology of brachial plexus injuries, Surg., Gynec. Obstet. *34*:351, 1922.

Adson, H. W., and Coffey, J. R.: A method of anterior approach for relief of symptoms by division of the scalenus anticus, Ann. Surg. *85*: 839, 1927.

Aitken, A. P., Smith, L., and Blackett, C. W.: Supracondylar fractures in children, Am. J. Surg. *59*:161, 1943.

Albee, F. H.: Orthopedic and Reconstructive Surgery, Philadelphia, Saunders, 1919.

Allen, P. D., and Gramse, A. E.: Transcondylar fractures of the humerus treated by Dunlop traction, Am. J. Surg. *67*:217, 1945.

Am. Orth. Assn. Committee: A survey of end results on stabilization of the paralytic shoulder, J. Bone Joint Surg. *24*:699, 1942.

Anderson, K. J., and LeCocq, J. F.: Rupture of the triceps tendon, J. Bone Joint Surg. *39-A*: 44, 1957.

Anton, J. I., and Reitz, G. B.: Ulnar nerve paralysis, complicating fracture of medial epicondyle of humerus, Am. J. Surg. *49*:89, 1940.

Arkin, A. M.: Habitual luxation of ulnar nerve, J. Mt. Sinai Hosp. *7*:208, 1940.

Aufranc, O. E., Jones, W. N., and Harris, W. H.: Complete acromioclavicular dislocation, J.A.M.A. *180*:681, 1962.

Badgley, C. E.: Brachialgia, Regional Orthopaedic Surgery and Fundamental Orthopaedic Problems, No. 11, p. 80, Ann Arbor, Mich., Edwards, 1948.

Bankart, A. S. B.: The pathology and treatment of recurrent dislocation of the shoulder-joint, Brit. J. Surg. *26*:23, 1938.

————: An operation for recurrent dislocation of the sternoclavicular joint, Brit. J. Surg. *26*:320, 1938.

Basnajian, J. V., and Latif, A.: Integrated actions and functions of the chief flexors of the elbow, J. Bone Joint Surg. *39-A*:1106, 1957.

Bennett, G. E.: Old dislocation of the shoulder, J. Bone Joint Surg. *18*:594, 1936.

————: Shoulder and elbow lesions distinctive of baseball players, Ann. Surg. *126*:107, 1947.

Bloom, F. A.: Wire fixation in acromioclavicular dislocation, J. Bone Joint Surg. *27*:273, 1945.

Blount, W. P.: Osteoclasis for supination deformities in children, J. Bone Joint Surg. *22*:300, 1940.

————: Conditions involving elbow, forearm, wrist and hand; progress in orthopedic surgery for 1942, Arch. Surg. *48*:169, 1944.

————: Progress in orthopedic surgery for 1943; conditions involving elbow, forearm, wrist and hand, Arch. Surg. *49*:258, 1944.

Bonney, G.: Prognosis in traction lesions of the brachial plexus, J. Bone Joint Surg. *41-B*:4, 1959.

Bost, F. C., and Inman, V. T.: The pathologic changes in recurrent dislocation of the shoulder —a report of Bankart's operative procedure, J. Bone Joint Surg. *24*:595, 1942.

Bosworth, B. M.: Muscular and tendinous defects of shoulder and their repair, Am. Acad. Orth. Surg. Lect., p. 380, 1944.

————: Acromioclavicular dislocation, Ann. Surg. *127*:98, 1948.

Boyd, H. B., and Stone, M. M.: Resection of the distal end of the ulna, J. Bone Joint Surg. *26*: 313, 1944.

Braimbridge, C. V.: Excision of the elbow joint, Lancet *1*:53, 1948.

Brooks, D., and Seddon, H. J.: Pectoral transplantation for paralysis of the flexors of the elbow, J. Bone Joint Surg. *41-B*:36, 1959.

Bunnell, S.: Fascial graft for dislocation of acromioclavicular joint, Surg., Gynec. Obstet. *40*: 563, 1928.

————: Restoring flexion to the paralytic elbow, J. Bone Joint Surg. *33-A*:566, 1951.

Burman, M.: Paralytic supination contracture of the forearm, J. Bone Joint Surg. *38-A*:303, 1956.

Campbell, W.: Operative Orthopedics, St. Louis, Mosby, 1939.

Carroll, R. E.: Restoration of flexor power to the flail elbow by transplantation of the triceps tendon, Surg., Gynec. Obstet. *95*:685, 1952.

Chaves, J. P.: Pectoralis minor transplant for paralysis of the serratus anterior, J. Bone Joint Surg. *33-B*:228, 1951.

Clark, J. M. P.: Reconstruction of biceps brachii by pectoral muscle transplantation, Brit. J. Surg. *34*:180, 1946.

Codman, E. A.: The Shoulder, Boston, Thomas Todd Co., 1934.

Cohn, B. N. E.: Painful shoulder due to lesions of the cervical spine, Am. J. Surg. *66*:269, 1944.

Corbin, K. B.: The anatomic basis for the more common types of mechanical brachial neuritis, Regional Orthopaedic Surgery and Fundamental Orthopaedic Problems, No. 11, p. 57, Ann Arbor, Mich., Edwards, 1948.

Cyriax, J. H.: The pathology and treatment of tennis elbow, J. Bone Joint Surg. *18*:921, 1936.

Darrach, W.: Surgical approaches for surgery of extremities, Am. J. Surg. *67*:237, 1945.

Davis, L., Martin, J., and Perret, G.: The treatment of injuries of the brachial plexus, Ann. Surg. *125*:647, 1947.

Deline, E.: Fractures at upper end of humerus, Surg. Clin. N. Amer. *25*:28, 1945.

Dickson, F. D.: Fascial transplants in paralytic and other conditions, J. Bone Joint Surg. *19*:405, 1937.

Dobbie, R. P.: Avulsion of the lower biceps bracii tendon, Am. J. Surg. *51*:662, 1941.

Dorling, G. C.: Fascial slinging of the scapula and clavicle for dropped shoulder and winged scapult, Brit. J. Surg. *32*:311, 1944.

Durman, D. C.: An operation for paralysis of the serratus anterior, J. Bone Joint Surg. *27*:380, 1945.

Eckhoff, N. L.: Cervical rib and brachial plexus lesions, Guy's Hosp. Gaz. *55*:135, 1941.

Eden, K. C.: Vascular complications of cervical ribs and first thoracic rib abnormalities, Brit. J. Surg. *27*:111, 1939.

Eyre-Brook, A. L.: The morbid anatomy of a case of recurrent dislocation of the should: Brit. J. Surg. *30*:32, 1942.

Finochiette, R., and Dickman, G. H.: Traumatic lesions of the brachial plexus in adults: Technique of surgical therapy, Arch. argent. neurol. *23*:30, 1940.

Flothow, P. G.: Cervical rib and the anterior scalenus syndrome, West. J. Surg. *44*:570, 1936.

Foerster, O.: Value of orthopedic fixation operations in nerve disease; compensation for combined serratus-trapezius paralysis by fixation of scapula to ribs with silver wire; compensation for thenar paralysis by fixation of first metacarpal in flexed position by a bone implant between first and second metacarpals, Acta chir. scand. *67*:351, 1930.

Frankel, E.: Humero-radial synostosis, Brit. J. Surg. *31*:242, 1944.

Gage, M.: Scalenus anticus syndrome: Diagnosis and confirmation test, Surgery *5*:599, 1939.

Garden, R. S.: Tennis elbow, J. Bone Joint Surg. *43-B*:100, 1961.

Gibbens, M. E.: An appliance for the conservative treatment of acromioclavicular dislocation, J. Bone Joint Surg. *28*:164, 1946.

Gilcreest, E. L., and Albi, P.: Rupture of muscles dislocation and elongation of long head of biceps brachii; analysis of 100 cases, Surg., Gynec. Obstet. *58*:322, 1934.

Gilcreest, E. L., and Albi, P.: Rupture of muscles and tendons, particularly subcutaneous rupture of biceps flexor cubit, J.A.M.A. *84*:1819, 1925.

————: Unusual lesions of muscles and tendons of shoulder girdle and upper arm, Surg., Gynec. Obstet. *68*:903, 1939.

Gill, A. B.: A new operation for arthrodesis of the shoulder, J. Bone Joint Surg. *13*:287, 1931.

Gotze, W.: Lesion of brachial plexus in peripheral nerve injuries, Arch. Psychiat. *112*:469, 1940.

Haas, S. L.: Longitudinal osteotomy, J.A.M.A. *92*:1656, 1929.

————: The treatment of permanent paralysis of the deltoid muscle, J.A.M.A. *104*:99, 1935.

Haggart, G. E.: Value of conservative management in cervicobrachial pain, J.A.M.A. *137*:508, 1948.

Hansson, K. G.: Scalenus anticus syndrome, Surg. Clin. N. Amer. *22*:611, 1942.

Henderson, M. S.: Habitual dislocation of the shoulder, J.A.M.A. *95*:1653, 1930.

————: Results following tenosuspension operations for habitual dislocation of the shoulder, J. Bone Joint Surg. *17*:978, 1935.

————: Tenosuspension operation for habitual dislocation of shoulder, Proc. Mayo Clin. *19*:5, 1944.

Henry, M. O.: Acromioclavicular dislocations, Minnesota Med. *12*:431, 1929.

Herzmark, M. H.: Traumatic paralysis of the serratus anterior relieved by transplantation of the rhomboidei, J. Bone Joint Surg. *33-A*:235, 1951.

Hill, R. M.: Vascular anomalies of upper limbs associated with cervical ribs; report of case and review of literature, Brit. J. Surg. *27*:100, 1939.

Howorth, M. B.: Calcification of the tendon cuff of the shoulder, Surg., Gynec. Obstet. *80*:337, 1945.

Jackson, R.: Cervical syndrome, Am. Acad. Orth. Surg. Instr. Course Lect., Vol. 10, Chap. 3, Ann Arbor, Mich., Edwards, 1953.

Jones, L.: Complete rupture of supraspinatus tendon; a simplified operative repair, Arch. Surg. *49*:390, 1944

Kaplan, E. B.: Tennis elbow, J. Bone Joint Surg. *41-A*:147, 1959.

Kelikian, H., and Doumanian, A.: Swivel for proximal radio-ulnar synostosis, J. Bone Joint Surg. *39-A*:945, 1957.

Kettlekamp, D. B., and Larson, C. B.: Evaluation of the Steindler flexorplasty, Paper No. 21, Am. Acad. Orth. Surg., January 31, 1962.

King, T., and Morgan, F. P.: Late results of removing the medial humeral epicondyle for traumatic ulnar neuritis, J. Bone Joint Surg. *41-B*:51, 1960.

Kleinberg, S.: Reattachment of the capsule and external rotators of the shoulder for obstetric paralysis, J.A.M.A. *98*:294, 1932.

Kolodney, A.: Traction paralysis of brachial plexus, Am. J. Surg. *51*:620, 1941.

Lowman, C. L.: Operative correction of old sternoclavicular dislocation, J. Bone Joint Surg. *10*: 740, 1928.

————: The use of fascia lata in the repair of disability of the wrist, J. Bone Joint Surg. *12*: 400, 1930.

MacAusland, W. R.: Mobilization of elbow by free fascia transplant, with report of 31 cases, Surg., Gynec. Obstet. *33*:223, 1921.

McLaughlin, H. L.: Lesions of the musculotendinous cuff of the shoulder. I. The exposure and treatment of tears with retraction, J. Bone Joint Surg. *26*:31, 1944.

Magnuson, P. B.: Treatment of recurrent dislocation of the shoulder, Surg. Clin. N. Amer. *25*:14, 1945.

Makowski, S. J.: Calcific deposits in supraspinatus tendon, Med. Times, N. Y. *70*:19, 1942.

Mayer, L.: Transplantation of the trapezius for paralysis of the abductors of the arm, J. Bone Joint Surg. *9*:412, 1927.

Mayer, L., and Greene, W.: Experiences with the Steindler flexor plasty at the elbow, J. Bone Joint Surg. *36-A*:775, 1954.

Meehan, A.: Treatment of late contractures resulting from Erb's palsy, Med. J. Australia *2*:464, 1940.

Merle d'Aubigne, R., Seddon, H. J., Hendy, A. M., and Brooks, D. M.: Symposium on reconstructive surgery of the paralyzed upper limb, Proc. Roy Soc. Med. *42*:831, Section 53-66, 1949.

Meyer, A. W.: Spontaneous dislocation and destruction of tendon of long head of biceps brachii, Arch. Surg. *17*:493, 1928.

Morrison, G. M.: Cast treatment of acromioclavicular dislocations, J. Bone Joint Surg. *30-A*:238, 1948.

Moseley, H. F.: Ruptures of the Rotator Cuff, Springfield, Ill., Thomas, 1952.

————: Disorders of the shoulder, Ciba Clinical Symposia *2*:251, 1950.

————: The inferior relations of the glenohumeral joint, Am. J. Surg. *83*:321, 1952.

Nachlas, I. W.: Brachialgia, J. Bone Joint Surg. *26*:177, 1944.

Nicholson, J. T.: Compound comminuted fractures involving the elbow joint, J. Bone Joint Surg. *28*:565, 1946.

Nicola, T.: Recurrent anterior dislocation of the shoulder, J. Bone Joint Surg. *11*:128, 1929.

North, J. P.: Tennis elbow—collective rview, Surg., Gynec. Obstet. *67*:176, 1938.

Ober, F. R.: An operation to relieve paralysis of the deltoid muscles, J.A.M.A. *99*:2182, 1932.

————: Transplantation to improve function of shoulder point and extensor function of elbow joint, Am. Acad. Orth. Surg. Lect., p. 274, 1944.

Ober, F. R., and Barr, J. S.: Brachioradialis muscle transposition for triceps weakness, Surg., Gynec. Obstet. *67*:105, 1938.

Omer, G. S., and Conger, C. W.: Osteochondrosis of the capitulum humeri (Panner's disease), U. S. Armed Forces M. J. *10*:1235, 1959.

Oppenheimer, A.: Arthritis of acromioclavicular joint, J. Bone Joint Surg. *25*:867, 1943.

Osmond-Clarke, H.: Habitual dislocation of the shoulder, the Putti-Platt operation, J. Bone Joint Surg. *30-B*:19, 1948.

Postlethwait, R. W.: Modified treatment for fracture of the head of the radius, Am. J. Surg. *67*:77, 1945.

Putti, V.: Obstetric and poliomyelitic paralytic syndromes of upper extremity: Surgical therapy with note on physiopathology of rotation of forearm, Chir. org. movimento *26*:215, 1940.

Reichert, F. L.: Compression of brachial plexus; the scalenus anticus syndrome, J.A.M.A. *118*: 294, 1942.

Ruhlin, C. W.: Clinical study of obstetric paralysis. J. Maine M. A. *32*:205, 1941.

Schottstaedt, E. R., Larsen, L. J., and Bost, F. C.: The surgical reconstruction of the upper extremity paralyzed by poliomyelitis, J. Bone Joint Surg. *40-A*:633, 1958.

Seddon, H. J.: The use of autogenous grafts for the repair of large gaps in peripheral nerves, Brit. J. Surg. *35*:151, 1947.

————: Transplantation of pectoralis major for paralysis of the flexors of the elbow, Proc. Roy. Soc. Med. *42*:837, 1949.

Segat, A., Seddon, H. J., and Brooks, D. M.: Treatment of paralysis of the flexors of the elbow, J. Bone Joint Surg. *41-B*:44, 1959.

Sever, J. W.: Results of a new operation for obstetrical paralysis, Am. J. Orth. Surg. *16*: 248, 1918.

————: Obstetric paralysis, J.A.M.A. *85*:1862, 1925.

————: Obstetric paralysis, Surg., Gynec. Obstet. *44*:547, 1927.

Snedecor, S. T., and Graham, W. C.: Severe war injuries of the elbow, J. Bone Joint Surg. *27*: 623, 1945.

Spira, E.: The treatment of dropped shoulder, J. Bone Joint Surg. *30-A*:229, 1948.

————: Replacement of biceps brachii by pectoral minor transplant, J. Bone Joint Surg. *39-B*:126, 1957.

Stammers, F. A. R.: Pain in the upper limb from mechanisms in the costoclavicular space, Lancet *1*:603, 1950.

Steindler, A.: Reconstructive Surgery of the

Upper Extremity, New York, Appleton, 1923.
———: Operations on the upper extremity: Problems in kinetics; end results, J. Bone Joint Surg. *9*:404, 1927.
———: Mechanics of Normal and Pathological Locomotion in Man, Springfield, Ill., Thomas, 1935.
———: Tendon transplantations in the upper extremity, Am. J. Surg. *44*:260, 1939.
———: Orthopedic Operations, Springfield, Ill., Thomas, 1940.
———: Transplantation of tendons at elbow, Am. Acad. Orth. Surg. Lect., p. 276, 1944.
Taylor, A. S.: Brachial birth palsy and injuries of similar type in adults, Surg., Gynec. Obstet. *30*:494, 1920.
———: Brachial Birth Palsy *in* Lewis, Dean (ed.): Practice of Surgery, vol. 3, Hagerstown, Md., Prior, 1929.
Telford, E. D.: Cervical rib and hyperhydrosis, Brit. J. Surg. *2*:96, 1942.
Theis, F. B.: Scalenus anticus syndrome and cervical ribs, Surgery *6*:112, 1939.
Thorndike, A., Jr., and Quigley, T. B.: Injuries to acromioclavicular joint, Am. J. Surg. *55*:250, 1942.
Toglar, J. L.: Operation for chronic dislocation of infected radio-ulnar articulation, Texas J. Med. *35*:278, 1939.

Tracy, J. F., and Brannon, E. W.: Management of brachial plexus injuries (traction type), J. Bone Joint Surg. *40-A*:1031, 1958.
Urist, M. R.: Complete dislocations of the acromioclavicular joint, J. Bone Joint Surg. *28*:813, 1946.
White, J. C., Poppel, M. H., and Adams, R.: Congenital malformations of first thoracic rib; cause of brachial neuralgia which simulates cervical rib syndrome, Surg., Gynec. Obstet. *81*:643, 1945.
Wickstrom, J.: Birth injuries of the brachial plexus, Clin. Orthop. *23*:187, 1962.
Wickstrom, J., *et al.*: Surgical management of residual deformities of the shoulder following birth injuries of the brachial plexus, J. Bone Joint Surg. *37-A*:27, 1955.
Wilson, P. D.: Capsulectomy for relief of flexion contractures of elbow following fracture, J. Bone Joint Surg. *26*:71, 1944.
Wright, I. S.: Neurovascular syndrome produced by hyperabduction of arms; immediate changes produced in 150 normal controls, and effects on some persons of prolonged hyperabduction of arms in sleeping, and in certain occupations, Am. Heart J. *29*:1, 1945.
Yeoman, P. M., and Seddon, H. J.: Brachial plexus injuries: Treatment of the flail arm, J. Bone Joint Surg. *43-B*:493, 1961.

Chapter 15

Wounds, Burns and Amputations

WOUNDS

GENERAL TREATMENT

Living things always have been subject to injury, but the present era might well be called the age of trauma. Each year industrial machinery and highway traffic cause more injuries than a war. Through the ages both plants and animals have developed methods of healing every type of tissue. The healing of fractures in prehistoric reptiles appears to have been the same as that seen in the bones of humans today. If circumstances are favorable, bones, tendons, nerves and ligaments rejoin, skin re-covers denuded areas, and arthritic joints splint themselves. An injured animal licks the wound clean and rests the injured part. The body tissues react with hyperemia to bring repair material to the damaged area, muscle spasm splints a painful part, and infection becomes walled off in abscesses which point and discharge the necrotic tissues.

As surgeons, we should build up these fundamentals, aid these processes and not interfere with the natural course of events. We should help to restore the favorable conditions and prevent the unfavorable. Certain fundamental principles in the treatment of all open wounds can be followed:

We can remove the contaminating material from the wound by thorough washing and irrigation.

We can refrain from introducing new contaminants or increasing the trauma to the tissues by using aseptic technics in handling the wound and not introducing mechanical or chemical agents to add to the injury.

We can cleanse the surrounding skin and prevent entrance of contaminated material into the wound.

We can excise the devitalized damaged tissues by removing mechanically the contaminated layer of tissue exposed by the wounding force.

We can cover all vulnerable structures, such as tendons, nerves, bones and joints, with viable tissue. In the presence of infection we can promote localization and drainage.

By these procedures we provide the optimal conditions for healing of the parts; rest and time assure the final repair.

Adequate circulation of the parts is essential. Ischemia results from joining deep tissues and skin under too much tension or from pressure dressings or unyielding plaster dressings over a swelling part. Stasis and congestive edema can result from a proximal constrictive bandage or from allowing the limb to hang too long. Elevation of the limb and splinting will aid healing. Generally, fractures are reduced early and immobilized until healed. Digits are not amputated unless there is loss of blood supply. The function of a finger may be damaged seriously, but later some of its tissue may be of value in reconstruction. All possible length of thumb is maintained.

THE WOUND AND THE LOSS OF FUNCTION

There are 2 elements in an injury: the wound and the loss of function. The wound breaks the protective skin barrier and opens the deeper parts to contamination and infection. The loss of function is the result of damage to structures which stabilize, nourish or innervate limbs. As surgeons, it is our primary responsibility to treat the wound, remove the contamination and restore the protective cover. If this can be done with assurance of prompt and uncomplicated healing, then the loss of function from severed deeper parts may be treated at the same time. A simple incised wound seen early and treated promptly should heal with little reaction. If this type of wound is accompanied by tendon or nerve injury, repair of the damaged tendon or nerve usually can be done at the same time. However, if there is severe crushing of the parts with avulsed skin and extensive tearing of the soft tissues, even the best wound treatment will not result in the type of healing required for ideal repair of the deeper structures in the hand. Primary treatment must be confined to closure of the wound, the loss of function being treated as a secondary procedure when the condition of the tissues will allow it.

FACTORS IN THE WOUND ITSELF

The time interval from wounding to operation, the type and the amount of contaminat-

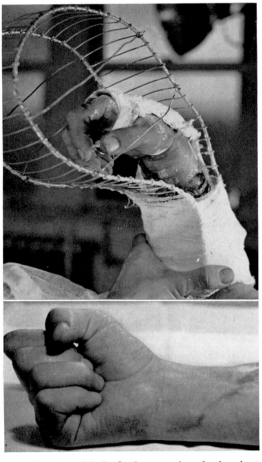

Fig. 721. Method of protecting the hand with the advantage of exposing wounds. Cramer wire incorporated in plaster dressing. (*Bottom*) After primary repair of all flexors in lower forearm.

ing materials present and the type and the location of the wound should be noted and recorded. All these factors must be considered in determining the proper treatment. The golden time for primary repair is that period before contamination changes to infection. All wounds are contaminated, and in the early period before the bacteria multiply and invade the tissues, one can excise the traumatized surface and convert the traumatic wound to a clean surgical wound. Open wounds should be covered with sterile dressings until examined in the hospital. The time interval during which primary excision and cleansing can be followed by normal healing processes varies with the amount of contamination and the type of wound. Though 6 hours is considered as being an orthodox time limit, there are many instances in which a longer interval can elapse and closure be carried out. Conversely, if there is gross virulent contamination of wounds, as from a human bite, closure of the wound should not be done even if the time lapse is only a few minutes. Thus, time and contamination factors must be considered together in judging the probability of primary healing.

The type and the location of the wound are also factors to be considered. Simple incised wounds from sharp cutting objects cause relatively little tissue damage. If approximated, the parts heal nicely. Lacerated and crushed tissues heal with more reaction, edema and fibrosis. Repair of deeper structures in wounds of this type means dense fibrosis binding all the intricate moving parts. The importance of the location of the wound as a factor in determining the scope of primary repair relates to flexor tendon injuries in the hand. (See Primary Tendon Repair.)

FACTORS IN THE FACILITIES OF TREATMENT

Even though the wound itself is such that primary repair of the deeper structures can be carried out with reasonable assurance of uncomplicated healing, such treatment requires adequate facilities. This means that proper operating room conditions, adequate assistance, instruments suitable for the work and a competent surgeon must be available. Lacking any of these, treatment should be confined to basic cleansing, removal of foreign bodies and devitalized tissues and closure of the wound. The wound and its care must be the primary

Fig. 722. In an automobile accident, most of the back of the hand had been ground off, including the tendons. The wrist joint was wide open. The wound was excised and closed primarily. Skin flaps from the side of the hand and the thumb were made to cover the wrist joint, and thin free graft was used to cover the remainder. Later, the dorsum was covered by good pedicle skin, and a new set of extensor tendons from the foot and a layer of paratenon fat from over the triceps tendon were placed between them and the bone. An excellent hand was obtained with full motion and flexibility.

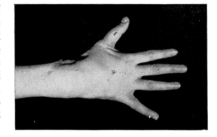

aim. The loss of function from severed tendons and nerves is secondary. The motto is "Treat the wound; prevent infection."

EXAMINATION

An open wound should make one suspicious of damage to the underlying parts. Keeping in mind the anatomy and the location of the various structures in the wounded area, examination is made to determine loss of function of these structures. Simple tests will suffice. For the long flexor or extensor tendons of the thumb, observe the action of the distal joint; for the abductor pollicis longus, the forward position of the thenar eminence, the dropping of the thumb arch and weakness of pinch. When an extensor or a flexor tendon of a

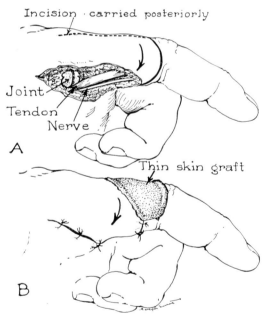

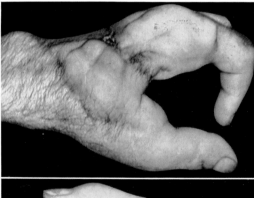

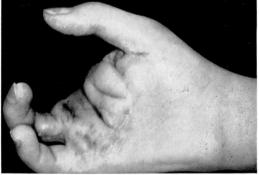

Fig. 723. Primary treatment of open wounds. After thoroughly debriding and cleansing, all exposed vulnerable tissues (such as nerves, tendons, bones and joints) are closed over with a primary plastic skin closure. In this case, a flap of skin is swung from the dorsum of the finger to cover the vulnerable tissues. A split-skin graft is used to cover the denudation left by swinging the skin flap.

Fig. 724. Two examples of double fillet. (*Top*) A crushing injury severely damaged the index and the middle fingers, and subsequent infection produced more damage. The index and the middle fingers were filleted, and their skin used to cover the cleft and the palm. (*Bottom*) A similar problem with much loss of palmar skin. A filleting of the 2 digits provided good cover for the palm.

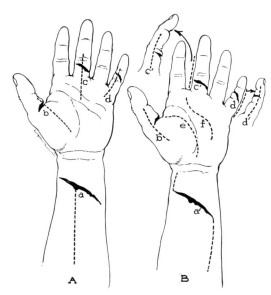

FIG. 725. (A) Incorrect incisions for obtaining exposure in treating lacerations as they cause flexion contractures and T scars. (B) Correct incisions for the same which are not harmful.

finger is severed, the finger rests in a position forward or behind the others.

Tests of nerve function are made by stroking the skin with a cotton swab and by pricking with a sharp point. Paralysis of the intrinsic muscles can be determined by palpating the thenar eminence on attempted opposition and the belly of the first interosseus on trying to abduct the index finger. Nerve supply to the hand is quite constant, and for injuries at or near the wrist, the standard patterns of sensory innervation and intrinsic muscle supply are dependable.

Roentgenograms are taken in at least 2 planes whenever fracture or dislocation is suspected.

Anesthesia

Local infiltration anesthesia is adequate in simple clean wounds. If used in a digit or for block at the base of a finger, epinephrine should be omitted. Hemostasis is secured with a blood pressure cuff tourniquet on the upper arm or by a catheter, not a rubber band,

around the base of the finger. Block anesthesia of the ulnar nerve at the elbow or of the median and the superficial radial nerves at the wrist can be done, or axillary or brachial block can be used. (See section on anesthesia, Chap. 5.) Extensive wounds require general anesthesia.

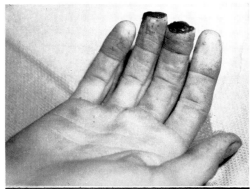

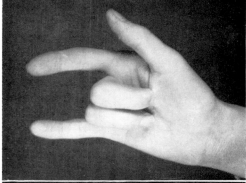

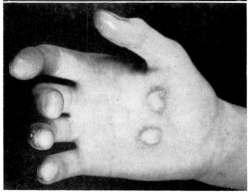

FIG. 726. Immediate palmar flaps to the ends of the amputated fingers. (L. D. Howard, M.D.)

FIG. 727. Immediate reconstruction for severe crush injury of index finger and dorsal skin. Metacarpal resected, and dorsum covered with split-skin graft.

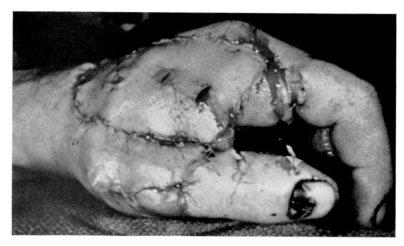

DECONTAMINATION OF THE WOUND

The wound is covered with sterile gauze, and the surrounding skin is cleansed thoroughly; the hairy parts are shaved. Soap and water or surgical detergents are used, and mechanical scrubbing similar to the surgeon's own hand scrub is continued until the parts are clean. Nails are cut short, and, if necessary, a brush is used on the thick horny epidermis of the palmar surfaces. Then the wound itself is washed and irrigated thoroughly with sterile normal saline. All the interstices of the wound are flooded with copious amounts of solution. An alternative method is to stain the wound surface with iodine, delineating the wound surface so that later the extent of excision can be determined. Either method is incomplete until a meticulous excision of the contaminated surface is carried out. This is done easily with fine double-pointed, curved-on-the-flat plastic scissors. All devitalized tissue is removed, including a narrow margin of the skin. In the bloodless field all tissues now stand out clearly, and exposed nerves, tendons and other structures can be inspected. Antiseptics should not be used in the wound unless the surface touched by them is excised later. The aim is to have a clean surgical wound free of foreign material of any kind. Local instillation of antibiotics is not indicated.

In spite of all efforts some contaminated surface will remain. Tissues have some protective power, and certain areas such as the face and the perineum have a high level of local resistance. Foreign bodies and particles of dead tissue may form a nidus for infection. Heavy clamps crush large bites of tissue, and ligatures of catgut are foreign bodies. Buried sutures and ligatures should be kept at a minimum. Dead spaces can be obliterated by careful compressive dressings. A small drain for 24 hours may prevent a hematoma.

After the decontamination has been completed, a decision must be made. Is this wound of such a type and in such a location that, judging by the surgeon's past experience, primary healing will result? Not just any type of healing, but healing by a process that produces the least amount of swelling and edema and minimal scarring in the deep tissues as well as the skin. If the answer is yes, then repair of the deeper structures such as bones, tendon and nerves can be carried out. If the answer is no, or if there is any doubt, the skin should be closed by suture, graft or flap, and restoration of the deep structures postponed.

COVER ALL VULNERABLE PARTS AND CLOSE THE WOUND

Tendons, nerves, joints and bone cannot be left exposed. These parts must be covered with protective soft tissue and skin. Free skin grafts should not be placed directly on such parts, but pedicle flaps of local skin can be swung over and the remaining denuded area covered with a split graft. Local flaps should be broad and long enough to cover the area easily and should have proximal pedicles. On the forearm, a parallel relaxing incision can be made, the intervening bridge of skin, being shifted to cover the vulnerable parts and the donor area grafted. Sometimes a finger is badly damaged but still has viable covering skin. Instead of amputating it, the bone is removed and the skin used as a pedicle flap. Skin which has been stripped from a part can be replaced after excising all the subdermal tissues, thus converting it to a free graft.

Some wounds should not be closed pri-

marily. Severe wounds from explosives or those that are first seen after infection is already beginning should be débrided and left open, secondary closure being carried out later. Fine-meshed gauze is packed loosely in the wound after all possible foreign material has been removed, and the whole involved part of the extremity is kept elevated and undisturbed. A week later, under strict operating room conditions, the wound is exposed and, if clean, closed by whatever means is suitable. If not clean, further débridement and

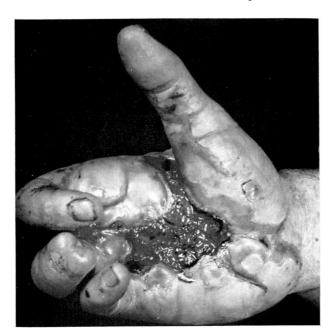

FIG. 728. (*Top*) Explosive wound in the palm covered by a fillet from the ring finger in the palm and a tubular pedicle for the thumb cleft. (*Bottom, left*) Hand is salvaged. (*Bottom, right*) Bed under tube pedicle is skin grafted. (W. B. Macomber, M.D.)

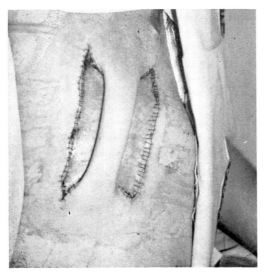

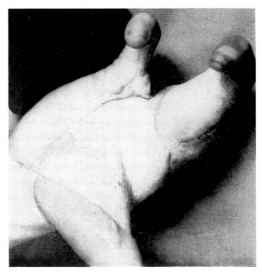

Fig. 729. Case J. M., age 2. (*Left*) From a birth tear in the ulnar border of the wrist, the holding of the scar distorted the growth of the hand, which was useless. The scar was excised, the ulnari elongated, the hand pinned in line with the forearm. A pedicle graft was applied. Two years later, osteotomy 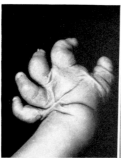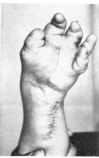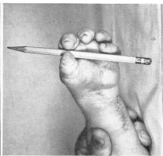 was done on the thumb metacarpal, the radius and each finger metacarpal. A pulley transfer was done for opposition, and the thumb cleft was deepened. All was pinned in place (*center* and *right*). Three years later, a letter stated that the hand was quite useful.

a few days of compress treatment usually allow final closure.

POSTOPERATIVE CARE

Dressings of fluffed gauze with moderate compression promote healing by preventing swelling, edema and hematoma. The term "pressure dressing" implies too much force. Compression should be distributed evenly and be moderate in degree. Including sponge rubber or, better, steel wool in the dressing maintains a more even pressure. After 24 to 48 hours some wounds can be left open to the air with simple protection provided by a wire-frame enclosure. The hand should be elevated with the hand higher than the elbow and the elbow higher than the shoulder. All joints not involved in the injury should be put through a normal range of motion at least once a day.

Injured tissues require immobilization. Movements break the newly forming capillaries of the reparative scar, letting loose exudate into the tissues. A siab of plaster on the outside of the dressings helps to maintain an even pressure and keeps the parts immobile. General body rest is useful to conserve energy.

Antibiotics of the broad-spectrum type are given until the danger of infection is over. Local chemotherapy or antibiotic therapy is not indicated, but in wounds involving much tissue damage a broad-spectrum antibiotic given for 3 to 5 days may forestall infection. Antibiotics are not a substitute for careful cleansing and decontamination of wounds.

TETANUS PROPHYLAXIS

The danger of tetanus is present in any wound, including burns, where devitalized tis-

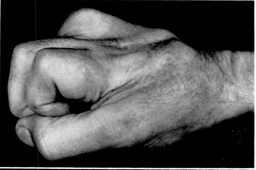

Fig. 730. Case S. M. (*Top*) The patient's hand had been caught in gears, fracturing the metacarpals of the index and the long fingers, lacerating the skin and resulting in infection. There were malalignment and nonunion, and the fingers did not move well. Excised the scar, placed iliac bone grafts in the metacarpals and capsulectomized the proximal finger joint. (*Bottom*) Good bony alignment and hence muscle balance were obtained. There was considerable improvement both cosmetically and functionally.

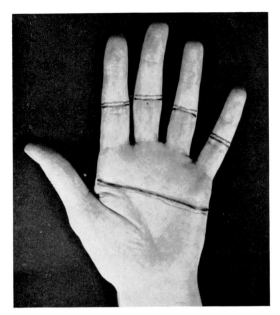

Fig. 731. "No-man's-land." The area between the distal palmar crease and the level of the middle finger joints where flexor tendon injuries frequently occur and repair is difficult.

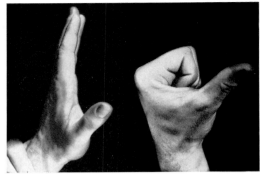

Fig. 732. Five hours after severance, by a broken bottle in the palm, of the flexor tendons to the index finger and the nerve to the second cleft, a primary suture of the nerve and each tendon was done using for the tendons removable stainless-steel wire. In 4½ months, sensation returned throughout, and the index finger had full range of motion, as shown in the illustration.

sue is present. The presence of a foreign body or dead tissue favors growth of the tetanus bacillus. Therefore, careful excision of the wound is prophylactic. Some judgment must be used, and antitetanic serum need not be given for every scratch or simple wound. Serious complications have followed its administration, such as peripheral neuritis, which often involves the brachial plexus. If the patient has not been immunized actively by toxoid and the wound has occured in a potentially contaminated area, and especially if it is a crushing type of wound, then passive immunization is necessary. After a negative skin test, 3,000 units of tetanus antitoxin are given. In severe injuries this should be repeated at the time of each subsequent reconstructive operation. Active toxoid immunization lasts many years, but a booster stimulating dose should be given at the time of injury. A course of

toxoid injections to provide future immunity may be started.

PRIMARY REPAIR OF SEVERED TENDONS

If seen early, the wound in which a tendon has been severed should be treated by careful cleansing and decontamination. If at the end of this part of the procedure the surgeon is certain that reactionless primary healing will occur on closure of the skin, then severed tendons can be repaired. Proper facilities for the operation must be available, and the technics

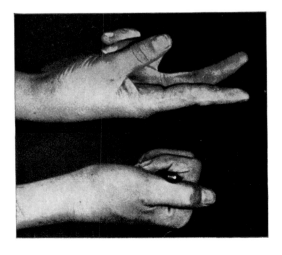

Fig. 733. Result of primary suture of the flexor tendon in the proximal segment of a finger with a stainless-steel wire removable suture. (Am. J. Surg. 47:508)

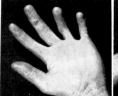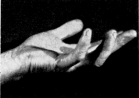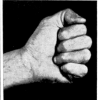

FIG. 734. Case P. G. Z. Primary repair of the flexor profundus tendon of the ring finger, using removable stainless-steel wire. The hand had been pulled into a lathe, gouging out the volar skin in the distal two segments of the fingers and severing the nerves and the tendons in the ring finger in the proximal segment. The pulley in this segment was slit; the flexor profundus united, fastening the wire to a button outside the skin. The nerves were sutured, and the denudations of the fingers were skin grafted. The illustrations show the return of range of motion 7 months later. Sensation returned to all but the extreme tip of the ring finger.

of the plastic surgeon must be used in handling the tissues in an atraumatic manner. If there is any danger of infection, tendons should not be sutured. The result will be a crippled hand; there will be no chance for later reconstruction. An occasional fortunate primary repair done under adverse conditions cannot justify one rampant infection. If during the first-aid treatment a futile attempt has been made to find and suture a tendon, the wound should be closed and repair done later when the danger of latent infection has passed. It is preferable to leave the severed tendon undisturbed so that it can be repaired or reconstructed later than to do what will make the hand worse.

Additional Exposure in Primary Tendon Re-

pair. A common fault in attempting to recover a retracted tendon end is to make an incision up the finger—the "pernicious median longitudinal incision" that cuts across creases and pulleys and damages the digit irreparably. Instead, a small transverse incision will suffice, or the wound can be extended along the midlateral line. Flexor creases should not be crossed at a right angle, and the digital nerves should be spared. A volar laceration can be extended by lengthening the wound proximally on one side of the finger in the midlateral line and distally on the other side, opening the digit in a bayonet fashion. Pressure on the muscle above will cause the cut proximal end to protrude in the wound. Blind searching with hemostats is traumatic. The use of a tourni-

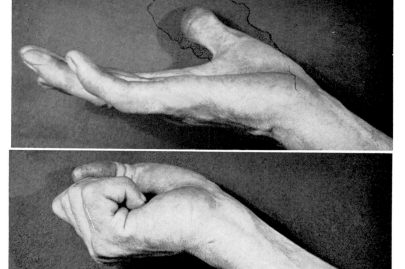

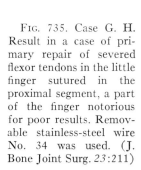

FIG. 735. Case G. H. Result in a case of primary repair of severed flexor tendons in the little finger sutured in the proximal segment, a part of the finger notorious for poor results. Removable stainless-steel wire No. 34 was used. (J. Bone Joint Surg. 23:211)

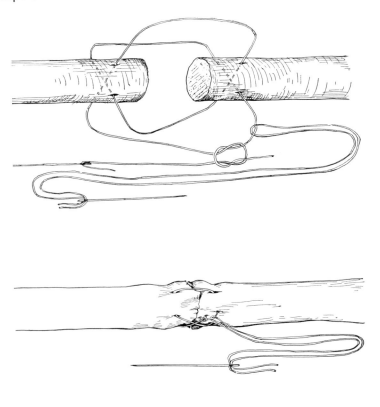

Fig. 736. Double right-angle stitch. This stitch is more than twice as strong as 2 simple through-and-through stitches because in each tendon end the stitch crosses a quadrant of tendon fibers diagonally. This displaces till somewhat on the bias as the stitch is pulled, all strands thus making for added strength. The 4 strands give a basket effect for better approximation of the tendon ends and divide the strain, so that a smaller strand of silk may be used. The stitch is simple and quickly placed. To prevent breaking, more reliance is placed on splinting the wrist in flexion to relax the flexor muscles than on the strength of this stitch. A pull-out wire is placed under the knot as shown, drawn out through the skin and left in place, if deemed advisable. If infection develops later, the stitch can be withdrawn as soon as the tendon unites, or if healing is *per primam*, the pull-out wire may be withdrawn. (J. Bone Joint Surg. *23*:209)

quet is essential as in all surgical procedures on the hand.

Healing of Tendons. Knowing how a tendon heals is of help in developing a concept of the technics of repair. There are 2 types of tendons, those within a sheath and those in paratenon formation. Sheathed tendons are present wherever a tendon passes over the concavity of a joint. The healing process is different in paratenon than in the sheath. If cut in a sheath, the proximal end retracts much farther than in paratenon, and the tendon ends become rounded over and sealed by epitenon, because a sheathed tendon has very little re-

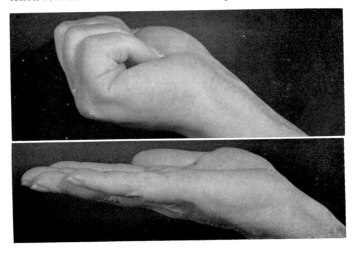

Fig. 737. Case E. M. Another case of primary repair of severed flexor tendons opposite the proximal phalanx. (J. Bone Joint Surg. *23*:212)

PLATE 11

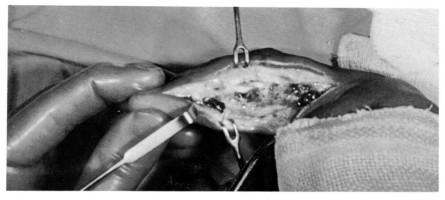

Grease under high pressure was accidentally injected into the finger on the flexor surface. The sheath is distended throughout its length. Immediate and thorough removal of all foreign material and involved tissue is the treatment of choice. (J. Bone Joint Surg. *43-A*:485)

PLATE 12

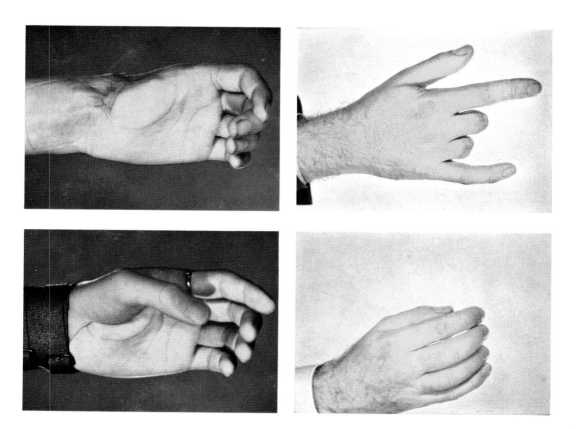

Lifelike plastic prostheses used for cosmetic purposes in cases of defects of part or a whole of hands, made of high-heat Vinyl resin with pigments to any tint of color laid in before processing. (L. W. Harris, D.D.S., Naval Dental School, Bethesda, Md.)

PLATE 13

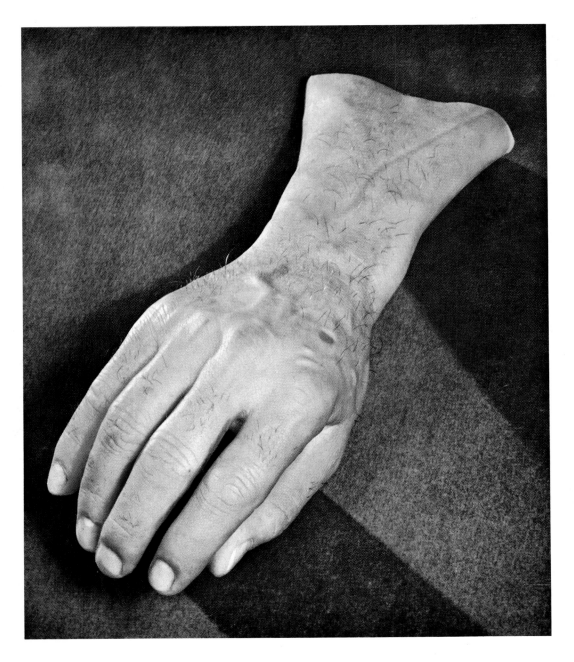

Flexible, hollow prosthesis of polyvinyl chloride with finger cores of malleable copper. Method of making learned in the Army Prosthetic Research Program. (C. O. Anderson, ceramist, San Francisco, Calif.)

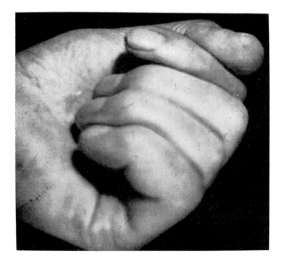

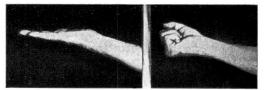

FIG. 739. Case E. M. Primary suture with removable stainless-steel wire of the flexor or the profundus tendon of the little finger severed with a knife at the middle crease. The pulley in the proximal segment was slit, and the sublimis tendon was removed. The nerves on the ulnar sides of the ring and the little fingers also were sutured. Sensation returned in 3 months. The illustrations show the degree of motion gained, 17 months later.

FIG. 738. Case C. C. As a knife slipped through the patient's hand, both the sublimis and the profundus tendons and the radial volar nerve were severed in the index finger as well as the profundus and one slip of the sublimis in the long finger, in the proximal segment of each.

Débridement and primary repair were done, using removable stainless-steel wire and "suturing at a distance"; namely, in the palm. In the index finger, the sublimis tendon was removed and the nerve sutured.

The photograph shows the degree of flexion in the fingers 7 months later. Sensation returned. He had 35° of voluntary flexion in the distal joint of the index finger and 40° in that of the long finger. With the index finger he touched the palm ¾ inch proximal to the distal crease in the palm and with the long finger touched the distal crease.

parative tendency. If the sheath is damaged, granulations grow into the tendon, much scar results, and the tendon end adheres to the sheath.

A tendon severed in paratenon heals in a different way. Each end seems to push out proliferative processes which may join, contract and draw the tendon ends together. These processes or pseudopodia arise not from the tendon cells but from the epitenon, the endotenon and the paratenon tissues. This reparative action is so great that when tendon ends are sutured, the juncture tends to grow fast to the surrounding tissues. If these tissues

are fixed, e.g., a fascial plane or ligament, the excursion of the tendon will be limited. The reaction of the tendon ends is aggravated by too early motion, infection and surgical trauma. Elaborate suture technics that leave large amounts of foreign-body suture material add to the reaction.

Materials for Suturing Tendons. Catgut is an unsatisfactory material for tendon suture. O'Shea found infection to be 6 times more frequent after catgut than after silk suture. Silk occasionally causes a reaction, though modern untreated silk is less prone to do so. Stainless steel wire provokes the least reaction. It glides easily and is strong for its diameter. Kinks in the wire weaken it and should be avoided. For many years 34-gauge wire has been used in all forms of tendon repair. It may be placed in such a way that it can be removed when tendon healing is complete. This is particularly important where tendons glide in sheaths or lie near a joint or just beneath the skin.

Type of Stitch. Suture material must be woven through a tendon end, or it will not hold. A single bite or pin through a tendon quickly cuts through on slight tension. A core suture inserted in such a way as to cause the least disturbance to the thin epitenon covering is placed, the slack of each loop is taken up, and the ends are joined so as to bunch the fibers in an accordion effect. If only approximated, the ends will separate as the suture cuts into the tendon substance.

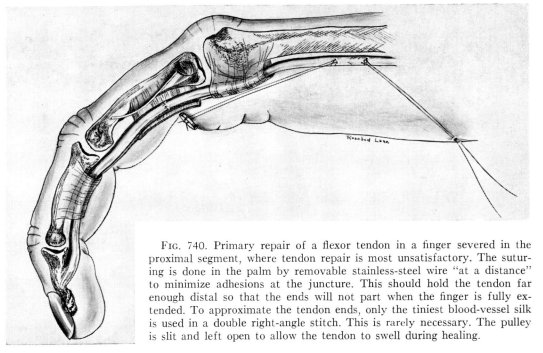

FIG. 740. Primary repair of a flexor tendon in a finger severed in the proximal segment, where tendon repair is most unsatisfactory. The suturing is done in the palm by removable stainless-steel wire "at a distance" to minimize adhesions at the juncture. This should hold the tendon far enough distal so that the ends will not part when the finger is fully extended. To approximate the tendon ends, only the tiniest blood-vessel silk is used in a double right-angle stitch. This is rarely necessary. The pulley is slit and left open to allow the tendon to swell during healing.

Splinting to relax the tendons by flexing the joints should be carried out instead of relying on strength or type of suture placement. Flexing the wrists relaxes the pull on digital flexors and robs the muscle of its power. Fingers should not be flexed to relax a flexor tendon; rather, the wrist is flexed to restrict the muscular pull. Relaxation of the suture line is maintained for 3 weeks; after this guarded active motion may be started. For extensor tendon repairs, the splint holds the wrist and the digits in extension. In this case a single approximating suture suffices. This is easily placed as a figure-of-eight with one loop

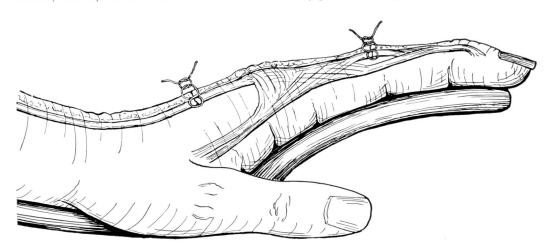

FIG. 741. For primary or secondary repair of the extensor tendons, a simple figure-of-eight stitch with No. 35 stainless-steel wire is used. One loop unites the tendon ends and the other the skin edges. The stitch is without strength and is merely for approximation of tendon ends. Splinting as shown prevents tendon ends from being pulled apart.

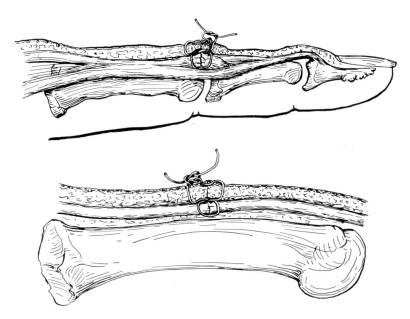

FIG. 742. (*Top*) Primary suture of the severed central slip of the extensor tendon with simple figure-of-eight stainless-steel wire, relying more on splinting to prevent parting. (*Bottom*) Similar method of primary suture of tendon on the dorsum of the hand. (Am. J. Surg. *47*: 503)

through the skin and the other through the tendon. It is withdrawn after 3 weeks. In primary repair of tendons, suture methods should be simple compared with those used in late reconstructions with grafts and transfers. Fewer crossings of the tendon fibers are made, and more reliance is placed on protective splinting.

Withdrawable Tendon Suture. A tendon pulls from its muscle end only. Therefore, if a suture is spliced securely in the end proximal to the point of severance and the 2 strands are passed through the distal end for some distance and out through the tissues to the surface, traction on these sutures will draw the proximal portion distally and approximate the severed ends. The 2 strands of suture are anchored outside by tying them over a button, a split shot or a bolster; if necessary, a fine apposition suture coapts the cut surfaces of the tendon. To remove the suture, after 3 weeks when tendon healing is complete, a pullout wire is left in place by passing a separate strand of wire through the first bite of the original tendon suture. Both ends of this are threaded on a single needle and passed through the skin. Traction on this wire, after the double wires are cut at the bolster, allows removal of all the suture material and thus diminishes the probability of a foreign-body reaction. This pullout method is applicable in many

areas, particularly in fastening a tendon to bone as in advancement procedures, opponens transfers and in any area where tendon must be held in firm approximation to a part.

Another form of withdrawable suture is a single figure-of-eight or vertical mattress type of stitch as used in repair of extensor tendons. One loop of wire holds the tendon ends in approximation while the second loop holds the

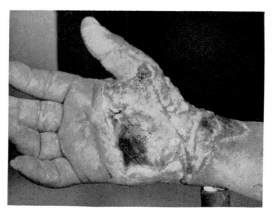

FIG. 743. A "degloving" injury tore the skin from over the wrist and the palm, leaving it attached by a distally based pedicle. When sutured back it became necrotic. Distally placed flaps sometimes can be replaced but only by converting the loose skin to a graft by excising all subcutaneous tissues.

FIG. 744. Another example of attempted replacement of a distally attached flap, here only by the first cleft skin. With such an injury an immediate free skin graft is indicated.

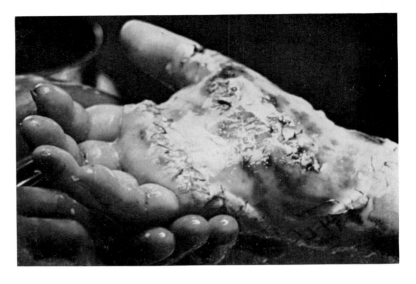

skin edges together. Deep fascial layers or long incisions through an aponeurotic layer may be closed with a running-wire withdrawable suture, each end passed through the skin and tied over a button. This is particularly useful in closing incisions or lacerations in the hood of the extensor mechanism over the metacarpophalangeal joints or a deep fascial or periosteal layer in the digit. When the tissues heal, all suture material is removed, and nothing is left to result in either a foreign-body reaction or a mechanical source of irritation.

Repair of Flexor Tendons in the Hand. Severed flexor tendons are common. To join a tendon by a surgical suture is easy, but to repair a flexor tendon and obtain a normal gliding structure is difficult. This varies with the region of the hand involved, and 3 zones can be defined.

PROXIMAL ZONE. In this area between the volar carpal ligament and the distal palmar crease, both sublimis and profundus tendons usually can be repaired. A core suture of No. 34 stainless steel wire is used and buried within the tendon. When both tendons are severed and the suture line of the sublimis lies directly

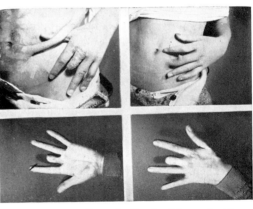

FIG. 746. Case A. B. Avulsion of skin from the long finger as the patient's ring caught on a nail when he fell off a fence. (*Top, left*) The distal portion of the finger was amputated as it had no blood supply, but the remainder was Thiersch-grafted until a tubular pedicle could be applied. (*Top, right*) Pedicle attached. (*Bottom*) Result.

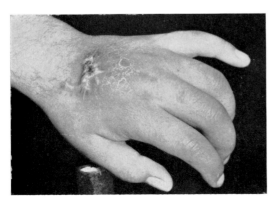

FIG. 745. Repeated drainage from the dorsum of this left hand was found to be from self-induced trauma.

over that of the profundus, the lumbrical muscle can be interposed. If this is not possible, the ends of the sublimis are excised, and only the profundus is repaired.

MIDDLE ZONE. This has been called "no man's land," the zone between the distal palmar crease and the middle flexion crease of the finger. In this narrow firm tunnel are 2 flexor tendons gliding over each other and through the snug pulleys. Any trauma results in swelling, and the tendon becomes ischemic, dies and is replaced by scar. Adherence of one tendon to the other limits both. Foreign suture material adds to the inflammatory reaction. Repair of a severed tendon in this area is attempted only under ideal conditions. If the wound is sharp and incised in type with minimal contamination and can be decontaminated thoroughly, and if adequate facilities are available, simple direct approximation of the tendon ends with either a withdrawable or a buried suture of fine wire can be done. The overlying sheath and the thick pulley structure at the level of the suture must be excised. Only the profundus tendon is repaired, the sublimis being excised. Isolated sublimis lacerations are not repaired. If there is laceration and crushing of the tissues or an accompanying fracture, or if good surgical facilities and an experienced surgeon are not available, then treatment should consist of simple wound decontamination and closure of the skin. Even under the best conditions, the results of pri-

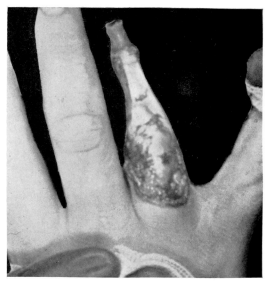

FIG. 747. Avulsion of skin from finger when a ring is caught. Can be covered with a split graft or buried in a single tubed pedicle.

mary repair of the profundus tendon in this area are poor.

DISTAL ZONE. Here, from the middle flexion crease of the finger to the insertion on the distal phalanx, only 1 tendon, the profundus, is involved. If the tendon is severed within 1 cm. of the insertion, tendon advancement is done. If the laceration is more proximal and

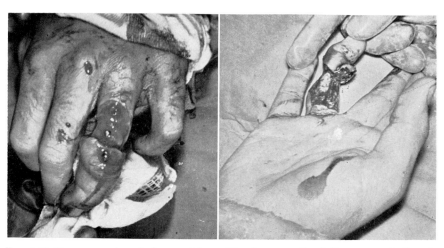

FIG. 748. Two examples of ring avulsions. The finger on the left was saved, though edema and swelling persisted for many weeks. The finger on the right was amputated.

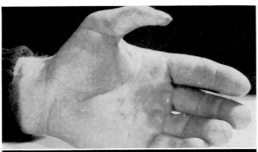

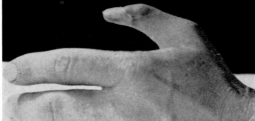

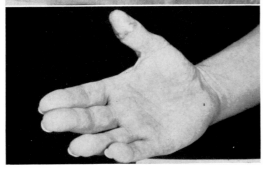

FIG. 749. (*Top* and *center*) Loss of pulp of thumb. Ideal for replacement with island pedicle flap as described in Chapter 10. (*Bottom*) The scar in the pulp prevents good use of the thumb. Either advancement of the volar skin (see Fig. 648) or an island pedicle transfer is indicated.

both ends of the tendon are present in the wound, direct approximation with a pullout wire suture is done. The pulley and the sheath in the vicinity of the junction must be excised. In some instances the proximal end of the tendon will have retracted into the palm due to the force of the muscle pull. When this happens, the mesentery of the tendon carrying the blood supply has been torn. It is technically difficult to rethread this tendon down its proper channel through the sublimis bifurcation without adding further trauma. In most cases it is better to tenodese the cut end to the middle phalanx with the distal joint in flexion and the fingertip in a pinching position. The intact and functioning sublimis will provide the power for grasp.

Repair of Flexor Tendons in the Wrist. A laceration across the wrist may damage all the digital as well as the wrist tendons. Since the median nerve lies within the flexor muscle mass of the forearm, becoming more superficial as it approaches the wrist, it is usually injured. Attempted repair of all the severed flexor tendons at the wrist results in a bulky mass of healing tissues in one small area. One tendon sticks to another, and the whole congeals into a solid cicatrix. This is particularly true of lacerations through the volar carpal ligament into the carpal tunnel. Here in this narrow channel are 9 digital flexor tendons and the median nerve. Even with the finest suture material and the most delicate technic, the resulting mass of scar is so great that little gliding can result. In lacerations at this level, only the essential structures—the 4 profundi, the flexor pollicis longus and the median nerve—are re-

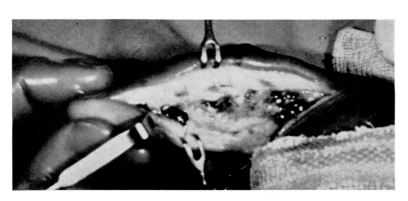

FIG. 750. Grease injected into the finger under high pressure here fills the flexor tendon sheath. (J. Bone Joint Surg. *43-A*:485-491, 1961)

FIG. 751. A high-pressure paint gun forced the toxic pigment and thinners into the index finger under extreme hydraulic pressure. This was not a spray paint gun using air mixed with the paint. Picture taken 6 days after injury and an ineffective attempt at "drainage." The index finger later was amputated. (H. H. Stark, M.D.)

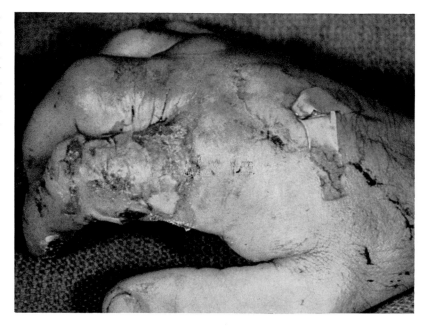

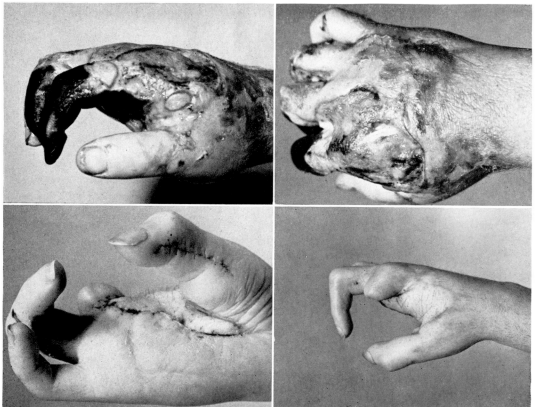

FIG. 752. Case J. B. M. (*Top*) Grease-gun injury. (*Bottom*) The necrotic tissue and most of the grease were excised, and a plastic closure using a pedicle graft was done.

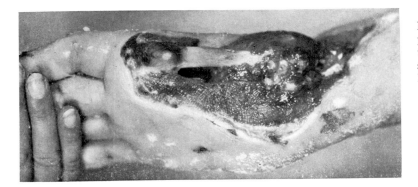

FIG. 753. Wound from high explosive. A direct pedicle was applied, and the exposed bone was saved. (Thomas Cronin, M.D.)

paired. Sublimi are sutured only if the level of the laceration is such that the suture lines will lie more proximal. Wrist flexors need not be repaired. The aim is to lessen the number of moving parts, provide room in the tunnel for the injured structures and restore essential function. Tendons severed more proximally in the lower forearm can be sutured with good results, using any acceptable technic. Successful suture of flexor tendons above the wrist is not a test of surgical skill or of a special technic.

Repair of Extensor Tendons. A single figure-of-eight wire passed through the skin and the tendon approximates the tendon ends. Splinting relieves the tension on the suture line, since these tendons do not tend to retract far when cut.

In the finger, a similar withdrawable figure-of-eight wire is used to appose the ends of the tendon. Splinting is mandatory for at least 3 weeks, though some protection against the pull of the powerful flexors should be maintained for an additional 2 weeks.

Repair of Nerves. Under ideal conditions and with perfect facilities, an experienced surgeon can obtain good results in primary nerve repair. Seldom are such ideal conditions found, and it is usually better to fasten the ends together with a single wire suture, which prevents retraction. Correct rotation of the nerve trunk is obtained by matching surface vessels. Accurate formal suture can be done when the wound is healed.

SPECIAL TYPES OF WOUNDS

Puncture Wounds. A cruciate incision at the wound of entrance is made, and the resulting 4 skin corners are clipped off. This provides adequate drainage. Grossly contaminated wounds, e.g., a human bite, should be débrided thoroughly and left open. The limb should be splinted, especially if a joint or a tendon sheath is involved. Deep structures may be severed, or a hematoma may form from damage to arteries. Aneurysms develop after partial lacerations of the major vessels.

Snake bites are puncture wounds and are treated as such. Unless there is definite evidence that the snake is not a poisonous variety, the part should be immobilized, a proximal tourniquet applied to block lymphatic return and each wound opened. Depth of penetration of fangs is approximately three fourths of the separation of the fang marks. Thorough suction, by mouth if necessary, must be started immediately; polyvalent antivenin is given after a skin test for sensitivity. Most rattlesnake venoms are hemorrhagic in action. Local swelling becomes severe in a few minutes, but some late signs occur up to 72 hours. Antitetanic measures and broad-spectrum antibiotics should be started. Rattlesnake and moccasin venoms contain enzymes that destroy tissues leading to local necrosis and sloughing. Early amputation of obviously necrotic parts is essential.

Some foreign bodies embedded in the hand are peculiarly damaging, e.g., indelible pencil punctures, palm thorns and redwood splinters. The tissue reaction is intense, and local necrosis occurs. One should excise the damaged tissue rather than simply pick out the foreign body.

Crushing Wounds. The effect of trauma is not limited to one type of tissue. All structures

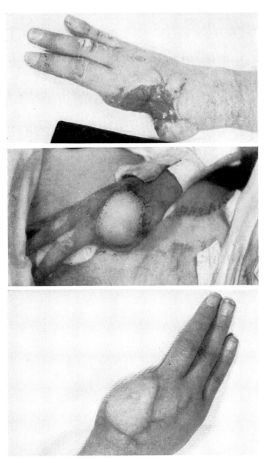

FIG. 754. Steps in closure of a gunshot wound (delayed a week) by direct application of an abdominal pedicle under the protection of chemotherapy. (Thomas Cronin, M.D.)

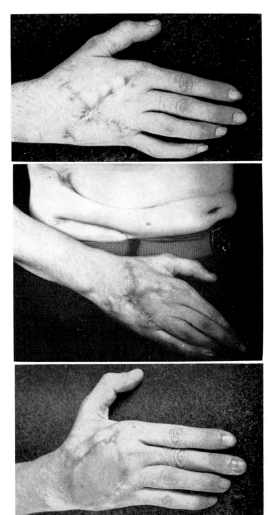

FIG. 755. X-shaped incision commonly seen after a gunshot wound through the palm. This makes repair difficult, as in this case a pedicle graft was necessary. In such wounds, extensor tendons are usually adherent or missing, and the proximal finger joints are stiff and straight. (L. D. Howard, M.D.)

are damaged when a hand is caught in punch presses, gears, or cornpickers or under heavy falling objects. Hemorrhage, swelling and edema follow quickly, and, later, thrombosis of the vessels occurs. Débridement is difficult because the vitality of the tissue cannot be determined at the time. Releasing the tourniquet and allowing the blood to fill the part may help to delineate the good tissue. Experimentally, an intravenous injection of a Disulphine Blue or Kitone fast-green stains all living tissue. Tempest reports that a free graft of stained skin loses its color in 12 to 15 hours. The dye is excreted by the kidney in 48 hours.

Treatment is confined to cleansing, decon-

taminating and closing the wounds. Skin grafts or local or abdominal flaps may be necessary. Fractures are treated by moulding into shape and dressing the hand with voluminous gauze and applying a moulded metal splint in the position of function. Small Kirschner wires for fixation may simplify the external splints. At the first dressing after 1 week areas of further

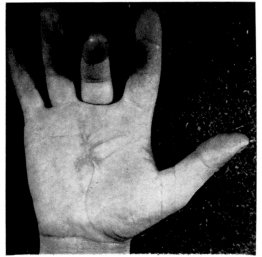

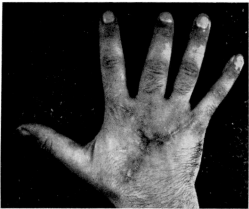

Fig. 756. Typical rifle wound through hand, some of which are self-inflicted wounds. The prevalent but unfortunate habit of making a stellate scar makes plastic repair difficult. (L. D. Howard, M.D.)

necrosis are excised, and skin grafts are applied. The aim of treatment is to preserve the circulation, prevent infection and maintain the position of function.

Roller, Wringer and Degloving Injuries. The force here not only crushes the tissues but may avulse the skin and the subcutaneous tissues, usually leaving a distal pedicle. A mangle injury adds the effects of burning to those of pressure.

Wringer injuries are common in children. The amount of damage is not apparent at first. Swelling occurs rapidly and, if unchecked, is followed by localized areas of thrombosis and patchy gangrene of the skin. More prolonged pressure or involvement of deeper tissues may result in muscle crush with late contractures. Treatment consists of thorough cleansing, application of a compression dressing and elevation. Necrotic areas are excised and skin grafted.

A degloving injury may involve the whole palm or a finger when a ring is caught. The skin with some subcutaneous tissue strips off and usually is left attached by a distal pedicle. Suturing the flap back is useless. Either sacrifice it and apply a split graft to the denuded

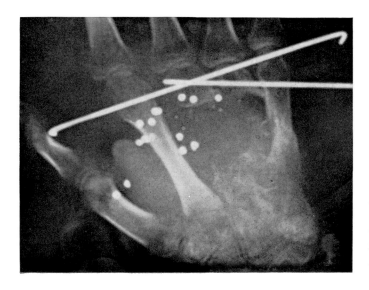

Fig. 757. A shotgun blew out the 2 central metacarpals. Primary débridement and closure of entrance wound in the palm, fixation of metacarpal heads to prevent displacement and coverage of dorsum by an immediate abdominal flap made it possible to replace the bones with iliac grafts within 6 weeks. (S. Blandford, M.D.)

area, or treat the avulsed portion as a skin graft by carefully excising all the subcutaneous tissues as one would in taking a full-thickness skin graft, then apply it to the denuded area. Excise all questionable areas, including most of the thick palmar skin. Ring avulsions often leave the terminal segment and the nailbed without blood supply. The viable portion of the finger can be covered with a split graft or set into a tubed pedicle prepared on the abdomen.

Grease-Gun Injuries. First described in 1937 by Rees, these wounds caused by grease or oil injected into the hand or the fingers occur more frequently in this modern machine age than they did formerly. These materials in a jet stream under high pressure penetrate the intact skin and fill the tissue spaces. First appearances are deceptive, and there is minimal pain. Within a few hours, pain and swelling develop, and the part then becomes numb and pale. Ischemia develops rapidly in closed spaces. Later damage is from chemical irritation and infection.

Treatment is immediate decompression through wide incisions of the involved area. Elective incisions as in reconstructive surgery are used. All possible foreign material should be removed, and infiltrated nonessential tissues excised. A damaged tendon sheath should be removed. The wounds are closed, and the hand immobilized in the position of function. Tetanus immunization should be started. A digit that is irreparably damaged should be amputated. With prompt and adequate care, much scarring will be prevented and disability lessened.

Gunshot Wounds. Most gunshot wounds in

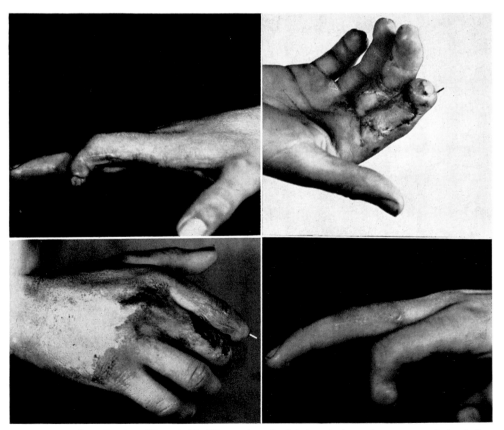

Fig. 758. Case W. D. (*Top, left*) The patient had injured the volar aspect of the index finger with a planer. (*Top, right*, and *bottom, left*) Cross finger flap covered defect. (*Bottom, right*) Skin graft on long finger.

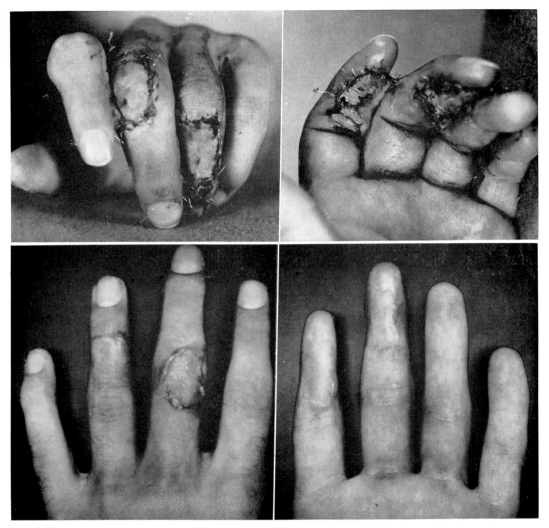

F<small>IG</small>. 759. Case K. C., age 18. A planer took the volar aspects of the index and the long fingers. Healed with flexion contractures with no sensation or flexion of the distal parts of the fingers. (*Top*) Two cross finger flaps were made. (*Bottom*) Good cover was provided.

civil life are from close range. There is wide destruction, especially in shotgun injuries, and shot, wad and particles of clothing may be deeply embedded in the wound. Infection follows frequently, and, because of the large skin loss, pedicle flaps are frequently required as the first step in reconstruction. Immediate treatment of the wound follows the principles used for crushing wounds. Careful excision of devitalized structures with early secondary closure by graft or flap will diminish the late disability. Nerve injuries are common.

BURNS

G<small>ENERAL</small> T<small>REATMENT</small>

A burn of the hand may be only one part of the total injury to the patient. The general principles of treatment of shock, fluid replacement and tetanus immunization all apply to burns of large body surfaces. The arm constitutes 9 per cent of the body surface.

The aim of treatment in burns of the hand is prevention of scarring, rapid re-covering with skin and maintenance of mobility of the

Fig. 760. The Rule of Nines:

Head and face	9%	Arms, each	9%
Neck	1%	Genitals	1%
Trunk, front	18%	Legs, each	18%
Trunk, back	18%		

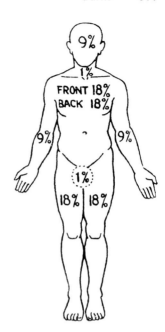

If 18% or more, in first 48 hours need of fluid:

Adult $\left\{\begin{array}{l}\text{1 bottle plasma}\\\text{1 bottle saline}\end{array}\right\}$ for each 9%

Children, age 9 $\left\{\begin{array}{l}\text{½ bottle plasma}\\\text{½ bottle saline}\end{array}\right\}$ for each 9%

Oral intake only $\left\{\begin{array}{l}\text{adult, 9 × 6 ml.}\\\text{child, 9 × 9 ml.}\end{array}\right\}$ per Kg. of weight

Urine $\left\{\begin{array}{l}\text{adult, 6 × 9 = 54 ml.}\\\text{child, 3 × 9 = 27 ml.}\end{array}\right\}$ per Kg. of weight

(Modified from Berkow, by Wallace, A. B.: The exposure treatment of burns, Lancet 260:502)

joints. Infection should be prevented, and the wound closed as quickly as possible. Numerous methods of treatment have been introduced and discarded. Tannic acid, alone, or with silver nitrate and gentian violet were used as sprays forming an eschar, but as the eschar hardened, constriction developed about the fingers and even the forearms. Constant irrigation with various solutions in plastic envelopes was popular because it allowed exercise. Ointments of infinite variety have been used. Wet dressings, either compresses or baths, are valuable in removing dead tissues, but to avoid waterlogging of the tissues, intermittent periods of exposure to the air or dry dressings are necessary.

LOCAL TREATMENT

A burn is a wound, and, just as for other wounds, decontamination, excision of devitalized tissue and protection from infection are the basic elements of treatment. First-aid consists of the application of a sterile dry dressing, medication for pain and transportation to a hospital for adequate treatment.

Primary Treatment. The burned skin and the surrounding area are cleansed with bland soap and water or surgical detergents. Grease and other foreign substances should be removed, and all devitalized tissue excised. Strict aseptic conditions must be maintained. In most burns it is impossible in the first hours to determine the exact depth of the burn, unless it is very circumscribed and deep. After thorough cleansing, a layer of nonadherent gauze, nylon or plastic is laid over the wound, and then several layers of dressings and gauze. Bandaging is done to cover all the surface evenly and with even compression. The hand must be in the functioning position. The hand and the arm are kept elevated. The compression dressing keeps down edema and lessens fluid loss. Compression dressings are essential in all hand injuries, but it is difficult to apply exactly the right amount of pressure. Care must be taken to avoid excessive pressure, because venous return must not be compromised. Antibiotics are usually given.

FIRST DRESSING. The original dressing is not changed for several days unless fever or local signs of infection occur. Subsequent dressings are done under aseptic conditions; any necrotic tissue present should be removed each time the dressing is changed. If the wound becomes dirty, compresses or baths of saline are used between dressings. At the earliest possible time, split grafts are applied to all areas of full-thickness loss.

SKIN GRAFTING is done just as soon as possible. The sooner that closure of the wound is

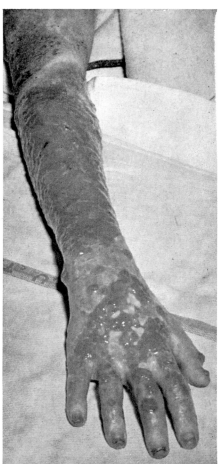
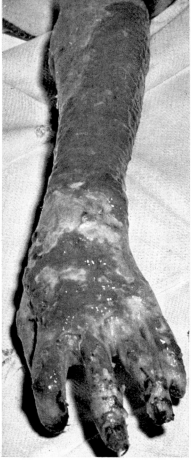

FIG. 761. Granulations from burns were scraped off with the handle of a scalpel, and skin grafts were applied under a pressure dressing. (W. B. Macomber, M.D.)

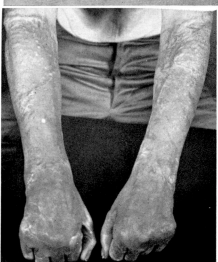

obtained, the less the contracture and stiffening of the hand. Usually, it can be done within the first 3 weeks. The longer the delay, the more scar is formed. Granulation tissue forms scar, which, if allowed to form, contracts in later stages. Granulations should be removed and the skin graft placed on the bed. With a tourniquet in place, they are scraped off down to the basic gray tissue layer, and the graft is applied with the hand in a position of function. A single layer of coarse meshed gauze is placed over the graft, and several small catheters are laid over this. Then the massive compression dressing is applied. The catheters must be placed directly over the graft, separated by only a single layer of dressing. Saline solution

FIG. 762. Heavy keloid from over the dorsum of the hand following burn.

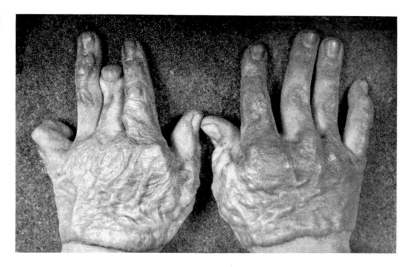

instilled through the catheters keeps the graft wet and mechanically flushes the surface. This dilutes the proteolytic enzymes liberated from the broken-down leukocytes in the wound area and allows the new epithelium to grow. Tissue cultures are made in liquid media; therefore, one cannot have too much solution; rather, the error is in not having enough so that the graft dries out or dissolves in the concentrated purulent secretions. Grafts can be applied to all raw surfaces. The aim is to provide skin cover as quickly as possible. The tourniquet is released only after the dressing is complete. Dressings are changed every 3 or 4 days, care being taken not to disturb the surface of the graft; after about a week or 10 days, ordinary dressing technic can be started.

MOVING THE HAND. Early movements of the hand serve to lessen the later disability. Occasional immersion in lukewarm baths and gentle passive or, better, voluntary motion should be encouraged. On concave surfaces, as in the palm, early movement may tend to crack the newly healing graft. Local splinting of this part and freedom of movement of all other joints improves nutrition. Contractures tend to occur after all but the most superficial burns. Prevention and treatment by splinting is essential and must be persisted in for many months. For late treatment of contractures and scarring, see Chapter 7, Skin and Contractures.

SPECIAL ASPECTS OF BURNS OF HANDS

Common burns are those of the thin skin over the dorsum of the wrist, the hand and the fingers. The palm is tougher and often is used to shield the face. Thus the exposed dorsum receives the brunt of the flash or flame. A severe burn may compromise the circulation of a digit so that gangrene occurs. On the dorsum of the finger the thin skin, especially that over the middle joint, has little resistance. Often the extensor tendon over the joint is burned, and when sloughed or excised, the joint is open. The bone may be charred. In selected cases the open joint can be covered with a flap and joint action preserved. Later, tendon transfers may help to restore function. Circulatory embarrassment due to swelling in the interosseus muscles can result in Volkmann's ischemia in the hand. Release of the tight intrinsics by splinting or tenotomy will be necessary. Splinting must be persisted in, because contracture develops slowly and gradually over a long period of time.

For severe burns of the upper extremity, Moncrief has recommended early release of the constricting tissue, even 2 or 3 hours after the burn. This is especially true of burns of the forearm. Early excision of the nonviable tissues can be carried out as soon as the patient's general condition permits, and the procedure may be repeated in 24 or 48 hours.

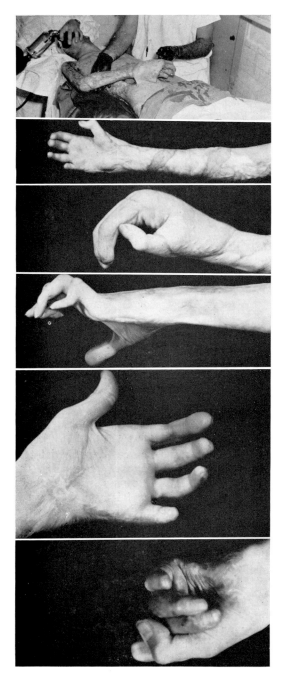

Fig. 763. Case H. F. B. Plane crash and multiple burns over body and both hands.

Right Hand. Such a severe dorsal burn as to require a pedicle graft. Fingers were clawed, thumb at side, proximal joints stiff and straight, could not grasp and hold any object. Upper arm hidebound. Operation: upper right arm slit longitudinally in 3 incisions, allowed to gap and skin grafted. Axilla tunnel grafted. Removed whole of dorsal skin of hand, did 4 capsulectomies, amputated the little finger, arthrodesed various interphalangeal joints and attended to finger webs.

Left Hand. Thumb good. Could use thumb and index. Borders of hand burned. Middle joints ankylosed in acute flexion. Needs better cover and positions of joints. Operation: split-skin graft over borders of hand. Pulley operation to oppose thumb. Result: better nutrition and cover for both, can open and close for grasp. Much greater function.

useless claw. Scars can draw the thumb to the side of the hand, and webs between the fingers limit their spread. Fibrous tissue thickens in response to intermittent tension. Scars at right angles to a flexion crease develop into keloids if there is motion. Slow gradual traction should be used to overcome contractures. Even minor losses of skin limit motions, for the hand covering must be sufficient in size and elasticity to allow great ranges of movement.

ELECTRIC BURNS

Burns from electricity differ from thermal burns in that the area of surface contact is relatively small, but the damage is severe. It is always greater than it appears. Even after the first few days it is difficult to determine the extent of the burn. Deceptive-looking small areas may appear to require immediate excision and skin grafting, but one must not give in to the temptation to operate. The current passing through the tissues causes blood vessel damage with later thrombosis or delayed hemorrhage. Common sites are the palms and the volar aspects of the wrists. Here the damage spares no tissue, and all the volar structures slough, necessitating pedicle grafts and nerve and tendon reconstruction. General treatment is the same as that for burns from any other source—prevention of infection, excision of devitalized tissue and skin closure.

Split-skin grafts applied in this way may salvage considerable function in the hand.

Contractures on the palmar surface can draw fingers so that the tips touch the palm; on the dorsum, the proximal joints can be dislocated, with the result that the compensatory flexion of the 2 distal finger joints makes a

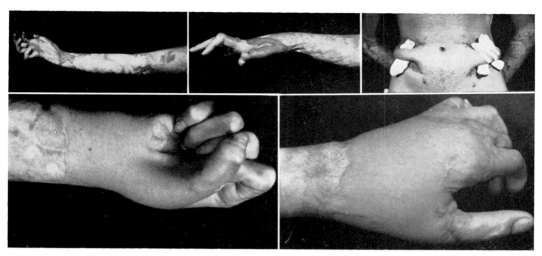

FIG. 764. Case I. T. V. (*Top*) Burn of both hands from an air crash. New cover by pedicle grafts was furnished each hand. Capsulectomies and establishment of thumb clefts were done and pulley operations for opposition of the thumbs. (*Bottom*) Could use both hands well.

FROSTBITE

Exposure to cold causes changes very similar to those caused by burns, and the basic treatment is the same. Rapid warming of the part is now the accepted practice. Immersion of the hand in a lukewarm whirlpool bath is the primary treatment. Pain is controlled with narcotics. When the frozen areas are thawed, the swollen erythematous parts are dressed with nonadherent gauze, and a compression dressing is applied. Thrombosis is the major damaging factor. General measures to

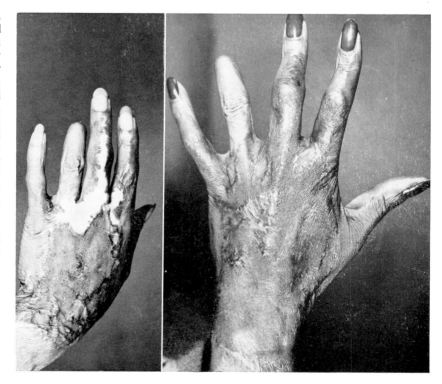

Fig. 765. Case S. W. (*Left*) Hand had been caught in a hot laundry press. One poor skin graft had been placed, but it did not allow flexion. Removed all dorsal skin and replaced with thick skin from thigh, paying attention to the borders so that they would not form contractures. (*Right*) The patient gained good function and made a good fist.

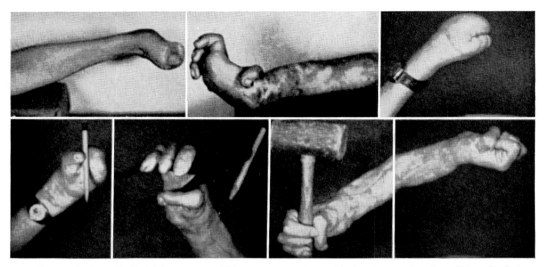

FIG. 766. Case D. P. This 13-year-old boy was sent from Alaska for repair of terribly crippled hands which had been burned in a gasoline fire 9 years previously. (*Top, left*) The left hand was a club with the digits folded up within the skin and in reverse direction, and flexion contracture of the wrist. (*Top, center*) The right hand showed digits in reverse direction and much cicatricial skin, making flexion contractures of the wrist and the digits.

Right Hand. Cuts were made across the strong contractures of wrist, thumb and proximal finger joints, the deep cicatrix being excised. This straightened out the joints somewhat. The thumb was repositioned and pinned in place. Capsulectomies of the proximal joints and lengthening of the extensor tendons allowed the fingers to come forward from the metacarpals, instead of backward, where they were pinned. Skin grafts were applied.

Left Hand. Flexion contractures of the wrist were cut across and that of the hand excised. This allowed the wrist to extend, where it was pinned. A thumb was carved from the hand, positioned in a forward position, and pinned there. For the cocked-back fingers, transverse scar excisions were made, and by capsulectomies and tendon lengthening the fingers were bent forward and pinned in position. The fingers in the left hand were not separated. The patient obtained quite good use of his hands. He could grasp objects of many sizes firmly.

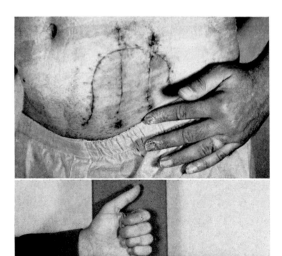

promote vasodilatation are used such as placing the patient in a warm room or giving him hot and/or alcoholic drinks. The damaged parts are not heated directly. Anticoagulant therapy has not proved to be of value.

As a late result of the effect of moderate frostbite in infants, epiphysial growth of the phalanges may be diminished or even stopped.

FIG. 767. Case H. G. (*Top*) After 5 years of office fluoroscopy, the backs of this patient's fingers were ruined by x-ray dermatitis. A pedicle flap was raised and replaced. In 10 days it was raised, interdigitated and replaced, and in 2 weeks more it was placed on 3 fingers. (*Bottom*) He obtained a good result.

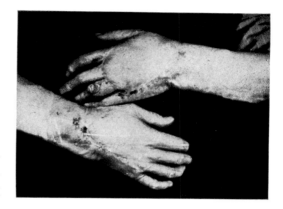

Fig. 768. Showing the prevalent error toward conservatism in treating x-ray burns as in this patient, a surgeon, in not making the pedicle grafts sufficiently large to include the borders of the burned area. These borders later had to be excised and covered with free skin grafts.

Radiation Burns

Prolonged exposure to sunlight causes hyperkeratotic changes leading to squamous cell cancers of the skin in susceptible individuals among the light-skinned races. The dorsum of the hand is a common area. Similar but more severe effects are seen following prolonged exposure to roentgen rays. Reducing fractures under a fluoroscope without protection has injured the hands of many surgeons. Dental technicians holding films in a patient's mouth characteristically burn the radial side of the index and the middle fingers from exposure to the intense rays. Often diagnosed as an allergic reaction to Novocain, these have been mistakenly treated with radiation.

Skin changes from less than erythema doses are late in developing. Changes in the vessels lead to atrophy of the skin with loss of hair and glands. Keratoses occur, and the parchmentlike skin breaks easily, forming fissures which crust over repeatedly and heal only to break open from the slightest trauma. Pain is present with ulceration. Telangiectases develop in the pale atrophic areas. More intensive radiation or prolonged exposure results in an acute burn with erythema, swelling and necrosis. Underlying tendons, bones and joints can be involved directly, but in the common type of radiation injury, changes in these tissues are usually secondary.

Treatment consists of complete excision and replacement with good skin. If the damaged area has a good base, split-skin grafts are accepted. Excision must be wide and into the normal skin. Junction lines of graft to normal skin must be in the correct anatomic areas to avoid later contractures. If deeper tissues are damaged, pedicle grafts are needed to carry skin and subcutaneous tissue to the part.

In the superficial types where the deeper tissues are good, split-skin grafts are applied at the time of excision. The removed skin must be examined microscopically. Many will show definite carcinomatous changes. Axillary gland dissections are done only when palpable glands are present. Amputation of one or more digits in the severely damaged hand may improve the over-all function of the hand by ridding it of a stiff and useless finger.

Indolent ulcerated areas can be excised and skin-grafted without waiting for complete healing. Placing a graft on the area and dressing it with the inserted-catheter wet-dressing technic explained under treatment of thermal burns has resulted in saving grafts applied on a poor foundation.

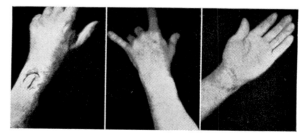

Fig. 769. Case W. R. P. X-ray burn. A chip of steel had entered the volar surface of the forearm. This was removed under a fluoroscope, the dorsal surface being toward the ray. (*Left*) Gangrenous ulcer already a year old, involving tendons. (*Center*) The ulcer was excised, covered at once temporarily with thin skin graft, and later with tubular pedicle graft. Drop fingers were corrected later by tendon graft. (*Right*) A similar case of prolonged ulceration acquired in the same way.

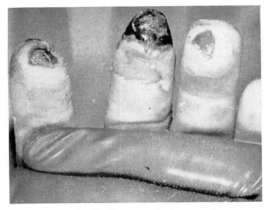

FIG. 770. Hydrofluoric acid burns of finger tips from industrial injury.

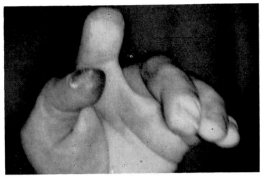

FIG. 771. Case J. R. The left thumb and the index finger had been amputated at their ends. In 4 hours, the index stump was closed and a cross finger flap from the dorsum of the index finger to the thumb was placed. This should give good sensibility.

CHEMICAL BURNS

Thorough washing with running water is the primary treatment of all chemical burns, whether acid or alkali. Following this, sodium bicarbonate solution or a weak acetic acid can be used to neutralize any remaining chemical and the area bandaged with compression and sterile dressings.

Chemical burns can occur from application of weak solutions in various forms of therapy when the solvent becomes more concentrated through evaporation. Carbolic acid, even in the ointment form, should not be applied to fingers.

AMPUTATIONS

GENERAL CONSIDERATIONS

Conservatism is the rule in amputations in the upper limb. All possible length is saved in the thumb, and in the other digits amputation is done only after careful study of the possible use of any part of the digit in later reconstructions. Even the skin of an otherwise useless finger may be used later to cover a defect in the hand. Only if the damage is too great to justify reconstructing tendons, nerves and joints and if none of these parts is of future use is amputation carried out. Loss of blood supply is the only real indication for primary amputation. In severe crush injuries, salvage of all viable tissue may provide enough for 2 opposable digits or a mechanism of crude grasp. Such a result is usually better than a prosthesis.

Skin Flaps. At the time of injury all possible skin is saved. Though volar skin may provide better padding for finger stumps, length need not be sacrificed to obtain it. Lateral or dorsal flaps can be used. It is best to err on the side of a bulky stump with loose pliable skin covering the bone than to close under tension. If possible, scars are away from the tactile surface and can be terminal or dorsal.

Special Tissues in Amputation. Amputations through the base of the nail should include all the matrix lest a troublesome nail horn grow later. If through the joint, removal of the cartilage will make the skin of the stump less mobile. The flare of the condyles of a phalanx makes wide bulbous stumps. Narrowing of the stump by shaving each side off makes a better appearance and, for the 2 central fingers, allows a better fist to be made. Flexor and extensor tendons are divided and allowed to retract; they are never sutured over the end of a finger, because this limits the adjoining fingers. In the middle, the ring and the little fingers, a common muscle activates the profundus tendons; holding back 1 tendon, as when sutured to a stump, limits the excursion of the other 2 tendons. If the ring finger is stiff and immobile for any reason, a similar restriction of the middle and the little fingers occurs.

In amputations of a finger, nerve ends should be dissected free from the accompanying artery, cut off and allowed to retract. Then one should resect a length of nerve sufficient to allow the end to lie in good soft subcutane-

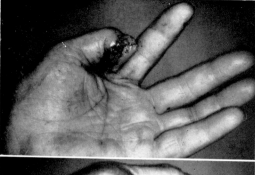

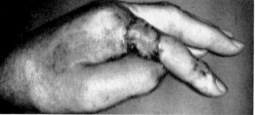

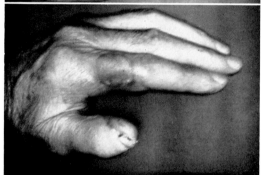

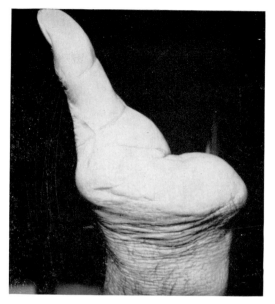

FIG. 773. Fingers lost through the metacarpals from mutilation by a corn picker, which greatly disables hands. Furnished patient with a useful prosthesis. By wrist motions, his hand worked against it and the thumb against the hook.

FIG. 772. Case M. L. The pulp of the thumb had been evulsed by a belt and pulley. Débrided and applied a cross finger flap, skin grafting the dorsum of the index finger and applying a stent. The phalanges are pinned together.

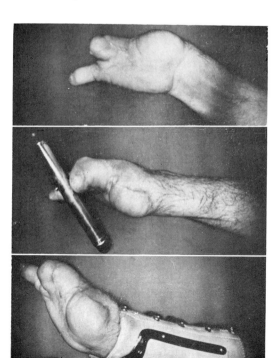

FIG. 774. Case L. D. (*Top*) The digits, especially on the radial side, had been amputated by a power saw. The cleft between the ring and the little fingers was not sufficient for function. The cleft was deepened and skin grafted. Tendons were grafted to adjoining sides of these digits to adduct them together. (*Center*) The patient obtained strong pinch for small objects. He also used a prosthesis against which his hand moved (*bottom*), as well as a cosmetic glove prosthesis.

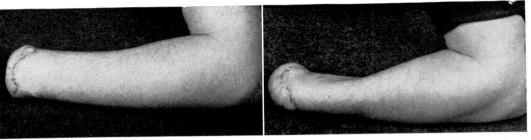

FIG. 775. Amputation through the carpus. (*Left*) Pronation. (*Right*) Supination. This is much better than an amputation through the radiocarpal joint.

ous tissues away from a pressure area. A severed nerve heals by forming a neuroma. If this is just beneath the skin or in scar tissue or if there has been delayed healing, it is painful. Such painful neuromata should be resected and the new neuroma allowed to form in good tissue away from scar.

FINGERTIP LOSSES. Exposed bone of the distal phalanx may be covered by a pedicle flap from palm, abdomen, pectoral region or an adjoining finger. Flexing the finger to obtain a palmar flap is not advisable in adults because joints stiffen easily. Unless it is taken from similar skin, pedicle skin will not have good stereognosis. Loss of soft tissue only, leaving a good base of subcutaneous tissue, can be replaced by a free graft of skin only. If only the tip of the pulp is lost, a split-skin graft will take well and contract, leaving a small terminal scar. Losses of part of the pulp can be replaced with full-thickness grafts that have come from the ear lobe or from toe pulp. In selecting the method of treatment some consideration should be given to the occupation of the patient, which finger is affected, and the loss of time and wages involved.

Levels of Amputation. There is no site of election for amputation of a finger, though certain general principles can be followed. All possible length of a finger that can be saved consistent with an adequate stump is a good general rule. The stump must be covered with nonsensitive durable skin. Disarticulations are satisfactory in most instances. A short segment of the base of the middle phalanx aids in gripping, and a short stub of proximal phalanx helps to maintain the length of the palm and prevent small objects from falling through the cleft.

MIDDLE AND RING FINGERS. Amputations in the region of the middle and the ring metacarpal heads have been controversial. If possible, it is best to leave enough of the base of the proximal phalanx so that the level of amputation is that of the distal edge of the finger webs. This preserves the length of the palm. Webs between the fingers are on the volar surface, sloping proximalward to the dorsum. Amputations through the joints of these 2 fingers are also satisfactory. Preserving the metacarpal head saves the transverse arch and ensures a broad surface for grasping. Removing a metacarpal head and allowing the other fingers to fall together makes the hand 25 per

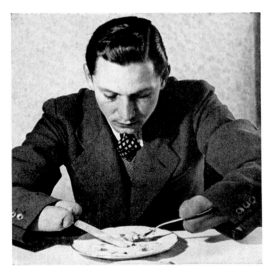

FIG. 776. Krukenberg amputationplasty. The great advantage is that prehension and the sense of touch are preserved. (G. F. Neubauer)

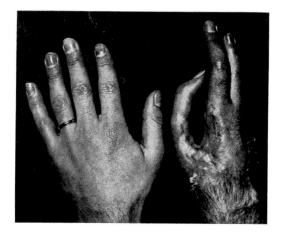

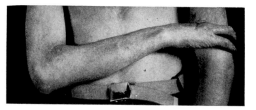

FIG. 777. (*Left, top*) Loss by gunshot wound of the 2nd and the 3rd rays and stiffening of the adjoining digits. (*Left, bottom*) Scar was excised, and a pedicle flap from the arm was laid in the cleft, skin grafting from where the graft came. (*Right, top*) New thumb cleft. (*Right, bottom*) Hand fitted with latex prosthesis made by Mr. Don Cash. (William H. Frackelton, Lt. Col., M.D.)

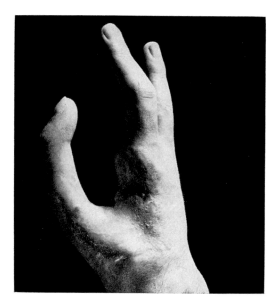

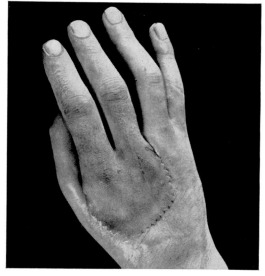

cent narrower. This impairs the leverage function of the palm in holding tools such as a hammer or a chisel. In women or in men in whom appearance is of more importance, the entire metacarpal except for the base can be removed and the adjoining marginal ray shifted over to take its place. This provides more stability and prevents a scissoring effect when the metacarpals roll toward each other and the fingers cross in flexion.

LITTLE FINGER. A short stub of the proximal segment of the little finger may be of considerable value to a workman using hand tools. When holding a hammer, the flare of the handle is grasped by the little finger, using the hypothenar muscles. Removal of this stabilizing influence places additional strain on the ring finger, and the balancing effect of the broad palm is lost. However, if this segment cannot be saved, then the head of the little finger metacarpal should be removed by an oblique cut through the bone. The hypothenar muscle mass makes a good pad.

INDEX FINGER. Loss of more than just the tip of the index finger creates a problem. If the index is amputated proximal to the distal segment, it is almost impossible to use this stump as a pinching mechanism against the

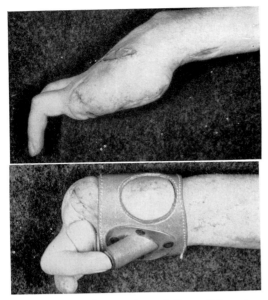

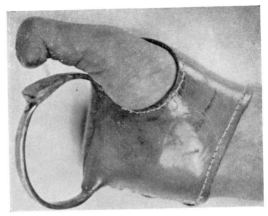

FIG. 779. Prosthesis for use when only the thumb remains. Devised by patient. Allows writing, grasping firmly of large and small objects and looping the ring over objects. (George S. Phalen, M.D.)

FIG. 778. Amputation of the radial part of the hand with a prosthesis substituting for the thumb. (L. D. Howard, M.D.)

thumb. Its length is inadequate, and the skin of the middle segment does not have the necessary sensibility. As a reconstructive procedure for skilled workers and especially where precision pinch is required, it is better to sacrifice the entire finger and remove the metacarpal in its proximal third. The 1st dorsal interosseus tendon is transferred to the 2nd on the radial side of the middle finger. This provides a satisfactory appearance and an adequate cleft for grasping. An index finger stump through the proximal segment may be useful in specific occupations, e.g., carpentry (the right hand), but when small tools or objects must be manipulated with the fingertips (screws, nuts and fine precision instruments), such a stub is in the way.

THUMB. There is no argument concerning the thumb. All possible length should be saved, even if the remaining bone must be covered with a pedicle flap. The skin of such a flap will not have stereognosis, but a good quality of sensation can be supplied to it as a later procedure by a neurovascular pedicled flap from a finger. (See Chap. 10 on Nerves.) Such reconstructive measures will not be needed in all cases; a well-padded sensible stump through the proximal phalanx is functional and needs no additional lengthening.

Amputations of the thumb through the metacarpal or involving the carpometacarpal joint should preserve not only all possible bone length but all local skin as well. Such skin may be valuable in later reconstructions.

METACARPALS AND CARPALS. Loss of all the digits by amputation through the distal portions of the metacarpals will leave a hand that can be made useful by adapting a simple prosthesis or phalangizing the fingers. Amputation through the bases of the metacarpals leaves a useful stump that can be controlled by the wrist motors. The motion of the wrist can be utilized to hold objects against a fixed post from a forearm cuff.

FOREARM AMPUTATIONS

The many advances in prosthetic design and manufacture during the last decade have changed the concepts of ideal amputation sites in the upper limb. Under present conditions, any length of stump adequately covered with well-nourished skin can be fitted with a prosthesis. This has made unnecessary the operations of elongating a stump by skin grafts and bone grafts. Even a short segment of ulna, provided that some elbow-joint function remains, can be utilized by the prosthetist to give reasonable function. Disarticulation at the radiocarpal joint, once considered an unfavorable site for amputation because of the flare of the distal radius and ulna, now can be fitted with a satisfactory prosthesis; the widened end of the stump aids in better fitting and control. Pronation and supination of the forearm are preserved when the distal radio-ulnar joint is intact.

KRUKENBERG AMPUTATION

In this the forearm is cleft to a radial and an ulnar portion, the 2 working together in an up-and-down pincer movement rather than a rotary one. It applies only to a forearm stump, and this must measure at least 17 cm. from the lateral epicondyle.

Tactile skin is placed over the 2 contact surfaces, i.e., in the bite, the 2 incisions being made one well ulnarward on the dorsum and the other somewhat radially along the volar surface. One jaw, the radial, is covered completely with normal skin; the deficit of the ulnar jaw is covered at once by a free or pedicle flap of skin, a strip of normal skin

with mainly the internal cutaneous nerve supply being left over the biting surface of this jaw. The muscles and the interosseus membrane are carefully separated high enough until the bones spread widely to 5 inches between their ends. The radius spreads from the ulna by the biceps, the extensors of the wrist and the brachioradialis. These are left with the radius. The flexor carpi radialis and the pronator teres are also left with the radius to help it squeeze against the ulna, which it does with moderate strength. Muscles are not removed because the jaws must be vascularized to keep warm.

Though the result is not cosmetic, the patients are pleased. There is the ability to feel, and also, if desired, a standard prosthesis may be worn. It is not suitable for a minor arm, because a patient will not use it, but it is suitable for an amputation of the major arm or

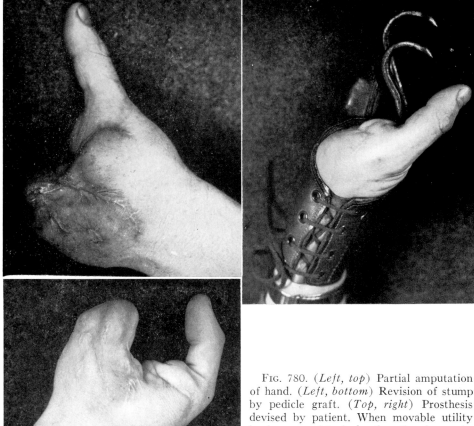

FIG. 780. (*Left, top*) Partial amputation of hand. (*Left, bottom*) Revision of stump by pedicle graft. (*Top, right*) Prosthesis devised by patient. When movable utility hooks are detached, the thumb works against leather stump cover. (L. D. Howard, M.D.)

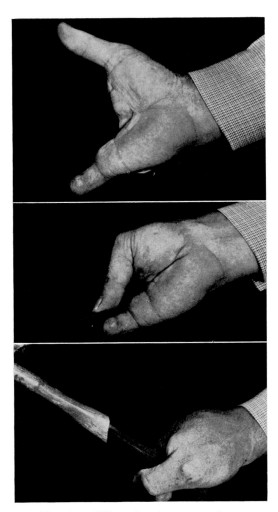

FIG. 781. When the thenar muscles are normal and some adductor function remains in the thumb, a good pinch and grasp can be accomplished against a portion of one other digit.

for bilateral amputations. It is used primarily for one side in a double amputee and for the blind who need to be able to feel. They cannot manage a prosthesis because they cannot see.

Swanson has performed the Krukenberg type of procedure on young children with congenital amputations. He uses the double-triangle skin-flap method to determine the depth of the cleft, attempts to get a 4-inch opening and carefully saves the pronator teres. A secondary osteotomy can provide a better pinching mechanism when desired.

The great advantage of the Krukenberg amputation over orthodox amputations with prosthesis is that there is natural sensation. Therefore, the Krukenberg double amputee works better, faster and more efficiently than does even the bilateral cineplasty amputee. Also, when desired for heavy work, a regular prosthesis with split hooks may be worn over the double stump.

PROSTHESIS

Artificial arms or parts of hands are too often discarded because of lack of sensation, for in the use of the hands sensation is equal in value to motion. In the dark they are useless. Leg prostheses are far more successful than arm prostheses. No matter how crippled, if a hand is painless, has sensation and slight opposing motion, it is far superior to an artificial hand. Most people select an artificial hand for appearance and lack what it takes to develop the ability to use the utilitarian attachments. By intelligence, ability and persistence, gifted people become very skillful and do remarkably well with prostheses. They must train their shoulders and elbows to synchronize and do the work of a hand. It is not a natural but a cultivated action. It is not the hook that has the skill, but the man behind it.

The artificial arm for amputations below the elbow is both useful and used; those for amputation above the elbow require more than average skill, are quite limited in practical use and are often discarded. This will change with improvements in prostheses.

Prostheses to substitute for hands are either in the shape of hands or else are made entirely for practical use, e.g., a metal split utility hook. The 2 hooks open by a shrug forward of the opposite shoulder and close by means of a powerful rubber band. They may have various projections for better grasp on the objects held. The Trautman and the Dorrance types are particularly useful.

The hook is interchangeable with the cosmetic hand as are also many types of devices such as a vise, a chuck, a grab hook or various tools for special work. It is an English custom for the amputee to carry these around in a well-arranged tool kit.

Cosmetic hands that look more or less like hands and over which a glove can be worn are less useful. Some have malleable digits that can be placed in any position. Many have joints, from 1 to 3 in each digit. Either the thumb or the fingers move, controlled by sleeve cables from the opposite shoulder. Generally, fingers are made parallel with each other so that they present a flat surface for the thumb, or they may be made to give a 3-point grasp. In some, the last 2 fingers may be set in any position, and the first 2 can be worked against the thumb (Hüfner). Hands are of wood, metal or plastic. Some have a whiffle-tree arrangement to equalize the force of the digits. Others move by levers, chains over pulleys or worm screws, and one has a force amplifier of 5:1 which works automatically to fit the need in grasping.

Various prostheses may be placed and set in several or any positions by the other hand. These include a swivel table above the elbow for rotation, an adjustment to set the elbow at any angle, or one to set the wrist for any angulation or rotation in pronation or supination. Also, digits may be set in various positions where they will maintain their grasp.

A man who has lost one arm will compensate by developing the use of his good arm, becoming left-handed if the right is gone. If ambitious, the patient develops much pride in these accomplishments, and if the amputation was done in childhood, his skill may be astonishing. With the development of compensatory ability there is a tendency to discard the prosthesis.

In amputations through the hand, no prosthesis will be used if there are 2 remaining digits that can feel and work against each other in a prehensile way. If, though, there is only 1 remaining digit, a prosthesis will furnish the necessary broad hook with a flat surface to work against. This is especially useful if the thumb remains and the fingers are off at the base of the palm. Semiflexed metal fingers are held by a metal and leather cuff laced on the forearm so that the thumb can work against them. If only the thumb is off, the patient usually discards the prosthesis furnished him. In contrast, a new digit produced by reconstruction or phalangization will be most useful. For an amputation through metacarpals or carpals the split utility hook may be used with the hinge action at the wrist. It projects lower than it should but is useful. If the hand remains but has only a few useless digits, a prosthesis may be built, based on the forearm, against which the hand can work.

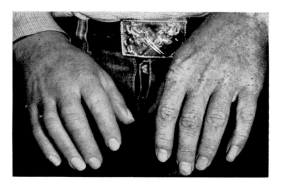

FIG. 782. For cosmetic purposes a simulated hand can be made to cover almost any deformity. This is the patient shown in Figure 781.

This prosthesis can terminate in a hook or a split hook. When a man has a partial hand with a little useful but weak prehension by a few digits, a prosthesis may be fitted onto what remains of the hand to make it possible to perform heavy work.

Beautiful imitations of hands have been made of vinyl chloride as a hollow glove $\frac{1}{8}$ inch thick. The texture, coloring and translucency are close to perfect. They fit on an amputated stump or onto a partial hand when part of the hand is missing.

CINEPLASTIC AMPUTATIONS

In 1898, Vanghetti, who was not a surgeon, conceived the idea of using the muscles in the stump to activate the hand, and Ceci, a surgeon, applied it. It is not suitable in the leg because stabilization instead of movement is more important. In succeeding years the method was advanced by Codivilla, Galeazzo, Pellegrini and Putti in Italy. During the First World War Sauerbruch in Germany improved the method, and later Bocchi-Arana in Argentina contributed a modification. In this country, Kessler, using the method of Sauerbruch, has had much success. Of his 78 cases, he found that after 2 to 6 years, 44 used their prostheses regularly, and 34 did so part of the time. He states that this is a greater porportion than used their orthodox artificial limbs, especially in upper arm amputations, and claims that in a survey in this country only 12 per cent of 276 cases used them, and in one in Germany only 1.8 per cent of 7,000 cases used them. In a case observed personally, a forearm amputee who had a cineplasty on one side, his major, and an orthodox hook on the other, used the latter so much more that this became the major hand. He then had the tunnels removed.

Main muscle groups were used as motors—for the upper arm, the biceps and the long head of the triceps; for the lower arm, the flexors and the extensors. Various plastic attachments for the muscles have been used, such as terminal loops or clubs; but later, the short, skin-lined canal through the muscle was adopted. There was much ulceration and necrosis until a satisfactory technic was developed. One advantage of cineplasty is that movements are natural, the opposing muscles being balanced in tone and movement, developing skill, and by muscle sense a conception of position, the size of objects and the right strength of grasp. Each muscle, by means of an ivory peg, pulls on the opposite arm of the lever, which is balanced by adjusting the attachments along the lever arms. This, in turn, opens and closes the hand. Another advantage over the usual artificial arm is that the apparatus in a forearm stump is lighter and shorter, not extending above the elbow except for a strap which loops about the upper arm above the elbow. For an upper arm prosthesis the strap fastens to the other shoulder.

Important disadvantages are that the motion is weak and the amplitude too small to be practical for other than very light usage.

The following is condensed from Nissen and Bergmann, who worked in Sauerbruch's clinic until 1933 and had subsequent experiences in this line. Cineplasty is not adapted to those who do heavy labor; it is useful for those in sedentary occupations who desire motion and skill even though it may be weak. They should have the mental equipment and perseverence to become adept. These authors claim that cineplasty is successful in perhaps over 68 per cent of cases (this is the figure given by Siegel in 1928).

Strength is proportional to cross-section area of muscle. Work equals force times length. A long muscle gives greater excursion and so is more adaptable than a short, thick muscle which has greater strength. A diagonal-fibered muscle is not suitable. The excursion gained from a biceps is 6 cm.; that from a triceps, 4 cm. A looped muscle pulls with only 5 to 20 per cent of its normal strength, and some of this is lost by friction of the prosthesis. In a short stump there is not sufficient excursion, and in the lower third of a limb segment the tendinous parts are unsuitable. Preferred sites for tunnels are the pectoral, the biceps and the triceps.

A canal is made by raising transversely to the limb a flap of skin 4 or 5 cm. square with, for vascularity, its base to the radial side of the forearm and the medial side in the upper arm. The flap is tubed, skin side in, passed through the muscle and sutured to the skin on the other side. The suture line in the tube is placed proximally, away from wear. The raw area in front of the muscle is closed by sliding skin or a free graft. The canal should be wide and short and at a right angle to the limb. If narrow, it ulcerates. It should penetrate the lower end of the muscle in a plane two thirds of the muscle thickness from the bone. If the vitality is doubtful, a 2-pedicled flap is used, splitting and suturing the muscle over it.

If the muscle is allowed to be contracted for long, it loses excursion and strength. Therefore, exercises and tension should be started at once and continued. Long excursion is furnished only by long muscle, and strength of pull is in proportion to the cross section of the muscle. To have muscle length it is better to have the tunnel in the lower portion of the segment than in the upper portion. As the muscle has its maximal strength only when under full tension (Inman), the motivating part of its excursion should be in that range. For this an improvement in apparatus is necessary. (For more details refer to Alldredge's article listed in the Bibliography).

Mazet recommended that cineplastic operations be done only after a conventional prosthesis has been worn for 6 months. The pin must be worn constantly, and daily skin cleansing is essential. In the biceps cineplasties he found 7 failures in 26, and, in a total of 56 tunnels of biceps and pectoral type, only 25 were used persistently. Poor patient selection, lack of cooperation, inadequate strength of the muscle and rotation of the prosthesis were the factors most often responsible for failure. Forearm tunnels are usually unsatisfactory, and, according to Brav, a survey of Army cineplasties revealed that only 35 per cent of the pectoral tunnels were used.

BIBLIOGRAPHY

WOUNDS

Aitken, G. T.: Lessons learned from review of hand cases evacuated from South Pacific, Am. Acad. Orth. Surg. Lect., p. 202, 1944.

Allen, H. S.: Crushing wounds of the hand, Am. J. Surg. *80*:780, 1950.

Bailey, H.: Surgery of Modern Warfare, Edinburgh, Livingstone, 1941.

Baker, J. M.: Molten plastic injuries of the hand, Plast. Reconstr. Surg. *15*:233, 1955.

Bardenwerper, H. W.: Serum neuritis from tetanus antitoxin, J.A.M.A. *179*:763, 1962.

Bell, J. L., Mason, M. L., and Allen, H. S.: Management of acute crushing injuries of the hand and forearm over a five-year period, Am. J. Surg. *85*:370, 1953.

Bell, R. C.: Grease gun injuries, Plast. Reconstr. Surg. *5*:138, 1952.

Bentley, F. H.: The treatment of fresh wounds by early secondary suture and penicillin, Brit. J. Surg. *32*:132, 1944.

Bisgard, J. D., and Baker, C. P.: Treatment of fresh traumatic and contaminated surgical wounds, Surg., Gynec. Obstet. *74*:20, 1942.

Bojsen-Møller, J., Pers, M., and Schmidt, A.: Finger-tip injuries: Late results, Acta chir. scand. *122*:177, 1961.

Boyes, J. H.: Principles of primary care of the injured hand, Texas J. Med. *52*:845, 1956.

———: The primary treatment of the injured hand, Kansas City M. J. *35*:14, 1959.

Boyes, J. H., and Melone, F. C.: Injuries to the hand from broken porcelain faucet handles, Western J. Surg. *59*:59, 1951.

Brocklehurst, T.: Pseudo-Raynaud's disease due to electric vibratory tools, Med. Press *213*:10, 1945.

Brooke, R., and Rooke, C. J.: Two cases of grease-gun finger, Brit. M. J. *2*:1186, 1939.

Brown, J. B., and Byars, L. T.: Spontaneous and surgical covering of raw surfaces, Lancet *60*:503, 1940.

Brownrigg, G. M.: Frostbite—classification and treatment, Am. J. Surg. *67*:370, 1945.

Bunnell, S.: Treatment of injuries of the hand, Calif. West. Med. *30*:1, 1929.

———: Traumatic surgery with special reference to certain principles of treatment, Indust. Med. *1*:24, 1932.

———: Primary repair of severed tendons: Use of stainless steel wire, Am. J. Surg. *47*:502, 1940.

———: Treatment of tendons in compound injuries of the hand, J. Bone Joint Surg. *23*:240, 1941.

———: Suggestions to improve the early treatment of hand injuries, Bull. U.S. Army Med. Dept., No. 88, p. 78, 1945.

———: The injured hand: Principles of treatment, Indust. Med. *22*:251, 1953.

Byrne, J. J.: Grease gun injuries, J.A.M.A. *125*:405, 1944.

Converse, J. M.: Early skin grafting in war wounds, Ann. Surg. *115*:321, 1942.

Cummins, R. C.: Dead hand, a lesion produced by rapid vibration, Irish J. M. Sci., 6 ser., p. 171, 1940.

Cutler, C. W., Jr.: Injuries of hand by puncture wounds and foreign bodies, Surg. Clin. N. Amer. *21*:485, 1941.

———: Early management of wounds of hand. Bull. U.S. Army Med. Dept., No. 85, p. 92, 1945.

Dudley, H. D.: Some facts about the hand, Western J. Surg. *55*:419, 1947.

Duncan, J. M.: Trauma of the hand, Brit. J. Surg. *35*:397, 1948.

Edgerton, M. T.: Immediate reconstruction of the injured hand, Surgery *36*:329, 1954.

Ender, J., Krotschek, H., and Simon-Weidner, R.: Die Chirurgie der Handverletzungen, Vienna, Springer, 1956.

Farmer, A. W.: Treatment of avulsed skin flaps, Ann. Surg. *110*:951, 1939.

Feil, A.: Symptoms in workmen who use compressed air tools, Presse méd. *43*:668, 1935.

Flynn, J. E.: Compound wounds of the hand, Ann. Surg. *135*:500, 1952.

Garlock, J. H.: Symposium: Industrial diseases and accidents to hand: Management of injuries of tendons and nerves of hand, New York J. Med. *36*:1740, 1936.

Graham, W.: Delayed tendon repairs, Am. J. Surg. *80*:776, 1950.

Haldemann, K. O., and Soto-Hall, R.: Injuries to muscles and tendons, J.A.M.A. *104*:2319, 1935.

Hauge, M. F.: The results of tendon suture of the hand: A review of 500 cases, Acta orthop. scand. *24*:258, 1955.

Hausman, P. F., and Everett, H. H.: Wringer injury, Surgery *28*:71, 1950.

James, J. I. P.: Le traitement précoce des blessures de la main, Rev. chir. orth. *46*:139, 1960.

Kitlowski, E. A.: The preservation of tendon function by use of skin flaps, Am. J. Surg. *51*:653, 1941.

Koch, S. L.: Treatment of compound injuries and infections resulting from them, Bull. Am. Coll. Surg. *16*:3, 1932.

———: Immediate treatment of compound injuries, Ill. Med. J. *67*:40, 1935.

———: Injuries of the hand—with particular reference to immediate treatment, Nebraska M. J. *21*:281, 1936.

————: Injuries of the hand, J.A.M.A. *107*:1044, 1936.

————: Treatment of compound injuries, with particular reference to hand, J. Mich. Med. Soc. *38*:27, 1939.

————: Treatment of hand injuries, New Engl. J. Med. *225*:105, 1941.

————: Division of flexor tendons within digital sheath, Surg., Gynec. Obstet. *78*:9, 1944.

Kyle, J. B., and Eyre-Brook, A. L.: The surgical treatment of flexor tendon injuries in the hand; results obtained in a consecutive series of 57 cases, Brit. J. Surg. *41*:502, 1954.

McCullough, N.: Rattlesnake bites; personal communication, 1962.

McDonald, J. J., and Webster, J. P.: Early covering of extensive traumatic deformities of the hand and foot, Plast. Reconstr. Surg. *1*:49, 1946.

Mason, M. L.: The treatment of injuries of the hand, Indust. Med. *15*:323, 1953.

Mason, M. L., and Allen, H. S.: Indelible pencil injuries to hands, Ann. Surg. *113*:131, 1941.

Mason, M. L., and Queen, F. B.: Grease gun injuries to hand; pathology and treatment of injuries (oleomas) following injection of grease under high pressure, Quart. Bull. Northwestern Univ. Med. Sch. *15*:122, 1951.

Mueller, R. F.: Management of compound injuries of hand, Minnesota Med. *27*:110, 1944.

Myers, M. B.: Prediction of skin sloughs at the time of operation with the use of fluorescein dye, Surgery *51*:158, 1962.

Orr, H. W.: Wounds and Fractures; A Clinical Guide to Civil and Military Practice, Springfield, Ill., Thomas, 1941.

O'Shea, M. C.: Treatment and results of 870 severed tendons and 57 severed nerves of hand and forearm (in 362 patients), Am. J. Surg. *43*:346, 1939.

Paradies, L. H., and Gregory, C. F.: Close range shot gun wounds of the extremities, Paper #16, Am. Acad. Orth. Surg., Jan. 30, 1962.

Posch, J. L., and Weller, C. N.: Mangle and severe wringer injuries of the hand in children, J. Bone Joint Surg. *36-A*:57, 1954.

Pratt, D. R.: Athletic injuries of the hand and digits, Clin. Orthop. *23*:100, 1962.

Rank, B. K., and Wakefield, A. R.: Surgery of Repair as Applied to Hand Injuries, ed. 2, Edinburgh, Livingstone, 1960.

Requarth, W. H.: Care of injured hand, U.S. Nav. Med. Bull. *41*:1329, 1943.

Robinson, D. W., and Hardin, C. A.: Corn picker injuries, Am. J. Surg. *89*:780, 1955.

Schink, W.: Handchirurgischer Ratgeber, Berlin, Springer, 1960.

Smith, F. H.: Penetration of tissue by grease under pressure of 7,000 pounds, J.A.M.A. *112*:907, 1939.

Snyder, R. D.: Snake bites, Am. J. Dis. Child. *103*:85, 1962.

Stark, H. H., Wilson, J. N., and Boyes, J. H.: Grease-gun injuries of the hand, J. Bone Joint Surg. *43-A*:485, 1961.

Stevenson, T. W., Jr.: Principles of treatment of avulsion of skin, Surg. Clin. N. Amer. *21*:555, 1941.

Stewart, S. F.: Traumatic and infectious tenosynovitis, Am. J. Surg. *56*:43, 1942.

Tempest, M. N.: Discussion, Spring Meeting, Brit. Orth. Assn., 1960, J. Bone Joint Surg. *42-B*:646, 1960.

Trueta, J.: Treatment of War Wounds and Fractures, New York, Hoeber, 1940.

Warren, L. H.: Leather buffers' nodes, J.A.M.A. *114*:571, 1940.

BURNS

Ackman, D., Gerrie, J. W., Pritchard, J. E., and Mills, E. S.: A report on the managemnt of burns. Ann. Surg. *119*:161, 1944.

Allen, H. S.: Treatment of superficial injuries and burns of the hand, J.A.M.A. *116*:1370, 1941.

Allen, H. S., and Koch, S. L.: Treatment of patients with severe burns, Surg., Gynec. Obstet. *74*:914, 1942.

Blocker, T. G.: Local and general treatment of acute extensive burns; open-air regime, Lancet *1*:498, 1951.

Brown, J. B., et al.: Surgical treatment of radiation burns, Surg., Gynec. Obstet. *88*:609, 1949.

Bunyan, J.: Method of treatment of burns and wounds, Med. Press *206*:103, 1940.

————: Envelope method of treating burns, Proc. Roy. Soc. Med. *34*:65, 1940.

Clarkson, P., and Lawrie, R. S.: The management and surgical resurfacing of serious burns, Brit. J. Surg. *33*:311, 1946.

Colebrook, L., and Colebrook, V.: Prevention of burns and scalds; review of 1,000 cases, Lancet *2*:181, 1949.

Conway H.: Surgical management of post radiation scars and ulcers, Surgery *10*:64, 1941.

Cope, O., Langohr, J. L., Moore, F. D., and Webster. R. C., Jr.: Expedious care of full-thickness burn wounds by surgical excision and grafting, Ann. Surg. *125*:1, 1947.

Dennison, W. M., and Divine, D.: Treatment of burns in war time, J. Roy. Army Med. Corps *77*:14, 1941.

Elman, R.: Therapeutic significance of plasma protein replacement in severe burns, J.A.M.A. *116*:213, 1941.

Enyart, J. L.: Treatment of burns from disaster, J.A.M.A. *158*:95, 1955.

Evans, E. I., and Bigger, I. A.: The rationale of whole blood therapy in severe burns, Ann. Surg. *122*:693, 1945.

Farmer, A. W., and Woolhouse, F. M.: Resurfacing of dorsum of the hand following burns, Ann. Surg. *122*:39, 1945.

Flemming, C.: Combination of burns and wounds; treatment, Proc. Roy. Soc. Med. *34*:53, 1940.

Gay, E. C.: Skin dressings in the treatment of débrided wounds, Am. J. Surg. *72*:212, 1946.

Glenn, W. W. L.: A physiologic analysis of the nature and of the treatment of burns, Ann. Surg. *119*:801, 1944.

Hannay, J. W.: Treatment of burns by envelope irrigation, Brit. M. J. *2*:46, 1941.

Harkins, H. N.: Treatment of Burns, Springfield, Ill., Thomas, 1942.

————: The fluid and nutritional therapy of burns, J.A.M.A. *128*:475, 1945.

Hudack, S. S.: Adaptation of structure to disturbed function following deep burns of hand, Amer. Acad. Orthop. Surg. Lect., p. 208, 1944.

Hull, H. C.: Treatment of burns of thermal origin, Arch. Surg. *45*:235, 1942.

MacCollum, D. W.: Burns of the hand, J.A.M.A. *116*:2371, 1941.

————: A practical outline for the treatment of burns, New Eng. J. Med. *227*:331, 1942.

McIndoe, A. H.: Burned hand, Med. Press *211*: 57, 1944.

Osborne, R. P.: The treatment of burns and wounds with skin loss by the envelope method, Brit. J. Surg. *32*:24, 1944.

Padgett, E. C.: Care of severely burned, with special reference to skin grafting, Arch. Surg. *35*:64, 1937.

————: Skin grafting in severe burns, Am. J. Surg. *43*:626, 1939.

Siler, V. E.: Primary cleansing, compression, and rest treatment of burns, Surg., Gynec. Obstet. *75*:161, 1942.

Wallace, A. B.: Treatment of Burns, London, Humphrey Milford, 1941.

————: The exposure treatment of burns, Lancet *1*:501, 1951.

Wilson, W. C.: Cause and treatment of lethal factors in burns (Honeyman Gillespie Lecture), Edinburgh M. J. *48*:85, 1941.

Woolhouse, F. M.: Reconstruction of hand, early surfacing of burns, Amer. Acad. Orthop. Surg. Lect., p. 187, 1944.

AMPUTATIONS

Alldredge, R. H.: The cineplastic method in upper extremity amputations, J. Bone Joint Surg. *30-A*:359, 1948.

Brown, A. M.: Prosthetic restorations after amputations about the hand, Am. J. Surg. *68*:338, 1945.

Kessler, H. H.: Amputation and prosthesis, Am. J. Surg. *43*:560, 1939.

————: Cineplastic amputation, Surg., Gynec. Obstet. *68*:554, 1939.

————: Symposium on reparative surgery; cineplastic amputations, Surg. Clin. N. Amer. *24*: 453, 1944.

Kirk, N. T., and Peterson, L. T.: Amputations *in* Lewis, Dean (ed.): Practice of Surgery, vol. 3, chap. 10, Hagerstown, Md., Prior, 1955.

McKeever, F. M.: Upper-extremity amputations and prostheses, J. Bone Joint Surg. *26*:660, 1944.

Mazet, R.: Cineplasty, J. Bone Joint Surg. *40-A*: 386, 1958.

Neller, J. L., and Schmidt, E. R.: Refrigeration amputation (in peripheral vascular disease), Wisc. M. J. *43*:936, 1944.

Nissen, R., and Bergmann, E.: Cineplastic Operations on Stumps of Upper Extremity, New York, Grune & Stratton, 1942.

Rank, B. K., and Henderson, G. D.: Cineplastic forearm amputations and prosthesis, Surg., Gynec. Obstet. *83*:373, 1946.

Slocum, D. B., and Pratt, D. R.: The principles of amputations of the fingers and hand, J. Bone Joint Surg. *26*:535, 1944.

Spittler, A. W.: Cineplastic muscle motors for prosthesis of arm amputees, J. Bone Joint Surg. *33-A*:601, 1951.

Steindler, A.: Artificial limbs, Military Surgeon *86*:560, 1940.

Woughter, H. W., and Myers, E. E.: Practical considerations in definitive amputation surgery, Surg., Gynec. Obstet. *80*:319, 1945.

Zanoli, R.: Krukenberg-Putti amputation, J. Bone Joint Surg. *39-B*:230, 1957.

Chapter 16

Fractures and Dislocations

SPECIAL FACTORS IN THE HAND

The principles used in the treatment of fractures of any long bones apply to those in the hand, but there are some special factors.

Healing of most fractures in the hand, except for some in the scaphoid, is usually prompt, and union is solid in a few weeks. immobilization aids healing and allows callus and bone to grow across the fracture line without disturbance. As in any bone, motion at

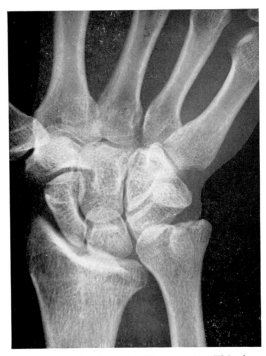

FIG. 783. Case A. W., age 17. This is not a Madelung's congenital deformity; the retardation of growth of the radius was due to a fall injuring the epiphysis at the age of 2 years. The patient complains of awkwardness in use of the hand.

the fracture site delays healing, but in addition, in the hand, pain may be marked, and osteoporosis and reflex vascular changes may arise. Attempts to hold the part still by reflex muscle action may pull the joints into nonfunctional positions, with marked stiffness of uninjured parts as the result.

There are two particularly important aspects of fractures in the hand. The hand mechanism is in delicate balance, and a minor deformity of angulation or dislocation can upset this balance and cripple other parts. Also, the balance can be upset by improper positioning of joints, such as the wrist. If the wrist is immobilized in palmar flexion and ulnar deviation, the Cotton-Loder position, as once used for lower radial fractures, the long flexors and extensors of the fingers are out of balance, and the fingers will be limited in action. The second way in which fractures of the hand differ is the close proximity of tendons to the bones. From the original trauma, which may damage the tendon or its sheath as well as the bone, or from the healing process, flexor or extensor tendons may adhere to the bone, most commonly in the proximal and the middle phalanges. This blocks the action of the common profundus or extensor muscle. Not only is the motion of that finger impaired, but the others are limited by the hold-back phenomenon, i.e., when one finger is held in either full flexion or extension it blocks the motion of the others.

Therefore, immobilization of the injured parts is necessary not only to hold the parts still, to avoid angular forces tending to displace the fragments, to place the joints in optimal position for muscle balance and the tension of their collateral ligaments but also must be applied in such a way that all uninjured parts can move through a full range. Prevention of stiffness by these measures is a fundamental part of the treatment of the fracture.

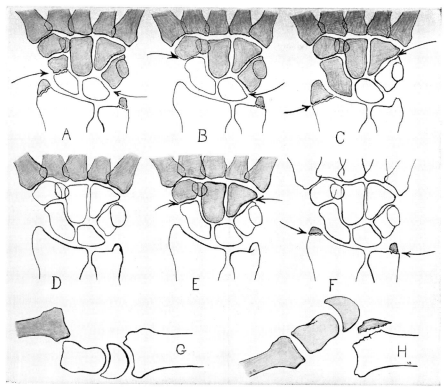

Fig. 784. Types of dislocations through the carpus with or without chip fractures of the 4 margins of the proximal socket of the wrist joint. (A) Carpus dislocates dorsally transscaphoid and perilunar with or without fracture of the styloids. (B) Radial oblique periscaphoid and lunar; dislocation of the carpus. (C) Ulnar oblique perilunar and triquetrous dislocation of the carpus. (D, G) Dislocation dorsally of the metacarpals from the carpus. (E) Midcarpal dislocation. (F, H) Radiocarpal dislocation, taking with it a marginal rim.

Fig. 785. Common dislocations through the carpus produced by a fall on the palm. (A, C) Dislocation of the lunate volarward from dorsiflexion and compression. The point of the lunate pierces the anterior capsule; the anterior radial lunate ligament holds, furnishing blood supply but turning the lunate about. (B, D) Dislocation dorsally of the carpus transscaphoid from the lunate, which remains in place.

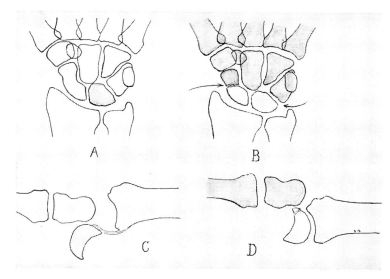

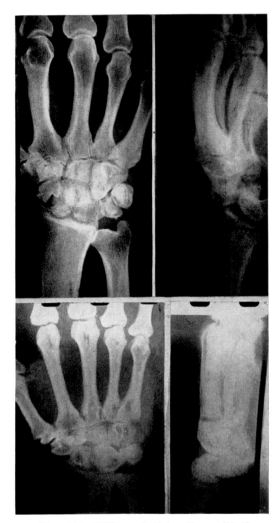

Fig. 786. Midcarpal dislocations. (*Top*) The distal row of carpals is dislocated posteriorly. (*Bottom*) The distal row of carpals is dislocated anteriorly.

IMMOBILIZATION

Immobilization must include all the parts that affect the movement of the injured part. Thus, to immobilize a proximal or a middle phalanx, the splint must extend above the wrist; for, if free, every motion changes the muscle pull on the fractured fragments. If the injured digit is held firmly and all others are active, stiffness of the joints adjoining the fracture will be the only late problem. This joint stiffness will be minimal if the fracture was aligned, firmly held and the joints put up in

slight flexion, which is the optimal position for the collateral ligaments.

In general, displaced long-bone fractures, as in other body regions, are reduced by placing the distal fragment in line with the proximal one and exerting traction. Traction is used to reduce the fracture—seldom is it needed to maintain reduction. Local injection into the hematoma or regional block of the nerves at the elbow and the wrist gives adequate anesthesia.

Dislocations and ligamentous ruptures are immobilized for 3 weeks. Rupture of a tendon, such as the extensor insertion into the distal phalanx, requires specific treatment (see Chap. 11, Tendons).

OPEN FRACTURES

Compound wounds involving the bones should be treated promptly, the wound closed, and reduction and immobilization carried out as for closed fractures. Closure by local or distant pedicle flaps may be required. The judicious use of a small Kirschner wire helps to provide immobilization and to avoid the use of bulky external splints.

Infected wounds are opened and drained as in soft-tissue wounds, and reduction of fractures is done by gradual traction to avoid spreading infection.

INJURIES OF THE WRIST

The wrist is a frequent site of injury. Colles' fracture is the commonest lesion; the next is fracture of the scaphoid. Then, in order of frequency, follow a variety of dislocations through the carpus and around the lunate and fractures of the carpal bones.

A strain of the wrist is infrequent. Therefore, in all wrist injuries, roentgenographic examination in several views is essential. Frequently, this will disclose chip fractures, fine cracks, carpal cysts, old arthritis, malalignment, semilunar dislocation and, often, fracture of the scaphoid. Another roentgenogram taken 10 days later often will show the last clearly.

In examining the exact structure damaged, comparison is made with the other wrist for deformity, swelling or limitation of motion. The area of injury is outlined exactly by local swelling or edema, pain and local tenderness. Tenderness about the complete joint circumference indicates arthritis or blood in the joint. Pushing on a digital ray may point to a certain carpal bone; moving the wrist in all directions —anteroposteriorly, laterally, in pronation and supination and to-and-fro, voluntarily and passively, with and without resistance and to the limit of range of motion—may disclose the exact ligament, bone or other structure involved—especially if at the same time the pain is accentuated by direct digital pressure. The diagnosis is made by listing and analyzing the positive findings.

COLLES' FRACTURE

Much impairment of function often follows a fracture of the lower radius. Injury to the soft tissues accounts for some of this, but inadequate treatment is the principal factor. Malunion results from incomplete reduction. The lower end of the upper fragment of the radius becomes a bony prominence that presses against the median nerve, and the flexor tendons are drawn tightly over it by the backward displacement of the end of the radius. This causes pain from pressure on the median nerve, and tenosynovitis and loss of function from pressure on the tendons. Malunion destroys the muscle balance—the flexors of the wrist, being tight, flex the wrist and the fingers, and because of the flexed wrist, the extensors are tight and extend the proximal finger joints. The angles of approach and the leverage of the tendons are disturbed at the wrist joint, since they are pulling out of line. The radial devia-

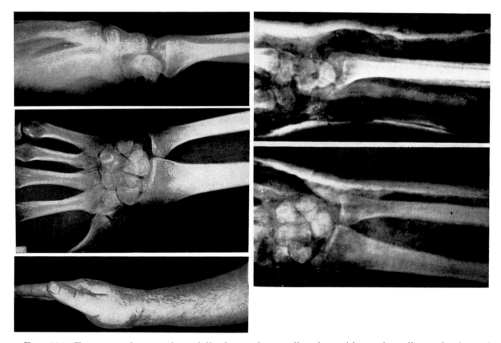

FIG. 787. Four months ago, in a fall, the patient suffered a midcarpal perilunar backward dislocation of his wrist with fracture of the scaphoid. Wrist movements were limited to one third. From muscle imbalance, the fingers lacked 2 inches of flexing to the distal crease in the palm.

(*Left, top* and *center*) Condition 4 months after the accident.

(*Left, bottom*) Deformity. The heel of the palm is displaced backward. Distal to the lunate, the dorsum of the hand is dorsal to the line of the forearm.

(*Right*) Operative reduction. After excising much scar, reduction was accomplished by traction with Kirschner wire through the metacarpal heads and a Davis skidder. On reduction, wrist movements were free again. The proximal fragment of the scaphoid, being dead, was removed because such a wrist would stiffen should immobilization be prolonged. Wrist motions are two thirds; finger motions are complete. He works steadily. There is slight lameness from arthritis. The bones remained in place.

tion angulates the carpal tunnel radially, weakening the grip. The head of the ulna becomes prominent dorsally from partial dislocation and projects distally. The lower ends of the radius and the carpus recede, deforming and limiting the motions of the wrist joint and those of pronation and supination.

It is never necessary to maintain reduction

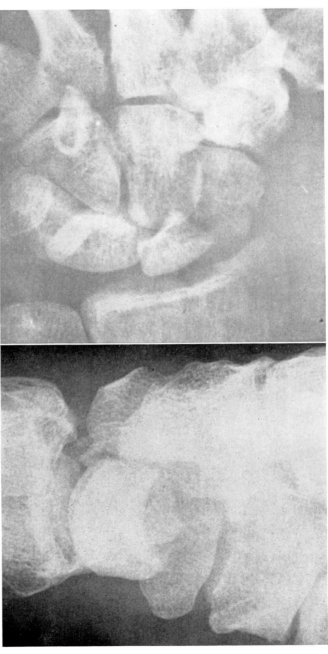

Fig. 788. Transscaphoid perilunar dislocation as seen 6 weeks after a fall.

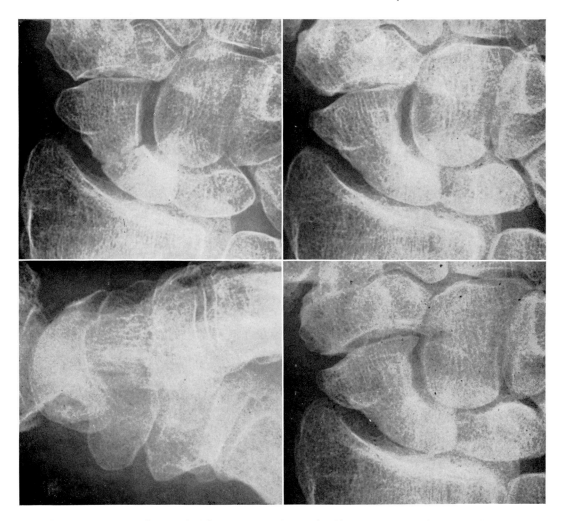

Fig. 789. Same patient as in Figures 788 and 790. (*Left*) After open reduction and removal of small central fragment of scaphoid. (*Right, top*) Nine months after reduction. (*Bottom*) Thirteen months after reduction. Healing is complete.

in Colles' fracture by placing the wrist joint in extreme flexion. The strain injures the joint. The digits should be entirely free, and the patient should be encouraged to use the hand in manual work during healing. The tendons will glide through the wrist with use, edema will not develop, and stiffening of joints is prevented.

Treatment. While traction is made by an assistant pulling on the thumb with one hand and on the index and the middle fingers with the other, the flexed elbow being held in a sling, the impaction is broken up, and the frac-

ture is reduced. There is no chance of over-reduction, because the unbroken dorsal and radial periosteum prevents it. The articular surface of the radius should face 30° ulnar-ward and at least 20° palmarward by drawing out the radial deviation and the longitudinal and backward displacement. This will restore the forward curve of the radius, the ulnar deviation of the hand and the position of the head of the ulna. The position is easily maintained by volar and dorsal nonpadded plaster slabs applied to the surface of the forearm and the hand with the wrist straight and in slight

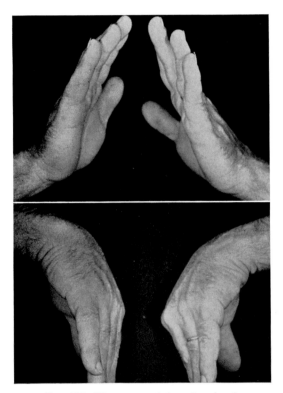

Fig. 790. The range of dorsal and palmar flexion thirteen months after open reduction of transscaphoid perilunar dislocation.

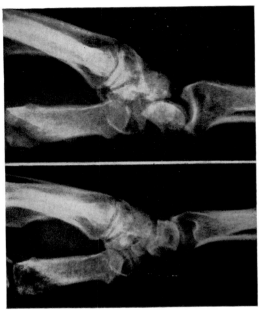

Fig. 792. Case M. R. (*Top*) Eleven days previously, in an automobile accident, the lunate dislocated forward, causing paralysis of the median nerve and much pain. (*Bottom*) Through a transverse volar incision and traction, the lunate was reduced easily. Dorsiflexing the wrist made its sharp point extrude through the capsule. The rent in the capsule was sutured. Causalgia followed but disappeared after 8 months.

ulnar flexion; the slabs should be separated from each other by waxed paper to make them bivalve easily. The cast should stop at the middle palmar crease. Colles' fracture involves the radio-ulnar joint, so that pronation and supination are painful. Therefore, much comfort can be given the patient by checking this motion for the first 2 weeks. To do this, a plaster strip is laid down the outer surface of the upper arm, around the elbow and up the inner surface and bandaged there. Fahey recommends that the forearm be supinated in all lower radial fractures. This part of the splint can be removed after 2 weeks and the

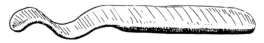

Fig. 791. The Davis skidder; useful in reducing old carpal dislocations.

remainder after 5 weeks. By stopping pronation and supination there will also be less radio-ulnar dislocation. For the first few days the arm should be kept elevated on an airplane splint. It should be inspected after 24 hours and the bivalve allowed to expand a little, if necessary, to allow for swelling. Later, as the swelling recedes, the bivalve should be tightened accordingly. To avoid stiffening, the patient should make full use of the hand from the first day.

Dislocation of Lower Radio-ulnar Joint

The head of the ulna may dislocate when the lower end of the radius is pushed away from it, as in fracture of the shaft or a Colles' fracture, or may do so from a severe twist, with or without fracture of the ulnar styloid. Dislocation with fracture is the more common, just as at the other end of the forearm the

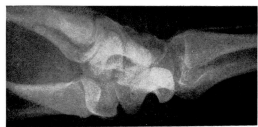

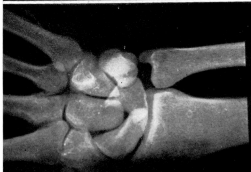

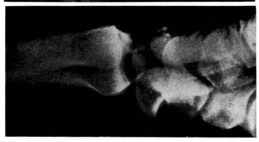

FIG. 793. Two examples of dislocations of the lunate. In the case shown in the center and the bottom illustrations, the median nerve was paralyzed. The paralysis cleared in a month after open reduction and suture of the rent in the anterior ligament.

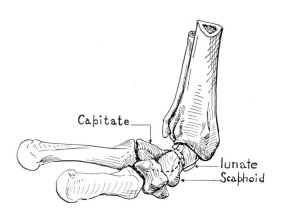

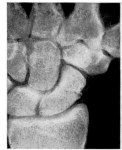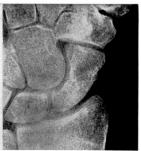

FIG. 795. (Left) Fracture of the scaphoid. Both fragments are nourished. Unites if immobilized. (Right) Same united, taken 1 year later.

head of the radius dislocates with fracture of the ulna; but dislocations of the ulnar head without fracture, except of styloid processes, are not rare. Forced supination on a fixed wrist causes it, and the forearm may be locked in supination. Rose-Innes immobilizes in pronation. After the dislocation is reduced, the head of the ulna is shoved tightly against the radius in the midposition or supination, and a nonpadded plaster-of-Paris dressing is applied from the distal crease in the palm to the axilla with the elbow at a right angle and is maintained for a month.

DISLOCATIONS: CARPAL, INTERCARPAL AND METACARPAL

The dislocation may be radiocarpal, midcarpal or, much less frequently, carpometacarpal. A midcarpal dislocation is often accompanied by a fracture of the scaphoid, the distal fragment going with the distal carpal row. As the carpus displaces, either partially or com-

FIG. 794. A fall on the palm when the wrist is dorsiflexed slightly may produce Colles' fracture. In complete dorsiflexion, the radius covers the lunate and half of the scaphoid. A fall on the palm then may produce any of the following: (1) It may drive the carpus dorsalward as a perilunar dislocation. If the forearm is oblique in the lateral plane, either of the 2 oblique perilunar dislocations may occur. (2) The dorsal edge of the radius may crack the scaphoid in two. (3) The lunate may be expressed forward from the carpus by dorsiflexion and the compression of the radius.

pletely, a part of the radius or the ulna usually is broken off with it, either by being shoved off or avulsed. The radial or the ulnar styloid may be avulsed in radiocarpal and midcarpal dislocations.

Reduction is made by traction and a direct shoving pressure. In radiocarpal dislocations, the carpus should be lifted and angulated around the flaring dorsal or volar border of the radius. Plaster from elbow to distal crease

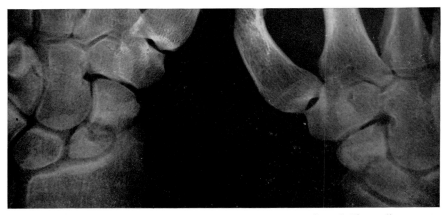

FIG. 796. Bilateral fracture of the scaphoid. A long radiostyloid predisposes to this fracture.

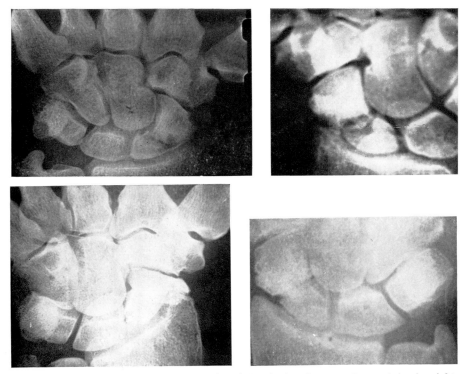

FIG. 797. Fractures of the scaphoid. (*Top*) Beginning degeneration and, in the right-hand illustration, some sequestration. (*Bottom*) Old ununited fractures with arthritis in adjoining parts.

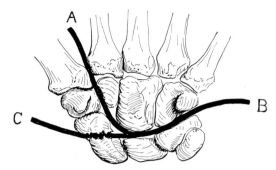

FIG. 798. Nonunion occurs after fracture of the scaphoid because both blood supply and immobilization are insufficient. The line of motion in lateral movement of the wrist is normally along A–B through the first cleft. When the scaphoid is fractured, it is along C–B, shearing the fracture line at every move.

in the palm is worn for 3 weeks, or longer if fracture is present.

Old dislocations upset mechanics and muscle balance so seriously that they should be reduced surgically. This can be done by using traction by Kirschner wire through the metacarpal heads and severing all the scar tissue that binds and prevents reduction.

DISLOCATIONS: LUNATE AND PERILUNATE

The articular surfaces of the radius face volarward, so that when a person falls on his palm with wrist dorsiflexed, the scaphoid and the lunate are covered by the jutting radius, and a fracture of the radius is produced. However, when the force happens to be against the palm or the more distal part of the carpus, as when the wrist is in strong dorsiflexion, it produces a dorsal dislocation of the distal row of carpal bones and may include the distal half of the scaphoid and the triquetrum. If the hand is in ulnar deviation, the triquetrum is held by the end of the ulna and remains in place with the forearm bones, along with the lunate. In that case, the whole scaphoid dislocates with the carpus. The capitate and the carpus are thrust backward over the lunate. Volar dislocation of the carpus is rare. The lunate remains with the radius. Its dorsal and volar radiolunate ligaments with their blood supply remain intact.

In the lateral view there is a midcarpal dorsal bulge, and, the heel of the palm, which

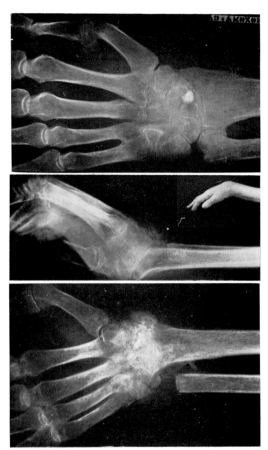

FIG. 799. End-result of nonunion of a fractured scaphoid. The patient related a history of "sprained wrist 20 years ago" and "rheumatism" in the wrist since. In the last year, he could not use the hand. (*Top*) The sequestrum of the upper end of the scaphoid is conspicuous, as also is the resulting arthritis, including the radioulnar joint. (*Center, inset*) The deformity. (*Center* and *bottom*) The wrist was arthrodesed, and the head of the ulna excised for free rotary movement.

has displaced backward, is flat rather than rounded.

Reduction is easy by straight traction and pressure. If the dislocation is several months old, reduction is difficult but can be done by open operation. Blood supply of the lunate is not a factor, as its dorsal and volar ligaments are preserved.

Sometimes, the capitate and the carpus in their backward thrust, instead of riding over

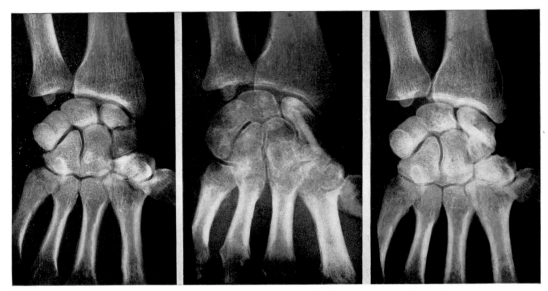

Fig. 800. (*Left*) Nonunion of fracture of the scaphoid after 3 months without treatment. The upper fragment has a lessened blood supply. (*Center*) X-ray appearance 4 months after pegging. Union is firm in spite of the avascular upper end. (*Right*) X-ray appearance 9 months later. The ends of the scaphoid are almost equal in density.

the lunate, pinch it against the radius in dorsi-flexion so that the lunate is shot volarward, like pinching a watermelon seed. With it may go the proximal half of the scaphoid or, less commonly, the whole scaphoid. Dislocation of the lunate alone is common and will be discussed separately.

The scaphoid alone may dislocate dorsally, causing tenosynovitis of the thumb extensors and limitation of motion, but is easily reduced under traction. The trapezoid alone may dislocate backward. The pisiform and the hamate alone rarely dislocate, but the latter with 2 metacarpals has been seen to be dislocated backward on the triquetrum, causing much pain. In this case, muscle balance of the fingers

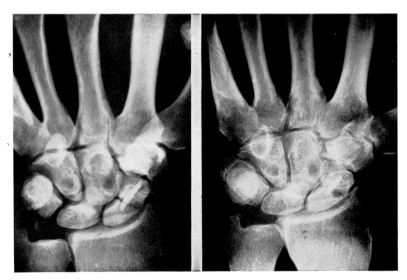

Fig. 801. (*Left*) After 4 months without splinting, the scaphoid was pegged with a piece from the ulna. (*Right*) Bony union followed. X-ray view taken 6 months later.

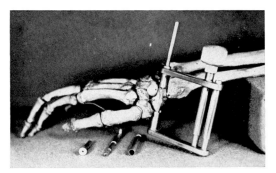

Fig. 802. Clamp for bone-pegging a fractured scaphoid. Through a short transverse incision over both the upper pole and the lower pole, the clamp is applied and screwed tight. The wrist is flexed to present the upper pole. A drill guided by the tubes of the clamp follows through the scaphoid exactly and is followed by a bone peg. The 3 gadgets below are, from left to right, a guide for a Kirschner wire, another drill with sleeve and an oscillating bone peg borer. The clamp is solidly free from weave. (H. Weniger, San Francisco, Calif.)

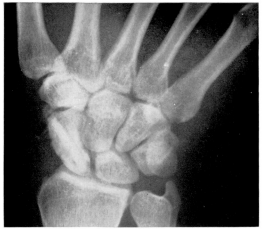

Fig. 803. Case R. B. For 1 year, the fracture of the scaphoid, which was not treated, had remained ununited. At operation, a bone peg from the ulna was placed by aid of the clamp. Bony union occurred in 3 months. As this radius had an unusually long styloid process, and since this is a factor in fracturing scaphoids, a centimeter of the styloid process was removed. This man also fractured his other scaphoid. Both radii had long styloid processes.

was upset, and the metacarpal heads projected in the palm. Replacement and lashing with palmaris longus tendon through drill holes relieved the disability. Dislocation of the trapezium with its metacarpal has accompanied a Bennett's fracture.

Minor displacements of the scaphoid are difficult to recognize. Lateral roentgenograms of both wrists with deviation in exactly the same angle will provide comparison. Laminagrams are of help. See Chapter 1 for normal scaphoid relationships in various positions of the wrist.

Dislocation of Lunate

In a fall with the wrist dorsiflexed, the weight of the body forces the radius against the head of the capitate, extruding the lunate volarward. The sharp, knifelike edge of its volar end penetrates the lunate-capitate ligament, the dorsal scapholunate ligament ruptures, and the bone escapes into the carpal tunnel, held only by its anterior radiolunate ligament. Further displacement rotates the lunate on this ligament until its concavity faces proximalward. Dorsal dislocation of the lunate by hyperflexion of the wrist is rare.

Lunate dislocation results in pain and limitation of motion. The bone presses against and diverts the flexor tendons, and the hand is held with the wrist and the fingers in semiflexion and the proximal finger joints fairly straight. Dorsiflexion of the wrist is painful. The wrist is thick and tender volarward between the 2 flexion creases which mark the lunate, and there is a dorsal hollow. The lunate also presses on the median nerve, causing intense pain, paresthesia, anesthesia, paralysis of the muscles of opposition and atrophy in the median area. In complete displacement such disability is permanent, but if the displacement is only partial, the permanent disability may be slight.

If unreduced, arthritis develops in the wrist joint from mechanical disarrangement rather than from lack of blood supply of the dislocated bone, which is still supplied through its anterior ligament. Strangely enough, Kienböck's disease has not been known to develop after dislocation of the lunate (Böhler).

Since the lunate retains its blood supply through its intact volar ligament, it will retain

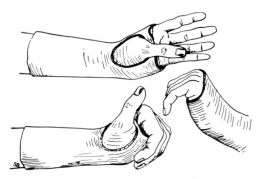

FIG. 804. *Correct* way to apply a cast to the hand and the forearm. All fingers are free to move because the cast does not extend farther than the distal flexion crease in the palm, and the thumb is free because the cast ends at the thenar crease. The wrist is in moderate dorsiflexion. The proximal finger joints can be flexed and the thumb opposed. (The Bulletin, U.S.A. Med. Dept.)

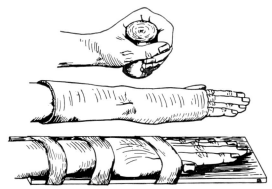

FIG. 805. Three *incorrect* ways of splinting a hand, all of which contribute to crippling. (*Top*) Bandaging all fingers over a roller bandage stiffens the hand as a whole and the joints of all fingers. Only the injured digit should be splinted and the others left free to move and be kept moving. (*Center*) A plaster cast should not be applied with the wrist and the fingers straight, and it should never include uninjured fingers beyond the distal crease in the palm. Result: The proximal finger joints will be stiff and straight, and the whole hand and forearm unexercised. Wrist, arches, thumb and fingers should be in the position of function. (*Bottom*) Strapping a hand to a board stiffens the whole member and in a position of nonfunction, namely, with the wrist straight instead of dorsiflexed, palm flat with loss of metacarpal arch, thumb at side of hand instead of in opposition and finger joints straight. (The Bulletin, U.S.A. Med. Dept.)

its vitality when reduced. Closed reduction is usually possible. The obstacle is the back of the posterior horn against the head of the capitate. Strong or prolonged traction, with fingers straight so that the taut flexor tendons will press on the lunate, will free the horn from the capitate and allow reduction. Böhler advises 10 minutes of steady traction. Closed reduction may be successful up to 2 weeks after injury.

If the closed method fails, reduction is easy by open operation under block anesthesia with traction supplied by Kirschner wire through the metacarpal heads. Using a pointed instrument, the posterior horn is tilted around the capitate head, and the lunate pops into place. It extrudes again on dorsiflexion but is held in place on flexion. After closing the ligamentous rent, the wrist is put up in a half plaster-of-Paris cast in slight flexion. After a week it is changed to the straight position, and after 3 weeks the cast is removed.

If accompanied by fracture of the scaphoid, the proximal scaphoid fragment should be removed if it is small; in this way convalescence will be shortened and long immobilization of a badly traumatized wrist will be avoided. If the fragment is larger, the immobilization should be maintained until the scaphoid unites.

Old Dislocations. Old unreduced dislocations of the lunate develop traumatic arthritis. If removed before arthritis develops, the disability will be slight, consisting of some weakness and limitation of motion. The gap between the carpal bones does not close. (We have had no experience with steel balls or plastic inserts reportedly used by others.) If removed after arthritis has developed, the arthritis will be permanent, but the pain will be less, and motion will be improved. If the lunate shows a relative excess of calcium indicating necrosis, or if 6 months have elapsed, immediate excision is advisable. If the x-ray appearance shows that the bone is viable and there is no arthritis, open reduction is advisable and possible under skeletal traction. The dislocation is reduced, great care being taken not to traumatize the carpal bones by leverage or to destroy the remaining blood supply of the lunate.

FRACTURE OF CARPAL BONES

Of all carpal bones, the scaphoid and the lunate are fractured most often, the scaphoid by far the most as the styloid acts as a wedge-like fulcrum against its center.

The relative frequency of fractures about the wrist is shown by the statistics of Schnek of Böhler's Clinic. Of 669 fractures and epiphysial separations of the lower end of the radius there were 437 cases of carpal injuries, consisting of the following:

Fracture of scaphoid	154
Fracture of lunate	23
Avulsion of posterior horn of lunate	59
Fracture of triquetrum	18
Fracture of trapezium	13
Fracture of pisiform	13
Fracture of hamate	8
Fracture of capitate	6

Snodgrass, from the Episcopal Hospital in Philadelphia, reports the order of frequency of carpal bone fractures as follows:

Scaphoid	144
Lunate	11
Triquetrum	7
Pisiform	1
Trapezium	3
Trapezoid	1
Capitate	2
Hamate	1

Fracture of Scaphoid. In fractures about the wrist, fracture of the scaphoid is next in frequency to Colles' fracture and is especially frequent in young adults. In military service its incidence was greater than that of Colles' fracture. In dorsiflexion the scaphoid is covered in its proximal half by the radius, its distal half projecting. In a fall, the scaphoid is extra vulnerable, since it spans the length of both rows of carpal bones and is fractured as the second carpal row bends backward on the first, imprisoned under the radius. Schnek pointed out that a large radial styloid predisposes to this fracture. In normal radial deviation of the wrist, the scaphoid must angulate forward to avoid the radial styloid. Fracture of the tuberosity is by avulsion.

SYMPTOMS. Swelling and edema are only moderate, and there is local pain on wrist motions and in grasping. Tenderness is present at the tubercle and in the snuffbox, and pain is elicited by shoving upward on the index or the middle digital rays. Wrist motions are moderately limited. Many fractures are over-

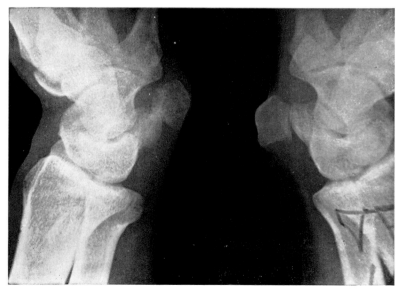

FIG. 806. Dislocation of the pisiform bone (*left*).

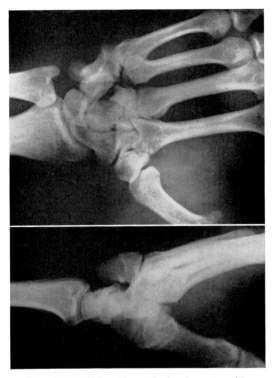

FIG. 807. Dislocation of the hamate. (B. Kahn, M.D.)

margins and patchiness or increased density in the proximal fragment if there has been a fracture. Subsequent roentgenograms show absence of the bone changes seen in fracture. Gollasch reported this rare condition in 10 members of a family.

NONUNION. There are 2 reasons why untreated fracture across the scaphoid does not unite: excess of movement and deficiency of blood supply.

Half of the lateral movement of the wrist is in the midcarpal joint, the cleavage plane of which normally curves to emerge through the first interdigital cleft. With a break across the scaphoid, this shearing movement takes place through the fracture line. Also, the scaphoid angulates forward with each radial deviation to avoid the radial styloid. Every advance of tissue growth toward union is sheared away until finally the 2 surfaces become eburnated. As in the head of the femur, the scaphoid receives most of its blood supply from the main bone, so that when broken there is insufficient circulation to allow union; thus, instead of sharing in the rarefaction of the surrounding bones, the fragment shines out with its original density.

Most of the surface of the scaphoid is cov-

looked; they may not show in the usual lateral and anteroposterior views because the long axis of the scaphoid is in an oblique position. To find an oblique fracture, slightly different angles may be needed. Unless views are taken in several directions, the tiny line indicating the crack through the scaphoid will be overlooked. Even so, if symptoms point to the fracture, new films should be taken after an interval of 3 weeks, since by then the fracture line will have spread and will show clearly.

BIPARTITE SCAPHOID is rare but when found may be confused with fracture; either of the 2 distal corners may be separate or cartilaginous; or there may be a separation at the waist, there having been 2 centers of ossification instead of the usual 1 for each carpal bone. Points to consider in differentiating are the presence of similar findings in the other carpus, the absence of history or signs of injury if it is an incidental finding, and the rounded, clear-cut edges, with equal bone density of each part, in contrast with the irregular

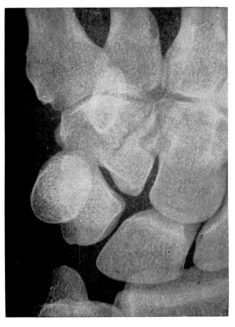

FIG. 808. Fracture of the hamatum.

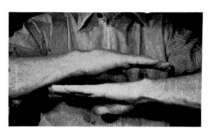
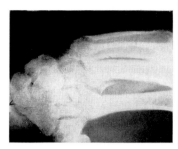
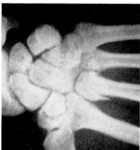

FIG. 809. Case R. D. A posterior dislocation of the 4th and the 5th metacarpals on the carpus and a fracture of the 3rd resulting from a punch to a chin. (*Top, left*) The deformity. Muscle balance was upset so that the fingers lacked 2 inches of flexing to the distal crease in the palm. (*Top, center* and *right*) X-ray appearance. (*Center* and *Bottom, left*) At operation 3 months later, adhesions were cut away, and the bones replaced and held there by a withdrawable stainless-steel nail and wire. On first withdrawing the nail, the wire is pulled out easily. The 3rd metacarpal was wired. (*Bottom, center* and *right*) Final result: correct approximation and complete motion.

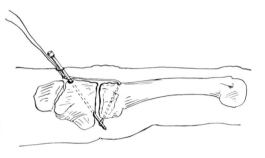

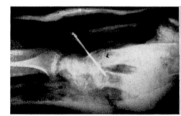
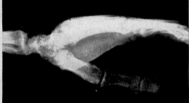
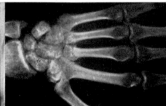

ered with cartilage, there being 5 articular surfaces, each of which moves on a different bone. The principal vessels enter along the ridge from the tubercle to the superior articular facet. They are distributed so that in a fracture through the waist each fragment may have some blood supply, but in the minority of cases, the proximal fragment will not. The more proximal the fracture line, the more avascular will be the upper fragment.

All fractures through the tubercle unite whether splinted or not. Most fractures through the waist will unite if immobilized for 8 to 10 weeks, since both fragments have circulation. Some more proximal fractures either do not unite or require, even with perfect immobilization, as long as a year for union. The time required is for gradual substitution, as in the case of the femoral head.

The proximal portion dies and is gradually replaced through ingrowing blood vessels. Barr tabulated 22 per cent of nonunions after all fractured scaphoids and claimed that 42 per cent of cases developed displacement, fragmentation, cysts, arthritic changes and functional

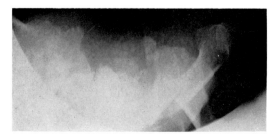

FIG. 810. Fracture of hook of hamate in tunnel view.

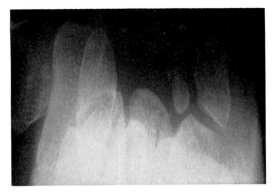

Fig. 811. Failure of fusion of hook process
to body of hamate.

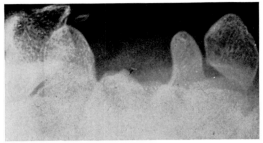

Fig. 812. Avulsion fracture of trapezial
ridge as seen in tunnel view.

impairment. In 220 fresh fractures Russe obtained 97 per cent union with a nonpadded
plaster, holding the middle metacarpal in line
with the forearm and including the first metacarpal but not the thumb. Increased density
developed in 30 per cent of all fresh fractures
during treatment. Seventy per cent of the
fractures were through the middle third, and
20 per cent were in the proximal third of the
bone.

If there is movement or displacement, the
fracture will never unite, even when through
the waist. In 1 or 2 months the gap becomes

wide and of cystic appearance. The distal fragment rarefies and may become cystic. The
proximal fragment, if avascular, will show as
a sequestrum. In a sedentary individual there
may not be much complaint from nonunion.
But in a manual worker, the hand will swell
and be painful. The inevitable result of nonunion, especially if one fragment has sequestrated, is arthritis, which gradually involves
the whole wrist. It shows in the radial styloid
and in the adjoining carpal bones as distortion, hypertrophic bone growth and erosion of
cartilage.

TREATMENT. *Immobilization in Nonpadded
Cast.* It has been shown conclusively that

Fig. 813. (*Top*) De-
formity with fracture of
the metacarpals. Three
extensor carpi dorsiflex
the proximal fragments,
and the intrinsic muscles
and the long flexors flex
the distal fragment. The
long extensor is tensed
over the fracture and
dorsiflexes the proximal
finger joints. There is a
hump in the dorsum of
the hand, and the head
of the metacarpal proj-
ects into the palm.

(*Bottom*) Deformity
with fracture of proxi-
mal phalanx is a buckling
forward because of the
dorsal aponeurosis which
is held taut by the in-
trinsic muscles and the
long extensor.

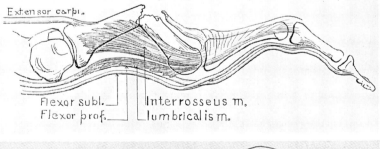

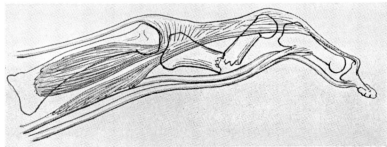

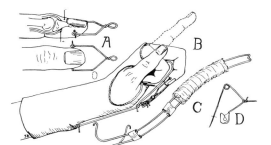 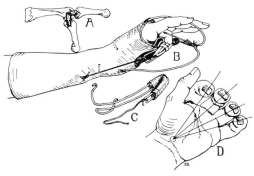

Fig. 814. Correct method of applying pulp traction for fracture of the phalanx or the metacarpal. (A) Pin transfixes at correct site, avoiding matrix (*upper arrow*), nail, phalanx and tendon sheath (*lower arrow*). (B) Plaster cast embraces the hand and the forearm, stops at the distal crease in the palm, leaving the uninjured fingers free to exercise throughout their range of motion and at the thenar crease, giving the thumb free motion of opposition. The finger whose phalanx or metacarpal is injured rests on a padded wire extension (as in C), which is incorporated into plaster. A cord from the wire to the cast at the forearm maintains the flexion. (C) Extension made of soft iron wire with 2 strips of tin and padding. A strip of duralumin may be used instead. (D) Method of using a steel safety pin for pulp traction. Point after transfixing is cut off. (The Bulletin, U.S.A. Med. Dept.)

Fig. 815. (B) Correct method of applying skeletal traction for fracture of the metacarpal. The wrist is dorsiflexed 20°, and the proximal finger joint is flexed 45°. Thin Kirschner wire transfixes the neck of the proximal phalanx and is bent, as shown, for traction to the stiff wire extension loop from the plaster cast. The finger is steadied by adhesive plaster on a wire extension (as in C) to maintain correct rotation. Skeletal traction on the fingers rarely is needed. (A) Shows the collateral ligaments of the proximal finger joint tight in flexion but relaxed in extension. If this joint is splinted in extension, these ligaments shorten so much that the joint cannot be flexed. If splinted in flexion and with skeletal traction, the joint remains limber. (D) Showing guides to correct rotation in setting fractures. In partial flexion, the planes of the fingernails form an arch. The planes of motion of the fingers converge to the tubercle of the scaphoid. (The Bulletin, U.S.A. Med. Dept.)

union will occur if immobilization is complete and prolonged. Immobilization is the key to success, not the position in which the limb is placed. With the bones exposed, it can be seen that abduction of the wrist or the thumb or any other position does not bring the fragments together. Nothing less than shoving up the 1st and the 5th rays will narrow the fracture line. The fact that union takes place with different positions of immobilization eliminates position as a factor. Even so, position may be used to stimulate union. A hand in the position of function will be used, and use without displacement provides optimal conditions for healing.

A padded cast or leather wristlet does not immobilize. A nonpadded cast fulfills the requirements of immobility if snugly molded and properly made. It should include three quarters of the length of the forearm and the hand, placed in the position of function of mild dorsiflexion and ulnarflexion and with the thumb in moderate opposition, not abducted. The fit about the head of the metacarpal of the thumb should be snug, leaving the distal two segments free to move, and the cast should end at the knuckles and the distal crease in the palm for free motion of the fingers. The hand should be used freely at work to keep it in good condition, preventing stiffness during the long period of immobilization of the wrist. Periodically, when the hand becomes loose in the cast, a new cast should be applied. One or 2 crossed Kirschner wires through the scaphoid have been used by Dehne to ensure immobility. Later, the wires are retrieved from beneath the skin. Similarly, a screw has been used (McLaughlin). Verdan

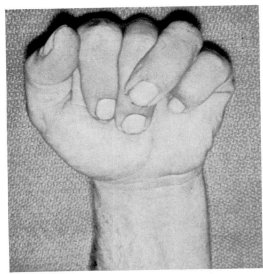

FIG. 816. Crossing of ring over middle finger from malrotation of metacarpal or proximal phalanx.

is reported to favor extending the immobilization to above the elbow in the early stages.

The average time for union is 12 weeks, but since the proximal fragment will be avascular in some cases, the rule should be to continue the immobilization until union is seen on roentgenograms, the criterion being obliteration of the fracture line, crossing of it by lines of force, and equal density in the ends of the bone.

Of course, the fragments must be in proper position. When properly immobilized and in position, practically all should unite. The patients seen with nonunion are usually those

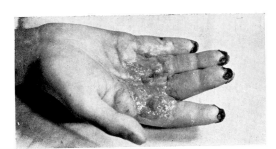

FIG. 817. Effect of overzealous pulp traction. Obviously a palm wound should have been closed before dense fibrosis had frozen the underlying tissues. (D. W. Macomber, M.D.)

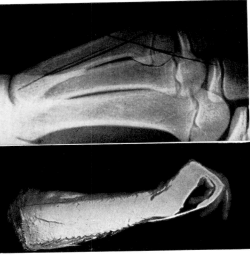

FIG. 818. (Top) Fracture of the neck of the metacarpal with usual deformity. The distal fragment is controlled through the phalanx after flexing the joint to a right angle. (Bottom) A pad under the middle knuckle and a cast as shown maintain position.

who were thought to have had sprains or were not treated or had inadequate treatment. In a survey, Donaldson found these to be the cause of nonunion in 85 per cent. If the fracture is several months old, immobilization may succeed, but it takes longer. In this way even a dead head has been made to unite in 1 or 2 years. McKim reports a case of nonunion of 2 years' duration which united well after immobilization for 9½ months.

Under certain conditions, when the chances for union by prolonged immobilization are poor or nil, or when long treatment is not advisable, an operative procedure is indicated. Thus, if the proximal fragment has sequestrated, it is best to excise it. If, in a complicated carpal injury involving the lunate and other bones, the proximal fragment of the scaphoid is small and loose, a long seige of stiffness will be avoided by excision of the loose fragment. In cases of wide separation with some relative increased density, one must decide on excision or bone graft.

If both fragments are rarefied or cystic, there is sufficient circulation, and long immobilization will suffice. Here, drilling to increase blood supply is superfluous. However, if the ends are eburnated or one fragment is denser, drilling may succeed in restoring circulation

FIG. 819. Fresh fracture pinned. Kirschner wire is cut beneath the skin to avoid infection. A cast is not necessary.

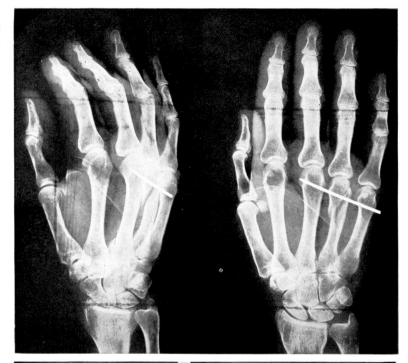

FIG. 820. Traction splint for fracture of metacarpals and phalanges. (*Left*) Made of duralumin for penetration by the roentgen ray, the splint is shaped to the hand and the wrist, as shown at the right. A steel safety pin bent as

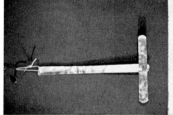

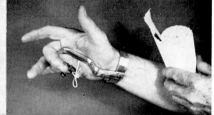

shown, with its point snipped off after being thrust through the finger pulp, serves for traction. (*Right*) The splint as shown is incorporated in plaster of Paris, enclosing the forearm and the hand to the distal palmar crease, after the first few layers of plaster are in place. This is similar to the splint of wire advised by Böhler.

and union, but a more positive course of action is to insert a bone graft.

Bone grafting is advisable in delayed cases to ensure quicker union by more complete immobilization and bony continuity. It is a short cut for slow-healing fractures and will bring blood supply to a partially dead head. It is indicated when the fragments are eburnated or even in a fresh case when they are separated. If, after 3 months or more, there is nonunion with pain and limited motion, grafting is justified.

In 100 cases of bone-grafted scaphoids, Gordon Murray found that 40 per cent showed aseptic necrosis of the upper end, but that

union was obtained in all except 1 case, and even this patient was able to return to work. In a later report of a larger series, 96 per cent fused. The proximal fragment became vascu-

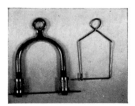

FIG. 821. Traction bows for fingers (Dupuy on *left*).

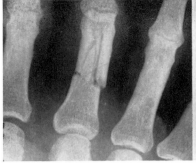
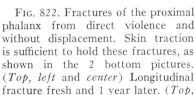
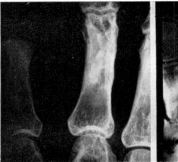
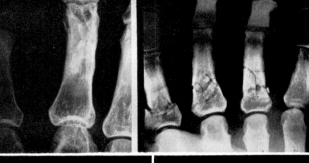
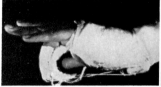
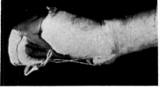

FIG. 822. Fractures of the proximal phalanx from direct violence and without displacement. Skin traction is sufficient to hold these fractures, as shown in the 2 bottom pictures. (*Top, left* and *center*) Longitudinal fracture fresh and 1 year later. (*Top, right*) These fractures solidified promptly, as in the *top center* illustration. Without displacement, tendons are not so likely to become adherent. (*Bottom*) Fixation for fractures of the proximal phalanx of the fingers. The plaster includes the forearm, stops at the distal crease in the palm to allow flexion of other fingers as shown in the *bottom right* picture. A padded wire loop extension, as used by Böhler, holds the injured finger, using skin or pulp traction.

larized and lived. Fractures through the waist, which constitute three fourths of the cases, should all unite if in position and properly immobilized. Similarly, most of those through the upper pole unite in time, though here the blood supply is doubtful. Of fractures of the tubercle, which constitute 10 per cent, all unite. It is the undiagnosed and, therefore, untreated fracture that results in nonunion.

In sequestration of the proximal fragment, excision should be done early to prevent arthritis.

It is usually the proximal fragment which is excised, but at the same time the sharp edges of the distal fragment should be rounded over. After excision of a part or all of the scaphoid there is usually some permanent weakness of grip and limitation of motion, and the hand deviates radially. Frequently, however, and especially in people who do not do manual work, there will be little or no complaint. Arthrodesis between the capitate and the 2 parts of the fractured scaphoid has been suggested by Sutro. Three of his 4 cases united. This will limit lateral motion of the wrist by one half. Arthrodesis with the lunate, as is normal in carnivores, has also been suggested to bring good blood supply to the scaph-

oid fragments. Bentzon interposed soft tissue across the fracture line in 6 cases. Waugh and Legge placed vitallium substitutes for scaphoids.

In an old case of fractured scaphoid, arthritis, if either progressive or crippling, calls for arthrodesis of the wrist. In such cases a bone graft is unnecessary, since broad approximation of the wrist bones can be obtained; otherwise, a flat graft of ilium is inserted. Gordon and King excise the styloid, fuse the radius, the scaphoid and the lunate and relieve pain, yet retain about 40° of anteroposterior and 30° of lateral motions.

Bone Grafting. Each pole of the scaphoid is exposed through an incision paralleling the skin creases. The tuberosity is felt and uncovered easily. It is just proximal to the ridge on the trapezium. To expose the upper pole in the snuffbox, the skin is first undermined superficially; then, through a longitudinal incision in the superficial fascia, the twigs of the radial nerve are drawn aside. The wrist must be strongly flexed to present the proximal pole. The extensor tendons of the fingers and the tendon of the extensor carpi radialis brevis are retracted ulnarward. Care is taken to avoid damaging the blood supply of the scaphoid,

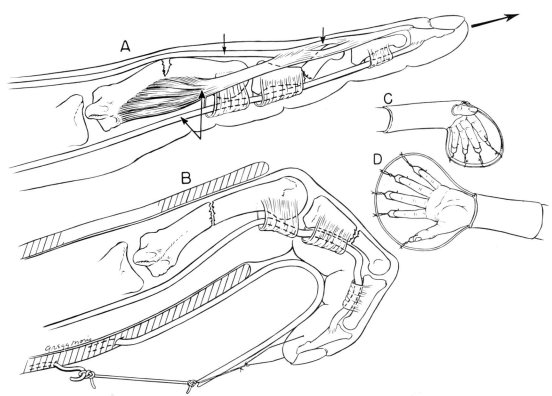

FIG. 823. (*Top*) *Incorrect* way to splint fractures of metacarpals and phalanges. They should never be pulled straight (A) or spread in flexion as by a banjo splint (C). The flexor tendon and the lateral band are pulled tight and straight, so that the fractures are cocked out of position.

(*Bottom*) *Correct* way to splint same (Böhler). The fingers are pulled around on an outrigger pulley in the semiflexed position of function. Note undulation of the flexor tendon. The banjo splint wrecks many hands. It pulls fingers in straight or wrong position which throws fractures out of line and stiffens all joints of digits. (C) Fingers in semiflexion should converge. Fingers are pulled straight and diverging. Thumb should not be enclosed in cast and wrist should be in dorsiflexion. (D) Digits are pulled in wrong or straight position and are not really splinted, since the hand flaps back and forth. Will result in much stiffening and malunion.

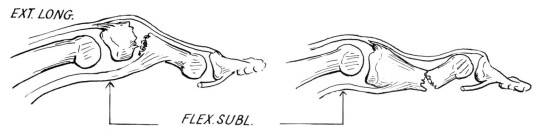

FIG. 824. Deformity with fracture of the middle phalanx, depending on whether or not the fracture line is proximal or distal to the insertion of the flexor sublimis tendon. This deformity is not constant.

which is along the dorsal ridge. A solid metal clamp with short spikes clasps the scaphoid from pole to pole and presses the fragments together. A hole is drilled through this clamp, which is used as a guide, and a bone graft is tapped into the hole.

Barnard exposed the scaphoid by excising the radial styloid, which he used for the graft.

Russe uses a volar incision, cleans out the fracture line and the soft inner part of each fragment and packs tightly with iliac bone. He reports 90 per cent union.

In the treatment of scaphoid fractures, there is still room for difference of opinions, though all agree that a fresh fracture should be immobilized. London feels that immobilization for six weeks is adequate, and, if there are no symptoms, regardless of the appearance in the roentgenogram, he removes all support. He reports 227 cases with 95 per cent union. In established nonunion, if there are minimal symptoms and the patient's age and occupation allow it, the fracture can be neglected and treatment advised only if the wrist becomes symptomatic. Occasionally, a scaphoid heals after a long period of delayed union. Mazet and Mason-Hohl reported a case, ununited after 3 years, that was healed 5 years later.

Simple styloidectomy is reported to relieve symptoms in 70 per cent of nonunions. If the Bentzon procedure is added, and radiocarpal arthritis has not developed, the results are even better. Frank sequestration of the proximal fragment requires excision, and with much arthritis, arthrodesis of the radiocarpal and the scaphoid-capitate joint is the best solution.

FRACTURES OF METACARPALS AND PHALANGES

Fractures of Metacarpals

Fractures of the metacarpals and the phalanges are the most common of all fractures. Distal to the radius, in order of frequency, are fractures of the phalanges, the metacarpals and the scaphoid. The 4th and the 5th metacarpals are subject to trauma because of their position and are fractured most often. The fracture may be near the base, in the shaft or through the neck, but the distal fragment always angulates volarward. Neck fractures are usually from blows, the 5th metacarpal being in the most vulnerable position. Shaft and base fractures are often from crushing by heavy objects or machinery and so are frequently

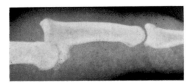

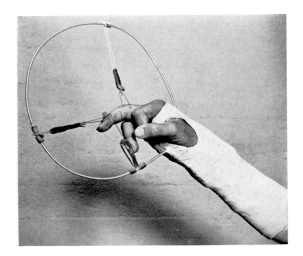

Fig. 825. Showing fracture-dislocation of the proximal interphalangeal joint. A simple method is to pin a semiflexed joint longitudinally. (*Top, left*) Before reduction. (*Top, right*) Apparatus used in treatment. (*Bottom, left*) Reduction with traction applied. (*Bottom, right*) Final result. (Robertson, R. C., Cawley, J. J., Jr., and Faris, A. M.: Treatment of fracture, dislocation of the interphalangeal joints of the hand, J. Bone Joint Surg. *28*:70)

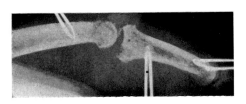

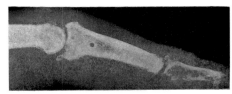

FIG. 826. (*Top*) Fracture of base of middle phalanx with dorsal subluxation on proximal phalanx. This type of fracture should be opened and reduced early. (*Bottom*) Open reduction with pinning of replaced fragment, and control of subluxation by Kirschner wire across joint.

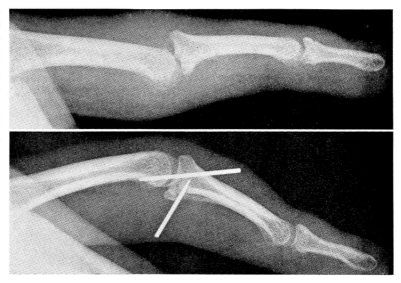

multiple, comminuted and open. Spiral shaft fractures are from rolling twists, with the fingers flexed at their proximal joints as levers. Malunion and nonunion are discussed in Chapter 8.

Malunion of a metacarpal upsets muscle balance, producing a clawed finger, and the head of the metacarpal projects in the palm and limits grasping because of pain. Malunion of rotation makes the fingers deviate or cross on flexion. Extensor and sometimes flexor tendons adhere in the callus. The interosseus muscles may be damaged, and often their tendons adhere to the firm parts beneath so that they cannot flex the proximal finger joint or extend the distal 2 joints. In open fractures, these important soft parts closely surrounding the bone may share in the injury and become embedded in the scar.

The most common complication is stiffening of the proximal finger joints in the straight position. This occurs not only from proximity of the fracture, but also because the collateral ligaments, when splinted in the straight position, become so contracted that they no longer will allow flexion. If splinted in the flexed position, these ligaments are kept long, and the joint is free to move.

Signs of the fracture are the hump on the dorsum of the hand and the prominence of the metacarpal head in the palm. On sighting along the knuckles, compared with the other hand, malalignment shows along the dorsum as a depression and along their ends as a re-

cession or shortening from bowing or overlapping. Shoving up that ray elicits pain, and there is tenderness over the fracture.

The deformity of dorsal buckling, with the distal fragment angulating volarward, is pro-

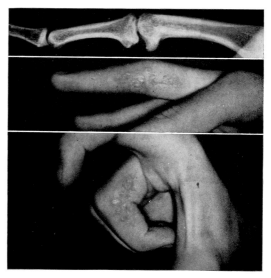

FIG. 827. Case E. G. While catching a baseball, this patient's long finger had hyperextended in its middle joint, causing an exostosis at each end of the volar ligament and greatly limiting the motion, as shown in the x-ray picture. Each exostosis was chiseled off smooth, allowing much motion (as shown in the remaining 2 pictures, taken 3 weeks later).

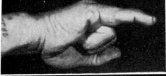

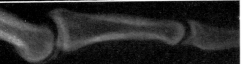

FIG. 828. Case W. K., age 42. While the patient was pushing a log, the little finger had bent backward, dislocating at the middle joint. It was pulled only partially in place and increasing pain followed. In making a fist, the finger stands straight forward. There is no flexion of the middle joint. The illustrations show the condition 6 months later. At operation, it was found that the whole of the anterior part of the capsule had evulsed from the proximal phalanx, and all was sealed by scar tissue. The capsule was resutured in place with removable stainless-steel wire. In 2 months, the joint flexed to 80° voluntarily and 92° passively, and the finger flexed to the proximal part of the palm, lacking ½ inch of the distal crease in the palm.

duced by the intrinsic hand muscles and the long flexor tendons of the fingers, all of which are in a plane volarward, flexing the distal fragments. Buckling of the metacarpals upsets the muscle balance from there distally, dorsiflexing the proximal finger joint and flexing the distal 2 joints.

Treatment. The wrist is dorsiflexed to restore the position of function. The fingers are flexed to relax the long flexor muscles and the interossei, and by traction and pressure on the dorsum the bone comes into alignment. The setting is done manually, and the position is maintained by a splint with the finger semiflexed.

The nonpadded plaster cast always should include the forearm and be molded against the metacarpals on the dorsum of the hand to the knuckles. Incorporated in the cast, over the palm and the wrist, is an extension curved to fit the volar surface of the finger. A cord from the end of this to the wrist maintains the curve. These extensions are for 1 or more fingers and may be of aluminum strip, but the long, padded, annealed iron wire loop popularized by Böhler is preferable. The curve is

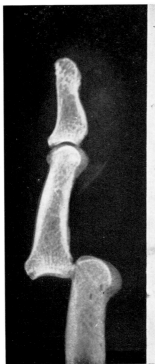

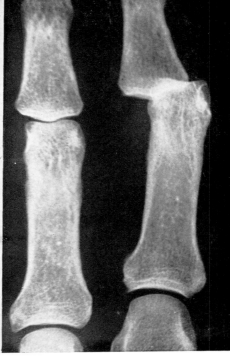

FIG. 829. Dislocation of the middle finger joint, necessitating open reduction. There will be some permanent limitation of motion if not reduced early.

FIG. 830. Dislocation of the distal finger joint.

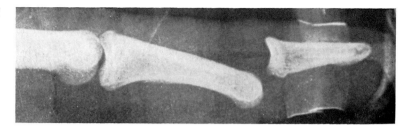

made so that the proximal finger joint is flexed from 20° to 45°, the middle to 90°, and the distal to about 45°. Too much flexion of the proximal joint cocks up the distal fragment; too little allows the proximal joint to stiffen in the straight position.

The metal extension is bent to maintain the fingers in the position of function. Midway in their range of motion the bones will have less tendency to displace. After the first manual setting, traction is applied by pulling the finger around the pulley, i.e., the metal extension.

If the fracture is transverse, the finger is held on the curved extension with adhesive plaster, but if traction is necessary, it is made by wire or pin through the tough finger pulp. Distraction resulting is nonunion is so frequent that skeletal traction is rarely necessary.

For pulp or skeletal traction, a fine Kirschner wire, cut off obliquely, is either inserted through the pulp or drilled through the head of the proximal phalanx, avoiding the joint and dorsal aponeurosis. Each end of the wire is bent down the finger to end ½ inch beyond the fingertip in a ring or a hook, to which the traction cord is attached. Special traction bows or steel safety pins may be used.

Traction has often been applied incorrectly, both in placing the wire and in pulling at the wrong angle, resulting in much damage. In the pulp, the pin should penetrate from side to side opposite the center of the nail just anterior to the phalanx. It should not penetrate the matrix, the joint or the flexor tendon sheath or be placed just under the flexor tendon, and it should not be placed anteroposteriorly. The pulp soon acquires a tough chitinlike coating. Nail traction pulls out the nail. The point of a large fishhook or heavy wire has been used for traction, hooking it into a drill hole on the dorsum of the proximal or the middle phalanx (Quigley).

Traction is obtained manually by the operator during reduction. Then the finger is pulled over the curved splint. The traction through pulp is just enough to maintain the position obtained by manipulation.

The dorsal hump is corrected by direct pressure and traction. Correct rotation is determined by observing that the plane of motion of each finger converges to the tubercle of the scaphoid. Immobilization is maintained for 3 to 4 weeks, according to the particular case, during which time all the uninvolved digits should be free and moved frequently by the patient through their full range passively and as much as he can move them voluntarily to keep the hand in condition and prevent stiffness. The finger should not be flexed over a roll of bandage because it increases the deformity and prevents exercise of the other fingers; nor should the finger be pulled straight in extension by a banjo splint or held so by a straight splint. Either displaces the fracture and stiffens the fingers. A flat splint straightens the arch.

Fractures through the metacarpal neck with angulation volarward and sometimes laterally are difficult to reduce.

The distal fragment is hard to control because it is short and the proximal joint is so mobile. If, though, this joint is flexed to a right angle, it is firm, and the fracture can be controlled through the phalanx. A thin piece of felt is placed over the middle knuckle, which is also bent to a right angle. By firm pressure on this the metacarpal is straightened and checked by its head's being in correct alignment. The forearm and the hand are encased in plaster, and the plaster strip is placed the full length along the dorsum of the finger, merging with the cast on the dorsum and in the palm to maintain the position. Care should be taken not to produce skin necrosis by this method. If for any reason the

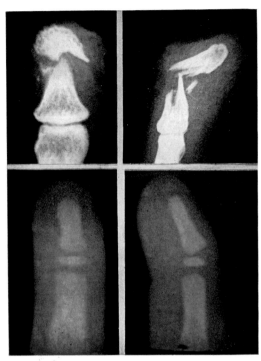

Fig. 831. (*Top*) Fractures of the distal phalanx. (*Bottom*) Slipped epiphysis of the distal phalanx.

A useful method suggested by Berkman and Miles to maintain position of a fractured metacarpal employs 1 or 2 narrow Kirschner wires, drilled at a right angle through 2 or 3 metacarpals. The need for a cast is eliminated, and the free exercise prevents joint stiffness. The wires should be cut off beneath the skin, thus eliminating a dressing and the danger of infection due to movement. They are removed later under local anesthesia.

In open fractures, good skin should be placed on the dorsum of the hand, at once if possible, by swinging a neighboring skin flap and split grafting or resorting to a pedicle graft.

Fractures of Phalanges

Finger fractures are common and often leave permanent impairment. Fractures of the proximal phalanx are twice as common as those of the middle and the distal phalanges. From direct or indirect force the shaft or either end of the proximal or the middle phalanx may be fractured and often comminuted. In the joints, an edge often is pushed off or torn off by overangulation in any direction, resulting in long-lasting, painful stiffness. If the shaft is realigned or the fragments replaced and immobilized for 3 weeks, most of this disability can be avoided. One painful finger may cause the whole hand to stiffen, but it will not do so if immobilized promptly, leaving the other fingers free to move.

Joint stiffening in fingers is a necessary evil, especially if the fracture is in or near the joint. This tendency to stiffen and the frequency with which the flexor and the extensor ten-

fracture does not remain in position, it may be held by a stainless steel pin, pinning it transversely to the other metacarpals.

If a fracture or a piece of bone, such as a fragment of phalanx or metacarpal head, or a dislocation cannot be held in place, there should be no hesitation in opening and fastening it firmly by a stainless steel pin.

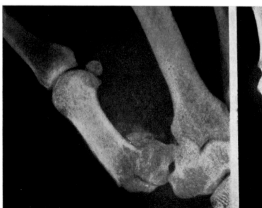

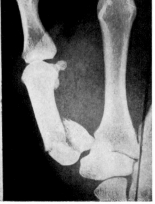

Fig. 832. Two fractures through the base of the thumb metacarpal, not Bennett's. Easily corrected by splinting with metacarpal well extended and the wrist in radial and dorsiflexion to relax the abductor pollicis longus.

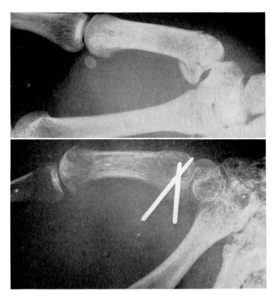

FIG. 833. A fracture through the base of the first metacarpal but with added fracture line through joint. Reduced under direct vision and pinned with Kirschner wire.

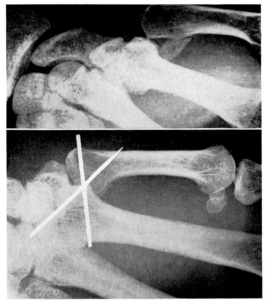

FIG. 834. Bennett's fracture. The hooklike process remains in place, but the shaft dislocates proximalward. Open reduction and pinning.

dons adhere in the callus of the proximal or the middle phalanx, especially if a projecting fragment of bone is against the tendon, accounts for the great disability from finger fractures. If there is no displacement, the tendons seldom adhere. If the fracture unites with dorsal angulation, the finger will be robbed of that same angle of flexion in making a fist. If there is rotary displacement, the finger flexes in the wrong plane.

Treatment of fractures of the proximal and the middle phalanges is by the same method of nonpadded plaster casts, including the forearm, and by the soft-wire extension holding the fingers semiflexed and under traction, as described for fractures of the metacarpals. The finger and the splint are not flexed together at the same time for fear of necrosis; instead, the finger is set, and the splint holds it so. Pulp traction is used or, if there is no displacement, spiral adhesive strips; often, even a curved gutter splint without traction will suffice. For fracture of the proximal phalanx, the proximal finger joint is placed at an angle of 45°, the middle 90° and the distal 45°. This places the distal phalanx parallel with the metacarpal. The strong angle at the

middle joint aids in maintaining the position on the splint.

If a finger is put up straight, as on a tongue blade or by a banjo splint, the fracture will displace, and the finger will stiffen. If one finger is too straight or too flexed, movement of the adjoining digits will be limited. These should be free for full movement by ending the cast at the distal crease in the palm and allowing full movement of the thumb.

In setting the fracture one should consider the natural lateral curves of the fingers, which bend slightly toward the middle finger. Under traction, in semiflexion the fingers should converge to the scaphoid tubercle. If fingers are pulled parallel or divergent, the bones will heal with angulation. In 3 or 4 weeks the union will be firm.

THE PROXIMAL PHALANX frequently is fractured transversely in its proximal half but may be much comminuted or fractured through either of its ends, often obliquely through the head. If the head is fractured off, it displaces backward. The deformity in shaft fractures is flexion of the proximal fragment because the interossei and the lumbricals flex the proximal finger joint by their transverse fibers, and

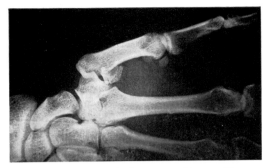

Fig. 835. Bennett's fracture with considerable dislocation of the main fragment.

dorsiflexion of the distal fragment by the pull of the dorsal aponeurosis through its lateral bands and central slip by the intrinsic muscles and the long extensor, respectively, thus buckling the phalanx volarward. There may also be some lateral and rotary displacement.

MIDDLE PHALANX. The deformity may be either volar or dorsal angulation depending on whether the fracture is proximal or distal to the insertion of the superficialis tendon. In the former case, the extensor tendon, which inserts at the base of the phalanx, extends the proximal fragment, and in the latter case the flexor which attaches at the middle of the phalanx flexes the proximal fragment. Reduction is by traction, placing the finger on the same curved splint as in fractures of the proximal phalanx and extending the cast well up the forearm. The splint should be straight only in that part crossing a fracture.

DISTAL PHALANX. Fractures here are from crushing and are usually comminuted with injury to the soft parts. Rarely, there is angulation. There is often a hematoma in the closed pulp space, with agonizing, throbbing pain. The pressure should be relieved at once by drilling a hole in the nail to remove the blood.

If the nail is split, it may be preserved as a splint. If the fracture is comminuted, removal of the nail allows drainage, inspection and the removal of loose fragments of bone.

Healing usually occurs after 2 weeks of simple splinting. If the break is across the shaft, healing may be slow, and after comminution a tip of bone may continue to cause pain from nonunion until removed.

Stubbing the finger, forcing the distal joint, often avulses the dorsal margin and, rarely, a volar triangle. Treatment is described under Rupture of Tendons (Chap. 11).

OPEN FRACTURES. The wound should be cleansed and closed promptly. Unattached fragments should be removed and, unless the wound is in the distal phalanx, pulp traction established.

Finger Sprains. Overangulation of a snugly fitting joint, such as the interphalangeal, ruptures part of the capsular ligament or avulses a fragment of bone. Immobilization on a curved splint stops pain, and the ligament heals promptly. Otherwise, for many months there will be tenderness, disability and stiffening of even the adjoining fingers. Some swelling and slight deformity may persist. The lateral and the dorsolateral ligaments are often torn, or there may have been a dislocation

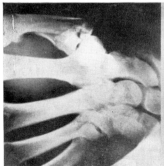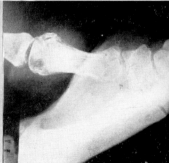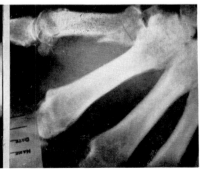

Fig. 836. (Left) Bennett's fracture with displacement. The loss of the hook action of the metacarpal on the greater multangular allows backward dislocation. (Center) Anteroposterior view. (Right) By skeletal pin traction through the head of the metacarpal, the hook united in perfect position, thus preventing dislocation.

FIG. 837. Treatment of Bennett's fracture with dislocation, primary and late. (*1, 2, 3*) For fresh fracture, skeletal traction and plaster cast are used. (*4, 5*) For a moderately late case not reduced, through an L incision stripping muscles from the metacarpal, the piece is chiseled off and replaced. Position is maintained by stainless-steel pins through the skin and a plaster cast. (*6, 7*) For an old case, backward dislocation is prevented by re-establishing the restraining hook of the metacarpal by a wedge osteotomy.

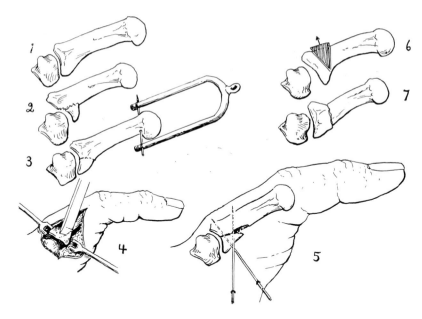

and immediate reduction. If the joint is hyperextended forcibly, the volar capsule may rupture. If rupture occurs at the proximal attachment and the finger not splinted, the rupture will heal with such thickening and shortening that a flexion contracture results which is impossible to correct surgically. If at the distal end, there will be hyperextension of the middle joint which may be remedied by suturing the capsule to the base of the middle phalanx.

DISLOCATIONS

DISLOCATION OF METACARPALS ON CARPUS

The metacarpals of the fingers are so firmly fixed to and move with the distal row of carpal bones that dislocation at this level is rare except by direct force as when crushed by heavy objects. Reduction is easy if done early but if late requires open operation and traction. Reduction is necessary to restore muscle balance and proper mechanics.

DISLOCATION OF PHALANGES

Proximal finger joints rarely dislocate. Usually, dislocation is of the index finger, from hyperextension; the head of the metacarpal

may be caught in the hole of the anterior capsule and the palmar fascia. The middle and the distal finger joints dislocate frequently, the distal phalanx of either joint displacing dorsally over the proximal one. Reduction under local anesthesia by traction is usually easy, and splinting for 3 weeks at 45° of flexion allows prompt healing of the ligaments and recovery.

Later, until the soreness leaves, the joint can be braced by wrapping 4 layers of adhesive plaster around it.

Some dislocations cannot be reduced without an open operation. It will be found that because of hyperextension, the head of the proximal bone has thrust through a hole in the anterior capsule and is caught there, so that the capsule prevents reduction. The hole can be seen through a lateral incision and, when it is enlarged longitudinally, the head of the bone will slip back into place. If done 2 weeks after injury, the capsule will be so organized by granulation tissue and scar that the joint will be permanently stiff.

In some interphalangeal dislocations it will be found that the anterior capsule has avulsed from the bone, either proximally or distally, and is turned in between the 2 bones. In an old case, it and the lateral ligaments may be found to be so thickened as to need excision. In others, the free distal edge of the anterior

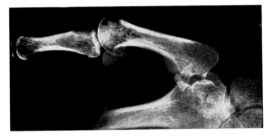

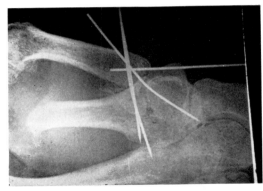

FIG. 838. (*Left*) Three months previously, the patient had received a Bennett's fracture as he braced his hands against the front seat in a head-on collision. Displacement of the hook and dislocation caused pain and crepitation on gripping. (*Right*) By open operation, the hook fragment was chiseled off, replaced and held so with 2 stainless-steel pins penetrating the skin. Another passing through the greater multangular keeps the dislocation reduced. Result: freedom from disability.

capsule can be reattached to the phalanx by catching it in a loop of stainless steel wire passed through a drill hole and on out the dorsal skin to be tied over a button. Maintenance of reduction is easy. The final result will be some limitation of movement.

INJURIES OF THE THUMB

The thumb is so important that whatever the injury, the surgeon should salvage every portion rather than amputate. Any of the bones of the thumb may be fractured, and any of its joints sprained or dislocated. Fractures of the phalanges are treated the same as those of the fingers. In the proximal phalanx, the thenar muscles, which are attached to the base of the phalanx, draw the proximal fragment into flexion and adduction, thus buckling this phalanx volarward, so that the distal fragment must be put in line with the proximal one, using a curved splint.

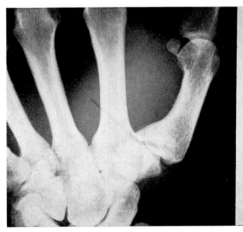
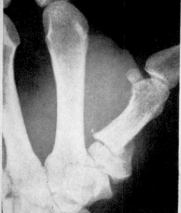
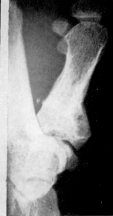

FIG. 839. Case A. C. Osteotomy for malunited Bennett's fracture. Three months ago, the patient had fallen, his hand striking a concrete floor. He complained of pain on pinching with the thumb or making a fist and could not bear the jar of using a hammer. (*Left*) The metacarpal dislocated freely, because the hook effect of the metacarpal on the greater multangular was lost. (*Center*) The metacarpal was angulated backward by a wedge osteotomy at its base to restore the hook effect. (*Right*) Final result. The hook and the dislocation are corrected. He is free from disability, though the tip of the thumb lacks ½ inch in flexion and adduction of reaching as far as does his other thumb.

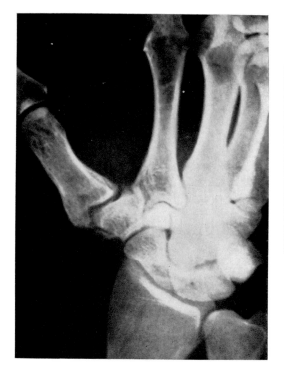

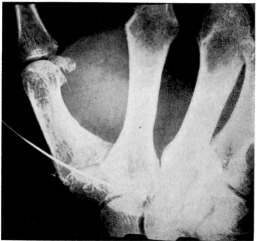

FIG. 840. Arthrodesis between thumb metacarpal and greater multangular with position maintained by a stainless-steel pin through the skin. The joint was painful and arthritic from an old unreduced Bennett's fracture. X-ray views before and after the arthrodesis.

METACARPAL FRACTURES, THUMB

Fractures of the 1st metacarpal are largely of 2 types—that which is transverse and near the base is easy to treat, and that through the carpometacarpal joint is difficult. In the former, the strong abductor pollicis longus cocks back the proximal fragment, and the thenar muscles and the long flexor tendon angulate the distal fragment volarward and ulnarward. In reduction, the metacarpal is grasped and forced into alignment with the proximal fragment. The metacarpophalangeal joint is allowed to flex so as to relax the long flexor tendon, and the wrist is supinated and dorsiflexed to relax the abductor pollicis longus. The angle between the first 2 metacarpals should be kept wide. Position is maintained easily by a nonpadded plaster cast, including the forearm and reaching to the distal joint of the thumb.

FRACTURE-DISLOCATION OF METACARPAL THROUGH CARPOMETACARPAL JOINT (BENNETT'S FRACTURE)

In this entity, commonly resulting from striking a blow with the clenched fist, the metacarpal is forced into flexion, and a tri-angular piece, including some of the joint surface, is pushed off the anterior margin. The small fragment remains in place, while the rest of the metacarpal displaces backward and proximally on the trapezium. Callus fills in between the 2 fragments, uniting them.

The joint remains tender and swollen, and the grasp is weak; in pinching there is pain, and the metacarpal is felt and seen to dislocate backward. Normally, the projecting volar lip of the base of the metacarpal hooks in front of the trapezium, preventing backward dislocation of the metacarpal. When broken off or malunited, this hook effect is gone, and there is nothing to check the backward dislocation. This to-and-fro extra mobility can be demonstrated easily. The hook shows best on roentgenograms taken at an angle of 20° to 30° from the vertical (Billing and Gedda).

Treatment. This fracture, being oblique, is quite unstable, and reduction cannot be maintained except by skeletal traction on the metacarpal or open pinning with Kirschner wire. A nonpadded cast should include the forearm and hold the wrist in radial flexion and supination. It should press firmly and flatly forward against the back of the metacarpal base to

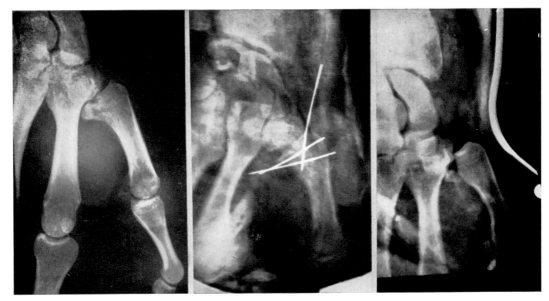

Fig. 841. Case W. G. (*Left*) Bennett's fracture and dislocation. Unreduced; reset by open operation 2 months later. (*Center*) Stainless-steel pins used to hold fracture and dislocation in place. Only 1 pin projects through the skin. (*Right*) The fragment was replaced enough so that excellent function was obtained.

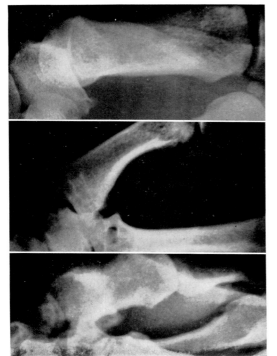

prevent dislocation backward. Projecting from the cast is a rigid wire extension for attachment of the skeletal traction, with the thumb in the direction of extension. Immobilization for 4 to 6 weeks is required. The criterion for

Fig. 842. Case H. H. M. (*Top* and *center*) While resting the hand on a railing 3 months previously, the base of the thumb had been forced volarward, dislocating the 1st metacarpal, rendering the carpometacarpal joint unstable. (*Top*) Shows instability of the joint, there being dislocation volarward. There were soreness and pain on gripping on using the hand. The first 2 metacarpals are wide apart. (*Center* and *bottom*) At operation, the debris was cleared from between the bones, and the metacarpal replaced. The 1st and the 2nd metacarpals were each drilled from front to back, and through these a tendon graft from the palmaris longus and a No. 28 stainless-steel wire were used to lash the bones together. The latter was to hold the bones in place until the graft was well established. The wire was placed so that it could be removed in 3 weeks. A good result was obtained with freedom from disability.

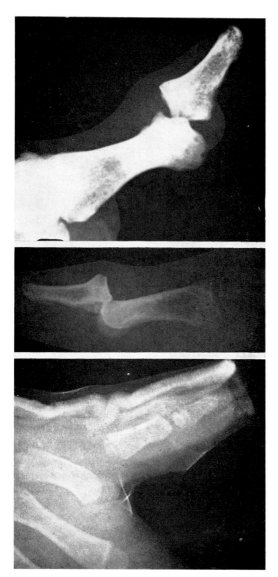

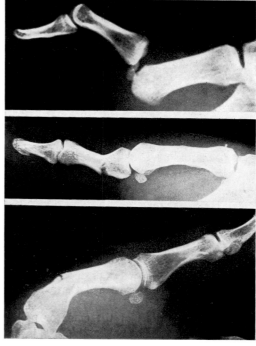

FIG. 843. Injuries of the thumb. (*Left, top* and *center*) Dislocation of the distal joint. (*Left, bottom*) Dislocation of the proximal joint with usual deformity (in child). (*Right, top*) Dislocation of the proximal joint with usual deformity. (*Right, center*) Usual angulation in fracture of the proximal phalanx. (*Right, bottom*) Usual angulation in fracture of the metacarpal.

adequate reduction is the reestablishment of a good hook.

An excellent method is to hold the fragments in anatomic position by pinning with removable Kirschner wires. The fracture is set manually by traction and pressure. The pins penetrate the metacarpal longitudinally and obliquely into the trapezium. The wires are cut beneath the skin, and a cast is applied to prevent movement. The best method is to pin the fracture with 2 Kirschner wires by the open method. By this an anatomic set may be assured.

In old cases of disability from malunion, several methods are available: (1) arthrodesis, (2) wedge osteotomy and (3) chiseling apart and refastening the fragments in place with 3 stainless steel pins. In arthrodesis, the other joints of the thumb will provide sufficient motion. In osteotomy, a wedge is removed with its base dorsally, so that the metacarpal bends backward after union. Then, when the metacarpal is flexed again, the hook effect will be reestablished, together with the articular ligaments that hold it snugly on the trapezium. In the open pinning of the fragment, 2 pins hold the fragment to the metacarpal, and 1 through the trapezium and the metacarpal prevents dislocation. The pins are withdrawn later. An excellent exposure is afforded by an incision along the dorsum of the metacarpal, turning volarward at the wrist to follow the flexion crease. The muscles attached to the metacarpal are stripped off volarward and replaced. In arthrodesing the carpometacarpal joint, a disk of ilium should be placed between the bones to prevent distraction, and the whole should be pinned together firmly.

Dislocation of Carpometacarpal Joint

Dislocation backward of this joint may occur without Bennett's fracture. If seen early, reduction and immobilization in a nonpadded plaster cast are sufficient. Later, it will be necessary to arthrodese the joint or to lash it in place by a free tendon graft placed through drill holes. Through a curved incision following the radial flexion wrinkles of the wrist, the twigs of the radial nerve and the artery are retracted backward; the bones are exposed between the tendons of the extensor pollicis longus and brevis. The palmaris longus tendon or a strip of fascia lata are placed so as to lash the metacarpal volarward on the trapezium. Passing laterally through a drill hole in the metacarpal from the radial to the ulnar side, the graft is drawn through and made to enter an anteroposterior hole in the trapezium from the volar to the dorsal side, emerging between the 2 dorsal prominences of that bone. Then it is passed with a carrier around under the oblique ridge of the trapezium and back, to be fastened to its other end at the metacarpal. Arthrodesis is usually preferable.

Injuries of Metacarpophalangeal Joint

From lateral sprains of the thumb, the ligament on the ulnar side or, more commonly, that on the dorsoradial side may rupture, causing pain, swelling, tenderness and abnormal mobility, and pain and weakness on pinching. If recent, splinting for a month will cure the condition; but if old, the capsular ligament should be sutured and reinforced by a graft of strip of fascia lata, well contacted to the bone.

A strain of the insertions of the adductor pollicis muscles causes pain on pinching. It may be splinted by a narrow web belt and buckle passed with one loop about the hand, crossing in the cleft of the thumb, and the other loop about the thumb.

One of the 2 sesamoid bones in the anterior capsular ligament of this joint of the thumb may be fractured across from direct violence. It will be sore for several months, but eventually the bone unites. A bipartite sesamoid may be confusing.

Dislocation of Metacarpophalangeal Joint.

If hyperextended, the capsular ligament yields, and the head of the metacarpal is shoved through the base of the anterior or glenoid ligament between the sesamoid bones and the tendons of the 2 heads of the flexor pollicis brevis. The proximal phalanx displaces backward until it stands at a right angle to and with its base resting on the dorsum of the metacarpal. Usually, the external collateral ligament is also ruptured, making the dislocation somewhat ulnarward, as well as backward. The 2 sesamoids are joined by the strong transverse glenoid ligament. This unruptured ligament and sometimes 1 of the sesamoids lie across the back of the metacarpal head, interposed between it and the phalanx, thus preventing reduction.

Reduction may be easy if done early and if one is mindful of the peculiar mechanism. The proximal phalanx is grasped as it stands at a right angle back of the metacarpal. It is shoved distalward at this angle, wiggling it in rotation so as to work the capsule over the head of the metacarpal until the joint flexes and snaps into place. It is immobilized in flexion for a month. If insufficiently reduced, the dislocation may recur, thus resulting in limitation of grasping power.

Open reduction may be necessary; through a lateral incision the anterior capsule is slit longitudinally sufficient to extricate the metacarpal head. If the joint is damaged too extensively, it may be fused.

BIBLIOGRAPHY

Adler, J. B., and Shaftan, G. W.: Fractures of the capitate, J. Bone Joint Surg. *44-A*:1537, 1962.

Aitken, A. P., and Nalebuff, E. A.: Volar transnavicular perilunar dislocation of the carpus, J. Bone Joint Surg. *42-A*:1051, 1960.

Barnard, L., and Stubbins, S. G.: Styloidectomy of the radius in the surgical treatment of nonunion of the carpal navicular, J. Bone Joint Surg. *30-A*:98, 1948.

Barr, J. G., *et al.*:Fracture of the carpal navicular (scaphoid) bone, J. Bone Joint Surg. *35-A*: 609, 1953.

Bartone, N. F., and Grieco, R. V.: Fractures of triquetrum, J. Bone Joint Surg. *38-A*:353, 1956.

Bjerre, B.: Bennett fracture, therapy, Boehler method and Moberg's osteosynthesis, Ugeskr. laeger *119*:931, 1957.

Blum, L.: Treatment of Bennett's fracture-dislocation of first metacarpal bone, J. Bone Joint Surg. *23*:578, 1941.

Böhler, L.: The Treatment of Fractures, Baltimore, Wm. Wood & Co., 1932.

Bonnin, J. G., and Greening, W. P.: Fractures of the triquetrum, Brit. J. Surg. *31*:278, 1944.

Cave, E. F.: Carpus, with reference to fractured navicular bone, Arch. Surg. *40*:54, 1940.

———: Retro-lunar dislocation of the capitate with fracture or subluxation of the navicular bone, J. Bone Joint Surg. *23*:830, 1941.

Clarke, H. O.: Bone-grafting the Scaphoid *in* Year Book of General Surgery, p. 770, Chicago, Year Book Pub., 1942.

Cordrey, L. J., and Ferrer-Torrella, M.: Management of fractures of the greater multangular; report of five cases, J. Bone Joint Surg. *42-A*: 1111, 1960.

Cravener, E. K., and McElroy, D. G.: Fractures of carpal (navicular) scaphoid, Am. J. Surg. *44*:100, 1939.

Darrach, W.: Colles' fracture, New Engl. J. Med. *226*:594, 1942.

Davis, G. G.: Treatment of dislocated semilunar carpal bones, Surg., Gynec. Obstet. *37*:225, 1923.

Deyerle, W. M.: Athletic injuries of the upper extremity, Clin. Orthop. *23*:84, 1962.

Dickison, J. C., and Shannon, J. G.: Fractures of the carpal scaphoid in the Canadian Army; a review and commentary, Surg., Gynec. Obstet. *79*:225, 1944.

Diveley, R. L.: Fracture of scaphoid bone, S. Afr. Orth. Assn. Proc., 1959; J. Bone Joint Surg. *42-B*:860, 1960.

Donaldson, W. F., Goodman, M. C., Rodriguez, E. E., Gartland, J. J., and Skovron, M.: Evaluation of treatment for non-union of the carpal navicular, J. Bone Joint Surg. *44-A*:169, 1962.

Edelstein, J. M.: Treatment of ununited fractures of carpal navicular, J. Bone Joint Surg. *21*:902, 1939.

Ghormley, R. K., and Mroz, J. R.: Fractures of wrist; review of 176 cases, Surg., Gynec. Obstet. *55*:377, 1932.

Goeringer, F.: Follow-up results of surgical treatment for non-union of the carpal scaphoid, Arch. Surg. *58*:291, 1949.

Gollasch, W.: Congenital bipartite carpal scaphoid bones, Arch. orthop. Unfall-Chir. *40*:269, 1939.

Gordon, L. H., and King, D.: Partial wrist arthrodesis, Am. J. Surg. *102*:460, 1961.

Greening, W. P.: Isolated fracture of carpal cuneiform, Brit. M. J. *1*:221, 1942.

Hart, V. L., and Gaynor, V.: Radiography of carpal canal, Radiog. Clin. Photog. *18*:23, 1942.

Heiple, K. G., Freehafer, A. A., and Van't Hof, A.: Isolated traumatic dislocation of the distal end of the ulna or distal radio-ulnar joint, J. Bone Joint Surg. *44-A*:1387, 1962.

Henry, M. G.: Fractures of the carpal scaphoid bone in industry and in the military service, Arch. Surg. *48*:278, 1944.

Howard, F. M.: Ulnar nerve palsy in wrist fractures, J. Bone Joint Surg. *43-A*:1197, 1961.

Howard, L. D.: The problems of metacarpal fractures of the hand due to war wounds, Am. Acad. Orth. Surg. Lect., p. 196, 1944.

Huet, P., and Huguier, J.: Frontal roentgen image in retrolunar luxations of carpus, Presse méd. *49*:860, 1941.

Jonasch, E.: Dislocations of first metacarpal bone, Mschr, Unfallh. *60*:154, 1957.

Kaplan, E. B.: Dorsal dislocation of the metacarpophalangeal joint of the index finger, J. Bone Joint Surg. *39-A*:1081, 1957.

———: Lateral subluxation of the metacarpophalangeal joint of the thumb; experimental study, Bull. Hosp. Joint Dis. *21*:200, 1960.

———: The pathology and treatment of radial subluxation of the thumb with ulnar displacement of the head of the first metacarpal, J. Bone Joint Surg. *43-A*:541, 1961.

Kaplan, L.: Treatment of fractures and dislocations of hand and fingers; technic of unpadded casts for carpal, metacarpal, and phalangeal fractures, Surg. Clin. N. Amer. *20*:1695, 1940.

Kuth, J. R.: Isolated dislocation of carpal navicular; case report, J. Bone Joint Surg. *21*:479, 1939.

Lewis, H. H.: Dislocation of the lesser multangular, J. Bone Joint Surg. *44-A*:1412, 1962.

London, P. S.: The broken scaphoid bone; the case against pessimism, J. Bone Joint Surg. *43-B*:237, 1961.

Lotsch, F.: Surgical therapy of subluxation in saddle-like joint of first metacarpal bone (i.e., dislocation of thumb metacarpal), Zbl. Chir. *66*:2060, 1939.

MacAusland, W. R.: Perilunar dislocation of the carpal bones and dislocation of the lunate bone, Surg., Gynec. Obstet. *79*:256, 1944.

McKim, L. H.: Fractures of the carpal scaphoid, Bull. Am. Coll. Surg., No. 142, p. 29, 1944.

McLaughlin, H. L.: Fracture of the carpal navicular (scaphoid) bone; open reduction and internal fixation, J. Bone Joint Surg. *36-A*:765, 1954.

Mazet, R., Jr., and Hohl, M.: Radial styloidectomy and styloidectomy plus bone graft in the treatment of old ununited carpal scaphoid fractures, Ann. Surg. *152*:296, 1960.

Meekison, D. M.: Some remarks on three common fractures, J. Bone Joint Surg. *27*:80, 1945.

Mondry, F.: Surgical therapy of posttraumatic

functional disturbance of proximal joint of thumb, Zbl. Chir. *67*:1532, 1940.

Murless, B. C.: Fracture dislocation of base of fifth metacarpal bone, Brit. J. Surg. *31*:402, 1944.

Murray, G.: End results of bone-grafting for non-union of the carpal navicular, J. Bone Joint Surg. *28*:749, 1946.

Nemethi, C. E.: The primary repair of traumatic digital skeletal losses by phalangeal recessions, J. Bone Joint Surg. *37-A*:78, 1955.

Nicholson, C. B.: Fracture dislocations of os magnum, J. Roy. Navy Med. Serv. *26*:289, 1940.

Nutter, P. D.: Interposition of sesamoids in metacarpophalangeal dislocations, J. Bone Joint Surg. *22*:730, 1940.

Obletz, B. E.: Fresh fractures of the carpal scaphoid, Surg., Gynec. Obstet. *78*:83, 1944.

Peterson, T. H.: Dislocation of lesser multi-angular; report of case, J. Bone Joint Surg. *22*:200, 1940.

Reitz, B. G.: Trauma to the sesamoid bones of the thumb, Am. J. Surg. *72*:284, 1946.

Rettig, H.: On habitual subluxation of the scaphoid bone of the hand, Arch. Orthop. Unfallchir. *53*:498, 1961.

Robertson, R. C., Cawley, J. J., and Faris, A. M.: Treatment of fracture-dislocation of the interphalangeal joints of the hand, J. Bone Joint Surg. *28*:68, 1946.

Roemer, F. J.: Hyperextension injuries to the finger joints, Am. J. Surg. *80*:295, 1950.

Rose-Innes, A. P.: Anterior dislocation of the ulna at the inferior radio-ulnar joint, J. Bone Joint Surg. *42-B*:518, 1960.

Rothberg, A. S.: Fractures of carpal navicular; importance of special roentgenography, J. Bone Joint Surg. *21*:1020, 1939.

Russe, O.: Fracture of carpal navicular, J. Bone Joint Surg. *42-A*:759, 1960.

Russell, T. B.: Intercarpal dislocations and fracture dislocations, J. Bone Joint Surg. *31-B*:524, 1949.

Sashin, D.: Treatment of fractures of the carpal Scaphoid, Arch. Surg. *52*:445, 1946.

Schnek, F. G.: The conservative treatment of total dislocation of the lunate bone, Beitr. klin. Chir. *161*:129, 1935.

Scobie, W. H.: Crush fracture of sesamoid bone of thumb, Brit. M. J. *2*:912, 1941.

Simon, P.: A contribution to fractures of the capitatum, Z. Orthop. *95*:365, 1962.

Sinberg, S. E.: Fracture of sesamoid of thumb, J. Bone Joint Surg. *22*:444, 1940.

Smith, C. H.: Compound fractures of fingers, Ann. Surg. *119*:266, 1944.

Speed, K.: Injuries of carpal bones, Surg. Clin. N. Amer. *25*:1, 1945.

Squire, M.: B. O. A. Meetings, J. Bone Joint Surg. *41-B*:1, 210, 1959.

Stener, B.: Displacement of the ruptured ulnar collateral ligament of the metacarpophalangeal joint of the thumb, J. Bone Joint Surg. *44-B*:869, 1962.

Vasilas, A., Grieco, R. V., and Bartone, N. F.: Roentgen aspects of injuries to the pisiform bone and pisotriquetral joint, J. Bone Joint Surg. *42-A*:1317, 1960.

Wagner, C. J.: Method of treatment of Bennett's fracture dislocation, Am. J. Surg. *80*:230, 1950.

———:Perilunar dislocations, J. Bone Joint Surg. *38-A*:1198, 1956.

Watson-Jones, R.: Fractures and Other Bone and Joint Injuries, Baltimore, Williams & Wilkins, 1940.

Waugh, R. L., and Ferrazzano, G. P.: Fractures of the metacarpals exclusive of the thumb; a new method of treatment, Am. J. Surg. *59*:186, 1943.

Waugh, R. L., and Revling, L.: Ununited fractures of carpal scaphoid; preliminary report on use of vitallium replicas as replacements after excision, Am. J. Surg. *67*:184, 1945.

Waugh, R. L., and Yancey, A. A.: Carpometacarpal fractures, J. Bone Joint Surg. *30*:397, 1948.

Webb, G., and Sheinfeld, W.: Reversed Colles' fracture with special reference to therapy, J.A.M.A. *104*:2324, 1935.

Wiggins, H. E., et al.: A method of treatment of fracture dislocation of the first metacarpal bone, J. Bone Joint Surg. *36-A*:810, 1954.

Woughter, H. W.: Carpal bone injuries; conservative treatment, J. Mich. Med. Soc. *39*:759, 1940.

Zaffaroni, A., and Tagliabue, D.: Fracture of the pyrimidal bone, Arch. ortop. (Milano) *73*:218, 1960.

Chapter 17

Infections

Under most conditions, a severely injured hand heals without infection if treated promptly, but a trivial scratch may go unnoticed and a virulent organism find its way into the lymphatics, a tendon sheath or fascial spaces. Though antibiotic therapy has resulted in a marked decrease in the number of these infections, knowledge of their course and treatment is still a basic part of surgery of the hand.

Infections may be from the pyogenic organisms, commonly a staphylococcus, or from the granuloma-producing group, e.g., the tubercle bacillus. Yeasts and fungi cause some chronic infections, and some unusual inflammatory reactions to foreign objects or animal tissue may be difficult to diagnose and treat.

PYOGENIC INFECTIONS

Any discussion of the suppurative infections of the hand must be based on the anatomy of the fascial spaces and the synovial sheaths.

ANATOMY

The study of the boundaries of tne various fascial spaces and the distribution of the synovial sheaths was an anatomic exercise for many years, but Kanavel, using an injection technic, showed the paths that infections would take and established the present concept of the palmar spaces. From these studies and the application of his findings to the treatment of infections of the hand, a logical systematic treatment developed. Kanavel's *Infections of the Hand* was published in many editions and represents a major contribution to the knowledge we now have of these infections. This work and later studies by Koch and Mason showed how infection spreads in a specific way—why from some areas it points to the surface and from others spreads rapidly up the forearm. A sheath infection is a serious problem with much resulting damage to the hand. Even with antibotics one must not delay proper surgical treatment, for in the closed spaces, swelling and edema can squeeze out the circulation so that the parts die of ischemia even though the infecting organism is controlled by its specific antibiotic.

SPECIFIC ENTITIES

Felon. The terminal pulp space of a digit fills and becomes distended when infected by a penetrating wound. If not drained, the blood supply of part of the diaphysis is blocked, and the diaphysis dies. The epiphysis is usually spared. Severe throbbing pain and a swollen

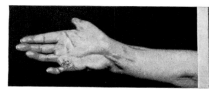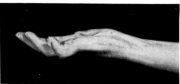

Fig. 844. Hand wrecked by infection starting in the pulp of the thumb and drained by a few tiny incisions. For 3 weeks the temperature was high, and it took 4 months to heal. Infection up the sheath of the thumb flexor, through the radial and the ulnar bursae and down the little finger. Midpalmar, thenar and forearm spaces became involved. Bare bone was present in the thumb. Tendons and nerves sloughed. Joints stiffened in positions of nonfunction.

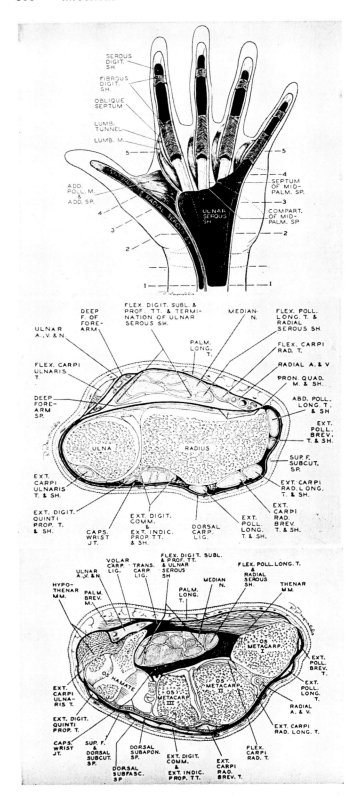

Fig. 845. Arrangement of fascial spaces and tendon sheaths in the hand.

(A) Diagrammatic drawing, showing the serous and the (partially) fibrous sheaths of the fingers and the palm, and their relation to the lumbrical tunnels and the midpalmar and the adductor spaces. The dotted lines indicate the natural creases, and the numbered, broken lines indicate the lines of section of (1) to (5), inclusive.

(*Note:* [1] to [5], inclusive, are line drawings made on bleached photographs of serial sections of human material.)

(1) Cross section through the forearm, just above the wrist, showing the relation of the radial and the ulnar serous tendon sheaths to the deep forearm space (proximal surface).

(2) Cross section through the junction of the wrist and the hand, showing the relation of the radial and the ulnar serous tendon sheaths to the transverse carpal ligament and the capsule of the wrist joint (proximal surface).

(*Continued on facing page*)

Fig. 845 (*Cont.*)

(3) Cross section through the proximal third of the hand, showing the relation of the radial and the ulnar serous tendon sheaths to the midpalmar and the adductor space (proximal surface).

(4) Cross section through the middle third of the hand, showing the individual compartments of the midpalmar space and their relation to the flexor tendons and the adductor space (proximal surface).

(5) Cross section through the distal third of the hand, showing the lumbrical tunnels and their relation to the flexor tendons and the sheaths (proximal surface). (Grodinsky and Holyoke: Anat. Rec. 79:435–451)

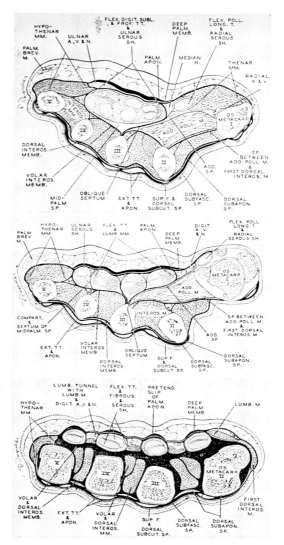

indurated pulp call for immediate treatment.

TREATMENT. Under general anesthesia the pulp space should be opened in a bloodless field. The space is traversed by multiple vertical septa from skin to periosteum, so that a vertical midline incision will not drain adequately. The incision should cut across these columns. Early, a short incision over the abscess will suffice, but in an advanced case it should pass along one side and around the tip. In the severe cases the alligator-mouthed incision dorsal to the tactile part of the pulp with a gauze strip laid across through it gives better drainage. This incision should be near the nail to leave the scar away from the tactile surface and, as soon as possible, should be drawn together to avoid a gutter scar. In incising a felon care must be taken not to cut through into the tendon sheath. The seques-

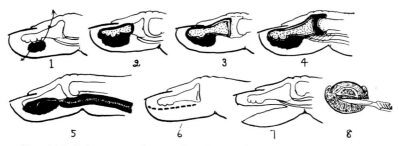

FIG. 846. Felon, extensions and drainage. (1) Simple felon points posteriorly or anteriorly. (2) Diaphysis has sequestrated. (3) Diaphysis and epiphysis involved. (4) Extension into distal joint. (5) Extends through tendon sheath, tenosynovitis. (6) Location of incision in one side only. (7) Alligator-mouth incision for severe involvement. (8) Incision in cross section intercepting vertical columns.

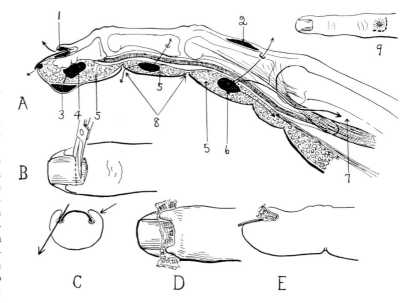

FIG. 847. (A) Diagram of locations of abscesses and where they point. (1) Paronychia. Perforates base of nail, preserves matrix. (2) Subcutaneous disk of septic necrosis. (3) Phlyctenular abscess indicative of felon beneath. (4) Felon. (5) Three fat pads of a finger separated from each other by the flexion creases which act as barriers to pus. (6) Abscess in fat pad. May perforate posteriorly through skin, proximally to subcutaneous tissue in palm or by lumbrical canal to palmar space (7). (7) Palmar space. (8) Puncture wounds in the flexion creases are dangerous, because they lead directly into the tendon sheath. (9) Method of draining abscess (2). The transverse arm of incision blocks upward extension.

(B) Treatment of paronychia. The proximal part of the nail is cut across and removed. Two lateral incisions are made so as to raise a dorsal flap.

(C) The knife cuts like the large, not the small, arrow to drain the pus at the depth of the sulcus.

(D) Now adherent gauze wick is laid across under the flap.

(E) The gauze should pack into the bottom of the angle but not tight enough to cause necrosis.

trum, if present, is removed. If the epiphysis is intact and the sequestrum is left for 2 weeks before removal, the bone will regenerate. If the distal joint is infected and the infection is progressing rapidly, the distal segment should be amputated, leaving the flaps open.

With the aid of antibiotics, a beginning abscess can be opened, the necrotic tissue excised and the wound sutured. Scott reported that the time of healing by excision and suturing was reduced to 2 weeks or less in half of the cases.

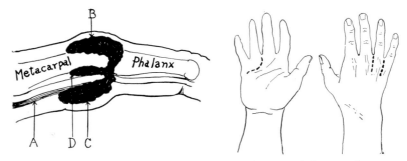

FIG. 848. Collar-button abscess. (A) Palmar fascia. (B) Posterior compartment on the dorsum opposite the cleft. (C) Anterior compartment of the subcutaneous and filling the web space. (D) Extension starting beneath the tendons toward the middle palmar space.

Caution and judgment must be used; open drainage is safer, now that many strains of staphylococcus are resistant to antibiotics.

Most infections of pulp and volar spaces in the fingers are caused by *Staphylococcus aureus*. They start as local cellulitis, and if the organism is sensitive to the antibotic, the infection may be controlled.

The argument, according to Gordon, for delayed surgery is that under this treatment, 23 per cent of 431 pulp-space infections resolved, as did 34 per cent of 228 cases of flexor cellulitis. With prompt surgery, pulp abscesses healed in 17 days, but with delayed surgery, they healed in 13; flexor cellulitis healed in 15 to 12 days.

Paronychia. The infection starts in the paronychium at the side of the nail with local redness, swelling and pain. Separation of the fold from the nail or a small incision from the depth of the sulcus outward, letting out a drop of pus, is adequate; but if untreated, the pus follows around the base of the nail under the eponychium, and at the angle infects the ungual bursa beneath the nail where the loose attachment corresponds to the lunula.

TREATMENT. When infection involves the whole eponychium, the base of the nail, including the lunula, should be removed by cutting across with pointed scissors. The fold should be kept packed widely open.

Only if both sides are involved should 2 incisions be made, one at each side of the nail, and the nail removed. The knife point is placed at the very depth of the base of the sulcus at the side where the nail curves in sharply and then is thrust on out through the soft parts, making a dog ear on each side. The whole flap of skin is lifted up, and a strip of packing is placed beneath it. The wound should be epithelized and healed in 2 weeks. If healing is delayed with adequate drainage, one suspects trichophytosis, moniliasis or syphilis.

Carbuncle. This typical lesion occurs in the hair-bearing areas on the dorsum of the wrist, the hand or the proximal segments of the digits.

TREATMENT. In addition to the stellate incision to as far as the borders of the induration, each flap should be undermined to cut the vertical columns.

Subcutaneous Abscess. In the volar aspect

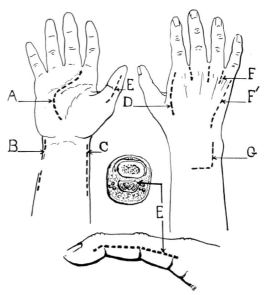

FIG. 849. Incisions for drainage. (A) For midpalmar space. (B) For ulnar bursa. (C) For radial bursa. (D) For thenar space. (E) For tenosynovitis, always midlateral behind the nerve and the vessels. In front of the latter, this leads to keloid contracture. The flexion creases end at the midlateral line, since to-and-fro stress stops here (F, F') For subaponeurotic space. (G) For subcutaneous abscess. Cross arm of incision blocks extension.

of a finger there are 3 fatty pads, separated by the 3 transverse volar creases which are attached to the tendon sheath. A subcutaneous abscess in any of these pulp spaces is limited by the creases. Infection in the middle pulp space may point out the side of the finger or may infect the tendon sheath. A subcutaneous abscess in the proximal pulp space may point at the side or the dorsum of the finger, may infect the tendon sheath, or may pass around the side of the proximal crease and enter the web space. It will not extend into the palm unless by way of the tendon sheath.

The pulp space should be opened at the site of the abscess, care being taken not to damage the volar digital nerves and vessels.

INFECTIONS FROM HUMAN BITES

Mouth organisms usually are introduced into the proximal finger joint areas when a

Fig. 850. Quadrilateral space in the forearm and cleavage for draining pus when present. Pus collects behind the flexor tendons and in front of the pronator quadratus; and, in draining laterally on each side, the posterior branch of the ulnar nerve is retracted forward and the radial nerve backward. The hemostat would expose the ulnar bursa for incision. (1) Abductor pollicis longus. (2) Radial nerve. (3) Drainage of radial side and for radial bursa. (4) Flexor pollicis longus. (5) Radial vessels. (6) Median nerve.

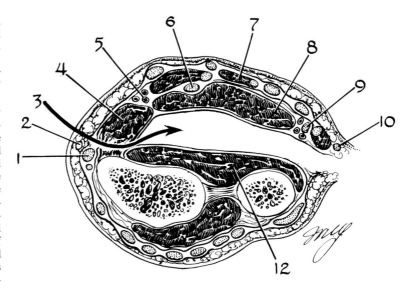

(7) Flexor digitorum sublimis. (8) Flexor digitorum profundus. (9) Ulnar nerve and vessels. (10) Posterior branch of ulnar nerve. (11) Hemostat in quadrilateral space. (12) Pronator quadratus.

person strikes someone in the teeth with his fist. The infection is commonly mixed, not only the usual combination of *Bacillus fusiformis* and the spirochetes of trench mouth but many forms of Streptococci and also Staphylococci, *B. coli*, diphtheroid bacilli and *B. proteus* as well. The organisms are human

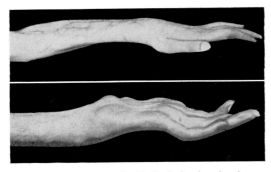

Fig. 851. Case G. T. J. Infection in the forearm which wrecked the hand. The patient's forearm had been squeezed between a moving ship and a wall, the lacerations being sutured at once. Severe infection in the forearm followed, resulting in sloughing of nerves and muscles. The remains of the flexor muscles have atrophied. The hand shows typical atrophy and deformity of paralysis of the median and the ulnar nerves.

acclimated, the tissues infected are ligamentous and, therefore, of low resistance, and the region is peculiar in that there radiate from it many fascial planes and passageways along which infection spreads to various parts of the hand and the fingers. Mason and Koch have made a careful study of these pathways of extension.

Pain and swelling commence after 1 to 2 days, sometimes accompanied by lymphangitis. In a few days a foul odor is noticeable and the inflammation extends. It spreads not only in the subcutaneous space but in the subaponeurotic space over the dorsum of the hand and distally over the proximal phalanx. The joint itself is usually infected. The infection extends into the web space, and by following along the interosseus and the lumbricalis muscles or by breaking through the anterior surface of the joint, the midpalmar or thenar space becomes involved, but only occasionally the sheath of the flexor tendons. From the joint, the metacarpal or proximal phalanx may become involved.

Treatment at the time of injury should be prompt and radical, consisting of excision and irrigation of the wound to its full depth with adequate incision so that the openings in the skin, the tendon and the joint will superimpose. Considering the potential danger from such a

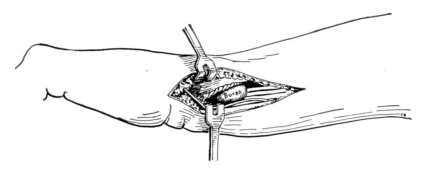

FIG. 852. Exposure of the pus-filled ulnar bursa for drainage. The dorsal branch of the ulnar nerve and the flexor ulnaris are retracted volarward. The distended bursa is seen between the flexor tendons and the pronator quadratus, which covers the bones.

wound, repair of tendon or joint capsule at this time is dangerous. The wound should not be closed. Immobilization, elevation, warmth and antibiotics systemically should prevent infection. If infection is already established, the necrotic tissue should be excised and the same measures used.

With vigilance, extension of infection along the various known pathways can be checked by prompt incision. Infections of this character will cross fascial planes readily. In advanced cases with necrosis, the finger should be amputated through the proximal joint and the wound left wide open. Even with efficient treatment the proximal finger joint probably will be limited in motion.

THREE MAIN FORMS OF INFECTION IN THE HAND

There are 3 systems of pathways of infection that are distinct from each other, though sometimes combined. One is infection in fascial spaces, another is through tendon sheaths, and the third is through the lymphatic system.

Fascial-space infections are more numerous, but synovitis accounts for the severely crippled hands, finger-joint and wrist-joint infections, osteomyelitis, extensions up the forearm, flexion contractures and some amputations. In extreme cases it may even result in death. Infections in the lymphatic system can progress rapidly.

Usually, each form of infection runs true to type, but infection may spread from space to sheath or vice versa, and from the deep lymphatics to the sheaths or the fascial spaces.

There is usually more swelling on the dorsum of a hand, because of the loose tissue, even though the infection is volar. One should refrain from incising the dorsum unless the pus is actually there.

Infections can be located accurately by outlining the tender area, starting away from and working toward it. The point of maximal tenderness is important. Other helpful signs are the local heat, the edema of the overlying skin and the pain on movement of the part. If tendons pass through an infected fascial space, movement of the tendons is painful—acutely so if through a sheath under tension.

Pain and tenderness are marked in the early stages of infection, but later they may lessen or disappear. They are greatest when the pus is under pressure and lessen temporarily as rupture occurs in another space. High temperatures mean absorption from infection

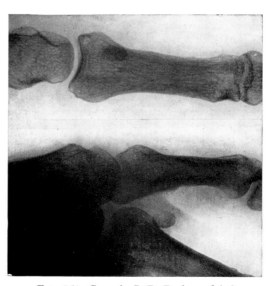

FIG. 853. Case A. J. B. Prolonged infection draining from a laceration in the palm for 6 months. X-ray picture shows the sesamoid to be in the wrong location. Therefore, it was removed with forceps as a sequestrum. The wound healed in 2 weeks.

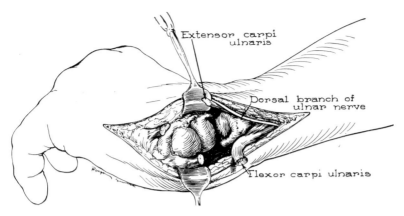

FIG. 854. Drainage for an infected wrist joint. Through a lateral incision, the dorsal branch of the ulnar nerve is retracted dorsally, and the insertions of the two carpus ulnari are severed. Cutting the capsule and abducting the wrist gives wide drainage. The carpi ulnaris re-establish their continuity.

in lymphatics, in a joint or a thrombus, or pus under pressure. A smear and culture should be made and the proper antibiotic selected.

Infections in Fascial Spaces. WEB SPACES. At the web interspaces are 3 small, triangular regions between the volar and the dorsal skin between divsions of the palmar fascia. When filled, the pus passes over the edge of the deep transverse ligament, and the abscess points dorsally.

Infection comes from skin cracks and under calluses that form on the distal fold in the palm, or it may extend up from the proximal pulp space or the side of the finger. As the space fills there is a tender, red bulging in the distal part of the palm which soon extends dorsally in the web, giving it the name collar-button abscess. The base of 1 finger is swollen, and the adjoining fingers are spread. The infection may extend laterally in the distal part of the palm to the adjoining webs. It may enter a lumbrical canal and extend into the palm.

Treatment. A curved incision is made over the swelling in the palm, and a longitudinal dorsal incision is made in the interspace.

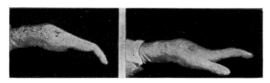

FIG. 855. Position of nonfunction from neglect following an infection of the wrist joint from a buzz-saw injury and removal of carpals. Limits of flexion and extension are shown.

MIDDLE PALMAR SPACE. This potential space has a floor of interosseus fascia, is covered on top by the flexor tendons of the fingers and extends from the line of the 3rd metacarpal to the hypothenar fascia. Distally, the space extends down the lumbrical canals of the ring and the little fingers and proximally to the carpal tunnel.

Infection in this space is direct by wounds or by extension from the sheaths of the index, the middle, the ring or the ulnar bursa, from the lumbrical canals or the subcutaneous tissues of the 4 fingers or the metacarpals or the proximal joints of the ulnar 3 digits.

Infection spreads to the distal palm or out through the skin at the base of the finger.

The normal concavity of the palm is lost from swelling beneath the flexor tendons, and tenderness outlines the borders of the space. Semiflexion of the fingers with pain on passive extension and dorsal swelling are signs of this space involvement.

Treatment. An incision is made paralleling the distal crease, starting at the middle metacarpal line, extending ulnarward and curving up inside the hypothenar eminence. The ulnar bursa should not be opened.

THENAR SPACE. This potential space is like a pantaloon straddling the transverse adductor muscle and thus involves the area of the first cleft; on the dorsum it is in the subcutaneous compartment.

It becomes involved from sheath infections of the index finger or the thumb or as an extension from the middle palmar space; from it infection can spread to the dorsum of the first cleft or down the index lumbrical canal.

It is characterized by tremendous swelling

FIG. 856. Case O. J. Hand wrecked by infection. Starting from a puncture in the thumb pulp into the tendon sheath, it traversed the tendon sheaths and the fascial spaces, including the arm, causing severe illness. The little fin-

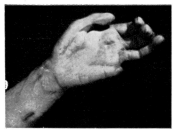 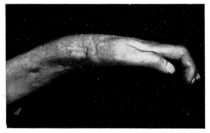

ger became gangrenous. Drainage was inadequate, lasting 5½ months, and position of function was not maintained.

of the first cleft that forces the thumb out into abduction.

Treatment. Two separate incisions are required: one on the dorsum over the radial border of the first interosseus muscle and the other in the palm parallel with the thenar crease. The motor branch of the median nerve should not be harmed, and through-and-through drains should not be used.

HYPOTHENAR SPACE. This is the fascial compartment enclosing the hypothenar muscles. It is unimportant and when infected points dorsally.

DORSAL SUBCUTANEOUS SPACE. This space is between the skin with its superficial fascia and the aponeurotic layer enveloping the extensor tendons on the back of the hand. Pus in it may point directly through the skin or

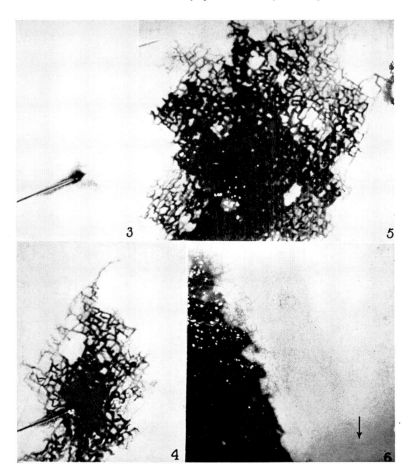

FIG. 857. Showing the free lymphatic flow in the skin immediately after injection with India ink (3). Shows how diffusely any lymphatic infection is spread. (Hudach, S. S., and McMaster, P. D.: J. Exp. Med. *57*: 774)

about the borders of the dorsum of the hand.

DORSAL SUBAPONEUROTIC SPACE. As its name implies, this is between the aponeurosis of the extensor tendons and the metacarpals. It extends down the dorsum of the fingers to each side of the insertion of the extensor tendon. Pus within it points at the webs and the periphery of the dorsum of the hand. From both the subcutaneous and the subaponeurotic spaces, pus can extend into the palm through the web spaces.

QUADRILATERAL SPACE IN FOREARM. PARONA'S SPACE. This space beneath the fascia of the profundus muscles lies on the pronator quadratus muscle and extends up the forearm where the profundus muscle is broadly attached on the interosseus membrane and the ulna. Extension of infection from here is over the profundus and the flexor pollicis longus muscles and under the superficialis muscle, coming to the surface of the forearm between the latter and the flexor ulnaris. It becomes involved usually from the radial or the ulnar bursa and occasionally from the wrist joint. A firm indurated swelling in the forearm, together with a bursal infection, is diagnostic.

Usually, the wrist is held flexed, and pain is produced when it is extended.

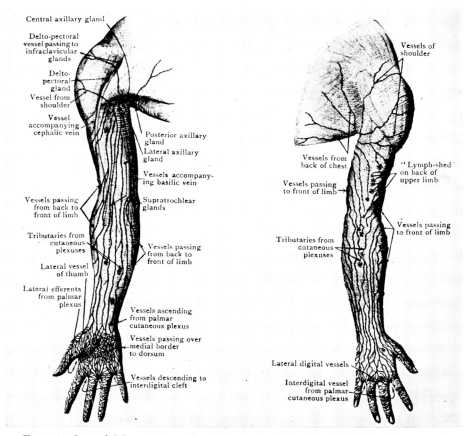

FIG. 858. *Superficial lymph vessels of the front of the upper limb.* The fingers on the ulnar side drain to the epitrochlear glands and on the radial side to the axillary glands. *Superficial lymph vessels of the back of the upper limb.* Drainage from the little and the ring fingers goes to the epitrochlear glands and from the fingers on the radial side to the axillary glands. Lymphatic vessels just below the elbow, like the veins, swing to the front around their respective sides. A small percentage from the long finger swing to the front in the upper arm along the cephalic vein to reach the subclavian gland. (Cunningham: Textbook of Anatomy, Oxford Univ. Press)

Treatment. In the lower part of the forearm an incision is made on each side, midlaterally volar to the radius and in front of the ulna. The radial nerve is displaced dorsally and the dorsal branch of the ulnar nerve volarward. The pus is always deep to the flexor tendons. If the pus extends high in the forearm, an incision should be made between the flexor

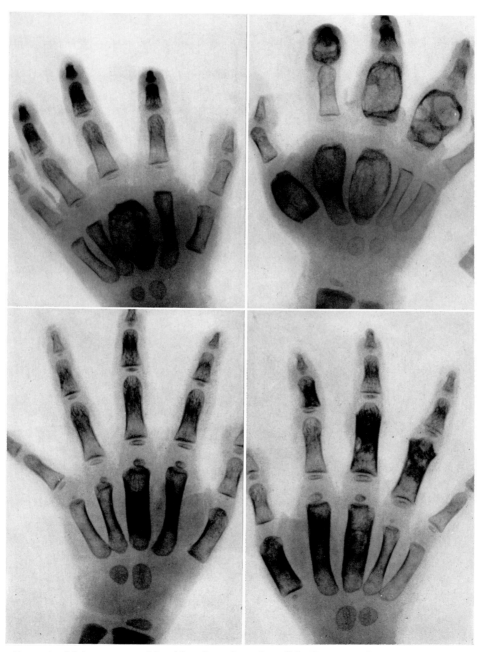

Fig. 859. Male, 3 years old, with tuberculous dactylitis. Lower 2 photographs show condition after conservative chemotherapy for 9 months. (Prof. A. Hodgson, University of Hongkong)

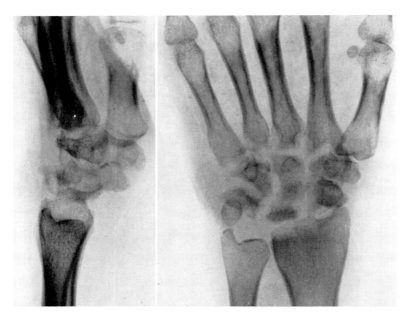

FIG. 860. A 34-year-old female with tuberculosis of the wrist of 1 year's duration. (Prof. A. Hodgson, University of Hongkong)

digitorum sublimis and the flexor ulnaris muscles.

Infection in Tendon Sheaths (Tenosynovitis). Tenosynovitis is more serious and more rapid in its progress than fascial-space infection. If it starts in the index or the middle or the ring finger, extension is into the thenar and the midpalmar spaces, respectively; if it starts in the thumb or the little finger, there is direct open connection to the radial or the ulnar bursae. If these are involved, it may extend into the thenar and the midpalmar spaces or break directly into the quadrilateral space of the forearm. From a sheath in a fin-

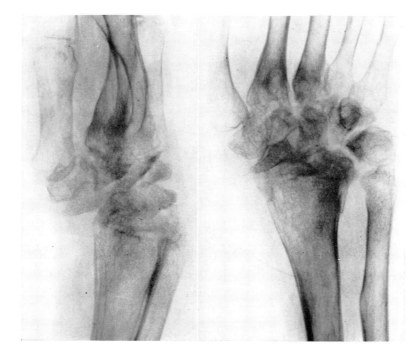

FIG. 861. A 30-year-old female with tuberculosis of the wrist of 2 years' duration. Multiple sinuses were present. (Prof. A. Hodgson, University of Hongkong)

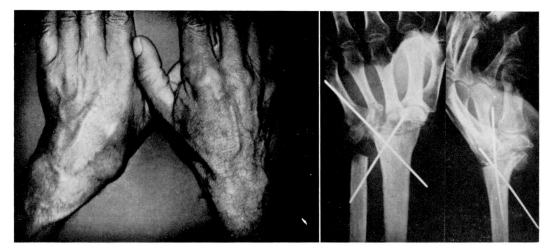

FIG. 862. Case A. C. (*Left*) Tuberculous tenosynovitis and wrist joint infection, soreness and stiffness of the fingers. Identified by culture. Removed the diseased tissues and fused the wrist, followed by streptomycin, PAS and isoniazid. Healing was uneventful. (*Right*) Wrist fusion is firm 3 months later. No recurrence after 3 years.

ger, the middle finger joint may become infected, and from the bursae the wrist joint.

ETIOLOGY. The usual cause is a puncture wound in a flexor crease of a finger where skin and sheath are close together, especially at the middle finger crease. Infection within the pulp space is a possible source, and a few result from infection in the palm or the dorsum of the fingers and the hand. The severe cases usually start in the thumb or the little finger.

TENOSYNOVITIS IN A DIGIT. In the index, the middle and the ring fingers the proximal cul-de-sac of the sheath usually ends at the distal crease in the palm. From the index finger, the infection breaks through into the thenar space, and from the middle and the ring finger sheaths, it spreads into the middle palmar space. From these spaces it travels through lumbrical canals to the finger and the web spaces and points dorsally. The sheaths of the thumb and the little finger flexors are usually continuous with their respective bursae, radial and ulnar. In rare cases, the sheath of the little finger or the thumb does not reach the bursa and must rupture into the fascial space, and occasionally the sheath about the ring finger flexor may reach the wrist. Sheath infection in a finger is prone to involve the middle finger joint.

Symptoms. The finger is held rigid and semi-flexed, the patient will not allow passive exten-

sion because of the great pain, and voluntary attempts to flex against resistance are painful. Tenderness can be outlined along the tendon sheath but is maximal over the proximal cul-de-sac of the sheath.

The whole finger and dorsum of the hand may be moderately swollen, though the finger is often not red. The course is usually rapid and may be as short as 6 hours.

Treatment. With antibiotics some sheath infections may be aborted, but a tendon is so poor in blood supply that when involved it may become a sequestrum beyond the reach of penicillin. Surgical drainage should be prompt to prevent tendon damage. A midlateral incision should be made from the distal crease of the finger to its base on one side only. Another curved incision, partially paralleling the distal crease in the palm, should drain the cul-de-sac of the sheath. In the thumb the incision is preferable down the ulnar side, so that it may be continued a little down the ulnar side of the thenar eminence posterior to the nerve. If a sheath and a joint infection are combined, except in the case of a thumb, it may be best to amputate through the joint.

ULNAR BURSA. There are 2 synovial sheaths under the transverse carpal ligament. One, the radial bursa, envelops the flexor tendon of the thumb, and the other, the ulnar bursa, envelops the flexor tendons of the fingers. The 2

A   B   C   D

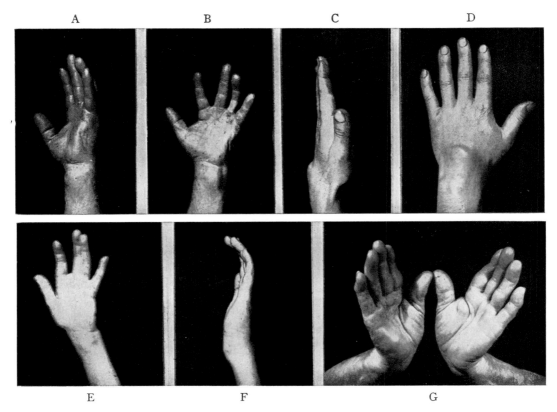

E   F   G

FIG. 863. Tuberculous tenosynovitis. (A, B) Case V. O. Ulnar bursa, palm and little finger. (C, D) Case H. R. Local, as shown. (E, F) Case S. C. Ulnar bursa, palm and index finger. (G) Case J. H. Bilateral ulnar bursae, left hand, palm and index finger.

bursae often communicate with each other, so that when tenosynovitis starts in one, the other becomes involved.

The ulnar bursa forms 3 longitudinal pockets: one volar of the tendons, one between the 2 tendon layers, and the third—the largest—under the profundus tendons. The mesotenons are on the radial side, which leaves the ulnar side free for drainage.

Distally, the ulnar bursa reaches to the distal crease in the palm, and here, just over the ring metacarpal, is a point of maximal tenderness in bursal infection. Proximally, it reaches to above the wrist level as a pouch lying on the pronator quadratus muscle. In the palm it partially overlies the midpalmar space and is beneath some of the hypothenar muscles.

Infections enter the bursa from the sheath of the little finger or the radial bursa or may come from the thenar space. After about 48 hours the bursa usually ruptures into the quadrilateral space in the forearm and also into the midpalmar space.

When the contents of the carpal tunnel swell and are under tension, the blood supply is squeezed out of the tendons and the nerves, and they necrose from the upper part of the annular ligament to the distal half of the palm.

Symptoms. The fingers are held semiflexed, the little finger the most and the index finger the least, and there is pain on passive extension—especially of the little finger. This is the hook sign.

There is pain on attempted voluntary flexion; the palmar concavity is not obliterated as it is in middle palmar space infections.

Tenderness is always maximal where the bursa almost reaches the distal palmar crease.

Motions of the wrist are restricted and painful.

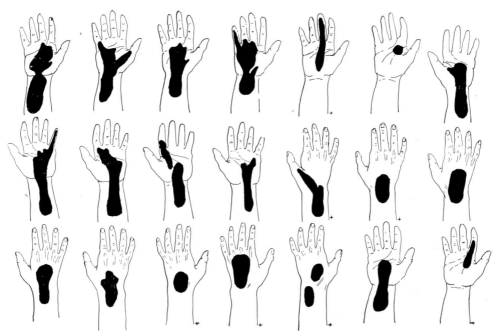

Fig. 864. Locations of the lesions in the 21 cases of tuberculous tenosynovitis reported. Of the 6 marked with +, the pathology seemed to be definitely that of tuberculosis, though the pathologist failed to find tubercles or organisms.

Treatment. The palm and the ulnar bursa are opened in a line paralleling the distal crease in the palm and curving at the tendon of the little finger proximally and centrally toward the heel of the palm. The ulnar bursa is opened in the forearm by a 3-inch incision just in front of the ulna. The dorsal branch of the ulnar nerve and the flexor carpi ulnaris muscle are retracted volarward. Entering along the pronator quadratus muscle, the bulge of the ulnar bursa is located and opened. If the quadrilateral space contains pus, a radial incision just in front of the radius should also be made. If the infection is far advanced, it is advisable to continue the palmar incision proximally, curving it as it crosses the wrist, and decompress and drain the carpal tunnel at its ulnar side.

RADIAL BURSA. The radial bursa is the sheath of the flexor tendon of the thumb; it reaches proximally to above the end of the radius but not quite so high as the ulnar bursa. It contains the flexor tendon of the thumb only, and in 85 per cent of cases communicates with the ulnar bursa. It is claimed that of the

2 bursae, the radial is more frequently responsible for wrist-joint infections.

Treatment. The radial bursa can be drained through the same 3-inch incision in front of the ulna that drains the ulnar bursa. This has the advantage of providing dependent drainage. A radial incision may be superfluous but can be added if the quadrilateral space in the forearm is involved.

Infection in Lymphatics. Lymphangitis. This usually starts from a superficial injury and spreads rapidly. Fever and toxemia are severe.

A dense meshwork of lymphatics in the palmar skin has a system of collecting trunks converging up the dorsum of the hand and the wrist. Two main groups extend up the forearm, from the radial side along the basilic vein to the axilla and from the ulnar border to the axilla, some through the epitrochlear glands but others direct. A few deep vessels follow the brachial artery.

Lymphangitis usually has a rapid onset, soon spreading up the arm to above the elbow. After a few days certain parts break down in abscess formation. This may be in the sheaths,

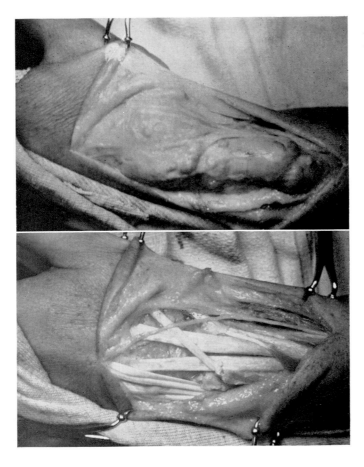

FIG. 865. Nonspecific tenosynovitis (? villonodular) involving wrist extensor sheaths. Note the superficial radial nerve coursing over the tumor.

the fascial spaces, the bones or the joints, or it may be in a lymph gland—cubital, axillary or subclavicular. Subcutaneous abscesses may form in the lymph vessels, as on the dorsum of the hand, the wrist or the flexor surface of the forearm. When lymphangitis has been intense, the infection spreads out into the surrounding tissue, and in this stage the tissues liquefy and break down to diffuse, progressive cellulitis. Thrombosis occurs in the veins, and often pyemia and septicemia follow.

The hand swells and is tender and red, but the fingers move painlessly, and there are no signs of sheath or fascial-space infection. The involved lymph glands are tender and swollen. General toxic symptoms are great for the appearance of the lesion: restlessness, headache, malaise, sweating, loss of appetite and vomiting. The patient looks sick and feverish, and the pulse is bounding.

The course may be fulminating, but most cases quickly respond to treatment. In some which do not subside promptly, an abscess localizes in a gland or at the lacunae in the course of the lymphatics, on the dorsum of the hand, the wrist or the forearm or in the flexor aspect of the wrist.

Some are more severe, and, after a week or 10 days during which time the whole arm swells and shows redness and blebs, the various complications mentioned arise. Tenosynovitis may run its course, extending to bones, joints and spaces, or the whole surface of the arm may break down in phlegmonous cellulitis. Thrombi from the clotted veins or even free pus in the veins may disseminate the infection to the lungs or throughout the body, causing multiple lung abscesses or pyemia. Such severe cases may need amputation and, if they do not die, will have a long, stormy convalescence. Involvement of the deep lymphatics must be suspected when the whole arm is greatly swol-

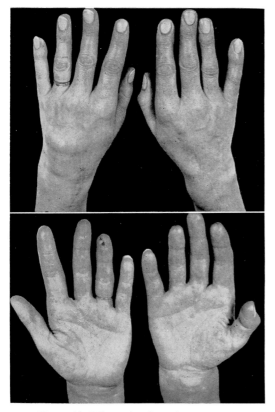

FIG. 866. Bilateral tuberculous tenosynovitis. History of tuberculous peritonitis at age 6 and pulmonary lesions present now.

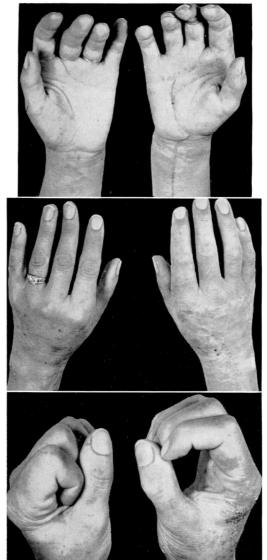

FIG. 867. Same patient as Figure 866. (*Top*) Postoperative view after excision of flexor sheaths on the right. (*Center*) After excision of extensor involvement. (*Bottom*) Four years after operation.

len and signs of abscess formation appear along the course of the arteries, as in the quadrilateral space in the forearm.

A more detailed description of lymphangitis may be found in the excellent article by Koch (see Bibliography).

TREATMENT. In lymphangitis there is often no apparent focus of infection, the infecting organism having spread so rapidly through the lymphatic system that the original focus has lost its identity. In such a case, incision for drainage is not only useless but decidedly harmful. Surgical incision has been castigated by Kanavel and Koch, who claim that most complicated cases have had ill-advised incisions. Undoubtedly, the best rule to follow is to avoid these incisions. However, there are cases which show a very definite focus, such as a drop of pus under a crust or blister or a pustule where lifting a lid or liberating the pus

very locally will eliminate the focus. Only such a focus should be attended to, but without cutting through an area of good tissue. Every patient with lymphangitis should be placed in bed in a hospital, and the hand and the arm should be elevated and wrapped in a volumi-

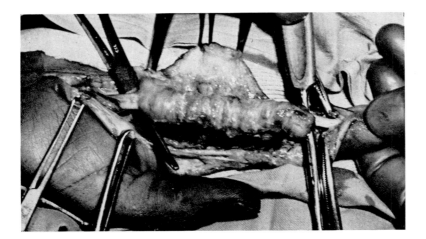

Fig. 868. Dissection of tubercular tenosynovitis of the flexors of the index finger. (Colonel Ernst Dehne)

nous warm compress reaching to the axilla. Broad-spectrum antibiotics should be given until a culture and sensitivity tests can be obtained. Water should be forced until the daily urine output is 1,000 ml., and blood transfusions should be given if necessary. Even when an abscess begins to form, one should err on the side of delaying surgical drainage, rather than rush in too quickly and disseminate infection. Tenosynovitis, joint and bone infections, abscesses and cellulitis demand drainage. In very severe cases, life-saving amputation must be considered.

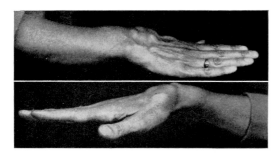

Fig. 869. Case A. D. A large lump came on the radial border of the wrist 2½ years ago. This was excised. It grew from the sheaths of the extensor tendons and the wrist and contained a few "melon seeds." The pathologist's report was "tenosynovitis, chronic, villiform," but considering that there were some calcified spots in the lung and a biopsy of some neck glands 10 years previously had showed tuberculosis, this is the probable cause.

Treatment of Infections. Treatment must be preceded by exact diagnosis of the type of infection—fascial space, tenosynovitis or lymphangitis—and of the exact boundaries of the infected areas. If it is a fascial-space infection, it should be drained soon, but tenosynovitis should be drained at once. In lymphangitis one should refrain from accelerating and spreading the infection by incising.

Also, one should be on guard for some underlying general disease such as diabetes.

If it is a case of fascial-space infection, tenosynovitis or lymphangitis, hospitalization is indicated, and all but trival cases and those of lymphangitis should be opened under general anesthesia and the ischemia of a tourniquet. Local anesthetic spreads infection and should not be used unless injected only in the line of the incision. Block anesthesia is dangerous in acute infection.

When using a tourniquet the blood should not be wound out of a limb with an Esmarch bandage, because this will express the infection into the circulation. Instead. after placing a blood pressure cuff loosely on the arm, the arm should be held vertical to empty it of blood. Then, the blood pressure band is filled rapidly before the arm fills with blood. Under ischemia the exact location of the infection can be seen and thorough drainage established.

If 3 or 4 days have elapsed, an abscess will be present, so that in such infections and in those of bone, tendon sheaths and joints, one should drain and at the same time, if feasible, excise necrotic tissue. Certain infections such as carbuncles and beginning abscesses have

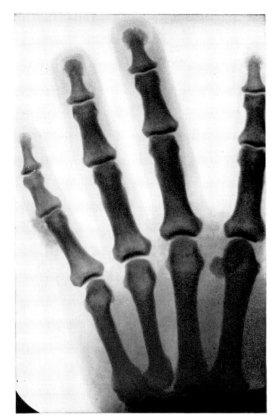

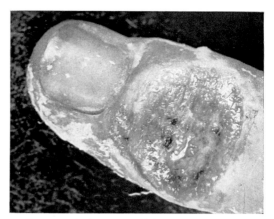

Fig. 871. Primary syphilitic chancre on the middle finger. Large axillary gland present.

Fig. 870. The calcareous deposit seen in the x-ray picture proved to be due to a local focus of tuberculosis in the sheath of the flexor tendons.

been checked by injecting the proper antibiotic into their centers and even around them if the area is indurated, without the necessity for surgical drainage. Whenever the antibiotic cannot reach or penetrate all of the tissues, drainage is necessary.

The area should be shaved and well cleaned with soap and water, all crusts and scales being removed, leaving only clean skin. Before expressing the pus from a sinus or an incision, one should carefully press around, starting at the periphery to determine the exact area of the abscess over which pressure will cause pus to escape. The incision should be chosen to drain widely, often through an L-shape or a flap, and to block by its cross arm the upward extension of infection. It should afford dependent drainage and not cross a flexion crease at

a right angle. If an annular ligament must be severed, it should be done laterally, not through its center. Drainage should never be through-and-through in either a digit or the hand. Suitable incisions are discussed in Chapter 7. The dorsum of the hand may be swollen, but rarely needs to be incised. Throughout the wound are placed slender catheters with fine mesh gauze folded about them. They should not contact either tendon or joint cavity. The catheters are led out of the dressing, and sterile normal saline is injected in each catheter every 3 hours. All is kept in place for at least 4 days, at which time the packing will be loose, the wound surface will be red, and a barrier will be established against infection. After that, drains usually are no longer necessary.

The first dressing should be done with strict asepsis. The wound is no longer packed open. A simple compress is applied with catheters leading into it for the local instillation of solution.

SUBSEQUENT CARE. From the beginning, the hand is kept on a metal cockup splint to keep the part at rest and to hold the wrist dorsiflexed, the proximal joints flexed, the thumb in oppositon, and the arches curved. The splint can be made from soft aluminum sheets cut to pattern.

The hand should be elevated, given rest, heat and moisture, and be kept clean. Parts of the hand that are not infected should be free

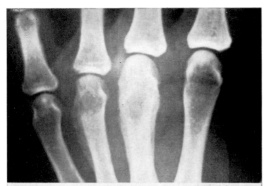

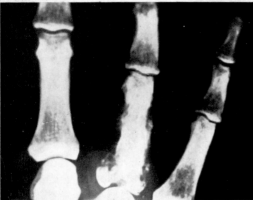

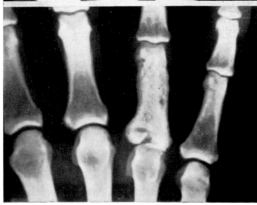

FIG. 872. Syphilitic dactylitis. (*Top*) Proliferation of the periosteal bone. (*Center*) Diffuse osteitis. (*Bottom*) Same, a year later after treatment.

to move. Elevation, by preventing edema, improves circulation. Heat should never be excessive, since sick tissue cannot tolerate it; lukewarm is a good expression. Moisture is added with each change of dressings, or the dressings may be changed once daily and the liquid injected every few hours. Wounds do much

better if kept clean. The surrounding skin should be kept clean.

Even an infected wound should be dressed with aseptic precautions to prevent adding a new infection. Baths are of doubtful value for this reason. Alternating with compresses, the wound and the hand do well if they are allowed to dry intermittently. Later, healing is hastened by exposure to sunlight.

The Orr treatment, though excellent elsewhere and in osteomyelitis of 1 bone in the hand, has not been satisfactory in extensive hand infection because of the tendency for the infection to extend to the various compartments within the hand.

If a finger is too badly damaged ever to be reconstructed, the infection may be terminated quickly by amputation. If infection is prolonged in 1 finger in an elderly person and is stiffening up the whole hand, amputation may be indicated—especially if it is the ring finger that is affected, for this finger especially, if stiff, prevents the adjoining fingers from flexing.

Joints should be maintained in the position of function by a simple volar metal splint, and as soon as the acute infection is over, motion should be started and persisted in. This will work out the edema and prevent stiffening of joints and adhesion to tendons. While the hand is incapacitated the arm should be raised frequently to the vertical at the shoulder, or eventually the patient will not be able to raise the arm. If an infection lasts too long, one suspects infection of a bone, a joint or a tendon, and if the fever and the symptoms seem to be too great, infection of a joint is suspected. In the course of infection, one or repeated severe hemorrhages may come from the superficial or the deep arch in the hand or the ulnar artery in the quadilateral space in the forearm. Such a hemorrhage comes from a lateral hole eroded into the vessel, which cannot be plugged by a terminal clot. The artery should be exposed at once, cut across, and each end ligated.

PHAGEDENIC INFECTION. In severe phagedenic anaerobic infection, after excising the necrotic tissue as advised by Meleney, the wound is packed with a 25 per cent suspension of zinc peroxide. Then it is covered with an impervious dressing, as described under gasbacillus infection. The treatment should be radical, as with gas gangrene.

FIG. 873. Primary cutaneous lesions in tularemia. (A) A primary papule on the 7th day. (B) A primary papule showing beginning liberation of the necrotic core on the 14th day. (C) A primary ulcer after liberation of the necrotic core on the 21st day. (D) A primary ulcer on the 42nd day. (Kavanaugh, C. N.: Arch. Int. Med. 55:70)

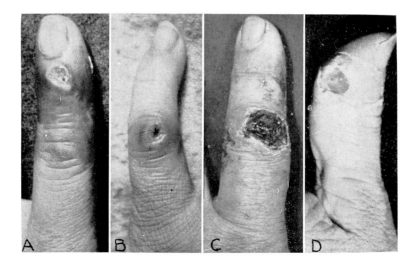

GAS-BACILLUS INFECTION. A necrotic field or one with a foreign body is essential for the growth of the anaerobes of gas infection. Therefore, such infection occurs in crushing or gunshot wounds and is more readily prevented than cured. Early complete surgical débridement of the wound is the best preventive. Next in importance are penicillin and polyvalent serum. Gas-bacillus infection is identified by the odor, the brick red or, later, bronzed appearance of the muscle, the gas in the tissue (sometimes seen on roentgenograms), pain, a rapid pulse and the Clostridia demonstrated in smears. The various bacteria should be identified specifically and the proper antibiotic determined. *Clostridium welchii* is the usual one found, but there may also be *Cl. sporogenes, Cl. tertium* or *Cl. histolyticum*. With these may be Staphylococcus, Proteus, *Escherichia coli, Pseudomonas aeruginosa* and nonhemolytic Streptococcus. Treatment should be immediate and radical. The wound should be excised widely, removing all necrotic tissue and packing the wound open. Penicillin is effective in lowering mortality in gas gangrene after adequate excision of devitalized tissue but is relatively ineffective without surgical excision (Lyons). Anti-gas-bacillus serum should be given in accordance with the direc-

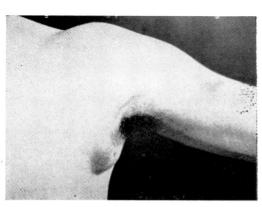

FIG. 874. Suppurating adenopathy in tularemia 4 weeks after onset. (Kavanaugh, C. N.: Arch. Int. Med. 55:71)

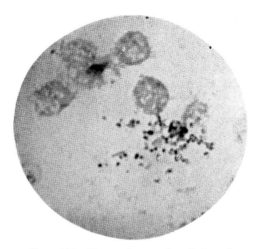

FIG. 875. Photomicrograph of *P. tularensis* in a dextrose broth-blood culture after 12 days. (Lufkin, N. H., and Evenson, A. E.: J. Lab. Clin. Med. 22:348)

tions on the individual package. X-ray treatment is of doubtful value. When gas gangrene is present, if a muscle group is involved the whole group should be excised; and if several groups, amputation is indicated. The wound may be filled with a creamy suspension of the medicinal grade of zinc peroxide. Over this is placed wet gauze, and all is covered with an impervious dressing of petrolatum gauze or cellophane to prevent evaporation. Every day or two the wound should be washed with normal salt solution and similarly redressed. Transfusions of whole blood are repeated as needed. Mortality from established and well-treated gas-bacillus infection is still in the neighborhood of 25 per cent.

OSTEOMYELITIS. Bone may become infected from a neighboring sheath or joint space. Drainage including the affected joint or sheath is necessary, but the bone should be allowed to sequestrate. In amputating through infected bone, care should be taken not to split the remaining bone and spread infection higher.

JOINT INFECTIONS. If fever persists and there is swelling around the circumference of the joint, infection within the joint space should be suspected. A felon spreads to the distal joint; sheath infections, to the middle joint. Joint infections treated by aspiration and instillations of antibiotics may subside, but in a finger especially, depending on the extent of damage to other structures, amputation should be considered early. To have only a stiff deformed and possibly painful finger as the result of months of treatment is not justifiable. One must consider the function of the hand as a whole.

Wrist Joint. Radial and ulnar bursal infections can spread to the wrist joint. The wrist is swollen, motions are painful, there may be excess mobility, especially if infection has been present for some time, and changes are present in the roentgenograms. Despite the anatomic separation of the radio-ulnar joint, when infection occurs in the radiocarpal and the intercarpal joints, it always becomes involved. Thus, instead of trying to drain through multiple incisions around the joint, it is better to open the ulnar side, divde the 2 ulnar wrist tendons and remove the lower end of the ulna. Involved carpal bones are excised, and the arm is immobilized in plaster to the axilla until healed.

SPECIAL INFECTIONS

TUBERCULOSIS

Direct inoculation of the skin may produce a chronic red papule which ulcerates. Bones and joints may become infected from blood-borne bacteria, especially in children. The phalanges and the metacarpals show a characteristic medullary involvement with marked enlargement of the shafts and secondary joint involvement. This dactylitis or spina ventosa can be distinguished from syphilitic infection by the lack of periosteal thickening. Biopsy, culture and guinea pig inoculation are needed for positive identification.

Specific chemotherapy with streptomycin, para-aminosalicylic acid and isoniazad (INH) usually will clear the lesion in children.

Wrist Joint. In children the wrist joint may be involved primarily from one of the carpal bones; but in adults, tuberculosis of the wrist joint is more commonly an extension of tenosynovitis.

Roentgenograms, aspiration and culture will

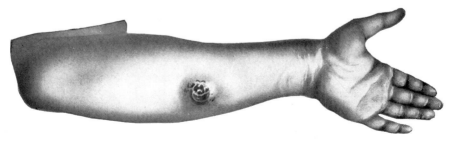

FIG. 876. Anthrax carbuncle showing the gangrenous crust surrounded by a zone of inflammation in which are vesicles filled with a serohemorrhagic fluid. (Hart, D.: Lewis' Practice of Surgery (after Lexer Bevan), vol. 5, p. 155, Hagerstown, Md., Pryor)

verify the diagnosis. Treatment is by long-time plaster immobilzation and chemotherapy. Persistent disease in an adult is an indication for resection and arthrodesis.

Tuberculous Tenosynovitis. This manifestation of tuberculosis, often the only apparent lesion in a patient, has been well described in a classic article by Kanavel. Modern chemotherapy has aided greatly in the treatment.

It is more common in adults and has been known to follow direct inoculation in certain occupations which deal with diseased cattle. It is seldom bilateral and is most often the only demonstrable active lesion of tuberculosis in the patient. Males predominate, and the average age is near 40. Twice as many cases involve the flexor as compared with the extensor tendon sheaths.

When the tendon sheaths are involved, the synovial reaction varies with the stage of the disease and the virulence of the organism. Serous effusions grading into granulomatous masses involve the radial and the ulnar bursae and invade the tendons. Untreated cases eventually may suppurate with multiple sinus formation. It may start in a digit and remain localized to that sheath or spread into a fascial space. In the extensor compartments, all the tendons become involved, but not below the dorsum of the hand. Villiform processes of the involved synovia loosen to form the "rice bodies." It is primarily an infection of the synovia and, if checked at this stage by chemotherapy or surgical excision, the tendons remain and function. Unchecked, the tendons themselves become involved as well as the annular ligaments and the neighboring joints, especially the wrist.

Tissue examination will disclose tubercules with typical giant cells and culture and guinea pig inoculation will verify the diagnosis. However, some will show only a nonspecific inflammatory reaction, and the cultures will be negative. Coccidioidomycosis can mimic tuberculosis in all its clinical and microscopic appearances, but a careful search will disclose the typical spherules in the giant cells. Rheumatoid disease usually includes involvement of synovia as well as joints.

In tuberculosis tenosynovitis the onset is insidious and the course slow, and pain and discomfort are not prominent. When the ulnar bursa is involved, there is a palmar swelling and another above the volar carpal ligament.

Pressure waves can be transmitted from one to the other if there is effusion. This is the historic "compound palmar ganglion." On the dorsum of the wrist there may also be a constriction in the swelling at the level of the dorsal retinaculum.

The typical swelling is not hot or indurated, and its consistency is usually described as doughy. There is no redness unless the disease is of long standing and rupture through the skin is imminent. Crepitus is a common finding. Limitation of motion is slight, but the grip is usually weak. Tendons rupture from direct involvement of their structure by the disease.

TREATMENT. Local therapy consists primarily of immobilization and, if required, surgical excision of all involved structures. Systemic chemotherapy and streptomycin are used as well as the usual general measures. Before chemotherapy was available, surgery, when properly done, resulted in complete arrest of the disease in approximately 70 per cent of the cases. Modern treatment is a combination of a short period of rest, antibiotics and chemotherapy followed by surgical excision of the involved tissues. The systemic therapy is continued.

Surgery consists of a complete excision and the removal of as much involved tissue as is technically possible. Incisions follow the rec-

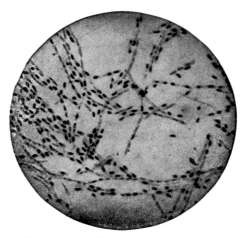

FIG. 877. *Bacillus anthracis* with spores; carbol fuchsin and methylene blue stain (× 1000) (Fränkel and Pfeiffer). (Jordan and Burrows: Textbook of Bacteriology, ed. 13, Philadelphia, Saunders)

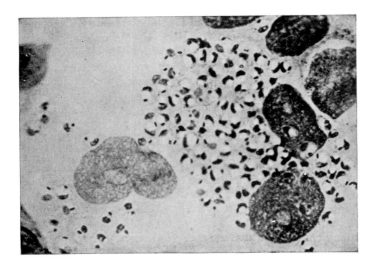

FIG. 878. Smear preparation from oriental sore. The ringlike bodies with white central portions and containing a larger and smaller dark mass are the micro-organisms. The dark masses stain lilac, and the peripheral portions pale robin's-egg blue, with Wright's stain. (Hart, D.: Lewis' Practice of Surgery, vol. 5, p. 219, Hagerstown, Md., Pryor)

ognized rules, leaving scars that will not make contractures. A block excision is made, removing the entire mass of diseased tissue. The mass of infected synovia must be incised to clear the material off the tendons by sharp dissection. Tendons that are frayed and diseased should be removed and their ends tapped into the adjoining tendons.

Closure is without drainage, and the limb is immobilized in plaster until the incisions heal.

In 21 cases varying in age from 11 to 64, there were 5 who had some contact with cattle: 2 tallow workers, 1 slaughterer, 1 milker and 1 dairyman. One tallow worker had an ulcerated lesion on a finger for 3 months before the tendon sheath of that digit became involved. The length of time from onset to treatment

varied from 1 month to 12 years. In 14 the flexor sheaths were involved, and in 9 of these both the radial and the ulnar bursae. In 1 patient the wrist joint was involved.

Tuberculosis was proved in 15. Some unusual findings were thick yellow creamy exudate and calcium of pastelike consistency.

Of 20 patients followed, there were 6 recurrences, and 2 died of generalized tuberculosis. Three of the other 4 recurrences were treated conservatively with good results. One wrist joint was fused.

SYPHILIS

Chancres occur especially on the index finger and may resemble a paronychia. Tertiary lesions are reported involving skin, tendon

FIG. 879. Oriental sore of 2 months' duration, appearing 3 months after exposure. The ulcer is covered with a firmly adherent, dirty, yellowish crust about $1\frac{1}{4}$ inches in diameter. Surrounding the crust is a reddish, firm, infiltrated zone covering twice the area of the central crust. There is a thin serous discharge, and the ulcer bleeds easily on traumatization. The lesion is painless, and there is no enlargement of the associated lymph nodes. Microscopic section of the skin showed edema, cellular infiltration, Langhans' cells and *Leishmania tropica*. (Hart, D.: Lewis' Practice of Surgery, vol. 5, p. 217, Hagerstown, Md., Pryor, from New York M.J. *116*:367)

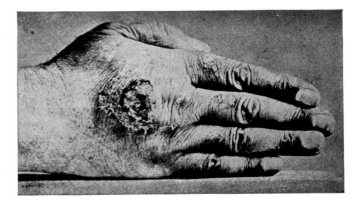

sheaths and bones. In the last, the typical lesion is periosteal thickening and increased bone density in metacarpals and phalanges. Charcot's painless destruction may involve the wrist or the proximal finger joints.

LEPROSY

Riordan described the changes in the hand in leprosy. Sensory losses out of proportion to the motor loss and especially of a glove or

sleeve type are seen and, later, bone absorption of the phalanges from loss of neurotrophic influences. Charcot-type changes are seen in the interphalangeal joints. Peripheral neuritis and traumatic nerve lesions should be differentiated easily.

TULAREMIA

Named after Tulare County, California, this disease often starts on the hand from infection with the organism *Pasteurella tularensis*) which is acquired by handling infected animals. The rabbit is the chief carrier. The lesion is a red granulomatous lesion of the skin which breaks down and is accompanied by lymphangitis and lymphadenitis. Suppuration in the glands is common. There are generalized toxic symptoms, and pneumonic and meningeal types are seen. Direct smears show the organ-

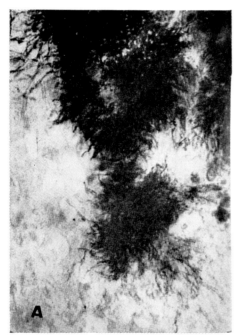

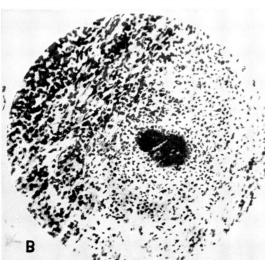

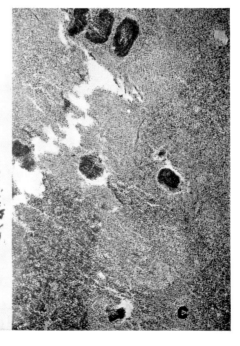

FIG. 880. (A) A sulfur granule (Gram's stain × 400); this is the typical ray fungus rosette. The conformation of the twisted mycelial threads is shown.

(B) A number of Actinomyces colonies surrounded by leukocytes.

(C) A Gram's stain of a sulfur granule, showing the intertwining mycelial threads of the Streptothrix (× 400). (After Wangensteen, O. H.: Ann. Surg. *104*:755)

Fig. 881. Actinomycosis of the hand. The infection had been present for 18 months and came on following a laceration which was treated with tobacco removed from the mouth. The original injury healed promptly. Two or 3 months later, small abscesses appeared about the scar, and these spread, despite the usual surgical treatment of incision and drainage, until most of the dorsum was involved. The surface of the affected area was irregularly nodular and crusted and showed areas of ill-defined scarring. The ulcers were irregular, and there were numerous sub-epidermal abscesses, some of which had opened and were discharging. The area was tender, the skin was bound down, and consider-

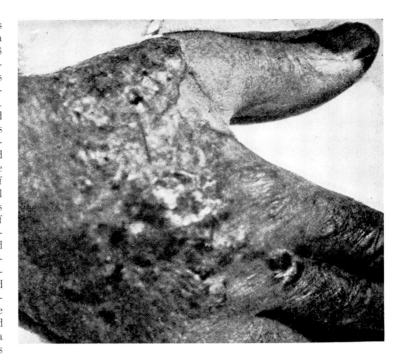

able induration was present but no lymphatic involvement. The patient was treated with large doses of potassium iodide internally and 25 per cent aluminum acetate and 10 per cent ammoniated mercury ointment locally. Three x-ray treatments were given; after 3 months healing was complete. The ray fungus was demonstrated in the pus. (Hart, D.: Lewis' Practice of Surgery, vol. 5, p. 202, Hagerstown, Md., Pryor)

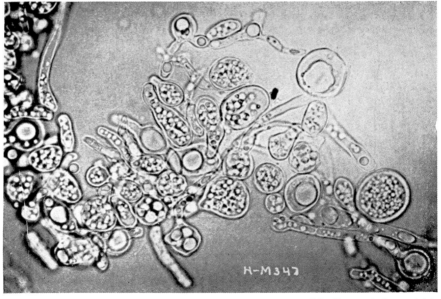

Fig. 882. Old culture of Blastomyces showing large round bodies and short, thick mycelium, containing sporelike bodies. (Montgomery, F. H., and Ormsby, O. S.: Arch. Int. Med. 2:25)

isms, and a positive blood culture can be obtained during the first week.

Chlortetracycline and streptomycin are said to be effective. The reports of Foshay and Kavanaugh are recommended reading.

ANTHRAX

Infection of the hand occurs through contact with the organism found in the hair and the hides of many domestic animals. The pustule has a typical vesicular center in a surrounding red swelling; when it ruptures, there is a black area in the base. Several pustules may be present and the disease may spread to the lungs, the meninges and the heart. Mortality is 15 to 20 per cent.

Direct smears show the typical bacillus. Several of the antibiotics such as penicillin, Chlortetracycline and Oxytetracycline seem to be effective.

GLANDERS

Contact with infected secretions of the horse and the mule and a break in the skin from an abrasion allows the organism *Malleomyces mallei* to infect the part. Small vesicles and pustules surround a granulomatous lesion,

and there is lymphangitis and lymphadenitis. The incubation is short (2 to 5 days), and the onset is acute with fever, vomiting and diarrhea. Later, lesions may break out in other areas and form draining sinuses. The mortality is high, and no specific treatment is reported to be effective.

GONORRHEA

Tenosynovitis and arthritis are the manifestations of blood-borne gonococcal infection in the hand. Lesions are acute or chronic, accompanied by swelling, redness and pain. Aspiration and identification of the organism by smear and culture is the only definite diagnostic procedure. Drainage is done only if a true abscess forms, antibiotics being the treatment of choice. Joints should be splinted. Ankylosis often follows arthritis.

LEISHMANIASIS

Oriental sore, Delhi boil or tropical ulcer from about the Mediterranean to India is also being found in the United States. *Leishmania tropica* is a spindle-shaped flagellated protozoa probably transmitted by a sandfly to exposed parts—especially the dorsum of the hand—

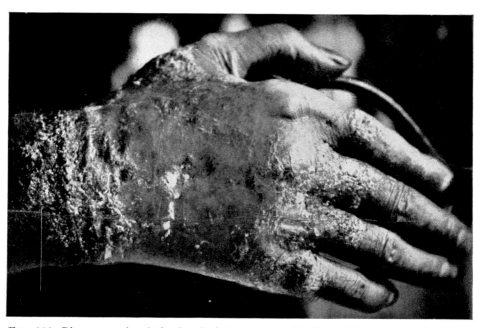

FIG. 883. Blastomycosis of the hand. (Montgomery, F. H., and Ormsby, O. S.: Arch. Int. Med. 2:5)

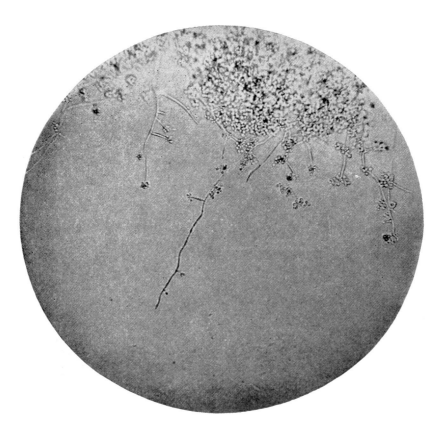

FIG. 884. *S. schenckii*; a low-power view of a culture on a slide. (Benham, R. W., and Kesten, B.: J. Infect. Dis. *50*: 442)

producing a sore. There is at first a papule which is red, raised and indurated and about 1 inch in diameter. In several months this breaks down to a crater which may last for years and leave a depressed scar. The ulcer teems with protozoa, many of which are intracellular, and these can be seen easily on a smear.

Tartar emetic is reportedly specific. Ball and Ryan in Africa successfully treated 500 cases with a preparation of antimony, Neostam, intravenously 0.05 to 0.2 Gm. 3 times a week until cured, the total amount of drug averaging 1.14 Gm. Neostibosan injected locally about the ulcer is the usual treatment in India.

Cures have been reported by J. Snapper from the diamidines, of which 2-hydroxystilbamidine is one, giving 225 mg. in 200 ml. of 5 per cent glucose up to 6.1 Gm.

MILKER'S GRANULOMA

This is a chronic red, painful, granulating nodule on the hand of a milker or one who works with cattle. It is caused by the presence of a cow's hair which, being provided with barbs, works in, remaining as a foreign body. The wound heals when the hair is removed and the nodule drained or excised.

Another entity known as milker's nodule occurs on the hands of milkers of cows that have crusted sores on their udders. Starting as an erythematous papule, the lesion develops to a bluish-red nodule, becomes depressed centrally and then granulates and heals in from 4 to 6 weeks. It is self-limited and resembles variola but is probably from a different virus (Becker).

BARBER'S HANDS—PILONIDAL SINUS

These consist of sinuses on the dorsum of the webs resulting from clipped hairs entering the skin and setting up a foreign-body reaction. Many short hairs are found in or protruding from the pits and the sinuses. A probe can be passed into one sinus opening and out the other, the epithelial-lined canals running through the subcutaneous tissue.

FIG. 885. *S. schenckii*; 5 colonies each from a single spore planted on a maltose agar plate. (Benham, R. W., and Kesten, B.: J. Infect. Dis. *50*:441)

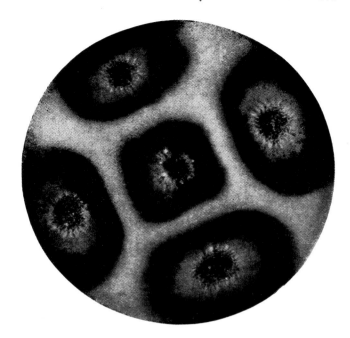

Treatment is to remove the hairs each night and to excise the pits and the sinuses.

ACTINOMYCOSIS

The ray fungus from infected cattle may enter the hand through an abrasion. The indolent granuloma resembles tuberculosis or syphilis, spreads gradually and eventually breaks down with many sinuses. It is chronic, and pain is not severe. Sulfur granules in the discharge when examined show the fungus.

Radical excision with administration of broad-spectrum antibiotics is recommended.

BLASTOMYCOSIS

This is essentially a skin disease caused by a yeast resulting in a spreading dermatitis and sometimes pulmonary involvement. It spreads slowly at the periphery, tending to heal in the center. A thick crust covers a rough surface with many ulcerations, abscesses and sinuses. Adenopathy is unusual. Yeast can be found in the exudate.

The systemic types involve organs and bones and have a high mortality rate.

Treatment with potassium iodide, carbosulfate or x-ray has been recorded. Elson says diamidines are fungistatic.

SPOROTRICHOSIS

Sporotrichum schenckii, a fungus, causes a local skin disease found usually on the hands and the forearms. It is seen especially in farmers and gardeners who work with plants and

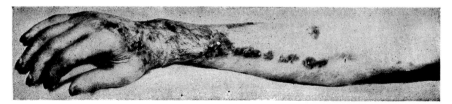

FIG. 886. Sporotrichotic lesions which gradually came on as nodules along a cord which followed the course of the lymphatic drainage. These nodules all went on to ulceration, with discharge of a gelatinous purulent material. (Hart, D.: Lewis Practice of Surgery, vol. 5, p. 196, Hagerstown, Md., Pryor)

become inoculated with the fungus through some trivial wound. It is also known in horses, dogs and rats and has been transmitted by a bite and also from one person to another and from man to plants.

The lesion, a pea-sized nodule, is in the skin and the subcutaneous tissue, only rarely involving bones and viscera. After a few weeks the nodule ulcerates or forms an abscess. After a remission of a week or a month, it extends along the lymph vessels, forming an indurated cord or chain of many firm nodules similar to the first. These are subcutaneous but later break down, attaching to the skin and forming abscesses, sinuses and ulcers. The picture with nodular lesions along an indurated cord is quite typical. Occasionally, a lymph gland is involved and progresses to abscess. The tissue is granulomatous with giant cells, but it is difficult to find organisms. There may be an eosinophilia of 8 per cent.

The fungus is readily cultured from an unopened nodule; it shows long threads with short branches, along both of which are clusters of small oval bodies called conidia. Only these, and not the threads, are found in tissue.

The lesions are painless and indolent, the disease remaining chronic for many months until treated.

With the history of occupation and the typical appearance of the lesion, a culture should be made. There is prompt response to potassium iodide, but this should be continued for 6 weeks after healing to prevent recurrence.

COCCIDIOIDOMYCOSIS

Coccidioidomycosis affects the hands in only a small portion of cases, either primarily through a break in the skin or secondarily in this unusual disease which in many respects resembles tuberculosis. It is found in California, where it is fairly common in the San Joaquin Valley. Also, a few cases have occurred in Arizona. Locally, a large percentage of the inhabitants react to the coccidioidin test (similar to tuberculin) without knowledge of having had the disease. Most recover from the initial respiratory infection in about 4 to 6 weeks. Erythema nodosum is a common manifestation. The course may be acute and short or may run on to the granuloma stage. Some cases show pulmonary, cutaneous and osseous lesions running a chronic course from mild to severe.

In the hands there are verrucous skin lesions, subcutaneous abscesses and granulomatous nodules which later become irregular indurated ulcers. In the secretions, cleared with 15 per cent potassium hydroxide, are seen many spherical bodies as large as 15 to 30 microns with refractive capsules; they are full of spores. The culture on glucose agar is fluffy white.

In an indolent tuberculous-appearing lesion, organisms should be searched for and found easily. The coccidioidin cutaneous test and the complement-fixation test are confirmatory.

Aside from excision and drainage, the treatment is general, as in tuberculosis. Potassium iodide does not help. A fungicide, ethyl vanillate, has been reported to be helpful in 3 cases (Fiese). Stilbamidine has been used. (See Bibliography.)

ERYSIPELOID

The fungus *Erysipelothrix rhusiopathiae* enters the skin of the hand through a trival wound, causing a local skin eruption somewhat resembling erysipelas, which seldom reaches above the wrist. It is usually contracted from handling fish or shellfish, though also from swine (hence, the name swine erysipelas), meat, poultry, game and cheese.

A dark bluish-red, slightly swollen area with an irregular papular border gradually spreads over a considerable area of the hand or the fingers, sometimes including the volar surface as it heals centrally. There may be lymphangitis and adenitis.

After an incubation of from 2 to 15 days, the disease runs its course in 2 or 3 weeks but does not confer immunity. Symptoms are slight, consisting of itching, burning, moderate pain and slight fever and malaise.

There is the typical appearance and history, and by smear and culture the threadlike organism can be identified. There is also an intradermal test showing a wheal in 24 hours.

Little if any treatment is needed. Cold compresses give relief. Sulfonamides are not effective, but penicillin acts within 48 hours. It should be continued for 3 days after apparent healing.

SPECIFIC PARONYCHIA

In chronic paronychia with redness, swelling, little or no pus and deformed or detached nails, a search should be made for *Epidermophyton*, *Trichophyton gypseum* and *Candida*

(*Monilia*) *ablicans*. The organisms of the above fungi may be found in skin scrapings. A detached nail should be clipped away. Ammoniated mercury ointment in gauze kept packed in next to the nail has cured without the necessity of avulsing the nail. *Candida albicans* is the yeastlike organism of thrush or vulvovaginal mycosis and is prevalent in hands long soaked in water; it may also be present on the dorsum of the webs. It can be grown in culture at room temperature. Use of the modern fungicide ointments applied daily and keeping the parts dry results in cure.

Syphilis is a possible cause of chronic indolent paronychia.

SEAL FINGER

This little known disease is endemic in Arctic Seas among seal hunters. It has been studied extensively by Candolin, who personally investigated 244 seal fingers in 193 patients in the Gulfs of Bothnia and Finland, where it is most common. It also occurs as far as Labrador in the North Atlantic, but not elsewhere, though 3 cases were reported from the Pribilof Islands in the Bering Sea and 2 from S. Georgia in the Antarctic. Most cases occur in the spring when seal hunters are active.

Infection occurs in fresh wounds in those who skin seals. The incubation is a week or less, and the disease lasts from a few weeks to a year, usually 4 months.

Pain is extreme, and the finger, which is red or livid, swells to 3 times its size. There are no general symptoms, fever or lymphangitis. In 63 per cent, an interphalangeal joint nearest to the entry was involved and often destroyed and ankylosed. Rarely was the metacarpophalangeal joint involved.

The appearance is like that of erysipeloid. The middle finger is involved in half of the cases, then the index finger, the thumb and the ring finger and last the little finger. Several may be affected, and it may recur.

Incision early may help by decompressing before bones are involved, but there is no abscess, and the results of incision are doubtful. Since there may be improvement for 2 years, amputation should be delayed. There is no medical treatment except that hot water lessens the pain. Penicillin has not helped, but apparently Aureomycin has. The finger should be immobilized in the position of function.

The organism is not known, though it comes from the true seals, the elephant seals and the fur seals but not from sea lions, whales or the fresh-water seals of Lake Ladoga.

CAT-SCRATCH GRANULOMA

An indolent papule or deep swelling may follow the bite or the scratch of a cat. Regional lymphadenitis 1 to 3 weeks later may break down to abscess. Fever up to 40° C. (104° F.) daily may last a month. The blood count is normal. There is some resemblance to tularemia, but the infecting agent in probably a virus like that of psittacosis. It can be transmitted to monkeys. An intradermal test with an antigen from an infected lymph gland produces a definite papular reaction. There is no specific therapy.

BIBLIOGRAPHY

PYOGENIC INFECTIONS

Andreasen, A. T.: Bone abscess from human bite, Brit. J. Surg. *34*:411, 1947.

Anson, B. J., and Ashley, F. L.: Midpalmar compartment, associated spaces and limiting layers, Anat. Rec. *78*:389, 1940.

Anson, B. J., Wright, R. R., Ashley, F. L., and Dykes, J.: The fascia of the dorsum of the hand, Surg., Gynec. Obstet. *81*:327, 1945.

Avent, C. H.: Anatomy and pathology of infections of the hand, Memphis Med. J. *15*:140, 1940.

Beck, C.: The Crippled Hand and Arm, Philadelphia, Lippincott, 1925.

Bolton, H., Fowler, P. J., and Jepsen, R. P.: Natural history and treatment of pulp space infection and osteomyelitis of terminal phalanx, J. Bone Joint Surg. *31-B*:499, 1949.

Bondi, A., Jr., and Diety, C. C.: Penicillin resistant staphylococci, Proc. Soc. Exp. Biol. Med. *60*:55, 1945.

Boyce, F. F.: Human bites; analysis of 90 (chiefly delayed and late) cases from Charity Hosp. of La. at New Orleans, South. M. J. *35*:631, 1942.

Brickel, A. C. S.: Surgical Treatment of Hand and Forearm Infections, St. Louis, Mosby, 1939.

Butler, H. M.: Bacteriological studies of Clostridium Welchii infections in man, Surg., Gynec. Obstet. *81*:475, 1945.

Caldwell, G. A.: Posttraumatic infections of the extremities, Am. J. Surg. *56*:64, 1942.

Cohn, R.: Infections of the hand following human bites, Surgery *7*:546, 1940.

Colebrook, L., and Hood, A. M.: Infection through soaked dressings, Lancet *2*:682, 1948.

Coleman, H. M., Bateman, J. E., Dale, G. M., and Starr, D. E.: Cancellous bone grafts for infected bone defects, Surg., Gynec. Obstet. *83*: 392, 1946.

Colson, P., and Houot, R.: Acute infections of the digital and digitocarpal sheaths; treatment by puncture-lavage of the sheath with penicillin; statistical study of 120 cases, Lyon chir. *53*:117, 1957.

Cooper, R. W.: Use of x-ray therapy in treatment of gas bacillus infection, Tri-State M. J. *13*: 2769, 1941.

Cutler, C. W.: The Hand: Its Disabilities and Diseases, Philadelphia, Saunders, 1942.

Cutler, E. C., and Sandusky, W. R.: Treatment of clostridial infections with penicillin, Brit. J. Surg. *32*:168, 1944.

Ellingsan, H. V., Kadull, P. J., Bookwalter, H. L., and Howe, C.: Cutaneous anthrax, J.A.M.A. *131*:1105, 1946.

Ferguson, L. K., Bush, L. F., and Kuehner, H. G.: Round-table conference on office surgery; office treatment of hand infections, Penn. M. J. *44*: 433, 1941.

Fifield, L. R.: Infections of the Hand, New York, Hoeber, 1927.

Flynn, J. E.: Clinical and anatomical investigations of deep fascial space infections, Am. J. Surg. *55*:467, 1942.

————: Acute suppurative tenosynovitis of the hand, Surg., Gynec. Obstet. *76*:227, 1943.

————: Surgical significance of middle palmar septum, Surgery *14*:134, 1943.

————: Medical progress; grave infections of hand, New Engl. J. Med. *229*:898, 1943.

Fritzell, K. E.: Infections of hand due to human mouth organisms, Lancet *60*:135, 1940.

Gordon, I.: Expectant treatment of pyogenic infections of the hand with special reference to infection of the flexor aspect of the fingers, Brit. J. Surg. *38*:331, 1951.

Grinnell, R. S.: Acute suppurative tenosynovitis of the flexor tendon sheaths of the hand, Ann. surg. *105*:97, 1937.

Grodinsky, M.: Pyogenic infections; lymphatic tendon sheath and fascial space infections of hand, Nebraska M. J. *27*:13, 1942.

Grodinsky, M., and Holyoke, E. A.: Fasciae and fascial spaces of palm, Anat. Rec. *79*:435, 1941.

Hall, I. C.: The value of antitoxin in the prevention and treatment of malignant edema and gas gangrene, Ann. Surg. *122*:197, 1945.

Handfield-Jones, R. M.: Hand; infections of tendons and tendon sheaths, Med. Press *211*: 53, 1944.

Heilman, F. R.: Streptomycin in treatment of experimental infections with micro-organisms of Friedlander group (Klebsiella), Proc. Mayo Clin. *20*:33, 1945.

Henry, A. K.: Medial approach to mid-palmar space and ulnar bursa, Lancet *1*:16, 1939.

Hudach, S. S., and McMaster, P. D.: The lymphatic participation in human cutaneous phenomena: A study of the minute lymphatics of the living skin, J. Exp. Med. *57*:751, 1933.

Iselin, M.: Tenosynovites digitales, Schweiz. med. Wschr. *62*:1159, 1932.

————: Surgery of the Hand, Philadelphia, Blakiston, 1940.

Jamieson, J. G.: The fascial spaces of the palm, with special reference to their significance in infections of the hand, Brit. J. Surg. *38*:193, 1950.

Jawetz, E., Melnick, J. L., and Adelberg, E. A.: Review of Medical Microbiology, Los Altos, Calif., Lange Med. Publ., 1954.

Kanavel, A. B.: Infections of the Hand, Philadelphia, Lea & Febiger, 1925.

————: Hand infections in industrial accidents, Surg., Gynec. Obstet. *60*:568, 1935.

Kanavel, A. B., and Mason, M. L.: Infections of the Hand *in* Encyclopedia of Medicine, Surgery and Specialties, Philadelphia, Davis, 1939.

Keefer, C. S.: Progress in the conquest of bacteria by new medicinal agents, Am. J. Pharm. *117*:12, 1945.

Kelley, R. P., Rosati, L. M., and Murray, R. A.: Traumatic osteomyelitis: The use of skin grafts —Part I, Ann. Surg. *122*:1, 1945.

Knight, M. K., and Wood, G. O.: Surgical obliteration of bone cavities following traumatic osteomyelitis, J. Bone Joint Surg. *27*:547, 1945.

Koch, S. L.: Felons, acute lymphangitis and tendon sheath infections; differential diagnosis and treatment, J.A.M.A. *92*:1171, 1929.

————: Diagnosis and treatment of major infections of the hand, Minnesota Med. *15*:1, 1932.

————: Acute rapidly spreading infections following trivial injuries of the hand, Surg., Gynec. Obstet. *59*:277, 1934.

————: Osteomyelitis of the bones of the hand, Surg., Gynec. Obstet. *64*:1, 1937.

————: Prevention and treatment of infections of the hand, J.A.M.A. *116*:1365, 1941.

————: Acute infections of hand, South. M. J. *37*:157, 1944.

Macey, H. B.: Paronychia and bone felon, Am. J. Surg. *50*:553, 1940.

McMaster, P. E.: Human bite infections, Am. J. Surg. *45*:60, 1939.

Mason, M. L.: Infections of the hand, Surg. Clin. N. Amer. *22*:455, 1942.

————: Pitfalls in the management of hand infections, Minnesota Med. *20*:485, 1937.

Mason, M. L., and Koch, S. L.: Human bite infections of the hand, Surg., Gynec. Obstet. *51*: 591, 1930.

Meleney, F. L.: Rational use of antibiotics in control of surgical infections, J.A.M.A. *153*:1253, 1953.

Milch, H.: Closed anterior space infections of finger, Med. Rec. *152*:361, 1940.

Moses, W. R.: The diagnosis of acute flexor tendon tenosynovitis, Surg., Gynec. Obstet. *82*: 101, 1946.

Orr, H. W.: Treatment of the infected wound in compound fractures, Surg. Clin. N. Amer. *22*: 1135, 1942.

Pratt, R., and Dufrenoy, J.: Antibiotics, ed. 2, Philadelphia, Lippincott, 1953.

Pulaski, E. J.: Surgical Infections, Prophylaxis, Treatment, Antibiotic Therapy, Springfield, Ill., Thomas, 1954.

Robins, R. H. C.: Infections of the hand, J. Bone Joint Surg. *34-B*:567, 1952.

Salsbury, C. R.: Contribution to anatomy of ulnar bursa, Canad. M. A. J. *43*:430, 1940.

Schatz, A., and Waksman, S. A.: Effect of streptomycin and other antibiotic substances upon *Mycobacterium tuberculosis* and related organisms, Proc. Soc. Exp. Biol. Med. *57*:244, 1944.

Scott, J. C., and Jones, B. V.: Results of treatment of infections of the hand, J. Bone Joint Surg. *34-B*:581, 1952.

Spaulding, J. E.: Fascial spaces of palm; contribution to their surgical anatomy, Guy's Hosp. Rep. *88*:432, 1938.

Stanley, M. M.: Bacillus pyocyaneus infections, Am. J. Med. *2*:347, 1947.

Stiles, G. W.: Chronic erysipeloid in man—the effect of treatment with penicillin, J.A.M.A. *134*:953, 1947.

Treves, F.: Applied Anatomy, Philadelphia, Lea Brothers & Co., 1901.

Trueta, J.: Principles and Practice of War Surgery, St. Louis, Mosby, 1943.

Umansky, A. L., Schlesinger, P. T., and Greenberg, B. B.: Tuberculous Dactylitis in the Adult *in* Year Book of General Surgery, 1947.

Weiner, J. J.: New incision for closed space infections (felon) involving distal phalanx of finger, Ann. Surg. *111*:126, 1940.

Welch, C. E.: Human bite infections of the hand, New Engl. J. Med. *215*:901, 1936.

Special Infections

Adams, R., Jones, G., and Marble, H. C.: Tuberculous tenosynovitis, New Engl. J. Med. *223*: 706, 1940.

Adamson, H. G.: Sporotrichosis, Brit. J. Derm. *20*:296, 1908.

Ayers, S., Jr., and Anderson, N. P.: So-called fungus infections of the hand, Calif. West. Med. *56*:63, 1942.

Benedek, T.: Fusospirochetal paronychia, Surgery *11*:75, 1942.

Benham, R. W., and Kesten, B.: Sporotrichosis, its transmission to plants and animals, J. Infect. Dis. *50*:437, 1932.

Bickel, W. H., *et al.*: Tuberculous tenosynovitis, J.A.M.A. *151*:31, 1953.

Birnbaum, W., and Callander, C. L.: Acute supportive gonococci tenosynovitis, J.A.M.A. *105*: 1025, 1935.

Candolin, Y.: Seal finger and its occurrence in the gulfs of the Baltic Sea, Acta chir. scand. Suppl. *177*:4, 1953.

Carson, D. R., and Solomon, F. A., Jr.: Sarcoidosis: A case with extensive metastatic calcification, renal failure and favorable response to steroid therapy, Calif. Med. *96*:114, 1962.

Currie, A. R., Gibson, T., and Goodall, A. L.: Interdigital sinuses of barbers' hands, Brit. J. Surg. *41*:278, 1953.

Curtis, A. C., *et al.*: The effect of stilbenes and related compounds on the mycoses, U. S. Armed Forces M. J. *5*:949, 1954.

Curtis, W. L.: Sulfanilamide in the treatment of tularemia, J.A.M.A. *113*:294, 1939.

Dickey, F. G.: Tularemia: A diagnostic and therapeutic study, Bull. Sch. Med. Univ. Maryland *24*:143, 1940.

Dickson, E. C.: Coccidioidomycosis, the preliminary acute infection with fungus coccidioides, J.A.M.A. *111*:1362, 1938.

Duran, R. J., Coventry, M. B., Weed, L. A., and Kierland, R. R.: Sporotrichosis, J. Bone Joint Surg. *39-A*:1330, 1957.

Fellander, M.: Tuberculous tenosynovitis of hand treated by combined surgery and chemotherapy, Acta chir. scand. *111*:142, 1956.

Fitzgerald, P., and Meenan, F.: Sarcoidosis of hands, J. Bone Joint Surg. *40-B*:256, 1958.

Foerster, H. R.: Sporotrichosis, an occupational dermatosis, J.A.M.A. *87*:1605, 1926.

Foshay, L.: Prophylactic vaccine against tularemia, Am. J. Clin. Path. *2*:7, 1932.

————: Tularemia treated by a new specific antiserum, Am. J. M. Sci. *187*:235, 1934.

————: Treatment of tularemia with streptomycin, Am. J. Med. *2*:467, 1947.

Fox, R. R.: Cat scratch fever, Arch. Path. *54*: 75, 1952.

Gillies, A.: Tuberculous tenosynovitis of palmar synovial bursa: "Compound palmar ganglion," case report, J. Bone Joint Surg. *13*:156, 1931.

Grebe, A. A.: Monostotic coccidioidal infection, J. Bone Joint Surg. *36-A*:859, 1954.

Guttman, P. H.: Pathology of cat scratch disease, Calif. Med. *82*:25, 1955.

Hamburger, W. W.: Sporotrichosis, J.A.M.A. *59*: 1590, 1912

Hamlin, E., Jr., and Sarris, S. P.: Acute gonococcal tenosynovitis; report of seven cases, New Engl. J. Med. *221*:228, 1939.

Hillman, C. C., and Morgan, T.: Tularemia: Report of a fulminant epidemic transmitted by the deer fly, J.A.M.A. *108*:538, 1937.

Houghton, G., *et al.*: Cat scratch fever, Stanford Med. Bull. *10*:157, 1952.

Howard, L. D., Jr.: Surgical treatment of rheumatic tenosynovitis, Am. J. Surg. *89*:1163, 1955.

Hyde, J. N., and Davis, D. J.: Sporotrichosis in man, J. Cutan. Dis. *28*:321, 1910.

Hyde, J. N., and Montgomery, F. H.: Cutaneous blastomycosis, J.A.M.A. *39*:1486, 1902.

Israel, H. L., and Jones, M.: Sarcoidosis, clinical observation on 160 cases, A.M.A. Arch. Int. Med. *102*:766, 1958.

Kanavel, A. B.: Tuberculous tenosynovitis of the hand, Surg., Gynec. Obstet. *37*:635, 1923.

Kavanaugh, C. N.: Tularemia—a consideration of 123 cases with observations at autopsy in one, Arch. Int. Med. *55*:61, 1935.

————:Tularemia (rabbit fever), Pub. Health Rep. *55*:65, 1940.

Kernahan, E. T., Jr., and Goldman, M. A.: Onchocerciasis of the hand, report of a case, J. Bone Joint Surg. *42-A*:575, 1961.

Knutsson, F.: Skeletal changes in sarcoidosis, Acta radiol. (Stockh.) *51*:429, 1959.

Lucchesi, P. E., and Gildersleeve, N.: Treatment of anthrax, J.A.M.A. *116*:1506, 1941.

Lufkin, N. H., and Evenson, A. E.: Tularemia diagnosed by routine blood culture, J. Lab. Clin. Med. *22*:346, 1937.

McCormack, L. J., *et al.*: Actinomycosis susceptible to penicillin in large doses, J. Bone Joint Surg. *36*:1656, 1954.

Mason, M. L.: Tubercular tenosynovitis of the hand, Surg., Gynec. Obstet. *59*:363, 1934.

Montgomery, F. H., and Ormsby, O. S.: Systemic blastomycosis, Arch. Int. Med. *2*:1, 1908.

Moses, W. R.: Diagnosis of acute flexor tendon tenosynovitis, Surg., Gynec. Obstet. *82*:101, 1946.

Olds, J. M.: Seal finger or speck finger: A clinical consideration observed in personnel handling hair seals, Canad. M. A. J. *76*:455, 1957.

Oppenheim, A., and Pollack, R. S.: Boeck's sarcoid (sarcoidosis), Am. J. Roent. *57*:28, 1947.

Orlow, G.: Specific monoarthritis of the fingers—"chinga," "speck-finger," "seal-finger," Zbl. Chir. *86*:2235, 1961.

Ormsby, O. S.: Diseases of the Skin, p. 104, Philadelphia, Lea & Febiger, 1934.

Parisu, H., *et al.*: Treatment of blastomycosis with stilbamidin, J.A.M.A. *152*:129, 1953.

Pearlman, H. S., and Warren, R. F.: Tuberculous dactylitis, Am. J. Surg. *101*:769, 1961.

Pernet, A.: Tendosinovite tuberculosa da mão, J. Internat. Coll. Surg. *28*:821, 1957.

Pinn, L. H., and Waugh, W.: Tuberculous tenosynovitis, J. Bone Joint Surg. *39-B*:91, 1957.

Potts, F. N.: Tuberculous tendons, tendon sheaths and bursae about the hand, N. Y. J. Med. *39*: 983, 1939.

Powell, H. D. W.: Interdigital sinuses in barber's hand, Brit. J. Surg. *43*:520, 1956.

Pulaski, E. J., and Amspacher, W. H.: Streptomycin therapy of tularemia in U. S. Army Hospital, Am. J. M. Sci *214*:144, 1947

Regan, J C.: Local and general serum treatment of anthrax, J.A.M.A. *77*:1944, 1921.

Riordan, D. C.: The hand in leprosy, J. Bone Joint Surg. *42-A*:661 and 683, 1960.

Riseborough, A. W., Joske, R. A., and Vaughan, B. F.: Hand deformities due to yaws in Western Australian aborigines, Clin. Radiol. (Lond.) *12*:109, 1961.

Santee, H. E.: Anthrax and its treatment, Ann. Surg. *78*:326, 1923.

Skinner, J. S.: Seal finger; the report of an occupational disease rare in the United States, A.M.A. Arch. Derm. *75*:559, 1957.

Sokoloff, L., and Bunim, J. J.: Clinical and pathological studies of joint involvement in sarcoidosis, New Engl. J. Med. *260*:841, 1959.

Sonnenschein, C.: Rotlaufinfektion; erysipeloid, Neue Deutsch. Klin. *11*:54, 1933.

Stein, G. N., Israel, H. L., and Sones, M.: Roentgenographic study of skeletal lesions in sarcoidosis, A.M.A. Arch. Int. Med. *97*:532, 1956.

Symmers, D.: Serum treatment of anthrax septicemia, Ann. Surg. *75*:663, 1922.

Symmers, D., and Cady, D. W.: Occurrence of virulent anthrax bacilli in cheap shaving brushes, J.A.M.A. *77*:2120, 1921.

Tempel, C. W.: Present status of specific drug treatment of tuberculosis, J.A.M.A. *150*:1165, 1952.

Walker, O. R., and Hall, R. H.: Coccidioidal tenosynovitis, J. Bone Joint Surg. *36-A*:391, 1954.

Wangensteen, O. H.: The role of surgery in the treatment of actinomycosis, Ann. Surg. *104*: 752, 1936.

Waters, W. J., Kalter, S. S., and Prior, S. T.: Cat scratch fever, Pediatrics *10*:316, 1952.

Wearne, W. M.: Actinomycosis of the finger, Proc. Roy. Soc. Med. *53*:884, 1960.

White, C. J.: Diseases of the nails, Clinical Symposia, Ciba Pharm. Products *1*:139, 1950.

Winship, T.: Pathological changes in so-called cat scratch fever, Am. J. Clin. Path. *23*:1012, 1953.

Young, H. H.: Tuberculous dactylitis, case report, Proc. Mayo Clin. *32*:381, 1957.

Chapter 18

Trophic and Vascular Conditions

TROPHIC CONDITIONS

Any serious injury to the limb results in some trophic changes distally. These may be the result of cicatrix acting as a block to the arterial supply or to the venous or the lymphatic drainage, or to direct division or thrombosis or spasm of the vessels, or to nerve damage resulting in paralysis of muscles, loss of sensation and vasomotor and sudomotor control.

If there is a strangling scar, excision and replacement of skin and soft tissues is usually the first step in treatment. An essential part of this is the deliberate excision of the deep binding scar, usually done as a separate procedure after the pedicle is applied. (See Chap. 7, Skin and Contractures.)

If the injury has been a direct one to a major vessel, the extensive collateral circulation in the forearm and the hand usually can maintain nutrition of the parts. The problem of nourishment of the hand arises when not only the major vessel is impaired but, in addition, there is damage to the collateral bed or vasospasm prevents its use. Even when the major vessel is intact, a generalized vasospasm may result in marked trophic changes.

When blood vessels are injured, reflex vasospasm in the accompanying uninjured vessels can lead to trophic and nutritional changes. Arterial injuries especially may be accompanied by this reflex spasm, which results in cool, glossy, tense skin from which blood gushes forth on pricking, and infiltrated tissues with nonpitting edema and with trophic, vasomotor and secretory disturbances. These signs may be due not to vessel injury but to the resulting vasospasm triggered by the injury of some other part.

Leriche, and later Ochsner and DeBakey, found that vasospasm accompanies venous thrombosis and arterial embolism, greatly ac-centuating the symptoms. A widespread venospasm and arteriospasm is set up, adding to the effects of vessel block with increased pain, lymph stasis, edema and fever. Procaine blocking of the sympathetic ganglia one or several times often removed the superimposed symptoms.

Following direct injury, and lasting 48 to 72 hours, a limb may go into shock from reflex vasospasm. It is pale, almost pulseless, and may even go on to gangrene. Sympathetic block 2 or 3 times a day may relieve the spasm and restore the circulation.

Trophic Effects From Injury of a Somatic Nerve

When a somatic nerve is divided, certain trophic changes take place in the muscles, the bones, the skin, the joints and all tissues supplied by it. Muscles undergo fibrous degeneration, the bones become porotic, the skin smooth and dry from lack of sudomotor activity, the joint cartilage thin, and the joint ligaments short. These effects are not due to vasospasm but to the loss of nerve fibers supplying the structures. In a somatic nerve are fibers of all kinds: motor, sensory, pilomotor, sudomotor and sympathetic. For the first 3 weeks after a major nerve injury there is vasomotor paralysis, and the limb is hot, flushed and dry. Later, it becomes cold and cyanotic, and its temperature is controlled not by vasomotor response but directly by the temperature surrounding it.

Disuse, whether caused by a lesion of motor nerves, fixation of joints or tendons, or even psychic disturbances, can result in a lowered blood supply. Some claim that the atrophy and tapering of the fingers from nerve lesions is from disuse, defective blood supply and lack of sensation. Whatever the exact mechanism, trophic changes follow nerve severance.

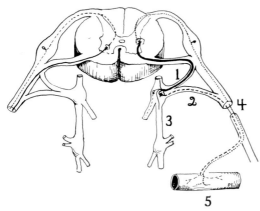

FIG. 887. Diagram indicating the connections in the vasomotor reflex arc between the spinal nerves and the sympathetic system. (*Dotted lines*) Afferent fibers. (*Dashed and solid lines*) Efferent fibers. (1) Preganglionic fibers in white ramus. (2) Postganglionic fibers in gray ramus. (3) Sympathetic trunk and ganglia. (4) Spinal nerve. (5) Peripheral artery. On the left, the somatic reflex is indicated.

The skin, the joints and other tissues no longer protected from the effects of trauma are easily injured and slow to heal. These painless injuries may set up a vicious reflex

vasospasm, resulting in much edema and degeneration of the tissues. Rough physiotherapy on insensitive parts quite commonly produces damage in this way.

The parts distal to a severed nerve are not painful unless reflex vasospastic changes occur at the site of neuroma formation. Partial injuries of nerves give rise to severe pain. It is an incomplete severance, a crushing or minor injury of a nerve that makes a painful lesion. These partial lesions of nerves cause trophic changes and pain of far greater intensity than result from complete nerve blockage.

Reflex Dystrophy. Normally, in the limbs and especially the hands, there is constant protective and regulatory reflex activity. Temperature is controlled by variations in the volume of blood and its rate of flow and the action of the sweat glands. Painful stimuli provoke the reflex actions of withdrawal as well as local changes in the specific area of time involved. Markee *et al.* showed that the vascular bed comprised 11.8 per cent of the total volume of the hand. Sixteen per cent of this bed is in the dermis.

Vasospasm is an abnormal state, an exaggeration of the normal way in which the vessels respond to various stimuli. It commonly occurs with trauma and can be incited by a painful stimulus in a distant part, or by emotional

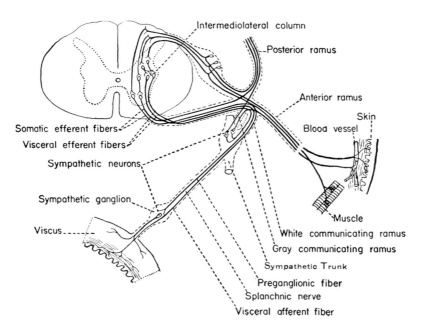

FIG. 888. Diagram illustrating the visceral and the somatic reflex arcs. (Kuntz, Albert: Textbook of Neuro-anatomy, p. 326, Philadelphia, Lea & Febiger)

FIG. 889. Diagram of the mechanism of vasomotility. (a) Cerebrobulbar vasomotor tract. (b) Bulbospinal vasomotor tract. (c) Spinosympathetic vasomotor tract. (d) Sympatheticomuscular vasomotor tract. (I–IV) Primary and subordinate centers. (R.A.) Radix anterior. (R.P.) Radix posterior. (R.C.A.) Ramus communicans albus. (R.C.G.) Ramus communicans griseus. (Bing, Robert: Compendium of Regional Diagnosis in Lesions of the Brain and Spinal Cord, p. 21, St. Louis, Mosby)

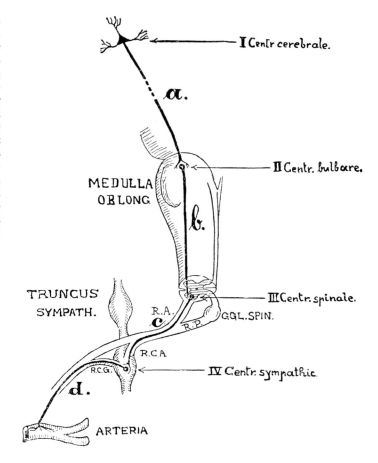

stimuli, particularly in susceptible individuals.

Vessels may be acted on by the nerves through reflex activity or by direct action on the vessel itself. Various reflex arcs, not always through the spinal cord synapses, have been postulated to explain some of the phenomena. The works of Leriche, Foerster, Benisty, Lewis, Southwick and White, Ochsner and De-Bakey, Livingston, de Takáts, Mayfield and Noordenbos have contributed much to a better, though still indefinite, understanding of the subject.

SYMPTOMS. Most dystrophies of this type have in common vascular phenomena, sweat disturbances, pain, osteoporosis, atrophy and edema. The symptoms vary in degree; in some, the vasospasm (as in Raynaud's phenomenon) may be the most striking feature, in others (e.g., causalgia), pain completely overshadows the other signs. In Sudeck's atrophy, osteoporosis is the outstanding sign. Hyperhidrosis

or a persistent edema may be the conspicuous feature. Almost all patients have some psychic disturbances or signs of constitutional biologic inferiority, whether they are the cause or the effect. Many times the symptoms are mild and transitory, or they may vary from one time to another. Once started, the process itself produces more dysfunction as if a vicious cycle of events was occurring.

In theory, the stimulus setting off this process arises from injury in one of the tissues. These stimuli reflexly activate peripheral receptors, causing the vascular disturbances. If the stimulus is continued or if the result of the first reflex act itself produces a noxious stimulus, a cycle of self-perpetuating symptoms arises.

Thus a damaged nerve may produce stimuli resulting in vasospasm. This by interference with nutrition causes more pain, which in turn causes more vasospasm. The focal point may

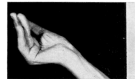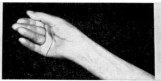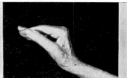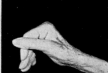

Fig. 890. Case A. M., age 78. (*Left*) Causalgia of 2 years' duration following a minor operation in the palm. Bitter complaint of burning pain in the palm and the fingers. Holds the hand immobile except for tremor, with a handkerchief between the atrophic, sweaty fingers. The distal joints are ankylosed, and the proximal and the middle ones have only a trace of motion. (*Right*) Some improvement in motion and feeling from several procaine injections of the upper 3 thoracic ganglia.

be a painful scar, a sprained ligament or a damaged nerve.

Occasionally, this self-perpetuating cycle may be interrupted by a temporary block with local anesthesia. Repeated blocks may be necessary to provide lasting relief. Sometimes the painful point can be relieved by splinting, and then the edema and the swelling can be dispersed by use of the other parts. The original injury heals, and the superimposed sources of stimulation formerly present are no longer able to provoke the reaction.

REFLEX MECHANISM. The peripheral receptors acted on by cold, trauma or infection send impulses through the main nerve trunks to enter the cord through the posterior roots. Efferent impulses through the anterior root then pass through the white rami to the sympathetic chain, ending there in a ganglionic synapsis. From the ganglion, fibers pass through gray rami to the cords of the brachial plexus and down the nerves, leaving the nerve to enter the vessel walls only a short distance away. Most of the nerves to the arm come from the 2nd and the 3rd thoracic ganglia.

This reflex arc can be influenced also by central fibers bringing impulses from the brain, and the sympathetic fibers themselves may cause adrenal and other endocrine organ activity which in turn sets free substances in the circulation that act on the vessel wall.

Stimulation of a sympathetic nerve causes vasoconstriction. Vasodilation can be produced by blocking the afferent or the efferent impulses by severing the somatic nerve, excising the involved vessel or performing sympathetic ganglionectomy. A sympathectomized part is more sensitve to the action of circulating epinephrine, and the vessels of the sympathecto-

mized part can still constrict by a local mechanism in response to direct stimuli.

FREQUENCY OF REFLEX DYSTROPHIES. With every injury there will be some vascular change, edema, pain and reflex spasm. These are the normal responses of tissues to trauma. In a few these become exaggerated and therefore abnormal. Considering the number of injuries to the upper limb that occur daily, only a few will progress to the pathologic state that we call reflex dystrophy. Usually, these dystrophies are found in people with emotional and vasomotor instability who are subject to various forms of neuroses. Often they have a history of angioneurotic edema, hyperhidrosis or acrocyanosis. Other stigmata of vasospastic phenomena may be present, such as transient cerebral symptoms from vasospastic areas in the cerebral vessels. De Takáts found electro-encephalographic changes in 4 patients and a degree of psychomotor epilepsy in 3 others among 66 patients presenting Raynaud's phenomena.

The mental state as well as local conditions has much to do with the perseverence of these dystrophies. Problems involving liability determinations or questions of compensation are at least aggravating factors. The severe dystrophies are not seen in children.

Causalgia is a form of dystrophy in which burning pain is the principal feature. Although the term has been used loosely to describe a condition in which the patient complains of severe pain, most authors prefer to limt the use of this term to a rather specific painful syndrome. It was described in 1813 in Denmark, but the classic description is that of S. Weir Mitchell who observed it during the Civil War and described it in 1865. Noordenbos questions the essential diagnostic criteria as given by Bonica:

. . . the presence of severe, constant, spontaneous pain, following partial or complete injury to a peripheral nerve, which is burning in nature, aggravated by emotional and peripheral stimuli, relieved by sympathetic block and which is often associated with vasomotor, sudomotor and trophic changes.

It occurs principally following partial injury to the median nerve. It is rare in civil practice and seldom follows lacerated wounds. It most often follows penetrating wounds of high velocity missiles as seen in military practice.

Pain is the predominant feature of causalgia and is aggravated by cold, touch and emotional stress. Vasomotor and sudomotor changes are usually present, but they may be either vasospasm or vasodilatation, and the skin may be dry or moist or clammy.

Sensory loss in the area supplied by the damaged nerve is present, but there is a wider area, following a dermatomal pattern, in which touch provokes a painful response, sometimes with a definite lag, which is explosive in nature. This "hyperirritability" (Trostdorf) in the zone beyond that of actual sensory loss has been said to be a distinguishing mark of causalgia.

The hand is held fixed with the fingers extended and the thumb adducted. The joints may even ankylose. The distal joints may be in hyperextension. The skin is thin, smooth, glossy and, in its volar parts, blotchy red. The hand is emaciated, atrophied and slender, not thick and edematous. There may be excessive perspiration or none, but the skin is often kept so wet by the patient that it macerates. The pain may commence suddenly or may build up gradually. In the early stage, according to de Takáts, blood flow increased 30 per cent as shown by the plethysmograph, the skin temperature is increased, and the pain and the hyperalgesia are local. This vasodilation, which is accompanied by progressive osteoporosis, is followed in the later stages by vasoconstriction with cyanotic skin, atrophy and stiffened joints. The hyperirritability may remain local or progress up the limb and expand over the trunk. Memory of the accident may play a part. Psychosis may overlap. The course reaches its maximum in a few months, and, though half of the cases recover spontaneously in about 2 years, others last many years.

The following quotation from Weir Mitchell paints the picture:

Its intensity varies from the most trivial burning to a state of torture, which can hardly be credited, but which reacts on a whole economy until the general health is seriously affected.

The part itself is not alone subject to a burning sensation but becomes exquisitely hyperesthetic, so that a touch or a tap of the finger increases the pain. Exposure to the air is avoided by the patient with the care that seems absurd and most of the bad cases keep the hand constantly wet, finding relief in the moisture rather than in the coolness of the application. Two of these sufferers carried a bottle of water and a sponge and never permitted the part to become dry for a moment.

As the pain increases the general sympathy becomes more marked. The temper changes and grows irritable. The face becomes anxious and has a look of weariness and suffering. The sleep is restless and the constitutional condition reacts on the wounded limb; exasperates the hyperesthetic state, so that the crackling of a newspaper, a breath of air, another step across the ward, the vibrations caused by a military band or the shock of the feet in walking give rise to increase of pain. At last, the patient grows hysterical, if we may use the only term which covers the facts. He walks carefully, carries the limb tenderly with his own hand, is tremulous, nervous and has all kinds of expedients for lessening his pain. In two cases, at least, the skin of the entire body became hyperesthetic when dry and the men found some ease from pouring water into their boots. They said when questioned that it made walking hurt less, but how or why, unless by diminishing vibration, we cannot explain.

The characteristic burning pain (hyperpathia), according to Doupe and his colleagues, flows up the sensory nerves from the periphery. The pain impulses arise at the point of nerve injury and flow distally through the sympathetic fibers to the periphery. Here, through the coinciding sympathetic and somatic fibers, the impulse is passed over to flow up the sensory nerves. The reflex causes trophic changes in the skin and the interchange of impulse takes place in the skin as a vicious circle. Barnes' theory is that an artificial connection at the point of injury allows crossing over of afferent, somatic and efferent sympathetic fibers. A conception based on selective damage to the large fast-conducting fibers, therefore causing an imbalance in the normal pattern and resulting in hyperesthesia, has been proposed by Noordenbos. He feels that this excess of slowly conducted impulses then influences the particular cord segment and, if persistent, breaks through the inhibitory effect of adjoining still-active fast fibers. This then accounts for the spread of the hyperesthesia beyond the zone of actual nerve damage and the finding that stimulus of this distant zone gives rise to pain in the region supplied by the injured nerve.

It is the skin of the hand that the causalgic wets and protects even though the point of nerve injury is in the shoulder or the upper arm region.

Sudeck's Post-traumatic Osteoporosis. The condition bearing Sudeck's name, which was first described by him in 1900, is less of an entity than a type of post-traumatic dystrophy in which osteoporosis is the prominent symptom.

In these hands the pain and the loss of function are out of proportion to the injury. The causative trauma is mild and often is limited to the wrist joint and the periarticular structures. Occurring less frequently in fractures or injuries where adequate splinting is used, it seems more often to follow where splinting has been omitted, and pain and edema have been great and long continued.

The pain, the swelling and the disability increase with paroxysms of greater intensity until the condition becomes chronic. It may pass in a year, or, in extreme cases, it may continue until, from fixation of attention, the patient's morale lowers to the point of request for amputation of the limb.

The swollen, painful hand, edematous and cyanotic, is held immobile and carefully guarded by the patient. The wrist and the fingers are usually semiflexed; the muscles are on guard to prevent any movement of the joints; the patient complains of tenderness to touch and of pain on movement and steadfastly refrains from moving the joints himself. There is edema throughout the limb and even in the joint capsules which thicken and shorten, limiting motion. Articular cartilages atrophy until in some cases ankylosis develops at the carpal and the finger joints. The state of mind influences the hand, and the

condition of the hand influences the patient until he seems to be content to be a charge on the community. Pain is always a conspicuous feature, but it is dull and aching and not accompanied by the marked hyperirritability of the skin to ordinary stimuli as seen in causalgia.

Plewes reported 37 cases, 21 of which followed fractures of the distal end of the radius, 2 a crushing of the finger, 3 a crushing wound of the hand without fracture, and 2 with brachial plexus injuries. Pain and swelling with hyperemia and limited movement were present over 8 weeks after injury. Roentgenographic changes were seen regularly after 6 to 8 weeks, showing the characteristic spotty rarefaction at the ends of phalanges and metacarpals, sometimes in the carpus and occasionally in the elbow and the shoulder. Plewes noted palmar fascial thickening in all except 1 patient.

Normally, following injury, there is vasoconstriction in the limb for a few hours and then vasodilatation as an aid to healing for several weeks. With chronic irritation, as from an unsplinted painful injury, vasodilatation is exaggerated, and there are edema and pain. In the acute bone atrophy of Sudeck there is an exaggeration of the normal reaction. Local temperature is increased, the oscillometer shows high waves, and the plethysmograph shows an average of 30 per cent rise in blood flow. There is a decrease in calcium in bones and especially in the metaphyses, the carpus and the heads of metacarpals where it is greatest. The limb is warm and flushed during establishment of the porosis but in the later stages is cyanotic and cold. Such bone is too weak and, like the joints, hurts so on stress that the limb is held useless. It is important to recognize the signs of excessive normal reaction to injury, to prevent them and to treat them as soon as they occur.

Paralysis With Contractures. Some hands, after injury, assume and maintain peculiar attitudes and seem to have no power of movement. These attitudes and contractures are quite varied: "accoucheur's hand," "fist hand," "holy water basin hand" with hollow palm and half-flexed fingers, flexed wrist with fingers extended, etc. They are painless unless the position is changed forcefully. Fixed vicious attitudes and contractures disappear under a tourniquet or an anesthetic but afterward are reassumed immediately. In some there is contracture, rigidity with contraction of both sets of muscles or contracture, tics and tremor and, in others, paralysis.

Vasomotor and secretory disturbances—tissue atrophy, coldness, cyanosis, hypotonia of some muscles and hypertonia of others without muscle atrophy—may be present. In these patients there seems to be a mixture of dystrophy and neurosis. The inciting cause may have been some pain at the onset, but later it may be only a flight from reality.

Edema in the hand and the forearm can be produced by self-inflicted contusions, a tight encircling bandage or simply hanging the arm immobile for several hours. Unless of long duration, when fibrosis has set in, elevation and sealing off of the suspected site of injury in plaster will relieve the signs. Elevation relieves the condition except in cases of long duration which become permanently stiffened in the joints.

Raynaud's phenomenon is not a disease but a sign of vasomotor instability. It is an exaggeration of the physiologic thermal control of the sympathetics. Cold is the usual irritant to start a paroxysm, placing the hand in water

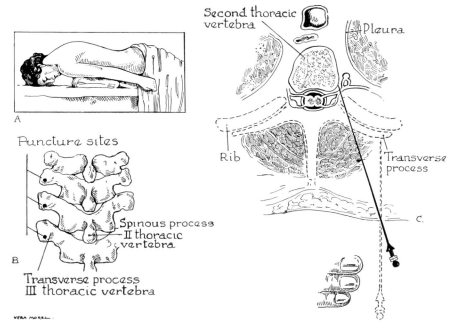

FIG. 891. Diagrammatic illustration of the technic of cervicodorsal sympathetic block by the posterior approach.

(A) Patient in the prone position with pillows beneath the chest.

(B) Cutaneous sites of puncture, lying immediately over the transverse processes of the 1st, the 2nd and the 3rd thoracic vertebrae. They may be determined by taking points approximately 2½ fingerbreadths lateral to and on a horizontal level with the spinous processes of the 7th cervical and the 1st and the 2nd thoracic vertebrae.

(C) Insertion of the needles. Each needle is inserted vertically until the transverse process, as shown by the dotted needle, is reached. The direction of the needle is then changed slightly toward the midline, and the needle is inserted 2½ fingerbreadths beyond the transverse process, so that the point of the needle is near the anterolateral surface of the body of the vertebra in the retropleural space, where the sympathetic chain lies. Five ml. of 1 per cent procaine hydrochloride solution is injected through each needle. (Ochsner and De Bakey: Arch. Surg. 40:227)

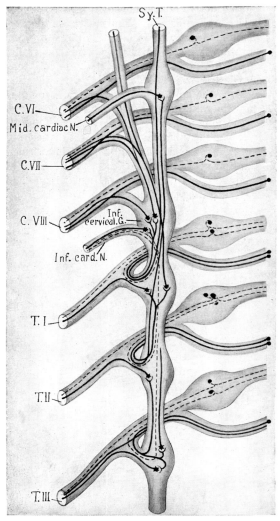

Sy. T.

C. VI —
Mid. cardiac N.

C. VII —

C. VIII —
Inf.
cervical. G. —

Inf. card. N.

T. I —

T. II —

T. III —

Fig. 892. Diagram showing the arrangement of the preganglionic and the postganglionic efferent and visceral afferent fibers in the upper thoracic and the lower cervical portions of the sympathetic trunk. (Kuntz, Albert: Textbook of Neuro-anatomy, p. 332, Philadelphia, Lea & Febiger)

and may be followed by a blister and then ulceration if thrombosis occurs. If more severe, gangrene follows, the line of demarcation forming anywhere in the length of 1 or more fingers. The changes are usually, but not always, symmetrical.

The first attack may be the only one, or attacks may come in great number until all 4 limbs, and even the nose, are affected. After repeated attacks there is osteoporosis, especially of the distal phalanges, and thickening of the arterial walls. Thrombosis is a secondary factor. The capillary pressure is low. This phenomenon may be an early sign of collagen disease such as lupus or scleroderma.

Pain in amputation stumps is a common complaint, especially from the 3rd month through the first 2 years. Neuromata that are bound in scar or pulled on by muscle action are painful but in a clean amputation are usually painless. The pain may be from anoxia of the nerve fibers in scar or from mechanical attachment and compression. Some individuals show excessive tendency to have persistently painful neuromata. Pain in stumps from ordinary neuromata is relieved by completely excising the scar and treating the neuromata, by excising, ligating and displacing it into good tissue. Disappointment follows if a nerve is merely freed or the block of scar tissue is not excised and the stump remodeled. Time alone remedies many painful stumps, as the consciousness of their presence fades.

Some excessively painful stumps resemble causalgia. The pain is steady or comes in paroxysms initiated by cold, emotional upsets or local trauma, or, at times, it is just cyclic without external cause. If it is not located in the amputated nerve as in painful neuroma but is throughout the whole limb, then it becomes a causalgia. Occurring in those with emotional and vasomotor instability, the pain is burning, gripping or shooting in character and is referred to the lost hand which feels twisted or cramped as in a vise. It feels as if the fingers

at 15° C. being the surest stimulus. Attacks can be initiated by trauma or from sudden emotion, such as fright, excitement or worry. In these patients there is real danger in operating on a hand, lest the operation incite an attack and be blamed for the loss of the fingers. In an attack there is first arteriospasm in 1 or several fingers, producing an ischemic appearance often described as alabasterlike and accompanied by great pain. This is of short duration, and soon the color becomes ashen and then cyanotic. As the attack ends the fingers are bluish-red and finally red, hyperemic and burning. This sequence is not always followed. The duration of an attack may vary from a few hours to several days

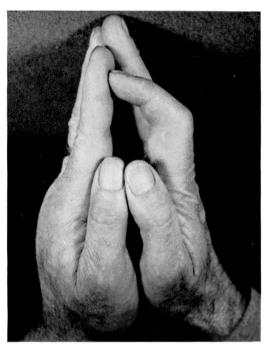

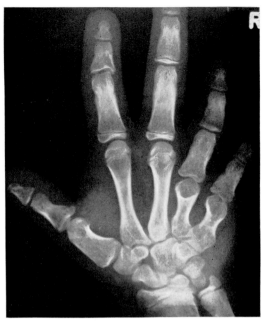

FIG. 893. Case W. M. The patient's hand had been crushed under a trunk. Drained spontaneously 5 months later and healed in 2 months. There was a swelling over the dorsum of 2 by 2 inches and tightness on making a fist as the fibrous reaction following hematoma.

FIG. 894. Pseudohypoparathyroidism. Shortening of the 4th and the 5th metacarpal bones is common in this condition, usually due to premature fusion of the epiphyses of these bones. The first radiant may also show the shortening. This patient exhibits premature closure of the epiphyses and shortening of the shafts of phalanges and metacarpals in the index, the ring and the little fingers, as well as partial premature closure of the epiphysis of the middle phalanx of the index finger with shortening of that structure and an abnormal proximal interphalangeal joint. No soft tissue calcifications are demonstrated here, although they may be present in this condition. Persons who exhibit the roentgen findings but not the chemical or the clinical findings of this condition have been confusingly termed "pseudo-pseudohypoparathyroidism."   (R. R. Schreiber, M.D.)

were in tight spasm and could not be moved, just as described by Livingston as the phantom-limb syndrome. Such torture lasts for months or years and breaks down the patient's morale. Scars and neuromata are resected, and reamputations performed. Whatever is done is successful for about 3 months, and then the pain returns. Finally, nerves or posterior roots are resected and even the lateral bundles severed in the cord, but with no better effect. Already the pain has worn a pathway to the brain which itself has become the seat of pain. If symptoms are not relieved by brachial plexus procaine block as a test, the pain comes from higher up.

If checked early, it may not become cerebral. There may be a trigger point that can be removed. This often is a neuroma in scar that has started the reflex. In a case in which 3 neuromata were removed from a forearm stump without relief, excision of a patch of cicatrix not near the nerves cleared the causalgia. By injections of local anesthetic agents the exact tender spot where the neuroma, the vessel or the scar which starts the reflex may be located and then remedied by excision. Surgical excision of the scar, treating and displacing neuromata and making a thorough

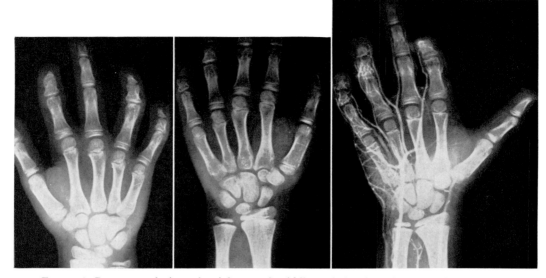

FIG. 895. Premature fusion of epiphyses of middle and distal phalanges in index, ring and little fingers from severe frostbite in infancy. The middle finger may escape damage. (*Bottom*) Arteriogram of same patient. (Dr. D. R. Bigelow, Winnipeg, Manitoba)

revision of the stumps is successful in many early cases. Repeated excision of neuroma or repeated amputation after 1 complete and thorough revision is useless. Subclavian peri-arterial sympathectomy has been used, but it is better first to block the upper several thoracic sympathetic ganglia. One to several injections may break the reflex permanently.

The limb becomes warm and flushed, the pain leaves, and the patient states that his fingers have relaxed from their spasm and he can move them. Encouraged by this, if the pain persists, severing of the rami or excision of the 2nd and the 3rd thoracic ganglia is indicated.

Phantom limb. Loss of a part of a limb or

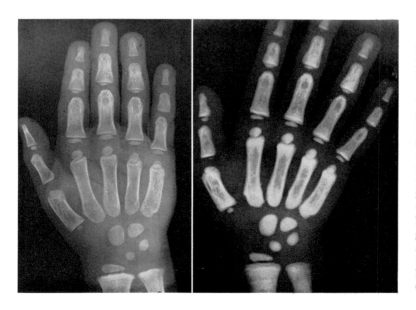

FIG. 896. Hypervitaminosis D and A. A 5-year-old male who was thought to have rickets 1½ years previously and was persistently given massive doses of vitamin D (and A) both at home and at school. Tremendous sclerosis of bone throughout the body to the extent that the diagnosis of osteopetrosis was made once on the basis of the roentgenograms. Patient eventually died because of renal damage. (R. R. Schreiber, M.D., Los Angeles Orthopedic Hosp.)

FIG. 897. Hyperpara-thyroidism. Subperios-teal resorption of bone gives a lacelike cortical pattern considered to be diagnostic. An 18-year-old female, before (*left*) and after treatment (*right*). This type of change usually is shown best in metacarpals and phalanges. (R. R. Schreiber, M.D., Los Angeles Orthopedic Hosp.)

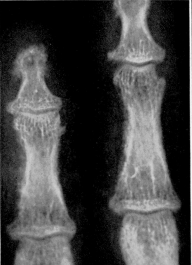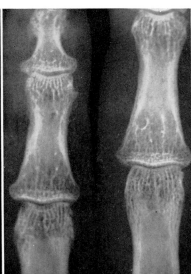

of the whole limb produces in most patients a temporary feeling of the presence of the absent part, often quite real, and sometimes painful and disturbing. The phantom limb usually disappears in a few weeks. S. Weir Mitchell, who is responsible for the term causalgia syndrome, used the term "sensory ghost." Painless phantom may disappear entirely or, if a major extremity is lost, only the intermediate part such as the forearm may go, leaving the phantom hand or fingers. If painful, it may be due to local stump changes which should be corrected, and a prosthesis should be worn. Sympathetic block may be of benefit. If not, surgical attacks on the more central part of the nervous system are probably of little use, and psychiatric measures should be used. Since the phantom-limb phenomenon is said not to occur in children with congenital absence of a limb, in those whose limbs were amputated before the age of 5 or, according to Rassek, in derelicts from the skid-row areas, there seems to be a reasonable basis for this approach.

Kallio, in performing the Krukenberg operation, reported that the phantom limb was also cleft, which would indicate some peripheral source of the pain.

A most interesting finding reported by Simmel was that in lepers in whom a digit has been lost by absorption, the phantom phenomenon never occurred, but, if one of these already shortened fingers was amputated, the phantom that appeared was the intact finger before absorption had taken place.

The phantom phenomenon is not a common complaint following the usual traumatic amputation of digits. Painful neuromata are quite common, and most respond to suitable surgical measures.

Secretan's Disease. In 1901 Henri Secretan described 11 patients who, following a simple contusion to the dorsum of the hand, showed "hard edema" of the dorsum, limited flexion of the fingers and a prolonged state of inability to work. He pointed out that fractures of the metacarpals in this area are quite common, heal readily and do not result in this brawny persistent swelling. In these cases, if mild, the swelling and the edema subside slowly. If more severe, an organizing mass of fibrous tissue embeds the extensor tendons. He warned against massage and felt that there should be complete recovery. No bony changes were ever seen. He explored one 11 months after injury, finding a peritendinous hard fibrous tissue tumor. Two weeks after healing, the wound ulcerated and persisted for 6 months. Disability for at least 6 months was present in most cases.

Occasional reports appear under the name of post-traumatic hard dorsal edema. In one study, excision of the mass disclosed evidence of old hemorrhage in the tissues. Secretan

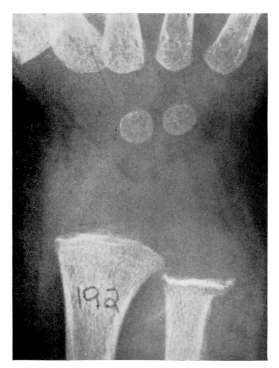

FIG. 898. Infantile scurvy. Ulnar epiphysial plate is dense and thick and extends to the sides beyond the usual limits. Small, marginal clefts are present at the corners just beneath these spurs. A faint line of diminished density, the "scurvy line," is present immediately beneath the sclerotic epiphysial plate. This combination of findings is essentially diagnostic. (R. R. Schreiber, M.D.)

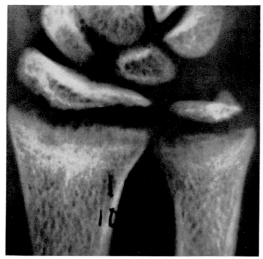

FIG. 899. Rickets. Widened epiphysial lines, coarse trabecular pattern, a little calcification along the metaphysial edges of the epiphysial lines, slight flaring and cupping of the metaphyses in a 10-year-old girl with resistant rickets. Simple vitamin D deficiency rickets is the usual type of rickets encountered in much of the United States today. (R. R. Schreiber, M.D.)

pointed out the lack of ecchymosis in his cases.

Severe crushing injuries to the dorsum of the hand can produce scarring and cicatrix and damage to the tendons and the bones and result in much crippling. In these cases there is no question that the amount of damage to the hand is proportional to the trauma. In this group of bizarre firm edematous hands that Secretan described, there is a characteristic history of relatively minor trauma. Ecchymosis does not appear, there is no break in the skin, and even when the hard edema has persisted for several weeks and the fingers have become limited in flexion, osteoporosis of the metacarpals and the phalanges is not present.

It can only be surmised that here is an example of reflex dystrophy in which edema is the major sign, just as in causalgia pain is the principal factor.

Treatment should consist of studious neglect in the sense that all passive manipulations, heat and massage are forbidden; however, an attempt should be made to have the patient exercise by voluntary means as much as possible. Never having seen a patient with this syndrome except where compensation from occupational injury was a possible factor, Secretan published his paper to call to the attention of the insurance companies the prolonged time away from work.

TREATMENT OF POST-TRAUMATIC DYSTROPHIES

The various post-traumatic dystrophies and vasomotor and secretory disorders are treated similarly, using physical methods, suggestion and measues to break the sympathetic nerve reflex. The first are especially essential in

Sudeck's atrophy and the various minor causalgias, where the reflex breaking is paramount for causalgia, hyperhidrosis and Raynaud's phenomenon.

Prevention. By recognizing potential problems early, prophylactic measures may prevent the development of the syndrome. The complaint of severe pain, often in paroxysms, is an early symptom, occurring as it does in the neurotic, vasomotor, unstable type of person. In a fracture or severe injury, the limb will be splinted, thus stopping the pain and the edema before they develop. It is the sprain, the crush, the laceration, the puncture and the minor vessel nerve injury that are usually not splinted that lead to Sudeck's atrophy and the causalgias. Therefore, all sprains and such minor injuries should be splinted. Only the injured painful part should be immobilized to stop pain, and the remainder of the limb should be used as usual. This functional treatment can be accomplished readily by a nonpadded cast, trimmed enough so that the motion of any uninjured part, especially the thumb and the fingers, is free. This determines whether the limb on removal of the cast will be stiff and painful or limber and painless. If minor injuries or sprains are not splinted, continuous movement causes swelling and pain which may increase the vasospasm and lead to Sudeck's atrophy or causalgia.

Treatment When Established. When the painful dystrophy has been established, the digit or the wrist or the painful involved part should be splinted, and active use of the arm and the hand started. Active use of the rest of the limb will reduce swelling and lessen the pain. When the cast is removed after a month or so, muscle tone and bone density will be restored, and the pain gone. The patient must be convinced that only by use can he toughen up his hand sufficiently to be able to work. Gurd and Fontaine report cures in Sudeck's atrophy by these measures in the average time of 6 months. Not all cases will respond easily. Already the pain may have spread, the joints stiffened, and the patient become discouraged and depressed. To refer such a patient to the physiotherapy department for treatment by heat, cold, massage and diathermy repeated each day is useless or even harmful and confirms his idea of serious disability. Forceful manipulation, with or without anesthesia, only increases the pernicious reflex, resulting in more pain, swelling and stiffness.

TRIGGER POINT. First, a search is made for the trigger point which started the vicious reflex. Location of tenderness is a guide, though the surer method is to inject the suspected area with local anesthetics. If the correct spot is reached, the pain disappears, spasm is relieved, and the joints can be moved. The relief may last for hours or overnight.

If the offending part is a joint, it should be immobilized; if a neuroma or a plaque of scar, it should be corrected surgically, as described under painful amputation stumps. If it is a deformity that has produced pain by strain, it should be corrected. In causalgia, operation should be undertaken with caution and not without good reason. Removal of a painful neuroma or a plaque of scar or the freeing of a nerve is justifiable once. If unsuccessful, then it is folly to repeat it. These measures often cure by removing the cause of the vicious reflex.

BREAK REFLEX ARC BY INJECTIONS OF LOCAL ANESTHETIC. Having eliminated the starter or trigger point, the reflex arc should be the site of the next attack. One may start with injections locally and then inject about the adjoining blood vessels or nerve.

The median and the ulnar nerves can be injected just above the wrist, and the ulnar nerve can be injected at the elbow.

The tissues about the radial or the ulnar arteries have been infiltrated for a distance of several inches opposite and just above the pain site.

Injections into the nerves or periarterially have failed so often that the routine custom now is to proceed at once with the ganglion block by either the posterior or the anterior approach.

The limb becomes warm and flushed from relaxation of the constrictor spasm. The burning pain disappears, the muscle spasm relaxes, and the joints can be moved voluntarily and passively as far as their intrinsic stiffness allows. The limb becomes dry, and the skin temperature is raised. Enophthalmos and miosis or Horner's syndrome shows on the affected side. Injection of ganglia has greater effect and lasts longer than the local nerve block.

A successful ganglion block is diagnostic. Occasionally, several such blocks suffice to make a cure, but in a goodly percentage there is improvement but not permanent relief. Direct surgical attack at the ganglion is the next step indicated. With the assurance furnished by a successful block, improvement or, in many, even cure may be anticipated by the preganglionic sympathectomy which at present is the method of choice.

Ganglion block and sympathectomy are used extensively to relieve persistent pain and to improve blood supply. Improvement has been seen in cases of painful Volkmann's contracture and in painful conditions of the arm and the shoulder. It has helped in hands with lowered vascularity from vessel obstruction or vasospasm. In Raynaud's syndrome there has been improvement, especially in the healing after necrosis of the digits and in lessening of the pain. However, color changes and susceptibility to cold are not entirely eliminated. The best results are attained in those with peripheral vascular disease and sympathetic hyperactivity. It is of no use in collagen disease and blood dyscrasias (deTakáts).

Tetraethyl ammonium chloride (Etamon) and Priscoline injected intravenously are supposed to block the autonomic nervous system. The fallacy lies in the lack of selective action on the limb involved and the possible effect of shunting blood away from ischemic areas.

After a severe injury of an extremity, sometimes there is a question as to whether or not the limb will survive due to a primary vasoconstriction which renders the limb pale and cold. Immediate improvement has been reported in these cases after several injections of the sympathetic ganglia.

Causalgia has been difficult to control. In World War II most were relieved temporarily, and a few permanently, by 1 or several ganglion blocks, and of those on which sympathectomy was performed many showed decided improvement. Cases with typical burning pain that were relieved by a test of procaine ganglion block responded well to pregangliectomy, almost all of them being relieved. The great majority of patients state that most of their pain was gone. Some retained local hyperesthesia. Many of those treated more conservatively also improved or were relieved, especially when encouraged to make active use of the hand, preferably at first under the protection of ganglion block. Some were cured by

excising the trigger point, whether a neuroma, a nerve in scar or just a patch of scar. It seems that any of the above procedures may serve to break the reflex. Some were cured suddenly; others after some procedure which started them on the road to improvement.

TECHNIC OF INJECTING GANGLIA. *Posterior Approach.* With the patient prone and a pillow under the chest to arch the neck forward, a spot is marked over the tip of each transverse process of the 1st, the 2nd, the 3rd and the 4th thoracic vertebrae. Injection locations are lateral to the spinous processes according to the size of the person, and each is opposite a spinous process, starting with that of the 7th cervical. The needle is thrust vertically to the tip of the transverse process and then is deviated medially about 35° and thrust about 2 inches farther to hit the anterior part of the body of the vertebra, just over which the ganglia rest. On the way, the ribs may be felt. If too medial, spinal fluid may come through the needle; and if too lateral, there will be cough from puncture of the pleura. If a nerve is hit, pain will extend around the chest. Draw the plunger back a little to test for blood or air and inject and repeat until each of the first 3 or 4 thoracic ganglia have 10 to 20 ml. of the solution distributed near them.

Anterior Approach. If the solution is injected in the neighborhood of the stellate ganglion, it will diffuse downward in the soft areolar tissue until the sympathetic ganglia supplying the arm are anesthetized. The stellate ganglion, with branches to C-7, C-8 and T-1 is 1 to 2 cm. long, consists of a fusion of the inferior cervical and the 1st dorsal ganglia and is located in front of the transverse process of C-7 and the neck of the 1st rib. It lies between the dome of the pleura and the great vessels of the neck. The vertebral artery is anterior. The ganglion rests on the prevertebral fascia covering the longus colli muscle just in front of the spine. It is in loose areolar tissue which extends down around the sympathetic chain.

Directions for injection have been given by Leriche, Fontaine, Lamont, Ochsner, De Bakey, Murphy and others as to how to avoid the vulnerable structures in the vicinity, but Pereira showed that by placing the finger on the palpable transverse process of the 6th cervical vertebra the great vessels were shoved

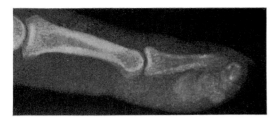

FIG. 900. Interstitial calcification with peripheral vascular symptoms.

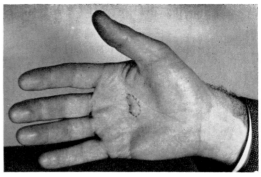

FIG. 901. Pulsating tumor in the palm of the right hand which had developed 2 years previously, following forceful driving of a chisel. An unconfirmed diagnosis of traumatic aneurysm of the superficial palmar arch was made.

away medially and a 24-gauge needle then could be inserted without danger, directly against the base, not the tip, of that process. The patient is sitting, so that gravity will help downward diffusion. Ganglia T-2 and T-3 should be anesthetized, since these supply the arm. Injection at the tip of the 6th transverse process anesthetizes the brachial plexus. The needle point is held against the base of the process, and the skin and the muscles are allowed to resume their former positions. The needle then angulates until it is in an almost transverse direction. Five ml. of the solution is injected at the bone. The needle is withdrawn 2 or 3 mm. until it is felt to be out of the prevertebral fascia, and 15 to 20 ml. more is injected. If in 15 minutes the arm does not react, Pereira advises injecting again after reinserting the needle tip $1\frac{1}{2}$ to 2 cm. lower against the 7th transverse process. This is also slightly deeper. Five ml. is injected there, and 10 ml. 2 to 3 mm. in front of it. If both sides are injected at once, there will be respiratory embarrassment.

PERIARTERIAL SYMPATHECTOMY. In this, the loose nerve-bearing tissue about a segment of an artery is excised, including not the adventitia but the veins and the tiny nerves passing from the tissues to the artery and from the artery to the main adjoining nerve. When the artery is in scar tissue or shows contraction, a segment of it has been removed in addition to its surrounding tissues. If the pain has spread too widely, the chances for success are less. The subclavian artery has been stripped for a high lesion and for vasospasm from cervical rib.

Herrmann and Caldwell report results in 34 cases of Sudeck's atrophy treated by periarterial sympathectomy. In all, pain disappeared in 24 hours and edema in a few days. They

averaged 3 months to return to work, compared with 9 months when treated by physiotherapy. Periarterial stripping has given way to sympathectomy.

SYMPATHECTOMY. This operation is done only after adequate response to injection of the ganglia. It is not necessary for the minor grades of dystrophy and should not be done

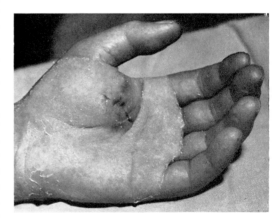

FIG. 902. False aneurysm of the hand which became evident 3 weeks following primary repair of a porcelain-faucet injury. At operation, a large organizing hematoma which filled the thumb web was evident. In the area volar to the adductor muscle, a false aneurysm sac approximately 2 cm. in diameter was found communicating with the deep palmar arch. (U.S. Public Health Hospital, San Francisco, Calif.)

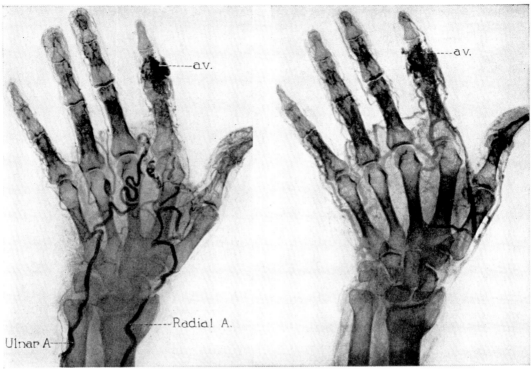

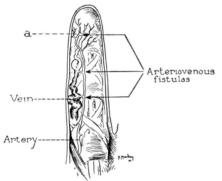

Fig. 903. (*Top, left*) Arteriogram of the right hand after injection of an opaque substance into the brachial artery: (a) the arterial tree is well outlined, but the opaque medium has not entered the distal portion of the right index finger. (*Top, right*) The venous tree is well outlined but the presence of fistulae in the index finger is evident: (av) showing the region in which the arteriovenous fistula was located. (*Bottom*) A dissection of the right index finger illustrating 3 arteriovenous fistulae. (Horton and Ghormley: Surg., Gynec. Obstet. *60*:979)

unless improvement from injection was definite. Removal of the stellate ganglion, formed by the inferior cervical and the 1st thoracic, has been found to be unnecessary because this did not affect the arm, and a Horner's syndrome is produced. As shown by Smithwick and others, sympathetic ganglia T-2 and T-3, and perhaps some below that by fibers running up the sympathetic trunk, are the only ones that affect the arm. Horner's sign is avoided, and regeneration—compared with other types of sympathectomy—is much delayed and lessened.

The approach (Smithwick) is through a paravertebral incision 7cm. long and 5 cm. from the midline opposite the 2nd and the 3rd dorsal spines. Muscles are split to allow removal of a part of the 3rd rib after cutting off the tip of the transverse process. On separating the pleura above and below, the 3rd and the 2nd thoracic nerves, the sympathetic trunk and ganglia and the spinal foramina are brought into view.

VASCULAR LESIONS

AXILLARY REGION

Injuries of the vascular supply in the axillary region are infrequent except when combined with nerve and gross soft-tissue trauma.

Fig. 904. (*Top*) Arteriovenous aneurysm of the superficial and the deep palmar arch, with marked hypertrophy of the 3rd and the 4th fingers. (*Bottom*) Arteriovenous aneurysm of the superficial and the deep palmar arch, showing overgrowth of the phalanges of the 2nd, the 3rd and the 4th fingers. (David, V. C.: Arch. Surg. *33*: 269)

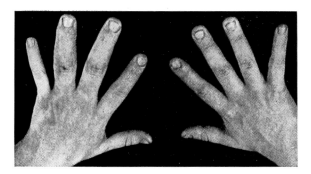

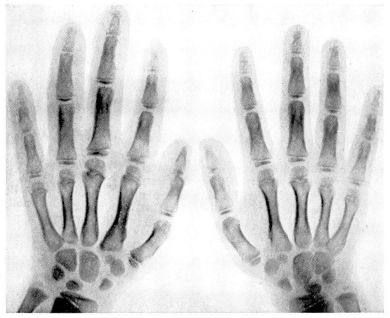

Repair of the damaged artery or insertion of a saphenous vein graft can be carried out. The technic of vascular repairs must be in the armamentarium of any surgeon dealing with trauma.

Long-standing crutch pressure has reportedly been responsible for gangrene of the fingertips. Stammers reported 4 cases (the thumb was not involved).

The Elbow Region

The collateral blood supply distal to the elbow is so great that injury to a radial or an ulnar artery at the wrist or to both simultaneously seldom results in impairment of the circulation to the hand. Complete rupture of the brachial artery has been reported several times without detriment to the hand. Dissections by Keen showed the brachial artery to be a single vessel in 55 per cent of the specimens. If, however, there is extensive soft-tissue injury in addition or if because of spasm the collateral vessels are constricted, then the distal parts cannot survive.

From trauma, as in supracondylar fracture, there may be a widespread spasm of the arteries, and the hand will appear cold and white. Pain, pallor and pulselessness are the 3 danger signs. Loss of the pulse alone is not an indication for major surgery, but if the hand is pale and cold and the artery is damaged, operative correction is indicated. If the collateral bed is involved with spasm, ligation and excision of the damaged segment of the artery, thus removing the trigger point, is the operation of choice (Lipscomb).

In the forearm direct repair of arteries can be carried out, for with modern sutures and technic Jacobsen has shown the possiblity of repairing vessels of only a few millimeters in diameter.

Certain technical points have been pointed out by Shaw. A good flow from the distal end of the artery is essential. Flushing with a warm solution of 10 mg. of heparin per 100 ml. to remove all thrombi is recommended, as is the use of a technic of oblique suture lines that avoid narrowing at the anastomosis. Fine silk sutures are used as a mattress type, and careful excision to prevent adventitial tissue from contacting the flow is practiced. Saphenous vein grafts are used to overcome defects. Postoperatively, the limb should be kept warm, and re-exploration and washing out the distal part should be repeated if thrombosis occurs.

Obstruction of venous outflow of the extremity is an important cause of death of the distal tissues. Though a plentiful number of veins allow for loss of many without jeopardizing the hand, obstruction of the flow, as by extreme swelling at the elbow, tight bandaging or unyielding plaster dressings, can cause the distal parts to fill with blood, increase the edema, and, when the blood collects in a closed space such as in the forearm fascial sleeve, cause ischemic necrosis. The difficulty is not lack of blood but too much blood and no way for it to circulate.

In surgery of the hand, this danger of venous obstruction is ever present, and being alert to the possibility will prevent many complications. More pedicled skin flaps are lost in transfer due to inadequate venous return than to lack of arterial supply. Edema is a big factor in accentuating the venous obstruction and is prevented by elevation, positoning and other measures.

Division of the brachial artery alone may produce few signs but, combined with damage to or spasm of the collaterals, can result in gangrene of the hand. Weeser and Hentschel reported gangrene of the hand from accidental injections of barbiturate into the brachial artery. Emboli lodged in the brachial artery should be removed promptly within 3 or 4 hours. Sympathetic block relieves the accompanying vasospasm. In a finger, lacerations commonly sever both volar digital arteries without loss of the digit, and if 1 artery is intact along with some venous return, a whole digit will survive. The pollicization operations

and the transfer of sentient skin by neurovascular pedicle methods both illustrate this capacity of tissues to survive with minimal blood supply. Yet, in a finger, local constriction at its base by a narrow tight band and a vasospasm induced by injecting the tissues around its whole circumference have resulted in loss of the tip.

THROMBOSIS AND THROMBOPHLEBITIS

Superficial or deep thrombophlebitis as a complication, postoperatively or post-traumatically, is rare in the upper extremity. Acute fulminating infections involving the forearm may spread to the veins as well as to the other tissues, and when this stage is reached the prognosis is poor.

Spontaneous deep venous thrombosis of the upper extremity, similar to that occurring in the calf, the thigh and the pelvis, does occur, but in only 17.6 per cent of a series reported by Matas. There is a special type which involves the axillary vein.

Axillary Thrombosis Caused by Strain. Schrötter in 1884 first described this syndrome; and by 1920, 27 cases had been reported. Gould and Patey added 8 cases, and Matas in 1934 gave the definitive description and diagnostic criteria.

A sudden onset of swelling of the upper extremity in a male between 23 and 40 years of age and following some muscular effort, usually with the arm abducted, is followed by dilatation of the superficial veins in the upper arm and the chest. There is very little fever. The axillary vessels are tender, and sometimes a thick cord can be felt. The pulse and the blood pressure are normal in the arm. In some cases, exploration has revealed only spasm, in others a thrombosis of the axillary vein. The causative factors appear to be a rupture of the intima or of a valve, due to back pressure in the vein from obstruction by the costocoracoid ligament or the subclavius muscle accompanying an expiratory strain. Matas recommended thrombectomy or excision of the involved segment.

A form of thrombosis, from direct trauma, is seen most often in the ulnar artery, distal to the pisiform where it is subject to repeated blows on the heel of the hand.

ANEURYSMS

Aneurysms in the hand may be true or false in type. The latter, from injury to the wall of the artery by direct trauma in a laceration or penetrating wound, has a fibrous capsule enclosing the extravasated blood, whereas the true aneurysm has a wall composed of the elements of the artery. True aneurysms are fusiform dilatations of the vessel weakened by disease or trauma. Most occur in the hypothenar eminence where the ulnar artery lies on the volar carpal ligament and is subject to repeated trauma. Another site is in the superficial branch of the radial artery over the thenar eminence. Aneurysms have been reported in the deep arch on the dorsum of the first cleft. The treatment is excision, done under the ischemia of a pneumatic tourniquet and with care being taken to preserve the other structures of the hand.

Arteriovenous fistulae appear in the hand in 2 forms—as a congenital cavernous hemangioma or, in the adult, from congenital remnants. Curtis described pain in ulcerated areas as an important symptom. Multiple abnormal communications are usually present, and complete surgical excision scarcely possible. Arteriograms may be of value in locating recurring fistulous connections. When one finger is involved, amputation is the procedure of choice.

BIBLIOGRAPHY

Abramson, D. I.: Resting blood flow and peripheral vascular responses in different portions, J. Mt. Sinai Hosp. 8:328, 1942.

Abramson, P. D.: Diagnosis and treatment of acral gangrene, Am. J. Surg. 57:253, 1942.

Al Akl, F. M., Singer, A., and Roesch, C. B.: Peripheral vascular surgery; lessons from six years' experience, Am. J. Surg. 55:520, 1942.

Atlas, L. N.: The role of the second thoracic spinal segment in the preganglionic sympathetic innervation of the human hand—surgical implications, Ann. Surg. 114:456, 1941.

Bailey, A. A., and Moersch, F. P.: Phantom limb, Canad. M. A. J. 45:37, 1941.

Barber, J. M., and MacIlwaine, Y. A.: Symmetrical peripheral gangrene as a toxic reaction to sulphamezathine and penicillin, Lancet 272:510, 1957.

Bisgard, J. D.: Traumatic neurocirculatory disorders, Am. J. Surg. 67:201, 1945.

Blain, A., III, et al.: Raynaud's disease, Surgery 26:387, 1951.

Blauth, W.: A contribution on traumatic edema of the back of the hand, Mschr. Unfallheilk. 63:189, 1960.

Bonica, J. J.: The Management of Pain, Philadelphia, Lea & Febiger, 1954.

———: Clinical Applications of Diagnostic and Therapeutic Nerve Blocks, Springfield, Ill., Thomas, 1959.

Burton, A. C.: Range and variability of blood flow in human fingers and vasomotor regulation of body temperature, Am. J. Physiol. 127:437, 1939.

Castro-Farinas, E., and Rivera-Lopez, R.: Arteriovenous fistulas of the hand, Angiologia 12:200, 1960.

———: Arteriovenous fistulas of the hand caused by intraosseous communication, Angiologia 13:332, 1961.

Cieslak, A. K., and Stout, A. P.: Traumatic and amputation neuromas, Arch. Surg. 53:646, 1946.

Cohen, S. M.: Traumatic arterial spasm; Hunterian Lecture, Lancet 1:1, 1944.

Coleman, S. S., and Anson, B. J.: Arterial patterns in the hand based upon a study of 650 specimens, Surg., Gynec. Obstet. 113:409, 1961.

Coller, F. A., Campbell, K. N., Berry, R. E. L., Sutler, M. R., Lyons, R. H., and Moe, G. K.: Tetra-ethyl-ammonium as an adjunct in the treatment of peripheral vascular disease and other painful states, Ann. Surg. 125:729, 1947.

Convert, P., and Mounier-Kuhn, A.: Arterial aneurysm of the ulnar artery of the hand, Lyon chir. 53:613, 1957.

Copley, A. C.: Causalgia in war wounds, S. Afr. Med. J. 17:343, 1943.

Costigan, D., Riley, J., and Coy, F.: Thrombosis of the ulnar artery in the palm, J. Bone Joint Surgery 41-A:4, 1959.

Creech, O.: Arterial injuries, Postgrad. Med. 29:581, 1961.

Curtis, R. M.: Congenital arteriovenous fistulas of the hand, J. Bone Joint Surg. 35-A:917, 1953.

DeBakey, M.: Traumatic vasospasm (technic of procaine hydrochloride block of regional sympathetic ganglion), Bull. U. S. Army Med. Dept. No. 73:23, 1944.

de Takáts, G.: Reflex dystrophy of the extremities, Arch. Surg. 34:935, 1937.

Nature of painful vasodilation in causalgic states, Arch. Neurol. Psychiat. 50:318, 1943.

———: Causalgic states following injuries to extremities, Arch. Phys. Ther. 24:647, 1943.

——— Sympathectomy in treatment of peripheral vascular diseases, Illinois Med. J. 84:373, 1943.

———: Causalgic states and neurotrophic lesions, Am. Acad. Orthop. Surg. Lect., p. 112, 1944.

———:Causalgic states, J.A.M.A. 128:699, 1945.

de Takáts, G., and Fowler, E. F.: Raynaud's phenomenon, J.A.M.A. 179:99, 1962.

———: The neurogenic factor in Raynaud's phenomenon, Surgery 51:9, 1962.

de Takáts, G., and Miller, D. S.: Post-traumatic

dystrophy of extremities; chronic vasodilator mechanism, Arch. Surg. 46:469, 1943.

Doupe, J. Cullen, C. H., and Chance, G. Q.: Posttraumatic pain and causalgic syndrome, J. Neurol., Neurosurg. Psychiat. 7:33, 1944.

Elkin, C.: The effect of vasodilator drugs on the circulation of the extremities, Surgery 29:323, 1951.

Estes, J. E.: Vasoconstrictive and vasodilative syndromes of the extremities, Mod. Conc. Cardiov. Dis. 25:355, 1956.

Felder, D. A.: et al.: Evaluation of sympathetic neurectomy in Raynaud's disease, Surgery 26: 1014, 1949.

Freeman, N. E.: Treatment of causalgia from gun-shot wounds of peripheral nerves, Surgery 22:68, 1947.

Fretheim, B.: Sympathetic denervation of the upper extremities in Raynaud's disease and secondary Raynoud's phenomenon, Acta chir. scand. 122:361, 1961.

Gairns, F. W., Garven, H. S. D., and Smith, G.: Digital nerve changes with ischemia, Scottish M. J. 5:382, 1960.

Goetz, R. H., and Marr, J. A. S.: Importance of second thoracic ganglion for sympathetic supply of upper extremities, with description of two new approaches for its removal in cases of vascular disease; preliminary report, Clin. Proc. 3:102, 1944.

Goidanichi, I. F., and Campanacci, M.: Congenital arteriovenous fistulae of limbs, Chir. org. movim. 50:263, 1961.

Gould, E. P., and Patey, D. H.: Primary thrombosis of the axillary vein; a study of eight cases, Brit. J. Surg. 16:208, 1928.

Gurd, F. B.: Posttraumatic acute bone atrophy (sudeck's atrophy), Ann. Surg. 99:449, 1934.

Hale, A. R., and Burch, G. E.: The arteriovenous anastomosis and blood vessels of the human finger; morphological and functional aspects, Medicine (Balt.) 39:191, 1960.

Hardy, W. G., Posch, J. L., Webster, J. E., and Gurdjian, E. S.: The problem of minor and major causalgias, Am. J. Surg. 95:545, 1958.

Herlyn, K. E.: Blood stasis in upper extremity, Beitr. klin. Chir. 169:299, 1939.

Herrmann, G.: Psychoneurocardiovascular disorders; peripheral vascular neuroses, Dis. Nerv. System 3:24, 1942.

Hillestad, L. K.: Dibenzylene in vascular disease of the hands, Angiology 13:169, 1962.

Homans, J.: Minor causalgia following injuries and wounds, Ann. Surg. 113:932, 1941.

———: Treatment of peripheral vascular disease, Med. Clin. N. Amer. 26:1457, 1942.

Horton, B. T., and Ghormley, R. K.: Congenital arteriovenous fistulas of extremities, Surg., Gynec. Obstet. 60:978, 1935.

Hunt, J. R.: Thenar and hypothenar types of neural atrophy of hand, Brit. M. J. 2:642, 1930.

Hyndman, O. R., and Wolkin, J.: Sympathectomy of the upper extremity, Arch. Surg. 45:145, 1942.

Jackson, J. P.: Traumatic thrombosis of the ulnar artery in the palm, J. Bone Joint Surg. 36-B:438, 1954.

Kallio, K. E.: Phantom limb of forearm stump cleft by kineplastic surgery, Acta chir. scand. 99:121, 1949.

———: Permanency of results obtained by sympathetic surgery in the treatment of phantom pain, Acta orthop. scand. 19:391, 1950.

Keen, J. A.: Arterial variations in the limbs, Am. J. Anat. 108:245, 1961.

Kirgis, H. D., and Kuntz, A.: Inconstant sympathetic neural pathways; their relation to sympathetic denervation of upper extremity, Arch. Surg. 44:95, 1942.

Kirgis, H. D., and Ohler, E. A.: Regeneration of pre- and postganglionic fibers following sympathectomy of the upper extremity, Ann. Surg. 119:201, 1944.

Kirtley, J. A.: Experiences with sympathectomy in peripheral lesions, Ann. Surg. 122:29, 1945.

Kuntz, A.: The Autonomic Nervous System, ed. 2, Philadelphia, Lea & Febiger, 1934.

Läwen, A.: Procaine hydrochloride blocking of stellate ganglion in therapy of traumatic hard edema of hand, Arch. klin. Chir. 201:687, 1941.

Learmonth, J.: Surgery of the sympathetic nervous system, Lancet 2:505, 1950.

Lehman, E. P.: Traumatic vasospasm—a study of four cases of vasospasm in the upper extremity, Arch. Surg. 29:92, 1934.

Leriche, R.: Surgery of Pain, London, A. Ballière, 1939.

———: Therapy of painful posttraumatic osteoporosis by lumbar infiltration with procaine hydrochloride, Presse méd. 49:609, 1941.

Leriche, R., Fontaine, R., and Dupertuis, S. M.: Arterectomy with follow-up studies on 78 operations, Surg., Gynec. Obstet. 64:149, 1937.

Lewis, T.: The Blood Vessels of the Human Skin and Their Responses, London, Shaw & Sons, Ltd., 1927.

———: The nocifensor system of nerves and its reactions, Brit. M. J. 1:431, 1937.

Lewis, T., and Pickering, G. W.: Circulatory changes in fingers in some diseases of nervous system, with special reference to digital atrophy of peripheral nerve lesions, Clin. Sci. 2:149, 1936.

Livingston, W. K.: The phantom limb, Arch. Surg. *37*:353, 1936.

————: Posttraumatic pain syndromes, an interpretation of the underlying pathologic physiology, West. J. Surg. *46*:341, 426, 1938.

————: Pain Mechanisms: Physiologic Interpretation of Causalgia and Its Related States, New York, Macmillan, 1943.

Lombardo, S.: Embolism of the brachial artery, Boll. soc. piemont. chir. *31*:369, 1961.

Markee, J. E., and Wray, J. B.: Circulation of the hand; injection-corrosion studies, J. Bone Joint Surg. *41-A*:673, 1958.

Markee, J. E., Wray, J., Norb, J., and McFalls, F.: A quantitative study of the vascular beds of the hand, J. Bone Joint Surg. *43-A*:1187, 1961.

Matas, R.: Primary thrombosis of the axillary vein caused by strain, Am. J. Surg. *24*:642, 1934.

Mayfield, F. H., and Devine, J. W.: Causalgia, Surg., Gynec. Obstet. *80*:631, 1945.

Mazet, R., Jr.: Elucidation of certain commonly disregarded neurovascular manifestations in war wounds and traumata, Am. Acad. Orthop. Surg. Lect., p. 190, 1944.

Merle d'Aubigne, R., and Benassy, J.: La sympathectomie preganglionnaire dans le traitement des maiguous douloureux et des causalgias, Mem. acad. Chir. *78-U*:1, 1952.

Mescon, H., Hurley, H. J., and Moretti, G.: Anatomy and histochemistry of arteriovenous anastomosis in human digital skin, J. Invest. Dermat. *27*:133, 1956.

Miller, D. S., and de Takáts, G.: Posttraumatic dystrophy of the extremities, Sudeck's atrophy, Surg., Gynec. Obstet. *75*:558, 1942.

Miller, H.: Post-traumatic reflex dystrophies, Am. J. Surg. *79*:814, 1950.

Moberg, E.: The shoulder-hand-finger syndrome as a whole, Acta chir. scand. *109*:284, 1955.

Montgomery, A. H., and Ireland, J.: Traumatic segmentary arterial spasms, J.A.M.A. *105*:1741, 1935.

Moore, R. M.: Some experimental observations relating to visceral pain, Surgery *3*:534, 1938.

Morton, J. J., and Scott, W. J. M.: Some angiospastic syndromes in the extremities, Ann. Surg. *94*:839, 1931.

Muller, S. A., Brunsting, L. A., Winkelmann, R. K.: Calcinosis cutis: Its relationship to scleroderma, A.M.A. Arch. Derm. *80*:15, 1959.

Murphy, R. A., *et al.*: The effect of priscoline, papaverine and nicotinic acid on blood flow in lower extremity of man, Surgery *27*:655, 1950.

Noordenbos, W.: Pain, Amsterdam, Elsevier, 1959.

Nwafo, D. C.: Congenital arteriovenous aneurysm of the right thenar eminence; report of a case, W. Afr. M. J. *11*:58, 1962.

Oberman, J. W.: Gangrene of fingers and toes accompanying Rocky Mountain spotted fever, Clin. Proc. Child. Hosp., Wash. *13*:3, 1957.

Ochsner, A., and DeBakey, M.: Therapy of phlebothrombosis and thrombophlebitis, Arch. Surg. *40*:204, 1940.

Oppenheimer, A.: The swollen atrophic hand, Surg., Gynec. Obstet. *67*:446, 1938.

Pataro, V. F., and Casal, M. A.: Effort thrombosis of the upper limb, or primary subclavioaxillary thrombosis, Prensa. méd. argent. *48*:1577, 1961.

Plewes, L. W.: Sudeck's atrophy in the hand, J. Bone Joint Surg. *38-B*:195, 1956.

Plewes, L. W., and Owen, J.: The swollen hand, Physiotherapy *45*:59, 1959.

Ray, B. S., Hinsey, J. C., Hare, K., and Geohegan, W. A.: Spinal origin of preganglionic sympathetic fibers to upper extremity in man, J. Am. Neurol. Assn. *68*:51, 1942.

Rein, H.: Organization of regulatory processes in in peripheral circulatory apparatus, Arch. Ges. Physiol. *244*:603, 1941.

Ribot, S.: Unilateral clubbing following traumatic obstruction of axillary vein; case, A.M.A. Arch. Int. Med. *98*:482, 1956.

Roberte-Jaspar, A., Heldenbergh, G., and Rogowsky, M.: A case of congenital arteriovenous fistulas of the hand, Acta Chir. Belg. *60*:530, 1961.

Ross, J. P.: The vascular complications of cervical rib, Ann. Surg. *150*:340, 1959.

Ruge, D., *et al.*: Gangrene of the hand as an initial sign of cervical rib, Arch. Surg. *81*:367, 1960.

Samitz, M. H., and Lisker, S.: Unusual skin lesions associated with thrombosis of subclavian artery, J.A.M.A. *161*:725, 1956.

Secretan, H.: Hard edema and traumatic hyperplasia of the dorsum of the metacarpus, Rev. Méd. Suisse Rom. *21*:409, 1901.

Sensory Ghosts, Pfizer Spectrum *9*:26, 1961.

Shaw, R. S.: Reconstructive arterial surgery in upper extremity injuries, J. Bone Joint Surg. *41-A*:4, 1959.

Shumacker, H. B., Jr.: Sympathectomy (dorsal or lumbar) in treatment of peripheral vascular disease, Surgery *13*:1, 1943

————: Causalgia, Surgery *24*:485, 1948.

Shumacker, H. B., Jr., Speigel, I. J., and Upjohn, R. H.: Causalgia, Surg., Gynec., Obstet. *86*:76, 1948.

Smith, J. W.: True aneurysms of traumatic origin in the palm, Am. J. Surg. *104*:7, 1962.

Smithwick, R. H.: Surgical intervention on the sympathetic nervous system for peripheral vascular disease, Arch. Surg. 40:186, 1940.

————: The problem of producing complete and lasting sympathetic denervation of the upper extremity by preganglionic section, Ann. Surg. 112:1085, 1940.

Smyth, E. H. J.: Primary rupture of brachial artery and median nerve in supracondylar fracture of the humerus, J. Bone Joint Surg. 38-B: 736, 1956.

de Sousa Pereira, A.: Blocking of the middle cervical and stellate ganglions with descending infiltration anesthesia: Technic, accidents and therapeutic indications, Arch. Surg. 50:152, 1945.

Speigel, I. J., and Milowsky, J. L.: Causalgia (following injuries of peripheral nerves); preliminary report of nine cases successfully treated by surgical and chemical interruption of sympathetic pathways, J.A.M.A. 127:9, 1945.

Stammers, F. A. R.: Peripheral arterial disease, J. Bone Joint Surg. 36-B:209, 1954.

Steindler, A.: Hysterical contractures, Internat. Clin. 4:221, 1935.

Stone, P. W.: Treatment of experimental acute arterial insufficiency (Priscolin), Surgery 27: 572, 1950.

Sudeck, P.: Über die akute entzündliche Knochenatropie, Arch. klin. Chir. 11:147, 1900.

————: Über die akute (reflektorische) Knochenatrophie nach Entzündungen und Verletzungen an den Extremitäten und ihre klinischen Erscheinungen, Fortshr. Geb. Roentgenstr. 5:277, 1901-1902.

Telford, E. D.: Technique of sympathectomy, Brit. J. Surg. 23:448, 1935.

Theis, F. V.: Anti-coagulants in acute frostbite, J.A.M.A. 146:992, 1951.

Ulmer, J. L., and Mayfield, F. H.: Causalgia, Surg. Gynec. Obstet. 83:789, 1946.

Van Demark, R. E.: Peritendinous fibrosis of the dorsum of the hand, J. Bone Joint Surg. 30-A: 284, 1948.

Van Der Elst, E.: Dorsal edema of the hand, so-called Secretan's edema, Z. Unfallmed. Berufskr. 53:112, 1960.

Wagner, W.: Das Sudeck-Syndrom, Vienna, W. Mandrich, 1960.

Warren, C. M.: Polycythaemia with gangrene of fingers, Brit. J. Derm. 69:104, 1957.

Washburn, B.: Frostbite treatment, New Engl. J. Med. 266:974, 1962.

Weese, K., and Hentschel, M.: Gangrene after injection of barbiturates into the cubital artery, Münch. med. Wschr. 103:1259, 1961.

White, J. C.: Painful injuries of nerves and their surgical treatment, Am. J. Surg. 72:468, 1946.

White, J. C., and Smithwick, R.: The Autonomic Nervous System, ed. 2, New York, Macmillan, 1941.

Wilkins, R. W., Doupe, J., and Newman, H. W.: Rate of blood flow in normal fingers, Clin. Sci. 3:403, 1938.

Williams, C.: Hysterical edema of hand and forearm, Ann. Surg. 111:1056, 1940.

Woollard, H. H., and Phillips, R.: Distribution of sympathetic fibers in extremities, J. Anat. 67: 18, 1932.

Woollard, H. H., and Weddell, G.: Composition and distribution of vascular nerves in extremities, J. Anat. 69:165, 1935.

Zancolli, E.: Peritendinous fibrosis of back of hand, Prensa. med. argent. 43:1867, 1956.

Chapter 19

Tumors

Tumors may arise as primary growths from any of the tissues present in the hand; most are benign. The presence of the tumor is often noted early. Excision is the procedure of choice.

Malignant tumors are uncommon, but when primary in the hand they offer a good chance for cure because of their location and early diagnosis.

THE COMMON TUMORS OF THE HAND

Studies based on material sent to hospital laboratories do not reflect the true incidence of tumors, since many obvious benign lesions such as inclusion cysts and ganglia are removed as office procedures and are never referred for histologic examination. Some series reflect a special interest of the author or the institution, such as Pack's extremely high percentage of melanomas and the studies of Butler *et al.* of specimens in 2 San Francisco hospitals, reporting a large number of squamous cell carcinomata.

Pack reported 389 tumors from the hand; 232 showed malignant changes, principally those of squamous cell carcinoma and melanoma. Such a predominance of malignancy is an indication of the selected group of patients. Butler *et al.*, from the specimens received over a 10-year period, found ganglia to represent 33 per cent and squamous cell carcinomata 24 per cent of the total series.

Some reports include lesions of inflammatory origin such as pyogenic foreign body or tuberculous granulomata, chronic synovitis of tendon sheaths and "precancerous" skin lesions, commonly the result of radiation. Therefore, a true picture of the incidence of tumor types is difficult to obtain.

My own series of 394 tumors of the hand, including ganglia, but excluding such lesions as tenosynovitis, exostoses, moles, warts and granulomata, shows the following incidences:

Ganglia	205
Xanthoma or benign giant cell tumors	52
Epithelial inclusion cysts	33
Mucous cysts, dorsum at base of nail	23
Fibromata	16
Vascular tumors	15
Neurofibromata	13
Epitheliomata, squamous cell	12
Lipomata	8
Chondromata	5
Glomus tumors	4
Dermatofibromata	3
Osteomata	2
Fibrosarcoma	1
Chondrosarcoma	1

Only 14 were malignant; and of these, 12 were squamous cell carcinomata resulting from radiation injury.

A survey of the characteristics of the most common tumors will be made, followed by a summary of other less common tumors that have been reported.

GANGLIA

This is the most common tumor seen in the hand and occurs principally at 1 of 3 sites—the dorsum of the wrist, the volar radial aspect of the wrist or in the tendon sheath over the flexor tendons at the proximal crease of the finger. Rare in children, it is common in young adults and more common in women than in men.

Many theories have been propounded as to the cause and the site of origin, e.g., that they are herniations of sheath or joint capsule or serous cysts, but it is now agreed that a ganglion represents a degeneration of fibrous tissue.

Etiology. Trauma is a factor in the history of approximately half the cases of ganglia, though a single direct injury is hardly a possible cause. Repeated minor trauma to the ligamentous connective tissues is accepted as a causative factor on the basis of the usual

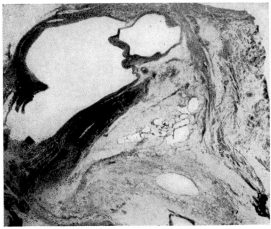
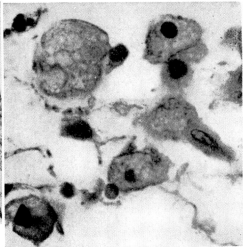

FIG. 905. (*Left*) Low-power photomicrograph of a ganglion. Above is the multicystic cavity surrounded by its dense fibrous wall with remnants of incomplete septa projecting into it. To the right is an accessory cyst cavity. Below it is an extensive area of mucinous degeneration with many tiny cavities scattered through it. (*Right*) A high-power photomicrograph showing some cells in an area of degeneration distended with vacuoles containing mucin. (Stout and Carp: Surg., Gynec. Obstet. 47:463)

location of the lesions and the fact that they occur predominantly in the wrist.

Pathology. Ganglia arise within the connective tissue near the joints or tendon sheaths but do not communicate with the synovial spaces. They may be single and large or multiple and small or a combination with many minute areas of cystic degeneration near the base of the tumor. There is no special cell lining the cavity, and the contents are clear, colorless and of jellylike consistency. There are no inflammatory changes, and malignant changes have not been reported in true ganglia.

Location. Ganglia occur most frequently on the dorsum of the wrist, arising from the scaphoid-lunate ligament; they present to the surface between the common digital extensor tendons and the long extensor of the thumb.

They are also found on the radial volar aspect of the wrist, arising from the ligamentous structures joining the distal radius to the trapezium. The third most common site is in the ligamentous tissues comprising the pulley mechanism of the flexor tendon over the proximal segment of the finger.

Ganglia may occur on any joint, especially the dorsum of an interphalangeal joint. At the middle finger joint they protrude through the fibers of the extensor aponeurosis to either side of the middle slip insertion and at the distal joint may be confused with the common mucous cyst or with Heberden's nodes. When present on the thumb, they present most often on the ulnar side of the proximal joint.

Ganglia have been noted arising from the wrist joint and extending into the carpal tun-

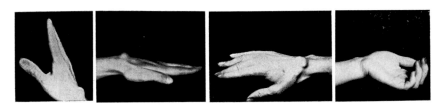

FIG. 906. Ganglia.

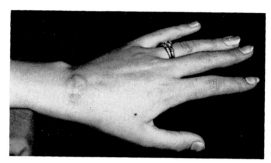

FIG. 907. Recurrence of a ganglion on the dorsum of the wrist a few months after incomplete excision.

nel where they cause symptoms of median nerve compression, or from the ulnar side of the carpus where they follow the course of the deep motor branch of the ulnar nerve and result in paralysis of the ulnar intrinsics. Seddon reported a series of these; an example is

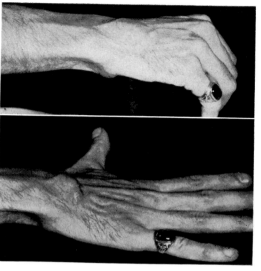

FIG. 909. This tumor on the dorsum of the wrist moves proximally when the fingers are extended. This is a thickening of the synovial sheath of the common digital extensor tendons and not a ganglion.

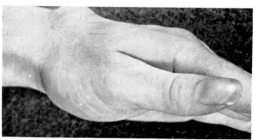

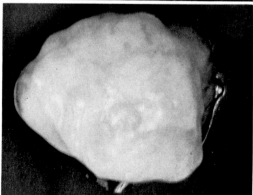

FIG. 908. (*Top*) Ossifying fibroma on the dorsum of the wrist simulating a ganglion. (*Bottom*) The removed specimen; on microscopic examination it showed abundant bone formation. (Wakeman, U.S. Army photograph)

recorded in Chapter 10, Nerves. In other cases, ganglia have arisen from the distal radio-ulnar joint region and compressed the dorsal sensory branches of the ulnar nerve.

Symptoms. The common dorsal carpal ganglion may be without symptoms except the local swelling, though usually there is the complaint of some weakness and occasional pain. Paradoxically, the small, barely palpable tumor may produce more discomfort than the large protruding type. Many patients report a sudden onset after a twisting or lifting strain, as if some overlying fascial plane had suddenly parted to allow a deep-lying tumor to protrude.

Usually, the diagnosis is made by noting the location and the typical appearance. Aspiration of the clear contents with the consistency of jelly will verify the diagnosis. Synovitis of the joint or a tenosynovitis of the surrounding tendon sheaths usually can be differentiated from the well-encapsulated, firm and well-demarcated ganglion.

The ganglia arising on the flexor surface of the fingers are more tender, quite firm to palpation, discrete and do not move with the tendon.

Treatment. Sometimes a ganglion disappears

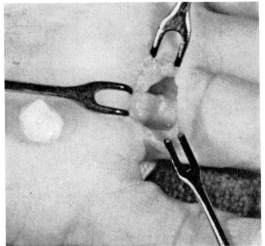

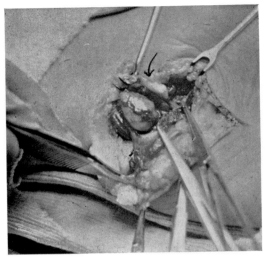

FIG. 911. Carpal ganglion projecting into the palm and displacing the motor branch of the ulnar nerve (arrow) with signs of paralysis of intrinsics.

Rupture by external force and injection by sclerosing agents such as iodine, carbolic acid and sodium morrhuate have been discarded. Caroid, a proteolytic enzyme, was tried by Ball but condemned by Kay. Hyaluronidase was popular temporarily, and now hydrocortisone is recommended by some authors.

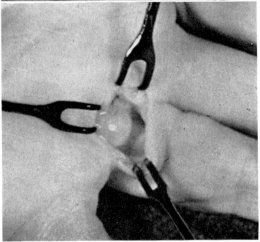

FIG. 910. Ganglion on flexor tendon sheath at typical location. It arises from the pulley, and, in the lower photograph, the slit-like opening in the fibrous tissue can be seen. It usually occurs on the middle or the ring finger.

spontaneously, but usually surgical excision is necessary to eliminate it. Many forms of non-operative treatment have been tried, and periodically reports appear extolling the results of local injection of material into the cyst cavity.

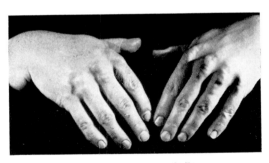

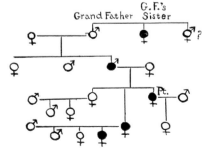

FIG. 912. (*Top*) Xanthomata, multiple over the body, hereditary, born with tumors over the proximal finger joints, increased in adolescence. (*Bottom*) Genealogy of patient.

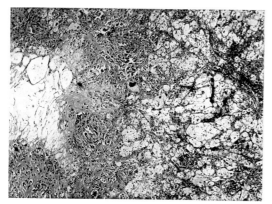

FIG. 913. Xanthoma showing large numbers of foam cells in the right side of the section and cholesterol clefts in the left side. Fibrous and cellular stroma and several foreign-body giant cells are present. (× 60) (Galloway, J. D. B., Broders, A. C., and Ghormley, R. K.: Arch. Surg. 40:516)

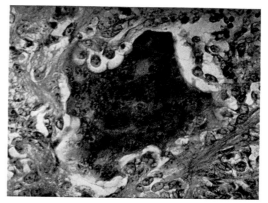

FIG. 914. Xanthoma, showing the shape and the structure of a foreign-body giant cell, with characteristic cytoplasm and many endotheliumlike nuclei. The surrounding tissue shows typical endotheliumlike stroma cells with their pale-staining nuclei and prominent nuclei. (× 440) (Galloway, J. D. B., Broders, A. C., and Ghormley, R. K.: Arch. Surg. 40:516)

Roentgen therapy is reported by Lyle and Woodburne to cause disappearance of a high percentage of ganglia.

Most authors agree that complete excision is the best treatment, but recurrence is frequent. If operative excision is done under the ischemia of a tourniquet with complete removal of the ligamentous tissue comprising the base, recurrences will be rare. Since the common dorsal ganglion arises from the scaphoidlunate ligament, a complete excision necessarily entails arthrotomy of the wrist joint for adequate exposure and excision. In the author's opinion this demands the use of major hospital operating-room facilities and adequate anesthesia. To open the wrist joint as an office procedure under local anesthesia is taking an unjustified risk of serious complications.

The small cysts on the flexor tendon sheaths can be incised with a sharp needle. Bruner has reported good results with this simple treatment.

Xanthoma

These tumors, also called benign giant cell tumor of tendon sheaths, benign synovioma or foreign-body giant cell tumor, are common in the fingers and occur as encapsulated firm multicolored growths with variable cell structure.

Some confusion results from an attempt to relate these tumors to the diffuse xanthochromic skin deposits on the dorsum of the hands and the feet, around the Achilles tendon, the elbows, the knees and the eyelids. As seen in the hand, a firm irregular painless nodule, usually on the finger, is a separate entity and can be treated as an isolated benign lesion. Studies of cholesterol metabolism and other tests that would be indicated in the systemic disease of xanthoma tuberosum are not necessary.

Since Chaissaignac in 1852 the site of origin has been said to be the tendon sheath. Phalen, McCormack and Gazale studied 56 tumors of this type, finding that most occurred in persons between 40 and 60; the sex incidence was almost equal.

The tumors occurred equally in the right and the left hands, most often in the index and the middle fingers and usually on the volar surface. Thorough local excision resulted in few recurrences.

Etiology. The origin of the tumor is unknown. An inflammatory lesion was suggested by Don, a cholesterin disturbance by Weber, and an origin from sesamoid bones by Geshickter and Copeland. Trauma cannot be excluded, and some authors indicate that trauma super-

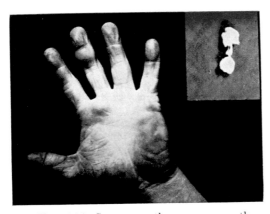

FIG. 915. Seven months ago, a month after striking the long finger with a hammer, the tumor appeared which now shows as a bulge in the finger and the palm. The insert shows the excised xanthoma. It grew from the annular ligament in the palm, extending down the tendon sheath, to form a 2nd nodule in the finger.

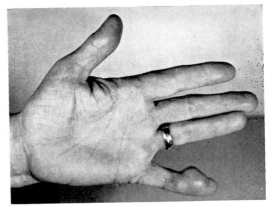

FIG. 916. Solitary xanthoma in the distal 2 segments of the little finger in a 63-year-old female. The tumor had been present for 1 year. Treatment was by surgical excision.

imposed on a disturbance of cholesterol metabolism is a likely cause.

Pathology. The tumor is benign and of variable size and consistency. It is encapsulated and grayish-yellow with brownish areas which may appear as streaks or clumps in the cut section. There is much variation in the number and the type of cells present. Foam cells with small nuclei and a granular cytoplasm full of lipoid globules are characteristic but vary in number. Carotene and xanthophyll pigment in the lipoid globules account for the color, and cholesterol crystals have been found. Foreign-body giant cells occur in varying number.

Symptoms. These tumors occur principally on the fingers, are painless and mechanically interfere with function. They may surround the nerves, erode the bones by pressure and fill the interstices of the interphalangeal joint. In my experience, with only a few exceptions, the one fixed site of the tumor from which it presumably arose has been the capsule of the middle or the distal joint. From here it may pass volarward or dorsalward, over or under the tendons and surround the neurovascular

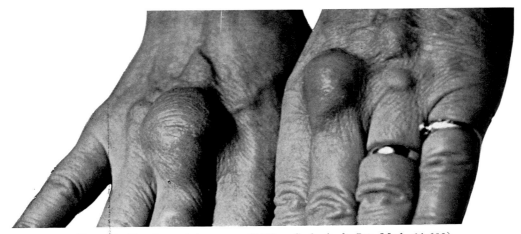

FIG. 917. Xanthoma tuberosum. (Miller, Carl: Arch. Int. Med. 64:680)

PLATE 14

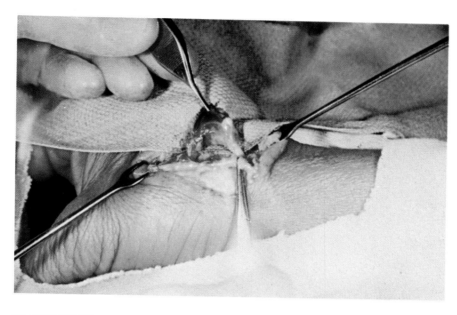

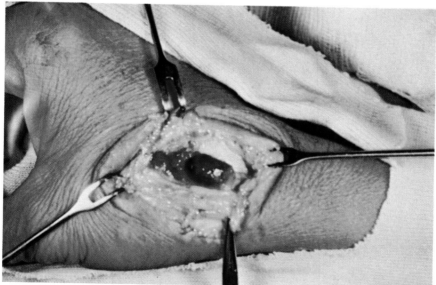

Aneurysm of the radial artery in the first cleft following trauma from closed injury.

PLATE 15

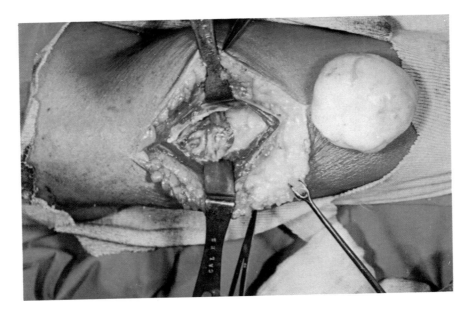

Solitary lipoma in area beneath supinator muscle causing complete posterior interosseus nerve palsy. Full recovery of motions within 3 months after removal of tumor.

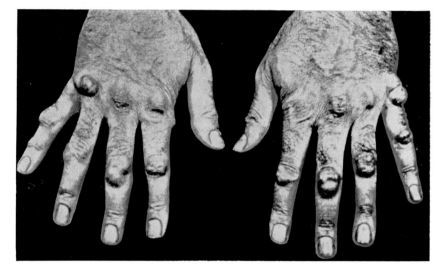

FIG. 918. Multiple xanthomas of the hands. Also of the feet. (Xanthoma tuberosum multiplex.) This condition may be related to a lipoid diathesis, as there is often an increase in the total lipids, cholesterol and cholesterol esters in the blood stream. (Pack, G. T.: Tumors of the Hands and Feet, St. Louis, Mosby)

bundles. In a few instances, multiple tumors occurred in the tendon sheath as if the tumor had seeded itself along the wall of the sheath. In each instance an incomplete excision of a clinically solitary tumor had preceded this development.

Diagnosis. Next to ganglia these tumors are the most common in the hand. They are firm, present usually away from rather than directly over the joint and usually can be moved laterally as contrasted with the ganglion. Once the tumor is exposed, the gross appearance is characteristic and makes it easy to distinguish it from lipoma or angioma.

Treatment. Excision done carefully under a tourniquet and with adequate exposure usually suffices. If a local recurrence takes place, local excision is again indicated, since the lesion is benign.

Adequate reports of roentgen therapy have not appeared, but there seems to be little reason to expect the results to be better than those from thorough local excision.

EPIDERMOID CYSTS

Epidermoid cysts were first described by Rizet in 1866 and have been recognized as clinical entities for over 60 years. They are commonly called inclusion cysts and are of special interest due to their occurrence in industrial workers and in some instances following operations. Because these cysts developed secondary to injury, the conception of implantation of epithelium gradually became evident. These cysts are known by various names, such as epidermal cyst, pearl tumors, dermal cysts, implantation dermoid, etc. King prefers to use the term "post-traumatic epidermoid."

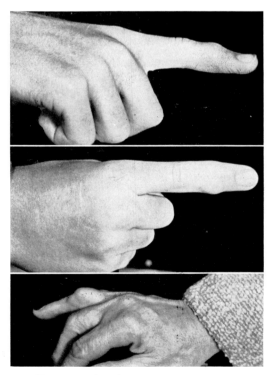

FIG. 919. (*Top*) Xanthoma from distal joint, extending beneath extensor tendon to opposite side. (*Bottom*) Xanthoma from middle joint of little finger.

Etiology. These are now generally accepted as implantation phenomena due to the frequency of a history of a wound preceding the development of the cyst, the fact that they are lined with squamous epithelium, that experimental implantation of the epidermis produces similar cysts (E. Kauffman), and also the observation that they occur postoperatively near scars.

Pathology. The cysts are round or ovoid with thick walls and are filled with a white material of a crystalline sheen which, on analysis, shows high cholesterol and low fat content, differing in this way from sebaceous cysts. On microscopic section, the wall is fibrous tissue with an inner lining of squamous epithelium which in areas shows laminated keratin. The epithelium is without papillae in its basal layer, and in the adjacent connective tissue some foreign-body giant cells usually are seen. At times the epithelial lining is not complete.

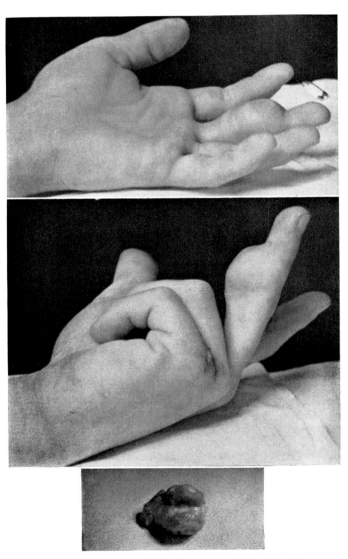

Fɪɢ. 920. Xanthoma of middle finger, straddling the flexor tendons. Origin from middle joint capsule.

Symptoms. These cysts occur most often in adults who traumatize their hands in their occupations. They occur frequently in males; while generally single, they may be multiple.

The palmar aspect of the hand and the fingers is the most common site. A history of crushing or laceration of the skin of this area or a history of penetrating wounds can be obtained in as many as half the cases. In rare instances the cysts may occur in the distal phalanx. Such cases are reported by Yachnin, Summerill, Pohlmann, Wachstein and Carroll.

There is generally a latent period of a few months to years between injury and the clinical manifestations of the cyst. First, a small nodule or thickening appears at the site of injury; this enlarges as the cyst increases in size. There is seldom pain, although tenderness may be present, especially during the growing period.

These cysts present as rounded, semifluctuant elastic tumors and generally are not adherent to other structures. They rarely become infected, and the principal differential diagnosis is between foreign-body granuloma, ganglion and xanthoma.

Treatment. Complete surgical excision of the entire cyst with its wall and contents ensures a cure.

SEBACEOUS CYSTS

Sebaceous cysts may occur on the hand, but they are quite unusual. They are limited in location to the dorsum of the hand and the fingers, since sebaceous glands do not occur in the palmar skin.

The gross appearance and the characteristics of this cyst on the hand are the same as those of cysts elsewhere on the body.

Mucous Cysts

Etiology. These cysts are believed to be due to mucoid degeneration in the cutis, or subcutaneous tissue. Trauma has been cited as a cause, but a history of specific injury is seldom obtained. The lesions which are degener-

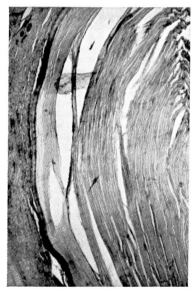

FIG. 921. Epidermoid cyst. Photomicrograph of a portion of the wall, showing excessive keratin formation. No doubt, cysts of this type were the reason for the term "cholesteatoma" formerly applied to these cysts ($\times$ 26). (King, E. S. J.: Brit. J. Surg. *21*:38)

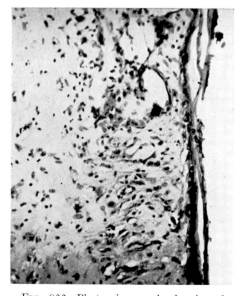

FIG. 922. Photomicrograph showing the wall of an epidermoid cyst with spaces and giant cells in the connective tissue, which is covered by a very low, poorly developed squamous epithelium, forming keratin ($\times$ 150). (King, E. S. J.: Brit. J. Surg. *21*: 38)

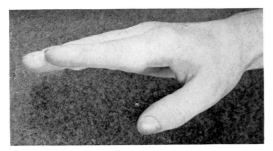

FIG. 923. A large epidermoid cyst in the proximal segment of the index finger. On removal, the specimen measured 18 x 9 x 7 mm. (Wakeman, U.S. Army photograph)

ative in type develop in some individuals with advancing age. Almost always they occur opposite a distal finger joint which shows clinical evidence of early degenerative or hypertrophic arthritis. This opinion is shared by such authors as Anderson, Stecher and Ormsby.

Pathology. Grossly, these are small cysts, usually in the skin, filled with a colorless gelatinous viscid fluid not unlike that found in ganglia. Microscopically, they are without epithelial lining, and there is no evidence of surrounding inflammation.

Incidence. Seventy-five per cent of cases occur in adult females.

These cysts occur on the dorsum of any of the fingers but most often on the middle finger. They usually lie in the region of the distal joint, generally to one side of the midline. They may be multiple on one or both hands.

Symptoms. Since they are small and occasionally tense, they may become tender due to trauma. As a rule, the patient complains

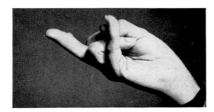

FIG. 924. A hard white tumor in the subcutaneous tissue for 2 years proved to be a many-layered skin inclusion cyst.

only of their presence. On occasions the fingernail may be grooved longitudinally as a result of direct pressure on the nail bed. Also, there may be a slight or moderate degree of dropfinger deformity of the distal joint if the overlying extensor tendon has undergone degeneration as well.

They are perhaps best described as "bleblike" in appearance. This is particularly true when they develop in the skin and have such a thin cover that they are translucent. Occasionally, a history of spontaneous rupture with extrusion of clear, jellylike material is given, or they may actually be opened by the patient in the belief that they are blisters. Grooving of the fingernail and the findings of degenerative arthritis of the distal joint, if present, support the diagnosis. In the differential diagnosis, Heberden's nodes, rheumatic nodule and periarticular ganglia must be considered.

Treatment. X-ray therapy has been advised and reported to be successful. Surgical excision will give a good result when the entire cyst is removed and the resulting denuded area covered by a split or full-thickness free skin graft. If the cyst is found to arise from the joint capsule or a ligament and thus is really a ganglion, a local rotational flap should be used to cover the site of origin, the donor area being split-grafted. Recurrences after surgical treatment are seen but probably are due to new areas of mucoid degeneration rather than to incomplete removal of the initial lesion. Conservative therapy consists of aspiration of the contents of the cyst with instillation of a small amount of hydrocortone. Then the distal joint is splinted in extension, and mild pressure is applied over the collapsed cyst. One or 2 treatments often result in prolonged relief. Spontaneous cure following rupture and mild infection has been seen.

VASCULAR TUMORS

Aneurysms following trauma to the major vessels of the hand occur from penetrating wounds or blunt trauma which weakens the vessel walls. (See Chap. 18 for discussion.)

True tumors of the vascular tissues consist of the angiomata, subdivided into endotheliomata, the benign tumor, and endotheliosarcomata, the malignant form.

Etiology and Pathology. All angiomata

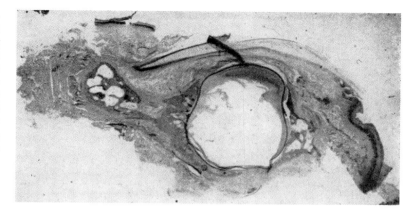

FIG. 925. Sagittal section of the terminal phalanx, demonstrating the position of the cyst within the phalanx. The tough membranous lining can be seen. The central caseous material fills the cyst. (Very low magnification.) (Carroll, R. E.: Am. J. Surg. *85*:329)

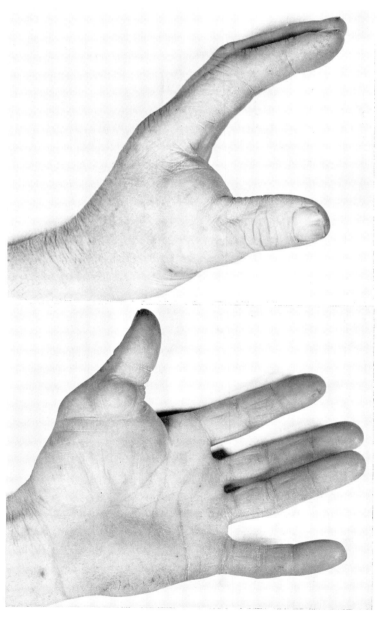

FIG. 926. Lateral (*top*) and anterior (*bottom*) views of a large epidermoid cyst in the thenar and the thumb web area of a 40-year-old male workman. The tumor had been present and growing for 10 years.

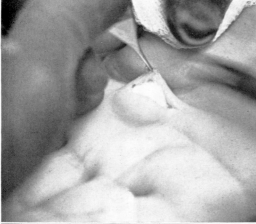

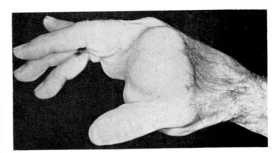

FIG. 928. Large inclusion cyst of many years duration in elderly dentist.

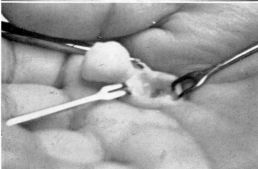

FIG. 927. Epithelial inclusion cyst in palm. The most likely cause is a penetrating wound.

probably are of congenital origin, though some first manifest themselves in later life. The common tumor may be present at birth and many regress spontaneously. All show endothelial proliferation in addition to the excessive number of vessels. Different forms are classified by their morphologic structure as capillary or cavernous or simply elongation and dilatation of existing vessels.

Symptoms. In the hand, angiomata can be present in practically any tissue from the skin, subcutaneous, nerve and muscle element, to involvement of bone and invasion of tendon sheaths. The thenar and the hypothenar eminences are favored locations, as are the deep spaces in the palms.

There is seldom pain, unless the lesion is located so as to cause pressure on nerves, or bone expansion is taking place. Complaint is of a small compressible tumor which seldom interferes mechanically with the function of the hand. If the tumor involves the skin, the cosmetic appearance often brings the patient to the doctor.

As a rule, diagnosis is not difficult. The tumor is compressible and enlarges when the venous return is obstructed. On clinical examination it is generally without definite limits.

Treatment. The capillary type needs little attention but if persistent can be treated by coagulation, excision, radiation or the application of carbon-dioxide snow. The cavernous type, on the other hand, requires a most careful and complete surgical dissection which is often difficult because of the ramifications of the tumor with involvement of important structures. The necessity of a bloodless field provided by a tourniquet is obvious; but, in a way, this is disadvantageous, because part of the lesion can be missed readily. Large lesions may require surgical removal in stages. In such cases the control of hemorrhage following the release of the tourniquet may be a problem. One method that has been found to be useful is to lower the cuff pressure momentarily, allowing a small amount of blood to enter the arm. Local pressure about the wound causes the blood to extrude from the open vessels, thereby identifying them for ligation or coagulation. This process may be repeated several times, thus controlling most of the opened vessels before final removal of the tourniquet. Careful attention to the wound is necessary, because the tissues often heal

FIG. 929. (*Top*) Photomicrograph of a myxomatous cyst. The cavity is formed by a myxomatous degeneration of the corium. The loose-textured connective tissue of the cyst wall merges gradually into the normal derma, as seen in the right lower portion of the picture. At the left, a downgrowth of the epidermal layer has surrounded a small part of the cyst. (× 20) (*Center, left*) Myxomatous cyst of the left middle finger. (*Center, right*) Same case as the top picture, 4 months after x-ray treatments. (*Bottom*) Photomicrograph of the roof of a cyst. The epidermis, *E*, and the corium, *C*, are essentially normal. The cyst cavity, which was filled with mucoid material, does not have any epithelial lining. (× 125) (Gross, R. E.: Surg., Gynec. Obstet. *65*:294–299)

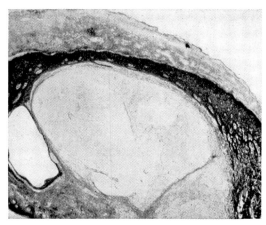

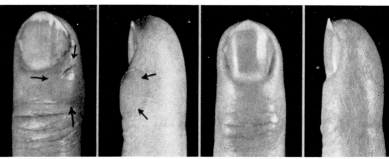

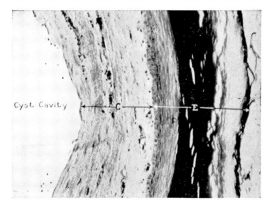

poorly in these cases. The use of sclerosing solutions as injections into the vessel-type of angioma has been advocated and may be of some value in selected cases. At times it is employed in obliterating small isolated portions of the angioma remaining after surgical removal.

The prognosis is guarded, since recurrences are prone to appear. The malignant form (angiosarcoma) may spread rapidly and be fatal.

Lymphangiectasis is an unusual condition of congenital origin; when a familial tendency is shown, it is known as Milroy's disease. It is doubtful if confusion between this condition and a tumor would occur. However, it is mentioned for the sake of completeness because there is some similarity to the angiomas. When the upper extremity is involved, generally the entire member is affected, and the condition is present at birth. The edema is due to replacement of the normal subcutaneous fat by dilated lymphatics and, later, fibrous connective tissue, as is readily demonstrated on microscopic section. Treatment is difficult and depends on excision of as much of the abnormal tissue as possible, utilizing salvaged skin and skin grafts to cover the resulting defect.

FIBROMAS

These tumors are common over the body but are not very frequent in the hand. They may occur at almost any site in the superficial or the deep structures. They are benign and, as a rule, grow slowly.

Pathology. The gross appearance is that of

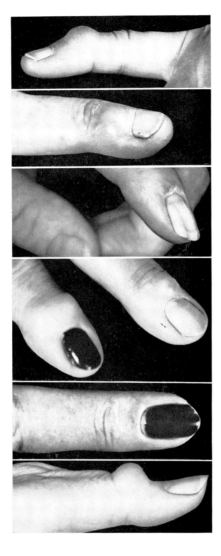

FIG. 930. (*From Top*) (1) Mucous cyst in female, age 48, with osteoarthritis. Relieved by splinting and local hydrocortisone injection. (2) Mucous cyst in male, age 63. Excised and skin-grafted. (3) Groove in fingernail from pressure of cyst removed recently. (4) Mucous cyst and osteoarthritis in female, age 48. (5) Postoperative view showing skin graft. (6) Cyst arising from the distal joint of the thumb is a ganglion rather than a mucous cyst.

believed to be hereditary and may represent an atavism. In the tendons, fibromata may lead to snapping finger, since the presence of the lesion increases the diameter of the tendon, producing the phenomenon as this area travels past the relative constriction of a pulley. Occasionally, a fibroma may be subungual in location, and, while they are not painful at this site due to their slow growth, they cause distortion of the nail and pressure atrophy of the distal phalanx. Levinthal and Kirschbaum report a case of a large fibroma of a metacarpal bone, but there is some question regarding the pathologic classification in that it could be regarded as an extreme case of a sclerosing type of giant cell tumor. Keasbey describes a type of fibroma arising in the palms and the soles of young children. The term "calcifying juvenile aponeurotic fibroma" is suggested for the 4 cases reported, 3 of which were in the hand. This fibroma is

a mass of variable size tending to be roughly spherical in shape and firm with an elastic resilience. The microscopic picture is that of dense fibrous connective tissue in sheets or whorls. At times calcification or even cartilage and bone formation may occur.

Location. Fibromata may occur in the skin or the subcutaneous tissue or may be connected with the deeper fascia or the ligaments of the hand. They have been described as tumors of the tendon sheaths and also of the tendon proper in rare instances. Occasionally, fibrous nodules are seen over the dorsum of the middle joints of all fingers, excluding the thumb. These are called Garrod's pads, are

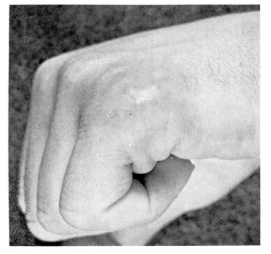

FIG. 931. Vessel type of angioma in the subcutaneous tissues overlying the proximal joint of the little finger. (Wakeman, U.S. Army photograph)

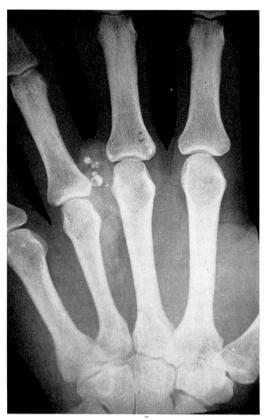

FIG. 932. Angioma growing from interosseus muscle. Tumor distinctive by presence of phleboliths.

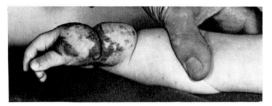

FIG. 933. Large-vessel type of hemangioma in a 10-month-old female. The tumor was confined to the skin and the subcutaneous tissues. Treatment was by excision and split-skin graft. Due to contracture of the graft, a pedicle type of cover will be needed later.

The diagnosis is generally made on the basis of the firmness of the tumor. Fibroma of the skin may be confused with neurogenous tumors. The deeper-seated fibromata offer a more difficult diagnostic problem in that they may be confused with ganglia, epidermoid cysts and other firm lesions.

The treatment is surgical excision, usually accomplished readily; prognosis for cure is good, because the tumors are benign.

NEUROFIBROMATA

This not uncommon small tumor occurs just beneath the skin and resembles a simple fibroma. However, on microscopic examination, it is seen to be of nerve tissue origin; it resembles the fibroma of von Recklinghausen's disease. Simple excision results in cure, because they are benign encapsulated masses, often on a tiny nerve fiber.

EPITHELIOMATA

A malignant tumor of the skin appears on the dorsum of the hands of dentists, physicians and other persons exposed to radiation.

characterized by its distinctive pathologic picture and infiltrating qualities and the marked tendency to recur.

Symptoms. As a rule, fibromata are symptomless unless their location and size are such that they interfere with function or press against nerves.

FIG. 934. Vessel type of hemangioma in the middle and the ring fingers of a 3-year-old male. Several operative procedures were necessary to reduce finger size. Spontaneous thrombosis in one area occurred while the patient was under observation.

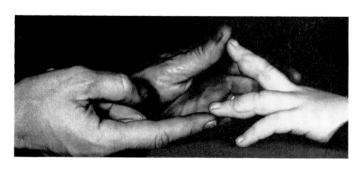

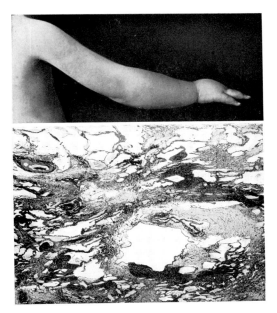

FIG. 935. (*Top*) Congenital lymphedema affecting the right arm of a girl, age 9. (*Bottom*) Microscopic appearance of tissue removed from the arm illustrated above. A remarkably large amount of the section is composed of lymph spaces surrounded by connective tissue. ($\times$ 16) (Mason, P. B., and Allen, E. V.: Am. J. Dis. Child. *50*: 945)

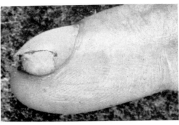
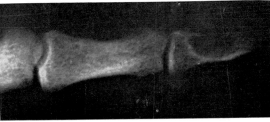

FIG. 936. (*Left*) Large subungual fibroma of 6 years' duration. Deformity of the nail, displacement of the finger pulp and erosion of the distal phalanx made amputation through the base of the distal phalanx necessary. (*Right*) X-ray picture showing erosion of the distal phalanx. (Wakeman, U.S. Army photograph)

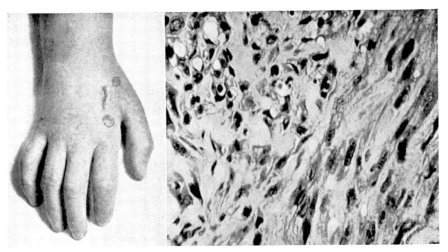

FIG. 937. Peripheral nerve tumor. Photograph and photomicrograph of a sub-epidermal spindle-cell sarcoma of the nerve sheath recurrent after excision and irradiation. The characteristic cells of Schwann are shown in the photomicrograph, with a large amount of collagen. (Geschickter, C. F.: Am. J. Cancer *25*:391)

FIG. 938. Tumor of the right thumb, probably attached to a digital branch of the radial nerve. Present for 12 years in a woman 28 years old. (Stout, A. P.: Am. J. Cancer 24:755)

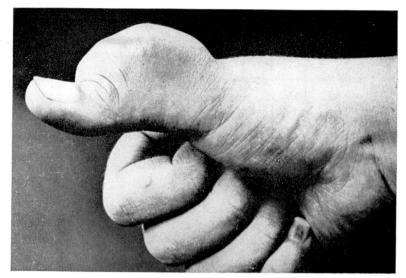

FIG. 939. Tumor nerve sheath of the right palm, attached to probably a branch of the n. cutaneus antibrachii lateralis. Present for 20 years in a woman 53 years old. (Stout, A. P.: Am. J. Cancer 24:755)

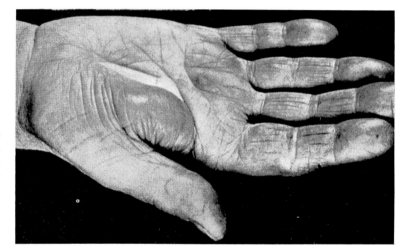

FIG. 940. Neurofibroma of median nerve with enlargement of branches to index and middle fingers and slight increase in size of these 2 digits. Resected involved nerve and did delayed repair by "bulb suture" technic.

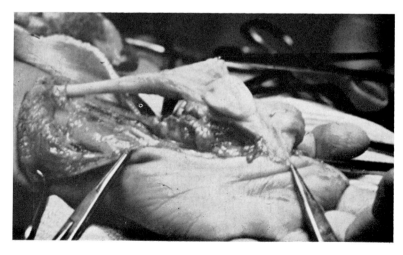

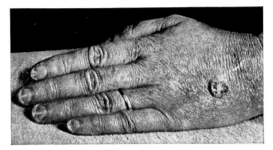

FIG. 941. Typical appearance of an early squamous-cell epithelioma of the dorsum of the hand; present 3 months. (DeBell and Stevenson: Surg., Gynec. Obstet. *63*:224)

It is the most common malignant tumor appearing in several series of cases.

Etiology. In no other malignant lesion does the role of chronic tissue irritation play such a prominent or so well-recognized part. This does not mean a single traumatism. While only 10 per cent of cutaneous carcinomas occur in the hands, Mason states that 40 per cent of these arise as a late result of injury, infection or scar. The particular susceptibility of radiation and thermal scars to undergo malignant changes is well known, and Ullman states that this type of scar is responsible for 80 per cent of the carcinomas developing in cicatrix. The type of trauma or tissue damage is of an irritative nature as a rule, and its action generally takes place over a period of time. The more common irritative agents are the roentgen rays, sunlight, contact burns and chronic infections with resulting scars and ulcerations. Chemical irritants such as acids, alkalies, tars, pitch, oils, paint, etc., likewise are offenders, and mechanical irritation over a prolonged period may also be cited as a cause. Chronic arsenic poisoning, resulting from repeated intake of small doses either internally or externally, is characterized by cutaneous keratoses which are highly susceptible to malignant change.

Pathology. The gross appearance varies from small fissures or cracks to areas of hyperkeratosis or actual tumor formation with or without ulceration. The microscopic picture is that of an epithelioma, of either the squamous or the basal cell types, and most of them are of low-grade malignancy. Lesions developing on the backs of the hands are almost entirely

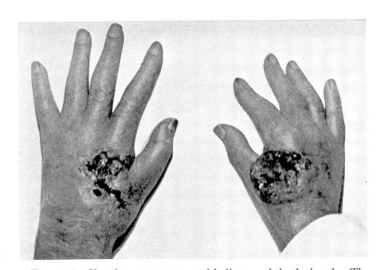

FIG. 942. Showing squamous epithelioma of both hands. The patient for 40 years had painted Pullman cars, using both hands and placing the paint brush between the thumb and the forefinger, at which site the epithelioma originated, growing upward over the dorsum of the hands. The right hand was amputated. The left hand was treated with radium rays. There is no evidence of any disease 4 years later. (Adair, F. E.: Surg. Clin. N. Amer. *13*:425)

of the squamous-cell type. In 1950, Johnson and Ackerman in their clinical study of 72 cases pointed out the pathologic changes in senile hand skin and the relation and the course of developing malignancy at this site.

Clinically and histologically, the cancer first spreads and involves the surrounding skin. In the later stages, fixation of the tumor to the deep fascia occurs, and the invasion of tumor cells extends deeply into the hand to involve all structures.

Metastases, which are reported as occurring in 10 to 20 per cent of all cases, usually come relatively late in the course of the disease and are detected first as enlargement of the axillary lymph nodes. The epitrochlear node may also be involved if the lesion is in this lymph drainage area. In fatal cases, lung metastases are evident, and the spread may occur elsewhere over the body.

Symptoms. Carcinoma of the hand occurs slightly more often in the male than in the female, various authors reporting a ratio of from 2.5 to 1 to 4 to 1, and individuals pre-

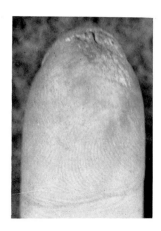

Fig. 943. Early skin changes on the volar surface of the tip of the index finger secondary to radiation. Note hyperkeratosis and marginal telangectasia. (Wakeman, U.S. Army photograph)

senting this lesion are mostly over 30 years of age. While the incidence of carcinoma is high among the malignant tumors of the hand, it is low when all tumors of the extremity are considered.

The great majority of lesions occur on the back of the hand. In a series of 61 cases on the upper extremity reported by De Bell and Stevenson, 84 per cent occurred at this site.

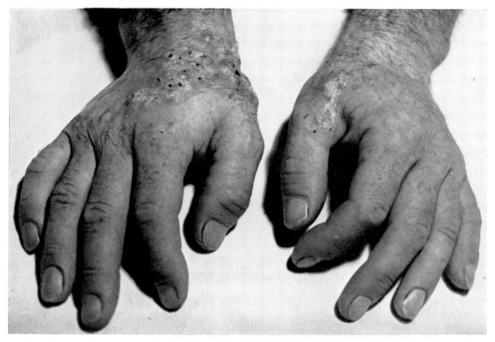

Fig. 944. Multiple carcinomalike lesions arising on the dorsum of the hands of a 35-year-old mechanic. A microscopic diagnosis of low-grade squamous type carcinoma could not be refuted; however, spontaneous healing occurred, indicating the diagnosis of keratocanthoma.

The right hand is involved a little more fre quently than the left, with the exception of carcinoma following roentgen dermatitis. In dentists, the area of involvement is mainly the thumb and the radial side of the index and the middle fingers where maximum x-ray exposure occurs while holding dental film in the patient's mouth.

Since the lesions appear on the surface they are always visible and accompanied by some pain. Ulcerations may be present and often secondarily infected.

Diagnosis. The possiblity of carcinoma in any chronic lesion of the skin on the dorsum of the hand in an individual over 30 years of age should be strongly suspected. Pain developing in a long-standing scar or sinus on the back of the hand is probably indicative of malignant change. Later in the course of the disease the tumor generally manifests itself as a hard nodular structure which may ulcerate and fungate. Metastasis to the regional lymphatics appears relatively late in the course of the disease, sometimes a matter of a year or 2 after the condition has been diagnosed. Biopsy is helpful in making the diagnosis, but it is perhaps best to excise the entire suspected lesion for microscopic study rather than to cut into the tumor for a sample of one part.

Recurrence locally following inadequate excision gives further evidence of the malignant nature of the lesion.

Treatment for carcinoma of the hands can be divided into 2 phases. First and most important, is prophylactic treatment of areas in which carcinoma is likely to develop; this consists of eradication of all types of chronic irritation or infection. If changes in the skin have already occurred and are likely to persist and result in malignant degeneration—such as scars from roentgen dermatitis—the

involved skin should be removed surgically and replaced by normal healthy skin by means of either a pedicle or a split-skin graft, as the need may be. The treatment of the cancer after it has developed is eradication of the local lesions by wide resection to include any other areas of skin which might later break down. In addition, Handley and other authors advised early and complete removal of the axillary and the epitrochlear glands for both treatment and prophylaxis. Other writers do not share this view of radical prophylactic treatment, feeling that in up to 75 per cent of cases the operation is not necessary. However, it seems to be advisable to do more than is necessary rather than to risk the fatal termination of the disease. When microscopic

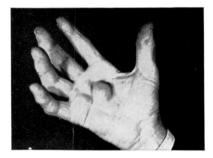

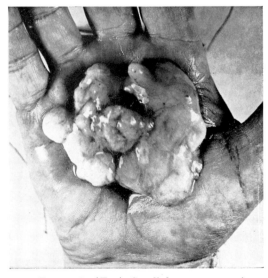

Fig. 946. (*Top*) Small lump present in the palm for 4 years, which proved to be a nodule on an extensive lipoma that filled the thenar and the palmar spaces. (*Bottom*) Tumor laid on a hand to show the location.

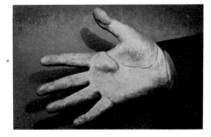

Fig. 945. Lipoma growing in the palm for 13 years.

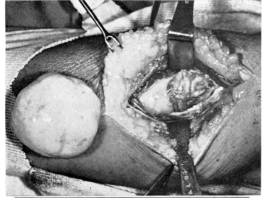

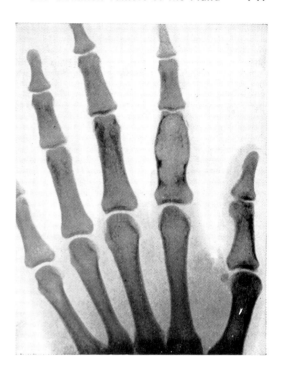

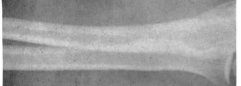

Fig. 947. Lipoma in supinator muscle in upper forearm producing paralysis of posterior interosseus nerve. Note the area of lessened density in the roentgenogram.

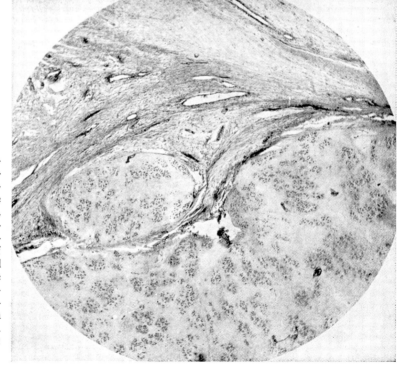

Fig. 949. (*Top*) Roentgenographic appearance of a benign chondroma situated in the phalanx of the forefinger. The chondroma is a central bone-destructive lesion and is composed of adult cartilage separated by strands of connective tissue. (*Right*) Microscopic appearance of benign chondroma shown in the upper illustration. (Geschickter, C. F.: Radiology 16:158–159)

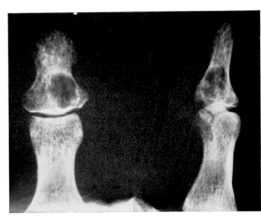

Fig. 949. Cyst of the phalanx of the thumb which proved to be a chondroma.

examination discloses definite malignant change in an area of radiation dermatitis, some authors recommend that axillary node resection be delayed until palpable nodes are present. Good reports on the treatment of the lesion by irradiation can be found. In a large published series by Braddon, unusually good results have been recorded. The author stresses accurate dosage, distribution and time of treatment. No form of radiation therapy is without danger, and certainly this method is contraindicated for carcinoma that has arisen from previously irradiated skin or from arsenical keratoses.

It is perhaps best to reserve radiation therapy for cases refusing surgical extirpation.

Naturally, the prognosis depends on the extent of the lesion at the time it is first seen. The local lesion in an early stage and without metastases offers an opportunity for cure. Once metastases are present, the outlook is poor.

LIPOMAS

The soft lipomas which occur mainly in the subcutaneous areas over the body are well known to the clinician and, as a rule, are easily diagnosed. Occasionally, they may occur in the hand; but in this location they are infrequent, and the diagnosis is often mistaken.

Pathology. On gross appearance these tu-

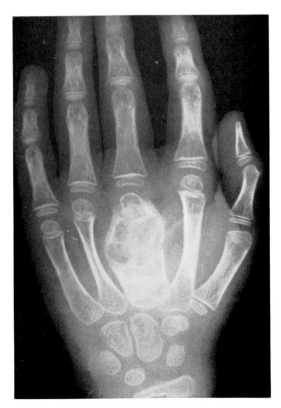

Fig. 950. Pseudotumor in a hemophiliac.

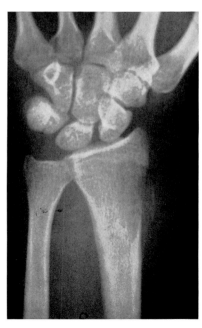

Fig. 951. Aneurysmal bone cyst of distal radius. (R. R. Schreiber, M.D.)

mors are soft, generally lobulated and surrounded by thin but definite capsules. The microscopic picture varies somewhat, depending on the amount of fibrous tissue associated with the fat. Some myxomatous tissue may also be present.

Location. Lipomas have been described in various locations on the hand. Those that involve the tendon sheaths as simple tumors or arborizing masses are considered by some authors to be basically synoviomas of the lipoid type. Other lipomas occurring outside the tendon sheaths may be superficial as found elsewhere in the body, or they may originate deep in the hand, usually in the palm from the retroflexor panniculus. At this site they become so bounded by the various ligaments, fascia and tendons that they take unusual form, insinuating themselves in the fascial planes and often presenting superficially in the distal palm or following the interosseus tendons to appear on the dorsum between the fingers. Lipomas may also occur in the thenar area. In general, they occur more frequently on the volar surface of the hand than on the dorsum.

The symptoms presented by lipoma in the hand are generally mechanical ones as a result of the size of the lesion.

Diagnosis. These lesions often are not diagnosed before operation; yet they have some characeristics that should lead to early recognition. Because they are soft and flabby in structure, they give a suggestion of fluctuation on physical examination. It has also been reported that the application of an ice bag over the tumor leads to an increase in the firmness as a result of chilling of the fat. The differential diagnosis includes hemangioma, synovioma, xanthoma and other soft lesions.

Treatment consists in surgical removal of the tumor. It is necessary to remove the lesion completely to avoid recurrence, and this is done best under the ischemia of a tourniquet, since perfect vision is essential.

Enchondroma or Chondroma

These are congenital tumors, almost entirely restricted to the hand, where they occur as single or multiple lesions in the phalanges and present a more or less characteristic picture.

Etiology and Pathology. The origin of these congenital tumors is believed to be cartilage rests where they represent potential joint carti-

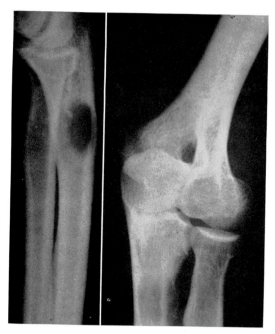

Fig. 952. Aneurysmal bone cyst in proximal ulna. (W. Heimstra, M.D., Department of Radiology, California Lutheran Hospital)

lages in the phalanges. This possiblity may explain their frequent occurrence in the hand where multiple joints are present.

The gross microscopic picture is that of

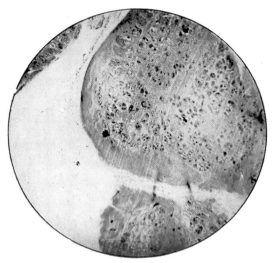

Fig. 953. Chondroma of the tendon sheath. ($\times$ 85) (Buxton, St. J. D.: Brit. J. Surg. *10*:471)

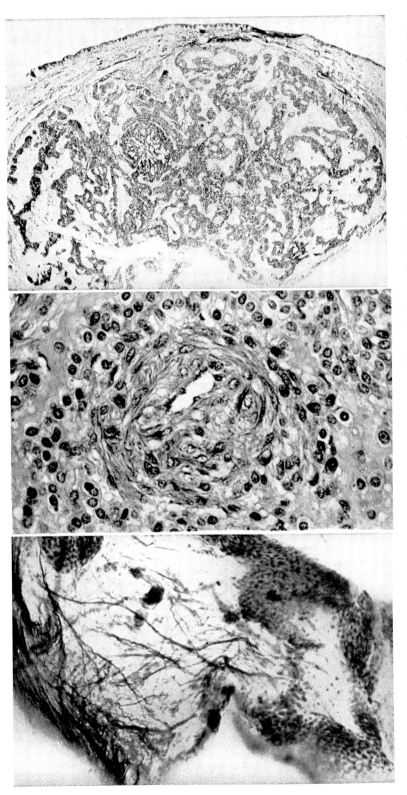

FIG. 954. (*Top*) Glomus tumor. Low-power photomicrograph of the encapsulated subungual tumor covered by the elevated nail bed. (*Center*) One of the tumor vessels cut somewhat tangentially, with a small, empty, endothelial-lined lumen surrounded by a somewhat irregularly arranged muscular coat, outside of which are the "epithelioid" cells with their clearly defined cell membranes. Each cell is separated from its neighbor by a delicate collagen fiber. (*Bottom*) Photomicrograph of a frozen section stained by a modified Gros technic, showing the large number of nerve fibers passing from the capsule along the stroma between the tumor vessels with their epitheloid cells. (Stout, A. P.: Am. J. Cancer *24*:261, 264, 267)

Fig. 955. (*Top*) Schematic reconstruction of a glomus: (A) Superficial preterminal artery. (Apa) Terminal branch entering capillaries. (L) The side branch is the afferent artery entering the glomus, dividing into 4 neuromuscular arterioles. The elastica of the afferent arteriole disappears as soon as the arteriole enters the glomus. The wall of the vessel becomes thick due to an increase in smooth muscle fibers, which terminate abruptly with the beginning of the venous segment. The efferent glomic vein leads into a collecting

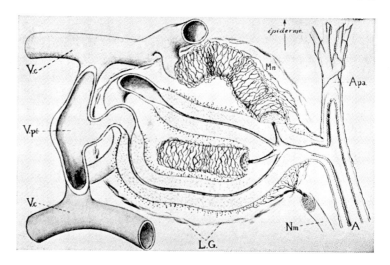

vein (V.pe.) which is dilated and thickened at the junction and in turn leads into the superficial veins (V.c.). Mn is the rich perivascular network of nerves, showing connections with the peri-arterial sympathetic nerves as well as myelinated sensory nerves to the skin. (After Masson) (Pack, G. L.: Tumors of the Hands and Feet, St. Louis, Mosby) (*Bottom*) Diagram of a glomus tumor.

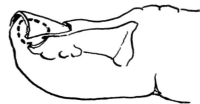

cartilage which at times may show some calcification within its substance and at times breaks out of the confines of the bone and extends into the soft tissues.

These tumors are generally recognized in individuals under 30 years of age, another factor indicating a congenital origin.

Symptoms. The phalanges are the primary site—particularly the proximal phalanges—though when multiple tumors appear, they may be in many of the phalanges and the metacarpals as well.

The symptoms are mild, if present at all. There is a uniform hard expansion of the phalanx that causes no disability. Pathologic fracture, which occurs in up to 25 per cent of cases, may be the first symptom, the tumor being discovered on x-ray examination.

The bone may be expanded, but a thin osseous covering is generally preserved. When multiple areas of such an appearance are present, the diagnosis is almost certain. In differential diagnosis xanthoma or bone cysts are the principal confusing lesions.

Treatment of these tumors, when indicated, is surgical, care being taken to remove all the cartilaginous material to avoid recurrence.

After excision, bone chips are packed in the resulting cavity. Small tumors may persist for years without appreciable increase in size, and treatment of these can be deferred.

GLOMUS TUMORS

This interesting tumor was recognized as a clinical entity long before it was given its present name by Masson, who identified the tumor by its structure as arising from the normal neuromyoarterial glomus. The first recorded cases are credited to William Wood who reported them in 1812 under the name of painful subcutaneous tubercle. In 1920, Barre outlined the clinical aspects of the tumor and emphasized the importance of surgical excision to effect a cure. Although seen infrequently, the tumor has been of interest to the profession as evidenced by 197 cases reported in the literature up to 1942 by Ottley. Some confusion in terminology has been apparent in the past, since cases of glomus tumor have been recorded under various names such as angioneuroma, glomangioma, Popoff tumor, *tumeur glominque*, angiomyoneuroma, angiosarcoma, etc.

The normal structure from which the glomus

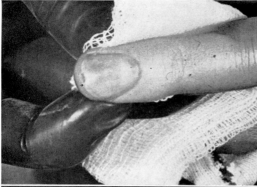

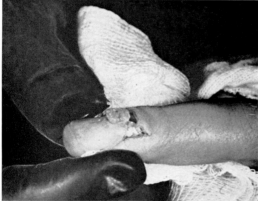

Fig. 956. Glomus tumor at base of nail, removed by turning back the cuticle as in a paronychia operation.

tumor arises is of greater scientific than clinical interest. This neuromyoarterial glomus lies in the stratum reticulare of the skin and serves as a controlled arteriovenous anastomosis or shunt between the terminal vessels, probably for thermal regulation by the vasomotor system. Such anastomoses were first described by Sucquet in 1860; he demonstrated direct connections between terminal arteries and veins by the injection method and noted their frequency in the palms, the soles, the fingers and the toes. Hoyer, in 1877, described similar arteriovenous anastomoses in animals. In 1902, Grosser described in detail these structures in man and other warm-blooded animals but found them to be absent in the poikilotherms. The latest and most detailed study of the neuromyoarterial glomus was made by Popoff, in 1934, using human material studied by serial section. He described the structure as consisting of an efferent arteriole from which branches the tortuous anastomotic vessel (Sucquet-Hoyer canal), which in turn opens directly into a primary collecting vein. The characteristic feature of this arteriovenous anastomosis lies in the structure of the anastomotic vessel which is endothelial-lined and surrounded by longitudinal and circular smooth muscle cells, among which appear the "glomal cells" which are epithelioid in appearance with oval or globular nuclei. The glomal cells have been described as embry-

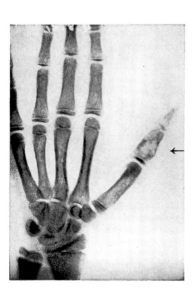

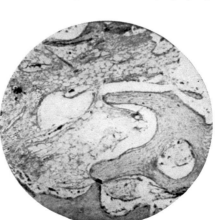

Fig. 957. (Left) Cyst of the proximal phalanx of the thumb (osteitis fibrosa), showing multicystic expansion of the phalanx. No sign of fracture. (Right) Cyst contents. Bone trabeculae undergoing erosion in the midst of delicate connective tissue. An early phase of osteitis fibrosa. (Platt, H.: Brit. J. Surg. 18:21)

FIG. 958. Multiple intra-osteal chondromata in a girl 8 years old, involving the whole skeleton. Heavy radiation gave only local improvement. (Kolodny, A.: Surg., Gynec. Obstet. *44*:94)

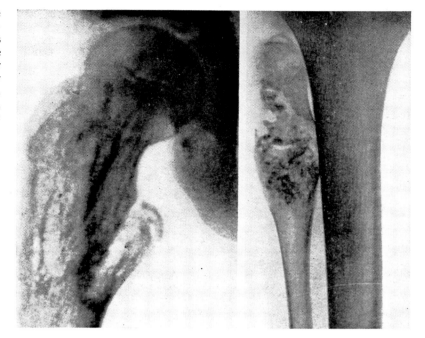

onic muscle cells, angioblasts and elastoblasts, although their true nature and function are not known. All parts of the glomus are bound together by a delicate collagenous reticulum in which nonmyelinated nerve fibrils are plentiful, and the whole is surrounded by a fibrous tissue capsule. This structure never exceeds 1 mm. in diameter.

The physiology of the normal glomus has been studied by Lewis and Pickering and by Grant and Bland in 1931, and it is their belief that these anastomoses serve to regulate peripheral blood flow and, therefore, the peripheral blood pressure and temperature. There is no known cause for a normal glomus to develop into a glomic tumor, although in the literature trauma has been cited as the activating agent in some cases.

Pathology. The glomus tumor represents a hypertrophy of the normal glomus. The gross appearance is that of a small encapsulated tumor and in its subungual location from 2 to 6 mm. in diameter. One of unusual size (4× 2.5×2 cm.) located near the elbow was reported by Riddell and Martin. It is generally of deep red or purple color and on cut section it exudes blood, following which it becomes gray. The microscopic appearance of the

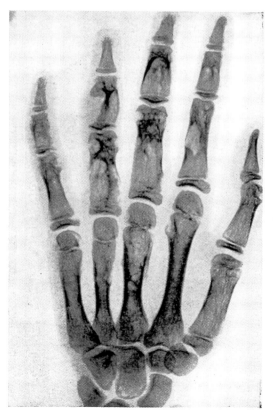

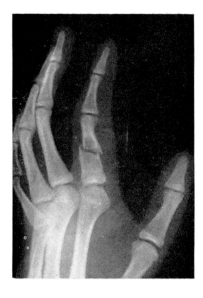

FIG. 959. Pathologic fracture through the central enchondroma of the proximal phalanx of the index finger. (Shellito, J. G., and Dockerty, M. B.: Surg., Gynec. Obstet. *86*:467)

tumor, by reason of its origin, closely resembles that of the normal glomus, the principal difference being a marked increase in the number of glomal cells and nonmyelinated nerves. Similarity of the microscopic picture to that of the glomus coccygeum is notable.

Incidence. This small tumor, which has a clinical picture characterized by pain, is found a little more frequently in males than in females. There is an increased incidence among Jewish people, due probably to their recognized susceptibility to sympathetic nerve disturbances. There is no special age group, cases being reported in individuals between 6 and 70 years old, with the majority falling in the 20- to 40-year-old period.

The glomus tumor is subungual in location in about half the cases and at this site shows a greater frequency in women than in men. However, the tumor may appear on any part of the surface of the body. It has been reported on both upper and lower extremities, on the trunk and even on the eyelids. The upper extremity is predominantly involved. Several cases of multiple tumors have been reported by Plewes. In one instance, 6 occurred on 1 foot, and in another instance 4 on 1 finger.

Symptoms. The constant and outstanding symptom of the glomus tumor is pain, and it is generally severe. It may be constant or intermittent and may arise spontaneously or by contact, or by change in temperature. The pain is described as stabbing or burning in character and often radiates up the extremity to the trunk.

As a rule, the diagnosis is not difficult if the examiner has the condition in mind. The clinical appearance of the tumor in the subungual location is quite characteristic. It is usually seen as a bluish or cyanotic discoloration 3 to 5 mm. in diameter under the fingernail. The lunula of the nail is often blurred, and the nail itself may be raised centrally with an increase in the convexity of the transverse plane. There may be associated vasomotor disturbances with vasodilatation of the affected member. In those suffering from exquisite pain and tenderness, a protective posture habit of the affected part may be assumed. In some cases, erosion of the distal phalanx may occur. and in 1 case reported by Lattes and Bull, the tumor was completely encased within the terminal phalanx, producing a cystic appearance. In such instances, the lesion can be detected roentgenographically. When the lesion occurs elsewhere, it is usually found in or just under the skin as a small painful nodule. The differential diagnosis in the subungual location includes subungual melanoma, exostosis, clavus, papilloma, fibroma and hemorrhage. In other locations it must be differentiated from many small tumors but particularly neuroma, neurofibroma and fibroma.

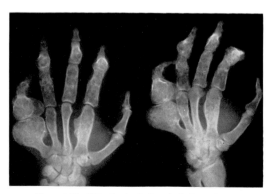

FIG. 960. Marked skeletal deformity resulting from multiple congenital enchondromata (Ollier's disease). (Col. Ernst Dehne, U.S. Army)

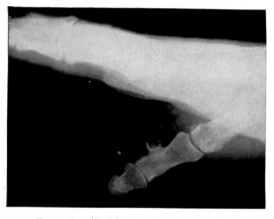
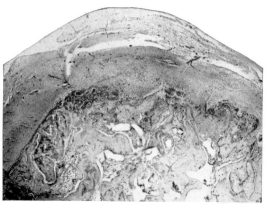

FIG. 961. (*Left*) Roentgenogram of an osteochondroma of the thumb. The tumor is arising at the insertion of the adductor pollicis. (*Right*) Photomicrograph of the same osteochondroma. (Geschickter, C. F., and Copeland, M. M.: Tumors of Bone, ed. 3, Philadelphia, Lippincott)

Treatment of this tumor consists of complete surgical removal; no other method—including roentgenotherapy—is of benefit. There are no reported cases of recurrence following adequate surgery. Relief of pain is prompt.

BONE TUMORS

Almost all tumors of bone which appear elsewhere in the skeleton may be present in the hand. Because of the small size of the hand bones these tumors appear in miniature, but in most instances they retain the characteristics that they have elsewhere. Malignant bone tumors are extremely uncommon distal to the forearm. The benign tumors are fairly well represented with only a few exceptions. Bone cysts are included with the tumors because of their similar radiologic appearance and the diagnostic difficulty that they present.

Cysts of Bone. The etiology of the cysts is unknown, but many causes have been advanced, such as traumatic hematoma, inflammation, faulty calcium metabolism and progressive osteoclastasia. The simple or solitary bone cysts are of the osteitis fibrosa cystica type. Some authors believe that there is a close relationship between the bone cyst and the giant cell tumor or xanthoma of bone, based on the finding of apparent transition stages between these 2 conditions. They point out that the cysts tend to occur in young individuals, the variants in the adolescent stage, and

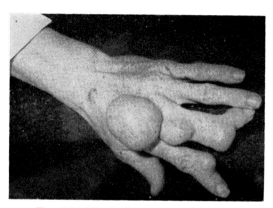
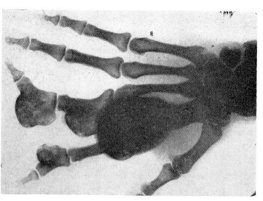

FIG. 962. Hand of a 33-year-old farm worker. The osteochondromata had been present for as long as he could remember. (Kyle, B. H., and Mundy, M. D.: Virg. Med. Month. 79:36, 37)

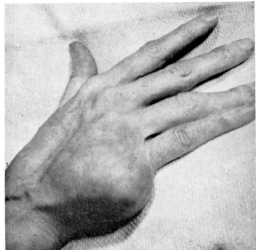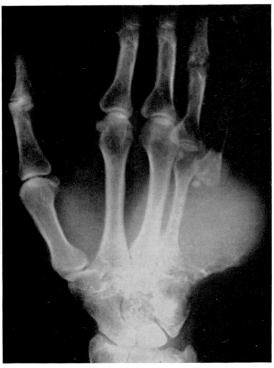

Fig. 963. Clinical (*left*) and x-ray (*right*) appearance of a benign giant-cell tumor of the 5th metacarpal. Note the "soap-bubble" appearance of the bone trabeculae. Excellent result obtained by amputation of the little finger with its ray, thus narrowing the hand. (Dr. Donald Wells, Hartford, Conn.)

the giant cell tumors after fusion of the epiphyses.

Platt divided bone cysts of the hand into 2 types. The simple or solitary cyst he classifies a osteitis fibrosa cystica. This cyst is incompletely filled with tissue, has a tough, fibrous lining and may show some xanthomatous tissue on microscopic section. The other type is the chondromatous or myxochondromatous cyst. In these there is a cavity filled with sagolike material mixed with a friable granulationlike tissue. There is no fibrous tissue lining, and some cartilage may be present. He admits that this type of cyst may belong with the enchondromas.

INCIDENCE. The sex incidence is about equal. Most of these cysts occur in persons under the age of 25 years, but they may occur at any age. In Silva's series of 97 bone cysts, 7 were in the phalanges and 1 in the metacarpal. The osteitis fibrosa cyst is quite rare, but when all cysts are included, Clapp found that 13 of 34 cases were in the miniature long bones, and Geschickter and Copeland found that 16 of 175 cases of the osteitis fibrosa type were of the smaller bones.

Bone cysts are found more frequently in the phalanges than in the metacarpals, and the majority are in the proximal phalanges. Most of these are located in the little finger; next in frequency is in the index finger.

Their presence is most apt to be detected when fracture occurs, often a result of a minor injury. It can be assumed that symptomless growth of the cyst has been going on for a long time before the bone becomes so weakened that it breaks. Other symptoms consist of local swelling of the bone and occasionally some mild pain.

DIAGNOSIS is principally by means of roentgenograms where it is seen that the cyst originates in the metaphysis near the growing end. In the hand, this is the distal end of a metacarpal or the proximal end of a phalanx. The cyst extends into the shaft, preserving the integrity of the epiphysis. The roentgen appearance may remain unchanged for a long time. The area of bone involvement is sharply demarcated with a smooth, well-defined wall. The differential diagnosis includes giant cell tumors and other neoplasms and infections.

TREATMENT consists in curetting out the material in the cyst and the cyst lining and obliterating the space by filling it in with bone chips. Indications for operations are active growth of the cyst or the presence of a very thin shell with impending danger of fracture. Cysts of the bone which are discovered roentgenographically by accident and have a very thick wall are probably quiescent, and treatment can be delayed.

The prognosis is good.

Exostoses. True exostoses of the bones of the hands are very rare, occur generally about a joint, and develop secondary to injury of that part. On occasion, a subungual exostosis of the terminal phalanx may occur. These generally appear on the index finger. Because of their location, they have been mistaken for other types of subungual tumors. They may continue to grow until they push up the nail and become quite painful. When removed,

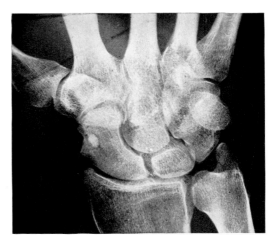

FIG. 964. Osteoid osteoma of the carpal navicular. Note the osteolytic area about the central zone of condensation. (Dr. Bradley L. Coley, New York, U.S. Army photograph)

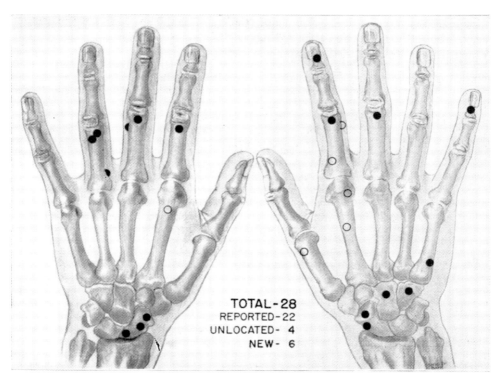

TOTAL - 28
REPORTED - 22
UNLOCATED - 4
NEW - 6

FIG. 965. Anatomic chart for location of the known cases of osteoid osteoma in the hand. The *solid dots* represent reported cases; the *circles* represent cases reported in the article cited in the reference at the end of this paragraph. The location of the tumor in 4 reported cases was not given specifically. (Carroll, R. E.: J. Bone Joint Surg. *35-A*:891)

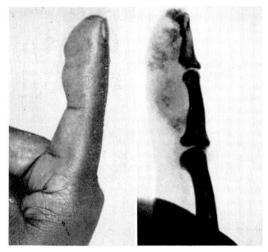

FIG. 966. Osteogenic sarcoma of the phalanx in a 37-year-old colored female. Treatment was by amputation through the metacarpocarpal joint. (Clark, C. E.: Am. J. Surg. *83*:112)

they are often observed to have a cap of cartilage, suggesting that they are closely related to, if not actually, osteochondromas. Treatment is simple excision of the exostosis, being certain to get all of the cartilage.

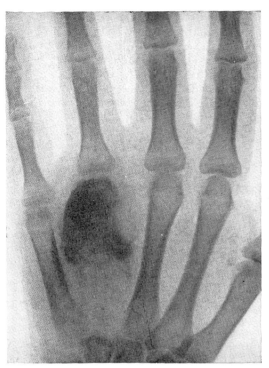

FIG. 968. An osteoblastic osteoid tissue-forming tumor of a metacarpal bone. (Jaffe, H. L., and Mayer, L.: Arch. Surg. *24*:500)

Giant Cell Tumors. These are benign tumors seen occasionally in the bones of the hands. They begin in the epiphyses but may spread rapidly to involve the whole bone, as a rule showing the characteristic soap-bubble appearance. The histologic picture is consistent with xanthomas elsewhere, and the diagnosis frequently can be established before surgery. The metacarpals are involved more commonly than other bones. As a rule, the symptoms are not pronounced unless pathologic fracture occurs. This latter may be the first indication of trouble. If the tumor is large, a diffuse increase in the size of the bone may be detected externally. Treatment depends on the extent of the lesion. Surgery is the preferred method and consists of careful removal of all tumor material and packing the resulting cavity with cancellous bone chips. Where resections of the

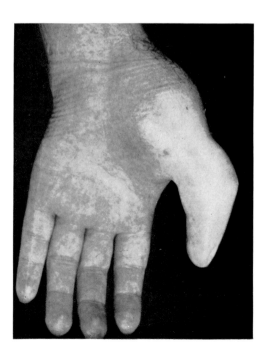

FIG. 967. Chondrosarcoma of 1st metacarpal and distal radius.

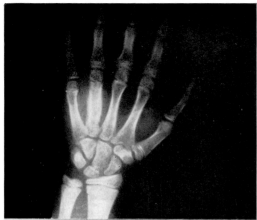

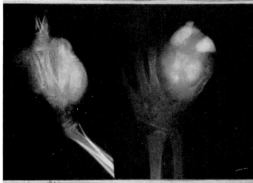

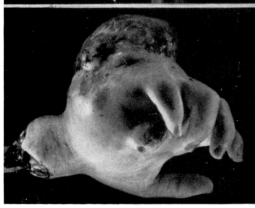

FIG. 969. Ewing's tumor of the metacarpal. (*Top*) Early stage. Proliferation of the periosteal layer of bone. (*Center* and *bottom*) Advanced stages. (Dr. F. M. McKeever, Los Angeles, Calif.)

made the distinction between this tumor and the enchondroma, giving it the name "perichondroma." This distinction is also emphasized by Geschickter.

The ecchondroma is also congenital in origin, usually making its presence known by the age of 25 years. Trauma has no true relationship to origin, although it may be cited as a cause by the patient.

In contrast with the enchondroma, the ecchondroma is peripheral in location, arising at or near the point of insertion of tendons at the base of the miniature long bones. The tumor itself has both cartilage and bone elements but has a cortical bone base and is capped by hyaline cartilage. When the tumor is large, some actual angular growth deformity of the short bone itself may ensue.

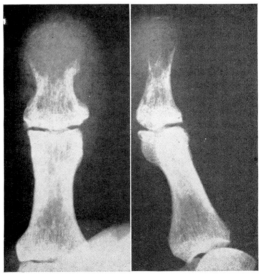

FIG. 970. Anteroposterior (*left*) and lateral (*right*) roentgenograms of the thumb, showing bone destruction of the distal phalanx due to metastatic epidermoid carcinoma. Grade 2, with the primary lesion in the left upper lobe of the lung. (Freni, D. R., and Averill, J. H.: Am. J. Surg. *83*:115)

bone are done, it is possible in most instances to make replacements by means of bone graft. X-ray therapy is effective but is not recommended for the treatment of hand lesions.

Ecchondroma or Osteochondroma. Osteochondroma represents the other type of cartilage tumor occurring in the hand but is less common (in a ratio of 1:3, Shellito, *et al.*) than the enchondroma. Virchow apparently

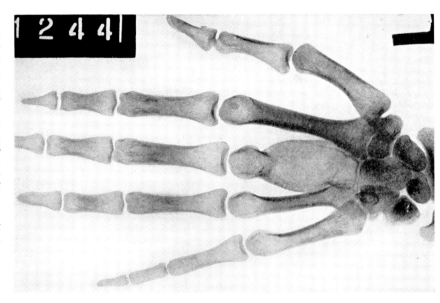

FIG. 971. (*Top*) Central metacarpal giant-cell sarcoma. Roentgenogram, anteroposterior, showing involvement of the 3rd metacarpal bone, the expanded and thinned-out cortex, the trabeculations and the limitation to one bone. (*Bottom*) Section of the tumor shown in the top roentgenogram, showing giant cells and stroma. (Duskes, Emile: Am. Surg. *85*:912)

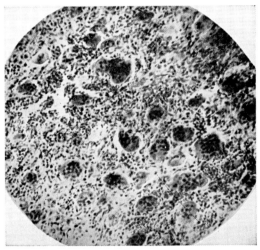

Ecchondromas are seen on both the phalanges and the metacarpals in about equal numbers. They tend to appear at the epiphysial ends of the bones and grow outward to form palpable protuberances. Multiple lesions have been reported and as such may represent a transition phase of the congenital chondrodysplasias.

In general, these tumors are symptomless except for the deformity. Function of the hand is not limited.

DIAGNOSIS AND TREATMENT. As a rule,

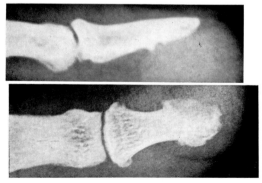

FIG. 972. Case J. A. Fibrosarcoma. Starting in the subcutaneous tissue 5 months previously, it grew to a firm, solid tumor. After amputation of this index finger and the distal two thirds of its metacarpal, the tumor did not recur.

roentgenograms promptly confirm the clinical impression. Because of the peripheral location, there is little chance to confuse the lesion with enchondroma or bone cyst.

When indicated, treatment is surgical excision. Special care should be taken to remove the entire base of compact bone. Recurrences are reported but are unusual when surgery has been adequate.

The prognosis for cure is good. Rarely, the ecchondroma, and even the enchondroma, can become malignant, but even then the grade of malignancy is low, and regional amputation is generally sufficient.

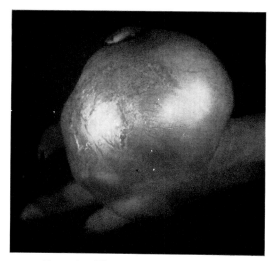

Fig. 973. Fibrosarcoma of the hand.

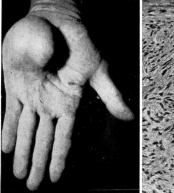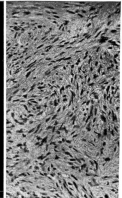

Fig. 974. (*Left*) Fibrosarcoma of the hand in 39-year-old white man. The tumor had enlarged gradually over a period of 30 years. (*Right*) The photomicrograph shows the similarity to simple fibroma. (Wilson, D. A.: Tumors of the subcutaneous tissue and fascia, Surg., Gynec. Obstet. *80*:502)

Osteoid Osteoma. This benign bone tumor may occur in adolescents and young adults, but it is rare in the hand. When present, the lesion is characterized by localized tenderness and pain. The pain is dramatically relieved by acetylsalicylic acid. Roentgenograms usually reveal a small, circumscribed, osteolytic area in the cancellous bone with or without associated bone condensation or calcification. The lesion is characterized by abundant osteoid tissue occupying the area of bone destruction. Calcification and new bone replacement are evident. The differential diagnosis includes both tumor and infection, the latter being suggested by the pain and local tenderness, although other signs of infection are absent. Although the natural course of the disease is probably self-limiting (Moberg), generally treatment is recommended for early relief of symptoms. A recent and complete review of osteoid osteomas of the hand is given by Carroll.

Surgical removal of the lesion is said to result in prompt and complete cure.

Malignant Bone Tumors. OSTEOGENIC SARCOMA. These tumors are very rare, although they do occur in the hand occasionally. Up to 1952, 6 cases of osteogenic sarcoma involving the phalanx had been reported (Clark). A history of trauma is obtained in approximately half the cases. Pain is an early and persistent symptom of this tumor which makes its appearance generally in the 2nd and the 3rd

decades of life. Early roentgen studies combined with biopsy should determine the diagnosis and facilitate early and radical amputation. Coley and Higinbotham believe that many of these tumors are secondary to benign chondromas and that osteogenic sarcoma in the hand offers a better prognosis than osteo-

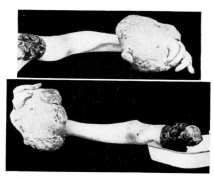

Fig. 975. Case A. B., age 31. Fibrosarcoma. When the patient was 17 years old, a toy cannon had exploded, leaving considerable débris in the hand. The tumor started in the thenar cleft and grew to 9 inches in diameter in 10 months, at which time the arm was amputated. The amputated limb is shown in the illustrations. The patient died from sarcomatosis 3 months later.

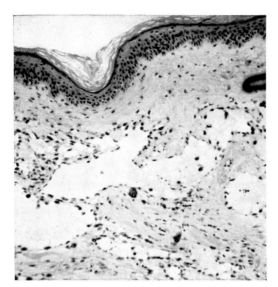

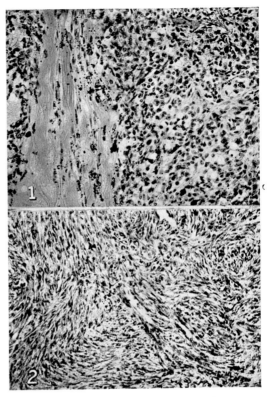

FIG. 976. (*Left*) Kaposi sarcoma in the skin. Photomicrograph of a section of skin. This is a very early lesion, showing the cavernous sinuses lined by endothelium. (*Right*) Later stages of the Kaposi sarcoma: (1) Photomicrograph of a section taken from a subcutaneous area. This is an older lesion than that shown in the left-hand photomicrograph. Now there is only a suggestion of sinus formation. There is proliferation of the endothelial lining cells, and some of them show spindling. (2) Photomicrograph of a well-developed lesion. There is almost no sinus formation. Practically all of the endothelial cells have undergone spindling, so that the tumor resembles neurofibroma or fibrosarcoma. (Aegerter, E. E., and Peale, A. R.: Arch. Path. *34*:415)

genic sarcoma elsewhere in the body, as evidenced by their survival figures. Carroll, in a recent exhaustive review of the literature, lists 8 recorded cases of osteogenic sarcoma of the hand and adds 2 personal cases. Five were in the metacarpal. He also is of the opinion that this tumor carries a better prognosis in the hand than elsewhere. He recommends wide local resection so that some functional portion of the hand will remain. When the clinical course of the tumor is not arrested, its metastatic manifestations are the same as those when the tumor originates elsewhere.

CHONDROSARCOMA. This form of malignant bone tumor should be mentioned for completeness, although it is very rare in the hand. In general, it occurs in older individuals and follows a more chronic course. It is believed to arise from mature cartilage such as is present

in a cartilage rest in bone, or capping an osteochondroma. When it is recognized, treatment is amputation, the extent or the level of the amputation being determined by the area involved.

EWING'S TUMOR. This tumor also may occur in the hand, but more cases are reported in the bones of the feet. It is characterized by pain, and frequently operation is performed for infection because of the low-grade fever which is usually present. Coley and Higinbotham state that the characteristic features of fusiform enlargement and periosteal splitting are less often present in small-bone involvement and recommend aspiration biopsy for diagnosis. Early and radical surgery perhaps offers the best chance for cure, but many factors are involved. Radiation therapy alone or combined with surgery has been used. The prognosis is

Fig. 977. Boeck's sarcoid in a 29-year-old male. The lesion had been present for 6 years. Also chest signs. (A. Schwartz, M.D.)

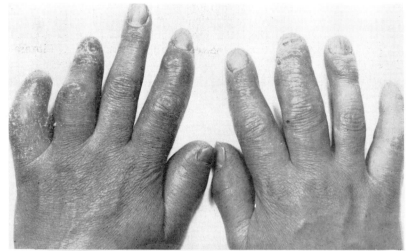

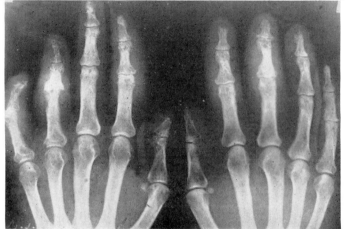

poor at best, but perhaps a little better than for the more centrally located lesions.

Metastatic tumors of the bones of the hand still may be considered to be rare, although in the past few years the literature on this subject has increased.

The terminal phalanx is involved most frequently, particularly that of the thumb. The offending carcinoma in most cases is bronchogenic in origin. The parotid and the breast also have been reported as primary sources for this metastasis.

From a diagnostic standpoint, a phalangeal metastasis resembles infection with pain, swelling and redness, but without local increase in heat. X-ray examination shows an osteolytic lesion which in some cases could be mistaken for infection.

Treatment, when indicated, is amputation proximal to the involvement. The microscopic examination may assist in the location of the primary lesion if this is not already evident.

Sarcoma implies a malignant tumor arising from cells of the mesothelial origin. Under this definition, all malignant tumors originating in the hand are sarcomas with the exception of those arising from the ectodermal components of the skin.

From a practical standpoint, sarcomas arising from specific structures, such as bone, nerve sheath, tendon sheath, muscle, etc., have been discussed with the tumors of these structures; similarly, the melanotic malignancies will be considered following the discussion of subungual melanoma.

This arrangement leaves the fibrosarcoma to

be considered separately; some authors would insist that many of the above-mentioned sarcomas really belong in the latter group, but the practical features outweigh the technicalities of classification.

Certainly, fiibrosarcoma is the most common mesodermal malignancy. Its many manifesta-tions and variable behavior make the condition difficult to treat from the standpoint of both the patient and the surgeon.

ETIOLOGY. Fibrosarcoma is considered to arise spontaneously from connective tissue elements or from benign tumors of fibrous tissue origin. It has been reported as developing in

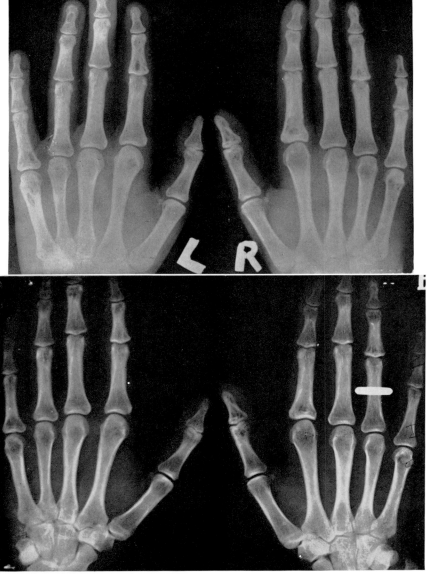

FIG. 978. (*Top*) Roentgenograms of both hands of a 26-year-old female complaining of pain for 6 years. No chest signs. (*Bottom*) Same patient 5 years later. (A. Schwartz, M.D.)

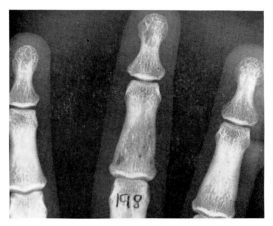

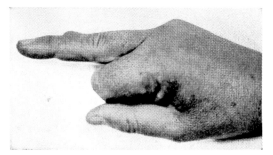

FIG. 980. Subcutaneous leiomyoma of the dorsal surface of the right middle finger. (Stout, A. P.: Am. J. Cancer *29*: 439)

FIG. 979. A 23-year-old Negro female. The combination of cystlike lesions and a coarse, reticular pattern in various areas in the middle and the distal phalanges is quite suggestive of sarcoid. Note the absence of periosteal new bone formation where the cortex of middle phalanx is involved. Changes in the distal phalanx must be differentiated from normal variations in pattern in distal phalanges. Joints are almost never involved.

scars, usually after many years, and in areas of tissue fibrosis following radiation therapy. Trauma as an etiologic factor is reported frequently, and in some cases convincing evidence is presented; however, most authors agree that there is little if any relationship. Carrol and Martin, in reporting their series, found that only 5 per cent gave a definite associated history of trauma. In another series of 60 cases reported by Heller and Sieber, only 6 had trauma as a definite part of the history, and of these only 1 fulfilled all of Ewing's postulates relative to trauma as a cause of malignancy.

PATHOLOGY. The microscopic picture of fibrosarcoma is so varied that there is little wonder that differences of opinion exist as to origin, type, classification and malignancy. From the clinician's standpoint, the acceptance of the views of one pathologist would seem to be more practical than becoming entangled in such a controversial subject. The common denominator is the fibroblast and the extracellular material that it produces. The cells vary in shape, maturity, and frequency of mitosis, and the extracellular material may

be scanty or abundant; giant cells may or may not be present. Necrosis, hemorrhage, calcification or mucoid degeneration may be evident. Other tissue elements such as muscle fibers or fat may be present, since the tumor is invasive in nature, and this often leads to confusion as to origin when a single biopsy specimen is examined.

INCIDENCE. The ratio of fibrosarcoma of the extremities to all admissions is reported as 1:2,400 by Wilson and as 1:4,000 by Meyerding, Broders and Hargrove. Of these, approximately two thirds arise in the lower extremities and one third in the upper extremities. Although exact statistics could not be obtained, the incidence of this lesion in the hand is a very small percentage of the total for the upper extremity. Thus, Beck, in a report of 42 cases in the extremities, states that 3 involved the hand, and, of these, 2 were neurogenous in origin. Wilson, reporting on a total of 111 cases in the extremities, found 7 on the hands and the feet.

Incidence is about equal in the sexes, although some authors give predominance to the male. The tumor may occur at all ages, but the greatest number occur during the 3rd, the 4th and the 5th decades., with an average age in the late thirties.

LOCATION. Hardly enough cases have been reported giving the exact site of origin in the hand to make it possible to draw any conclusions as to predilection of site. Presumably, the tumor may arise in any area.

DIAGNOSIS. The presence of a tumor or an increase in the size of an existing tumor is what usually causes the patient to seek medical advice. Pain is unusual unless the disease is advanced.

The diagnosis is sometimes difficult and often remains obscure until microscopic section is made. A history of rapid growth of a small existing tumor, often several years' duration, is significant. Also, the infiltrating nature of the growth as determined on physical examination is characteristic. Wilson states that 90 per cent of fibrosarcomas are 5 cm. or over in diameter when seen, whereas 85 per cent of fibromas are under 3 cm. in diameter. However, this dictum does not necessarily apply to the hand.

The tumor may vary greatly in consistency and in fixation. It is more commonly superficial than deep. Excluding microscopic section, the most conclusive evidence of its malignant nature is the tendency for local recurrence within 1 year after excision.

Such features as anemia, leukocytosis and sometimes fever, which may be associated with other types of malignancies, are seldom present early. Biopsy of the tumor, although not entirely without risk, gives the best basis on which to formulate treatment.

Metastases may be late, but when they occur they are usually by way of the blood-stream to the lungs, although regional lymphatic spread may also be present.

The differential diagnosis includes all soft-tissue tumors, but fibroma, lipoma, xanthoma and synovioma are probably the most important.

TREATMENT. When positive proof of the nature of the tumor has been obtained, amputation well above the lesion offers the best chance for cure. Local excision can be performed for the more common well-differentiated types if wide excision does not prove to be too crippling. A recurrence after local excision is definite evidence of the need for amputation. X-ray therapy is reserved for palliative treatment in advanced cases with metastases and may be used on cases refusing surgery. Coley's toxin has been used but is not of proved curative value.

Survival figures for fibrosarcoma of the hand are not available; but judging from the statistics on fibrosarcoma of the extremities, the prognosis is poor. Wilson reports a mortality rate of 66 per cent in his series. Meyerding, Broders and Hargrove observed that all of their cured cases had a low grade of malignancy and concluded that cure of a given case is perhaps more dependent on the type of tumor than the amount or the type of surgery.

Kaposi's Sarcoma. In 1872, Kaposi described this lesion and named it idiopathic multiple pigment sarcoma. It is rare, but occasionally the lesions appear as tumors on the hand.

The disease appears spontaneously, although occasionally trauma is noted prior to the development of some of the lesions.

The disease is characterized by the fact that all stages can be seen in a single lesion. The lesion developing in the skin first appears as a macule which is hyperemic but later becomes cyanotic due to stasis of the blood; finally, hemorrhage occurs, followed by pig-

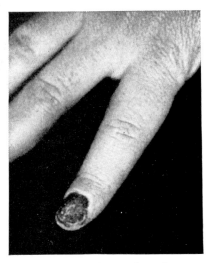

FIG. 981. Subungual melanoma. Note the pathognomonic border or halo of black pigment at the edge of the involved nail. (Pack, G. T.: Tumors of the Hands and Feet, St. Louis, Mosby)

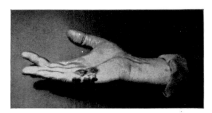

FIG. 982. Melanosarcoma of hand.

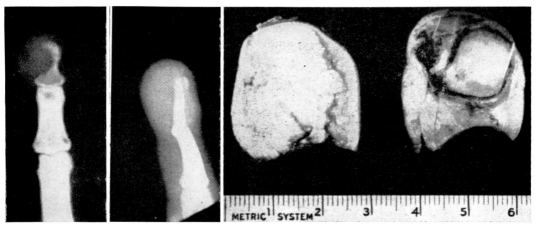

FIG. 983. (*Left*) Roentgenograms of the index finger, showing swelling of the soft tissue and destruction of the bone of the terminal phalanx. (*Right*) The distal portion of the amputated finger. At the left is a longitudinal section showing the tumor mass, which has eroded the bone. On the right, an incision has been made along the edge of the nail to show the craterlike lesion in the sulcus. (Russell, L. W.: J.A.M.A. *144*:19, 20)

mentation. The microscopic appearance of the first stage resembles a cavernous hemangioma. Following this, fusiform cells make their appearance and proliferate rapidly, sometimes resembling a fibrosarcoma. Some inflammatory reaction and round-cell infiltration are seen. This led early writers to question whether the disease was neoplastic or inflammatory. The tumor cells are believed to arise from the endothelium, and the late picture of the disease is one of invasion of every organ.

INCIDENCE. Most of the cases occur within a geographic area—from central and southeastern Europe to include Russia, northern Italy and Poland. It occurs from the 5th to the 7th decades of life and is much more common in males than in females, the incidence being approximately 20 to 1. Laborers and outdoor workers are particularly affected. Some authors report a higher incidence in Jewish people.

LOCATION. The disease is primarily in the skin and most often begins on the lower extremity. Lesions may occur on the hand as well as on any other part of the body.

SYMPTOMS. There is an occasional local pruritis. The symptoms are principally those associated with the disease in general; namely, wasting, debility and edema. Diagnosis is made by observation of the development of a typical nodule. The lesion never regresses, although

it may remain stationary for some period of time. It looks like a neoplasm in the way it extends to the adjacent skin and the subcutaneous tissues, blocking the lymphatics and producing edema. A biopsy of a lesion will confirm the diagnosis histologically. Persons suffering with this disease almost always present anemia with monocytosis.

TREATMENT. Radiation has been the best treatment for this condition. Small doses of low voltage are given as necessary. Arsenicals are also said to be of some help.

PROGNOSIS. This disease lasts from 8 months to 25 years, but it usually runs its course over a period of 5 to 10 years and is always fatal, although the patients often die of intercurrent disease.

Boeck's Sarcoid. This tumor is considered to be a disease of the reticuloendothelial system and in many respects resembles tuberculosis. The disease is manifested most commonly in the lungs, although lesions of other organs and tissues may be associated with or independent of pulmonary involvement.

The new growth is composed of epithelioid and giant cells and replaces normal tissue. On the hand, raised nodular lesions may be present in the skin. A biopsy is diagnostic. Certain bone changes may be present in the small hand bones and often are looked for as a diagnostic aid. These consist of condensation of the tra-

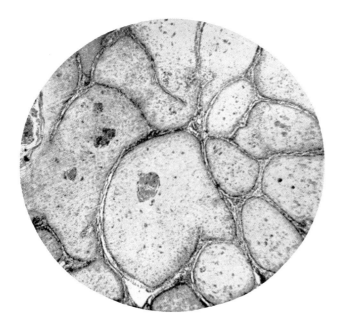

Fig. 984. High-power photomicrograph of the tissue shown in Figure 983, showing the typical picture of a squamous-cell carcinoma with cornification. (Russell, L. W.: J.A.M.A. *144*:20)

beculae of the phalanges and small cystic structures, usually near the joints.

Treatment consists mainly of supportive measures to improve the general health. X-ray therapy has been advocated by some authors. The prognosis is good, although the course of the disease may be prolonged.

MUSCLE TUMORS

Tumors of both skeletal and smooth muscle can occur in the hand, though the latter are more common.

Rhabdomyosarcomata show a predilection for the extremities, and of the 12 cases reported by Potenza and Winslow as occurring in the hand, 4 arose in the thenar eminence, 4 in the hypothenar eminence and 4 on the dorsum from the interosseus muscles. The age of the patients varied from 5 months to 35 years, and one fourth were females. All were fatal.

Credit is given to Forster in 1858 for the first published account of the solitary superficial leiomyoma.

These tumors are believed to arise from superficially situated smooth muscle as indicated by their frequency about the perineum and the nipples. In other locations such as the hand, they probably arise from vascular smooth muscle or from the erector pili muscles.

The solitary leiomyoma is generally a small tumor, well encapsulated and rounded in contour, lying just beneath the skin. It is of a firm to hard consistency.

The microscopic picture shows the smooth muscle cells to be irregularly arranged with varying amounts of interposed fibrous connective tissue and varying numbers of blood vessels.

Stout collected 95 cases including his own 15, and in this group 19 were on the upper extremity. Of his personal cases, 2 were located on the hand.

The distribution as to sex was about equal, and most of the tumors appear after the 30th year.

On the extremity, the extensor surfaces are the most usual locations, and of the 2 cases on the hand reported by Stout, 1 was on the extensor surface of the middle finger and 1 was on the extensor surface of the thumb. They may arise in the skin, or they may be subcutaneous.

Aside from the presence of the tumor, pain is the only other symptom complained of and is present in only a small proportion of cases. When pain occurs, it may amount only to local tenderness, or it may be of more severe paroxysmal type—either spontaneous or induced—and in this respect resembles the glomus tumor.

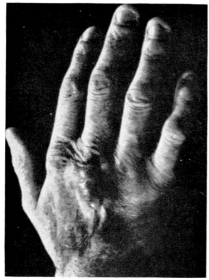

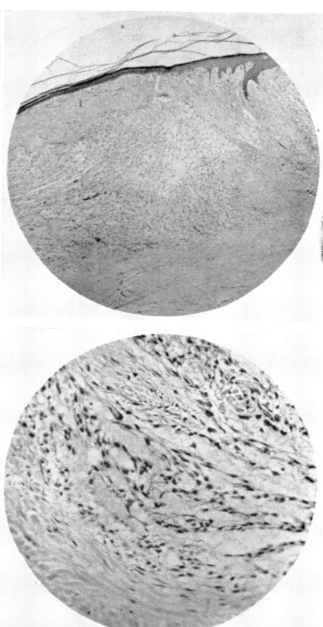

FIG. 985. (*Left*) Recurrent malignant synovioma on the dorsum of the hand after 2 operative excisions. (*Right*) Photomicrographs of sections of the removed tumor. (Crampton, R. F.: Brit. J. Plastic Surg. 4:57, 59)

The diagnosis may be difficult, since there is little to distinguish them from other small subcutaneous tumors unless the paroxysmal type of pain is present. However, they never occur subungually.

Treatment is surgical excision. The prognosis for cure is good because they are benign lesions.

SUBUNGUAL MELANOMA

Subungual melanoma, or "melanotic whitlow," is a malignant lesion requiring urgent treatment. It was first described by Jonathan Hutchinson in 1886 and is due to pre-existing inflammation. There is apparent limitation of the lesion to the distal segment of the affected digit. He described the "narrow band of black bordering the inflamed part" and called it a pathognomonic sign of the disease.

Since this time, considerable literature has accumulated on the subject, and the lesion has been given various names such as onychial melanoma, melanosarcoma, melanocarcinoma and melanoblastoma.

Etiology. Trauma has been given a prominent role as an etiologic factor, a history of such being obtained in 50 per cent of cases. In most instances there is no history of a mole prior to development of the tumor, although in some reported cases a pigment spot has been present under the nail for years. The genesis of the tumor is attributed to cells associated with the tactile end-organs of the nail bed, and for this reason many authors include it in the group of neurogenous tumors.

Pathology. The gross appearance of the tumor is that of a pigmented, fungating mass, often ulcerated, involving the sulcus of the nail and the nail matrix. There is frequently a coal-black border at the junction of the tumor with the normal tissue.

Microscopically, evidence of moderate inflammatory reaction may be present in addition to the tumor tissue. The latter is composed of 2 types of cells: one is a fusiform spindlelike cell with infrequent mitosis, hyperchromatic nuclei and both intracellular and extracellular pigment; the other is a spherical or polygonal cell in sheets or pseudo-alveolar arrangement, with more mitoses and less pigment.

Thus, the first type of cell resembles sarcoma and the second carcinoma. Although this has aroused much discussion and difference of opinion as to the actual origin of the melanin-producing cell, it is primarily of academic interest, because the tumor runs much the same clinical course regardless of its histologic appearance. There is marked variation in the amount of pigment present, ranging from no pigment to so much that the lesion has a coal-black appearance. Similarly, metastases may be pigmented or nonpigmented and occur through the lymphatic and the blood streams.

Incidence. Subungual melanomata occur in white individuals (rarely in Negroes) during the latter part of adult life. Average age is 58.7 years, according to Pack. The sex incidence is about equal. When all melanomas are considered, the incidence of the subungual type is

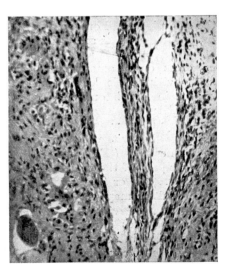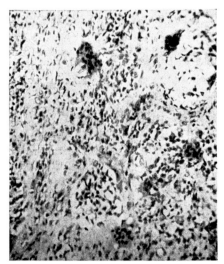

FIG. 986. (*Left*) Photomicrograph of a section of a synovioma removed from the thumb. The tissue lining the space resembles that of synovial membrane, and is of the fibrous type. (× 80) (*Right*) Photomicrograph of another portion of the growth shown in the left-hand illustration. Giant cells and foam cells are present. (× 80) King, E. S. J.: Brit. J. Surg. *18*:599)

not high, being variously reported from 1 to 3 per cent for both the hand and the foot.

Location. The tumor on the upper extremity is practically always found on the thumb and makes its appearance under the nail or protruding from the sulcus at the edge of the nail. When the tumor is present on the foot, the great toe is the usual location.

Symptoms. Although almost always associated with infection and in an ordinarily tender area, pain is never a conspicuous symptom, even in the late stages of the local disease. The patient complains principally of the presence of the lesion and of the discharge if ulceration has occurred.

Diagnosis. In the early stages, a black spot only may be noted under the fingernail. With growth of the tumor, the nail splits or is decompressed surgically and a funguslike growth makes its appearance. A common site for the tumor is the sulcus along the margin of the nail. Here it presents a granulated surface, usually with a pigmented border. Sooner or later the tumor ulcerates and weeps a thin brown fluid which stains clothing. The entire nail is lost as the lesion progresses, and some degree of infection is common. Differential diagnosis must be made from the infections that occur about the nail (these are usually acute in onset) and also from other subungual lesions such as subungual hematoma, fibroma, glomus tumor and carcinoma of the nail bed. Benign tumors do not break through the nail; therefore, this point becomes of diagnostic significance. The fungating lesion may not be pigmented. However, the narrow pigment border is usually present.

Treatment. For such a malignant lesion as a subungual melanoma, early and adequate surgery offers the only hope of cure, and most authors advise amputation well proximal to the tumor and, at a later date (approximately 2 weeks), extirpation of the regional lymph nodes. Roentgen therapy has been used, but in most instances the response is poor.

Prognosis. In general, the prognosis is poor, although the subungual melanoma offers the best chance of all the malignant melanomas for cure, due to slow growth, late dissemination and the location.

Local recurrences are common, and metastases occur along the lymphatics and in the regional lymph glands. Generalized dissemina-

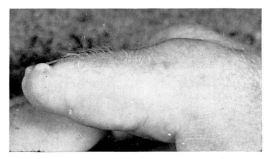

Fig. 987. A fibrillary neuroma terminates each volar digital nerve and has grown into the scar of the amputation stump, producing a visible tumor. (Wakeman, U.S. Army photograph)

tion of the tumor follows with its resulting effects. The absence of metastases at the time of treatment of the initial lesion is favorable but does not ensure a cure. Figures given by Pack for 5-year survival with no evidence of recurrence are 18.75 per cent for all subungual melanomas.

Malignant melanomas may appear elsewhere on the hand. Bickel, Meyerding and Broders, in reporting 107 cases of malignant melanoma of the extremities, noted 7 cases subungual (finger) in location, 3 cases arising elsewhere on the fingers, and 2 cases arising from other locations on the hand.

The pathology, the course and the treatment are essentially those outlined for the subungual variety.

CARCINOMA OF NAIL

This neoplasm is of extremely infrequent occurrence. Up to 1939, 19 cases were reported in the literature, 13 of which were on the hand. Since then Ellis has reported 3 cases, and Russell and Branson each 1 case. The lesion is distinguished from the malignant melanoma described elsewhere.

Most cases report a history of trauma or infection which is resistant to treatment. Silverman reports a case following a chronic paronychia of over 1 year's duration on the thumb. Pardo-Castello records the origin of the condition in association with Bowen's disease.

This squamous cell epithelioma arises from the nail bed or groove and is of prickle-cell type. As a rule, it is of low-grade malignancy,

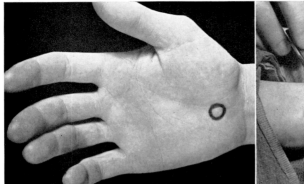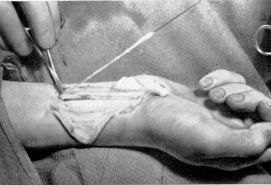

FIG. 998. (*Left*) Ink outline of a palpable but not visible tumor overlying the deep carpal ligament. The tumor is firm, round and slightly tender on pressure. (*Right*) Same tumor at operation, showing its origin from the palmar branch of the median nerve. Microscopic study showed proliferating nerve sheath cells and myxomatous connective tissue surrounded by a well-developed fibrous capsule. The diagnosis is neurilemmoma (benign nerve sheath tumor). (Wakeman, U.S. Army photographs)

involves the structures locally and may even invade or erode the bone.

The commonest site is on the thumb, and the next commonest on the index finger. The right side is involved more frequently than the left.

Symptoms and Diagnosis. Pain is usually a symptom, since the lesion is expanding in a tender area. This seems to be in contrast with the symptoms of melanotic whitlow.

The diagnosis is based on the appearance of a wartylike growth in the sulcus of the nail. It resembles a chronic paronychia which is resistant to treatment. Ellis emphasizes the frequency of bone destruction by direct invasion as disclosed by x-ray examination.

The treatment of this condition is amputation. Mason advises amputation and dissection of the glands in the axilla.

The prognosis for cure is good. There is seldom a recurrence unless metastasis has occurred already.

TENDON-SHEATH TUMORS—SYNOVIA

This specialized connective-tissue structure lines all open joints, with the exception of the articular surfaces, and forms the lining of tendon sheaths. Therefore, tumors that arise from the synovia occur in the joints and the sheaths. Most develop from the tendon sheaths. They may be benign or malignant.

Much confusion is apparent as to the nature of these tumors. King attempts to clarify the subject by stressing that most authors classify the tumor by the predominating cell, when in reality—since these tumors all arise from the synovia—the basic cell is the same, and their variable gross and microscopic appearance is due to cell structures closely associated with the tissues underlying the true synovial covering. Thus, such terms as angioma, arborizing lipoma, endothelioma, myeloma, fibroma, chondroma, etc., of the tendon sheaths appear in the literature.

The synovial cell is a modified connective-tissue cell of mesodermal origin and is spindle or spheroidal in shape. In certain instances, transition to cartilage cells or even bone cells is not uncommon and evidences its potentialities. Projections of synovial membrane, as a result of inflammation or infection, occur, forming villi in tendon sheaths. These villi are covered by synovial cells, but their internal structure takes on the character of the underlying tissues in that region. When tumors form, the type cell of the synovia is always present, and within the tumor spaces appear which are lined with synovia. The outward appearance varies in accordance with the other cells present, accounting for the wide diversity of forms. The term "sarcoma" is properly applied to the malignant form of the tumor.

Haagensen and Stout in 1944 reported on synovial sarcoma, and their series included 3

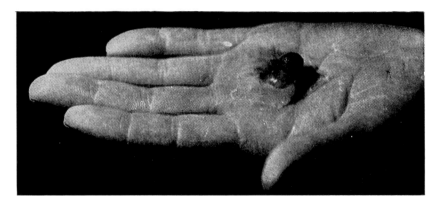

Fig. 989. Granuloma pyogenicum: sessile and pedunculated growths. They were removed by surgical excision, an undesirable scar resulting. (Michelson, H. E.: Arch. Dermat. & Syph. *12*:498)

of the hand, 4 of the fingers and 4 about the wrist. They stated that this malignant tumor is slightly more common in males than in females and usually occurs in early adult life. Pain is an early symptom in contrast with the benign form, and, while the early course of the disease may be chronic, metastasis occurs sooner or later through the blood and the lymph streams. In 1951, 2 cases of synovial sarcoma in the hand were reported in the literature. One occurred on the dorsum, the other in the palm. Both had recurred after local removal. Although apparently rare in the hand, the possibility of this malignant type of synovioma must be kept constantly in mind.

Pathology. The pathology of synoviomas is characterized by the diversity of cell forms,

and many sections through the tumor are needed to show all types of cells present. The synovial type of cell is always present, and spaces in the tumor so lined generally can be found. In addition, there may be fibrous tissue, cartilage, foam cells, giant cells and fatty tissue which appear in variable amounts and arrangement with one or another type of cell predominating, leading to a specific name for that particular tumor. The giant cells of foreign-body type and the foam cells characteristic of the xanthoma may be present in abundance and are almost always present in some degree. The xanthomas of the tendon sheaths and the joints which have been described separately probably represent one variant of this group. In the malignant forms of the

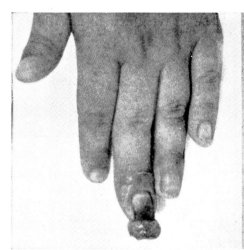
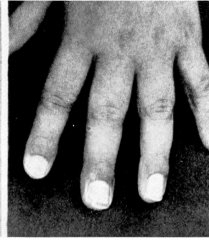

Fig. 990. Pyogenic granuloma (*left*) before and (*right*) after radiation therapy. (Pack, G. T.: Tumors of the Hands and Feet, St. Louis, Mosby)

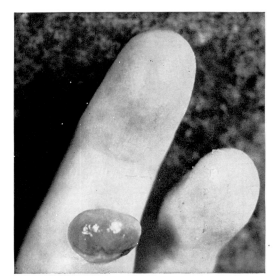

FIG. 991. Pyogenic granuloma which developed in the flexion crease of a finger following a burn. Cured by excision and cauterization of the base with silver nitrate and splinting the finger until healed. (Wakeman, U.S. Army photograph)

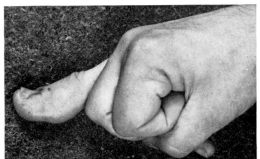

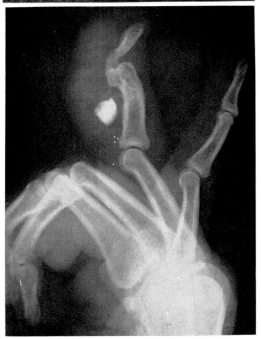

FIG. 992. Tumor of the finger due to a foreign-body granuloma. (*Bottom*) Roentgenogram of the tumor, showing a single large metallic foreign body and other finely divided foreign material which casts a faint shadow. At operation, amputation was necessary due to the extensive spread of fine foreign bodies throughout the soft parts. (Wakeman, U.S. Army photograph)

synovioma, the spindlelike cells are densely packed and have round or ovoid nuclei with numerous mitotic figures. In gross appearance the benign tumors are generally soft and lobulated, extending a variable distance up and down the sheath; they may become adherent at numerous points. In contrast, the malignant synovioma rarely projects into a joint or a sheath but invades the surrounding structures. Benign forms do not show the invasive tendency of the malignant variety. In color the tumors are most commonly grayish-white but have a light to dark-yellowish tint if fat or xanthoma cells predominate.

Symptoms. Because these are slow-growing tumors as a rule, they do not give rise to much in the way of symptoms until they have become of considerable size. Then they may interfere with motion or appear as visible swellings on the hand.

Diagnosis may be difficult but usually can be made on the basis of the physical examination. The tumor may follow along the course of one of the tendons for a variable distance, or it may remain localized. Some interference with function may be present.

Treatment. The benign forms of synovioma can be removed locally with good results if a careful and complete operation is performed. Like other tumors, they are prone to recur. In the malignant forms early amputation is advisable. The site of amputation can be judged most satisfactorily by the surgeon at the time of operation.

The prognosis is good for the benign forms, but the malignant synoviomas tend to recur locally and metastasize readily through the blood or the lymph channels.

PERIPHERAL NERVE TUMORS

The best basis for a study of these tumors is a knowledge of the histologic elements of a peripheral nerve with recognition of the fact that tumors may arise from each element or from combinations of elements. Present in a peripheral nerve are the neuraxon, which may give rise to fibrillary neuromas, and the sheath structures, including the sheath of Schwann and the connective-tissue endoneurium, which may give rise to several types of new growths classed as tumors of the nerve sheath. In addition to the nerve fibers and their sheaths, specialized end-organs of nerves are present, and tumors arising or believed to arise from these end-organs are also classed as nerve tumors.

Sometimes included in this group are the glomus tumors, melanosarcomata or carcinomata, some types of xanthomata and the leiomyomata.

Fibrillary Neuromas. The most commonly encountered neuroma in the hand is that resulting from traumatic injury or severance of a peripheral nerve. Foot calls this tangle of neuraxons and sheath cells a false fibrillary neuroma, and states that some authors are hesitant about classifying neuromas with true tumors. They result from the efforts of the severed nerve ends to reunite.

The etiology is always clear, since there is a history of injury which involves one or more of the peripheral nerves. The gross pathologic picture is that of a bulbous termination of the proximal end of a severed nerve, or a bulbous enlargement of a nerve at the point of injury. These tumors are encapsulated unless they are buried in dense scar. Microscopically, all elements of the nerve are seen in one tangled mass.

The symptoms are tenderness and pain, the latter being shocklike or burning in nature and referred over the course of the sensory distribution of the nerve. Small neuromata of the sensory branches of the radial nerve in the hand are particularly bothersome.

The diagnosis of these traumatic neuromata is based on the history, the local signs of neuroma, often including the palpable tumor, and the area of disturbed cutaneous sensation. Treatment is discussed under nerve suture, but when this cannot be accomplished —as in amputation stumps—resection of the neuroma is advisable. The prognosis in general is good, although some cases prove to be refractory.

True fibrillary neuromata, as contrasted with the post-traumatic type discussed above, have been described as enlargements in excess to need of peripheral nerves. They may be localized areas in a nerve, or they may form plexiform structures. When they involve the deeper nerves they are sometimes associated with localized hypertrophy of a part (elephantiasis nervorum). They are usually considered to be congenital in origin.

Nerve-Sheath Tumors. In this group are numerous, small, usually benign tumors which occur in the hand.

Various classifications of these tumors have been suggested. Geschickter advises that they be grouped on the basis of their differentiation, and this method is as practical as any.

The well-differentiated forms show varying degrees of fibrosis, and the type cell has a small nucleus with peripherally located chromatin, the cytoplasm being abundant and syncytial. They are well encapsulated and generally occur on the flexor surface of the upper extremity in the subcutaneous tissue where they are attached to a peripheral nerve branch, often in the vicinity of a flexion crease. Most cases appear in the age period of 30 to 50 years. They are usually symptomless and do not often become malignant, so that they are cured readily by surgical removal. The term neurilemmoma has been suggested for them.

The less-differentiated forms, characterized histologically by a loose reticular structure, spindle cells and considerable myxomatous tissue, are not encapsulated and occur most frequently in the subepidermis or deep along the main nerve trunks.

The subepidermal types are quite common and may be multiple. They vary in form and appearance, and removal of some tumors of this type often is sought for cosmetic reasons. In general, they are called neurofibromata and include the multiple neurofibromata of von Recklinghausen.

The more deeply situated tumors are present along nerve trunks and involve the nerve to varying degrees. They are poorly demarcated from the surrounding structure, grow fast and are prone to recurrence and malignant degeneration. In contrast with the well-differentiated types, they may occur in young individuals.

In the series reported by Geschickter, 30 per cent recurred, and of these half became malignant. Fortunately, they do not occur frequently in the hand.

Neurogenous sarcoma may arise from any of the nerve-sheath tumors but most frequently develop in the poorly differentiated types. Histologically, they show bundles of interlacing plump spindle cells with frequent mitoses and tumor giant cells. They are highly malignant and invasive, extending up and down the course of the nerve. They are prone to occur in the 3rd and the 4th decades, and the only satisfactory treatment is prompt and radical amputation. It has been reported that in 13 per cent of the cases of von Recklinghausen's disease one or more of the tumors undergo malignant degeneration.

The differential diagnosis of all forms of nerve-sheath tumors necessitates consideration of many other varieties of tumors. The superficial ones may be confused with fibroma or lipoma, while the deeper ones may resemble ganglion, xanthoma, synovioma and other tumors. In general, the incidence of correct preoperative diagnosis is low except in cases which show dysfunction of a specific nerve.

BIBLIOGRAPHY

TUMORS OF THE HAND IN GENERAL

Butler, E. D.: Tumors of the hand, a ten-year survey and report of 437 cases, Am. J. Surg. *100*:293, 1960.

Düben, W.: Tumors of the hand, Chirug. *31*:494, 1960.

Mason, M. L.: Tumors of the hand, Surg., Gynec. Obstet. *64*:129, 1937.

Pack, G. T.: Tumors of the Hands and Feet, St. Louis, Mosby, 1939.

Posch, J. L.: Tumors, J. Bone Joint Surg. *38-A*: 517, 562, 1956.

Stack, H. G.: Tumors of the hand, Brit. M. J. *1*:919, 1960.

SPECIAL TUMORS

Epidermoid Cysts

Carroll, R. E.: Epidermoid (epithelial) cyst of the hand skeleton, Am. J. Surg. *85*:327, 1953.

Dolce, F. A., and Clark, R. L.: Epithelial cysts (of hand), N.Y. J. Med. *44*:2358, 1944.

Galli, G., and Davalli, C.: Intraosseous epithelial cysts of phalanges, Chir. org. movimento *42*· 50, 1955.

Kelly, A. P., Jr., and Clifford, R. H.: Epidermoid cysts of bony phalanges, Plast. Reconstr. Surg *17*:309, 1956.

King, E. S. J.: Post-traumatic epidermoid cysts of hands and fingers, Brit. J. Surg. *21*:29, 1933

Kotcamp, W. W., and Cesarno, F. L.: Epidermoid cyst of the terminal phalanx of the finger; report of a case, J. Bone Joint Surg. *44-A*:377 1962.

Oehlecker, F.: Beitrag zur traumatischen Epithelcyste der Lingerendphalanx, Mschr. Unfallheilk. *55*:332, 1952.

Pohlman, H. F., and Wachstein, M.: Epidermoid (squamous epithelial bone cysts of phalanx, Ann. Surg. *119*:148, 1944.

Wien, M. S., and Caro, M. R.: Traumatic epithelial cysts of skin, J.A.M.A. *102*:197, 1934.

Yachnin, S. C., and Summerill, F.: Traumatic implantation of epithelial cyst in a phalanx, J.A.M.A. *116*:1215, 1941.

Mucous Cysts

Anderson, C. R.: Longitudinal grooving of nails caused by synovial lesions, Arch. Dermat. Syphilol. *55*:828, 1947.

Arner, O., Lindholm, A., and Romanus, R.: Mucous cysts of fingers; 26 cases, Acta chir. scand. *111*:314, 1956.

Gross, R. E.: Recurring myxomatous cutaneous cysts of fingers and toes, Surg., Gynec. Obstet. *65*:289, 1937.

King, E. S. J.: Mucous cysts of the finger, Aust. New Zeal. J. Surg. *21*:121, 1951.

MacKee, G. M., and Andrews, G. C.: Pathologic histology of synovial lesions of skin, Arch. Dermat. Syph. *5*:561, 1922.

Montgomery, D. W., and Culver, G. D.: Pathologic anatomy of synovial lesions of skin, Arch. Dermat. Syph. *5*:329, 1922.

Ormsby, O. S.: Synovial lesions of skin, J. Cutan. Dis. *31*:943, 1913.

Stecher, R. M., and Houser, H.: Heberden's nodes, Am. J. Roentgenol. *59*:326, 1948.

Ganglia

Carp, L., and Stout, A. P.: Study of ganglion with especial reference to treatment (with references from 1746 to 1928), Surg., Gynec. Obstet. *47*:460, 1928.

DeOrsay, R. H., McCray, P. M., and Ferguson, L. K: Pathology and treatment of ganglion, Am. J. Surg. *36*:313, 1937.

Kaplan, E. B.: Treatment of ganglion by injection of sodium morrhuate, Am. J. Surg. *34*:151, 1934.

King, E. S. J.: The pathology of ganglion, Aust. New Zeal. J. Surg. *1*:367, 1932.

Lyle, F. M.: Radiation treatment of ganglia of wrist and hand, J. Bone Joint Surg. *26*:162, 1941.

McEvedy, B. V.: The simple ganglion, Lancet *1*:135, 1954.

Meyer, M.: Über das Ganglion, Helv. chir. acta *17*:155, 1950.

Seddon, H. J.: Carpal ganglion as a cause of paralysis of the deep branch of the ulnar nerve, J. Bone Joint Surg. *34-B*:386, 1952.

Sonnenschein, A.: Zur Pathologie und Therapie der Ganglien, Med. klin. Berlin *48*:1431, 1953.

Woodburne, A. R.: Myxomatous degeneration cysts of skin and subcutaneous tissue, Arch. Dermat. Syph. *56*:407, 1947.

Fibromas

Compere, E L.: Bilateral snapping thumbs, Ann. Surg. *97*:773, 1933.

Keasbey, L. E.: Juvenile aponeurotic fibroma (calcifying fibroma), Cancer *6*:338, 1953.

Kyle, B. H.: Ossifying fibroma—thenar space, Virginia Med. Monthly *68*:165, 1941.

Levinthal, D. H., and Kirschbaum, J. D.: Fibroma of middle metacarpal bone, Surg., Gynec. Obst. *68*:936, 1939.

Whitesides, T. E., and Ackerman, L. V.: Desmoplastic fibroma, J. Bone Joint Surg. *42-A*:1143, 1960.

Lipomas

Bosch, D. T., and Bernhard, W. G.: Lipoma of palm, Am. J. Clin. Path. *20*:262, 1950.

Straus, F. H.: Deep lipomas of hand, Ann. Surg. *94*:269, 1931.

Strauss, A.: Lipoma of tendon sheaths, Surg., Gynec. Obstet. *35*:161, 1922.

Sullivan, C. R., Dahlin, D. C., and Bryan, R. S.: Lipoma of the tendon sheath, J. Bone Joint Surg. *38-A*:1275, 1956.

White, J. F.: Arborescent lipoma of tendon sheaths, Surg., Gynec. Obstet. *38*:489, 1924.

White, W. L., and Hanna, D. C.: Troublesome lipomata of the upper extremity, J. Bone Joint Surg. *44-A*:1353, 1962.

Xanthomas

Galloway, J. D. B., Broders, A. C., and Ghormley, R. K.: Xanthoma of tendon sheaths and synovial membranes—a clinical and pathologic study, Arch. Surg. *40*:485, 1940.

Mason, M. L., and Woolston, W. H.: Isolated giant cell xanthomatous tumors of fingers and hands, Arch. Surg. *15*:499, 1927.

Miller, C.: Angina pectoris in hereditary xanthomatosis, Arch. Int. Med. *64*:675, 1939.

Phalen, G. S., McCormack, L. J., and Gazale, W. J.: Giant-cell tumor of the tendon sheath (benign synovioma) in the hand, evaluation of 56 cases, Clin. Orthop. *15*:140, 1959.

Stevenson, T. W.: Xanthoma and giant cell tumor of the hand, J. Plast. Reconstr. Surg. *5*:75, 1950.

Stewart, M. J.: Benign giant-cell synovioma and its relation to "xanthoma," J. Bone Joint Surg. *30-B*:522, 1948.

Weber, F. P.: Cutaneous xanthoma and xanthomatosis of other parts of the body, Brit. J. Dermat. *36*:335, 1924.

Tendon-Sheath Tumors

Anderson, K. J., and Wildermuth, O.: Synovial sarcoma, Clin. Orthop. *19*:55. 1961.

Berger, L.: Synovial sarcomas in serous bursae and tendon sheaths, Am. J. Cancer *34*:501, 1938.

Briggs. C. D.: Malignant tumors of synovial origin, Ann. Surg. *115*:413, 1942.

Bussebaum, G.: A contribution on inflammatory tumors presenting the picture of malignant tumors. with a consideration of so-called giant cell sarcoma of tendon sheaths, Halle-Wietenberg, Dissertation, 1935; abstract Surg., Gynec. Obstet. *62*, 1936.

Buxton, St. J. D.: Tumours of tendon and tendon sheaths, Brit. J. Surg. *10*:469, 1923.

Cramptom, R. F.: Malignant synovioma of the hand, Brit. J. Plast. Surg. *4*:56, 1951.

DeSanto, D. A., Tennant, R., and Rosahn, P. O.: Synovial sarcoma in joints, bursae and tendon sheaths; clinical and pathologic study of 16 cases, Surg., Gynec. Obst. *72*:951, 1941.

Foster, L. N.: The benign giant cell tumor of tendon sheaths, Am. J. Path. *23*:567, 1947.

Geiler, G.: Die Synovialome, Morphologie und Pathogenese, Berlin, Springer, 1961.

Haagensen, C. D., and Stout, A. P.: Synovial sarcoma, Ann. Surg. *120*:826, 1944.

King, E. S. J.: Malignant tumors of tendon sheaths, Aust. New Zeal. J. Surg. *10*:338, 1941.

Lewis, D.: Tumors of the tendon sheaths, Surg., Gynec. Obst. *59*:344, 1934.

McShane, K. L.: Malignant synovioma of the hand, J. Int. Coll. Surg. *15*:373, 1951.

Morton, J. J.: Tumors of tendon sheaths; their close biological relationship to tumors of joints and bursae, Surg., Gynec. Obstet. *59*:441, 1934.

Ragins, A. B., and Shively, B. S.: Further observations on benign tumors of the tendon sheath, Ann. Surg. *109*:632, 1939.

Schnepper, E., and Menges, G.: The diagnosis, clinical picture, and treatment of synovioma,

Langenbeck Arch. klin. Chir. *297*:147, 1961.

Shepherd, J. A.: Osteochondromata of tendon sheaths, Brit. J. Surg. *30*:179, 1942.

Stewart, M. G.: Benign giant cell synovioma and its relation to "xanthoma," J. Bone Joint Surg. *30-B*:522, 1948.

Strauss, A.: Lipoma of the tendon sheaths; with report of a case and review of the literature, Surg., Gynec. Obstet. *35*:161, 1922.

Tumors of Nerves

Cutler, E. C., and Gross, R. E.: Surgical treatment of tumors of peripheral nerves, Ann. Surg. *104*:436, 1936.

Foot, N. C.: Histology of tumors of the peripheral nerves, Arch. Path. *30*:772, 1940.

Geschickter, C. F.: Tumors of peripheral nerves, Am. J. Cancer *25*:377, 1935.

Grant, G. H.: Methods of treatment of neuromata of the hand, J. Bone Joint Surg. *33-A*:841, 1951.

Patterson, T. J. S.: Pacinian corpuscle neuroma of thumb pulp, Brit. J. Plast. Surg. *9*:230, 1956.

Penfield, W.: The encapsulated tumors of the nervous system; meningeal fibroblastomata, perineural fibroblastomata, and neurofibromata of von Recklinghausen, Surg., Gynec. Obstet. *45*:178, 1927.

Stout, A. P.: The peripheral manifestations of the specific nerve sheath tumor (neurilemmoma), Am. J. Cancer *24*:751, 1935.

Aneurysm

Curtis, R. M.: Congenital arteriovenous fistulae of the hand, J. Bone Joint Surg. *35-A*:917, 1953.

David, V. C.: Aneurysms of hand, Arch. Surg. *33*:267, 1936.

Horton, B. T., and Ghormley, R. K.: Congenital arteriovenous fistulas of extremities "visualized" by arteriography, Surg., Gynec. Obstet. *60*:978, 1935.

White, J. A.: A case of congenital multiple arteriovenous fistulae of the hand, Brit. J. Surg. *34*:209, 1946.

Angioma

Geschickter, C. F., and Keasbey, L. E.: Tumors of blood vessels, Am. J. Cancer *23*:568, 1935.

Thomas, A.: Vascular tumors of bone; pathological and clinical study of 27 cases, Surg., Gynec. Obstet. *74*:777, 1942.

Lymphangiectasis

Mason, P. B., and Allen, E. V.: Congenital lymphangiectasis (lymphedema), Am. J. Dis. Child. *50*:945, 1935.

Glomus Tumors

Blanchard, A. J.: The pathology of glomus tumors, Canad. M. A. J. *44*:357, 1941.

Lattes, R., and Bull, D. C.: A case of glomus tumor with primary involvement of bone, Ann. Surg. *127*:187, 1948.

Lewis, T., and Pickering, G. W.: Vasodilatation in the limbs in response to warming the body with evidence for sympathetic vasodilator nerves in man, Heart *16*:33, 1931.

Love, J. G.: Glomus tumors, diagnosis and treatment, Proc. Mayo Clinic *19*:113, 1944.

Mason, M. L., and Weil, A.: Tumor of subcutaneous glomus, Surg., Gynec. Obstet. *58*:807, 1934.

Murray, R. M., and Stout, A. P.: The glomus tumor; investigation of its distribution and behavior and identity of its "epithelioid" cell, Am. J. Path. *18*:183, 1942.

Ottley, C. M.: Glomus tumour, Brit. J. Surg. *29*:387, 1942.

Pietrabissa, G.: Multiple intraosseous glomus tumors of phalanges of hand; case, Minerva ortop. *7*:458, 1956.

Plewes, B.: Multiple glomus tumors; four in one finger tip, Canad. M. A. J. *44*:364, 1941.

Radasch, H. E.: Glomal tumors, Arch. Path. *23*:615, 1937.

Riddell, D. H., and Martin, R. S.: Glomus tumor of unusual size, Ann. Surg. *133*:401, 1951.

Stout, A. P.: Tumors of the neuromyo-arterial glomus, Am. J. Cancer *24*:255, 1935.

Subungual Melanoma

Bickel, W. H., Meyerding, H. W., and Broders, A. C.: Melanoepithelioma (melanosarcoma, melanocarcinoma, and malignant melanoma) of the extremities, Surg., Gynec. Obstet. *76*:570, 1943.

Engman, M. F., Mook, W. H., and Engman, M. F., Jr.: Melanotic whitlow, Arch. Dermat. & Syph. *23*:1174, 1931.

Lausecker, H.: Melanosarkom der Hohlhand, Der Hautarzt *4*:81, 1953.

Scannell, R. C.: Subungual melanoma, Am. J. Surg. *53*:163, 1941.

Womack, N. A.: Subungual melanoma; Hutchinson's melanotic whitlow, Arch. Surg. *15*:667, 1927.

Carcinoma of Nail

Branson, T. W., *et al.*: Secondary carcinoma of the phalanges, Radiology *57*:864, 1951.

Ellis, V. H.: Squamous-celled carcinoma of the nail bed, J. Bone Joint Surg. *30-B*:656, 1948.

Levine, J., and Lisa, J. R.: Primary carcinoma of the nail, Arch. Surg. *38*:107, 1939.

Pardo-Castello, V.: Diseases of Nails, pp. 47-50, Springfield, Ill., Thomas, 1936.

Russell, L. W.: Primary carcinoma of the nail, J.A.M.A. *144*:19, 1950.

Silverman, I.: Epithelioma following chronic paronychia, Am. J. Surg. *29*:141, 1935.

Carcinoma

Adair, F. E.: Epitheliomas of hand: Type and treatment, Surg. Clin. N. Amer. *13*:423, 1933.

Bick, E. M.: Primary carcinoma of the extremities, Am. Surg. *102*:410, 1936.

Braddon, P. D.: Treatment of carcinoma on dorsum of the hand, Med. J. Australia *1*:368, 1944.

Caulfield, P. A.: Common premalignant and malignant lesions of the hand *in* Symposium on the diagnosis and treatment of premalignant conditions, Surg. Clin. N. Amer. *30*:1675, 1950.

Clark, P. J., and Johnson, T. M.: Epidermoid carcinoma of the hand, J. Kansas M. A. *49*:100, 1948.

DeBell, P. J., and Stevenson, T. D.: Squamous cell epithelioma of the extremities, Surg., Gynec. Obstet. *63*:222, 1936.

Handley, W. S.: The treatment of x-ray carcinoma and x-ray dermatitis, Lancet *1*:120, 1934.

Johnson, R. E., and Ackerman, L. V.: Epidermoid carcinoma of the hand, Cancer *3*:657, 1950.

Mason, M. L.: Carcinoma of hand, Arch. Surg. *18*:2107, 1929.

Schreiner, B. F., and Wehr, W. H.: Primary new growths involving the hand, Am. J. Roentgenol. *32*:516, 1934.

Bone Tumors

Bell, J. L., and Mason, M. L.: Metastatic tumors of the hand, Quart. Bull. Northwest. Univ. Med. Sch. *27*:114, 1953.

Carroll, R. E., Godwin, J. T., and Watson, W. L.: Osteogenic sarcoma of phalanx after chronic roentgen-ray irradiation, Cancer *9*:753, 1956.

Coley, B. L.: Neoplasms of Bone, ed. 2, New York, Hoeber, 1960.

Dahlin, D. C.: Bone Tumors, Springfield, Ill., Thomas, 1957.

Freni, D. R., and Averill, J. H.: Metastatic carcinoma of the lung to the thumb, Am. J. Surg. *83*:115, 1952.

Gatewood: Enchondroma of hand, Surg. Clinics, Chicago *3*:1199, 1919.

Geschickter, C. F.: Roentgenologic diagnosis of bone tumors, Radiology *16*:111, 1931.

Greene, M. H.: Metastasis of pulmonary carcinoma to the phalanges of the hand, J. Bone Joint Surg. *39-A*:972, 1957.

Guy, R., Langevin, R., Raymond, O., and Martineau, G.: Phalangeal aneurysmal bone cyst, Union Med. Canada *86*:866, 1957.

Jaffe, H.: Tumors and Tumorous Conditions of Bones and Joints, Philadelphia, Lea & Febiger, 1958.

Karten, I., and Bartfeld, H.: Bronchogenic carcinoma simulating early rheumatoid arthritis; metastases to the fingers, J.A.M.A. *179*:162, 1962.

Kerin, R.: Metastatic tumors of the hand, J. Bone Joint Surg. *40-A*:263, 1958.

Lichtenstein, L.: Bone Tumors, ed. 2, St. Louis, Mosby, 1959.

Strong, R.: Phalangeal metastasis of bronchogenic carcinoma, first sign, Brit. J. Surg. *39*:372, 1952.

Bone Cysts

Coley, B. L., and Higinbotham, N. L.: Solitary bone cyst, Ann. Surg. *99*:432, 1934.

Freund, E.: The use of bone chips in the treatment of localized osteitis fibrosa, J. Bone Joint Surg. *19*:36, 1937.

Platt, H.: Cysts of the long bones of the hands and feet, Brit. J. Surg. *18*:20, 1930.

Exostoses

Probstein, J. G., and Brooks, B.: Subungual exostoses, J. Missouri M. A. *21*:211, 1925.

Cartilage Tumors

Geschickter, C. F., and Copeland, M. M.: Tumors of Bone, ed. 3, Philadelphia, Lippincott, 1949.

Heiple, K. G.: Carpal osteochondroma, J. Bone Joint Surg. *43-A*:861, 1961.

Jakobson, E., and Spjut, H. J.: Chondrosarcoma of bones of hand, Acta radiol. *54*:426, 1960.

Kyle, B. H., and Mundy, B. K.: Multiple osteochondromata of hand, Virginia Med. Monthly *79*:36, 1952.

Lausche, W. F., and Spjut, H. J.: Chondrosarcoma of the small bones of the hand, J. Bone Joint Surg. *40-A*:1139, 1958.

Sbarbaro, J. L., Jr., and Straub, L. R.: Chondrosarcoma in a phalanx; report of a case, Am. J. Surg. *100*:751, 1960.

Shellito, J. G., and Dockerty, M. B.: Cartilaginous tumors of the hand, Surg., Gynec. Obstet. *86*:465, 1948.

Xanthoma of Bone

Cole, W. H.: Giant cell tumor involving phalanges, Ann. Surg. *83*:328, 1936.

Goldner, J. L., and Forrest, J. S.: Giant cell tumor of bone, South. Med. J. *54*:14, 1961.

Meyerding, H. W., and Johnson, R. E.: Benign giant cell tumors, Surg. Clin. N. Amer. *30*:1201, 1950.

Platt, H.: Cysts of long bones of hands and feet, Brit. J. Surg. *18*:20, 1930.

Osteoid Osteoma

Carroll, R. E.: Osteoid osteoma in the hand, J. Bone Joint Surg. *35-A*:888, 1953.

Dunitz, N. L., Lipscomb, P. R., and Ivins, J. C.: Osteoma, osteoid, of the hand and wrist, Am. J. Surg. *93*:65, 1957.

Jaffe, H. L.: Osteoid osteoma, Arch. Surg. *31*: 709, 1935.

Jaffe, H. L., and Mayer, L.: An osteoblastic osteoid tissue forming tumor of a metacarpal bone, Arch. Surg. *24*:550, 1932.

Moberg, E.: Further observations on "cortical-isosteoide" or "osteoid osteoma," Acta radiol. *38*:279, 1952.

Ponsetti, I., and Barta, C. K.: Osteoid osteoma, J. Bone Joint Surg. *29*:767, 1947.

Osteogenic Sarcoma

Carroll, R. E.: Osteogenic sarcoma in the hand, J. Bone Joint Surg. *39-A*:325, 1957.

Clark, C. E.: Osteogenic sarcoma of the finger, Am. J. Surg. *83*:112, 1952.

Drompp, B. W.: Bilateral osteosarcoma in phalanges, case report, J. Bone Joint Surg. *43-A*: 199, 1961.

Kolodny, A.: Bone sarcoma; primary malignant tumors of bone and giant cell tumor, Surg., Gynec. Obstet. *44*:1, 1927.

Lichtenstein, L., and Jaffe, H. L.: Chondrosarcoma of bone, Am. J. Path. *19*:553, 1943.

Olson, A. E.: Sarcoma of second metacarpal bone, Minnesota Med. *17*:24, 1934.

Sarcomas

Brick, E. M.: Fibrosarcoma of the extremities, Ann. Surg. *101*:759, 1935.

————: Fibroblastic tumors of the extremities, Arch. Surg. *35*:841, 1937.

Carrol, G. A., and Martin, T. M.: Fibrosarcoma of the extremities, Surg. Clin. N. Amer. *24*: 1220, 1944.

Heller, E. L., and Sieber, W. K.: Fibrosarcoma: A clinical and pathological study of 60 cases, Surgery *27*:539, 1950.

Kleinberg, S.: Soft tissue sarcoma of the hand, Bull. Hosp. Joint Dis. *9*:81, 1948.

Meyerding, H. W., Broders, A. C., and Hargrove, R. L.: Clinical aspects of fibrosarcoma of the extremities, Surg., Gynec. Obstet. *62*:1010, 1936.

Snedecor, S. T.: Sarcomata of the hand subsequent to trauma, J. Bone Joint Surg. *25*:907, 1943.

Stout, A. P.: Fibrosarcoma, the malignant tumor of fibroblasts, Cancer *1*:30, 1948.

————: Sarcomas of the soft tissues, CA *2*:210, 1961.

Wilson, D. A.: Tumors of the subcutaneous tissue and fascia, Surg., Gynec. Obstet. *80*:500, 1945.

Kaposi's Sarcoma

Aegerter, E. E., and Peale, A. R.: Kaposi's sarcoma; a critical survey, Arch. Path. *34*:413, 1942.

MacKee, G. M., and Cipollaro, A. C.: Idiopathic multiple hemorrhagic sarcoma (Kaposi), Am. J. Cancer *26*:1, 1936.

Muscle Tumors

Potenza, A., and Winslow, D.: Rhabdomyosarcoma of the hand, J. Bone Joint Surg. *43-A*: 700, 1961.

Stout, A. P.: Solitary cutaneous and subcutaneous leiomyoma, Am. J. Cancer *29*:435, 1937.

Thompson, G. C. V.: Rhabdomyosarcoma of skeletal muscle, Clin. Orthop. *19*:29, 1961.

Sweat Gland

Potter, C. M.: Pleomorphic tumor of sweat gland in hand, J. Bone Joint Surg. *39-B*:102, 1957.

Index

Abduction, index finger, by tendon transfer, 507
    transfer of proprius, 505
Aberrant tendon, thumb, 473
Abnormalities, arteriovenous, congenital, 93
Abscess, subcutaneous, 669
Absence, congenital, of radius, 62
    treatment, 70
Achondroplasia, 51
Acromioclavicular dislocation, 578
Acromioclavicular separation, 568
Acrosyndactylism, 87
Actinomycosis, 693
Adaptation, hand in animals, 42-45
  weight-bearing of arm, 33
Adduction contracture, thumb, 536
Adduction, thumb, in cerebral palsy, 395
    loss of, 511
    restoration of, 511
    tendon transfers for, 515
Adherence of tendons, diagnosis of level of lesion,
    108-109
  effect on motion, 108
Age, as factor in treatment of congenital deformities, 94
Aims of reconstruction of hand, 122
Ambiguity in records, how to avoid it, 112
Amelia, types, 60
Amphibia, intrinsic muscles, 28
Amplitude of tendons, 12-15
  digits, 14-15
  importance in tendon transfers, 441
  method of increasing, 15
  wrist, 14
Amputation(s), 616-624
  arm, for brachial plexus lesions, 574
  cineplastic, 623
  congenital, 622
  finger tips, 618
  forearm, 620
  general considerations, 616
  index finger, 619
  for infection, 684
  Krukenberg, 621
  levels, 618
  little finger, 619
  megalodactylia, 93
  metacarpals, 620
  middle and ring fingers, 618

Amputation(s)—(*Cont.*)
  painful stump, 706
  radiocarpal joint, 620
  skin flaps, 616
  special tissues, 616
  thumb, 620
  in treatment of mirror hand, 79
  treatment of neuromata, 392
Anatomy, comparative, 24-48
  surgical, 20
    dorsum of hand, 22
    fingers, 22
    forearm, 21
    palm, 20, 21
    wrist, 20
Anesthesia, axillary block, 136
  block, 135
    digit, 139
    median nerve, 138
    radial nerve, 138
    ulnar nerve, 137
  brachial plexus, 136
  local, 140
    in reflex dystrophy, 711
  for primary wound treatment, 590
  selection of, 135
Aneurysm, arteriovenous, 715
  hand, 716
Angioma, 730-732. *See* Tumors, vascular.
Antagonism in tendon transfer procedures, 443
Anthrax, 691
Antibiotics in treatment of infections, 683
Aponeurosis, extensor tendon, 487
  shift mechanism, 488
Arachnodactylia, 91
Arches, of hand, effect on finger motions, 6
  transverse, 6
Arm, embryology, 48
  phylogenetic development, 32
  transfer of nerves, 567
Arsenic poisoning and epithelioma, 738
Arteriovenous aneurysm, 715
Arteriovenous fistula, 717
Artery, axillary thrombosis, 716
  brachial, rupture of, 247
  median, and compression syndrome, 363
  ulnar, thrombosis, 716
Arthritis. *See specific joints*

Arthritis, rheumatoid, 327-348
  arthrodesis, 336
  arthroplasty, finger joints, 338
  artificial syndactyly in treatment, 338
  buttonhole deformity, 329
  carpal tunnel syndrome, 335
  deformities, 327
  dislocation, extensor tendons, 333
    lower radio-ulnar joint, 329
  electromyography, 334
  metacarpophalangeal joints, 329
  release of intrinsic contracture, 341
  relocation of extensor tendons, 343
  rupture of tendons, 328, 330
  subcutaneous nodules, 328
  swan-neck deformity, 329
  synovectomy, 335
  synovitis flexor sheaths, 328
  tendon lesions, 328
  tendon ruptures, 330
  thumb deformities, 337
  thumb joints, 330
  treatment, 334
  ulnar drift, 331, 333
  wrist joint, 329
Arthrodeses, combined with tendon transfers, 444
  distal finger joint, 324
  finger joints for clawing, 501
  intercarpal for scaphoid fracture, 648
  joints, in rheumatoid arthritis, 336
  metacarpotrapezial, 326
  middle finger joint, 324
  for opposition, 531
  shoulder, Gill's, 572
    deltoid paralysis, 578
    optimum position, 561
    technic, 579
  value of, in combination with tendon surgery, 305
  wrist, 302
    indications, 306
    with involvement of radio-ulnar joint, 304
    in mirror hand, 80
    optimum position, 307
    in rheumatoid arthritis, 336
    technic, 307
Arthroplasty, elbow, 582
  finger joints in rheumatoid arthritis, 338
  metacarpophalangeal joints, 314, 316
  middle finger joint, 321
  wrist, 309
Assistant, role of, in surgery, 131
Atavism, relation to congenital deformities, 63
Atlas of skeletal maturation, Todd, 52
Atrophy, bone, Sudeck, 704
Avulsion, spinal nerves, 562
Axon flare test in brachial plexus injuries, 562
Axonotemesis, 398

Balance of tendon action, from bony deformity, wrist, 265
Barber's hand, 692
Bennett's fracture, 659
  old, treatment, 327
Bentzon, fasciaplasty for fracture of scaphoid, 648
Biceps, rupture distal tendon, 575
Bifid thumb, 93
Blastomycosis, 693
Block, local for painful states, 707
  sympathetic nerve in Volkmann's, 253
Blocker, stemless pedicle graft, 210
Blount osteoclasis of forearm, 274
Board for arm as operating table, 130
Boeck's sarcoid, 761
Böhler splint for finger, 153
Bone(s), 265-297
  achondroplasia, 51
  aneurysmal cyst, 742
  attaching tendon by pull-out wire technic, 418, 420
  carpal, arthrodesis, 302
    correction of deformities, 265
    degeneration, 293
    excision of proximal row, 306, 309
    fractures, 641
  cysts of, 749
    carpus, 294-296
  deformity, bone carpentry, 266
  delayed union after osteotomy, 266
  ecchondroma, 753
  forearm, comparative anatomy, 34
    correction of deformities, 273
    operations, 277
    secondary operations, 278
  giant cell tumor, 752
  hand, amphibia and reptiles, 37
    birds, 37
  infection from sheaths or spaces, 686
  loss of in thumb, reconstruction, 548
  malignant tumors, 755
  malunion, correction by bone graft, 266, 267
    effect on motions, 265
  metacarpal(s), correction of deformities, 267
    defect of shaft, treatment, 290
    fibroma of, 734
    losses, 282
    shortening to release intrinsic contracture, 341
  metastatic tumor, 757
  omovertebral, in scapular deformity, 65
  os centrale, 36
  osteochondrodystrophy, 50
  osteochondroma, 753
  osteogenesis imperfecta, 51
  osteoma, 755
  osteotomy of ulna, 274
  reptile hands, 34

Bone(s)—(*Cont.*)
  sarcoma, 756
  sources of grafts, 269
  stabilization by pinning, 269
  tumors, 749-756
  ulna, excision of lower end, 311
  wing of duck, 36
  wrist, comparative anatomy, 37
Bone block for opposition, 531
Bone grafts, for delayed union, 266
  for defects, 269
  forearm, 278
  scaphoid, 648
  sources, 269
  stabilization by pinning, 269
  technic, in phalanges, 267
  thumb for stabilization, 535
  from ulna, 267
Boss, metacarpal, 288, 292
Boutonnière deformity, 502
Brachial plexus, deformities, late operation, 568
    diagnostic points, 562
    Erb-Duchenne palsy, 359
    injuries, diagnosis, 562
      findings at operation, 565
      locating lesion, 355
      prognosis, 566
      salvage procedures, 573
    Klumpke palsy, 359
    palsy, transfers for, 452
    traction injuries, 562
Brachioradialis transfer for adduction of thumb, 514
Brachydactylia, 91
Brachyphalangia, 90
Bracing, functional, 180
Bracing as part of operative technic, 145
Brisement forcé, danger of use, 303
Brooks, studies on vascular occlusion related to Volkmann's ischemic contracture, 250
Bunnell operation for claw fingers, 499
Bunnell pulley operation for opposition of thumb, 527
Burns, 608-616
  chemical, 616
  contracture, axilla, 571
  dressings, 609
  electric, 612
  general treatment, 608
  local treatment, 609
  radiation, 615
  special aspects, 611
    early excision, 611
  treatment of contracture, 184
  wet dressing technic, 610
Buttonhole rupture of extensor tendon, 469

Calcification, periarticular, 345
  in tendons, 474
Calcinosis circumscripta, 345, 474
Campbell's operation, for malunion of Colles' fracture, 280
Capsulotomy, finger joints, 313
Carbuncle, 669
Carcinoma, bronchogenic, metastatic to hand, 757
  of nail, 765
    symptoms and diagnosis, 766
  skin, 735. *See* Epithelioma
Care, postoperative, 147
    after tendon operations, 460
Carpus, absence of, partial, 67
  bony development in animals, 35
Casts, plaster of Paris, application, 152
  errors in application, 152
Cat, clawing mechanism, 28
Cat-scratch granuloma, 695
Causalgia, 702
Center(s) of ossification, appearance, 49
Cerebral palsy, 394
  contraindications to surgery, 394
  selection of patients, 394
  tenodesis of sublimis tendons, 395
Chemical burns, 616
Chondrosarcoma, 756
Cicatrix, effect of, on contractures, 182
Cineplasty, 623
Clavicle, comparative anatomy, 32
  delayed ossification, 50
Claw-hand, knuckle-bender splint, 169
Clawing of fingers in ulnar palsy, 369
Cleft hand, 77
  treatment, 79
Clinarthrosis, general, 72
  incidence, 72
  treatment of, 72-73
  wrist, 68
Closure of epiphyses, normal times, 50
Coccidioidomycosis, 687, 694
Cock-back of proximal joints, prevention, 501
Colles' fracture, 631
  malunion of, treatment, 280
  tendon rupture following, 470
  treatment, 633
Compression dressing for wounds, 593
Contracture, adduction of thumb, 536
  axilla from burns, 571
  from burns, 228
    treatment, 184-230
  correction of before tendon transfer, 438
  Dupuytren's, 231-244
    changes in fascia, 237
    diagnosis, 235
    etiology, 231
    extent of involvement, 234
    heredity, 231

Contracture, Dupuytren's—(*Cont.*)
    incidence, 231
    pathologic changes, 236
    postoperative care, 244
    relation to trauma, 232
    splint, 164
    symptoms, 233
    treatment, 239
        conservative, 239
        limited excision, 241
        operative technic, 241
        radical, 241
        subcutaneous fasciotomy, 241
    effect of infection, 182
    effect of push and pull, 187
    finger, excision of scar, 191, 192
    flexion, 182
        from cicatrix, 301
        of digits, diagnosis, 110
        middle finger joint, 321
        repair of, 187
    intrinsic muscles, 256, 497
        release of in rheumatoid arthritis, 341
        in rheumatoid arthritis, 332
        of thumb, 531
    ischemic, local in the hand, 256-260
        symptoms, 258
        treatment, 258, 259
    pronation, transfers for, 454
    recording of, 104
    role of tendons in, 183
    secondary effects of, 183
    shoulder from disuse, 578
    of skin from burns, 228
    splinting to overcome, 159
    thumb, adduction, 531
    thumb cleft, 197
        treatment by sliding flap, 200
    treatment, conservative, 183
        general principles, 183
        skin replacement, 183, 184
    Volkmann's ischemic, definition, 244
        etiology, 245
        of forearm, 244-260
        history, 244
        mechanism, 248
        pathologic findings, 247
        symptoms, 251
        treatment, 253
Creases in hand in primates, 46
Creases, of skin, finger, 1, 2
    importance of locating incisions, 141
    palm, 2
Cyst(s), aneurysmal bone, 742, 743
    bone, 749
        diagnosis, 750
        incidence, 750

Cyst(s)—(*Cont.*)
    treatment, 751
    epidermoid, 727
        symptoms, 729
        treatment, 729
    inclusion, 727
    mucous, 729
        pathology, 730
        symptoms, 730
        treatment, 730
    sebaceous, 727

Darrach operation, 311
Defect, congenital ulnar bud, 71
    filling of with fat, 196
Deficiencies, congenital skeletal, classification, 55
        intercalary, 60
        paraxial, 60
Deformities, acquired, 64
    boutonnière, 502
    brachial plexus lesions, late operations, 568
    cerebral palsy, 394
    congenital, 55-97
        absence of radius, operation, 66
        absence of ulna, 71
        arm, 65
        classification of skeletal deficiencies, 60
        from diet, 64
        effect of heredity, 56
        etiology, 56
        forearm, 65
        hands, 77
        incidence, 55
        neurogenic theory, 63
        principles of treatment, 94
        shoulder, 65
        skeletal deficiences, 55
        terminology, 55
        time of development, 49
    distal joints, in rheumatoid arthritis, 330
    fingers from tendon injuries, 457
    finger tips, repair, 194
    hand, from ulnar palsy, 368
    intrinsic minus, 494
    intrinsic plus, 497
    Madelung, 280
    middle finger joints in rheumatoid arthritis, 329
    "swan-neck," 337
    thumb, intrinsic plus, 531
        in rheumatoid arthritis, 330, 337
    ulnar drift, in rheumatoid arthritis, 332
    from ulnar palsy, 369
    wrist, in cerebral palsy, 395
Degeneration, carpal bones, 293
    Wallerian, 351
Deltoid paralysis, 578
Dermatomes, diagram, 359
De Quervain's disease, 472

Diagnosis of impaired function, 107
Digit(s), comparative anatomy, 37
    transfer to thumb, 553
    variation in mammals, 39
Dimelia, ulnar, 78. *See* Mirror hand
Direction of tendon pull in tendon transfer operations, 442
Disability, rating of, 116
Dislocation, acromioclavicular joint, 578
    carpal, 635
    congenital, 74
    extensor tendons, repair of, 343
        in rheumatoid arthritis, 333
    finger joints, 324
    head of radius, correction, 273
    lower end of ulna, treatment, 312, 315
    lower radio-ulnar joint, 634
        in rheumatoid arthritis, 329
    lunate, 637, 639
    metacarpals, 657
    metacarpophalangeal joint of thumb, 324, 662
    metacarpotrapezial joint, 326
        operative treatment, 307
    perilunar, 637
    phalanges, 657
    recurrent shoulder, 580
    tendons, 470
    thumb, carpometacarpal joint, 662
    wrist, surgical treatment, 306
Dissection, technic of, 141, 143
Dogiel's nerve endings in skin, 19
Dominance, of hand, 1
Dorsal subaponeurotic space infection, 674
Dorsal subcutaneous space infection, 673
Dressings for burns, 609
    postoperative, 146
Drop finger, 467
Dupuytren's contracture, 231, 244. *See* Contracture, Dupuytren's
Dyschondroplasia, hand, 92
Dysostosis, cleidocranial, 50
Dysplasia, chondro-ectodermal, 79
    metaphysial, Pyle's disease, 51
Dystrophy, reflex, frequency, 702
        prevention, 711
        Raynaud's, 705
        Sudeck's, 704
        symptoms, 701
        treatment, 711
        use of local anesthetic, 711

Ecchondroma, 753
    diagnosis and treatment, 754
Ectrodactylia, 64
Ectromelia, 64-65
Edema, hand, dorsal, 709
    prevention of, 299

Elbow, arthroplasty, 582
    danger of tight casts, 152
    excision of, 582
    flexion by tendon transfer, 581
    incisions, 577
    nerve injuries, 581
    osteochondritis, 582
    paralysis of flexors, 580
    prosthesis, 581
    rupture of brachial artery, 715
    Steindler flexor plasty, 580
    surgical aspects, 582
    vascular lesions, 715
Elbow and shoulder, 561-585
Electric burns, 612
Electromyography, lumbrical muscles, 483
    in recovering muscles, 398
    in rheumatoid disease, 334
Elevation, congenital, of scapula, 65
        treatment, 65
    importance of in postoperative care, 147
Ellis-Van Creveld syndrome, 79
Embryology, arm and hand, 48
    hand, 48
Enchondroma, 743. *See* Tumor(s), enchondroma
Endorotation of metacarpal, 493
Endothelioma, 730. *See* Tumors, vascular
Entrapment syndrome, median nerve, 362
Epicondylitis, tennis elbow, 582
Epiphyses, arrest in megalodactylia, 93
    premature closure from frostbite, 614, 708
    time of appearance, 50
    transplant of fibula for absence of radius, 69
Epitenon, 404
Epithelioma, 735
    diagnosis, 740
    etiology, 738
    pathology, 738
    symptoms, 739
    treatment, 740
Erysipeloid, 694
Esmarch bandage, use of, 134
Evaluation of results of tendon reconstruction, 463
Ewing's tumor, 756
Examination of the hand, 98-119
Exercise for stiff joints, 303
    following tendon operations, 461
Exorotation of metacarpal, 493
Exostoses, 751
    subungual, 751
Extension, of thumb, splint to maintain, 170
Extremity, upper, sensory distribution, 358

Facilities as factors in wound treatment, 588
Factors affecting prognosis after hand surgery, 148
Fascia, graft in arthroplasty of finger, 317

Fascia—(*Cont.*)
  subcutaneous fasciotomy in treatment of Du-
    puytren's contracture, 241
  thickening in Dupuytren's contracture, 236
  used as a tendon graft, 437
Fascial grafts, technic of suturing, 426
Fascial space infections, 672
Fasciaplasty, Bentzon, for scaphoid fracture, 648
Fasciotomy in Volkmann's ischemic contracture,
  253
Felon, 665
Fibroma(s), 733. *See* Tumor(s), fibroma
Fibrosarcoma, 758
  diagnosis, 759
  etiology, 758
  incidence, 759
  location, 759
  pathology, 759
  treatment, 760
Field, operative, control of motion, 145
Fillet of digit, technic of, 196
Finger(s), amputation, levels of, 619
  crossed from bony deformity, 265
  fillet of, 196
  incisions, 141
  index, abduction by tendon transfer, 507
  recording measurements of function, 101
  splints for, 164
  stenosing tenosynovitis, 474
  surgical anatomy, 22
  tendon transfer, for extension, 455
    for flexion, 456
Finger prints, primates, 46
Fistula, arteriovenous, 717
Flaps, cross finger, 195
Flexor plasty, Steindler, at elbow, 580
  modifications, 580
Foot, fascial thickening in Dupuytren's contracture, 232
Fowler transfer for middle joint extension, 503,
  504, 508
Fractures, 628
  Bennett's, 659
    treatment, 327
    use of Kirschner wire, 180
  carpal bones, 641
  cervical vertebra with cord lesion, transfers for,
    453
  Colles', effect of malunion, 265
  distal phalanx, 656
  immobilization by splints, 630
  metacarpal of thumb, 659
  metacarpals, 650
  middle phalanx, 656
  open, 630
  pathologic, in enchondroma, 745
  phalanges, 654
  proximal phalanx, 655

Fractures—(*Cont.*)
  scaphoid, 641
    nonunion, 642
    treatment, 644
  special factors in the hand, 628
  supracondylar of humerus, in Volkmann's
    ischemic contracture, 245
  wrist, 630
Fracture(s) and dislocation(s), 628-662
  carpus, 629
Fracture-dislocation of metacarpotrapezial joint,
  659
Frostbite, 612
Function, appraisal of impairment, 118
Function of hand, importance of nerves, 377

Game-keeper's thumb, 324
Ganglia, carpal, 721
  as cause of ulnar palsy, 372
  causing nerve compression, 723
  compound palmar, 687
  etiology, 721
  flexor tendon sheath, 722
  location, 722
  pathology, 722
  sympathetic blocking by local anesthesia, 712
  sympathetic block in Volkmann's, 253
  symptoms, 723
  treatment, 723
    excision, 725
    injection, 724
Gangrene of finger from block anesthesia, 139
Gargoylism, 50
Garrod's pads, 734
Gas-bacillus infection, 685
Giant cell tumor of bone, 752
Gillies' cocked-hat operation, 538
Gill's arthrodesis, shoulder, 572
Girdle, pectoral, 29-31
  amphibia, 30
  birds, 31
  fish, 28, 29
  mammals, 32
  reptiles, 31
Glanders, 691
Glomus, anatomy, 745
  tumor, 745
    incidence, 748
    pathology, 747
    symptoms, 748
    treatment, 749
Glove as traction splint, 168
Goldner, tendon transfer for thumb in cerebral
  palsy, 396
Gonorrhea, 691
Gout, 348
Grafts, bone. *See* Bone graft
  fascia for metacarpotrapezial joint, 327

Grafts—(*Cont.*)
  nerve, 391
  partial and whole joints, 318
  pedicle for first cleft, 134
  skin. *See* Skin grafts
  sources of for gliding material, 424
  tendon, 432. *See* Tendon grafts
  tubed pedicle, for first cleft, 134
Granuloma, pyogenic, 767
Grasp, forms of, 10, 11
    power, 12
    precision, 12
Grease gun injuries, 607
Green, W. T., transfers in cerebral palsy, 395
Grip, loss of, in ulnar palsy, 371
Grooves, annular, in extremities, 92
Gunshot wounds, 607

Hair follicle(s), nerve supply, 19
Hand, adaptation in animals, 42-45
  congenital deformities, classification, 55
    incidence of, 55
  dorsum, surgical anatomy, 22
  embryology, 48
  examination of, 98-119
  imitation plastic, 623
  importance of tactile sensation, 185
  incisions, 141
  normal, 1
  primate, 45-48
  primitive, 35
    compared with human, 35
  tumors, 721-774
  variation in muscles of primates, 47
Healing, effect of trauma, 144
Heat, avoidance of when using tourniquet, 133
Hematoma, effect of, in healing, 143
Hemimelia, radial, 60-68
  types, 60
  ulnar, 60, 68
Hemophilia, pseudo tumor, 742
Hemostasis, importance of, 143
Heredity in congenital deformities, 56
History, importance of in examination of the hand, 98
Horner's syndrome in brachial plexus injuries, 562
Human bite infections, 669
Hyperparathyroidism, 709
Hyperphalangia, 91
  definition of, 56
Hypervitaminosis, 708

Imbalance of muscles in deformity, 121
Impairment, evaluation of, 117
Impairment of function, rating of, 116
Incisions, elbow, 577
  for exposure after lacerations, 590

Incisions—(*Cont.*)
  finger, technic, 141
  in the hand, 127-128
    technic, 141
  for metacarpals, 271
  mid-lateral, value of in finger, 141
  palm, 142
  for phalanges, 271
  shoulder, 570
Index, pollical, 45
Infections, 665-695
  anatomy, 665
  effect on contractures, 182
  forms of, dorsal subaponeurotic space, 674
    dorsal subcutaneous space, 673
    fascial space, 672
    in hand, 671
    hypothenar space, 673
    middle palmar space, 672
    quadrilateral space, 674
    radial bursa, 679
    thenar space, 672
    ulnar bursa, 677
  gas-bacillus, 685
  human bites, 669
  joints, 686
  lymphatic, 679
  osteomyelitis, 686
  phagedenic, 684
  postoperative care, 683
  pyogenic, 665
  response of tendons, 405
  special, 686
    actinomycosis, 693
    anthrax, 691
    blastomycosis, 693
    cat-scratch granuloma, 695
    coccidioidomycosis, 687, 694
    erysipeloid, 694
    glanders, 691
    gonorrhea, 691
    leishmaniasis, 691
    leprosy, 689
    seal finger, 695
    sporotrichosis, 693
    syphilis, 688
    tuberculosis, 686
    tularemia, 689
  specific entities, 665
    carbuncle, 669
    felon, 665
    paronychia, 669
    subcutaneous abscess, 669
  stages of healing, 182
  tendon sheath, 676
  treatment of, 682
  use of antibiotics, 683
Injury, nerves, symptoms and signs of, 351

Interosseus muscle, stripping for release of intrinsic contracture, 260
Intrinsic-minus hand, 494
Intrinsic muscles, 482-533
    origin, 24
    paralysis from infection, 182
    of thumb, 508
Intrinsic-plus hand, 497
Intrinsic plus, in rheumatoid arthritis, 332
    thumb, 531
Island flap for thumb, 543, 553
Island pedicle transfer, 392

Jepson, studies on vascular supply in Volkmann's ischemic contracture, 250
Joint(s), 298-349
    acromio-clavicular dislocation, 578
    arthrodesis in rheumatoid arthritis, 336
    arthroplasty in rheumatoid arthritis, 338
    capsular advancement, to prevent cock-back, 501
    carpometacarpal of thumb, dislocation, 662
    changing position by splints, 159
    contracture of capsule, 184
    distal finger, arthrodesis, 324
        in rheumatoid arthritis, 330
        surgery, 324
    distal radio-ulnar dislocation, 634
    elbow, incisions, 577
        paralysis of flexors, 580
        surgical aspects, 582
    exercising for stiffness, 303
    finger, dislocation, 324
        partial excision, 321
        rupture of volar plate, 321
        surgery of, 313
        use of prosthesis, 319
    flexing to obtain nerve length, 388
    graft of, 318
    infections, 686
    interphalangeal, sprains, 656
    metacarpophalangeal, in rheumatoid arthritis, 329
        of thumb, dislocation, 662
    metacarpotrapezial, dislocation, 327
        fracture dislocation, 659
        operation for dislocation, 307
        surgery, 326
    middle, arthrodesis, 324
        for clawing, 501
        arthroplasty, 321
        deformities in rheumatoid arthritis, treatment, 337
        extension by tendon transfer, 504
        in rheumatoid arthritis, 329
        shift of extensor tendon, 490
        surgery of, 320

Joint(s)—(Cont.)
    mobilization of, 300
        by elastic or spring splints, 303
        position when splinted, 151
        proximal, advancement of volar plate for clawing, 497
            arthroplasty, 316
            relation to clawing, 501
    radio-ulnar, in pronation and supination, 310
    repair of, 305
    shoulder, arthrodesis, 572
        contracture from disuse, 578
        incisions, 570, 579
    sternoclavicular, operation, 570
    stiffening of, causes, 298
        prevention, 299
    subluxation in rheumatoid arthritis, 329
    thumb, surgery of, 324
    wrist, arthroplasty, 309
        in rheumatoid arthritis, 329
        surgery of, 305
        tuberculosis, 686

Kaposi's sarcoma, 760
Keloid(s), 187
    excision of, 190
Kienböck's disease, 291-295
    etiology, 294
Kirschner wire in Bennett's fracture, 180
    fixation of radius and ulna, 275
    as internal splint, 177
    in stabilization of bone grafts, 271
    use in cleft contractures, 197
Klippel-Feil syndrome, 67
Knuckle-bender splint, 168
Knuckle pads, 93
Krause nerve endings in hand, 19
Krukenberg amputation, 621

Lead poisoning and metaphysial dysplasia, 51
Leiomyoma, 762
Leishmaniasis, 691
L'Episcopo's operation, 568
Leprosy, 689
Leriche, theory of ischemic contracture, 251
Leverage as part of operative technic, 145
Ligament(s), collateral, fingers, excision of, 313
    in rheumatoid arthritis, 329
        role in joint stiffness, 298
    thumb, rupture, 324
Limbs, origin, 24
Lines of Langer in hand, 141
Lipoma, 742. See Tumor(s), lipoma.
Lipscomb, treatment of Volkmann's ischemic contracture, 251
Lobster-claw hand, 77
Lunate, dislocation, 637, 639
Lunate-scaphoid fusion, congenital, 74

Lunate-triquetral fusion, congenital, 74
Luxation of tendons, 470
Lymphangiectasis, 732
Lymphangitis, 679

Madelung's deformity, 280
Malingering, diagnosis, 111
Mallet finger, 467
Malunion, radius and ulna, 276
Maturation, skeletal, 49-52
Mayer, artificial tendon sheath, 429
    operation for deltoid paralysis, 578
    rule for tension in tendon suture, 422
    transfer of pronator teres in cerebral palsy, 395
Median nerve, course, 359-362
    neurectomy, 397
    paralysis, splint for, 160
        treatment, 450
    repair of, 363
    signs of damage, 363
    tendon transfer for paralysis, 450
    and ulnar paralysis, 375
Megalodactylia, 93
Meissner corpuscles, in hand, 19
Melanoma, subungual, 763
        diagnosis, 765
        etiology and pathology, 764
        incidence, 764
        treatment, 765
Merkel-Ranvier nerve endings in hand, 19
Mesotenon, 404
Metacarpals, absence of, 68
    defect of shaft, treatment, 290
    dislocation, 657
    fractures, 650
    loss of head, 287
    losses, treatment, 282
    resection of head, in rheumatoid arthritis, 335
    shifting after ray excision, 286
    shortening in release of intrinsic contracture, 341
    sign in Turner's syndrome, 51
Metatarsal, graft to hand, 318
Middle palmar space infection, 672
Middle slip tendon rupture, treatment, 469
Milch osteotomy of ulna, 274
Milgrim, artificial tendon sheath, 429
Milker's granuloma, 692
Milker's nodule, 692
Mirror hand, 78, 82, 102
    treatment, 71
Moberg's sliding flap for tactile surface of thumb, 538
Mobility of hand, importance of, 185
Motions, automatic, 444
    fingers, 6, 8
        metacarpophalangeal joints, 7
    lateral of fingers, test for, 493

Motions—(Cont.)
    shoulder, 561
    thumb, 7-9, 510
    wrist, primates, 47
Movements, arm, 3
    carpal bones, 4, 5
    control of in operative technic, 145
    forearm, 3
        pronation and supination, 3, 4
    hand, 6
        from intrinsic muscle action, 493
    limitation of, diagnosis, 107
    wrist, 3, 6
        anteroposterior, 4
        lateral, 4
        measurement, 100
Muscle(s), aberrant, dorsum of hand, 29
    action of, importance of coordination, 9
    artificial, 179
    balance in normal hand, 121
    contrahentes, 29
    deltoid, paralysis, 578
    differentiation from amphibia to mammals, 40
    electrical reactions, 354
    forearm, amphibia, 28
        mammals, 29
        reptiles, 28
    hypothenar, anatomy and function, 491
    importance of splints for paralysis, 379
    integrity in tendon transfers, 442
    interossei, 485
        comparative anatomy, 29
        function, 491
        insertions, 485
        variations, 485
    intrinsic, amphibia, 26, 28
        amphibia through primates, 29
        anatomy and function, 483
        in diagnosis, 109
        effect on finger motions, 493
        hand, 482-533
        paralysis, 494
        release of in rheumatoid arthritis, 341
        reptiles, 27
        thumb, 508
        treatment of paralysis, 498
    lumbrical, 483
        variation, 485
    mechanics of action, 9
    paralysis, serratus anterior, treatment, 565
    pectoral, rupture, 566
    pectoralis to biceps transfer, 581
    phylogeny of intrinsic muscles, 24
    power required for tendon transfer, 439
    primate hand, 47
    scapulothoracic, paralysis, 576
    segmental innervation, 355, 357
    sternocleidomastoid to biceps transfer, 581

Muscle(s)—(*Cont.*)
  supraspinatus, rupture, 566
  system of recording activity, 353
  testing function, 353
  transfer, to restore opposition, 526
    at shoulder, 577
  triceps, paralysis, 581
  tumors, 762

Nail, carcinoma, 765
  function, 2
  primates, 46
  rate of growth, 2
  treatment of, in syndactylia, 86
Nerve(s), 351-403
  arm, area of sensory distribution, 358
  brachial plexus injuries, 562
    locating lesion in, 355
  bulb suture, 389
  changes in motor function following injury, 351
  classification of injury, 398
  combined lesions of median and ulnar, 375
  condemned procedures, 386
  dermal network, 18
  endings in hand, 352
  examination for loss of function of, 106, 107
  freeing of, 390
  hand, 377
    comparison in primates, 48
  importance of correct rotation in suture, 385
  importance in hand function, 377
  importance of splinting for paralysis, 379
  indication for repair, 381
  injury at elbow, 581
  injury, location of lesion, 355
  involvement in Volkmann's ischemic contracture, 253
  loss of sensation following injury, 355
  median, 359
    compression in carpal tunnel in gout, 348
    compression of in rheumatoid arthritis, 335
    compression syndrome, 362
    in lunate dislocations, 639
    neurectomy, 397
    overcoming gap in repair, 363, 387
    repair of, 363
  neurectomy, 396
    in cerebral palsy, 396
  painful neuromata, 392
  partial injury, 390
  pedicled graft, 392
  peripheral, injury to, 359
  primary repair, 604
  primary vs. secondary repair, 383
  prognosis following injuries, 397
  radial, 364
    paralysis, 445
    surgical repair, 366

Nerve(s)—(*Cont.*)
  rate of regeneration, 378
  reflexes, upper extremity, 357
  repair, special procedures, 387
    in infected wound, 382
    technic, 383
  segmental innervation of muscles, 355, 357
  sensory changes following injury, 351
  sheath tumors, 769
  signs of recovery of function, 398
  in skin of hand, 355
  sympathetic, block, 712
    periarterial, 713
  symptoms and signs of injury, 351
  technic of suturing, 371, 374
  timing of operation, 381
  transfer of, 390, 567
  transfer with island pedicle flap, 392
  treatment, in amputations, 616
    of injuries, 379
  trophic signs following injury, 354, 699
  tumors, 769
  ulnar, 366
    course, 366
    repair of, 371
    tardy palsy, 582
    transplantation at elbow, 582
Neurilemmoma, 769
Neurofibroma, 735, 769
Neurolysis, technic, 390
Neuroma, excision of in dystrophy, 711
  fibrillary, 769
  treatment of, 392
Neuropraxia, 398
Neurotomesis, 398
Nodules, rheumatoid, 328
No man's land, 600
Nonunion, radius and ulna, 276
Nutrition of hand, importance in results of operation, 148

Oppenheimer splint, 171
Opposition, by arthrodesis, 531
  return of following nerve suture, 364
  by tenodesis, 530
  thumb, 516, 531
    definition, 518
    measurement, 104
    methods of restoring, 521
    muscle transfer, 526
    in primates, 45
    splint to maintain, 170
    splinting, 519
Order of operative procedures, 126
Origin of limbs, 24
Ossification, embryonic and fetal life, 49
Osteochondritis, elbow, 582
Osteochondrodystrophy, Hurler's, 50

Osteochondroma, 753
Osteoid osteoma, 755
Osteogenesis imperfecta, 51
Osteoma, osteoid, 755
Osteomyelitis, following infection of hand, 686
Osteoporosis, post-traumatic, 704
Osteotomy, first metacarpal, 327
Osteotomy, thumb, for rotation, 538

Pain, amputation stump, 706
Palm, incisions, 142
    blood supply, 240
    surgical anatomy, 20
Palmar flap for finger tip losses, 618
Panner's disease, elbow, 582
Paralysis, adductors of thumb, 511
    deltoid, 578
    flexors of elbow, 580
    intrinsic muscles, 494
        from infection, 182
        treatment, 498
    median and ulnar, 177
    muscles, splints for, 159
    obstetrical, 568
    radial, splint, 174, 176
        treatment, 445
    scapulothoracic muscles, 576
    serratus anterior, treatment, 565
    spastic, 396
    thenar muscles, from median nerve injury, 363
    from tourniquet, 133
    triceps, 581
    ulnar, splint, 177
Paraplegia(s), tendon transfers for, 453
Paratenon, 404
    sources for gliding material, 424
Parkinson's disease, intrinsic muscle action, 497
Parona's space infection, 674
Paronychia, 669
Patterson's maneuver, 273
Pectoral girdle, 29-31. See Girdle, pectoral
Pectoralis major muscle, congenital absence of, 90
Pedicle grafts, 202
    neurovascular in hand, 392
    tubed, to lengthen thumb, 540
Pentadactylia, origin, 24
Peyronie's disease, association with Dupuytren's
    contracture, 232
Phalanges, dislocation, 657
    fractures, 654
Phalangization of metacarpals, 539
Phantom limb, 708
Phocomelia, 63
    from thalidomide, 64
    types, 60
Phylogeny and comparative anatomy, 24-48
Phylogeny, hand, 24
Pilonidal sinus, 692

Pinch, mechanics of, 8, 9, 12
Plan of reconstruction, 123
Plaster, nonpadded for forearm, 152
Plaster of Paris, dressing for pedicle grafts, 216
    splints, 151
Pollicization, Bunnell's operation, 546
    for congenital absence of thumb, 550
    historical, 543
    little finger, 550
    middle finger, 549
    on neurovascular pedicle, 547
Polydactylia, 80
    treatment, 81
Polyphalangia, definition of, 56
Polythene as gliding mechanism, 429
    interposition in forearm synotosis, 276
Position, intrinsic plus, 256
Postion of function, 10
    importance of, 123
    importance of wrist, 10
    restoration of, 125, 301
Position of wrist in arthrodesis, 307
Posture, upright, change in bone development, 33
Pouce flottant, treatment, 552
Power, of muscle, 12
Preiser's disease, 293
Preparation of skin before operation, 129
Primate hand, 45-48
Principles of reconstruction, 121-149
Principles, thumb reconstruction, 553
    wound treatment, 587
Prognosis after operations on hand, 147
    in nerve injuries, 397
Pronation, forearm in cerebral palsy, 395
    restoration of, 273
    and supination, measurement, 99
Prosthesis, after amputation for brachial plexus
        injury, 574
    elbow flexion, 581
    for finger joint, 319, 325
        in rheumatoid arthritis, 340
    upper extremity, 622
Pseudohypoparathyroidism, 707
Pseudo tumor of hemophilia, 742
Pulley, advancement for clawing, 497
    construction of in transfers for opposition, 529
    importance in tendon function, 404
    reconstruction of, 429
    repair of, 407
Pull-out-wire suture in tendon repair, 416
Pyle's disease, 51

Radial bursa, infections, 679
Radial nerve, 364
    paralysis, 445
    repair of, 366
    symptoms of injury, 365
Radial palsy, 365

Radial palsy—(*Cont.*)
  operative procedure, 448
  splints for, 160, 174
  tendon transfers for, 438, 444
Radiation, as cause of epithelioma, 738
Radius, congenital absence of, 67
    use of fibular graft, 279
    treatment, 68
  defect of, incidence, 67
  dislocation of head, correction, 273
  fracture, Colles', 631
Ray, excision of, 282
  shifting of, for metacarpal losses, 283
Raynaud's phenomenon, 705
Receptors, sensory, in skin, 19
Reconstruction, principles of, 121-149
  of thumb, 535, 560
Records of examination, 111
Reflex dystrophy, 700
Reflex mechanism, arm and hand, 702
Reflex(es), upper extremity, 357
Regeneration of nerve(s), 378
Repair of nerves in hand, 377
Reptiles, intrinsic muscles, 28
Results, of operations on hands, 148
  of tendon reconstruction, 463
Rhabdomyosarcoma, 762
Rheumatoid arthritis, 327-348. *See* Arthritis,
  rheumatoid
Rickets, 710
Rixford's operation for malunion of Colles' frac-
  ture, 280
Roentgen ray, as cause of congenital deformities,
  59
Rotation of forearm, control of, in applying pedicle grafts, 215
Rotator cuff tears at shoulder, 589
Rupture, distal biceps tendon, 575, 581
  extensor tendon, splint, 153, 158
  extensor tendon of thumb, 470
  ligaments of thumb, 324
  long head of biceps, 579
  pectoral muscle, 566
  serratus anterior muscle, 565
  supraspinatus, 566
  of tendons, 464
    in rheumatoid arthritis, 328, 330
  volar plate, finger, 321

Sarcoid, Boeck's, 761
Sarcoma, 757
  Kaposi, 760
    incidence, 761
  nerve sheath, 770
  nerve in Von Recklinghausen's disease, 770
  osteogenic, 755
  synovial, 766
Scalenus anticus syndrome, 575

Scaphoid, absence of, 68
  bipartite, 63, 642
  fracture, 641
Scapula, failure of descent, 65
  symptoms, 65
Scar, excision of, 190
  with skin graft, 191
  with Z-plasty, 191
  finger tip, plastic repair, 192
  importance of excision, 126
Scleroderma, Raynaud's sign, 706
Scurvy, 710
Seal finger, 695
Secretan's disease, 709
Seddon, classification of nerve injuries, 398
  coin test, for sensibility in fingers, 20
  interpretation of lesion in Volkmann's ischemic
    contracture, 248
  test for nerve suture, 386
Sensation, areas of loss following nerve injury,
  355
  changes following nerve injury, 351
  definition of, 18
  loss from median nerve lesion, 363
  recovery in tubed pedicle, 541
  restored by island pedicle flap, 392
  tests for loss of, 106
  thumb, restoration, 538
Sensibility, cutaneous, 18
  deep, in hand, 19
  in hand, 18
  importance of in thumb, 543
  Moberg's test, 104
  testing of, 18, 20
Separation, acromioclavicular, 568
  sternoclavicular, 570
Sever's operation, 568
Shift, of aponeurosis of extensor tendon, 488
  of extensor tendon at middle joint, 490
Shoulder, arthrodesis, 572
  contracture from disuse, 578
  incisions, 570, 579
  measurements of motion, 561
  motions, 561
  optimum position for arthrodesis, 561
  recurrent dislocation, 580
  rotator cuff tears, 579
Shoulder and elbow, 561-585
Shoulder girdle, embryonic development, 63
  fish, 63
Skin closure in wounds, 591
Skin and contractures, 182-263
Skin, finger, nerve supply, 19
Skin flaps in amputations, 616
  sliding for thumb pulp, 538
  technic of dissection, 193
Skin graft(s), 200
  abdominal pedicle, 206

Skin graft(s)—(*Cont.*)
    delayed, 210
    dressing, 208
    for burns, 609
    in children, 95
    choice of, 123, 201
    for contracture of thumb cleft, 260
    in cross finger flaps, 195
    dermal, 195
    dressings for, 227
    for fingertip losses, 618
    flap, technic, 207
    free, 220
        placing of, 227
        full thickness, 220
            choice of donor site, 221
            technic, 222
    operating beneath, 220
    pedicle, blood supply, 203
        to cover all fingers, 218
        errors, 185
            common, 204
        to fill defect, 195
        pocket flap, 204
        thinning of excess fat, 199
    in primary care of wounds, 592
    split thickness, 222
        variation with age, 225, 227
    stemless pedicle, 210
    in syndactylia, 84
    tubed pedicle in one stage, 219
        fixation of, 216
        pancake extension, 214
        technic, 211, 213
            using split skin graft, 219
        transfer of, 215
Skin, plastic repair of flexion contractures, 187
    preparation before operation, 129
    suturing of, 197
    transposition of, to cover finger tips, 195
    use of local flap in closure, 192
Smith-Petersen arthrodesis of wrist, 304
Spasm, brachial artery, in Volkmann's ischemic
    contracture, 251
Splints and functional bracing, 150, 181
    active, by spring or elastic, 160
    for adduction of thumb, 170
    after nerve suture, 389
    following operation, 147
    for paralysis, 172
    for radial palsy, 366
    after tendon repair, 423
    after tendon surgery, 461
    in treatment of rheumatoid hand, 334
    in Volkmann's ischemic contracture, 254
Splints, Böhler for fingers, 153
    to change position of joints, 159
    cockup for wrist, 157

Splints—(*Cont.*)
    dorsal wrist, 163
    for Dupuytren's contracture postoperative, 164
    dynamic to gain supination, 161
    effect of prolonged use, 125
    elastic or spring, use in treatment of stiff joints,
        303
    to extend thumb, 170
    finger, 164
    fitting, 161
    to flex finger, 166
    to flex metacarpophalangeal joints, 167
    to flex proximal joints, 163
    flexor hinge, 178
    gutter, 166
    hand spreading, 164
    historical, 154, 155
    to immobolize, 150
    internal, 177
    for mallet finger, 467
    median palsy, 160
    median and ulnar palsy, 177
    Oppenheimer, 173, 175
    for opposition of thumb, 170
    to overcome contracture, 159
    for palm, 164
    plaster of Paris, 150
        for continuous traction, 301
        nonpadded, 151
    postoperative for syndactylia, 86
    to prevent deformity, 150
    to promote extension of fingers and wrist, 171
    to protect tendons, 156
    radial palsy, 160, 173
    ruptured extensor tendon, 153
    safety-pin type, 166
    spring cockup, 156
    to straighten finger, 165
    as substitute for paralyzed muscles, 159
    Thomas for radial palsy, 174, 176
    types of, 167, 172
    ulnar palsy, 160, 177
    wrist cockup, 162
Sporotrichosis, 693
Sprains, interphalangeal joints, 656
Sprengel's deformity, 65
    omovertebral bone, 63
Steel wool as compression dressing material, 143
Steindler's flexor plasty at elbow, 580
    transfer of flexor carpi ulnaris in cerebral palsy,
        395
Sternoclavicular joint separation, 578
    operation, 570
Stiffening, prevention of, 125
Stiles' operation, intrinsic imbalance, 498
Stoffel, neurectomy, 396
Strap and buckle splint, 170
Styloidectomy for fracture of scaphoid, 650

Subluxation, metacarpophalangeal joints, in rheumatoid arthritis, 329
Sucquet-Hoyer canal, 746
Sudeck's dystrophy, 704
Supination, importance of in postoperative dressings, 147
    restoration of, 273
    splint to regain, 161, 164
Supraspinatus, rupture, 566
Suture material for nerves, 386
    in tendon repair, 414
Swan-neck, deformity in rheumatoid arthritis, 329
Swanson tenodesis, 342, 395
Swelling, role of in hand stiffening, 125
Sympathetic block, 712
    in Volkmann's ischemic contracture, 253
Sympathectomy, periarterial, 713
    Smithwick, 714
Symphalangia, 91
Syndactylia, 81
    in monkeys, 47
    splints after operation, 164
    treatment of, 82
    use of skin flaps, 85, 89
Syndactyly, artificial, in treatment of rheumatoid arthritis, 338
    use of skin grafts, 85
Syndrome, carpal tunnel, 362
    compression, median nerve, 362
    scalenus anticus, 575
Synergism in tendon transfer procedures, 443
Synostoses, congenital, 74
        radius and ulna, 63
    of forearm, treatment, 275
    treatment of, 76
Synovectomy, in rheumatoid arthritis, 335
Synovia, tumors of, 766
Synovioma, 767
    benign, 725. See xanthoma
    treatment, 768
Synovitis, flexor tendon sheaths, in rheumatoid arthritis, 328
    rheumatoid, 328
Syphilis, 688

Table, operating, for hand surgery, 130
Technic, atraumatic, 144-147
    in hand surgery, 123
    importance of, 144
    importance in nerve repair, 397
    nerve secondary repair, 383
    operative, 129-146
    order of procedures, 146
Tendon(s), 404-481
    action of, on joint, 16
    available as motors for opposition, 528
    balance, effect of bony deformity, 265
    calcification in, 474

Tendon(s)—(*Cont.*)
    distal biceps, rupture, 575
    extensor, dorsal aponeurosis, 487
        at middle joint reconstruction, 508
        repair of dislocation in rheumatoid arthritis, 343
        rupture, 465
    extensors of toes, technic of removal for use as grafts, 436
    fibromas of tendon sheath, 734
    function of, in finger, test for, 110
    healing process, 407-411
    insertion for opponens transfer, 527
    lesions of, in rheumatoid arthritis, 328
    mechanics of action, 9
    morphology, 404
    preserved for grafting, 437
    primary repair, exposure, 595
        indications, 594
    problem of gliding, 424
    reconstruction of gliding mechanism, 406
    response to injury, 405
    rheumatoid arthritis, repair of ruptures, 346
    role of, in contractures, 183
    rupture, biceps at shoulder, 579
        distal biceps, operative technic, 581
        etiology, 465
        extensors, 465
        extensor tendon at insertion, 466
            at middle joint, 469
        extensor of thumb, 470
        flexors, 470
        middle slip extensor, splint for, 166
        in rheumatoid arthritis, 330
            repair of, 346
    sheaths in rheumatoid arthritis, 328
    special situations, 467
    splinting after repair, 423
    stenosing tenosynovitis, 472
    tenodesis in cerebral palsy, 395
        for clawing, 498
    tension after suturing tendons, 422
Tendon grafts, 432-437
    fate of, 432
    as pulley, in finger, 430
    sources, 433-436
    technic of suturing, 416
    for tendon rupture, 346
Tendon healing, importance of rest and activity, 412
Tendon loop operation, 512
Tendon luxation, 470
Tendon repair, postoperative care, 460
    primary, advancement of profundus, 601
        demarcation of zones in hand, 600
        exposure, 595
        extensor tendons, 604
        in the hand, 600

Tendon repair, primary—(*Cont.*)
  healing process, 596
  indications, 594
  suture materials, 597
  tenodesis profundus, 602
  type of suture, 597
  withdrawable wire suture, 599
  at wrist, 602
  secondary, 412-424
    to bone, 418
    buried-wire technic, 415
    end-to-end technic, 418
    flexor to distal phalanx, 421
    removable wire technic, 416
    running wire technic, 417
    selection of site of junction, 427
    side-to-side suture, 421
    silk suture technic, 409, 415
    splinting, 423
  technic, 412
Tendon sheath, infection, 676
  inflammation following trauma, 471
  making artificial, 429
  structure, 404
Tendon transfers, 438-460
  for abduction of thumb, 459
  for adduction of thumb, 511
  brachioradialis to adduct thumb, 515
  for clawing of fingers, 502
  combined median and radial palsy, 452
  for extension of fingers, 455
  for extension of thumb, 457
  for extension of wrist, 455
  for flexion of fingers, 456
  for flexion of thumb, 457
  for median palsy, 450
  for middle joint extension, 503
    Fowler, 503, 504, 508
  for opposition, basic considerations, 524
  for paraplegia, 453
  principles, 438
  for pronation deformity, 454
  proprius of fingers for clawing, 497, 502
  proprius to first interosseus, 507
  radial palsy, 444
  requirements for success, 438
  to restore opposition, 521
  role of synergists and antagonists, 443
  selection of donors, 14
  sublimi to lumbricals, 499
    through interosseus membrane, 449
  superficialis to adduct thumb, 514
  thumb in cerebral palsy, 396
  timing of operations, 442
  triceps to biceps, 575
  ulnar palsy, 451
  use of arthrodeses and tenodeses, 444
  value of arthrodeses, 305

Tendon T operation, 513
Tennis elbow, 582
Tenodeses, combined with tendon transfers, 444
  for clawing, 498
  long extensor tendon in rheumatoid arthritis, 342
  for opposition, 530
  for relief of cock-back, 501
  sublimi in cerebral palsy, 395
    in finger, 340
  Swanson's operation, for hyperextension of middle joints, 342
  Tsuge's method for ulnar drift, 342
Tenosynovitis, digit, 677
  flexor tendons as cause of median nerve compression, 363
  in rheumatoid arthritis, 328
  stenosing, finger, 474
    radial styloid, 472
    thumb, 473
  traumatic, 471
  tuberculous, 687
Tenotomy, pronator teres for cerebral palsy, 395
Test, for intrinsic contracture, 257
  for tendon function, 110
Tetanus, prophylaxis, 593
Thalidomide, as cause of phocomelia, 64
Thatcher, artificial tendon sheath, 429
Thenar space injection, 672
Thomas splint for radial palsy, 174, 176
Thrombophlebitis, 716
Thrombosis, axillary vein, 716
  ulnar artery, 716
  venous, 716
Thumb, aberrant tendon, 473
  adduction contracture, 531
  amputation levels, 620
  congenital absence, treatment, 550
  contracture, of cleft, 197
    of intrinsic muscles, 531
    from ischemia, 260
  deformity in cerebral palsy, 395
    in rheumatoid arthritis, treatment, 337
  dislocation, carpometacarpal joint, 662
    metacarpophalangeal joint, 662
  effect of ulnar palsy, 370
  extension by splints, 170
  floating, treatment, 552
  fracture of metacarpal, 659
  importance of abduction in transfers for radial palsy, 447
  increasing stability by arthrodesis, 540
    by bone graft, 540
  injuries to bones, 658
  intrinsic muscles, 508
  joint deformities in rheumatoid arthritis, 330
  joints, surgery of, 324

Thumb—(*Cont.*)
  lengthening by tubed pedicle, 540
  limitation of motion, diagnosis, 108
  local skin flap for covering, 538
  loss of adduction, 511
  loss of, partial, 536
  measurement of motion, 101, 102
  metacarpophalangeal joint, dislocation, 324
  metacarpotrapezial joint, surgery, 326
  opposability in primates, 45
  opposition, definition, 518
    methods of restoring, 521
    by splints, 170
  primates, 45
  reconstruction, 535-560
    principles, 553
  relative lengthening by Z-plasty, 538
  restoration of tactile surface, 538
  restoring sensation by island flap, 393
  rotation osteotomy, 538
  sliding flap to improve spread, 538
  splint to maintain adduction, 170
  stabilization by bone graft, 535
  tendon transfer, for abduction, 459
    for extension, 457
    for flexion, 457
    for opposition, 521
  trigger phenomenon, 473
Timing of operations, 126
Tinel's signs, 398
Toe to hand transfer, 553
Tophi, excision of, 348
Tourniquet, application of, 133
  dangers of, in use on finger, 139
  pneumatic, 133
  technic in surgery of vascular tumors, 732
  use of, in infections, 135
    in overcoming contractures, 301
    in surgery, 132
Transfer of digit, 553
  finger skin for restoring sensation, 392
  flexors at elbow, Steindler, 580
  nerve(s), 390
    arm, 567
  pectoralis to biceps, 581
  pronator teres and flexor carpi ulnaris in cerebral palsy, 395
  of ray for metacarpal losses, 283
  sternocleidomastoid to biceps, 581
  tendons, see tendon transfer, 438
  toe to hand, 553
  triceps to biceps, 580
Transplant of epiphysis in treatment of congenital absence of radius, 69
Transplantation, metacarpal, 283
  ulnar nerve, at elbow, 373
    at wrist, 368
Trapezium, absence of, 68

Trauma, in etiology of fibrosarcoma, 759
  relation to epithelioma, 738
  role in etiology of melanoma, 764
Trigger finger, 474
  in rheumatoid arthritis, 328
Trigger point in reflex dystrophy, 711
Trigger thumb, 473
Trophic effects from nerve injury, 699
Trophic and vascular conditions, 699-717
Tsuge, tenodesis for ulnar drift, 342
Tuberculosis, 686
  tendon sheaths, 687
Tularemia, 689
Tumor(s), 721-774
  bone, 749-756
    ecchondroma, 753
    malignant, 755
    osteochondroma, 753
    osteoid osteoma, 755
  chondroma, 743
  common types, 721
  enchondroma, 743
    etiology, 743
    pathology, 743
    symptoms, 745
    treatment, 745
  epidermoid cysts, 727. *See* Cysts, epidermoid
  epithelioma, 735
  fibroma, 733
    location, 734
    metacarpal, 734
    pathology, 733
    subungual, 734
    symptoms, 735
  fibrosarcoma, 758. *See* Fibrosarcoma
  ganglia, 721. *See* Ganglia
  giant cell, of bone, 752
    of tendon sheath. *See* Xanthoma, 725
  glomus, 745. *See* Glomus
  lipoma, 742
    diagnosis, 743
    location, 743
  malignant, incidence, 721
  metastatic, 757
  mucous cysts, 729
  muscle, 762
  nail, 765
  neurofibroma, 735
  peripheral nerve, 769
  synovia, 766
  tendon sheath, 766
  vascular, 730
    etiology, 730
    symptoms, 732
    treatment, 732
  xanthoma, 725. *See* Xanthoma
Turner's syndrome, 51
Twinning, as cause of congenital deformity, 61

Ulna, congenital absence of, 71
    treatment of, 72
    nonunion, treatment, 276
    shortening in Kienböck's disease, 294
Ulnar bursa infections, 677
Ulnar drift, operation for, 347
    See also Arthritis, rheumatoid, 331
Ulnar nerve, 366
    clawing, 369
    and median paralysis, 375
    neurectomy, 397
    paralysis, splints for, 160
    recovery following suture, 369
    repair, 372
    symptoms of injury, 367
    transplantation at wrist, 368
    treatment of paralysis, 451
Ulnar palsy, from carpal ganglia, 373
    operative treatment, 451

Vascular changes after nerve injury, 699
Vascular lesions, 714
    elbow, 715
Vasospasm, following nerve lesions, 354
Vater-Pacini corpuscles in hand, 19
Vein(s), antecubital, compression of in Volk-
    mann's ischemic contracture, 246-249
    thrombosis, 716
Volkmann's ischemic contracture. *See* Contrac-
    ture, Volkmann's ischemic, 244-260
V-Y plasty, after scar excision, 191

Wallerian degeneration, 351
Weber, 2-point discrimination test, 20
Webs, development in flying animals, 44
    interdigital, in syndactylia, 82
Wire, suture technic, in tendon repair, 415
Work, of muscles, 12
Wounds, 587-608
    closure by relaxing incision, 193
    covering with skin, 591
    decontamination, 591
    effect of on hand motion, 126
    examination of, 589
    factors controlling treatment, 588
    frostbite, 613
    general treatment, 587
    infected, with nerve damage, 382
    postoperative care, 593

Wounds—(*Cont.*)
    special types, 604
        crushing, 604
        degloving, 606
        grease gun, 607
        gunshot, 607
        puncture, 604
        roller, 606
        snake bite, 604
        wringer, 606
Wrist, absence of extensors in mirror hand de-
    formity, 80
    arthrodesis, 302
        with involvement of radio-ulnar joint, 304
        technic, 307
    arthroplasty, 309
    axis of motion, 10
    deformity in cerebral palsy, 395
    effect of bony deformity on tendon action, 265
    fractures, 630
    importance of in muscle balance, 123
    importance in splinting, 150
    measurement of motion, 100
    motions of, 13
        primates, 47
    in rheumatoid arthritis, 329
    splints, 158
    spring cock-up splint, 163
    surgical anatomy, 20
    tendon transfers for extension, 455
    volar cock-up splint, 162
Wrist joint, infection, 686
    surgery of, 305
    tuberculosis, 686
Wryneck, in scapular deformity, 65

Xanthoma, diagnosis, 727
    etiology, 725
    historical, 725
    pathology, 725
    symptoms, 726
    treatment, 727
X-ray burns, 615

Z-plasty, for cleft hand, 81
    to deepen thumb cleft, 538
    after excision of scar, 191, 192
    thumb web, 133
    in treatment of club hand, 68